European Manual of Medicine

Otorhinolaryngology, Head and Neck Surgery

M. Anniko, M. Bernal-Sprekelsen, V. Bonkowsky,
P. Bradley, S. Iurato
Editors

W. Arnold
U. Ganzer
Series Editors

M. Anniko
M. Bernal-Sprekelsen
V. Bonkowsky
P. Bradley
S. Iurato
Editors

Otorhinolaryngology, Head and Neck Surgery

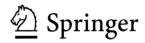 Springer

Series Editors

Wolfgang Arnold, MD
Department of Otorhinolaryngology,
Head & Neck Surgery
Technical University of Munich
Klinikum rechts der Isar
81675 München
Germany
Email: w.arnold@lrz.tum.de

Uwe Ganzer, MD
Department of Otorhinolaryngology,
Head & Neck Surgery
University of Düsseldorf
40225 Düsseldorf
Germany
Email: uwe.ganzer@arcor.de

Volume Editors

Matti Anniko, MD, PhD
Professor of Otolaryngology and Head & Neck Surgery
Department of ORL-HNS Uppsala
University Hospital (Akademiska sjukhuset)
SE-751 85 Uppsala
Sweden
Email: matti.anniko@akademiska.se

Manuel Bernal-Sprekelsen, MD, PhD
Director, Dept. of Otorhinolaryngology
Hospital Clinic Universitari
calle Villarroel, 170, Esc. 8, 2A
08036 Barcelona
Spain
Email: mbernal@clinic.ub.es

Viktor Bonkowsky, MD
Director, Department of Otorhinolaryngology and Head & Neck Surgery
Klinikum Nürnberg
Prof.-Ernst-Nathan-Str. 1
90340 Nürnberg
Germany
Email: viktor.bonkowsky@klinikum-nuernberg.de

Patrick J. Bradley, MB, MBA, FRCS
Professor of Head and Neck
Oncologic Surgery
Department ORL-HNS
Nottingham University Hospitals
Queens Medical Centre Campus
Nottingham NG7 2UH
UK
Email: pjbradley@ zoo.co.uk

Salvatore Iurato, MD
Professor and Past Chairman
Department of Ophthalmology and Otorhinolaryngology
Faculty of Medicine
University of Bari
70214 Bari
Italy
Email: iurato@bluewin.ch

ISBN   978-3-540-42940-1
e-ISBN   978-3-540-68940-9

DOI   10.1007/978-3-540-68940-9

Library of Congress Control Number: 2008942109
Springer Heidelberg Dordrecht London New York
© Springer-Verlag Berlin Heidelberg 2010

Cover design: eStudio Calamar, Figueres/Berlin
Typesetting and Production: le-tex publishing services oHG, Leipzig, Germany

Printed on acid-free paper

Springer is part of Springer Science + Business Media
(www.springer.com)

Foreword of the Series Editors

The *European Manual of Medicine* was founded on the idea of offering residents as well as specialized clinicians the latest and most up-to-date information on diagnosis and treatment in Europe. In contrast to existing textbooks, the *European Manual of Medicine* aims to find a consensus on the demands of modern European medicine based on the "logbooks" recommended by the Union of European Medical Societies (UEMS).

To fulfil these demands we—together with Springer—recruit editors who are well established and recognized in their specialities. For each volume at least three editors from different European countries are invited to bring the high clinical and scientific standards of their discipline to their book.

Wherever possible the book editors were asked to follow a standardized structure for each chapter so as to guarantee the reader easy and quick access to the material. High-quality illustrations and figures should provide additional useful information. For the interested reader, detailed references allow him or her to further investigate areas of individual interest.

The Series Editors are deeply grateful to Springer-Verlag, especially to Gabriele Schroeder, Waltraud Leuchtenberger and Stephanie Benko for their support and assistance in the realization of this project from the early stages.

The third volume of the *European Manual of Medicine* series is *Otorhinolaryngology, Head & Neck Surgery*. The aim is to provide ENT trainees with a comprehensive yet condensed guide to the core knowledge required in our speciality and to give them the ability to work in their speciality in the whole of the EU.

The volume editors (Matti Anniko, Uppsala, Manuel Bernal-Sprekelsen, Barcelona, Viktor Bonkowsky, Nuremberg, Patrick J. Bradley, Nottingham, and Salvatore Iurato, Bari), leading European experts in their discipline, recruited more than 71 contributors from 13 European countries as well as one colleague from the USA to compile a textbook that fulfils our original concept for the *European Manual of Medicine*.

Munich   **Wolfgang Arnold**
Düsseldorf   **Uwe Ganzer**
Autumn 2009

Preface

Despite some regional differences there is a vast consensus among the European nations as to what should be included in the training programmes for residents in Otorhinolaryngology-Head & Neck Surgery. These programmes are promoted by national institutions, such as Academies, Medical Schools at the Universities and national Societies. However, the duration of these training programmes continues to differ depending on the country.

For this reason, the ORL-section of the Union of European Medical Societies (UEMS) has proposed that each trainee should have a log-book registering his/her training progress. The log-book also offers guidelines for standard training, in an attempt to achieve a homogeneous level of resident training programmes all over Europe. More recently, the UEMS ORL-section has created the European Board Examination (EBE) in ORL-HNS.

This 3rd issue of the European Manual Series has been written for residents in Otorhinolaryngology-Head & Neck Surgery, with the aim of providing the most recent information on our discipline. The section on each organ contains concise chapters on clinical anatomy and physiology, the principles of clinical examination, technical diagnostic procedures and imaging. For each disease definition, the aetiology, symptoms, diagnostic procedures, complications, conservative and surgical treatment are described, as well as elements of differential diagnosis. The philosophy underlying this new edition is to supply all the relevant information in a clear, concise style. References are limited, and there are a few suggested readings.

We hope that this book will provide residents with a comprehensive tool helping them to prepare for the board examination at national or international (EBE) level, and finally to provide our patients with the best quality care.

The volume Editors are grateful to Springer, Ms. Gabriele Schroeder, Ms. Stephanie Benko, Ms. Martina Himberger, Ms. Petra Moews and Mr. Patrick Waltemate for their work, support and assistance.

Uppsala, Sweden	**M. Anniko**
Barcelona, Spain	**M. Bernal-Sprekelsen**
Nuremberg, Germany	**V. Bonkowsky**
Nottingham, UK	**P. Bradley**
Bari, Italy	**S. Iurato**

Contents

Diseases of the Nose and Paranasal Sinuses

Edited by Manuel Bernal-Sprekelsen

Diseases of the Nasopharynx
Edited by Uwe Ganzer and Andreas Arnold

Diseases of the Oral Cavity, Oropharynx, Hypopharynx, Cervical Esophagus

Edited by Viktor Bonkowsky

Diseases of the Larynx
Edited by Patrick J. Bradley

Voice Disorders

Edited by Patrick J. Bradley

Diseases of the Thyroid Gland: Diagnostics and Treatment

Edited by Matti Anniko

Head and Neck Tumors

Edited by Matti Anniko

Ear, Nose and Throat Anaestesia
Edited by Matti Anniko

List of Contributors

Acosta, Rafael
University Hospital
Dept. of Plastic and Reconstructive Surgery
781 85 Uppsala
Sweden
E-mail: *acostaplastikkirurgi@telia.com*
rafael.acosta@akademiska.se

Alobid, Isam
Hospital Clinic Universitari
Servicio de ORL
Villarroel, 170
0836 Barcelona
Spain
E-mail: *32874iao@comb.es*

Anniko, Matti
Uppsala University Hospital
Department of Otolaryngology
75185 Uppsala
Sweden
E-mail: *matti.anniko@akademiska.se*

Arnold, Andreas
Universitätsklinik für HNO Hals- und Kopfchirurgie
Inselspital
3010 Bern
Switzerland
E-mail: *andreas.arnold@insel.ch*

Arnold, Wolfgang
Department of Oto-Rhino-Laryngology
Klinikum rechts der Isar
Technische Universität München
Ismaningerstraße 22
81675 Munich
Germany
E-mail: *w.arnold@lrz.tum.de*

Aygun, Nafi
The Russell H. Morgan Department of Radiology
and Radiological Sciences
The Johns Hopkins Medical Institution
600 N. Wolfe Street / Phipps B-126-A
21287 Baltimore, MD
USA
E-mail: *Naygun1@jhmi.edu*

Bernal-Sprekelsen, Manuel
Hospital Clinic Universitari
Servicio de ORL
calle Villarroel, 170, Esc. 8, 2A
0836 Barcelona
Spain
E-mail: *mbernal@clinic.ub.es*

Blomquist, Erik
Department of Oncology
Akademiska sjukhuset (University Hospital)
75185 Uppsala
Sweden
E-mail: *erik.blomquist@akademiska.se*

Bockmühl, Ulrike
Universitätsklinikum Giessen und Marburg
Dept of ORL, Head and Neck Surgery
Klinikstraße 29
35392 Giessen
Germany
E-mail: *ulrike.bockmuehl@hno.med.uni-giessen.de*

Bodestedt, Åke
Australian Telemedicine Clinic
20/4 Chaplin Drive, Lane Cove
NSW 2066 Sydney
Australia
E-mail: *ake.bodestedt@vattnet.com*

Bonkowsky, Viktor
Klinikum Nürnberg
Hals-, Nasen- Ohrenklinik
Professor-Ernst-Nathan-Straße 1
90419 Nürnberg
Germany
E-mail: *viktor.bonkowsky@klinikum-nuernberg.de*

Bossolesi, Paolo
Ospedale di Circolo Fondazione Macchi
University of Insubria
ENT Department
Viale Borri 57
21100 Varese
Italy
E-mail: *pbossol@libero.it*

Bovo, Roberto
Audiology and Phoniatrics Unit
University Hospital of Ferrara
Corso Giovecca, 203
44100 Ferrara
Italy
E-mail: *bvorrt@unife.it*

Bradley, Patrick J.
Department ORL-HNS
Nottingham University Hospitals
Queens Medical Centre Campus
Nottingham NG7 2UH
UK
E-mail: *pjbradley@zoo.co.uk*

Caballero, Miguel
Hospital Clinic Universitari
Servicio de ORL
Villarroel, 170
08036 Barcelona
Spain
E-mail: *mcaba@clinic.ub.es*

Cambria, Cristian
Ospedale di Circolo Fondazione Macchi
University of Insubria
ENT Department
Viale Borri 57
21100 Varese
Italy
E-mail: *criscambria@ngi.it*

Castelnuovo, Paolo
Clinica Otorinolaringoiatrica
Azienda Ospedaliera
Universitaria Ospedale di Circolo
Viale Borri 57
21100 Varese
Italy
E-mail: *paologc@tin.it*

Chevalier, Dominique
University Hospital Claude Huriez
ENT and Head and Neck Surgery Department
Rue Michel Pononovski
59037 Lille
France
E-mail: *d-chevalier@chru-lille.fr*

Coca, Andrés
Department of Otolaryngology
Hospital Universitario Central de Asturias
Universidad de Oviedo
33006 Oviedo
Spain
E-mail: *andrewlane8@hotmail.com*

Coste, André
Hôpital Intercommunal de Créteil
Service ORL et Chirurgie Cervico-Faciale
94010 Créteil
France
E-mail: andre.coste@chicreteil.fr

Darrouzet, Vincent
Department of ENT
Univ. Hospital of Bordeaux
Place Amélie Raba-Léon
33076 Bordeaux Cedex
France
E-mail: *vincent.darrouzet@chu-bordeaux.fr*

de Bernardi, Francesca
Ospedale di Circolo/Fondazione Macchi
ENT Department
21100 Varese
Italy
E-mail: *francescadebernardi@hotmail.com*

de Haro, Josep
Hospital Municipal de Badalona
Department ENT
Maria Cristina 16
8911 Barcelona
Spain
E-mail: *15583jhl@comb.es*

Dejonckere, Philippe H.
The Institute of Phoniatrics
University Medical Center Utrecht
3508 GA Utrecht
The Netherlands
E-mail: *Ph.deJonckere@kmb.azu.nl*

Dobritz, Martin
Klinikum rechts der Isar
Technische Universität München
Abt. Radiologie
Ismaningerstraße 22
81675 Munich
Germany
E-mail: *dobritz@roe.med.tu-muenchen.de*

Dufour, Xavier
CHU Poitiers, Hôpital Jean Bernard
Service d'ORL et de Chirurgie Cervico-Faciale
86021 Potiers
France
E-mail: *x.dufour@chu.poitiers.fr*

Eckel, Hans Edmund
A. ö. Landeskrankenhaus Klagenfurt
HNO-Abteilung
St. Veiter Straße 47
9027 Klagenfurt
Austria
E-mail: *hans.ecke@kabeg.at*

Friedrich, Gerhard
Universitäts-HNO-Klinik Graz
Augenbrugger Platz 20
8036 Graz
Austria
E-mail: *gerhard.friedrich@kfunigraz.ac.at*

Ganzer, Uwe
Klinikum der Heinrich-Heine-Universität
Hals-Nasen-Ohrenklinik
Moorenstraße 5
40225 Düsseldorf
Germany
E-mail: *uwe.ganzer@arcor.de*

Garcia, Jacinto
Servicio ORL del Hospital de la Sta Creu i St Pau
C/ Mas Casanovas s/n
Barcelona
Spain
E-mail: *jgarciaL@santpau.cat*

Garcia-Piñero, Alfonso
Hospital Clinic Universitar
Service de ORL
Villaroel, 170
0836 Barcelona
Spain
E-mail: *algarp2000@yahoo.es*

Gavilán, Javier
Hospital Universitario la Paz
Pº de la Castellana, 261
28046 Madrid
Spain
E-mail: *jgavilan.hulp@salud.madrid.org*

Gerdemann, Petra
Klinikum Nürnberg
Prof.-Ernst-Nathan-Straße 1
90419 Nuremberg
Germany
E-mail: *petra.gerdemann@klinikum.nuernbeg.de*

Gertzén, Hans
University Hospital
Department of Otolaryngology and Head and Neck Surgery
22185 Lund
Sweden
E-mail: *Hans.gertzen@orebroll.se*

Gras-Cabrerizo, Juan-Ramon
Department ENT
Hospital Sant Pau
0825 Barcelona
Spain
E-mail: *jgras@hsp.santpau.es*

Grénam, Reidar
University Hospital Turku
Department of ORL, Head and Neck Surgery
Turku
Finland
E-mail: *reidar.grenman@tyks.fi*

Guilemany, Jose-Maria
Department ENT
Hospital Clinic
Villaroel 170
0836 Barcelona
Spain
E-mail: *33785jgt@comb.es*

Guntinas-Lichius, Orlando
Friedrich-Schiller-University Jena
Department of Otorhinolaryngology
Lessingstraße 2
07740 Jena
Germany
E-mail: *orlando.guntinas@med.uni-jena.de*

Haman, Karl-Friedrich
HNO-Universitäts-Klinik der Technischen Universität
Klinikum rechts der Isar, TUM
Ismaningerstraße 22
81675 Munich
Germany
E-mail: *m.stobrawe@lrz.tu-muenchen.de*

Herranz, Jesús
Rúa Courel 6
15179 – Oleiros
A Coruña
Spain
E-mail: *Jesus.Herranz.Gonzalez.Botas@sergas.es*

Hierholzer, Johannes
Klinikum Ernst von Bergmann
Abt. für Diagnostische und Interventionelle Radiologie
Charlottenstraße 72
14467 Potsdam
Germany
E-mail: *jhierholzer@klinikumevb.de*

Iurato, Salvatore
Department of Otorhinolaryngology and
Ophthalmology
University of Bari – Policlinico
70124 Bari
Italy
E-mail: *iurato@bluewin.ch*

Jungehuelsing, Markus
Klinikum Ernst von Bergmann
Klinik für HNO-Heilkunde
Charlottenstraße 72
14467 Potsdam
Germany
E-mail: *mjungehuelsing@klinikumevb.de*

Kiefer, Jan
Klinik und Poliklinik für Hals-Nasen-Ohrenheilkunde
Klinikum rechts der Isar
Technische Universität München
81675 Munich
Germany
E-mail: *j.kiefer@lrz.tum.de*

Kleinsasser, Norbert
Klinik- und Poliklinik für HNO der
Bayr. Julius-Maximilians-Universität
Josef-Schneiderstraße 11
97080 Würzburg
Germany
E-mail: *kleinsasser_n@klinik.uni-wuerzburg.de*

Klossek, Jean Michel
CHU Poitiers Hôpital Jean Bernard
Service d'ORL et de Chirurgie Cervico-Faciale
86021 Poitiers
France
E-mail: *j.m.klossek@chu-poitiers.fr*
j.m.klossek@wanadoo.fr (private)

Lamm, Kerstin
Clinic for Oto-Rhino-Laryngology
Hearing and Vestibular Disorders and Tinnitus
Candidplatz 9
81543 Munich
Germany
E-mail: *contact@prof-dr-lamm.de*

Lefèbvre, Jean Louis
Centre Oscar Lambret
Department of Head and Neck Surgery
Rue F Combemale, BP 307
59020 Lille
France
E-mail: *jl-lefebvre@o-lambret.fr*

Lichtenberger, György
State Healthcare Center
Department of ORL, Head and Neck Surgery
Podmaniczky u. 109–111
1062 Budapest
Hungary
E-mail: *Orl.rokus@mailbox.hu*

Livi, Walter
ENT Department, University of Siena
Policlinico "Le Scotte"
V. le Bracci
53100 Siena
Italy
E-mail: *livi@unisi.it*

Llorente Pendás, José Luis
Hospital Central Universitario Asturias
ENT Department
c/JM Caso 14
33006 Oviedo, Asturias
Spain
E-mail: *llorentependas@telefonica.net*

Lombardi, Davide
Department of Otorhinolaryngology
University of Brescia
P.zzale Spedali Civili 1
25100 Brescia
Italy
E-mail: *davinter@libero.it*

Maldonado-Fernández, Miguel
c/Oviedo, 12
33400 Salinas
Asturias, Spain
E-mail: *mmaldonadof@mixmail.com*

Marchal, Francis
Department of Otolaryngology Head and Neck Surgery
University of Geneva
Bd du Pont-d'Arve 40
1211 Geneva 4
Switzerland
E-mail: *francis.marchal@bluewin.ch*

Martin, Christian
Service ORL
CHU de Saint-Etienne
42023 Saint-Etienne, Cedex 2
France
E-mail: *christian.martin@chu-st-etienne.fr*

Martin, Lourdes
Jaras 49
28230 - Las Rozas
Madrid
Spain
E-mail: *lourdesmartinmendez@yahoo.es*

Martinez-Vidal, Brígida
Hospital Clínic
Servicio de ORL
c/ Villarroel, 170, Esc.8, 2A
08036 Barcelona
Spain
E-mail: *brigidamartinez@hotmail.es*

Martini, Alessandro
Dipartimento di Discipline Medico-Chirurgiche
della Comunicazione e del Comportamento
Sezione di Otorinolaringoiatria
Corso Giovecca, 203
University of Ferrera
44100 Ferrara
Italy
E-mail: *alessandro.martini@unife.it*

Massegur, Humberto
Department of ENT
Hospital Sant Pau
0825 Barcelona
Spain
E-mail: *hmassegur@hsp.santpau.es*

Montserrat, Joan-Ramon
Department of ENT
Hospital Sant Pau
0825 Barcelona
Spain
E-mail: *jmontserrat@hsp.santpau.es*

Mullol, Joaquim
Unitat de Rinologia, Servei d'ORL ICEMEQ
Hospital Clinic
Villarreol 170
0836 Barcelona
Spain
E-mail: *jmullol@clinic.ub.es*

Suarez Nieto, Carlos
Department of Otolaryngology
Hospital Universitario Central de Asturias
Universidad de Oviedo
33006 Oviedo
Spain
E-mail: *csuarezn@seorl.net*

Obando, Andrés
Hospital Clinic Universitari
Servicio de ORL
08036 Barcelona
Spain
E-mail: *drobandov@gmail.com*

O' Donoghue, Gerard M.
Professor of Otology and Neurotology
Co-Director, National Biomedical Unit in Hearing
Department of Otolaryngology
Queen's Medical Centre
NG7 2UH Nottingham
UK
E-mail: *g.o'donoghue@nottingham.ac.uk*

Önerci, Metin
Hacettepe University
Faculty of Medicine
Sihhga
06100 Ankara
Turkey
E-mail: *metin@tr.net*

Paiva, António
Serviço de ORL
Hospitais da Universidade de Coimbra
Praceta Mota Pinto
3000-075 Coimbra
Portugal
E-mail: otorrino@huc.min-saude.pt

Palma, Pietro
Ospedale di Circolo/Fondazione Macchi
ENT Department
Viale Borri, 57
21100 Varese
Italy
E-mail: mail@pietropalma.it

Papon, Jean-François
Service d'ORL et de Chirurgie Cervico-Facial
des Hôpitaux Intercommunal
et Henri Mondor de Créteil
94010 Créteil
France
E-mail: jean-francois.papon@hmn.aphp.fr

Percodani, Josiane
Service d'ORL et de Chirurgie-Faciale
CHU Rangueil-Larrey
31059 Toulouse Cedex 9
France
E-mail: percodani.j@chu.toulouse.fr

Peretti, Giorgio
Department of Otorhinolaryngology
University of Brescia
P.zzale Spedali Civili
25100 Brescia
Italia
E-mail: g.peretti@tin.it

Piazza, Cesare
Department of Otorhinolaryngology
University of Brescia
P.zzale Spedali Civili
25100 Brescia
Italia
E-mail: ceceplaza@libero.it

Pistochini, Andrea
Ospedale di Circolo/Fondazione Macchi
ENT Department
21100 Varese
Italy
E-mail: docpisto@mac.com

Remacle, Marc
Clinic Universitaire UCL d'Mont Godinne
Service d'ORL et chirurgie cervico-facial
5530
Mont Godinne
Belgium
E-mail: remacle@orlo.ucl.ac.be

Ribeiro, João Carlos
Serviço de ORL, 10° piso
Hospitais da Universidade de Coimbra
Praceta Mota Pinto
3000-059 Coimbra
Portugal
E-mail: jcarlosribeiro@gmail.com

Rusieka, Michalina
Hospital Clinic
Servicio de ORL
c/ Villarroel, 170, Esc.8, 2A
08036 Barcelona
Spain
E-mail: rusiecka@clinic.ub.es

Mariño, Franklin Santiago
Hospital Clinic Universitari
Servicio de ORL
08036 Barcelona
Spain
E-mail: fmarino@clinic.ub.es

Serrano, Elie
CHU Hôpital Larrey TSA 300 30
Service d'ORL et de Chirurgie Cervico-Faciale
24, Chemin de Pouvourville
TSA 30030 -31 059
Toulouse Cedex 9
France
E-mail: serrano.e@chu-toulouse.fr

Sittel, Christian
HNO-Klinik der Universität Heidelberg
Im Neuenheimer Feld 400
69120 Heidelberg
Germany
E-mail: christian_sittel@med.uni-heidelberg.de

Somers, Thomas
Sint-Augustinus Hospital
University ENT Department
Oosterveldlaan, 24
2610 Wilrijk, Antwerp
Belgium
E-mail: thomas.somers@gza.be

Sterkers, Oliver
Hôpital Beaujon
Service d'ORL et de Chir. Cervico-Faciale
100 Bd. du Général Leclerc
92110 Clichy Cedex
France
E-mail: *olivier.sterkers@bjn.aphp.fr*

Suárez, Carlos
Hospital Central Universitario
ENT Department
33006 Oviedo, Asturias
Spain
E-mail: *csuarezn@seorl.net*
carlos.suarez@sespa.princast.es

Tomás-Barberán, Manuel
Hospital Son Dureta
ENT Department
Andrea Doria, 54
07014 Palma de Mallorca
Spain
E-mail: *mtomasb@hotmail.com*

Vázquez, Carlos
University Hospital Juan Canalejo
Department of ORL
A Coruna
Spain
E-mail: *carlos.vasquez.barro@sergas.es*

Wennerberg, Johan
University Hospital
Department of Otolaryngology, Head, and Neck Surery
22185 Lund
Sweden
E-mail: *johan.wennerberg@onh.lu.se*

Werner, Jochen A.
Universitäts-Klinik für HNO-Heilkunde
Deutschhausstraße 3
35037 Marburg
Germany
E-mail: *wernerj@med.uni-marburg.de*

Wiklund, Lars
University Hospital
Department of Anesthesiology
75185 Uppsala
Sweden
E-mail: *Lars.Wiklund@akademiska.se*

Zinreich, S. James
The Russell H. Morgan Department of Radiology and Radiological Sciences
The John Hopkins Medical Institution
600 N. Wolfe Street / Phipps B-126-A
21287 Baltimore, MD
USA
E-mail: *sjzinreich@jhmi.edu*

List of Abbreviations

A(B)VD	**a**driamycin [doxorubicin], **b**leomycin, **v**inblastine, **d**acarbazine
3DCRT	three-dimensional conformal radiotherapy
AILT	angioimmunoblastic lymphoma
ALCL	anaplastic large cell lymphoma
ALL	acute B-/T-cell lymphoblastic leukaemia
ANA	antinuclear antibody
ANA	antinuclear antibodies
BEACOPP	**b**leomycin, **e**toposide, **a**driamycin, **O**ncovin, **p**rocarbazine, **p**rednisolone
BFM	Berlin–Frankfurt–Münster Group
c-ANCA	cytoplasmic-staining antineutrophil cytoplasmic antibodies
CAVE	cyclophosphamide, adriamycin, vincristine, etoposide
CBF	ciliary beat function
CHOP chemotherapy	**c**yclophosphamide (Cytoxan), doxorubicin (adriamycin, **h**ydroxydaunomycin), vincristine (**O**ncovin) and **p**rednisone chemotherapy
CLL	chronic lymphatic leukaemia
COS	chronic obstructive sialadenitis
cP	centipoises
cysLT	cysteinyl leukotriene type
DHAP	cisplatin, cytarabine, dexamethasone
DLBCL	diffuse large B-cell lymphoma
DMFT	decayed, missing and filled teeth
EA	early antigens
EBV	Epstein-Barr virus
ENT	ear, nose and throat
ESR	erythrocyte sedimentation rate
FDG-PET-CT	^{18}F-2-deoxyglucose– positron emission tomography–computed tomography
FL	follicular lymphoma
FNAC	fine-needle aspiration cytology
FSOT	frontal sinus outflow tract
GAN	greater auricular nerve
G-CSF	granulocyte colony-stimulating factor
HCV	hepatitis C virus
Ig	immunoglobulin
IMRT	intensity-modulated radiotherapy
IPI	international prognostic index
LEL	lymphoepithelial lesions
M component	abnormal monoclonal immunoglobulin
MALT	mucosa-associated lymphoma
MMF	maxillomandibular fixation

MPO	myeloperoxidase
MRSA	methicillin-resistant *Staphylococcus aureus*
NMCC	nasal mucociliary clearance
NOE	naso–orbital–ethmoid
PBC	primary biliary cirrhosis
PCP	*Pneumocystis jiroveci* (formerly *Pneumocystis carinii*) pneumonia
PDS	polydioxanone
PNIF	peak nasal inspiratory flow
PPS	parapharyngeal space
PR3	proteinase 3
PTCL	peripheral T-cell lymphoma
PTLD	posttransplantation lymphoproliferative disorders
RA	rheumatoid arthritis
RF	rheumatoid factor
SCM	sternocleidomastoid muscle
SLE	systemic lupus erythematosus
SS	Sjögren's syndrome
SSc	systemic sclerosis
TNF	tumour necrosis factor
TNM	tumour–node–metastasis
U-SMAS	U-shaped, superficial musculoaponeurotic system
VCA	virus capsid antigens
ZMC	zygomatic–maxillary complex

Otology and Neurotology

Edited by Salvatore Iurato and Wolfgang Arnold

1.1 Basics

SALVATORE IURATO

1.1.1 Clinical Anatomy

SALVATORE IURATO

1.1.1.1 External Ear

The external ear includes the auricle and the external auditory canal (Fig. 1.1.1):
- The shape of the *auricle* is quite complex and is determined by the shape of the aural cartilage.

- The *external auditory canal* (meatus) measures approximately 2.5 cm in length and is about 9 mm high by 6.5 mm wide. The lateral third consists of the elastic cartilage of the auricle (Fig. 1.1.1). Superiorly the cartilage is lacking between the tragus and the helical crus. This *incisura terminalis* is used by the surgeon when making an extracartilaginous endaural incision (see Sect. 1.4.6.8) without cutting into the cartilage. The *fissures of Santorini* in the cartilage of the external auditory canal (Fig. 1.1.1) are a potential route for the spreading of infection to the infratemporal fossa and

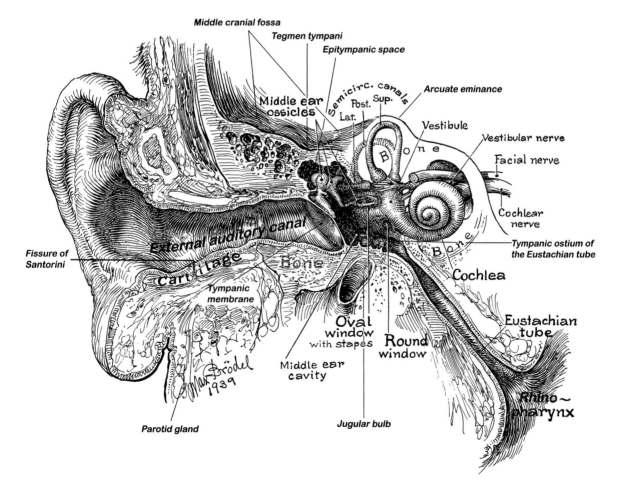

Fig. 1.1.1 Coronal view of the temporal bone (Modified from Brödel [2])

skull base. The medial third of the external auditory canal is osseous (Fig. 1.1.1).

The narrowest part of the external auditory canal (*isthmus*) is located between the fibrocartilaginous and the bony canal. The skin of the fibrocartilaginous canal is bound to the perichondrium without a subcutaneous layer. In the osseous part the skin is much thinner and closely adherent to the periosteum, and is devoid of hair follicles and ceruminous glands, whereas these are present in the cartilaginous part. Therefore, furuncles occur only in the cartilaginous meatus. Owing to its thinness, the skin of the osseous canal is easily traumatized during manipulations (e.g. wax removal with cotton tips).

The sensory innervation of the external ear comes from the greater auricular nerve (C^3), lesser occipital nerves (C^2 and C^3), the auricular branch (Arnold's) of the vagus nerve (X) and the auriculotemporal nerve (V). For local anaesthesia, firstly infiltrate the skin, the soft tissues and the periosteum of the lateral surface of the mastoid, up to incisura terminalis, then the posterior, superior and inferior walls of the canal and, finally, the anterior wall.

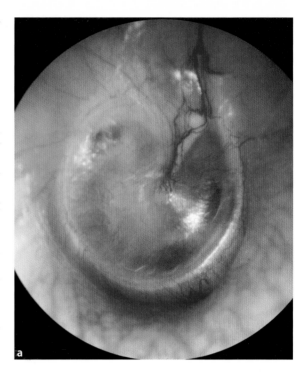

1.1.1.2   Middle Ear and Mastoid

Tympanic Membrane
- Elliptical in shape, slightly conical like a loudspeaker, pale grey in colour, the tympanic membrane forms an acute angle with the inferior wall of the auditory canal (Fig. 1.1.1). This angle should be respected in myringoplastic procedures (blunting strongly reduces the vibratory capacity of the tympanic membrane).
- Landmarks visible at **otoscopy** (Fig. 1.1.2): the lateral or short process and the handle of the malleus, the pars flaccida (Shrapnell's), and the pars tensa with the umbo and the triangular cone of light (*light reflex*). In the thin, transparent tympanic membrane: the chorda tympani, the long process of the incus with its *lenticular process* and its articulation with the head of the stapes (Figs. 1.1.1, 1.1.2).
- Histologically, the tympanic membrane is formed by an outer epidermal layer which is continuous with the skin of the external auditory canal, a fibrous middle layer (radial and circular fibres) and an inner mucosal layer which is continuous with the mucosal layer lining the middle ear cavity.
- The fibrous layer thickens peripherally to form the *annulus* (Fig. 1.1.2), which is inserted in a bony groove (*tympanic sulcus*). The fibrous layer is missing in the pars flaccida, which does not have the annulus.
- **Innervation**: of the anterior part, from the auriculotemporal branch of the V nerve; of the posterior part, from the auricular branch (Arnold's) of the X

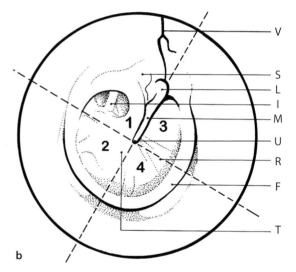

Fig. 1.1.2 a Otoscopic view of a normal thin tympanic membrane (right ear). The long process of the incus is just visible as a shadow in the posterosuperior part of the tympanic membrane. Note the vascular strip and the blood vessels along the handle of the malleus. The thickness of the tympanic membrane between the handle of the malleus and the anulus amounts to 0.1mm. **b** The tympanic membrane subdivided into four parts: *1* posterosuperior; *2* posteroinferior; *3* anterosuperior; *4* anteroinferior. *V* vascular strip, *S* pars flaccida (Schrapnell's), *L* lateral (or short) process of the malleus, *I* long process of the incus, *M* handle of the malleus, *U* umbo, *R* triangular cone (light reflex), *F* fibrous tympanic annulus, *T* pars tensa

nerve; of the inner surface, from the tympanic branch (Jacobson's) of the IX nerve.

Surgical Landmarks

1. On the lateral surface of the temporal bone
   - Suprameatal spine of Henle
   - Cribriform area
   - Posterior root of the zygomatic process and temporal line
   - Tympanomastoid suture
2. On the superior surface of the temporal bone (middle fossa approach)
   - Arcuate eminence (superior semicircular canal) (Fig.1.1.1).
   - Facial hiatus and greater petrosal nerve
   - Meatal plane
   - Superior petrosal sinus

Middle Ear Ossicles

- The average height of the stapes is 3.26 mm.
- The average size of the stapes footplate is 2.99 mm × 1.41 mm.

- The approximate distance (Fig. 1.1.3) between the stapes footplate and the utricle is 2.0–3.0 mm and the stapes footplate and the saccule is 1.0–1.5 mm.
- The weakest part of the ossicular chain is the long process of the incus at the level of its lenticular process, which articulates with the head of the stapes (Fig. 1.1.1).

Middle Ear Muscles

- Tensor tympani, innervated by a branch of the mandibular nerve (V)
- Stapedius muscle, innervated by a branch of the VII nerve

Other Important Anatomical Features of the Middle Ear

- Notch of Rivinus where the tympanic sulcus and the annulus tympanicus are both absent.
- *Promontory* (corresponding to the basal turn of the cochlea, Fig. 1.1.1) with the tympanic nerve (Jacobson's; Fig. 1.4.8c), which arises from the inferior ganglion

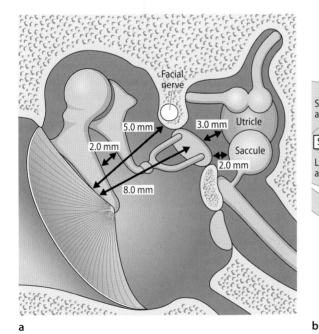

a

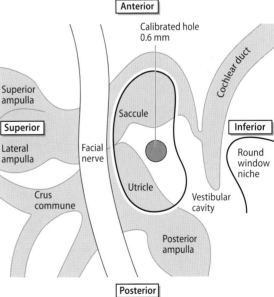

b

Fig. 1.1.3 a Average measurements in the middle and inner ear according to Anson and Donaldson [1]. Tympanic membrane – footplate = 8.0 mm; Tympanic membrane – facial nerve (FN) = 5.0 mm; Malleus handle – long process of incus = 2.0 mm; Foot-plate – utricle (U) = 3.0 mm; Footplate – saccule (S) = 2.0 mm; Stapes height = 3.26 mm; Footplate length = 2.99 mm; Footplate width = 1.41 mm. **b** Oval window surgical anatomy (right ear) in relation to stapedotomy calibrated hole 0.6 mm diameter

of the IX nerve and is joined by the caroticotympanic nerve.
- *Cochleariform process* (mind cholesteatoma matrix remnants!).
- Oval window, ponticulus, sinus tympani, subiculum and round window (Fig. 1.1.1).
- Footplate of the stapes which articulates with the oval window by the *annular ligament*.
- Facial nerve in the *Fallopian canal* (labyrinthine portion; first turn; tympanic portion with its relation with the bony lateral semicircular canal and the stapes; second turn with its relation with the short process of the incus; vertical or mastoid portion). The facial nerve is dehiscent in its tympanic course (oval window region) in about 30% of individuals.
- Round window membrane which plays an important role in the transmission of acoustic energy to the inner ear, and as a site through which toxic substances and therapeutic principles may enter the inner ear.
- *Chorda tympani* containing sensory (taste) fibres from the geniculate ganglion, directed to the anterior two thirds of the tongue.
- Epitympanic space (Fig. 1.1.1) containing the head of the malleus and the body of the incus. Bone defects in the roof of the tympanic cavity (*tegmen tympani*; Fig. 1.1.1) are present in about 35% of individuals. These bony dehiscences are sometimes associated with meningoencephaloceles.
- Floor of the tympanic cavity (*hypotympanum*) overlying the jugular bulb (Fig. 1.1.1) (individual variations).
- Anterior wall (*protympanum*) with (1) the semicanal of the tensor tympani, (2) the ostium of the Eustachian tube (Figs. 1.1.1, 1.4.8d) and (3) the vertical segment of the petrous carotid artery.
- Anterior epitympanic recess (area to be explored as cholesteatoma may penetrate and be hidden).
- Posterior wall with (1) the pyramidal eminence and stapedial tendon (Fig. 1.4.9a), (2) the chordal eminence and (3) the facial recess between the pyramidal eminence and the chordal eminence.

Mastoid

- Normal mastoids may be *fully pneumatized*, *diploic* or *sclerotic*. Pneumatization may extend (beyond the mastoid, perilabyrinthine and petrous apex regions) into the root of the zygomatic process and into the squamous part of the temporal bone.
- Mastoid cavities (the main cavity is called the "antrum") are lined with a very thin mucosa and communicate with the epitympanic space of the middle ear via the *aditus ad antrum*. Mastoid cavities play a role in pressure regulation and gas exchanges.

Eustachian Tube

- The bony part (11–14 mm) opens into the protympanum (tympanic ostium), and the fibrocartilaginous part (20–25 mm) opens into the lateral wall of the rhinopharynx (Fig. 1.1.1).
- Lined with respiratory ciliated mucosa, the tube connects the rhinopharynx with the middle ear and permits ventilation of the pneumatized temporal bone spaces. It opens on swallowing.
- Blockage of the Eustachian tube is responsible for otitis media with effusion, middle ear atelectasis, retraction pockets and failures in middle ear surgery.
- The *patulous tube syndrome* seems to be caused by a defect in the mucosal valve located within the cartilaginous portion of the Eustachian tube.

1.1.1.3   Inner Ear

The Bony Labyrinth

- The osseous portion (otic capsule, the densest bone in the body) consists of the vestibule, the three semicircular canals, the cochlea and the two aqueducts: the *vestibular aqueduct*, which contains the endolymphatic duct, and the *cochlear aqueduct* connecting the scala tympani in the basal turn with the subarachnoid space. A patent cochlear aqueduct (or small defects in the fundus of the internal auditory canal) is responsible for profuse outflow of the perilymph/cerebrospinal fluid from the oval window ("gusher") in stapes surgery. A large vestibular aqueduct is the most common inner ear anomaly, and is associated with a congenital hearing impairment.
- The cochlea makes 2.5 turns around the modiolus and contains the *cochlear duct* or *scala media*.
- The three semicircular canals lie at right angles to each other. The lateral (external) semicircular canal forms a 30° angle with the horizontal plane.

The Membranous Labyrinth

- The membranous labyrinth consists of the cochlear duct, the saccule, the utricle and the membranous semicircular canals. The *cochlear duct* communicates with the saccule via the *ductus reuniens*. The utricular duct and the saccular duct form the *endolymphatic duct*, which ends in the *endolymphatic sac* in the posterior fossa.
- The ampullae of the semicircular canals contain sense organs (*cristae ampullares*). The sense organs contained in the utricle and saccule are called *maculae*. The cristae ampullares and the maculae contain the vestibular hair cells and their supporting cells.
- The cochlear duct (*scala media*) is separated from the *scala tympani* by the *basilar membrane*, which con-

nects the bony spiral lamina with the spiral ligament. *Reissner's membrane* separates the scala media from the *scala vestibuli*. The *organ of Corti* (Fig. 1.1.4) is situated on the basilar membrane and consists of the sensory (hair) cells and of the supporting cells (pillars, Deiters', Hensen's, inner and outer supporting cells).

Endolymph and Perilymph

The scala media contains endolymph (with a high potassium and a low sodium concentration) and has a positive resting potential of 80 mV (endocochlear potential), maintained by the stria vascularis. The scala tympani and scala vestibuli contain perilymph (with a low potassium and a high sodium concentration similar to that of extracellular fluid).

Inner and Outer Hair Cells

- There are 3,500 *inner hair cells* (IHCs) and 12,000 *outer hair cells* (OHCs).
- The stereocilia of the OHCs are firmly embedded in the tectorial membrane, those of the IHCs are only loosely connected to the tectorial membrane or have no connection at all (Fig. 1.1.4).
- The OHCs contain contractile proteins. They are able to shorten and lengthen like muscle cells in response to neural signals. This active mechanism plays an important role in excitation of the IHCs.

Innervation: Peripheral

Vestibular Sensory Organs

- Superior vestibular nerve: n. utricularis + superior and lateral ampullary nerves + saccular branch (Voit's)

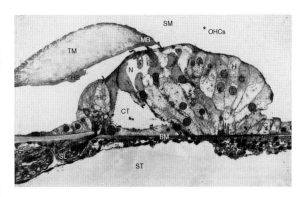

Fig. 1.1.4 Human organ of Corti (semithin section from W. Arnold) TM tectorial membrane; MB Marginal band; HS Hensen's stripe; IHC inner hair cell; OHCs outer hair cells; BM Basilar membrane; SL Spiral lamina; CT Corti's tunnel; N Nuel's space; H Hensen's cells; Claudius cells; SM Scala media (endolymphatic space); ST Scala tympani (perilymphatic space)

- Inferior vestibular nerve: n. saccularis + posterior (singular) ampullary nerve

Cochlea

- *Afferent innervation*: About 35,000 ascending first-order neurons convey signals from the cochlea to the CNS. They are components of the *spiral ganglion (cochlear ganglion)*, which is located in Rosenthal's canal, spirally arranged in the modiolus, the central support of the bony cochlea; 90–95% of them (bipolar cochlear type I neurons) innervate the IHCs (each IHC is innervated by ten to 15 type I neurons); 5–10% of them (pseudomonopolar cochlear type II neurons) innervate the OHCs (each type II neuron innervates about ten OHCs) (Fig. 1.1.5).

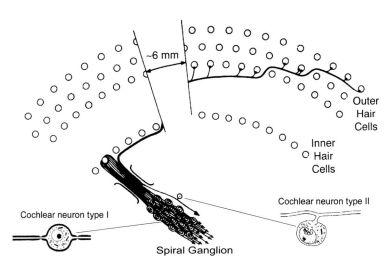

Fig. 1.1.5 Afferent innervation to the inner and outer hair cells; 90–95% of the neurons of the spiral ganglion (bipolar cochlear type I neurons) innervate the inner hair cells; 5–10% (pseudomonopolar type II cochlear neurons) innervate the outer hair cells (Adapted from Spoendlin [3])

- *Efferent innervation*: A much smaller population (approximately 1,600) of descending neurons sends signals from the CNS to the cochlea. Efferent fibres synapse directly with the OHCs but not with the IHCs. Most of the fibres from the lateral olivocochlear bundle (uncrossed efferents) synapse in the inner spiral bundle with the afferent fibres associated with the IHCs. Most of the fibres from the medial olivocochlear bundle (crossed efferents) synapse directly with the OHCs.
- *In summary*: The 3,500 IHCs have a mainly afferent innervation. The 12,000 OHCs have a mainly efferent innervation.
- *Adrenergic innervation*: A perivascular adrenergic plexus supplies the branches of the modiolar artery and a second adrenergic plexus, independent of the blood vessels, supplies the habenula perforata.

Innervation: Central

There is an increasing order of complexity from the cochlea/auditory nerve to the central auditory nervous system (Fig. 1.1.6).

- The cochlear nerve fibres (*first-order neurons*) leave the temporal bone through the internal auditory canal, pass through the cerebellopontine angle and enter the brainstem at the *ventral cochlear nucleus* or the *dorsal cochlear nucleus*, where they synapse with the second-order neurons.
- Some fibres from *second-order neurons* extend to the superior olivary complex on the same side, but a majority cross to the contralateral side via the trapezoid body. Some of the fibres that cross over synapse in the contralateral superior olivary complex and some of them ascend to the contralateral lateral lemniscus. The superior olivary complex receives information from both ears (bilateral representation). The acoustic stapedial reflex and the aural-palpebral reflex mediate at this level.
- *Third-order neurons* arise from the superior olivary complex and lateral lemniscus. They may synapse at the inferior colliculus or terminate at the medial geniculate body of the thalamus like the fibres originating from the inferior colliculus.
- The medial geniculate body of the thalamus is the subcortical station in the auditory pathway. Fibres from the medial geniculate ascend along the auditory radiations to the auditory cortex. *Tonotopic organization* is present at each level of the auditory system from the cochlea up to the cortex.

References

1. Anson BJ, Donaldson JA (1981) Surgical anatomy of the temporal bone, 3rd edn. Saunders, Philadelphia
2. Brödel M (1946): Three unpublished drawings of the anatomy of the human ear. Saunders, Philadelphia
3. Spoendlin H (1975) Neuroanatomical basis of cochlear coding mechanisms. Audiology 14:383–407

Suggested Reading

1. Gelfand SA (2001) Essentials of audiology, 2nd edn. Thieme, New York
2. Spoendlin H (1978) The afferent innervation of the cochlea. In: Naunton RF, Fernandez C (eds) Electrical activity of the auditory nervous system. Academic Press, New York
3. Schuknecht HF, Gulya AJ (1986) Anatomy of the temporal bone with surgical implications. Lea & Febiger, Philadelphia

1.1.2 Physiology

SALVATORE IURATO

The external ear (auricle and external auditory canal) and the middle ear (tympanic membrane and ossicular chain) are called the "conductive system" because their function is to conduct the sound signals from the air to the inner ear. The term "sensorineural apparatus" comprises the hair cells (sensory) and the cochlear nerve (neural).

1.1.2.1 Auricle and External Auditory Canal

The auricle and external auditory canal collect, amplify and convey sound to the tympanic membrane.

1.1.2.2 Tympanic Membrane and Ossicular Chain

These structures efficiently transfer sound energy from the air to the inner ear fluids:
- *Hydraulic effect*: the area of the tympanic membrane is much larger than that of the footplate (17:1).
- *Lever effect*: the malleus handle is longer than the long process of the incus (1.3:1).
- The approximate total gain is 27.5 dB.

1.1.2.3 Oval and Round Windows

Sound waves reach the two windows in different phases. The round window is protected by the intact tympanic membrane and by the margin of the round window niche. Large perforations of the tympanic membrane and those exposing the round window are often associated with a

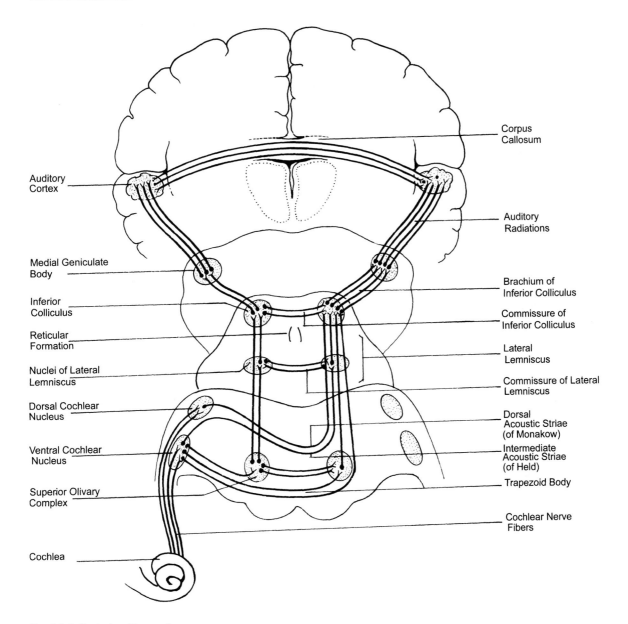

Fig. 1.1.6 Central auditory pathways

high degree of hearing loss. In surgical procedures, the round window membrane must be protected from the direct impact of sound.

1.1.2.4   Basilar Membrane and Travelling Waves

The basilar membrane is narrower and stiffer in the basal turn than in the middle and apical turns. The mechanical stimulation of the cochlea results from a travelling wave. The maximum displacement of the basilar membrane is related to the frequency of the stimulus: near the base of the cochlea for high-frequency tones, near the apex for low-frequency tones. This *tonotopic organization* is preserved along the auditory pathway from the cochlea to the auditory cortex.

1.1.2.5   Inner and Outer Hair Cells

- There are shearing forces between the tectorial membrane and the stereocilia of the hair cells. The hair cells respond when their stereocilia are bent towards the basal body (towards the lateral wall of the cochlear duct). There are cross-links (filaments) between the stereocilia. Pulling of the filaments opens a pore which permits ions to flow (activation); bending of the filaments in the opposite direction closes the pore (inhibition).

- The inner hair cells (IHCs) are the mechanoelectrical transducers of the inner ear. They synapse with dendrites of cochlear type I neurons. Glutamate is accepted to be their main neurotransmitter.
- The outer hair cells (OHCs), with cilia connected to the tectorial membrane, receive neural signals from the efferent olivocochlear bundle. The efferent innervation controls the contractile activity of the OHCs (**cochlear amplifier**), which enhances the movements of the basilar membrane (travelling waves) that stimulate the IHCs. The contractile activity of the OHCs is responsible for the ability of the cochlea to produce sounds (otoacoustic emissions). The nerve endings of the efferent olivocochlear bundle have vesicles containing the neurotransmitter acetylcholine. The ability to hear soft sounds and fine frequency distinctions is dependent on the integrity of the OHCs; without the OHCs, the hearing threshold is raised by 40–50 dB and frequency discrimination deteriorates.
- The stria vascularis provides the high concentration of potassium necessary to maintain the endocochlear potential (80 mV).

1.1.2.6 Semicircular Canals, Utricle and Saccule

- The semicircular canals with their ampullae provide information about angular acceleration.
- The receptor organ contained in each ampulla is called the "crista". It contains the vestibular hair cells, the supporting cells and a gelatinous mass called the "cupula". The stereocilia of the vestibular sensory cells extend into the cupula and are bent by deflection of the cupula. Deflection of the cupula is caused by the flow of endolymph.
- Like the cochlear hair cells, the vestibular hair cells are polarized: when the stereocilia are bent towards the kinocilium the response is excitatory; it is inhibitory when they bend away from the kinocilium. In the lateral semicircular canal, bending towards the utricle is excitatory, bending away is inhibitory. The opposing arrangement of the kinocilium in the two vertical canals is responsible for their opposite response (excitatory away from the utricle, inhibitory towards the utricle).
- The maculae of the utricle and saccule are covered by the *otolithic membrane*, on the top of which there are calcium carbonate crystals called "otoliths". They provide information about linear acceleration and the position of the head in space. Spontaneous de-

generative changes of the otoliths, particularly in geriatric patients, or their traumatic displacement, are responsible for their release into the endolymph (see Sect. 1.6.15).

- The endolymphatic sac has a pressure-regulation role because of its capacity to absorb water. Its content is markedly hyperosmolar in comparison to the osmolarity of the endolymph contained in the other parts of the membranous labyrinth. In patients with the *large vestibular aqueduct syndrome* pressure changes may cause reflux of hyperosmolar endolymph from the endolymphatic sac into the cochlear duct, and damage to the cochlear hair cells. The epithelium of the endolymphatic sac is metabolically active and plays an important role in the immunological defence of the inner ear. It has properties similar to those of the epithelium of the mucosa-associated lymphatic tissue system. According to whether antigen stimulation is systemic or local (inner ear), there is a cellular reaction as well as specific local antibody production.

Suggested Reading

1. Dallos P (1988) Cochlear neurobiology: revolutionary developments. ASHA 30:50–56

1.1.3 Ear-related Questions

SALVATORE IURATO AND WOLFGANG ARNOLD

No otologic symptom alone is diagnostic and therefore the otologic history must include questions about hearing loss, earache, otorrhoea, tinnitus and dizziness, plus a careful medical history. "It has been said that if you will listen to what a patient says, he will give you the diagnosis" [1].

1.1.3.1 Hearing Loss

- Bilateral or unilateral, which side?
- Recent or long-standing?
- Sudden? Stable? Progressive? Fluctuating?
- Continuous or intermittent?
- Is it associated with autophony?
- Is the speech discrimination poor?
- Is there a family history of hearing loss?
- Is the onset associated with a specific event (e.g. noise exposure, head trauma or disease)?
- What is the patient's occupation? Is there occupational or recreational (e.g. hunting, discotheque, rock concert, fireworks) noise exposure?

- Is there a history of diseases such as meningitis, parotitis, measles or syphilis, or of high fever of unknown origin? Is there a history of head trauma or unconsciousness?
- Is there a history of ototoxic drugs (e.g. streptomycin, gentamicin, diuretics, quinine, cytostatic drugs)? Diabetes, hypertension ?
- Is there a history of previous ear surgery?

1.1.3.2 Earache (Otalgia, Ear Pain)

See also the algorithm for earache in Fig. 1.1.7.
1. Bilateral or unilateral, which side?
2. Continuous or intermittent?
3. Is it associated with a discharge and/or movement of the pinna, pressure on the tragus?
4. Is it associated with swimming or diving?
5. Is it associated with a recent infection of the upper respiratory airways?
6. In normal otoscopic findings (referred ear pain)
   - Dental problems, dentition difficulties
   - Irritation of the temporomandibular joint (temporomandibular joint syndrome)

- Cervicofacial syndrome (patients with a history of cervical trauma or elderly patients with cervical arthritis)
- Neuralgia of the auriculotemporal branch of the trigeminal nerve (diagnosis of exclusion), neuralgia of the auricular branch of the vagus nerve (Arnold's) in acute tonsillitis or following tonsillectomy, neuralgia of the tympanic branch of the glossopharyngeal nerve (Jacobson's) in oropharyngeal carcinoma
- Aerodigestive malignancies (detectable with an accurate endoscopic examination in cases of mucosal lesions and with X-rays in cases of submucosal lesions), neoplasia of the infratemporal fossa (MRI with gadolinium)
- Elongated styloid process syndrome (Eagle): irritation of the glossopharyngeal nerve

1.1.3.3 Otorrhoea (Aural Discharge)

See also the algorithm for otorrhoea in Fig. 1.1.8.
- Bilateral or unilateral, which side?
- Character (mucous, mucopurulent, purulent, bloody, foul, clear)

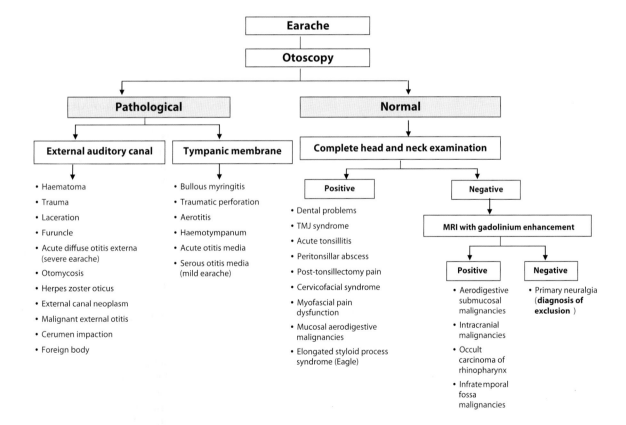

Fig. 1.1.7 Earache. Basic diagnostic procedures: case history, otoscopic examination, complete head and neck examination including endoscopy, dental and temporomandibular joint (*TMJ*) evaluation

- Continuous or intermittent?
- Recent or long-standing?
- Is the onset associated with a specific event (e. g. swimming or diving or an episode of upper respiratory airways infection?)

1.1.3.4   Tinnitus (Head Noise)

See also the algorithm for tinnitus in Fig. 1.1.9.
- Bilateral or unilateral, which side?
- Time of onset (recent or chronic)
- Continuous or intermittent, pulsating?
- Character of the tinnitus (low-pitched like the noise of the sea, high-pitched like a whistle)
- Is the onset associated with a specific event or noise exposure? With ototoxic drugs (aspirin, aminoglycoside antibiotics, quinine)?

1.1.3.5   Dizziness/Vertigo

See also the algorithm for vertigo in Fig. 1.1.10.

Vertigo of otologic origin implies a sensation of motion (spinning), is usually accompanied by rhythmic eye movements (nystagmus) and may be due to peripheral or central vestibular disorders. If peripheral in origin, it causes episodic attacks with normal equilibrium between the spells. The episodic attacks may last from a few seconds, as in the case of benign paroxysmal vertigo, to some hours, as in the case of Ménière's disease. Central non/

vestibular dizziness begins insidiously and lasts longer. *It is essential to collect a detailed clinical history:*
- Is the dizziness continuous (often described as unsteadiness) or does the patient experience the walls of the room whirling around him/her only during the attacks?
- What is the interval between the spells?
- Does head motion incite the attacks of vertigo?
- Are there accompanying symptoms such as nausea and vomiting?
- Are there associated cochlear symptoms such as unilateral hearing loss, hearing fluctuation, ear fullness and/or tinnitus?
- Is vertigo and/or oscillopsia evoked by sounds of high intensity (**Tullio's phenomenon**) or tragal compression (**Hennebert's sign**) or the **Valsalva manoeuvre**?
- Are there ocular symptoms such as double vision, or neurological symptoms such as numbness of the face or extremities, altered consciousness, difficult swallowing, speech problems, loss of memory?
- Is there a history of chronic ear infection?
- Is there a history of previous ear operations?
- Is there a history of disorders such as diabetes, syphilis, arteriosclerosis, cardiac problems, head trauma, and flulike symptoms?

References

1. Sheehy JL (1967) The dizzy patient. Eliciting his history. Arch Otolaryngol 86:44–45

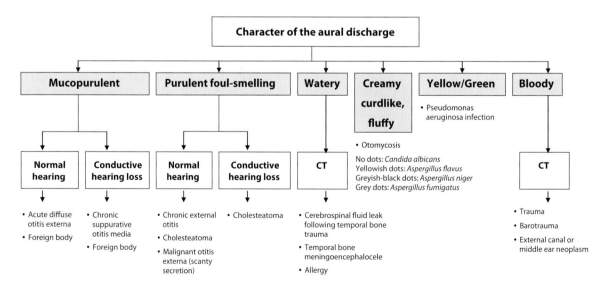

Fig. 1.1.8 Otorrhoea. Basic diagnostic procedures: case history, otoscopic examination, aspiration, rough hearing assessment with tuning fork tests, pure-tone audiometry

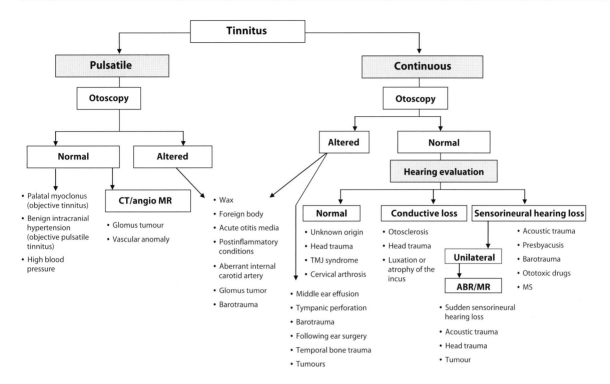

Fig. 1.1.9 Tinnitus. Basic diagnostic procedures: case history, ENT examination, otomicroscopy, hearing evaluation (pure-tone audiogram, tympanometry, stapedial reflex), tinnitus mea- surement, masking tests of tinnitus, blood pressure. *ABR* audi- tory brainstem response

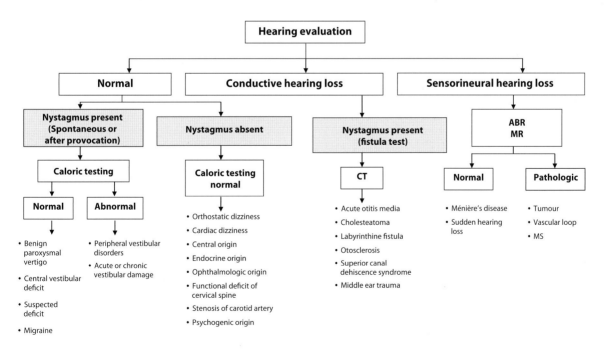

Fig. 1.1.10 Vertigo. Basic diagnostic procedures: case history, ENT examination, hearing evaluation (pure-tone audiogram, speech perception test, tympanometry, stapedial reflex), ves- tibular examination (nystagmus spontaneous, after provocation, vestibulospinal reflex, fistula symptoms, caloric testing), func- tional testing of the cervical spine, blood pressure, and blood sugar

1.1.4   Principles of Clinical Examination

SALVATORE IURATO

1.1.4.1   Inspection and Palpation

Gross inspection and digital palpation of the external ear and surrounding structures may reveal the presence of inflammatory processes, congenital malformations and neoplastic diseases.

Otoscopy

See also the algorithm for otoscopy in Fig. 1.1.11.

The *electric otoscope* (magnification ×2.5) is adequate for a routine otolaryngological examination (patient sitting) but when an otologic disease is suspected, examination at ×6–10 with the binocular *operation microscope* (patient supine) is recommended.

1. The largest speculum which can be inserted into the canal without pain should be used.
2. For a right-handed examiner using the microscope, the ear speculum is held between the thumb and forefinger of the left hand, with the ring finger in the concha, pulling the external ear posteriorly (conveniently straightening the external auditory canal) and the little finger on the patient's head to stabilize the speculum. The right hand is free to move the microscope and to manipulate instruments and exert suction.
3. The external auditory canal is inspected for wax, foreign bodies, mycosis, secretions, granulations, exostoses, growths and ulcerations. The quality of the skin should be noted.
4. *Often only a portion of the tympanic membrane is visible at one time.* The speculum and the microscope should be adjusted to *make a mental reconstruction* of the entire tympanic membrane. To facilitate orientation, the non-expert otologist should begin by identifying the short process of the malleus (Fig. 1.1.2).
5. Through a thin tympanic membrane, the long process of the incus may be seen posteriorly as a shadow (Fig. 1.1.2), as may the round window, although this is less common. Anteriorly, the opening of the Eustachian tube may be seen by transparency. Also the chorda tympani may be seen in the upper posterior part.
6. An intact pars tensa does not necessarily mean a healthy middle ear.
7. Systemic inspection must be made of the tympanic membrane both in the pars tensa and in the pars flaccida for:
   - Variations in colour, texture, thickness, vascularization (acute otitis, myringitis, tympanosclerosis, otitis media with effusion), pulsation (glomus tumour).
   - Variations in shape (see light reflex), retraction pockets, atelectasis (the result of chronic dysfunction of the Eustachian tube). Distinguish between stable (self-cleaning) and unstable retraction pockets.
   - Perforations (central, marginal, of the pars flaccida).
   - Secretion: clear, purulent, mucopurulent, bloody, foul. Fetid secretion indicates cholesteatoma or osteitis, odourless secretion indicates chronic otitis media without cholesteatoma but odourless secretion turns fetid if retained.
   - Crusting: dry secretion masking perforations, retraction pockets, osteitis, cholesteatoma. The crusts can be removed with a small round ear hook to reveal the underlying disease.
   - Middle ear mucosa (in cases of perforation): normal, with granulations or polyps, with keratin.
   - Cholesteatoma: marginal perforations, bony erosions, attic perforations.
   - Ossicular disease through a perforation.
8. The 0°, 4 mm **tele-otoscope** enables the observer to photograph the external canal and the whole tympanic membrane with excellent optical resolution (Fig. 1.1.2). Good-quality TV pictures may also be obtained for documentation and/or teaching purposes.
9. The 30° and the 70°, 1.9 mm **tele-otoscopes** enable the observer to examine the retrotympanum through a perforation. **Warning**: take care not to damage the stapes while using the 70° otoscope!
10. **Pneumatic otoscopy,** increasing and decreasing the pressure in the external ear canal with the pneumatic Siegle speculum with plain glass to:
    - Evaluate the mobility of the tympanic membrane and malleus
    - Identify middle ear effusions
    - Identify small perforations
    - Distinguish between fixed and mobile retraction pockets
11. Paper **patch test**: Under microscopic control, place a wet paper patch over the perforation and repeat the audiogram. An improvement of hearing with closure of the air–bone gap means that tympanic membrane perforation is the only problem. If after application of the patch the hearing is the same or worse, the problem involves the ossicular chain.
12. **Stapedial reflex**: Mobility of the stapes can be evaluated directly under the microscope when the stapes is visible through a perforation, by stimulating the opposite ear with a Barany noise box (crossed stapedial reflex).
13. **Toynbee's manoeuvre**: The patient is asked to swallow with the nose firmly closed: an inwards movement of the posterior half of the tympanic membrane (ob-

Otoscopy

Interpretation of the otoscopic picture

Colour	Perforation/s	Other changes

Colour

- White chalky patches: Tympanosclerosis
- Yellowish/golden: OME
- Pink (Schwartze's sign): Active otosclerotic focus
- Whitish underneath: Congenital cholesteatoma Recurrent cholesteatoma
- Blue: Haemotympanum Barotrauma Cholesterol granuloma High jugular bulb
- Red: Glomus tumour Ectopic ICA

Perforation/s

- Central "safe": COM Trauma Previous AOM
- Marginal "unsafe": Pars tensa cholesteatoma
- Attic: Pars flaccida cholesteatoma
- Multiple: Recurrent otitis media Tuberculosis

Other changes

- Haemorrhagic blisters: Acute bullous myringitis Herpes zoster oticus
- Granular aspect: Chronic myringitis
- Dry cast: Recent AOM
- Vascular changes, redness: AOM (earliest sign)
- Bulging, *Pis de vache*: AOM (stage of impending suppuration)
- Retraction (partial or complete): Atelectasis Adhesive otitis media Retraction pockets Potential cholesteatoma
- Polyp/s: Inflammatory (COM) Cholesteatoma Squamous cell carcinoma
- Keratinising squamous epithelium Cholesteatoma
- Air-fluid level/air bubbles: Serous otitis media Barotrauma
- False fundus: postinflammatory EAC stenosis

Fig. 1.1.11 Otoscopy. *AOM* acute otitis media, *ICA* internal carotid artery, *COM* chronic otitis media, *OME* otitis media with effusion (serotympanum, glue ear), *EAC* external auditory canal

served with the microscope) means that the Eustachian tube opens regularly.

1.1.4.2 Fistula Test

A Politzer bag is used to apply pressure to the ear canal. In the case of a bony fistula, pressure changes are transmitted through the fistula to the labyrinthine fluids. A positive fistula test is associated with deviation of the eyes towards the contralateral ear, followed by nystagmus towards the involved ear, if the pressure is held. If the pressure is released, the eyes return towards the midline. In fistula of the lateral semicircular canal (the most common), nystagmus is horizontal, whereas it is rotatory if the fistula is present in the superior canal and vertical if it is in the posterior canal. A positive response in the presence of an intact tympanic membrane (**Hennebert's sign**), originally described in congenital syphilis, may be seen in perilymphatic fistula, in labyrinthine hydrops and in the superior semicircular canal dehiscence syndrome.

- *False-positive fistula test result*: owing to an abnormally mobile stapes.

- *False-negative fistula test result*: owing to loss of labyrinthine function.

1.1.4.3 Tube Inflation

Tube inflation can be carried out (1) by Valsalva manoeuvre (autoinflation) or (2) by politzerization with a Politzer bag or (3) by using a catheter to:
- Evaluate a retraction pocket (fixed or mobile?) or a tympanic membrane atelectasis
- Detect a tiny perforation
- Confirm the presence of a serous effusion in the middle ear

1.1.4.4 Patulous Eustachian Tube

Synchronous movements of the tympanic membrane with respiration may be observed under the microscope. Otoscopy should be carried out with the patient in the sitting position, during forced inspiration and expiration through the nose while occluding the contralateral nostril.

1.1.5 Technical Diagnostic Procedures

SALVATORE IURATO

1.1.5.1 Subjective Tests

- Tuning fork tests
- Pure-tone audiometry
- Speech audiometry

1.1.5.2 Objective Tests

- Tympanometry
- Acoustic reflex
- Evoked response audiometry
- Otoacoustic emissions

Tuning Fork Tests

The 512-Hz (c²) aluminium tuning fork is struck on the examiner's elbow or knee.

Weber Test

Firmly place the stem of the vibrating tuning fork in the middle of the forehead or on the teeth.
- Lateralization to the ear with a hearing loss or with the greater hearing loss (advise the patient that this apparently strange possibility exists): *conductive* loss.
- Lateralization to the better hearing ear or no lateralization suggests that the problem in the involved ear is *sensorineural.*

Rinne Test

Comparison of bone conduction (stem of the fork firmly pressed on the mastoid) and air conduction (2–3 cm lateral to the tragus with the tines oriented parallel to the frontal plane of the skull):
- If the tone is louder on bone (negative Rinne test finding), this indicates conductive hearing loss or greater conductive hearing loss.
- If the tone is louder by air (positive Rinne test finding), this indicates sensorineural hearing loss.
- **Warning**: To minimize the risk of operating on a non-hearing ear always confirm the negative Rinne test finding by masking the contralateral ear with a Barany noise box!

Bing Test

Firmly place the stem of the vibrating tuning fork on the mastoid and then occlude the meatus by pushing the tragus:
- In conductive hearing loss there is no change.
- In sensorineural loss the turning fork is heard louder.

Comment: The tuning fork tests are not an optional but a standard part of the otologic evaluation. The results **must** be in agreement with those of the pure-tone audiometry.

Basic Audiologic Evaluation

See also the algorithms for hearing loss and steps in audiologic evaluation in Figs. 1.1.12 and 1.1.13.

Pure-tone Audiometry

- Determination of the air-conduction and bone-conduction thresholds at frequencies from 125 to 8,000 Hz, beginning with 1,000 Hz.
- The patient responds by raising an index finger or lighting a signal light when she/he hears the tone.
- The bone-conduction vibrator should be applied with a force of 400 g to the midline of the forehead or to the mastoid. At low frequencies, more energy (10–15 dB) is needed in frontal placement to reach the threshold as compared with mastoid placement.
- The hearing thresholds obtained with an audiometer are reported in decibels and registered on a graph (audiogram).
- The air-conduction pure-tone average is the average of the hearing levels at the frequencies 500, 1,000 and 2,000 Hz.
- **Masking**: It is essential to avoid interference of the opposite ear. For air-conduction testing using standard earphones, masking should be applied to the opposite ear whenever the threshold of the test ear exceeds the threshold of the non-test ear by 40 dB (value of interaural attenuation for air conduction) or more. For bone-conduction testing, interaural attenuation practically does not exist; therefore, during bone-conduction testing, masking should always be applied to the non-test ear. There is no need to mask when no air-bone gap is present in either ear and when the Weber test is lateralized to the test ear. The amount of effective masking should be evaluated to avoid both under-masking and overmasking. The masking rules apply for both pure-tone and speech audiometry.
- **Interpretation**: Air conduction tests the entire hearing system. Bone conduction tests only the inner ear and auditory nerve, bypassing the conductive mechanism. Comparing the air-conduction with the bone-conduction thresholds allows us to differentiate *conductive* (problem located in the external auditory canal or middle ear), *sensorineural* (problem located in the cochlea or auditory nerve [retrocochlear lesion]) and *mixed* hearing loss. A difference between the air-conduction and air-conduction thresholds (A/B gap) implies that there is a problem with the conductive mechanism (Figs. 1.1.14, 1.1.15). When the sensorineural part accounts for the total amount of loss (bone conduction is

equivalent to air conduction), it means that the whole loss is sensorineural and the conductive mechanism is normal (Figs. 1.1.16, 1.1.17). An example of a bilateral mixed hearing loss (conductive and sensorineural) is shown in Fig. 1.1.18: both the conductive mechanism and the cochlea are impaired.

Speech Audiometry

Lists of two-syllable words with equal stress on both syllables are administered by air conduction through earphones or in free-field to both ears. The intensity of the words is varied through the audiometer attenuator. The patient is asked to repeat the words and the results are plotted on a special graph (*speech audiogram*).

At the speech reception threshold the patient repeats correctly approximately 50% of the words. In conductive hearing loss there is a good agreement between the speech reception threshold and the pure-tone average obtained at the frequencies 500, 1,000 and 2,000 Hz. When the speech reception threshold is much better than the pure-tone average, the examination should be repeated (suspected *non-organic hearing loss*). Patients with a conductive hearing loss and normal cochlear function reach a discrimination of 100%. Patients with a moderate sensorineural loss generally also have a good speech

discrimination. Speech discrimination is not so good in patients with a severe sensorineural loss and in patients with a high tone loss. In lesions of the cochlear nerve and in those of the auditory central pathways, the speech discrimination is often poorer than expected from the pure-tone average (*tone–speech dissociation*). In some of these patients, discrimination decreases when the lists of words are administered at a higher intensity (*helmet curve* in the speech audiogram): this indicates the possible presence of a retrocochlear lesion.

Impedance Audiometry

Tympanometry

Tympanometry is an objective method serving to evaluate the mobility of the tympanic membrane and the functional condition of the middle ear, as pressure is altered in the external auditory canal from +400 to –600 daPa. A tympanogram is its graphic representation (Fig. 1.1.19):

- **Type A** curve in patients with a normal tympanic membrane, good tube function (normal patients and patients with a sensorineural loss).
- **Type A$_S$** curve (Fig. 1.1.14) in patients with reduced compliance (associated with otosclerosis, tympanosclerosis, fixed malleus).

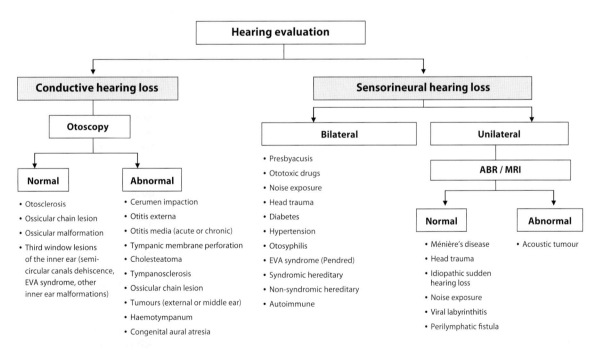

EVA = enlarged vestibular aqueduct

Fig. 1.1.12 Hearing loss. Basic diagnostic procedures: family history, case history, otoscopic examination, complete hearing evaluation (pure-tone audiometry, speech audiometry, tympanometry, acoustic reflex). *ABR* auditory brainstem response, *EVA* enlarged vestibular aqueduct

Steps in audiological evaluation

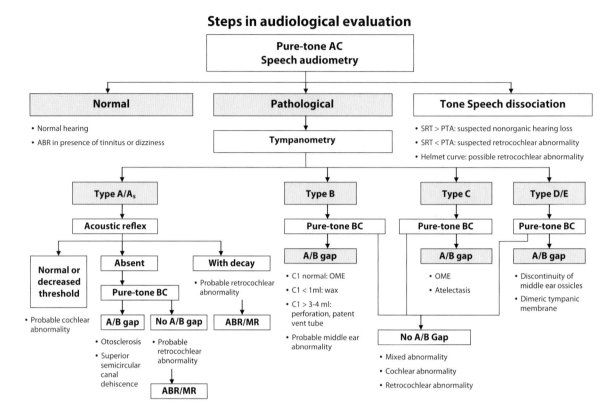

Fig. 1.1.13 Steps in audiologic evaluation. *AC* air conduction, *BC* bone conduction, *SRT* speech reception threshold, *PTA* pure-tone average, *OME* otitis media with effusion, *A/B gap* air/bone gap

- **Type A$_D$** pattern in patients with an abnormally flaccid tympanic membrane (discontinuity of the ossicular chain, dimeric tympanic membrane).
- **Type B** (Fig. 1.1.15) hypomobile or non-mobile tympanic membrane owing to the presence of fluid in the middle ear (otitis media with effusion), tympanic perforation, patent transtympanic drainage (vent tube) or ear canal totally occluded by wax.
- **Type C** (Fig. 1.1.15) mobile tympanic membrane with poor Eustachian tube function (in some cases, with a small amount of fluid in the middle ear).
- **Type D/E** hypermobile tympanic membrane (e. g. ossicular disruption).
- **Importance of C$_1$** (volume of the external canal). Normal values are 1.0–1.5 ml. Values less than 1 ml may be due to wax occluding the canal or may indicate that the probe tip is occluded or pushed against the walls of the canal. A volume exceeding 2.5 ml may indicate perforation of the tympanic membrane or a patent ventilating tube.

- Movements of the tympanic membrane due to a *patulous Eustachian tube* may be registered.

Stapedial Reflex (Acoustic Reflex)

The stapedial muscles contract bilaterally when one of the two ears is stimulated with a sufficiently loud sound.

- In the normal ear the contraction reflex occurs at an intensity of 70–100 dB SL (mean value 82.2 dB SL for pure tones and 65 dB SL for white noise). The lowest signal intensity capable of eliciting the reflex is recorded as the acoustic reflex threshold for the stimulated ear (and not for the probe ear).
- In cochlear sensorineural hearing loss the reflex threshold decreases (positive recruitment).
- In retrocochlear hearing loss (e. g. acoustic tumour) the acoustic reflex may be absent or decline (Fig. 1.1.17) under continued pure-tone stimulation (**acoustic reflex decay**).

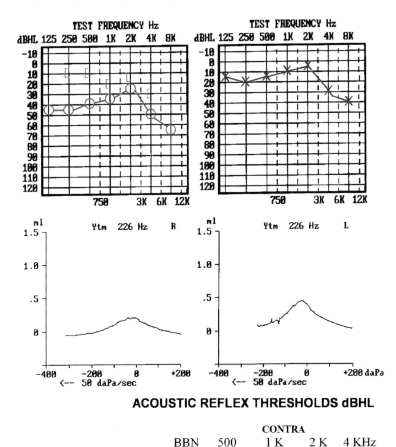

Fig. 1.1.14 An example of a conductive hearing loss in the right ear (stapes fixation due to otosclerosis). Note that in the right ear the tympanogram is type A$_s$ and the acoustic reflex is absent

ACOUSTIC REFLEX THRESHOLDS dBHL

		CONTRA		
	BBN	500	1 K	2 K	4 KHz
PROBE RIGHT EAR	nr	nr	nr	nr	nr
PROBE LEFT EAR	95	95	100	100	100

- In bilateral conductive hearing loss the reflex is absent bilaterally. In unilateral conductive hearing loss of 30 dB HL or more the reflex is also absent bilaterally. This occurs because when the sound is presented to the ear with a conductive loss of 30 dB or more, the loss itself prevents the sound from being heard loudly enough to elicit the reflex. When the sound is presented to the normal ear, with the probe in the ear with unilateral hearing loss, the disease prevents the change in compliance.
- **Warning**: Avoid measuring the reflex in cases of acute sensorineural hearing loss or recent tinnitus, to avoid the risk of further damage.

Evoked Response Audiometry

The main applications of evoked potential audiometry are (1) to diagnose hearing impairment in non-cooperative patients (infants and handicapped adults) and (2) to identify retrocochlear disorders (site-of-lesion tests). The principle is that of algebraic summation of the electrical events following repeated stimulation, thus discriminating stimulus-related electrical potentials from spontaneous activity. Depending on their latencies in milliseconds, first (0–2 ms), early (2–10 ms), middle (10–50 ms), slow (50–300 ms) and late (300 ms or more) potentials have been described (Fig. 1.1.20).

Electrocochleography

The *cochlear microphonics*, *summating potentials* and *action potentials* are electrical potentials that occur before the auditory brainstem response (ABR) potentials. They are recorded with a needle electrode through the tympanic membrane (transtympanic electrocochleography) or with distant electrodes and indicate the function of the inner ear and auditory nerve.

Electrocochleography is used in the evaluation of patients with suspected Ménière's disease (a significant enhancement of the summating potential to action potential amplitude ratio occurs in 60% of patients with Mé-

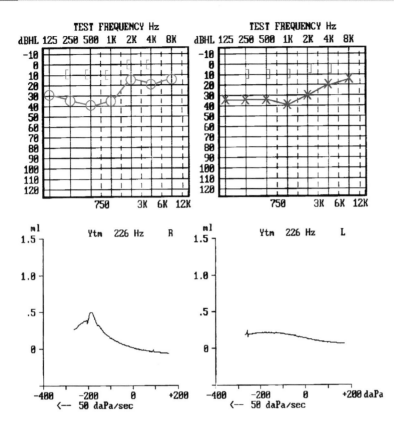

Fig. 1.1.15 An example of a moderate bilateral conductive hearing loss—middle ear atelectasis in the right ear (tympanogram type C) and otitis media with effusion (OME) in the left ear (tympanogram type B)

nière's disease), patients with a suspected perilymphatic fistula and to exclude residual cochlear function before performing a cochlear implant.

Auditory Brainstem Response

1. Latency is between 1.5 and 10 ms. Peaks following wave I occur at approximately 1-ms intervals and are indicated as I–VII (Jewett). Wave I Jewett corresponds to wave N1 of electrocochleography (Fig. 1.1.20). The sources of the waves are:
   - I and II: eighth nerve
   - III: cochlear nucleus
   - IV: olivary complex
   - V: lateral lemniscus
   - VI: inferior colliculus
2. Latency measurements to differentiate retrocochlear from cochlear lesions are the interwave interval (usually measured between waves I and V), the interaural latency and the absolute latency (Fig. 1.1.17).
3. A I–V interval longer than 4.4 ms is considered abnormal (however, each centre should have its own normative data).
4. A difference greater than 0.4 ms between wave V latency in the two ears (interaural latency) is considered an indication of retrocochlear abnormality (Fig. 1.1.17). Latency is corrected by subtracting 0.10 ms for

every 10 dB of hearing loss greater than 50 dB HL at 4 Hz.
5. ABR should be present at high-intensity levels if the pure-tone threshold at 4 kHz does not exceed 70 B HL.
6. Absent ABR in a patient with a mild sensorineural hearing loss is an indication of retrocochlear abnormality.

Cortical Evoked Response Audiometry

The late components (evoked response audiometry and vertex potentials of the old terminology) are not used routinely in clinical hearing evaluation, mainly because the results are very variable.

Otoacoustic Emissions

Small sounds from healthy outer hair cell activity (motility) transmitted back into the external auditory canal (echoes) and picked up by the probe tip microphone.
- *Spontaneous otoacoustic emissions* are present in 50% of normal young individuals.
- *Evoked otoacoustic emissions* in response to acoustic stimulation are present if hearing loss is equal to or better than 30 dB HL, and are absent if the hearing loss is greater than 30 dB HL.

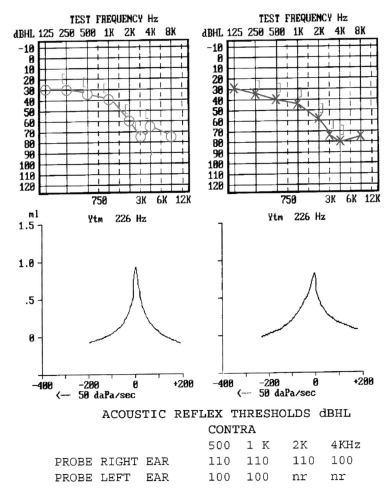

Fig. 1.1.16 An example of bilateral sensorineural hearing loss (Pendred's syndrome). The air-conduction and bone-conduction thresholds are equal and the acoustic reflex is present on both sides (From Arnold et al. [1])

ACOUSTIC REFLEX THRESHOLDS dBHL
CONTRA

	500	1 K	2K	4KHz
PROBE RIGHT EAR	110	110	110	100
PROBE LEFT EAR	100	100	nr	nr

- Otoacoustic emissions are frequently used in screening of newborns and to monitor the status of the cochlea during treatment with ototoxic drugs.
- *Distortion product otoacoustic emissions.* On simultaneous stimulation with two tones of different frequency, the cochlea generates another tone. Distortion product otoacoustic emissions are absent when there is a sensorineural hearing loss of about 50–60 dB HL or greater.

Assessment of Infants and Children
For details see Sect. 1.6.12. The hearing assessment of neonates and infants during the first 3–4 months of life is mainly based on physiological tests (otoacoustic emissions and ABR). After 5 months, the use of both behavioural and physiological tests is recommended.

Behavioural Audiometry
Behavioural audiometry involves watching the responses to sudden and intense stimulus sounds presented in the sound field. It is used for infants in the 5–24 months age range, in combination with impedance audiometry.

Conditioned Orientation Reflex
A visual reinforcement acts as a reward, increasing the chances that the child will continue to respond to subsequent sound presentations. It is used for infants in the 25–36 months age range, together with impedance audiometry.

Warning: Behavioural audiometry and conditioned orientation reflex are free-field tests, so they do not reveal the status of each ear.

Play Audiometry
The child is trained to answer with a motor response (game). Thresholds should be obtained before habituation occurs.

Examination of the Vestibular Organ
A complete clinical and medical history is essential in the evaluation of a patient complaining of dizziness.

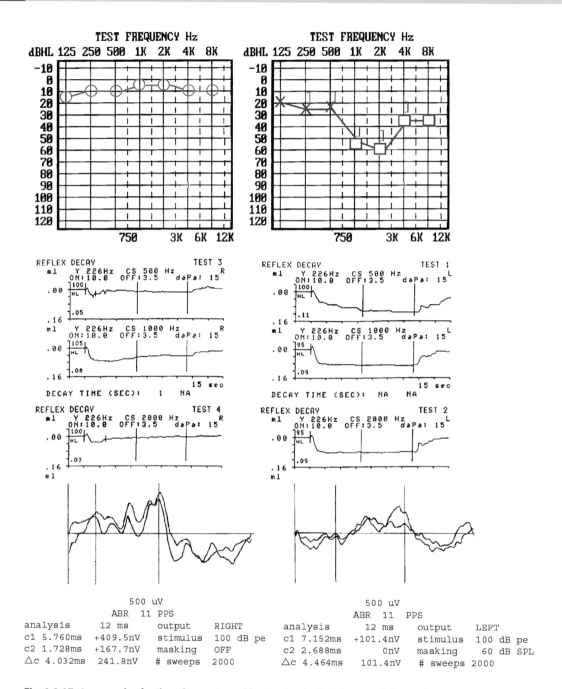

Fig. 1.1.17 An example of unilateral sensorineural hearing loss in the left ear (with decay of the acoustic reflex and pathological ABR). The retrocochlear abnormality (vestibular schwannoma) was confirmed by MRI and at surgery (From Arnold et al. [1])

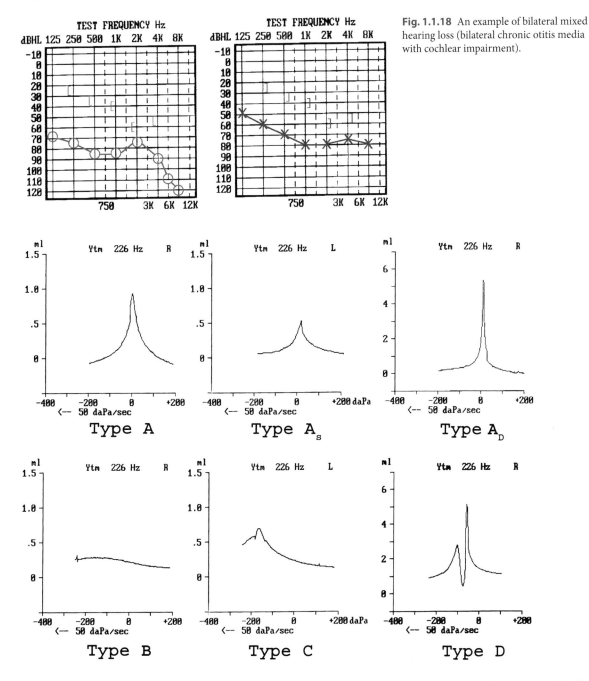

Fig. 1.1.18 An example of bilateral mixed hearing loss (bilateral chronic otitis media with cochlear impairment).

Fig. 1.1.19 Classification of tympanograms: type A, normal; type As, reduced compliance (e.g. otosclerosis)—see also Fig. 1.1.14; type A_D, flaccid /scarred tympanic membrane; type B, non-mobile tympanic membrane (e.g. OME)—see also Fig. 1.1.15; type C, poor Eustachian tube function—see also Fig. 1.1.15; type D, hypermobile tympanic membrane (e.g. ossicular disruption). (From Arnold et al. [1])

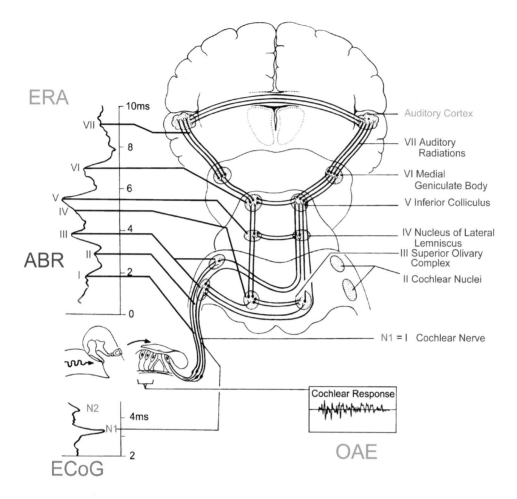

ERA

ABR

ECoG

OAE

Auditory Cortex

VII Auditory
   Radiations

VI Medial
   Geniculate Body

V Inferior Colliculus

IV Nucleus of Lateral
   Lemniscus
III Superior Olivary
   Complex

II Cochlear Nuclei

N1 = I Cochlear Nerve

Cochlear Response

Fig. 1.1.20 Otoacoustic emissions (*OAE*), electrocochleography (*ECoG*), ABR, cortical evoked response audiometry (*ERA*): topographical map

- Does the patient experience a spinning sensation (this means a disease of the vestibular system) or a sensation of unsteadiness (non-vestibular dizziness)?
- Is the vertigo episodic, with a normal equilibrium between the attacks? The spells last seconds in the case of benign paroxysmal vertigo and hours in the case of Ménière's disease. Short episodes associated with nausea and vomiting suggest a peripheral labyrinthine abnormality. Acute rotational vertigo lasting several days with slow recovery is characteristic of viral, traumatic or vascular labyrinthitis or vestibular neuronitis.
- Does a rapid head movement, particularly when turning over in bed, incite vertigo? If so, benign paroxysmal vertigo is likely.
- Does vertigo occur with neck motion? If so, cervical vertigo is likely.

- Central non-vestibular disease begins insidiously and lasts days or months. The sensation of dysequilibrium is usually chronic.
- Are there associated cochlear symptoms? Hearing loss, fullness, tinnitus? These symptoms suggest a cochlear (Ménière) or a retrocochlear (vestibular schwannoma) abnormality.
- Are there other otologic symptoms, acute otitis media, cholesteatoma, perilymphatic fistula?
- Are there other disorders, including cardiovascular disease, cerebrovascular disease, neurological disorders, visual impairment and diabetes?
- Does the patient use alcohol, medications or other drugs (ototoxic antibiotics, antihypertensive, antidepressant, sedative-hypnotic drugs)?

Nystagmus

This is rhythmic, involuntary movements of the eyes. The slow phase is vestibular, the quick phase central. The direction of the quick component, which is more evident at visual inspection, is used to define the direction of nystagmus.

Spontaneous Nystagmus

As visual fixation may suppress spontaneous nystagmus, movements of the eyes are observed without and with illuminated *Frenzel glasses* (20-diopter lenses that magnify the eyes and eliminate fixation). Spontaneous nystagmus may result from peripheral or central disorders (Table 1.1.1).

- **Peripheral**: attack of Ménière, labyrinthitis, temporal bone fracture, sudden unilateral loss of the vestibular function, benign paroxysmal vertigo.
  Horizontal or horizontal-rotatory, visually suppressed, often associated with auditory symptoms and vertigo, directed towards the irritated labyrinth, away from the paretic labyrinth.
  Degree I occurs only with the eyes pointing in the direction of the quick phase. It should be differentiated from physiological positional nystagmus. Degree II also occurs with the eyes looking straight ahead. Degree III also occurs with the eyes pointing in the direction of the slow phase.
- **Central**: head trauma, encephalitis, multiple sclerosis, brain tumour, drugs, alcohol.
  Any direction, often vertical, not visually suppressed, may or may not occur with vertigo, points towards the side of lesion, unusual auditory symptoms.

Positional Nystagmus

Patient supine with Frenzel glasses, slow changes of position.
- Head in mid position
- Head turned to the right
- Head turned to the left
- Head hanging over the edge of the bed

Postural Test (Hallpike Manoeuvre)

Patient seated (with Frenzel glasses) on the examining couch in such a way that when moved into the supine position, the head and neck will extend beyond the edge of the couch. The head is held by the physician, who rapidly moves the patient into the following nine positions (time of observation, 20–30 s per position):
1. Patient seated, head in mid position
2. Patient supine, head hanging
3. Patient seated, head in mid position
4. Patient seated, head to the right
5. Patient supine, head hanging turned to the right
6. Patient seated, head to the right
7. Patient seated, head to the left
8. Patient supine, head hanging turned to the left
9. Patient seated, head to the left

The postural test evaluated as follows:
- *Peripheral*: fixed direction of the nystagmus (beats in the same direction in different positions), occurs after a latent period, lasts less than 60 s, undergoes fatigue (weaker and shorter responses when repeating the manoeuvre). Classic finding of benign paroxysmal positioning vertigo.
- *Central*: changing direction of the nystagmus, no latency, lasts more than 60 s, does not undergo fatigue.

Vestibulospinal Reflexes

Abnormalities in the vestibulospinal pathways are revealed by the following tests:
- Finger-to-nose test (dysmetria)
- Heel-to-toe
- Dysdiadochokinesis (inability to rapidly turn the hand prone and supine)
- Pointing test
- Romberg test (standing with eyes closed, feet together and arms to the side)
- Posturography (objective Romberg test) with Luzern platform
- Unterberger test (stepping in place with eyes closed).

Caloric Test

The minimal caloric test is performed in the office setting with the patient sitting with head tilted backwards by 60°, and 5 ml of water injected in the ear at a temperature of 23°C. The opposite ear is tested in the same way. The length of the nystagmus is recorded. The **ice-water caloric test** is administered if no response is obtained with the 23°C test.

Electronystagmography/Videonystagmography

Nystagmus can be recorded electrically (electronystagmography), by means of an infrared photoelectric system, or by a video camera (videonystagmography).
- The patient is placed supine with the head raised by 30°, with the lateral semicircular canal placed in the optimal position for stimulation. A *heat irrigator* containing a pump system is used for irrigation (70–100 ml water per 30 s) with water at 7°C above and 7°C below body temperature. The caloric test sequence consists of right cold, left cold, left warm and right warm irrigation. The speed of the slow phase of nystagmus can be measured with a computer.
- Cold caloric stimulation means nystagmus beating away from the stimulated side.
- Warm caloric stimulation means nystagmus beating towards the stimulated side.

Table 1.1.1 Features in the history that help distinguish between peripheral and central causes of vertigo (from Kesser and Friedman [2])

	Peripheral	Central
Imbalance	Mild–moderate	Severe
Nausea and vomiting	**Severe**	Variable; may be minimal
Auditory symptoms	Common	Rare
Neurological symptoms	**Rare**	Common
Compensation	Rapid	Slow

- A "weaker" response on one side by 20% or greater is interpreted as a sign of a peripheral vestibular lesion (on that side).

Vestibular Evoked Myogenic Potentials (VEMP)

- *Definition*: Sound-induced vestibular evoked myogenic potentials are a valuable clinical tool for evaluation of vestibular function (functional status of the saccule and inferior vestibular nerve).
- *Principles*: To obtain information on its function, the saccule is acoustically stimulated by means of clicks at an intensity of 120 dB SPL and its response is registered at the level of the sternocleidomastoid muscle.
- *Indications*: In Ménière's disease, in vestibular neuritis, vestibular schwannomas originating from the inferior vestibular nerve, in forensic medicine, in rare isolated functional disorders of the saccule and when a superior canal dehiscence is suspected (see Sect. 1.5.2.10).

References

1. Arnold W, Ganzer U, Iurato S (2007) Checklist otorinolaringoiatria, CIC, Rome
2. Kesser BW, Friedman RA (2002) Functional disorders. In: Seiden AM, Tami TA, Pensak ML, Cotton RT, Gluckman JL (eds) Otolaryngology: the essentials. Thieme, Stuttgart, pp 33–43

Suggested Reading

1. Glasscock ME, Jackson CG, Forrest Josey A (1987) The ABR handbook: auditory brainstem response. Thieme, Stuttgart
2. Northern JL (1984) Impedance audiometry. In: Northern JL (ed) Hearing disorders. Little Brown. Boston
3. Poe DS (2007) Diagnosis and management of the patulous tube. Otol Neurotol 28:668–677
4. Robinette MS, Glattke TJ (2007) Otoacoustic emissions. Clinical applications, 3rd edn. Thieme, Stuttgart
5. Welgampola MS, Colebatch JG (2005) Characteristics and clinical applications of vestibular-evoked myogenic potentials. Neurology 64:1682–1688

1.1.6   Imaging of the Temporal Bone

MARTIN DOBRITZ

This section provides an overview of the principles of conventional radiography, computed tomography (CT) and magnetic resonance imaging (MRI) as well as details of their use in the practice of otology (Table 1.1.2). The physics of CT and MRI is beyond the scope of these guidelines.

1.1.6.1   Conventional Radiography

Although conventional radiography more and more has been replaced by CT, it is still worthwhile summarizing the principles and indications of some conventional techniques. The reason is that the Schüller and the transorbital projections are still useful to identify some preoperative and postoperative details, as well as for the recognition of large lesions in or around the temporal bone.

One of the most frequent indications for the *Schüller projection* is the preoperative assessment of the mastoid size and degree of pneumatization (Fig. 1.1.21a), the course of the sigmoid sinus, fracture lines and bony defects, e. g. caused by a cholesteatoma (Fig. 1.1.21b).

One of the most frequent indications for the *transorbital projection* is the postoperative demonstration of the correct position and integrity of the cochlear implant electrodes (Fig. 1.1.22). Note that CT techniques are not able to show the continuity of the electrodes in one image.

Schüller Projection

Projection:
- Lateral view of the mastoid
- Sagittal plane of the head parallel to the tabletop
- X-ray beam rotated 30°

What can be visualized:
- Extent of pneumatization of the mastoid

- Distribution/degree of aeration of the air cells
- Status of trabecular pattern
- Position and course of the sigmoid sinus

Notes:
- The sinus plate casts a sharp radiodense vertical line (Fig. 1.1.21) behind the external auditory canal (EAC).
- The oblique line crossing the radiolucency of the EAC is the superior ridge of the petrous bone.
- The internal auditory canal (IAC) is superimposed to the EAC.
- The temporomandibular joint can be seen directly anterior to the EAC (Fig. 1.1.21).

Transorbital Projection
Projection:
- Occiput facing the film
- Head flexed on the chin (15°)
- Each side obtained separately
- Beam directed to orbit centre

What can be visualized:

- Petrous apex, which appears foreshortened
- IAC in its full length
- Lateral to the IAC the vestibule and the semicircular canals
- Apical and middle coils of the cochlea superimposed upon the IAC, the basal turn underneath the vestibule (Fig. 1.1.22)

1.1.6.2 Computed Tomography

Since its introduction in the 1970s, CT has developed to the widely accepted gold standard for evaluating most of the diseases of the temporal bone for the following reasons.

The high contrast between air and osseous structures in connection with the high spatial resolution leads to easier differentiation and excellent recognition of inflammatory or neoplastic changes of the bone as well as fractures. In addition to that, the ossicular chain and the status of pneumatized cells can be determined in an excellent way.

Multislice techniques produce isotropic 3D datasets to perform excellent multiplanar reformations. Besides re-

Table 1.1.2 Computed tomography (*CT*) versus magnetic resonance imaging (*MRI*)

Pathologic conditions	CT (bony structures)	MRI (soft tissues)
Temporal bone fractures	+++	–
Exostosis, osteoma of external auditory canal	++	–
Congenital malformations of middle and inner ear	+++	+
Inflammatory conditions (mastoiditis, chronic otitis media, malignant external otitis)	++	+
Otosclerosis	+++	–
Cholesteatoma	+++	+
Petrous apex lesions	+++	+++
Cerebral abscess	++	+++
Labyrinthitis, meningitis	+	++
Schwannoma	–	+++
Sinus thrombosis	++	++
Endolymphatic sac tumour	++	+++
Arterial and venous variants	++	++
Tumour of cerebellopontine angle	–	+++
Paraganglioma	++	+++
Malignant neoplasms	++	+++
Postoperative imaging:		
Cochlear implant, position of the prosthesis following stapedectomy, status of mastoid following "close" tympanoplasty	+++	–
Follow-up vestibular schwannoma surgery, skull base surgery	–	+++

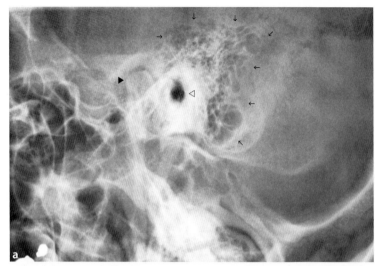

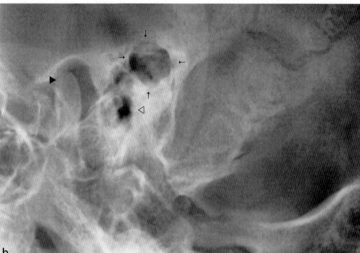

Fig. 1.1.21 a Schüller projection left side, normal anatomy. External auditory canal (◁), pneumatized area (→), temporomandibular joint (▶). **b** Schüller projection left side. Reduced pneumatization and bony defect (→) caused by cholesteatoma (*arrows*). External auditory canal (◁), temporomandibular joint (▶)

ducing radiation exposure for the patient, the secondary reconstruction helps to localize abnormalities in vertical and horizontal planes as well as to define the relationship to adjacent intracranial and extracranial lesions.

The following list gives the reader an update of the actual CT technique and its limitations:

- Slice thickness less than 1 mm, multiplanar reformations (axial slices, coronal plane, paracoronal plane), imaging of calcified structures
- Multislice spiral CT (64 slices)
- Isotropic datasets (primary axial data acquisition)
- Multiplanar reconstructions possible
- Bone reconstruction algorithm/high-resolution osseous structures.
- Window, width 4,000 HU, centre 500 HU

What can be visualized:

1. Anatomy of the temporal bone (Figs. 1.1.23, 1.1.24).
2. Tympanic membrane and tensor tympani muscle.
3. Auditory ossicles (Fig. 1.1.23; Fig. 9.3.1b). Note that the whole stapes is visible only in the axial projection (Figs. 1.1.23a, 1.5.5b).
4. Bony labyrinth
   - Cochlea, e. g. congenital malformations (Fig. 1.2.2)? Ossification of the cochlear turns (Fig. 1.1.25) following meningitis, prior to cochlear implantation? Cochlear otosclerosis?
   - Vestibule (air bubbles? Fig. 1.5.5a)
   - Semicircular canals (fistula?)
5. Round and oval windows (Fig. 9.3.1a)
6. Vestibular aqueduct (Fig. 1.1.23, normal; Fig. 1.1.26, enlarged).

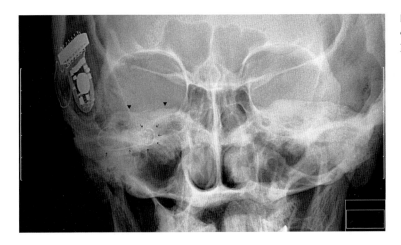

Fig. 1.1.22 Transorbital projection, cochlear implant (→), superior edge of petrous portion (▼)

7. Intratemporal facial nerve (labyrinthine, tympanic and mastoid segments).
8. Defects of the temporal bone (Fig. 1.4.17b).
9. Fractures (Figs. 1.5.5b, 1.5.8b, 1.7.4).

Notes:
- No contrast media.
- No useful information in cases of vestibular schwannoma.
- The reconstructed images are not always as satisfactory as the native sections in coronal or lateral projections, which, on the other hand, are sometimes difficult to obtain (children, traumatized patients, older people).

1.1.6.3 Magnetic Resonance Imaging

As CT is the gold standard for bony lesions, MRI is an excellent modality for imaging of the cranial nerves (Fig. 1.2.3), the vestibulocochlear system, soft tissue lesions of the temporal bone and the cerebellopontine angle (see Table 1.1.1).

Otologists ordering MRI should be aware of the following basic principles:
- Compatibility with certain implanted medical devices; cave, a pacemaker and a cochlear implant are contraindications; titanium implants and modern stapes prosthesis are compatible.
- In MRI there is no involvement of ionizing radiation.
- After a high-frequency impulse, the resonance of the protons provides the signal used for the images.
- Visualization of water and soft tissue.
- Air and cortical bone do not have protons and therefore these components are not visible in any sequence. Consequently, MRI does not delineate bony anatomy (Fig. 1.2.3).

- Differences in relaxation properties among tissues cause typical contrast between different tissues. Fat appears as bright areas in T1-weighted images (Fig. 1.1.27a, 1.4.18a,b) and fluids (CSF, inner ear fluids) appear as bright areas in the T2-weighted images (Figs. 1.1.27b, Fig. 1.4.18c). Vessels containing flowing blood emit no or low signal (Fig. 1.5.6c) because the excited protons move out of the area before detection of the emitted signal (most sequences). See Sect. 1.5.5 for the differential diagnosis of congenital cholesteatoma, cholesterol granuloma and mucocele.
- A variety of techniques can be employed in MRI of lesions of the temporal bone area.
- 3D T2-weighted sequences (3D constructive interference in steady state and 3D fast spin echo) offer submillimetre isotropic high-resolution datasets.
- Intravenous contrast agents (Fig. 1.1.27a) can be employed to enhance MRI (most commonly gadolinium as a T1-positive contrast agent is used).
- Enhancement is commonly observed in neoplasms (Fig. 1.1.27a) and inflammatory conditions (Fig. 1.7.2).

Suggested Reading

1. Ahuja AT et al. (2003) Computed tomography imaging of the temporal bone—normal anatomy. Clinic Radiol 58:681–686
2. Chan LL et al. (2001) Surgical anatomy of the temporal bone. An atlas. Neuroradiol 43:797–808
3. Harnsberger R et al. (2004) Diagnostic imaging. head and neck, 1st edn. Amirsys, Altona
4. Swartz JD et al. (1997) Imaging of the temporal bone, 3rd edn. Thieme, Stuttgart
5. Valvassori GE et al. (2004) Imaging of the head and neck, 2nd edn. Thieme, Stuttgart

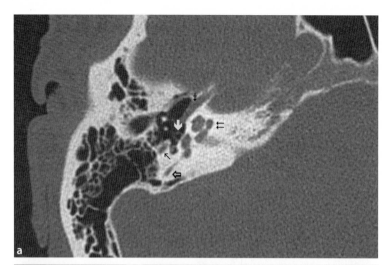

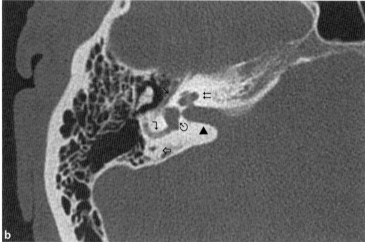

Fig. 1.1.23a,b Axial computed tomography (CT) slice, right ear. Tensor tympani muscle (⇅), stapes (⇩), cochlea (⇆), facial nerve (↖), vestibular aqueduct (⇐), internal auditory canal (▲), vestibule (↻), lateral semicircular canal ⌐). Note the incudomalleal joint and the "ice-cream cone" (body of the incus with the malleus head)

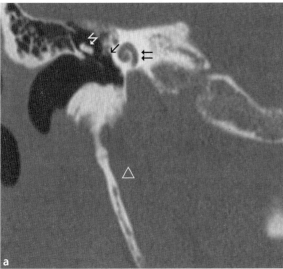

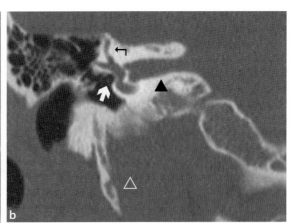

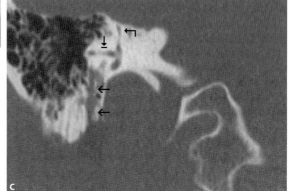

Fig. 1.1.24a–c Coronal CT reformations, right ear. Cochlea (⇌), styloid process (◁), facial nerve (↖), malleus head (↯), superior semicircular canal (↩), lateral semicircular canal (⊥), stapes (⇩), internal auditory canal (▲)

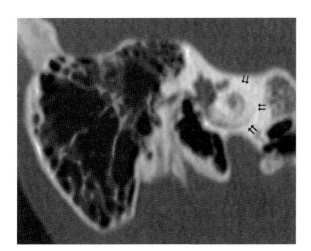

Fig. 1.1.25 Coronal CT reformation right side. Labyrinthine ossification (⇊)

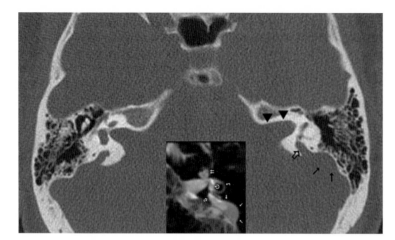

Fig. 1.1.26 Large endolymphatic sac anomaly with progressive deafness in a 1 year-old girl (large vestibular aqueduct syndrome). Axial CT: internal auditory canal (▼), vestibular aqueduct (⇔), endolymphatic sac area (↑). *Insert*: magnetic resonance imaging (MRI), T2-weighted: cochlea (⇔), lateral semicircular canal (⌐), endolymphatic duct (⇔), endolymphatic sac (↑), vestibule (↺)

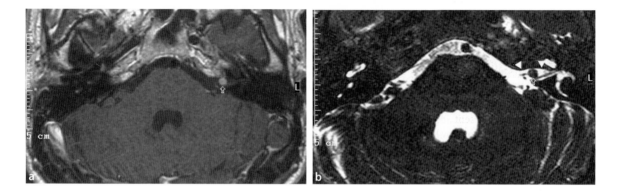

Fig. 1.1.27a,b Vestibular schwannoma (⇑) left side. Internal auditory canal (▽). **a** MRI, T1-weighted contrast enhanced. **b** MRI, T2-weighted

1.2 Malformations of the Ear

JAN KIEFER, THOMAS SOMERS, AND WOLFGANG ARNOLD

1.2.1 Synonyms

Congenital, hereditary, developmental defects of the external, middle and/or internal ear. Synonyms for outer and middle ear malformations are congenital aural atresia, ear atresia, microtia, anotia and major malformations of the ear.

1.2.2 Definition

Congenital malformations of the external, middle or inner ear are, by definition, present at birth. They can be caused by *genetic defects* (chromosomal abnormalities, spontaneous single gene mutations, polygenic inheritance) or by *acquired* factors that disturb the embryonic development of the ear. Intrauterine influences may be extrinsic in origin (drugs, nutritional deficiencies, viral infections, hormonal) or may be the result of maternal influences such as autoimmune reaction or metabolic disorders.

Malformations of the outer ear and the middle ear are often combined, whereas malformation of the inner ear occurs independently from outer ear malformation in most cases.

Malformations of the **outer and middle ear** can be graded according to the severity of malformations and functional impairment:

- *Minor auricular malformations*: small malformations of the cartilage of the auricle (Fig. 1.2.1a), in rare cases associated with malformed or fixed middle ear ossicles, good pneumatization of the middle ear and mastoid.
- *Middle grade auricular malformations* (Fig. 1.2.1b): microtia, stenosis or atresia of the outer ear canal, normal or slightly reduced pneumatization of the middle ear and mastoid, malformations or fixation of the ossicles.
- *Severe auricular malformations* (Fig. 1.2.1c): anomalia or aplasia of the auricle, atresia of the external auditory canal, severely reduced or missing pneumatization of the middle ear cavity or the mastoid, replacement of parts of the middle ear by a bone plate or connective

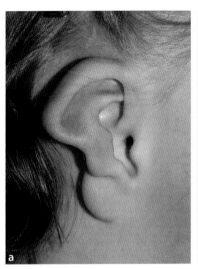 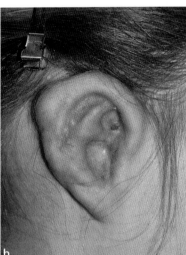 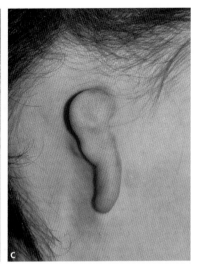

Fig. 1.2.1 a Minor auricular malformation (in a case of Goldenhar syndrome). **b** Middle grade auricular malformation. **c** Severe microtia

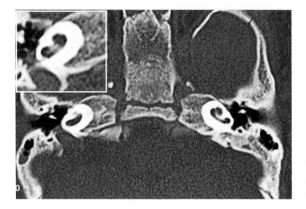

Fig. 1.2.2 Mondini–Alexander dysplasia of the cochlea with enlarged basal turn (*insert*) combined with vestibular aplasia

tissue, severely malformed, not differentiated or missing ossicles, missing one or both cochlear windows. In 20% of cases there is an anomalous course of the facial nerve.

Malformations or dysplasia of the **cochleovestibular system** mostly occur isolated from malformations of the outer or middle ear; however, they can also be associated with other craniofacial abnormalities and hereditary syndromes. Typical morphological forms of cochleovestibular dysplasia can be related to a disturbed or arrested intrauterine development of the labyrinth, resulting in various forms and degrees of malformations. They may be caused by viral infection, hypoxia, intoxication or exposition to X-rays during the third to eighth gestation weeks or by genetic defects.

Clinically, the following forms of malformations can be distinguished:

- *Michel dysplasia*: total aplasia of the bony and membranous labyrinth, no inner ear development.
- *Cochlear aplasia*: missing cochlea with vestibular parts present.
- *Cochlear hypoplasia*: mild or severe hypoplasia of the cochlea, vestibular parts are present.
- *Common cavity*: single cavity, no partition between cochlear and vestibular parts.
- *Mondini–Alexander dysplasia*: dysplasia of the bony and membranous labyrinth with reduced number of cochlear turns, incomplete partition between turns, enlarged vestibule and anomalies of the semicircular canals (Fig. 1.2.2).
- *Bing–Siebenmann dysplasia*: dysplasia of the membranous vestibular labyrinth, normal anatomy and function of the cochlea.
- *Large vestibular aqueduct syndrome*: frequent isolated malformation (enlargement) of the endolymphatic spaces of the cochlea and the vestibular aqueduct (Fig.

1.1.26), often associated with Mondini dysplasia, part of *Pendred* syndrome (Fig. 1.1.16); progressive hearing loss during childhood, also fluctuating in most cases, resulting in deafness. In 60% of cases there are attacks of vertigo.

- *Aplasia/malformation of the cochlear/vestibular nerve*: a missing cochlear or cochleovestibular nerve (Fig. 1.2.3).

Malformations of the cochleovestibular nerve are rare. They may occur as isolated forms with normal cochlear anatomy (Fig. 1.2.3), or in conjunction with malformations of the inner ear, e.g. in a common cavity. In these cases, a common cochlear and vestibular nerve may be present.

1.2.3 Epidemiology

The incidence of syndromic and non-syndromic malformations of the external and middle ear is 1:10,000 to 1:20,000 live births per year. The incidence of cochleovestibular malformations is around 1:80,000 per year. A unilateral major ear malformation is 3 times more common than a bilateral malformation. These malformations occur more commonly in males and more often on the right side. Non-syndromal (sporadic) congenital malformations of the ear are more common than syndromic cases that are associated with other symptoms.

In summary, the incidence of congenital hearing defects is a follows:

- Severe hearing loss or deafness of any origin 1:1,000
- Hereditary sensorineural hearing loss 1:4,000

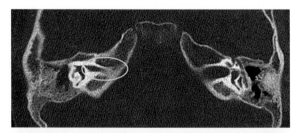
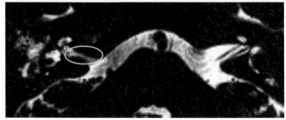

Fig. 1.2.3 Unilateral narrow internal auditory canal and missing cochleovestibular nerve (*ovals*) with normal cochlear anatomy

- Syndromic and non-syndromic external and middle ear malformations 1:10,000–20,000
- Malformations of the cochleovestibular system 1:80 000

Common craniofacial syndromes with involvement of the ear are:

- *Waardenburg syndrome*: sensorineural hearing impairment, partial albinism (white forelock), heterochromia of the iris, lateral displacement of the medial canthi
- *Pierre Robin syndrome*: micrognathia with glossoptosis, cleft soft palate, anomalies of the heart, blood vessels, skeletal system, eyes and ear
- *Treacher Collins–Franceschetti syndrome*: malformed external ear, malar hypoplasia, antimongoloid slant, coloboma of the lower eyelid, conductive hearing loss, caused by stenotic or atresic external auditory canal, small middle ear space, deformed and ankylosed malleus, fused incudomalleolar junction, stapes malformation, poorly pneumatized mastoid, anomalous course of the facial nerve
- *Goldenhar syndrome*: facial asymmetry, unilateral malformed external ear (Fig. 1.2.1a) with retroauricular tags and sinuses, conductive hearing loss, microphtalmia, epibulbar lipodermoid, macrostomia with mandibular hypoplasia, vertebral anomalies

1.2.4 Symptoms

Malformations of the external ear are visible at birth. In patients with a severe external deformity a middle ear abnormality is to be expected. Only in rare instances atresia of the outer ear canal may be seen in patients with normal pinna.

Craniofacial abnormalities in syndromic cases should draw attention to possible malformations of the external, middle or inner ear. Usually, malformations of the auricle or outer ear canal give early indications of conductive, mixed sensorineural hearing loss or deafness.

Inner ear malformations in general are accompanied with severe or profound sensorineural hearing loss. The main symptoms are missing reactions to sound and delayed development of language (see Sect. 1.6.12). Inner ear malformation will often be unrecognized at birth; therefore, routine newborn hearing screening is recommended for early detection of hearing loss caused by isolated inner (or middle) ear malformations.

1.2.5 Complications

Especially in cases of bilateral external malformations, early evaluation of hearing and continuous follow-up is necessary as well as early adaptation of conventional bone-conduction hearing aids. A delay in a proper diagnosis and auditory rehabilitation will have an impact on the entire development of the individual because of delayed or insufficient speech and language acquisition. Also in unilateral cases, a missed diagnosis of an associated hearing problem at the normal looking side (e.g. sensorineural hearing loss, malformation of the ossicles, serous otitis media, etc.) can lead to deficits in the development of speech and cognitive retardation.

1.2.6 Diagnostic Procedures

1. Assessment of auricular deformity and atresia at birth.
2. Early postnatal paediatric counselling with general physical examination to search for other congenital anomalies.
3. Early evaluation of the auditory function in both unilateral and bilateral atresia.
4. Newborn hearing screening is the most efficient method for early detection of hearing loss (see also Sect. 1.6.12). Otoacoustic emission screening in unilateral cases is performed at the normal side followed by an air-conduction auditory brainstem response if no emissions are found. We should bear in mind that even a total sensorineural hearing loss may occur in the normal-appearing ear.
5. A bone-conduction auditory brainstem response is performed for bilateral cases of congenital aural atresia within the first few weeks of life. The incidence of an association of an inner ear abnormality with a congenital aural atresia is uncommon but must be excluded.
6. In case of bilateral cochleovestibular malformation, early imaging is mandatory, as cochlear implantation in a deaf-born baby should be performed at the end of the first year of life (see also Sect. 1.6.12). MRI visualizes the fluid spaces of the cochlea and identifies the presence of the cochlear and vestibular nerves (Fig. 1.2.3). A high-resolution CT scan in both the axial and the coronal planes is obligatory to show the bony structures of the petrous bone.
7. Imaging in the case of aural atresia can be postponed until surgery is planned. Reconstruction of the outer ear canal and middle ear can recommended to be performed between the fifth and the tenth years of life. Reconstruction of the auricle with autogenous rib car-

tilage is usually possible from age 8–10 years upwards, when sufficient cartilage is available.

8. For reconstruction of the outer ear canal or middle ear high resolution CT scans in both the axial and the coronal planes are important. Critical information for an eventual repair is:
   – The presence of sufficient space to create a new ear canal
   – The degree of pneumatization of the temporal bone
   – The course of the facial nerve, both the relationship of the horizontal portion to the oval window and the location of the mastoid segment
   – The existence of the oval window and stapes footplate
   – The presence and appearance of the ossicular chain
   – The existence of a round window and its relation to the facial nerve
   – The anatomy of the cochleovestibular system

1.2.7 Therapeutic Management

1.2.7.1 Malformations of the Outer and Middle Ear

- The management of severe malformations of the external and middle ear (as well as the inner ear) and their surgical treatment should be centralized and performed by experienced surgeons seeing a reasonable number of patients.
- The therapy varies according to whether the abnormality is unilateral or bilateral.
- In unilateral cases priority is usually given to the aesthetical aspect (if hearing is normal at the contralateral side), whereas in bilateral cases attention should be primarily focused on the auditory aspect.

1.2.7.2 Management of Hearing Impairment

- Early amplification with a classic bone-conduction hearing aid is mandatory in bilateral cases of aural atresia with useful cochlear function (Fig. 1.2.4a). If there is a demand for better speech discrimination especially in noise, bone-conduction hearing aids or active middle ear implants can be valuable also in unilateral atresia.
- Amplification with a bone-anchored hearing aid (Fig. 1.2.4b, c) can only be envisaged when the mastoid bone has reached sufficient thickness (not sooner than the age of 2–3 years). Sufficient bone thickness is necessary to allow a good osseous integration of the im-

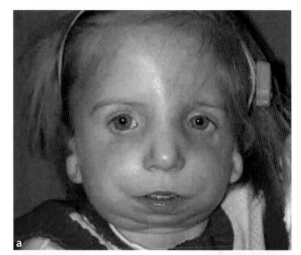

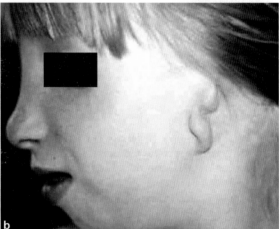

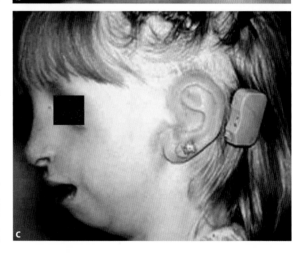

Fig. 1.2.4 **a** Child with bilateral atresia with a bone-anchored hearing aid mounted on a soft headband. **b** Child age 6 years, before surgery. **c** The same child after placement of a bone-anchored hearing aid and bone-anchored auricular prosthesis

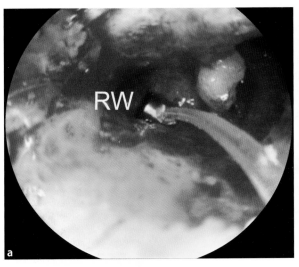
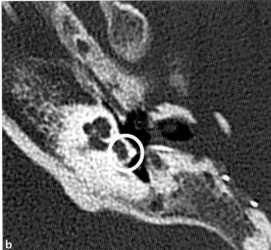

Fig. 1.2.5 Intraoperative view (*left*) and postoperative CT scan (*right*) showing the vibrating element (FMT) placed on the round window membrane

planted titanium screw. In comparison with a classic bone-conduction hearing aid, a bone-anchored hearing aid offers the patient a better sound input (especially at higher frequencies) and less distortion. This system is also experienced by most patients as being more comfortable than the conventional aid. If bone conduction is normal (which is usually the case) it ensures quasi-normal hearing. Bilateral bone-anchored hearing aid adaptation in bilateral cases has been shown to be beneficial to bilateral atresia patients.

- Implantable hearing aids (such as the Vibrant Soundbridge® produced by MED-EL and the MET® middle ear transducer produced by Otologics) have been implanted with excellent results in patients with atresia. In cases of congenital aural atresia, the ossicular chain is often severely malformed and/or fixed. Under these circumstances, the active element of the implantable hearing aid can be coupled to the round window membrane (Fig. 1.2.5). The implantation can be combined with reconstruction of the auricle using a cartilaginous framework (Fig. 1.2.6).

Surgical repair of the external auditory canal and middle ear is reserved for ideal cases (Fig. 1.2.6) where good postoperative hearing (within 30 dB AC) can be expected.

1.2.7.3   Management of Aesthetic Deficits

- To improve the aesthetic appearance and to restore self-confidence, the patient with the family should be counselled in an unbiased way regarding the two contemporary surgical options: the auricular reconstruc-

tion using rib cartilage (or alloplastic material) and the fitting of an auricular prosthesis. The pros and cons of each technique are extensively discussed and the new candidates are presented to patients having undergone one or the other procedure. Realistic presentation of pre- and postoperative pictures of one's own patients is an alternative.

- If an auricular reconstruction is performed, it is delayed until the costal cartilage has developed sufficiently. There has to be enough cartilage available to construct a cartilaginous framework of a normal size (Fig. 1.2.7). The first operative step of microtia repair should be done between the fifth and the tenth year of age before or simultaneously with any functional operation because scar formation, due to prior functional surgery in the region, compromises the aesthetical result.

- The alternative for an auricular reconstruction is an epithesis attached to two bone-anchored percutaneous titanium fixtures (Fig. 1.2.4b, c). This procedure can be combined with a bone-anchored hearing aid implantation. This gives excellent cosmetic results but the patient has to accept the wearing of an epithesis, the possible occurrence of skin reactions and the fact that the epithesis needs regular care and annual or biannual renewal.

1.2.7.4   Malformations of the Inner Ear

- Children with inner ear malformation generally suffer from a sensorineural hearing impairment, in most cases severe or profound. Providing early amplifica-

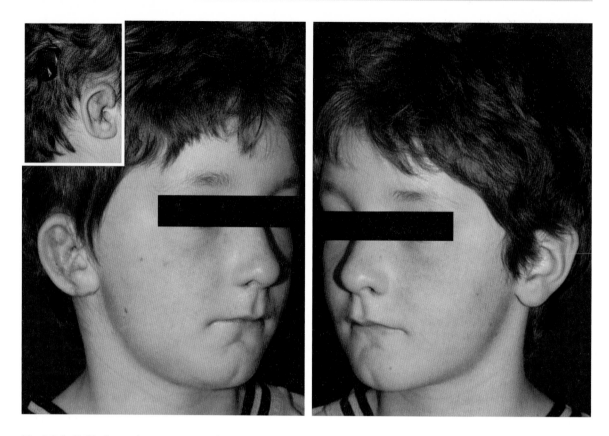

Fig. 1.2.6 Child after total reconstruction of the right auricle and implantation of an active middle ear implant. The *insert* shows the external audioprocessor

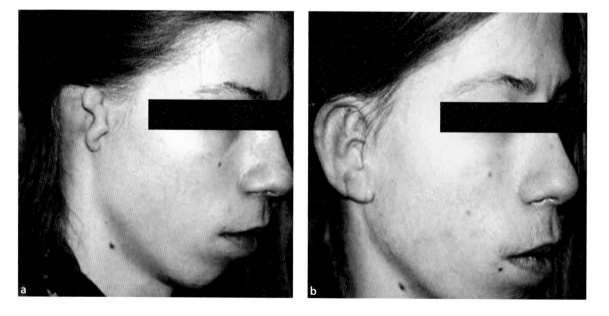

Fig. 1.2.7a–c Young man before (**a**) and after (**b**) auricular reconstruction according to the Nagata technique using rib cartilage; the retroauricular sulcus is preformed in a second stage (**c**)

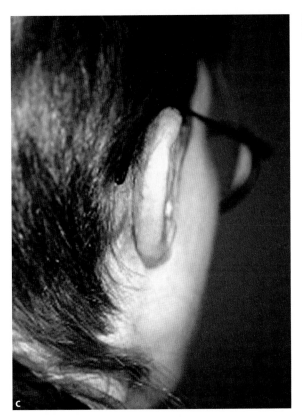

Fig. 1.2.7 *(continued)* **a–c** Young man before (**a**) and after (**b**) auricular reconstruction according to the Nagata technique using rib cartilage; the retroauricular sulcus is preformed in a second stage (**c**)

tion with hearing aids and, if necessary, cochlear implantation is essential to avoid the sequelae of auditory deprivation. The therapeutic management of children with sensorineural hearing impairment is described in detail in Sect. 1.6.12.

- Cochlear implantation is possible in most cases of inner ear malformations with the exception of cochlear aplasia/severe hypoplasia or a missing cochlear/vestibular nerve. However, the types of electrode and surgical access have to be tailored to the individual type of malformation as diagnosed by CT and MRI.
- Complications such as intraoperative reflux of liquor (gusher), facial nerve stimulation, or meningitis after implantation have a slightly higher incidence.
- The outcome after cochlear implantation is generally reduced in severe malformation in comparison with a morphologically normal cochlea. Patients with an isolated large vestibular aqueduct have prognosis comparable to that of patients with normal cochleae.

1.2.8 Surgical Principles

1.2.8.1 Cochlear Implantation

See Sect. 1.6.12.

1.2.8.2 Bone-Anchored Hearing Aid (Tjëllström Technique)

- Local (adults) or general anaesthesia (children).
- Marking of the implant site about 55 mm behind the anticipated external canal.
- Retroauricular split-thickness skin flap elevation with dermatome leaving hair follicles in the dermis or straight incision with subdermal elevation.
- Wide subcutaneous tissue reduction with removal of dermis and hair follicles to establish a hairless region and a reaction-free penetration of the abutment through the skin. A periosteal layer is preserved.
- A hole is made with the 4-mm guide drill under abundant irrigation for cooling.
- Widening of the hole with a countersink drill.
- The self-tapping fixture with premounted abutment (coupling element) is screwed into the hole.
- The skin flap is perforated to allow passage of the abutment, laid back on the periosteum, and the wound is closed.
- A healing cap is snapped onto the abutment keeping an ointment-soaked gauze down to eliminate bleeding.
- Mastoid dressing for 1 day.
- Fitting of the sound processor after healing, usually after 1 month.

1.2.8.3 Functional Surgery for Ear Atresia (Jahrsdoerfer Technique)

- General anaesthesia.
- Installation of facial monitoring.
- Retroauricular incision and mastoid periosteum reflection.
- Revelation of a large temporalis fascia free graft for tympanic repair.
- Anterior approach behind the glenoid fossa with drilling along the middle fossa plate towards the epitympanum.
- Careful removal of the atretic plate and freeing of the ossicular mass in the epitympanum (Fig. 1.2.8).
- Ossicular reconstruction with the patient's intact, although malformed, ossicular chain is preferred to use of an ossicular prosthesis.

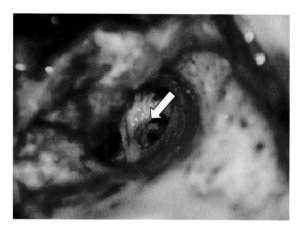

Fig. 1.2.8 Intraoperative view after drilling of a new ear canal and exposure of the (incomplete) atresic plate (with the incudo-stapedial joint behind it)

- Tympanic membrane repair with fascia.
- Coverage of the new auditory canal and the drum with a very thin split-thickness skin graft.
- Meatoplasty and suturing of the lateral end of the skin graft to the skin of the concha.
- Silicone button on the drum and packing of the ear canal.
- Closure of the retroauricular incision.
- Mastoid dressing.

1.2.8.4   Bone-anchored Epithesis

- The procedure is similar to the placement of a fixture for a bone-anchored hearing aid (see Sect. 1.2.8.2) but two fixtures are placed instead of one.
- The bridge construction for attachment of the silicone epithesis as well as the epithesis itself is made by a prosthetic technician after complete healing (1 month).

1.2.8.5   Implantation of Active Middle Ear Prosthesis

- The first steps until identification of the ossicular chain are similar to the Jahrsdoerfer technique for functional reconstruction of the atresic ear.
- Approach may be transmastoid (if pneumatized) or postglenoid for total atresia.
- Identification of the epitympanic space, ossicular chain and facial nerve.
- Opening of facial recess (in transmastoid approach) or transcanalicular identification of the round window niche.

- Removal of the bony overhang until the round window membrane is well identified.
- Preparation of the bony implant bed.
- Placement of the active vibrating element, e.g. the floating mass transducer, in contact with the round window membrane with interposition of a piece of temporalis fascia.
- Fixation of the implant, wire and the vibrating element.
- If the implantation is combined with reconstruction of the external ear, the retroauricular sulcus may be covered with a well-vascularized temporoparietal fascial flap.
- Wound closure and light compressive dressing.

1.2.8.6   Reconstructive Surgery of the Auricle (Nagata Technique)

1. Stage 1: insertion of auricular framework and lobule transposition
   - General anaesthesia.
   - Preparation of two surgical fields (in the auricular and thoracic regions).
   - Thoracic incision and retrieval of rib cartilage: the floating rib is used for the helix, the synchondrotic area of ribs 6, 7 and 8 is used for the framework body.
   - Carving and assembling of the three-dimensional auricular framework (helix, anthelix, scapha, triangular fossa, tragus and antitragus).
   - Careful dissection and excision of malformed vestigial cartilage.
   - The incision in the auricular area allows for transposition of the lobule usually in the posterosuperior direction.
   - A large skin pocket is developed and the framework is inserted.
   - Two silicone drains ensure vacuum suction essential for good cooptation of the skin.
   - Dressing.
2. Stage 2 (3–6 months after stage 1): elevation of the auricle from the head and grafting of posterior aspect of the new auricle
   - General anaesthesia.
   - Incision along the helix.
   - Elevation of the auricle.
   - A semilunar piece of cartilage is placed under the auricular framework to form the posterior conchal wall and to elevate the new auricle.
   - Coverage of this cartilage with a pedicled superficial temporalis flap or a mastoidal musculoperiosteal flap.
   - Grafting of the rear aspect of the auricle with a thin split-thickness skin graft.
   - Closure of the incision.

Suggested Reading

1. Bosman AJ, Snik AF, van der Pouw CT, Mylanus EA, Cremers CW (2001) Audiometric evaluation of bilaterally fitted bone anchored hearing aids. Audiology 40:158–167
2. Colletti V, Soli S.D, Carner M, Colletti L (2006) Treatment of mixed hearing losses via implantation of a vibratory transducer on the round window. Int J Audiol 45:600–608
3. De la Cruz A, Chandrasekhar SS (1994) Congenital malformation of the temporal bone. In: Brackmann DE, Shelton C, Arriaga MA (eds) Otologic surgery. Saunders, Philadelphia, pp 70–84
4. Firmin F, Guichard S (2001) La reconstruction auriculaire en cas de microtie. Principes, méthodes et classification. Ann Chirurgie Plast Esthet 46:447–466
5. Jahrsdoerfer RA, Yeakley JW, Aguilar EA et al. (1992). Grading system for the selection of patients with congenital aural atresia. Am J Otol 13:6–12
6. Jackler RK, Luxford WM, House W (1987) Congenital malformations of the inner ear. A classification based on embryogenesis. Laryngoscope 97(Suppl 40):2–14
7. Kiefer J, Arnold W, Staudenmaier R (2006) Round window stimulation with an implantable hearing aid (Soundbridge®) combined with autogenous reconstruction of the auricle-a new approach. ORL J Otorhinolaryngol Relat Spec 68:378–385
8. Marquet JF, Declau Fr, De Cock M et al. (1988) Congenital middle ear malformations. Acta Otorhinolaryngol Belg 42:117–302
9. Somers T, De Cubber J, Govaerts P et al. (1998) Total auricular repair: bone anchored prosthesis or plastic reconstruction. Acta Otorhinolaryngologica Belg 52:317–327
10. Weerda H (2007) Surgery of the auricle. Tumors—trauma—defects—abnormalities, Thieme, Stuttgart

1.3 Diseases of the Auricle and of the External Auditory Canal

SALVATORE IURATO

1.3.1 Trauma/Otohaematoma

Owing to its position, shape and prominence, the auricle is at risk of sharp and blunt trauma, lacerations, bite wounds, burns and damage from extreme cold.

1.3.1.1 Sharp Trauma, Lacerations and Bite Wounds

Diagnostic Procedures
- History (accident, assault, animal bite, human bite)
- Inspection (sharp wound, loss of tissue, avulsion)
- Photographic documentation for legal purposes
- In cases of infection, bacterial cultures to isolate the offending organism

Therapy

Conservative Treatment
Early treatment is essential for optimal cosmetic results and to prevent infection! Treatment involves:
- Jet washing with 4% H_2O_2 or iodopovidone (10% solution) or benzalconiochloride.
- Removal of debris and all devitalized tissues, sterile medication.
- Antibiotics: amoxicillin plus clavulanic acid or cephalosporins. Antimicrobial therapy directed at specific organisms detected in the laboratory.
- Steroids in the case of lacerations.

Useful Additional Therapeutic Strategies
- Rabies prevention for animal bites
- Tetanus prevention for all contaminated wounds
- Hyperbaric oxygen following large avulsion injuries

Surgical Treatment
Surgical treatment involves surgical repair depending on the severity of the wound and the time interval between injury and treatment.

1.3.1.2 Blunt Trauma and Auricular Haematoma

Synonyms
Otohaematoma, haematoma of the auricle, traumatic seroma.

Definition
Serous fluid or blood accumulation between the perichondral layer and the underlying auricular cartilage (subperichondrial haematoma).

Aetiology/Epidemiology
A blunt trauma (contact sports, assaults) to the external ear is the main cause (boxer ear) (Fig. 1.3.1).

On the outer surface of the auricle, a layer of subcutaneous connective tissue is missing and therefore a tan-

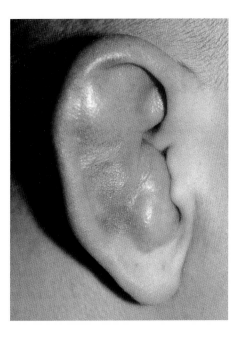

Fig. 1.3.1 Subperichondrial seroma over the lateral surface of the auricle (result of blunt trauma)

gential force is directly transmitted to the perichondrium and the underlying cartilage. The small blood vessels of the perichondrium are ruptured, causing a blood leak which raises the perichondrium away from the underlying cartilage.

Symptoms
Soft fluctuating mass on the outer surface of the auricle, feeling of tension and warmth, pain.

Therapy
Treatment is aimed at the aseptic drainage of the blood or serous fluid and prevention of its reaccumulation.
- Simple aspiration is not sufficient (risk of a high rate of recurrence and/or infection).
- Local injection of lidocaine, small retroauricular skin incision, fenestration of the cartilage and drainage of the blood. Placement of a pressure dressing covered with ointment and fixed into the concha with through-and-through mattress sutures using monofilament nylon.

Complications
- Recurrences needing repeat drainage procedures.
- The most frequent complications are necrosis of the cartilage, organization of the haematoma by ingrowth of fibrocytes and infection (perichondritis) with chondroneogenesis. The end result is a "cauliflower ear".

1.3.1.3   Frostbite

Following very low temperature exposure, the superior part of the auricle is the most affected area.

Symptoms
There is no symptom at the beginning owing to the anaesthesia of the affected part caused by the very low external temperature. At the beginning the skin of the affected area is pale and numb, then it is blue-reddish with serum-filled blisters.

Therapy
- Mild rewarming (infrared light at 38–42°C). Direct heat or snow massage is not recommended.
- Medication of the serum-filled blisters with iodopovidone solution.
- Sterile dressing to prevent the development of secondary infection.

1.3.1.4   Burning

- When the skin is still present, medication with antibiotic ointment
- Surgical treatment if the cartilage is exposed

1.3.2   Infections of the Auricle and of the External Auditory Canal

1.3.2.1   Infections of the Auricle

Aetiology
Infections of the auricular skin are caused by *Staphylococcus aureus* or *Streptococcus pyogenes*. Trauma (wounds, surgical incisions, bites) or microtrauma (scratching) can introduce pathogenic organisms. Chronic bacterial or fungal infections of the external auditory canal (external otitis) can progress and involve the auricle. *Pseudomonas aeruginosa* is the main agent responsible for the infection of the perichondrium of the auricle.

Symptoms
The auricle is swollen, erythematous, indurated, painful (bacterial infection) or itching (mycosis, allergy). The skin weeps a serous or purulent exudate.

Complications
Extension of the infection into the perichondrium and cartilage (chondritis).

Diagnostic Procedures
It is important to check whether the perichondrium and the underlying cartilage are involved.

Differential Diagnosis
- *Erysipelas*: the whole auricle, ear lobe included, is painful, reddish and swollen (Fig. 1.3.2a).
- *Perichondritis*: bacterial infection of the auricular cartilage without involvement of the ear lobe (Fig. 1.3.2b).
- *Allergic reaction* to insect bite.
- *Relapsing polychondritis* (Fig. 1.3.2c): autoimmune disorder (see Sect. 1.6.7). In 90% of cases it begins at the level of the auricle and later extends to other cartilages (nasal septum, laryngeal, tracheal and bronchial cartilages). The main symptoms are local pain, oedema, erythema, articular pain often associated with fever, sensorineural hearing loss, iritis, conjunctivitis,

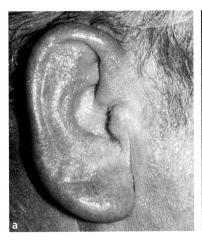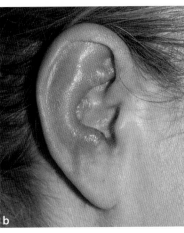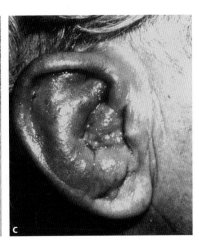

Fig. 1.3.2 a Erysipelas; **b** perichondritis; **c** relapsing polychondritis. Note that in erysipelas (**a**) the whole auricle, ear lobe included, is involved, while in perichondritis (**b**) the ear lobe is normal

elevated sedimentation rate, and involvement of the septal cartilage and tracheal cartilage, with cartilage destruction and respiratory problems.

- *Chondrodermatitis nodularis chronica*: unknown cause.
- *Gouty tophi.*

Treatment
1. Bacterial infection
   - Local disinfection
   - Antibacterial treatment (orally): amoxicillin plus clavulanic acid, sulphamethoxazole plus trimetropin
   - Antiphlogistic treatment: diclofenac
2. Erysipelas: antibiotic treatment directed at *Streptococcus pyogenes* (penicillin) continued for 10–14 days
3. Relapsing polychondritis (see Sect. 1.6.7)

1.3.2.2 External Otitis

Synonym
Otitis externa

Definition

Bacterial and/or fungal infection of the EAC, generally without involvement of the tympanic membrane (myringitis).

Aetiology/Epidemiology
Frequent after microtrauma (cotton tips, foreign objects, fingernail), in the presence of exostoses or chronic otitis media. Following swimming or bathing in a warm humid climate; these factors raise the pH of the EAC from its normal acidic value (pH 4–5) to a neutral or alkaline pH that is more favourable to bacterial proliferation. Different types of external otitis can be observed.

Acute, Diffuse External Otitis (Swimmer's Ear)
Often public swimming pools are pools of infections agents, but water immersion is not always the cause as the disease occurs frequently in humid warm conditions. The most common agents responsible for acute diffuse external otitis are *Pseudomonas aeruginosa* followed by *Staphylococcus aureus*, *Proteus vulgaris*, *Streptococcus* species, *Candida albicans*, *Aspergillus niger* and mixed infections. Allergens are soaps, hair spray, ear plugs and some ear drops.

Symptoms
It begins with itching, a sensation of fullness, auricular pain and pain in the EAC. Pain is exacerbated by movements of the temporomandibular joint (chewing) and by touching the tragus. There is secretion and hearing loss.

Diagnosis
- Inspection: diffuse oedema of the skin of the EAC with accumulation of debris and secretion. Secretion is from clear to cloudy and then purulent greenish-yellow. Intense pain is elicited when pulling the auricle backwards and upwards. The skin of the bony part of the canal and of the tympanic membrane is mostly not

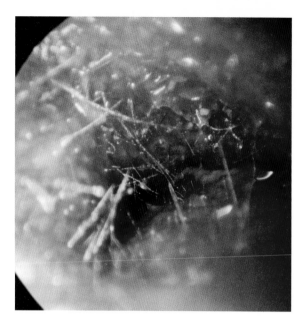

Fig. 1.3.3 Acute external otitis. The cartilaginous external auditory canal is oedematous and the size of its lumen is reduced

affected by inflammation, but this is difficult to evaluate owing to the generalized pain and the reduced size of the lumen (Fig. 1.3.3).

- Otomicroscopy: following local anaesthesia with cotton wool soaked with 4% lidocaine plus 1:1,000 adrenalin in equal parts, inspection with a small speculum under the microscope and cleaning by suctioning with a thin suction tube.
- Bacteriology (in cases resistant to treatment): identification of the pathogenic organisms.
- Laboratory tests: blood glucose to exclude diabetes.

Differential Diagnosis
- Furunculosis.
- Chronic otitis media.
- Malignoma of the EAC.
- External fibrous otitis.
- Benign osteitis of the EAC: limited ulceration of the skin of the floor of the EAC with osteitis, granulations and accumulation of keratin debris. A complication of microtrauma, in elderly patients. Treatment consists in the removal of the granulations and debridement of the ulceration in the outpatient clinic.
- Malignant external otitis.
- Keratosis obturans (see Sect. 1.3.3.6).
- Inflammation of the temporomandibular joint.
- Glossopharyngeal neuralgia.

Treatment
After thorough cleaning of the ear canal under the microscope, a gauze strip or a Pope Oto-Wick with a solu-

tion containing 70% alcohol and steroid (such as Volon A tincture or Kenacort-A tincture or betamethasone plus sulphacetamide sodium) is inserted. The wick can be left in situ for 2–3 days and drops should be applied several times daily. After reduction of inflammatory skin swelling, a wick with a moderate amount of antibiotic or antimycotic cream with steroid is inserted and left for 1–2 days. The patient should be instructed to avoid any manipulation of the ear. *Antibiotic drops with steroids may be useful, but the major drawback of their uncontrolled use is the possible overgrowth of fungi (otomycosis).* After the oedema has been reduced, topical drying agents such as Castellani solution, gentian violet or iodopovidone should be applied. Oral antibiotics are indicated only in cases of severe external otitis with cellulitis or lymphadenitis, and always in diabetic patients. Oral analgesics are indicated.

Complications
Recurrence in non-compliant patients who continue to manipulate the EAC with their fingers or foreign objects to alleviate itching; ear canal stenosis with a false fundus (Fig. 1.3.8).

Prevention
The key to prevention is to instruct the patient to avoid the use of cotton tips to clean the ear, explaining that the ear will be best protected against infection if the EAC is not overcleaned.

Furunculosis (Acute Localized External Otitis)
This is acute, localized infection of the outer cartilaginous part of the EAC arising from a hair follicle and its sebaceous and ceruminous gland. The pathogenic organism is usually *Staphylococcus aureus*. The symptoms are pain, itching and oedema. The aspect of the furuncle depends on the stage of infection. The treatment also depends on the stage of infection: a diffuse infection is treated like external diffuse otitis plus oral antibiotics such as amoxicillin with clavulanate or cephalosporins. A superficial furuncle is treated with drainage followed by topical and oral antibiotics.

Otomycosis (Fungal External Otitis)
Mycotic infections of the EAC are seldom primary, and more frequently follow treatment of bacterial otitis externa with antibiotic and steroid drops. The most frequent pathogenic organisms are *Aspergillus niger, Aspergillus fumigatus, Aspergillus flavus* and *Candida albicans*.

Symptoms are dull pain, itching and thick secretion. Examination under the operating microscope is diagnostic as it reveals a creamy secretion (see the algorithm for otorrhoea in Fig. 1.1.8). Frequently it is possible to identify the tiny mycelia (hyphae and fruiting heads, Fig. 1.3.4).

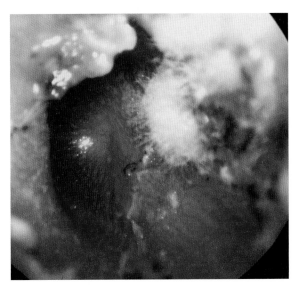

Fig. 1.3.4 Otomycosis: a creamy whitish exudate covers the skin of the external auditory canal. Fungal hyphae and conidiophores are visible. In this case the tympanic membrane (see the light reflex) is not affected

Treatment involves thorough cleaning by suction under the microscope with complete removal of the infected material and debris followed by application of a topical antimycotic lotion (e. g. clotrimazole or miconazole). Repeated applications are often necessary. Ear irrigation is not recommended.

Chronic Otitis Externa

Definition
Low-grade chronic inflammatory disorder of the skin of the EAC.

Aetiology
Incomplete treatment of acute diffuse external otitis, repeated contamination with water, allergens, self-manipulation and infected pus from chronic otitis media.

Symptoms
Itching and fullness. At inspection, the skin is dry and hypertrophic, similar to eczema. There is a lack of wax. Sometimes there is a partial or complete stenosis of the ear canal.

Differential Diagnosis
Eczematous external otitis (chronic dermatitis, eczema): dermatological disorder of the auricle and EAC in patients with a history of atopic dermatitis, psoriasis or eczema. Symptoms and signs are intense itching, scaly skin,

crusts, fissuring and oozing of the skin of the auricle and of the ear canal.

Treatment
The underlying cause must be removed, and then a repeated, thorough toilet of the external canal made, using 70% alcohol solution and topical medication with an antimycotic cream.

Complications
The most frequent complication is false fundus (Fig. 1.3.8) (see Sect. 1.3.3.5)

Prevention of External Otitis
- Patients should be informed that ear wax protects the skin of the EAC from infections. Overcleaning or microtrauma damages the normal protective barrier of the delicate canal skin.
- Avoid scratching with a foreign body, Q-Tips or a finger nail. *Hands-off is the rule.*
- In a warm, humid climate dry the ear after swimming or bathing using a blow dryer. Paper towels should not be used.

1.3.2.3   Malignant External Otitis

Synonyms
Necrotizing external otitis, otogenic cranial base osteomyelitis

Aetiology
Invasive, necrotizing infection of the EAC *and* later skull base in elderly patients with diabetes mellitus and in patients with a generalized immunodeficiency. The causative organism is *Pseudomonas aeruginosa* in 100% of cases.

Symptoms
- Intermittent otalgia, mainly at night, with headache and temporomandibular joint pain (spontaneous and with chewing)
- Scanty foul purulent otorrhoea
- Hearing loss
- Swelling of the parotid gland

Complications
Complications are cranial nerve palsies (nerve VII owing to diffusion to the parotid gland and stylomastoid foramen, nerves IX, X and XI owing to diffusion to the jugular foramen, nerve XII at the hypoglossal canal), meningitis, epidural abscess and thrombophlebitis (fatal complications).

Diagnostic Procedures
Physical Examination
- External otitis not responsive to standard treatment.

- Granulation tissue in the floor of the EAC and/or ulceration at the cartilage-bone junction, diffuse swelling of the soft tissues.
- The surface of the bone may be palpated with a small hook.

Laboratory
- Biopsy (to exclude a diagnosis of squamous cell carcinoma)
- Glycaemia, glucose tolerance test
- Erythrocyte sedimentation rate (often greater than 80 mm/h)
- Bacteriology: to confirm the pathogenic organism

Imaging
- CT is the best imaging technique for defining the extension of the disease and evaluating the integrity of cortical bone ("CT scan of the ear" *and* of the skull base).
- MRI may be useful in evaluating soft tissue changes.
- Bone scanning with ^{99m}Tc may be useful to study the sites of osteoblast activity and for classifiying the grade of lesion
- Gallium-67 scanning citrate may be useful to study the sites of granulocytes and bacteria accumulation.

Therapy
- Continuous control of diabetes.
- Topical antibiotic ear drops are of very limited value in the treatment of this pseudomonal infection which should be considered as an osteomyelitis of the bone of the EAC *and* skull base.
- Systemic long-term (6–8 weeks) treatment with antibiotics in high dosage (quinolones—for example, 750 mg ciprofloxacin per day orally; third-generation cephalosporins—e. g. 1–2 g ceftriaxone per day intravenously; 1–2 g ceftazidime per day intravenously in combination with an aminoglycoside.

Useful Additional Therapeutic Strategies
- Analgesics/anti-inflammatory drugs: e. g. 75–150 mg diclofenac orally/suppository
- Hyperbaric oxygen in patients with extensive osteomyelitis of the skull base
- Surgery: limited to biopsy and to removal of necrotic fragments of bone

Differential Diagnosis
Squamous cell carcinoma of the EAC: biopsy.

Prognosis
Although this disease after control of diabetes is treated successfully with quinolones, cephalosporins and aminoglycosides, complications and/or recurrences of the disease can still be fatal.

Prevention
Aural irrigation with tap water (which may contain bacteria) to remove wax must be avoided in elderly people with diabetes and in HIV patients. Tap water should be boiled before use to kill bacteria.

Suggested Reading

1. Arnold W, Ganzer U, Iurato S (2007) Checklist: otorinolaringoiatria (edizione Italiana). CIC, Roma, pp 1–645
2. Bojrab DI, Bruderly TE (1997) External otitis. In: Johnson JT, Yu VL (eds) Infections diseases and antimicrobial therapy of the ears, nose and throat. Saunders, Philadelphia, pp 301–313
3. Franco-Vidal V, Blanchet H, Bebear C et al. (2007) Necrotizing external otitis: a report of 46 cases. Otol Neurotol 28:771–773
4. Grandis JR (1997) Necrotizing (malignant) external otitis. In: Johnson JT, Yu VL (eds) Infections diseases and antimicrobial therapy of the ears, nose and throat. Saunders, Philadelphia, pp 314–320

1.3.3   Obstructions of the External Auditory Canal

1.3.3.1   Impacted Ear Wax (Cerumen)

Wax can be removed:
- *By aural irrigation:* Wax can be removed by ear rinsing with warm tap water (patient seated). A prior check that the tympanic membrane is normal must be made, and sterile water must be used in elderly patients with diabetes (risk of inducing malignant external otitis). It is important to make sure that the syringe muzzle is firmly screwed into place (risk of damage to the tympanic membrane and ossicles). Care must be taken to avoid any trauma to the tympanic membrane and the skin of the external auditory canal (EAC).
- *By instrumentation:* Wax can be removed under direct microscope control (patient supine) with a curette and suction tip.
- *With ceruminolytics:* 4% H_2O_2, olive oil, 25% sodium bicarbonate. Ceruminolytics should be avoided in cases of tympanic membrane perforations, external otitis and contact dermatitis. Ceruminolytics containing skin irritants should not be used.

1.3.3.2   Foreign Bodies

Diagnosis
- A variety of foreign bodies may be discovered in the EAC (Fig. 1.3.5).

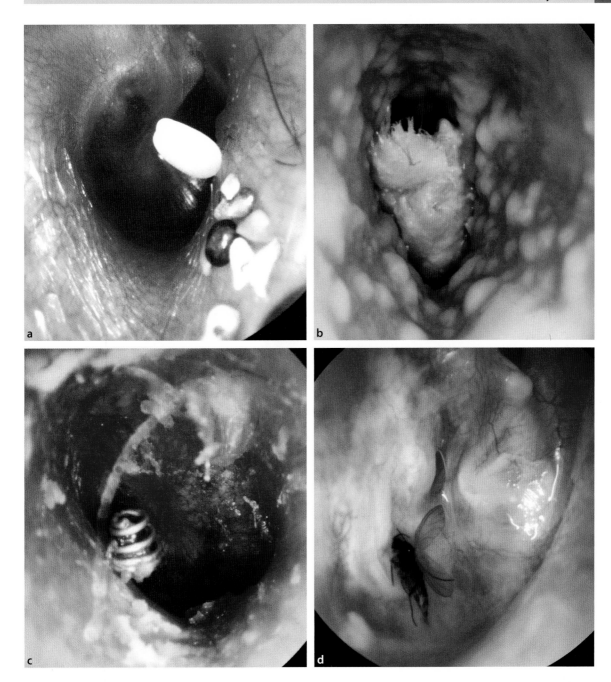

Fig. 1.3.5 a Sand particles can be seen along the anterior wall of the external auditory canal. **b** A piece of paper has been "forgotten" inside this external auditory canal; secondary infection (external otitis) of the skin. **c** A metallic hearing aid component, with secondary infection of the skin of the external auditory canal. **d** A deceased insect on the surface of this tympanic membrane

• Diagnosis is easy using the operating microscope and a small blunt hook.

Removal

Removal is done with a small blunt hook or aural crocodile forceps without anaesthesia or under general anaesthesia (in children). Syringing is effective for small plastic or metallic foreign bodies but not for organic foreign bodies, which may swell with water.

• *The main harm by a foreign body in the EAC is caused by its careless removal!*
• Removal under general anaesthetic with the help of the microscope may be necessary in children.

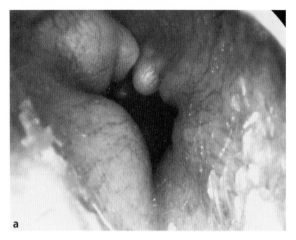

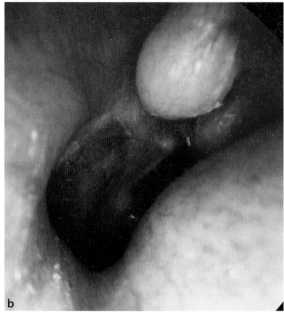

Fig. 1.3.6 a Coalescent exostoses with subtotal occlusion of the external auditory canal (left ear). Debris due to manipulation with cotton-tipped applicators. **b** Right ear of the same patient: one pedunculated superior exostose and a large sessile anterior exostose. The tympanic membrane with malleus is partly visible behind the exostoses

1.3.3.3   Exostoses

Definition
Areas of localized new bone growths in the osseous part of the EAC, usually multiple and bilateral (Fig. 1.3.6).

Aetiology/Epidemiology
They appear in patients with a history of frequent aquatic activities (swimming in cold water, diving, surfing) and may be caused by asymptomatic chronic periostitis.

Diagnosis
They appear as discrete round or ovoid bony tumours, sometimes pedunculated, or as diffuse bulges of bone covered by very thin, normal skin (Fig. 1.3.6). Very gentle palpation under the microscope with a blunt ear hook is usually painful but will confirm the diagnosis.

Symptoms and Therapy
Generally asymptomatic, they require surgical treatment in rare cases of subtotal occlusion of the EAC with retention of wax or in individuals who have problems in drying the EAC owing to the retention of water between the exostoses and the tympanic membrane.

1.3.3.4   Osteomas

Definition
Benign bony tumour of the EAC extending beyond its limits (e. g. into the mastoid).

Symptoms
Conductive hearing loss due to accumulation of keratin and wax between the osteoma and the tympanic membrane, and recurrent otitis externa.

Diagnosis
Solitary bony mass covered by normal skin (Fig. 1.3.7). CT scan shows the extension of the mass.

Therapy
Surgical removal by drill, avoiding injury to the tympanic membrane, ossicles and temporomandibular joint. As much skin as possible should be preserved.

1.3.3.5   External Fibrous Otitis

Synonyms
False fundus, lateralization of the tympanic membrane, acquired external (post inflammatory) canal stenosis, blunt meatus, postinflammatory acquired atresia of the

EAC, postinflammatory medial canal fibrosis, meatal fibrotizing otitis, medial meatal fibrosis

Definition
The EAC is short and ends blindly at the isthmus (junction between the outer cartilaginous third and the bony inner two thirds).

Aetiology
Chronic myringitis, chronic self-manipulation, chronic or recurrent external otitis with exuberant granulomatous tissue covered by skin, following ear operations, spontaneous or of unknown origin.

Symptoms
Itching, secretion following manipulation and moderate to severe conductive hearing loss.

Diagnosis
At otoscopy the EAC has a short, rounded end (Fig. 1.3.8). The normal landmarks of the tympanic membrane (e.g. the malleus handle) are lacking and the angle between the tympanic membrane and the anterior part of the bony canal is obliterated.

Additional Useful Diagnostic Procedures
CT is required to evaluate the thickness of the stenotic part and to check that no hidden cholesteatoma is present.

Therapy
In early cases the granulations should be removed under microscope control, and medication with steroid creams should be applied. The patient must be instructed to avoid *any* manipulation.

In stabilized cases, surgery is possible but it is not an easy task and there is a high risk of recurrence.

1.3.3.6 Keratosis Obturans

Definition
Rare entity characterized by exaggerated accumulation of keratin in the bony part of the EAC with gradual erosion of the bony walls of the canal.

Aetiology
Altered mechanism of lateral epithelial migration. In the young, it is frequently associated with sinusitis or bronchiectasis.

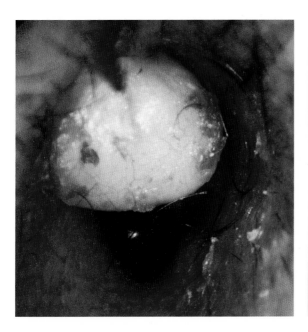

Fig. 1.3.7 Solitary osteoma of the external auditory canal covered by normal skin

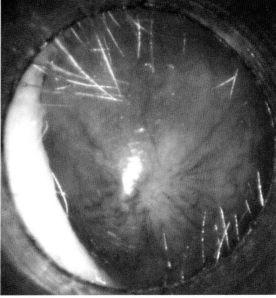

Fig. 1.3.8 External fibrous otitis: the auditory canal ends blindly at the isthmus (stabilized "false fundus" normally epithelized)

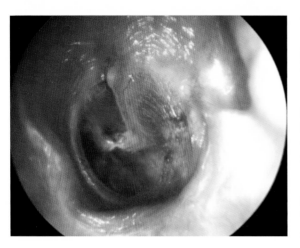

Fig. 1.3.9 Keratosis obturans (left ear). After keratin plug removal the external auditory canal appears wider than normal

Diagnosis

A large plug of compressed keratin occluding the external canal. The plug should be softened with olive oil and the layers of keratin removed under the operating microscope. After plug removal (Fig. 1.3.9), the canal appears wider than normal (probably from the pressure effect of the keratin plug). Keratosis obturans should be differentiated from the **cholesteatoma of the EAC**, which is defined as an invasion of squamous tissue into a localized area of bony erosion; it is associated with intermittent otorrhoea and a dull, chronic otalgia. CT scan reveals the extension of the invasion of the EAC.

Therapy

Frequent (every 6 months) cleansing under the microscope. The patient must be instructed to avoid self-cleaning.

1.3.3.7   Postoperative Cholesteatoma of the External Auditory Canal

Definition

White, soft epidermic cyst covered by normal skin (Fig. 1.3.10). More frequently it appears as small white "pearls" (epidermal inclusion cysts).

Aetiology

Incorrect repositioning of the skin flaps in overlay myringoplasty and in tympanoplasty procedures.

Treatment

Surgical removal.

1.3.3.8   Collapsing Canal

Synonym

Lateral stenosis of the EAC.

Definition

Stenosis of the external opening of the canal, spontaneous (due to aging), related to recurrent external otitis, or more frequently following ear operations, especially otopexia.

Diagnosis

The external opening of the canal is reduced to a narrow, elongated opening.

Therapy

Meatoplasty.

Suggested Reading

1. Chole RA (1988) A color atlas of ear disease. Wolfe, London
2. Hawke M, Keene M, Alberti PW (1990) Clinical otoscopy. Churchill Livingstone, Edinburgh
3. Hopsu E, Pitkäranta A (2002) Idiopathic inflammatory medial meatal fibrotizing otitis. Arch Otolaryngol Head Neck Surg 128:1313–1316
4. Sanna M, Russo A, De Donato G et al. (2002) Color atlas of otoscopy. From diagnosis to surgery. Thieme, New York

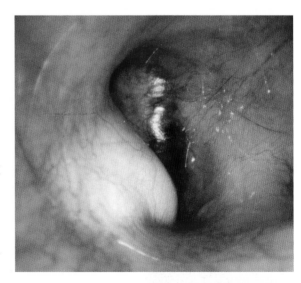

Fig. 1.3.10 Postoperative cholesteatoma of the external auditory canal, the result of incorrect repositioning of the skin flaps in "overlay" tympanoplasty

1.3.4 Tumours of the Auricle and of the External Auditory Canal

1.3.4.1 Tumours of the Auricle

Benign Lesions

- *Keloids*: hypertrophic scars secondary to surgical incisions, ear piercing or cutaneous injuries in keloid-prone individuals
- *Chondrodermatitis nodularis chronica (Wrinkler's nodule)*: one or several tender nodules located on the apex of the helix
- *Gouty tophus*: a painless sodium urate concretion on the margin of the helix in gouty persons
- *Keratoacanthoma*: a benign squamous epithelial neoplasia characterized by a rapid development (maximum dimension 1–2 cm) followed by a spontaneous involution (within 6–12 months)
- *Epidermal inclusion cysts*: round cystic masses located along the retroauricular sulcus which may become infected

Malignant Lesions

Malignant tumours of the auricle account for roughly 6% of all malignant tumours of the skin. The main predisposing factors are prolonged sun exposure, chronic skin infections, psoriasis, burning with chemical agents or X-rays.

1. Basal cell carcinoma (Fig. 1.3.11a)
   - Slowly growing dry or ulcerated lesion with local infiltration of the subcutaneous tissues and late invasion of the perichondrium and periosteum of the external auditory canal (EAC).
   - Preferred localizations: dorsal skin surface of the auricle, margin of the helix, area between tragus and crus helices.
   - Secondary infection.
   - Various histological patterns.
   - A second cancer of the skin of the face in roughly 33% of patients.
2. Squamous cell carcinoma (Fig. 1.3.11b)
   - Accounts for roughly 85% of the tumours of the auricle.
   - Rapidly growing ulcerated lesion frequently fixed to the underlying structures. Painful and bleeding.
   - Preferred localizations: margin of the helix, triangular fossa, entrance of the EAC.
   - For lesions extended to the EAC, see Sect. 1.5.4.1.
3. Malignant melanoma (Fig. 1.3.11c): accounts for roughly 7% of malignant melanomas of the head and neck.

Aetiology/Epidemiology

More common in males (80%) than in females, occur later in life. Sun-exposed areas of the head and neck, burns following radiotherapy.

Diagnostic Procedures (for More Details See Sect. 9.3.2.5)

- History.
- Inspection.

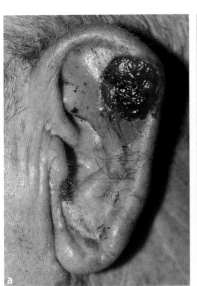 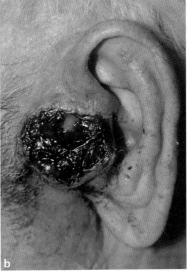 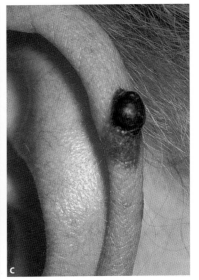

Fig. 1.3.11 a–c Malignant lesions of the auricle: **a** basal cell carcinoma; **b** squamous carcinoma; **c** malignant melanoma

- Palpation of the tumour and of the lymphatic drainage pathways: preauricular and parotid lymph nodes, infra-auricular lymph nodes, postauricular lymph nodes and lymph nodes in the jugulodigastric area or the spinal accessory lymph node chain.
- Echography.
- Biopsy (if possible with complete surgical excision). When malignant melanoma is suspected, complete surgical excision with a margin in healthy tissue of at least 1 cm.

Therapy

Conservative Treatment

There is no conservative treatment of malignomas of the skin!

Surgical Treatment

- Squamous cell carcinoma: wide "in sano" excision of the primary lesion. Histological control of the margins. Its tendency to metastasize to the parotid gland and cervical lymph nodes makes their inclusion in the treatment programme necessary. Postoperative radiation therapy should be scheduled.
- Basal cell carcinoma: wide surgical excision of the lesion.
- Malignant melanoma: radical excision of the auricle and adjacent tissues, including the parotid gland and lateral neck dissection. Radiation therapy. Immuno-chemotherapy (interdisciplinary discussion).

1.3.4.2 Tumours of the External Auditory Canal

Benign Lesions

- Osteoma (Fig. 1.3.7). See Sect. 1.3.3.4.
- Cerumen gland adenoma: benign tumour of the apocrine glands located in the lateral third of the EAC. Covered by skin, often pedunculated. Symptoms (fullness, tinnitus and hearing loss) appear when the EAC is occluded.

- Squamous papillomas: benign tumours associated with human papilloma virus. They tend to recur if not excised completely.
- Rarer benign lesions : neurofibromas, paragangliomas (see Sect. 1.5.4.3), angiomas.

Malignant Lesions

- Squamous cell carcinoma (see Sect. 1.5.4.1) accounts for over 60% of the malignant tumours of the EAC and it is frequently associated with chronic otorrhoea.
- Basal cell carcinoma: the EAC is rarely the primary site of origin, more frequently the EAC is invaded by a lesion originating in the auricle (see Sect. 1.3.4.1).
- Ceruminous gland tumour: it accounts for about 15% of malignant lesions of the EAC.
- Rarer malignant lesions (adenocarcinoma, adenoid cystic carcinoma, rhabdomyosarcoma, melanoma).

Diagnostic Procedures (for More Details See Sect. 9.3.2.1)

- Palpation of the lymphatic drainage pathways
- Otoscopy
- Echography
- CT scan
- Biopsy

Management

For all malignant tumours of the EAC radical surgical removal is the method of choice. Since the lymphatic drainage from the EAC is diffuse, postoperative radiotherapy is strongly recommended. The surgical resection margins depend on the extent of tumour growth and on vital barriers in the skull base area. Indication of radical surgery depends on tumour localization and extension, age of the patient, his/her health conditions and possible postoperative quality of life.

1.4 Middle Ear

SALVATORE IURATO, CHRISTIAN MARTIN,
OLIVIER STERKERS AND WOLFGANG ARNOLD

1.4.1 Traumatic Perforations of the Tympanic Membrane

SALVATORE IURATO

1.4.1.1 Definition

Perforations of the tympanic membrane caused by a direct penetrating injury or by indirect trauma.

1.4.1.2 Aetiology

- *Direct trauma:* insertion of a cotton-tipped applicator (frequently it is a second person who hits the hand or the elbow of the patient causing the trauma) (Fig. 1.4.1a), hairpins or matchsticks, accidental penetration of the spike of a leaf or a twig and accidental penetration of a drop of welding metal.

- *Indirect trauma:* abrupt change of air pressure in the external auditory canal produced by an explosion (Fig. 1.4.1b), a violent blow with the cupped hand, diving (Fig. 1.4.1c) and other underwater activities, barotrauma and temporal bone fracture.

1.4.1.3 Symptoms

Earache, haemorrhage, fullness, tinnitus, hearing loss.

1.4.1.4 Diagnostic Procedures

- Otoscopy with the binocular operation microscope. Photographic documentation
- Hearing examination: tuning fork (c^2), lateralization to the affected side
- Audiogram: light (10–30 dB) conductive hearing loss; severe mixed hearing loss and often complete deafness

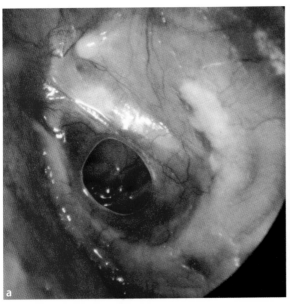 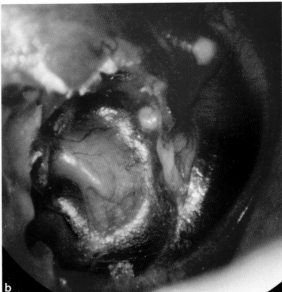

Fig. 1.4.1 a Penetrating injury of a left tympanic membrane caused by improper use of a cotton-tipped applicator. **b** Right ear. Severe damage to the tympanic membrane and ossicular chain (stapes) caused by an explosion (complete hearing loss)

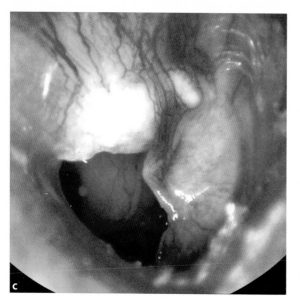

the microscope. The area is then covered with a cigarette paper patch moistened with Ringer's solution.
The paper patch is left in place for 3–4 weeks.

- Small perforations that do not heal spontaneously can
  be treated with "fat graft myringoplasty" (see Sect.
  1.4.6).
- In cases of large mesotympanic perforations, standard
  underlay myringoplasty is recommended (see Sect.
  1.4.6).

1.4.1.6   Prognosis

The prognosis is generally very good, as many traumatic
perforations heal spontaneously within 3 months. It is
not so good in cases of drops of welding metal, when the
middle ear ossicles are damaged and when the inner ear
is affected.

Fig. 1.4.1 *(continued)* **c** Traumatic perforation caused by diving (5 years ago). A tympanosclerotic plaque can be seen in the
posterosuperior part of this right tympanic membrane

1.4.2   Myringitis

SALVATORE IURATO

when the perforation is caused by an explosion (Fig.
1.4.1b)
- Vestibular examination

1.4.1.5   Treatment

- Small, recent perforations: replacement of the displaced
  flaps in their original position (avoiding any introflec-
  tion) under local anaesthesia and under the control of

1.4.2.1   Definition

A distinct form of external otitis limited to the tympanic
membrane. Different types of myringitis can be observed:
- *Viral myringitis* (flue myringitis, bullous myringitis,
  myringitis bullosa): acute, painful inflammation of
  the thin epidermic layer of the tympanic membrane
  caused by influenza viruses. Red vesicles (serohae-
  morragic content) under tension between the epider-

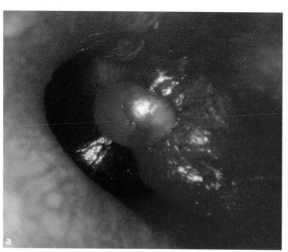

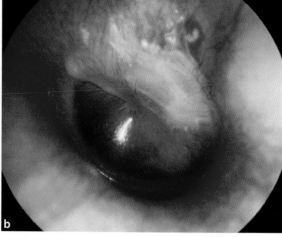

Fig. 1.4.2 **a** Acute bullous myringitis (left ear). Notice multiple bullae filled with serohaemorrhagic exudate. **b** Bullous myringitis
(same patient) 30 days later recovered without any hearing problem

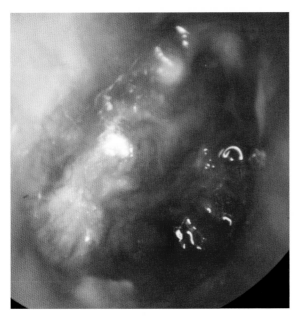

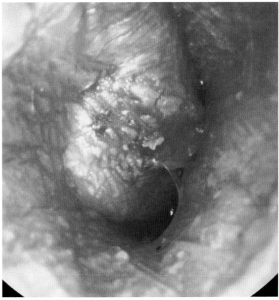

Fig. 1.4.3 Granular myringitis: a portion of the tympanic membrane (right ear) and of the external canal is covered with granulation tissue

Fig. 1.4.4 Acute otitis media before perforation. The posterior half of this right tympanic membrane shows severe outward bulging. Notice keratin patches on the surface

mis and the fibrous layer of the tympanic membrane (Fig. 1.4.2a). A serous fluid collection may be present in the middle ear.

- *Granular myringitis* (chronic myringitis, myringitis granulosa): small pyogenic granulations on the external surface of the tympanic membrane (Fig. 1.4.3) following manipulation/local trauma (often with cotton tips).
- *External myringitis:* bacterial inflammation involving the epidermic and fibrous layers of the tympanic membrane during the course of an external otitis.
- *Tympanogenic myringitis:* during an acute otitis media the tympanic membrane will bulge, resulting in loss of landmarks. The outer layer may undergo desquamation (Fig. 1.4.4) and eventually the tympanic membrane may perforate (see Sect. 1.4.3).

1.4.2.2 Diagnostic Procedures

- Ear microscopy: red vesicles under tension are diagnostic for viral otitis (Fig. 1.4.2a), in the same way as a bulging and pulsating tympanic membrane with a serous or blood-stained discharge is diagnostic for acute otitis media (Fig. 1.4.4), and pyogenic granulations for chronic myringitis (Fig. 1.4.3).
- Audiogram: mild or no hearing loss. Sensorineural loss in cases of inner ear involvement during viral otitis.

1.4.2.3 Therapy

- *Viral myringitis:* contact anaesthesia and puncture of the vesicles to release tension and alleviate pain. Medication with anaesthetic drops or with a strip of gauze with chlortetracycline and triamcinolone; analgesics (diclofenac). In cases of inner ear involvement, treatment is as for idiopathic sudden hearing loss.
- *Granular myringitis:* contact anaesthesia and removal of the infected granulations using fine double-cup forceps. Acetic acid (1.5% solution) regimen. *Stop any manipulation!* Note that if left untreated, granular myringitis can lead to lateralization of the tympanic membrane (see Sect. 1.3.3.5).
- *External myringitis:* see treatment for external otitis.
- *Tympanogenic myringitis:* see treatment for acute otitis media.

1.4.3 Acute Otitis Media

WOLFGANG ARNOLD AND SALVATORE IURATO

1.4.3.1 Synonyms

AOM, purulent otitis media.

1.4.3.2   Definition

Acute, in most cases purulent inflammation of the mucous membrane of the middle ear cavity, caused by viruses and/or bacteria from the nasopharynx reaching the middle ear cleft via the Eustachian tube.

1.4.3.3   Aetiology/Epidemiology

- An acute upper respiratory tract infection and/or a chronic or acute infection of the nasopharynx are presuppositions for the development for the disease. About 80% of all cases of acute otitis media are caused by viral infections (rhinoviruses accounting for most illnesses, followed by influenza A and respiratory syncytial viruses). In 20% of cases, next to the causal virus infection there is a complicating bacterial secondary infection. The bacteria responsible for acute otitis media are *Streptococcus pneumoniae* (40–50%), *Haemophilus influenzae* (30–40%), *Moraxella catarrhalis*, *Staphylococcus pyogenes*, and *Staphylococcus aureus* (10–20%). The most frequent viruses causing otitis media are rhinovirus, respiratory syncytial virus, influenza virus, parainfluenza virus and adenovirus.
- In children, enlarged chronically inflamed adenoids are the most common cause next to recurrent tonsillitis, influenza, coryza of measles, scarlet fever or whooping cough.
- More than 60% of all children under the age of 6 years experience one or more episodes of acute otitis media.

1.4.3.4   Symptoms

- Sudden onset of severe and pulsating earache. The child may cry and scream inconsolably, he/she is flushed and ill; the temperature may be as high as 40°C. In children often unspecific side symptoms such as irritability and stomach ache are present.
- Nasal congestion, sore throat, cough, runny nose.
- Hearing loss of conductive nature is always present in acute otitis media and adults may report tinnitus sensation.

1.4.3.5   Complications

- Acute otitis media must be managed with care to prevent subsequent complications such as mastoiditis (inflammation of the mastoid cell system), acute labyrinthitis (dizziness, vertigo, deafness), facial palsy, thrombosis of the sigmoid sinus, meningitis and subdural-epidural abscess (Fig. 1.4.16).

- Gradenigo syndrome: palsy of the abducent nerve and trigeminal neuralgia (first and second branch) when the destructive inflammatory process in acute otitis media spreads to the apex of the temporal bone (petroapicitis).

1.4.3.6   Diagnostic Procedures

- Body temperature.
- Inspection (red, prominent auricle? swollen skin over the mastoid surface?).
- Palpation (pain when touching or pressing on the mastoid surface, when pulling the auricle forwards?).
- Inspection of the oral cavity, nasal cavity and nasopharynx (signs of inflammation, purulent secretion?).
- Otoscopy or ear microscopy: injection of small vessels around the periphery and along the handle of the malleus; redness and fullness of the drum, the malleus handle becomes more vertical; bulging of tympanic membrane with loss of landmarks. Purple colour. The outer layer of the tympanic membrane may desquamate causing blood-stained serous discharge (Fig. 1.4.4).
- Early necrosis may be recognized, heralding imminent perforation. Perforation with otorrhoea which—at the beginning—will often be blood-stained. Profuse and mucoid at first, later becoming thick and yellow.
- Hearing examination: tuning fork, audiogram.
- Frenzel glasses: to exclude vestibular irritation.

1.4.3.7   Additional/Useful
Diagnostic Procedures

- Endoscopy of the nose/nasopharynx (adenoids, nasopharyngeal tumour)
- Microbiology: culture taken from the nose/nasopharynx
- Blood cell differentiation, blood sedimentation rate
- Ultrasound of the paranasal sinuses
- Schüller X-ray (see Sect. 1.1.6.1), paranasal sinuses
- Paediatric counselling

1.4.3.8   Therapy

Conservative Treatment
- Antibiotics: (e.g. 1.5–3 g amoxicillin orally per day for adults, 50–100 mg/kg body weight orally for children, or 1–2 g erythromycin orally or intravenously per day for adults, 30–50 mg/kg body weight orally or intravenously for children). Sensitivity reports from the laboratory should be used as a guide! Note that as acute otitis media in 80% of the cases is a complication of a viral upper respiratory tract cold-like infection, a watchful waiting period of 48–72 h may be considered

in selected cases (age more than 6 months, light earache, temperature under 39°C, reliable parents) before beginning the treatment with antibiotics.

- Analgesics/antiphlogistics: e.g. 75–150 mg diclofenac orally/suppository for adults, 2 mg/kg body weight orally/suppository for children.
- Mefanaminic acid: 750–1,500 mg orally/suppository for adults; 6.5 mg/kg body weight orally or 12 mg/kg body weight suppository for children. Avoid the use of aspirin in children.
- Nasal vasoconstrictors: nose spray/nose drops, e.g. 0.1% xylomethazoline for adults, 0.05% for children, several times per day.

Useful Additional Therapeutic Strategies
- Application of local hyperthermia twice a day for 5–10 min.
- In children: cold bandages around the legs to reduce fever.
- Note: that ear drops containing antibiotics are of questionable value in acute otitis media with an intact ear drum. The use of drops containing local anaesthetics can reduce pain but may cause allergic reactions.

Surgical Treatment
The recommended European standard is:
- Myringotomy (paracentesis): indicated when bulging of the tympanic membrane persists, for immediate relief of pain (!).
- Adenoidectomy: in recurrent acute otitis media, in most cases accompanied by myringotomy and insertion of grommets.
- Antrotomy/mastoidectomy: in cases of present or imminent mastoiditis, labyrinthitis, thrombosis of the sigmoid sinus or endocranial complications. Usually simultaneous insertion of grommets.

1.4.3.9   Differential Diagnosis

1. Usually acute otitis media shows very characteristic clinical features.
2. Earpain in normal otoscopic findings: see also the algorithm for "Earache" in Fig. 1.1.6.
   - Neuralgia of the auricular branch of the vagus nerve, e.g. in acute tonsillitis, neuralgia of the glossopharyngeal nerve following tonsillectomy or in carcinoma of the lateral wall of oropharynx and hypopharynx
   - Eagle syndrome: irritation of the glossopharyngeal nerve by an abnormally long processus styloideus
   - Irritation of the temporomandibular joint (temporomandibular joint syndrome)
   - Cervicofacial syndrome (C4–C5)

   - Costen syndrome: otodental syndrome (malocclusion causing irritation of the mandibular joint)

1.4.3.10   Surgical Principles

Myringotomy
- Surface anaesthesia of the tympanic membrane with, e.g., lidocaine in dimethyl sulphoxide (1:10), or lidocaine 4% plus ephinephrine 1:1000 in equal parts or local anaesthesia of the ear canal in adults and general anaesthesia in children.
- Incision of the tympanic membrane in the area of the lower anterior quadrant (Fig. 1.4.5a) parallel to the radial fibre structure of the pars tensa (right ear at 5 o'clock, left ear at 7 o'clock).
- In the case of accumulation of serous or mucous effusion in the middle ear spaces, irrigation with saline solution or xylomethazolin (0.25%) and suction of the diluted middle ear fluid.
- To avoid prompt healing of the myringotomy incision, a small sheet of silicone or a ventilating tube (Fig. 1.4.5b) may be placed through the incision using microforceps and a needle.

Adenoidectomy
See Sect. 3.4.12.

Antrotomy/Mastoidectomy
See Sect. 1.4.5.

1.4.3.11   Prognosis

- Correct high dosage antibiotic therapy over a period of at least 1 week, combined with antiphlogistic therapy of the blocked Eustachian tube will heal the disease

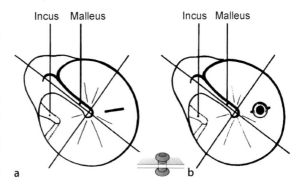

Fig. 1.4.5 a Right ear, surgical position. Incision of the tympanic membrane in the area of the lower anterior quadrant. **b** Insertion of a grommet (ventilating tube) through the incision

in most cases. In some cases there may be a slight high tone sensorineural hearing loss.

- In cases of recurrent acute otitis media in children, adenoidectomy and paracentesis/grommets will solve the problem in about 85% of cases.

1.4.3.12   Special Remarks

For special cases of recurrent acute otitis media (e. g. immunodeficient individuals) vaccination for *Streptococcus pneumoniae* is recommended.

Suggested Reading

1. American Academy of Pediatrics and American Academy of Family Physicians (2004) Diagnosis and management of acute otitis media. Pediatrics 113:1451–1465
2. Bluestone CD (1997) Otitis media. In: Johnson JT, Yu VL (eds) Infections diseases and antimicrobial therapy of the ears, nose and throat. Saunders, Philadelphia, pp 273–291

1.4.4   Otitis Media with Effusion

CHRISTIAN MARTIN, OLIVIER STERKERS, SALVATORE IURATO, AND WOLFGANG ARNOLD

1.4.4.1   Synonyms

Serous otitis, seromucotympanum, glue ear, serous otitis media, secretory otitis media, salpingitis.

1.4.4.2   Definition

Accumulation of *non-purulent* fluid of various viscosities within the middle ear cavity usually accompanied by malfunction (occlusion) of the Eustachian tube.

1.4.4.3   Aetiology/Epidemiology

- Recurrent virus infections of the upper respiratory tract, especially of the adenoids, predispose individuals to the inflammatory changes which develop Eustachian tube dysfunction and otitis media with effusion.
- Functional disturbance of the Eustachian tube during nasopharyngeal inflammation or in nasopharyngeal tumour growth (e.g. inflamed adenoids, nasopharyngeal tumours, Wegener's granulomatosis, cysts).
- Allergy, chronic rhinosinusitis.

- Cleft palate, skull base fracture, transnasal intubation, nasogastric tube.
- Nasopharyngeal package.
- Radiotherapy in the area of the ear/nasopharynx.
- The highest incidence of otitis media with effusion is the age group between 2 and 5 years (20%).
- Bilateral otitis media with effusion is reported in 84% of cases, mainly in young children.
- Environmental smoking.

1.4.4.4   Pathophysiology

- Inflammatory (also allergic) conditions of the nasopharynx cause dysfunction of the Eustachian tube and reduced or missing aeration of the middle ear cavity. This causes negative pressure to develop within the middle ear cavity, leading to formation of serous effusion, metaplasia of the middle ear mucous membrane epithelium to a secretory active epithelium and formation of viscous effusion (mucotympanum).
- In addition to infective conditions and allergy, irritation from cigarette smoke is a proven factor.
- Mucous effusion is mostly seen in children; serous effusion is mostly seen in adults.
- Precondition for recurrent otitis media.

1.4.4.5   Symptoms

- Pressure feeling, short episodes of earache
- Changing conductive hearing loss
- Tinnitus
- Often asymptomatic, only detected during hearing screening

1.4.4.6   Complications

- Recurrent acute otitis media caused by viral or bacterial infection of the effusion
- Chronic or subacute masked mastoiditis
- Retraction pockets, atelectatic ear (adhesive otitis media), cholesteatoma
- Tympanic membrane perforation
- Tympanosclerosis
- Fibrous otitis media and cholesterol granuloma
- Toxic labyrinthitis

Special remarks: developmental impairments in children have been attributed to persistent middle ear effusions in the early years of life.

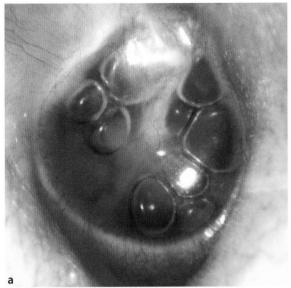
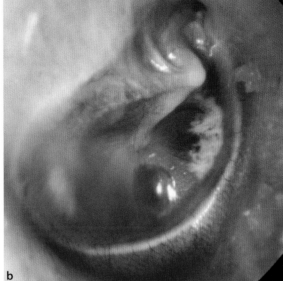
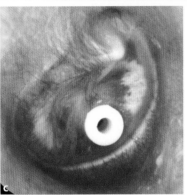

Fig. 1.4.6 a Serous otitis media with bubbles following air inflation, right ear. **b** Mucous otitis media. **c** Same ear after insertion of a Teflon grommet

1.4.4.7   Diagnostic Procedures

Recommended European Standard

- Endoscopic investigation of the oropharynx, nose and nasopharynx: nasopharyngeal endoscopy is mandatory!
- Ear microscopy: in *serous effusion* retracted tympanic membrane. Fluid disc or air bubbles behind the ear drum following a Valsalva manoeuvre (Fig. 1.4.6a).
- Retracted bluish, grey or brown tympanic membrane in *mucous effusion* (Fig. 1.4.6b).
- Reduced mobility of the tympanic membrane and malleus during pneumatic otoscopy.
- Hearing examination (tuning fork, audiogram, conductive deficit up to 40 dB; Fig. 1.1.15).
- Tympanometry: flat curve (type B, Fig. 1.1.19).

Additional/Useful Diagnostic Procedures

- Politzer manoeuvre
- Otoacoustic emissions

- Schüller X-ray: reduced pneumatization, detection of masked mastoiditis
- Allergy tests (prick test, immunoglobulin E, intranasal provocation, radioallergosorbent test)
- CT/MRI to exclude nasopharyngeal neoplasia
- Gastro-oesophageal reflux screening
- Biopsy from nasopharyngeal tissue augmentation

1.4.4.8   Therapy

The recommended European standard follows.

Conservative Treatment

- As pathogenic bacteria cause the nasopharyngeal infection, a trial of antibiotic therapy as for acute otitis media is beneficial.
- To relieve Eustachian tube obstruction, nose drops with a vasoconstrictive effect in combination with

orally given antihistamines, such as 10 mg loratadine per day for adults and children older than 12 years.

- Eustachian tube ventilation exercises (Valsalva). In children blowing up a balloon with the nose following application of a nasal decongestant or blowing up a balloon with the nostrils closed with fingers.

Special remark: the use of ear drops is senseless!

Surgical Treatment

- Myringotomy with fluid aspiration (Fig. 1.4.5a).
- Insertion of ventilating tubes (grommets; Figs. 1.4.5b, 1.4.6c): indicated in cases of more than 30 dB hearing loss unresponsive to medical treatment for 3 months or more and in cases of formation of retraction pockets. Under general anaesthesia in children; under local anaesthesia in teenagers and adults.
- Adenoidectomy (see Sect. 3.4.12).
- Antrotomy or mastoidectomy in cases of persistent and refractory middle ear effusion or in cases of long-standing chronic secretion through ventilating tubes (Schüller X-ray!).
- Nasopharyngeal tumour: surgical or radio-oncological therapy depending on the histopathologic result from biopsy and from tumour extension.

1.4.4.9   Differential Diagnosis

- *Eosinophilic otitis media:* extensive accumulation of eosinophils in the middle ear effusion and middle ear mucosa. Progressive mixed hearing loss ending in profound hearing loss. Frequently associated with bronchial asthma.
- *Otoliquorrhoea* (see Sect. 1.6.4)
- *Haemotympanum:* accumulation of blood within the middle ear cavities following temporal bone fracture or barotrauma (Fig. 1.5.1)
- *Otitis nigra:* inflammation of the middle ear mucous membrane caused by paramyxovirus of the parotitis epidemical group causing microhaemorrhages and subepithelial as well as epithelial deposits of haemosiderine
- *Glomus tympanicum tumour* (Fig. 1.5.16): see Sect. 1.5.4.3
- *Wegener's granulomatosis* of the middle ear: autoimmune disease, inflammatory blockage of the Eustachian tube, combined conductive/sensorineural hearing loss, antineutrophil cytoplasmic autoantibodies titre positive

1.4.4.10   Prognosis

- Insertion of a ventilating tube usually results in a dramatic hearing gain.
- Long-term outcome will depend on the quality and continuity of the treatment and on the different factors influencing the disease (allergy, diseases of the upper respiratory system, nasopharynx).

Suggested Reading

1. Bluestone CD (1997) Otitis media. In: Johnson JT, Yu VL (eds) Infectious diseases and antimicrobial therapy of the ears, nose and throat. WB Saunders, Philadelphia, pp 273–291
2. Cunningham MJ, Eavey RD (1993) Otitis media with effusion. In Nadol JB, Schuknecht HF (eds) Surgery of the ear and temporal bone, Raven Press, New York, pp 205–221
3. Friedmann RA, Kesser BW (2001) Surgery of ventilation and mucosal disease. In: Brackmann DE, Shelton C, Arriage MA (eds) Otologic surgery. WB Saunders, Philadelphia, pp 68–81

1.4.5   Acute Mastoiditis

CHRISTIAN MARTIN,
OLIVIER STERKERS, AND WOLFGANG ARNOLD

1.4.5.1   Synonym

Tympanomastoiditis.

1.4.5.2   Definition

Bacterial infection of the bony cell system of the mastoid in the course or as an extension of an acute, subacute or chronic otitis media.

1.4.5.3   Aetiology/Epidemiology

In most cases acute mastoiditis occurs in young children. During acute otitis media the bacteria spread via the antrum into the mastoid air cell system, causing hyperaemia and oedema of the mucous membrane of the pneumatized cells. Accumulation of serous effusion is followed by a purulent effusion, demineralization of the bony cellular walls and necrosis of the bone. Formation of an abscess cavity with possible penetration into neighbouring structures is regarded as a severe complication.

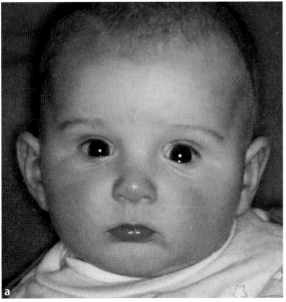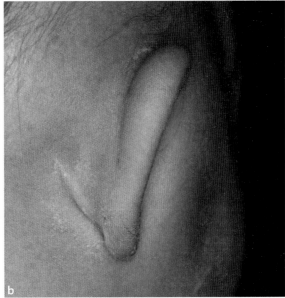

Fig. 1.4.7 a An infant with acute right mastoiditis. **b** Deflected auricle in the same infant

The bacteria responsible for acute mastoiditis are similar to those of acute otitis media: *Streptococcus pneumoniae* (30%), *Streptococcus pyogenes* (5%), *Haemophilus influenzae* (20%), *Staphylococcus aureus* (20%), *Pseudomonas aeruginosa*, *Escherichia coli* and *Proteus mirabilis*. In Europe the incidence of acute mastoiditis due to *Streptococcus pneumoniae* is increasing because of species with limited sensitivity to penicillin.

1.4.5.4 Types/Symptoms

Types

- *Masked mastoiditis*: chronic inflammation of the mucous membrane lining of the pneumatized cells without abscess formation, e.g. in children with a chronic mucous effusion of the middle ear or chronic secretory otitis media. Clinically there are unspecific complaints, rarely pain or fever.
- *Acute mastoiditis*: acute mastoiditis becomes clinically apparent a few days to 1 or 2 weeks after the onset of untreated acute otitis media. A postauricular subperiosteal abscess (Fig. 1.4.16) may develop as the lateral mastoid cortex is destroyed (*subperiosteal abscess*). Redness, swelling, tenderness and fluctuation develop in the area of the planum mastoideum; the pinna is displaced laterally and inferiorly (Fig. 1.4.7). With exacerbation of aural pain, fever and otorrhoea usually occur. The pain tends to be persistent and throbbing; a creamy profuse discharge is common. Next to the lat-

erally displaced pinna, pulling the pinna is very painful. There is leucocytosis, subfebril or septic temperature, and sometimes shivers.

Symptoms

- Otalgia with pain over the mastoid by palpation or spontaneously
- Fever
- Hearing loss

These symptoms can be masked by insufficient previous antibiotic therapy (masked mastoiditis). However, the tympanic membrane fails to return to normal and there may be persistent tenderness over the mastoid in association with low grade fever, elevated blood sedimentation rate and general malaise.

1.4.5.5 Complications

See Fig. 1.4.16. Complications are:
- Facial palsy
- Meningitis
- Labyrinthitis
- Thrombosis of the sigmoid sinus
- Bezold descending abscess (perforation of the tip of the mastoid and spreading of the abscess into the neck muscles)
- Petrositis (osteomyelitis of the temporal bone)

1.4.5.6   Diagnostic Procedures

Recommended European Standard

- *Inspection*: postauricular erythema, tenderness, swelling. The pinna is pushed forwards and inferiorly (Fig. 1.4.7b).
- *Otoscopy*: red, bulging tympanic membrane or opacity due to a middle ear effusion. Central perforation of the tympanic membrane with purulent secretion can be seen. One of the most important otoscopic findings in acute mastoiditis is sagging of the posterosuperior meatal wall.
- *Rhinoscopy*: swollen turbinates, signs of rhinopharyngitis, purulent nasal secretion.
- Tuning fork, audiogram.
- *Frenzel glasses*: spontaneous nystagmus?
- *X-ray*: Schüller projection shows reduced pneumatization, cloudiness of the mastoid air cell system and the formation of abscess cavities.
- *CT scan*: the mastoid air cells are opaque while filled with fluid and a CT scan may show a soft tissue density due to purulent fluid, swollen mucous membrane and granulation tissue. In coalescent mastoiditis, cell partitions become indistinct.

Additional/Useful Diagnostic Procedures

- Swab for bacterial culture taken from the nose/nasopharynx
- Blood cell differentiation, blood sedimentation rate
- X-ray: paranasal sinuses

1.4.5.7   Therapy

Conservative Treatment

The initial antibiotic given should provide coverage for the common pathogens and be stable to β-lactamase. Antibiotic penetration into the CNS is desirable if a complication seems impending. A sample of otorrhoea is taken for culture and for determination of antibiotic sensitivities. Subsequent intravenous therapy depends on cultures, sensitivities and the clinical course. Antibiotic therapy should be continued for at least 2 weeks.

Surgery

Recommended European Standard

- Myringotomy with or without insertion of grommets.
- Cortical mastoidectomy is required as a surgical emergency if there is no improvement after initial antibiotic therapy or in the case of a subperiosteal abscess.

Additional Useful Surgical Procedure

Adenoidectomy is an additional useful surgical procedure (see Sect. 3.4.12).

1.4.5.8   Differential Diagnosis

- Subacute or acute otitis externa
- Meatal furunculosis
- Suppuration of postauricular lymph nodes
- Erysipelas of the pinna

1.4.5.9   Prognosis

In most cases acute mastoiditis resolves without sequelae when early treatment is well adapted to the causing pathogens.

1.4.5.10   Surgical Principles

1. Myringotomy/grommets (Fig. 1.4.5)
2. Mastoidectomy
   - Retroauricular incision through the skin and periosteum to the planum mastoideum, sampling of pus for microbiological testing if there is a cortical perforation
   - Elevation of the periosteum up to the spine of Henle and the posterior bony margin of the meatus
   - Exposure of the whole planum mastoideum
   - Removal of the mastoid cortex with a large cutting burr
   - Exposure of the antrum and enlargement of the aditus ad antrum as well as identification of the incus
   - Removal of all inflammatory mastoid cells
   - Closure of the wound with in most cases a soft drain left in the lower part of the cavity for 3 days

Suggested Reading

1. McKenna MG, Eavey RD (1993) Acute mastoiditis. In Nadol JB, Schuknecht HF (eds) Surgery of the temporal bone. Raven, New York, pp 145–154

1.4.6   Chronic Otitis Media (Without Cholesteatoma)

SALVATORE IURATO, CHRISTIAN MARTIN, AND OLIVIER STERKERS

1.4.6.1   Definition

Chronic inflammation of the middle ear mucosa characterized by a *long-standing central perforation* of the tympanic membrane with permanent or intermittent drainage (active and inactive stages).

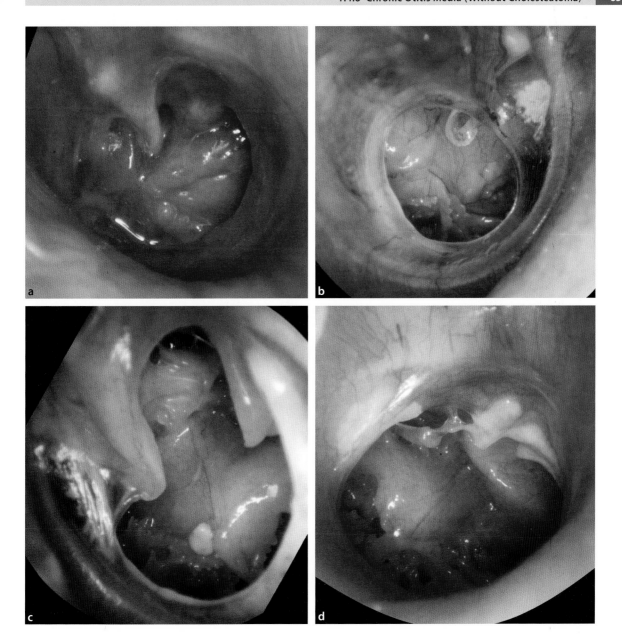

Fig. 1.4.8 a Chronic otitis media, left ear, active stage. Granulation tissue on the promontory in contact with the tip of the malleus handle. **b** Chronic otitis media, right ear, dry perforation. Note the tip of the malleus handle. **c** Kidney-shaped dry perforation, left ear. Note the long process of the incus and Jacobson's nerve along the promontory. **d** Subtotal perforation with atrophy of the long process of the incus and of part of the malleus handle in this right ear. Note the semicanal of the tensor tympani, the ostium of the Eustachian tube and the round window niche

1.4.6.2 Aetiology/Epidemiology

Perforations resulting from acute otitis media (and most traumatic perforations) generally heal in a few days. Central long-standing perforations occur in patients who have experienced repeated infections owing to Eustachian tube problems, such as adenoid hypertrophy and recurrent adenoid infections, impaired nasal respiration (septal deviation, allergy), chronic infections of the paranasal cavities, cleft palate, collagen diseases and ciliary paresis of tubal mucosa as in Kartagener syndrome, severe traumatic perforations, acute necrotizing otitis media (rare) and immune deficiency.

The most frequent pathogenic organisms cultured from chronically draining ears are *Pseudomonas aeruginosa* (60–80%), *Staphylococcus aureus* (10–25%), *Proteus*

(10–20%), *Streptococcus viridans* and *Enterobacter*. Other multiorganisms are cultured. Mycotic superinfection is possible.

1.4.6.3   Symptoms

Recurrent episodes of drainage (otorrhoea). In the **active stages** the secretion is mucopurulent, odourless, and may be very profuse particularly when the mastoid mucosa is involved (Fig. 1.4.8a). These episodes of reactivation are initiated by upper respiratory infections, or by external auditory canal manipulations, or by penetration of water in the ear. In **inactive stages** the only symptom is some degree of conductive hearing loss and a dry central perforation (Fig. 1.4.8b, c).

1.4.6.4   Complications

- **Ossicular resorption** (most frequently the long process of the incus) and/or **ossicular fixation** (most frequently the malleus head) are rather frequent (Fig. 1.4.8d). In a few cases the ossicular lesion may be present under an intact (repaired) tympanic membrane.
- **Tympanosclerosis**: hyalinized collagen changes of the middle ear mucosa limited to the tympanic membrane with (Fig. 1.4.9a, b) or without (Fig. 1.4.9c) perforation

or, less frequently, extended to the ossicles (fixation and conductive hearing loss) and to the promontorium. The white plaques may be thickly calcified. Small tympanosclerotic plaques confined to the tympanic membrane do not affect hearing, but a severe conductive hearing loss and even a severe mixed hearing loss may be present in extensive forms (with promontorial and stapes involvement). When tympanosclerosis blocking the stapes cannot be easily removed at surgery, a second-stage operation is necessary to avoid the risk of labyrinthitis and dead ear. In some cases of extensive tympanosclerosis, surgery is not recommended at all owing to the high risk of sensorineural hearing loss.

- Conductive or mixed hearing loss (inner ear toxic involvement).
- Other complications are external otitis and eczema.

1.4.6.5   Diagnostic Procedures

- **Otoscopy (ear microscopy)**: location and size—from a central hole (Fig. 1.4.8b) to a kidney-shaped (Fig. 1.4.8c) or subtotal (Fig. 1.4.8d) perforation—of calcifications, presence of the annulus, integrity of the ossicular chain. In **inactive stages** the middle ear may be perfectly dry with the margins of the perforation covered with a healed epithelium (Fig. 1.4.8b–d). When the middle ear is infected (**active stage**) the central

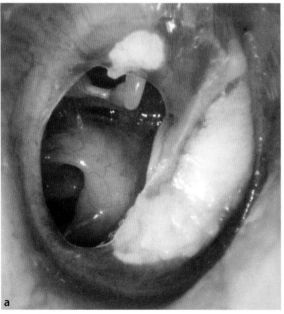
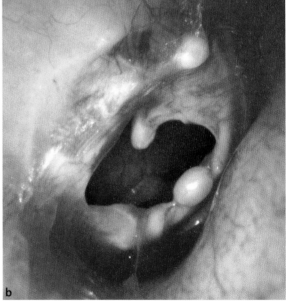

Fig. 1.4.9 a Chronic otitis media, right ear, dry perforation (inactive stage). Notice a tympanosclerotic plaque involving the anterior half of the tympanic membrane. A smaller plaque is located at the level of the long process of the incus. Note the incudostapedial articulation, the stapedial tendon emerging from the tip of the pyramidal eminence and the round window niche. **b** Chronic otitis media, right ear, inactive stage: tympanosclerotic tissue along the margin of the perforation

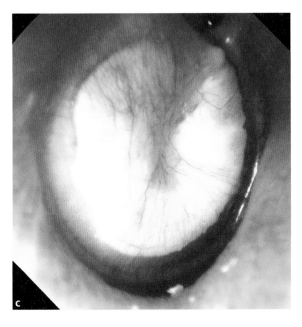

Fig. 1.4.9 *(continued)* **c** Tympanosclerosis may be present without perforation of the tympanic membrane

perforation is surrounded by a ring of granulation tissue and a yellowish mucopurulent exudate can be seen draining in the external auditory canal (Fig. 1.4.8a).

- **Hearing examination** (tuning fork tests and audiometry): conductive hearing loss; sensorineural impairment not common but possible (Fig. 1.1.18).

1.4.6.6 Additional/Useful Diagnostic Procedures

- X-ray (Schüller) examination to assess the degree of mastoid pneumatization (Fig. 1.1.21)
- High-resolution CT (hidden cholesteatoma?)
- Paranasal sinuses X-ray
- Nasopharyngeal fibroscopy

1.4.6.7 Therapy

Recommended European Standard: Conservative Therapy
- Periodic cleaning of the ear by local suction under the microscope.
- Topical treatment: quinolone eardrops are routinely applied twice for 7–10 days. In cases of bacterial resistance to this antibiotic, other eardrops containing mainly aminoglycosides could be used.
- Oral (e.g. trimethoprim–sulphamethoxazole, 15 mg/kg twice per day) or parenteral antibiotics: may be

occasionally beneficial for treating particularly active and resistant drainage.

Note that in presence of a tympanic membrane perforation, a conventional air-conduction hearing aid is not recommended, even if the perforation is dry: it will not remain dry any longer! It is necessary to close first the perforation surgically.

Additional/Useful Therapeutic Options
- Treatment of the nose, paranasal sinus or nasopharynx
- Elimination if possible of allergic factors

1.4.6.8 Surgery

1. **Myringoplasty and tympanoplasty without mastoidectomy**: if the perforation is dry, repair the drum (myringoplasty) and eventually the ossicular chain (ossiculoplasty). Alternatively, the patient may choose to live with the perforation and hearing loss. Precautions must be taken against water entering the middle ear during swimming or showering.
2. **Tympanoplasty with mastoidectomy**: if suppurative drainage persists and the mucosa of the mastoid is involved.
3. Myringoplasty and tympanoplasty without mastoidectomy can be accomplished through either the endaural or the retroauricular approach.
   - The **endaural approach** (see Sect. 1.1.1.1) is preferred when the ear canal is large, the perforation is located posteriorly, the area of major interest is around the oval window and the anterior half of the tympanic membrane does not need to be repaired.
   - The **retroauricular approach** is preferred when the ear canal is narrow, the perforation is located anteriorly and it is masked by a prominent anterior wall.

The technique is as follows:
1. Local anaesthesia (lidocaine with 1:100,000 epinephrine) or general anaesthesia in combination with local anaesthesia.
2. Skin incision (retroauricular or endaural).
3. Exposure and removal of the temporalis fascia (or perichondrium) in the desired quantity.
4. The margin of the perforation is refreshed removing the epidermic rim with the help of the sickle knife and microforceps. Note that bony canalplasty may be required when the bulging of the anterior canal wall does not permit the control of the whole border of the perforation.
5. The tympanomeatal flap is elevated and the tympanic cleft is controlled from behind. All the abnormality,

e. g. granulation tissue, polypoid disease, localized epidermization, can be removed. The chorda tympani is spared whenever possible.

6. The integrity and the mobility of the ossicular chain (incudostapedial joint and stapes included) are controlled. A small amount of the bony annulus is removed when needed.

7. The fascial graft is used as an **underlay graft** (under the anterior tympanic annulus and under the malleus handle). Note that a thin silastic sheet may be necessary when the promontorial mucosa is missing or damaged.

8. When the perforation is 4 mm or smaller in diameter and control of the tympanic cleft is not needed, a "**fat graft myringoplasty**" can be carried out. Following contact anaesthesia, the margin of the perforation is refreshed through an ordinary ear speculum without skin incision. The perforation is closed by inserting a fat graft obtained from the ear lobule. The size of the graft should be slightly larger than the perforation: half of the graft will be inserted through the perforation and half will remain outside. This office procedure is particularly convenient in cases of anterosuperior perforations which are treated with some difficulties with a standard underlay myringoplasty.

9. When the ossicular chain is eroded or fixed, **ossiculoplasty** can be carried out using the patient's incus or the head of the malleus as a sculpted autograft or using a titanium prosthesis. There are three main conditions.

   a. *Stapes present, mobile*: the incus or the head of the malleus (Fig. 1.4.10a) or a titanium partial ossicular replacement prosthesis may be interposed.

   b. *Stapes superstructure missing*: a hydroxyapatite–titanium (Fig. 1.4.10b) or a titanium total ossicular replacement prosthesis is the best solution (generally in two stages and with the protection of a film of cartilage between the reconstructed tympanic membrane and the titanium).

   c. *Footplate fixed*: a titanium total ossicular replacement prosthesis after removal of the footplate and protection of the oval window with perichondrium (always staged).

1.4.6.9   Differential Diagnosis

• **Middle ear atelectasis and retraction pockets**: Complete or partial (pocket) invagination of the tympanic membrane (Fig. 1.4.11a, c) caused by chronic Eustachian tube dysfunction, by sniffing or by an old perforation repaired with loss of the fibrous layer. The symptoms are fullness and hearing loss. On otoscopy the tympanic membrane appears retracted, sometimes draped over the incus and stapes and in contact with promontorium (Fig. 1.4.11a). It is not always easy to distinguish at the first glance an atelectatic ear from a dry perforation (Fig. 1.4.11c), but a successful Valsalva manoeuvre blows the thin atelectatic membrane outwards (Fig. 1.4.11b, d).

Retraction pockets are frequently located in the posterosuperior part of the tympanic membrane. Some of them may become *non-self-cleaning* and therefore potentially dangerous (formation of a cholesteatoma). Pneumatic otoscopy with a Siegle speculum is helpful in distinguishing between fixed and mobile retraction

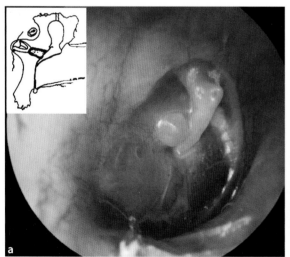

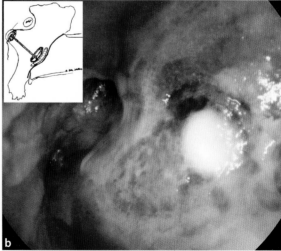

Fig. 1.4.10 a Ossiculoplasty: the sculpted incus has been inserted between the mobile stapes and the malleus handle (autograft). **b** A hydroxyapatite–titanium total ossicular replacement prosthesis has been inserted between the reconstructed tympanic membrane and the mobile footplate

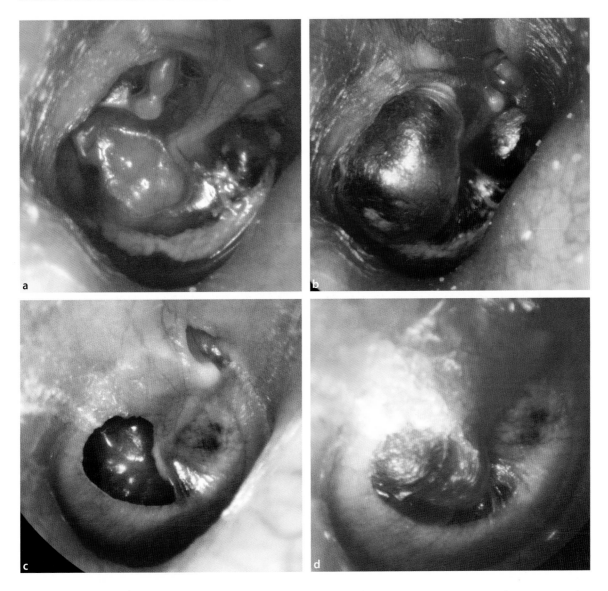

Fig. 1.4.11 a Middle ear atelectasis. The tympanic membrane is retracted and contacts the promontorium. Notice the long process of the incus and the stapedial tendon. **b** Same following inflation (Politzer). The tympanic membrane has been blown outwards (reversible atelectasis). **c** Central retraction pocket simulating a central perforation. **d** Following autoinflation (Valsalva manoeuvre) the retraction pocket has blown out

pockets. Complications are cholesteatoma when dead keratin debris accumulates in the pocket.

- **Adhesive otitis media**: In cases of long-standing middle ear atelectasis or fixed retraction pockets, the whole tympanic membrane or part of it is plastered on the promontorium, ossicles and the medial wall of the tympanic cavity (Fig. 1.4.12). Indications for surgery should be carefully and individually evaluated (cartilage and perichondrium instead of fascia will be used to reconstruct the tympanic membrane). A bone-anchored hearing aid or the Vibrant Soundbridge onto the round window (Colletti) may be a good solution in some cases.

Suggested Reading

1. Bluestone CD (1997) Otitis media. In: Johnson JT, Yu VL (eds) Infections diseases and antimicrobial therapy of the ears, nose and throat. Saunders, Philadelphia, pp 273–291

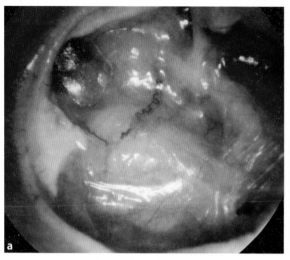 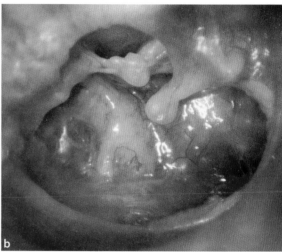

Fig. 1.4.12 a Severe adhesive otitis media with the thinned tympanic membrane adherent to the medial wall of the middle ear. Ossicles are missing. **b** Adhesive otitis media with irrevers- ible retraction of the tympanic membrane. Keratin patches along the stapedial tendon

2. Glasscock ME, Shambaugh GE Jr (1990) Surgery of the ear. Saunders, Philadelphia
3. Gross CW, Bassila M, Lazar RH et al. (1989) Adipose plug myringoplasty: an alternative to formal myringoplasty techniques in children. Otolaryngol Head Neck Surg 101:617–620
4. Hawke M, Keene M, Alberti PW (1990) Clinical otoscopy. An introduction to ear diseases, 2nd edn. Churchill Livingstone, Edinburgh
5. Nadol JB Jr, Schuknecht HF (1993) Surgery of the ear and temporal bone. Raven, New York
6. Tos M (2000) Surgical solutions for conductive hearing loss. Thieme, Stuttgart

1.4.7   Cholesteatoma of the Middle Ear

CHRISTIAN MARTIN, WOLFGANG ARNOLD, OLIVIER STERKERS, AND SALVATORE IURATO

1.4.7.1   Synonyms

Chronic otitis media with cholesteatoma, epidermoid cyst, epidermal cyst, keratosis, keratoma.

1.4.7.2   Definition

Cholesteatoma implies the presence of keratinizing stratified squamous epithelium within the middle ear cleft. It consists of a *matrix* which continually desquamates and of sheets of exfoliated *keratin debris* which accumulate and form the bulk of the cholesteatoma. The simplest definition of cholesteatoma is that of "skin in the wrong place". It is considered as the "unsafe" chronic otitis media owing to the high risk of complications.

1.4.7.3   Aetiology/Epidemiology

Cholesteatoma of the middle ear is relatively frequent and may arise all through the life. It is rarely a primary lesion (**congenital cholesteatoma**), originating from epithelial rests of ectodermal origin in the petrous bone, which may spread in and around the labyrinth and extend into the middle ear cleft. In the great majority of the cases, cholesteatoma is secondary to an inflammation and/or infection of the middle ear (**acquired cholesteatoma**). Acquired cholesteatomas usually develop owing to a chronic Eustachian tube dysfunction which is responsible for a prolonged negative pressure inside the tympanic cleft with retraction of the tympanic membrane (which may perforate). Retractions are mostly located in the upper part of the tympanic membrane (*pars flaccida cholesteatoma* or *Shrappnell's cholesteatoma* or *attic cholesteatoma* or *epitympanic cholesteatoma*; Fig. 1.4.13a, b) or in the posterosuperior part (*pars tensa cholesteatoma*) (Fig. 1.4.13c).

Local inflammation processes (Fig. 1.4.13a), mainly due to *Pseudomonas aeruginosa* and *Bacillus proteus*, stimulate the keratin production and exfoliation and thus the cholesteatoma growth. As far as the size of the cholesteatoma increases inside the middle ear cavities, it will

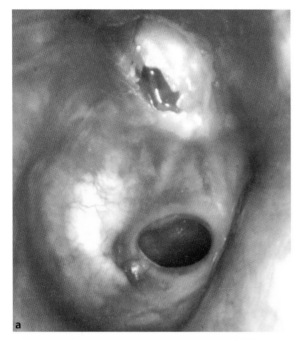

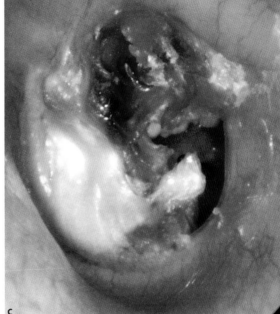

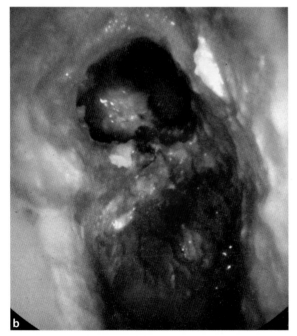

Fig. 1.4.13 a Suppurated attic cholesteatoma (right ear) combined with a central perforation. **b** Large erosion of the attic, with cholesteatoma. **c** Pars tensa cholesteatoma invading the posterior half of mesotympanum (**b** From Arnold et al. [1])

the fibrous annulus (Fig. 1.4.13c). This allows the keratinized epithelium of the external auditory canal to migrate inside the tympanic cavity and grow into the middle ear by the already mentioned mechanism.

1.4.7.4 Symptoms

Cholesteatoma is often asymptomatic for years as the accumulation of keratin in dry cholesteatoma (Fig. 1.4.13b) is slow. However, infection increases the exfoliation rate and the mass of keratin in infected cholesteatomas (Fig. 1.4.13a, c) may grow quickly. The main symptoms are:

- *Otorrhoea*: Usually the discharge is not profuse, but always smelly.
- *Bleeding*: It occurs from granulation or polyps and may alarm the patient.
- *Earache*: It is due to inflammation of the meatal skin or rarely it may indicate an extradural abscess.
- *Hearing loss*: It may vary from normal hearing threshold to total deafness.
- *Tinnitus.*
- *Dizziness*: It may indicate the presence of a labyrinthine fistula.
- *Headache*: It is highly suggestive of intracranial extension.

demineralize the different bony structures, accounting for complications such as destruction of ossicles, fistulization or invasion of the labyrinth, erosion of the Fallopian canal, and cortical bone erosion with intracranial complications (Fig. 1.4.16). Acquired cholesteatoma may also originate following a middle ear infection with an *"unsafe" marginal perforation* located in the posterosuperior part of the tympanic membrane with destruction of

1.4.7.5   Complications

See Fig. 1.4.16. Complications are:
- *Ossicular chain lesions*
- *Sensorineural hearing loss*
- *Labyrinthine fistula*
- *Acute labyrinthitis*
- *Facial palsy*
- *Intracranial complications*: extradural or epidural abscess, subdural abscess, localized or diffuse meningitis, lateral sinus thrombosis, and temporal lobe or cerebellar abscess

1.4.7.6   Diagnostic Procedures

Recommended European Standard
- *Otoscopy (ear microscopy)*: In most cases, cholesteatoma is visualized through attic or marginal perforation (Fig. 1.4.13).
- *Audiometry*: Pure tone and speech audiometry are performed to assess the degree of conductive and sensorineural impairment.
- *High-resolution CT scan* (see Sect. 1.1.6.2) defines the size and location of the cholesteatoma and provides important information on the integrity of the ossicular chain, lateral semicircular canal, cochlea, antroattical tegmen and cortical bone of the middle and posterior fossa. On a coronal CT scan blunting of the scutum (the upper bony edge of the external auditory canal) is often observed. A CT scan may also detect intrapetrous extension (apical, supralabyrinthine, infralabyrinthine and translabyrinthine).

Additional/Useful Diagnostic Procedures
- *MRI*: in the case of suspicion of intrapetrous extension or intracranial complications
- *Vestibular testing with fistula sign* (see Sect. 1.1.4.2): in the case of suspicion of labyrinthine fistula

1.4.7.7   Special Forms

- *Congenital cholesteatoma* (rare): A spherical white cyst may be seen by transparency underneath an intact tympanic membrane, often in a young child (Fig. 1.4.14).
- *Post-traumatic cholesteatoma*: Following a temporal bone fracture the epithelium of the external auditory canal may remain entrapped within the fracture line.
- *Cholesteatoma from ventilating tubes*: This is a very rare complication due to invagination of the epithelium at the edge of the myringotomy.
- *Iatrogenic cholesteatoma*: See Fig. 1.3.10.

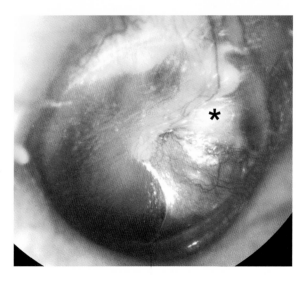

Fig. 1.4.14 Congenital cholesteatoma (*asterisk*) in the middle ear of a young child located behind the anterosuperior quadrant of the tympanic membrane (one site of predilection)

1.4.7.8   Differential Diagnosis

- Active chronic otitis media with polyps in the external auditory canal
- Tuberculous otitis media: sensorineural deafness, facial palsy
- Cholesterol granuloma

1.4.7.9   Therapy

Recommended European Standard

Conservative Therapy
Periodic observation may be indicated in limited cases of a dry cholesteatoma in the only ear or in elderly patients, or in individuals in very poor health.

Surgical Treatment
Cholesteatoma requires surgical treatment usually with mastoid exploration. The priority is to remove the disease and close the middle ear cleft. The reconstruction of the ossicular chain may be feasible immediately or at a later stage. Cholesteatoma can be removed through a canal wall up (close technique) or a canal wall down (open technique) procedure:
- *Close technique*: particularly indicated in children with a well-pneumatized mastoid.
- *Open technique*: particularly indicated in sclerotic mastoids and in revision surgery for recurrences.

Canal Wall Up Technique

See Fig. 1.4.15a. The technique involves:

- General anaesthesia.
- Postauricular incision.
- Musculoperiosteal flap with an anterior pedicle.
- Drilling of the mastoid cortex over the antrum.
- Exposure of the posterior extension of the cholesteatoma.
- Completion of the mastoid cavity to the tegmental and sinus plates.
- Identification of the lateral semicircular canal. If a fistula is suspected on CT, removal of the matrix will be performed at the end of the procedure to avoid any traumatic suction.
- Anterior elevation of the remnants of the tympanic membrane and evaluation of the incudostapedial joint.
- Anterior extension of the mastoidectomy behind the preserved posterior canal wall to perform the anterior tympanotomy. Removal of the incus and section of the head of the malleus are usually necessary to have access to the anterior attic.
- Posterior tympanotomy by opening the facial recess (Fig. 1.4.15a).
- Removal of the cholesteatoma by elevating it and dissecting it towards the epitympanum and middle ear,

working on both sides of the preserved canal wall and through the posterior tympanotomy (Fig. 1.4.15a).

- Once removal of the disease has been accomplished, reconstruction of the tympanic membrane and eventually of the ossicular chain is performed.
- Reinforcement of the attical defect and of the tympanic membrane by thinned cartilage harvested from the concha or tragus.
- Postauricular closure in two layers without drain and packing of the ear canal.

Canal Wall Down Technique (Modified Radical Cavity)

See Fig. 1.4.15b. The technique involves:

- General anaesthesia.
- Postauricular incision.
- *Mastoidectomy*: a canal wall up mastoidotomy may be done first to determine whether the canal wall down technique is necessary; alternatively, if a canal wall down mastoidectomy has already been planned, the drilling over the mastoid antrum is extended anteriorly to include the posterior canal wall.
- In removal of the posterior canal wall, the "bridge" overlying the aditus ad antrum is removed first, providing a wide exposure of the facial nerve, which will

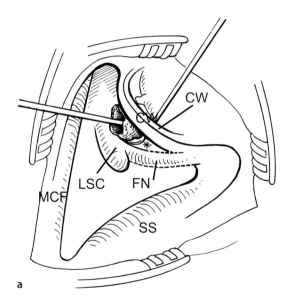
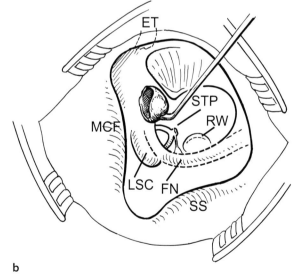
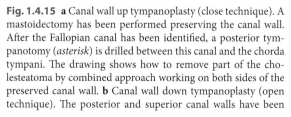

Fig. 1.4.15 a Canal wall up tympanoplasty (close technique). A mastoidectomy has been performed preserving the canal wall. After the Fallopian canal has been identified, a posterior tympanotomy (*asterisk*) is drilled between this canal and the chorda tympani. The drawing shows how to remove part of the cholesteatoma by combined approach working on both sides of the preserved canal wall. **b** Canal wall down tympanoplasty (open technique). The posterior and superior canal walls have been removed and the cavity has been saucerized to obtain smooth walls and rounded margins. The facial ridge has been lowered down to the level of the Fallopian canal and the tip of the mastoid removed when necessary. *CW* canal wall, *FN* Fallopian canal, *LSC* lateral semicircular canal, *MCF* middle cranial fossa, *SS* sigmoid sinus, *ET* Eustachian tube, *STP* stapes, *RW* round window niche

be followed inferiorly. With the facial nerve identified used as a landmark, the posterior canal wall is lowered to the level of the Fallopian canal (Fig. 1.4.15b).

- Canalplasty is performed without violation of the temporomandibular joint; the superior aspect of the canal and scutum are removed to expose the anterior attic. The tympanic bone anteriorly and inferiorly is removed to further expose the middle ear, hypotympanum and sinus tympani.
- Cholesteatoma is removed according to its extension in the mastoid and the middle ear. Usually, malleus and incus have been removed.
- Tympanic membrane is repaired by fascial graft reinforced by cartilage; the fascial graft should extend largely into the mastoid cavity, covering the lateral semicircular canal. Ossiculoplasty is usually performed.
- Partial obliteration of the mastoid cavity could be eventually performed.
- Meatoplasty is crucial for the success of the procedure.
- Skin closure in two layers and packing of the mastoid cavity.

Fistula of the Lateral Semicircular Canal

- If a fistula of the lateral semicircular canal is suspected on CT or identified at surgery, removal of the matrix over the fistula site will be performed at the end of the procedure to avoid any traumatic suction.
- The fistula is covered with a fascial graft and then with cartilage or bone, sealed with fibrin glue.

1.4.7.10 Prognosis

- A long-term clinical otoscopic follow-up is necessary to detect *residual* cholesteatomas and *recurrences*.
- In canal wall down mastoidectomy, serial otoscopic examinations with eventual cleaning of the mastoid cavity are needed.
- In the canal wall up technique residual cholesteatoma or recurrence occurs in 10–20% of cases. A second-look surgery is advocated after at least 1 year to disclose residual cholesteatomas and to restore hearing, if necessary. A CT scan can help with the follow-up.

References

1. Arnold W, Kau R, Niedermayer HP (1999) Ohr. In: Seifert G (ed) HNO-Pathologie, Nase und Nasennebenhöhlen, Rachen, Tonsillen, Ohr, Larinx, vol 4. Springer, Berlin, pp 265–546

Suggested Reading

1. Brackmann DE, Shelton C, Arriaga, MA (2001) Otologic surgery. Saunders, Philadelphia
2. Glasscock ME, Shambaugh GE Jr (1990) Surgery of the ear. Saunders, Philadelphia
3. Nadol JB Jr, Schuknecht HF (1993) Surgery of the ear and temporal bone. Raven, New York
4. Schuknecht HF (1993) Pathology of the ear. Lea & Febiger, Philadelphia
5. Tos M (2000) Surgical solutions for conductive hearing loss. Thieme, Stuttgart

1.4.8 Intratemporal and Intracranial Complications of Otitis Media

SALVATORE IURATO

1.4.8.1 Definition

Infection spreading to adjacent structures outside the defence barriers (mucoperiosteum and intact bony walls) of the middle ear and mastoid. Note that coalescent mastoiditis (see Sect 1.4.5) is considered as a stage in the development of acute otitis media and not as a complication.

1.4.8.2 Aetiology/Epidemiology

Complications occur in association with cholesteatoma and less frequently in association with chronic otitis media without cholesteatoma and acute otitis media. Their incidence has substantially declined with the availability of antibiotics; nevertheless they are still frequent in developing countries.

1.4.8.3 Pathways

- *Without bone erosion* through a progressive thrombophlebitis of small venules, as in acute otitis media or in acute exacerbation of chronic otitis media
- *By bone erosion* as result of coalescent mastoiditis or cholesteatoma
- *By preformed pathways*, e.g. oval window, round window, internal auditory canal, endolymphatic duct and sac, developmental dehiscences of the tegmen or the hypotympanum, over the jugular bulb, the result of a skull fracture or previous aural surgery

1.4.8.4   Complications

Note that in approximately one third of the cases, two or more otogenic complications are present concomitantly:
1. Intratemporal (Fig. 1.4.16)
   – *Labyrinthitis, serous or purulent* (the most frequent intratemporal complication). Note that a dead labyrinth is the consequence of a purulent labyrinthitis
   – *Labyrinthine fistula* (with or without simultaneous labyrinthitis)
   – *Petrositis or petrous apicitis*
   – *Facial paralysis.*
2. Intracranial (Fig. 1.4.16)
   – *Extradural (or epidural) abscess*: collection of pus between the dura and the bony wall, and *perisinus abscess* (pachymeningitis), the most frequent complication
   – *Meningitis.* There are two clinical types or degrees:
      (a) Localized, without invasion of CSF
      (b) Diffused, generalized
   – *Lateral sinus thrombophlebitis*, rarely seen today
   – *Brain abscess*

Note that diffuse meningitis and brain abscess are the two most important complications.

1.4.8.5   Symptoms

Signs and symptoms of impending complications in the course of acute otitis media or chronic otitis media with or without cholesteatoma are as follows:
1. Early signs
   – Malodorous (fetid) discharge from the ear.
   – Deep and constant pain. Note that earache in chronic otitis media means that something is going wrong and if pus is under pressure in the middle ear cleft, an intracranial complication may be impending.
   – Headache and drowsiness.
   – Visual field defect (one of the earliest signs of brain abscess).
2. Signs generally occurring later but that may be present at the time of diagnosis: elevated temperature, suggesting meningitis or lateral sinus thrombosis. Note that lateral sinus thrombosis should be considered in a patient with suppurative acute otitis media who begins to run even a slight or intermittent fever because chronic otitis media even with a large infected cholesteatoma rarely causes an elevation in temperature.
3. Rarer findings
   – Disequilibrium

INTRATEMPORAL and INTRACRANIAL COMPLICATIONS

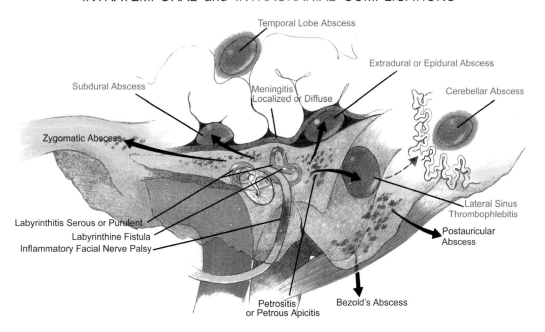

Fig. 1.4.16 Pathways of the intratemporal [ossicular chain lesions, labyrinthine fistula, labyrinthitis (serous or purulent), facial paralysis, petrositis or petrous apicitis] and intracranial (extradural or epidural abscess, perisinus abscess, meningitis, lateral sinus thrombophlebitis, temporal lobe or cerebellar abscess) complications of otitis media (Adapted from Harris and Darrow [1])

– Hearing loss
– Nucal rigidity
– Cranial nerve neuropathies
– Seizures

1.4.8.6 Diagnosis of Established Specific Complications

1. **Labyrinthine fistula**: The patient often complains of dizziness when he/she exerts pressure on the tragus or manipulates the auricle (Hennebert's sign).
   – Fistula test: see Sect 1.1.4.2.
   – Tullio's phenomenon: see Sect. 1.1.3.5.
2. **Serous inflammatory labyrinthitis.**
   – Vestibular symptoms: spontaneous (irritative) nystagmus towards the infected ear becomes a paralytic nystagmus towards the opposite ear. Vertigo, nausea, vomiting, ataxia.
   – Cochlear symptoms: hearing impairment greater for high-pitched tones, diplacusis.
3. **Suppurative inflammatory labyrinthitis**: signs similar to those of serous labyrinthitis but with a more abrupt onset.
4. **Dead labyrinth**: absence of caloric responses and deafness.
5. **Petrositis**.
   – Pain, frontal or behind the eye in anterior petrositis; occipital, parietal or temporal in cases of posterior petrositis.
   – Persistent aural discharge following a simple mastoidectomy. Note that the three symptoms, e.g. persistent otorrhoea, pain around the eye in the trigeminal distribution and diplopia, due to nerve VI paralysis, constitute **Gradenigo's syndrome.**
6. **Facial paralysis**: may be a complication of either acute otitis media (through a dehiscence of the Fallopian canal) or chronic otitis media (onset of symptoms often slow and progressive). For facial nerve testing see Sect. 1.7.1.
7. **Subperiosteal abscess**: a relatively uncommon complication of otitis media in the antibiotic era. It is usually associated with the development of acute mastoiditis following an episode of acute otitis media.
8. **Extradural (and perisinus) abscess** (with risk of extension to produce lateral sinus thrombophlebitis, subdural abscess, meningitis or brain abscess).
   – Persistent headache on the side of otitis media.
   – Profuse or intermittent pulsating otorrhoea accentuated by compression of the internal jugular vein.
   – Low-grade fever of unknown origin following acute otitis media.
   – Signs of meningismus (Kernig's, Brudzinski's).
   – Recurrent attacks of generalized non-meningococcic meningitis.

– Lumbar puncture: increased white cell count, but usually with lymphocyte predominance. Glucose level normal, no organisms.
– MRI: epidural collection with a contrast-enhancing periphery.

Note that the majority of perisinus and extradural abscesses produce no symptoms and are a chance finding at operation.

9. **Localized meningitis.**
   – *Symptoms*: headache, increased temperature (the two more constant). Patient irritable or drowsy. Convulsions (in infants).
   – *Signs*.
     • Neck rigidity, slight to moderate (chin does not touch the chest).
     • Kernig's sign (inability to extend the leg completely with the thigh flexed on the abdomen).
     • Brudzinski's sign (flexion of the hip and knee when the neck is bent).
     • Babinski's sign (extension of the toes instead of flexion on stimulating the sole of the foot).
     • CSF clear or slightly opaque, 10–1,000 cell/mm^3 with lymphocytes predominating, glucose level normal, no organisms in cultures.
10. **Generalized meningitis**: pyogenic infection of the pia arachnoid over the entire brain and spinal cord with viable organisms in CSF. It results from chronic otitis media in adults, and from acute otitis media in the paediatric age group. The symptoms are similar to those of the localized variety but greater in degree. A chill may accompany the initial rise in temperature. Pulse is rapid, and temperature is high to very high (41–42°C). There is constant headache and the pain may become excruciating. Photophobia. Neck retracted, spine stiff. Sensorium clouded, ocular paralyses, other paralyses. Kernig's, Brudzinski's, Babinski's. CSF: high pressure, grossly cloudy, containing 1,000 cells/mm^3 or more (predominantly polymorphonuclear), elevated protein concentration, reduced glucose level, organisms on stained smear and culture (in 85% of cases, provided antibiotic therapy has not been started prior to lumbar puncture). Differentiate otitic meningitis from meningitis due to meningococcus.
11. **Lateral sinus thrombophlebitis**: Although rarely seen today, this complication does occur and is very easily overlooked because of the masking effect of antibiotics on fever, the most constant symptom. Characteristically caused, in order of frequency, by haemolytic streptococcus or type III pneumococcus or staphylococcus.
    – Septic-type fever ("picket-fence" temperature chart), seen rarely owing to the use of aggressive antibiotic therapy. Chills usually precede the sharp rises in temperature and profuse sweats accompany the downward swings. Between the bouts of fever, the

patient is alert with a sense of well-being in contrast to the apathy of the patient with a brain abscess and the prostration of the patient with meningitis.
– Headache.
– Progressive anaemia, especially rapid and pronounced in haemolytic streptococcal infection.
– Progressive emaciation, not so rapid and pronounced as in cerebellar abscess.
– Eye-ground changes (papilloedema).
– CT/MRI.
– Oedema over the posterior aspect of the mastoid process due to thrombosis of the mastoid emissary vein (**Griesinger's sign**: less common symptom).
Note that today the final diagnosis depends on surgical exploration as both the fever and the blood culture are masked by antibacterial medication.

12. **Otitic hydrocephalus**: increased intracranial pressure (without a brain abscess) several weeks or more after acute otitis media. This condition occurs more often in children and adolescents. Symptoms are headache (the more constant symptom) often with nerve VI paralysis on the same side and vomiting.
– Papilloedema, which may reach 5 or 6 dioptres.
– CSF pressure exceeding 300 ml water; CSF is clear, without increase in cells or protein (unlike localized meningitis).
– No localized neurological signs, in contrast to brain abscess.
– CT shows no space-occupying lesions.
– MRI.

13. **Cerebrospinal otorrhoea.**

14. **Brain abscess.**
– *First stage* (initial encephalitis): symptoms mild and evanescent but sufficiently characteristic; they may often mimic an exacerbation of chronic otitis media or even a viral syndrome.
   • A chill or a chilly sensation followed by a slight or moderate rise in temperature (lasting several days) frequently heralds the invasion of the brain.
   • Headache and nausea, sometimes with nonprojectile vomiting.
   • The patient may appear apathetic, drowsy or irritable.
   • Convulsions may be the first sign (in children).
   • In the case of a localized meningeal reaction, slight stiffness of the neck and moderate increase in cells and protein with normal glucose content.
– *Second stage* (latent or quiescent): lasts from 10 days to several weeks or, rarely, several months. Symptoms may be minimal or absent. In other cases
   • Malaise, poor appetite.
   • Intermittent headache.

   • Slight temperature elevation with listlessness, drowsiness, slowed cerebration, irritability due to continued encephalitis.
– *Third stage* (of manifest expanding abscess).
   • As the encephalite and oedema fluctuate from hour to hour and day to day, so the symptoms and signs may come and go.
   • Headache severe and usually continuous, refractory to symptomatic therapy.
   • Projectile vomiting (common and characteristic).
   • Intermittent slowing of the pulse, due to pressure on the vagus centre in the brain stem.
   • Temperature slightly elevated, normal or subnormal.
   • Apathy, drowsiness, disorientation.
   • Jacksonian convulsions (30–50% of patients) and ocular paralyses with pupillary changes.
   • Eye-ground signs of increased intracranial pressure occur in about half of the cases, with blurring of the disc margins, hyperaemia or papilloedema.
   • CSF is rarely normal, with usually a slight increase in cells and protein. Caution should be taken when withdrawing spinal fluid; only small amounts should be withdrawn and only by ventricular puncture in the case of suspected cerebellar abscess to avoid herniation of the brain stem into the foramen magnum.
   • Cheyne–Stokes respiration, elevation of the blood pressure.
   • Less constant focal symptoms: aphasia (left temporal lobe abscess in a right-handed patient), paresis of face and mouth on the opposite side (central type, not affecting the frontal muscle), visual field defects.
   Note that the symptoms and signs of increased intracranial pressure are more constant and definite in a cerebellar than in a temporal lobe abscess because of the restricted space and its proximity to the brain stem. In cerebellar abscesses, there is ataxia on the same side (finger-to-nose test), adiadochokinesia (decreased ability to alternate movements rapidly), coarse intention tremor, gait is ataxic with tendency to fall towards the diseased side, spontaneous fluctuating (in degree and direction) nystagmus and emaciation despite a fair appetite.
– CT: On a contrast-enhanced scan, a brain abscess appears as a hypodense area surrounded by an enhanced ring (the so-called ring sign) (Fig. 1.4.17).
– MRI: There is better contrast between the area of the peripheral oedema and the surrounding brain (Fig. 1.4.18).

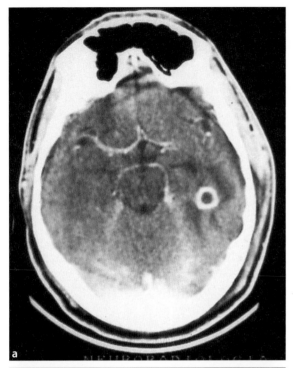

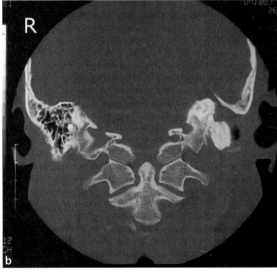

Fig. 1.4.17 a Axial CT scan of an otogenic brain abscess which appears as a hypodense area surrounded by an enhanced ring (ring sign). **b** Same patient, bone programme coronal CT demonstrating the bone erosion caused by cholesteatoma in the left tegmen

- Subdural infection (rare): neurological findings are more focal than would be found in meningitis and more rapid in onset than in brain abscess.
  - Severe headache.
  - Drowsiness.

- Meningeal signs.
- Hemianopsia and deviation of the eyes.
- Focal seizures in some 60% of cases.
- MRI for definitive diagnosis.

1.4.8.7   Treatment of Specific Complications

1. Labyrinthine fistula: see Sect. 1.1.4.2
2. Serous labyrinthitis: if the cause is an early suppurative acute otitis media, antibacterial treatment and myringotomy. If the cause is a perilabyrinthine osteitis or a cholesteatoma, mastoidectomy plus antibacterial treatment.
3. Suppurative labyrinthitis: in bed under close and continuous observation and antibacterial medication. At the first appearance of any meningeal sign, CSF examination, and the labyrinth should be drained surgically as an emergency operation. Suppurative labyrinthitis secondary to meningitis does not require drainage of the labyrinth.
4. Petrositis: preliminary complete simple mastoidectomy. If no sign of meningitis wait 8–10 days before further surgery. If the symptoms and signs of petrositis persist, cell tracts should be explored systematically.
5. Facial paralysis: immediate operation in chronic otitis media, only myringotomy in acute otitis media.
6. Subperiosteal abscess: abscess should be drained and a simple mastoidectomy performed.
7. Perisinus and extradural abscesses: simple or radical mastoidectomy with cautious exploration of a necrotic lead to a subdural abscess or a brain abscess. Specific antibacterial medication to prevent postoperative spreading of infection.
8. Localized otic meningitis: immediate surgical exploration with wide dural exposure (when secondary to suppurative labyrinthitis, the labyrinth should be drained). In the case of meningismus in acute otitis media, a myringotomy with antibacterial medication for the causative organism may suffice.
9. Generalized otic meningitis
   - First, examine every patient with fever for stiffness of neck and Kernig's sign.
   - Second, lumbar puncture. Note CSF pressure, fluid gross clarity or cloudiness, glucose and protein levels. Centrifuged sediment should be stained with Gram's stain and acid-fast stains.
   - Third, adequate and appropriate antibacterial treatment. Ampicillin (200–400 mg/kg per day) plus chloramphenicol (75 mg/kg per day). Third-generation cephalosporin, 2 g intravenously every 12 h for 7–10 days. Dexamethasone. Lumbar or ventricular punctures. Search for a suppurative focus.

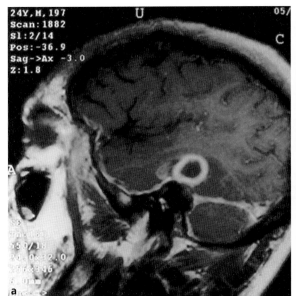

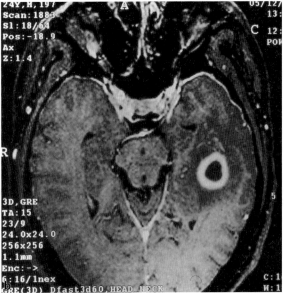

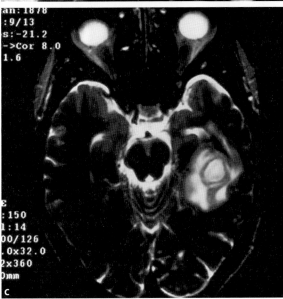

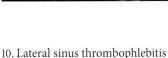

Fig. 1.4.18a–c Same patient as for Fig. 1.4.17. With MRI a much better contrast is achieved. a Sagittal plane, b axial plane, T₁, c axial plane, T₂. Note the cerebral oedema surrounding the abscess in T₂-weighted sections

10. Lateral sinus thrombophlebitis
    - Intravenous antibiotics.
    - A complete simple mastoidectomy or a radical mastoidectomy if the patient had chronic otitis media with cholesteatoma.
    - Inspection and palpation of the exposed wall of the sinus (small-gauge needle first, if no blood, surgical extralumen packing before incision). Note that today internal jugular vein ligation is reserved for cases with continued sepsis after mastoidectomy and sinus exploration and in those in which septic emboli are developing. Use of anticoagulant therapy is controversial.

11. Otitic hydrocephalus
    - Repeated lumbar or ventricular punctures or placement of a lumbar drain.
    - Diuretics, hyperosmolar dehydrating agents.
    - Steroids.
    - Subtemporal decompression if necessary to prevent optic atrophy from prolonged papilloedema.
12. CSF otorrhoea: if not surgically corrected, the patient sooner or later develops meningitis.
13. Brain abscess
    - After MRI, intravenous antibiotic therapy (aqueous penicillin G combined with metronidazole and a third-generation cephalosporine, such as ceftriaxone, combined with metronidazole.
    - Dexamethazone intravenously.
    - Mannitol.
    - Surgical approach through a craniotomy (not through the ear). Repeated aspirations–irrigations of the abscess cavity.
    - Ear is approached surgically 3–4 days after craniotomy.

References

1. Harris JP, Darrow DH (1993) Complications of chronic otitis media. In: Nadol JB, Schuknecht HF (eds) Surgery of the ear and temporal bone. Raven, New York, pp 171–191

Suggested Reading

1. Neely JC (1986) Complications of temporal bone. In: Cummings CU, Fridrickson GJ, Harker L et al. (eds). Otolaryngology—head & neck surgery, 4th edn. Mosby, St Louis, pp 2988–3015

1.5 Middle Ear/Inner Ear

WOLFGANG ARNOLD, VINCENT DARROUZET, CHRISTIAN MARTIN, OLIVIER STERKERS AND SALVATORE IURATO

1.5.1 Barotrauma

SALVATORE IURATO

1.5.1.1 Synonyms

Aerotitis media, barotraumatic otitis media, otitic baro-trauma, inner ear decompression illness.

1.5.1.2 Definition

Acute, mono- or bilateral loss of ventilation in the middle ear caused by a sudden increase of atmospheric pressure not compensated for by the Eustachian tube function. In patients with acute rhinitis, barotrauma may occur during descent in an aircraft: the external pressure increases rapidly, collapsing the tympanic membrane inwards. Divers may experience barotrauma on deep descent.

1.5.1.3 Symptoms

Sudden onset of a sensation of pressure inside the ear, earache which can often be severe, tinnitus (continuous or pulsatile), hearing loss, vertigo.

1.5.1.4 Complications

Rupture of the round window membrane with perilymphatic fistula (severe hearing loss with strong vertigo).

1.5.1.5 Diagnostic Procedures

Otoscopy or ear microscopy: retracted tympanic membrane with injection of the vessels; clear or haemorrhagic fluid (haemotympanum) may be evident behind the tympanic membrane (Fig. 1.5.1).
- Nose and nasopharynx inspection.
- Evaluation of the Eustachian tube function.
- Hearing examination: tuning fork, audiogram. The tuning fork is lateralized in the affected ear. When barotrauma is complicated by rupture of the round window membrane or bleeding into the labyrinth, the tuning fork is heard in the unaffected ear.
- Tympanometry: negative pressure inside the middle ear, with reduced compliance.
- Fistula test (see Sect. 1.1.4.2).
- Study of spontaneous nystagmus with Frenzel glasses: often directed towards the involved labyrinth; in cases of rupture of the round window membrane it is possible to observe nystagmus towards the irritated labyrinth as well as nystagmus towards the contralateral labyrinth (paretic nystagmus).

1.5.1.6 Therapy

- Nasal decongestants: nose spray/drops, e.g. 0.1% xylometazoline hydrochloride, several times per day. Val-

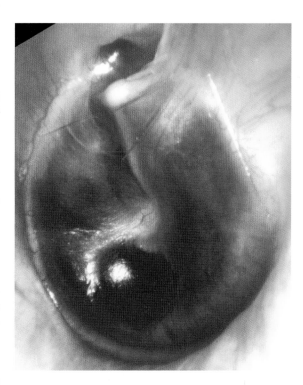

Fig. 1.5.1 Haemotympanum. The left middle ear of this patient has filled with blood following a recent barotrauma

salva manoeuvre, politzerization with a Politzer bag or tube inflation using a catheter.

- In cases of persistent negative pressure in the middle ear, myringotomy with insertion of a grommet (Fig. 1.4.5).
- In cases of inner ear involvement, high doses of corticosteroids and rheologic therapy (the same treatment as for idiopathic sudden hearing loss).
- In cases of nasal bacterial infection, antibacterial treatment, e.g. trimethoprim plus sulphamethoxazole.
- In cases that occurred in a compression chamber, immediate decompression.
- In cases of suspected rupture of the round window membrane, exploratory tympanotomy and closure of the fistula.

1.5.1.7   Differential Diagnosis

- Inner ear decompression illness

1.5.1.8   Prognosis

- Good in cases of middle ear barotrauma without inner ear damage.
- In cases of rupture of an inner ear window, persistent vertigo and fluctuating sensorineural hearing loss or deafness with tinnitus.

1.5.1.9   Suggestions

- Avoid air travel during severe upper respiratory airways infections.
- In the case of chronic Eustachian tube dysfunction, apply decongestant nose drops 20 min before takeoff and landing.

1.5.2   Otosclerosis

WOLFGANG ARNOLD, CHRISTIAN MARTIN, OLIVIER STERKERS AND SALVATORE IURATO

1.5.2.1   Synonym

Otospongiosis.

1.5.2.2   Definition

- Inflammatory disease of certain genetically determined topographic regions of the otic capsule strongly associated with a local measles virus infection of bone cells.

- Sites of predilection according to frequency: oval window/stapes footplate, round window, promontory, enchondral ossification zone of the cochlea.
- The inflammatory resorptive bone process (otospongiosis) is followed by a remineralization and formation of new bone. If this very hard new bone (sclerosis) gradually invades the annular ligament and stapes, *bony ankylosis of the stapes* (Fig. 1.5.2a) *and therefore impairment of hearing* results.

1.5.2.3   Aetiology/Epidemiology

Molecular biology investigations from different research centres in Europe and the USA have proven that the inflammatory phase of the disease (otospongiosis) is strongly associated with a local measles virus infection. The genetically determined very specific sites of predilection may have special receptors for measles viruses, which could explain the hereditary (autosomal dominant) aspect of the disease. Measles virus vaccination significantly influences the incidence of otosclerosis, in the course of which the decline is much greater in men than in women. A relation between the local renin angiotensin system activity and otosclerosis has been recently described.

1.5.2.4   Incidence

- Histologically (autopsy findings): 8–12% of the white population (Caucasians), 1% of the black or Chinese population.
- The prevalence of clinical otosclerosis is approximately 15–20 cases per 100,000 inhabitants per year (Europe).
- The disease becomes clinically manifest after the 20th year of age (third decade) and in central Europe today the highest incidence is seen in the fifth decade. About half of clinical otosclerosis patients report a family history of this condition. Clinically females are affected twice as often as males (USA 2:1; Denmark 2:1; Israel 2:1; Switzerland 1.84:1; Germany 1.64:1).
- According to recent investigations it is questionable if pregnancy has some influence on the clinical outbreak of otosclerosis.

1.5.2.5   Symptoms

- Progressive unilateral (70%) or bilateral (30%) conductive hearing loss with/without additional sensorineural component. In severe otosclerosis hearing loss can be subdivided into *far-advanced otosclerosis* (patients with air-conduction thresholds in excess of 85 dB and nonmeasurable bone conduction) and *very far advanced otosclerosis* (patients with a blank audiogram with

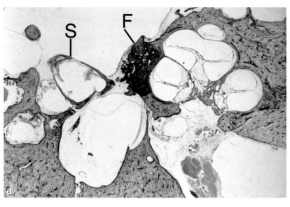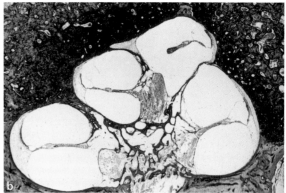

Fig. 1.5.2 Otosclerosis. **a** The focus (F) involves the anterior part of the oval window with fixation of the footplate and the adjacent bony labyrinth (basal turn) S=stapes. **b** Cochlear otosclerosis involving all three turns of the cochlea

both bone-conduction and air-conduction thresholds not measurable with a clinical audiometer).
- Otoscopy and X-ray control of pneumatization are usually normal. Missing history or signs of local inflammatory middle ear diseases are characteristic for otosclerosis patients.
- Tinnitus of variable intensity (60%).
- Sometimes vertigo.

1.5.2.6   Complications

- Pulsation or fluctuating tinnitus.
- Progressive deafness in the cochlear otosclerosis.

1.5.2.7   Diagnostic Procedures

1. Otoscopy (ear microscopy): usually clean outer ear canals, tympanic membrane without any postinflammatory signs. In cases of florid otosclerosis (otospongiosis), thickened, hyperaemic middle ear mucous membrane can be seen by transparency through the ear drum in the area of the oval window (Schwartze sign).
2. Hearing tests.
   - Tuning fork (Gellé test).
   - Audiogram (Fig. 1.1.14): pure conductive hearing loss (30%), combined hearing loss (70%). In 20% of patients with otosclerosis there is an elevation of 20–30 dB of the bone conduction threshold called Carhart's notch. It is thought to be caused by disturbed micromechanics of the cochlea and disappears after successful surgery. In cases of severe cochlear otosclerosis (Fig. 1.5.2b), there is pure sensorineural hearing loss.
3. Tympanometry: generally normal (type A, Fig. 1.1.19), sometimes type A$_s$ (Figs. 1.1.14, 1.1.19).

4. Stapedius reflex is absent because of stapes fixation (Fig. 1.1.14).

1.5.2.8   Additional/Useful Diagnostic Procedures

- Speech audiometry.
- Imaging: High-resolution CT can visualize the otospongiotic foci (irregular zones) of decalcification/resorption, typically located at the anterior part of the oval window niche, fissula ante fenestram or as perichlear demineralization "halo".

1.5.2.9   Therapy

Conservative Treatment
- No treatment when conductive hearing loss is less than 20 dB.
- Hearing aid if the affected ear is the patient's last hearing ear or if the patient is deciding against surgery.

Surgical Treatment
- Stapedotomy or stapedectomy with or without laser. Indicated especially in young patients usually when the threshold reaches more than 20 dB.
- Cochlear implantation in selected cases of severe/profound deafness due to otosclerosis.

1.5.2.10   Differential Diagnosis

- Postinflammatory/aseptic necrosis of the long process of the incus.
- Interrupted or fixed ossicular chain (post-traumatic, luxation of the incus).

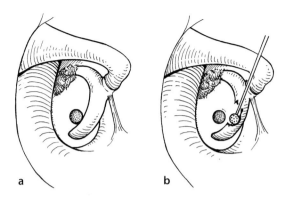
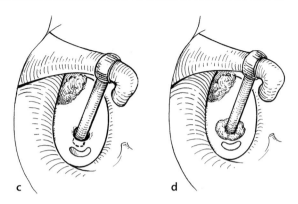

a   b   c   d

Fig. 1.5.3 a–d Stapedotomy. **a** A calibrated hole (0.6–0.8-mm diameter) is prepared (Skeeter or laser) in the footplate. **b** The crural arch is drilled and removed and the stapedial tendon is cut. **c** Teflon piston in place, the remnant of the posterior crus and the anterosuperior otosclerotic focus which has not been disturbed by the procedure are visible. **d** Small pieces of connective tissue and a drop of blood seal the aperture in the footplate

- Tympanosclerosis.
- Malleus head fixation, calcification of the anterior malleus ligament.
- Minor malformations of the middle ear.
- Osteogenesis imperfecta (van der Hoeve syndrome): stapes footplate fixation in association with blue sclerae, pathologic bone fractures. Stapedius reflexes can be present when the stapes crura are weak or fractured.
- Paget disease of the bone: ear symptoms are identical to otosclerosis.
- **Superior semicircular canal dehiscence** is a recently described condition resulting in a low frequency "inner ear" conductive hearing loss with autophony and ear blockage associated with vertigo and oscillopsia induced by loud sounds (Tullio phenomenon), changes in pressure in the ear canal (Hennebert sign) or Valsalva manoeuvre (with evoked nystagmus). Weber tuning fork is laterized to the affected ear. Acoustic reflexes and responses to the vestibular evoked myogenic potentials (VEMP) are normal. ECoG abnormalities: elevated SP/AP ratio. Torsional/vertical vibration induced nystagmus. Diagnosis is confirmed with temporal bone computed tomography and surgical repair can be carried out via a middle cranial fossa approach similar to that described in Fig. 1.5.9.

1.5.2.11 Surgical Principles

Stapedotomy
- Local or general anaesthesia.
- Transcanal or endaural approach.
- Elevation of the tympanomeatal flap.
- Exposure of the stapes and oval window by removal of the posterior bony rim.

- Assessment of the mobility of the malleus to rule out malleus fixation as a cause for conductive impairment.
- Calibrated platinotomy (creating a small perforation of the footplate) using either a laser or a microdrill (Fig. 1.5.3a).
- Removal of the stapes suprastructure (Fig. 1.5.3b).
- Insertion of a commercial prosthesis into the calibrated platinotomy and fixation of the prosthesis to the long process of the incus (Fig. 1.5.3c). The length of the prosthesis must be perfectly adapted and the platinotomy should be sealed with a drop of blood or with connective tissue (Fig. 1.5.3d).
- Reapplication of the tympanomeatal flap.

Stapedectomy
- Access to middle ear identical to stapedotomy (Fig. 1.5.4a)
- After removal of the stapes suprastructure and careful fracture of the footplate with a needle, partial (hemiplatinectomy; Fig. 1.5.4b, c) or total removal of the footplate
- Covering the open oval window with a venous or connective tissue graft
- Prosthesis is placed on the graft and fixed to the incus
- Alternatively a hand-made prosthesis is used consisting of connective tissue from the temporal fascia and stainless steel wire (Fig. 1.5.4d; Schuknecht prosthesis)

1.5.2.12 Prognosis

- Surgery usually results in a dramatic and prolonged hearing gain. The success rate as measured by closure

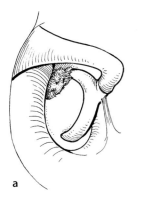
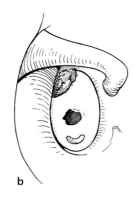
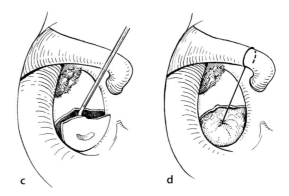

Fig. 1.5.4 a–d Stapedectomy. **a** Anterosuperior otosclerotic focus. **b** After a safety hole has been prepared in the central part of the footplate, the crural arch is fractured and removed. **c** The posterior half of the footplate is removed. **d** A Schuknecht connective tissue and wire prosthesis is inserted. There are many variants, e.g. total stapedectomy instead of haemiplatinectomy, protection of the oval window with perichondrium, different types of prostheses

of the air–bone gap to within 10 dB is approximately 95%.
- Surgery has a small but definite risk of high tone sensorineural hearing loss.
- Postsurgical vertigo usually lasts for 2 or 3 days.
- If a prosthesis is too long, it can touch the wall of the saccule (for anatomical details see Fig. 1.1.3), causing permanent vertigo. In such cases postoperative high-resolution CT should be performed to identify the exact localization of the prosthesis, immediate revision surgery should be performed and the too-long prosthesis should be carefully either changed or shortened with special instruments.
- In cases of a conductive postoperative hearing loss, revision surgery is possible with a slightly higher risk depending on the cause of failure and the technique previously used.

Suggested Reading

1. Arnold W, Häusler R (eds) (2007) Otosclerosis and stapes surgery. Advances in Oto-rhino-laryngology, vol 65. Karger, Basel
2. Arnold W, Busch R, Arnold A et al. (2007). The influence of measles vaccination on the incidence of otosclerosis in Germany. Eur Arch Otorhinolaryngol 264:741–748
3. Brackmann DE, Shelton C, Arriaga MA (1994) Otologic surgery. Saunders, Philadelphia
4. Schuknecht HF (1993) Otosclerosis. In: Pathology of the ear, 2nd edn. Lea & Febiger, Philadelphia, pp 365–379
5. Shea JJ JR (1998). A personal history of stapedectomy. Am J Otol 19:2–12

1.5.3 Traumatisms of the Temporal Bone

VINCENT DARROUZET

1.5.3.1 Definition

Blunt or open trauma to the temporal bone resulting in a simple concussion or a fracture crossing one, two or three of the three components of the temporal bone: *pars petrosa* (petrous bone) including the otic capsule, *pars squamosa* (squamous bone) and *tympanic bone*. More so than in bone lesions themselves, which heal spontaneously, severity resides in lesions and damage of temporal bone-resident organs and structures: external auditory canal, middle ear cleft, inner ear, meninges, internal carotid artery, venous system and cranial nerves.

1.5.3.2 Aetiology/Epidemiology

Trauma of the temporal bone can be blunt, open (associated with a wound) or ballistic. Incidentally, a blast mechanism can be combined with the direct trauma of the bone, leading to severer lesions of the tympanic membrane and labyrinth.

Blunt trauma results more often than not from a road traffic accident (60–80%), aggression or sport accidents. Motorcycle accidents are usually severe and temporal bone lesions are associated with severe and life-threatening head traumas. These are becoming rarer and rarer thanks to seat belts, airbags and helmet use. Gunshot lesions are much more severe, combining the effects of loss of substance, heating and burning, blast and lesions to the brain.

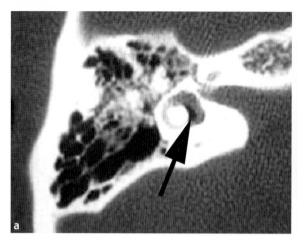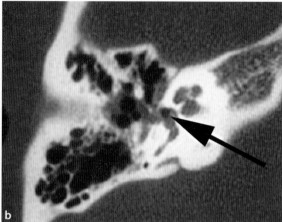

Fig. 1.5.5 a,b High-resolution CT of the right petrous bone (axial view, bone algorithm). **a** An air bubble (pneumolabyrinth) is visualized within the vestibule (*arrow*). **b** A fracture of the stapes is observed, associated with a pneumolabyrinth

1.5.3.3 Symptoms

Pain to the ear is commonly associated with otorrhagia and swelling of the ear region. Deafness is constant, usually of conductive nature. A wound or a haematoma can be found near the auricle. In the case of total loss of consciousness, a common situation in head trauma, otorrhagia is the only symptom evoking the diagnosis.

1.5.3.4 Complications

They must be systematically looked for:
- A peripheral facial nerve paralysis which can be immediate owing to the trauma itself or after 2–12 days owing to neural oedema or to herpes virus reactivation in the geniculate ganglion; it can be complete or incomplete (see Sect. 1.7.2). It occurs in 10–30% of cases.
- A CSF fistula is evoked facing an abundant clear or pink ear discharge (15–35% of cases).
- Meningitis may occur some months or years following a temporal bone fracture (late complication).
- A perilymphatic fistula is difficult to diagnose. Symptoms are a sloping hearing level associated with vertigo, dizziness and nystagmus beating to the opposite side of the traumatized ear (see Sect. 1.6.5). High-resolution CT is helpful in this context (Fig. 1.5.5).
- A labyrinthine concussion (see also Sect. 1.6.3) results in a non-worsening moderate to severe sensorineural hearing loss, unsteadiness and tinnitus to the trauma without any fracture line near the inner ear. Its incidence seems to be higher in the paediatric population.
- A sensorineural hearing loss is common, going from a high-frequency hearing loss to a dead ear. A dead ear

is systematically observed in transverse translabyrinthine fractures.
- Ossicular dislocation or fracture is associated with longitudinal or oblique fractures. A persistent conductive deafness of more than 30 dB or a mixed severe hearing loss is observed after resorption of haemotympanum. Incudostapedial joint disjunction is the most common lesion. Stapes fracture is less frequent. The diagnosis can be made by high-resolution CT (Fig. 1.5.5).
- Abducens nerve palsy is uncommon (less than 1%), as are vascular compromises (carotid cavernous fistula, sigmoid sinus thrombosis, internal carotid artery rupture; Fig. 1.5.6).

1.5.3.5 Diagnostic Procedures

See the algorithm for trauma to the skull in Fig. 1.5.7. Clinical examination and workup involve:
- Inspection: ear canal discharge (blood, CSF, mixture of both), haematomas, wound, bullet penetration.
- Otoscopy and ear microscopy: blood and clots in the ear canal; aspiration and cleaning up help one recognize the structures and check the tympanic bone (bone fragments? stenosis) and finally the tympanic membrane (perforation? size? location? haemotympanum 85%).
- Hearing examination: tuning fork in emergency. A standard audiogram is done as early as possible, depending on the patient's neurological status, to look for hearing and exclude associated sensorineural hearing loss. Hearing disorders are observed in 70% of cases.
- Frenzel glasses: to look for nystagmus if not spontaneously visible and exclude vestibular irritation or loss.

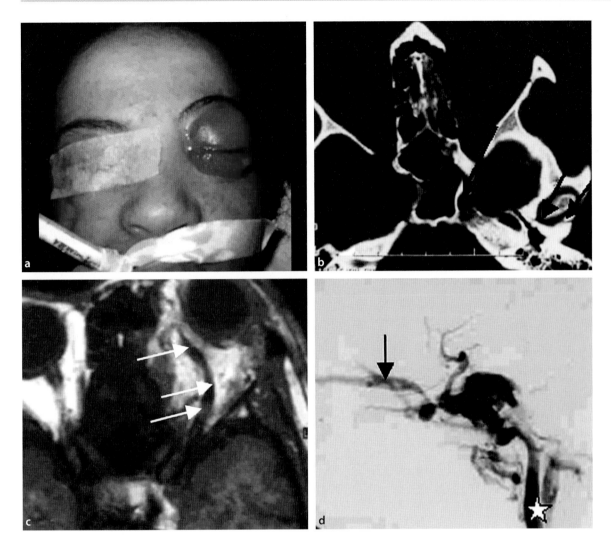

Fig. 1.5.6 a–d Left-sided carotid cavernous fistula. **a** Chemosis and pulsatile exophtalmus of the left eye. **b** The fracture line crosses the glenoid fossa and goes towards the cavernous sinus (*arrows*). **c** T1-weighted MRI showing exophtalmus and huge dilatation of the ophthalmic vein (*arrows*). **d** Internal carotid artery (*star*) angiography showing the arterial-venous fistula, feeding the cavernous sinus (*CS*) and the ophthalmic vein (*arrow*)

- Examination of cranial nerves with a specific attention to the facial nerve function. Abducens and last cranial nerves are also checked.
- Eye examination: look for dry eye and pulsatile exophtalmos (carotid cavernous fistula). Horner's syndrome is also looked for.
- Complete neurological examination and evaluation of the level of consciousness (Glasgow score) is mandatory, as is looking for meningitis symptoms (fever, headache, vomiting and nausea, neck tenderness).
- Examination of the temporomandibular joint function.

A radiological workup of the temporal bone is to be done. Plain skull radiographs cannot exclude a fracture. A CT scan using a brain and bone algorithm and less than 1 mm slices is the standard examination. Native axial and coronal scan planes are optimal but may not be possible in acutely traumatized patients. The brain algorithm looks for intracranial haematomas and pneumocephalus; iodine enhancement is not necessary in non-complicated temporal bone traumas and can worsen brain oedema. The fracture line is usually classified as *oblique* (75%), *transverse* (13%) or *longitudinal* (12%), with regard to the great axis of the petrous bone. It can also be described as *labyrinthine* (more often than not transverse, crossing the otic capsule) or *extralabyrinthine* (Fig. 1.5.8). More complex fractures (comminute) can be observed. In cases of gunshot trauma, lesions are complex and the diagnosis may be limited by metallic streak artefacts.

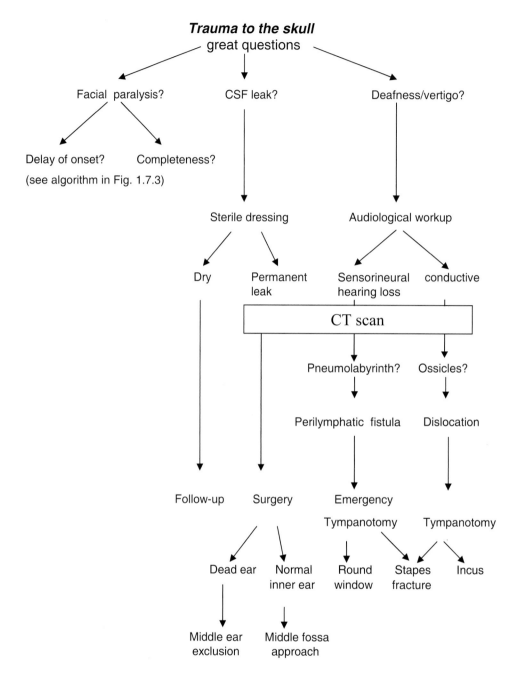

Fig. 1.5.7 Algorithm for trauma to the skull

1.5.3.6   Additional/Useful Diagnostic Procedures

- X-ray of the mandible (fracture of the condyles).
- MRI scan in rare cases of complications (prolonged loss of consciousness, persistent CSF fistula, facial paralysis).
- Intrathecal contrast combined to temporal bone high-resolution CT may be useful to define the site of a CSF leak.
- EMG in cases of facial paralysis (see Sect. 1.7.1).
- Videonystagmography in cases of persistent vertigo and dizziness.

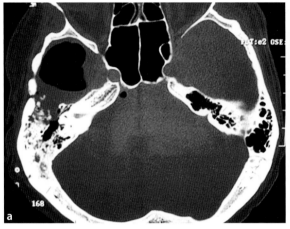

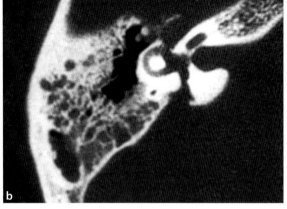

Fig. 1.5.8 a High-resolution CT of the skull base (axial view, bone algorithm). An extralabyrinthine fracture is associated with a pneumoencephalus. **b** High-resolution CT of the right petrous bone (axial view, bone algorithm). Displaced translaby-rinthine fracture following the vestibular aqueduct, crossing the vestibule and lateral canal ampulla. The fracture divides the tympanic segment of the Fallopian canal

- Internal carotid artery angiography in cases of carotid cavernous fistulas (Fig. 1.5.6d).
- Ophthalmologist counselling (facial paralysis).
- Neurologist counselling (severe head trauma and brain concussion associated with high risk of seizure).

1.5.3.7   Therapy

Conservative Treatment
- Analgesics: paracetamol.
- Collection of ear discharge: a graduated plastic sterile disposable collector sealed to the ear enables one to harvest, quantify and evaluate daily discharge volume and characteristics. It is of paramount importance in the case of suspicion of CSF leak.
- Close clinical survey (including otomicroscopy) for a minimum of 3 days, looking for secondary onset of facial paralysis, deafness or vertigo.

Note that ear drops or ear canal disinfectants are of no value in this context. Moreover their use can be dangerous for inner ear function.

Useful additional procedures are:
- Cleaning of the ear canal using a microscope and aspiration.
- Calibration of the meatus using Pope Oto-Wicks in the case of stenosis.
- Antibiotics can be indicated in the case of CSF leak, using non-blood–brain-barrier-crossing drugs (e.g. roxithromycine). But there is no consensus.

Surgical Treatment
- Exploration of an external auditory canal stenosis under general anaesthesia to remove bone fragments occluding the lumen due to tympanic bone fracture usually associated with mandibular fracture.
- Emergency exploratory tympanotomy is advisable in the case of suspicion of perilymphatic fistula (vertigo, dizziness, sloping hearing level, air bubble in the labyrinth at CT scan or MRI).
- Surgical treatment of CSF fistulas is rarely necessary since they heal and dry spontaneously within 1 week in 95% of cases. This is the rule in the case of trauma to the roof. In contrast, translabyrinthine fractures can cross the internal auditory canal and lead to a very productive leakage that must be sealed using a middle ear exclusion technique. This is also the case in gunshot trauma.
- Closure of a tympanic membrane perforation is not done as a short-term surgical procedure, with the exception of excessive epidermal middle ear penetration (blast trauma).
- Treatment of facial paralysis (see Sect. 1.7.2).

1.5.3.8   Differential Diagnosis

Traumatisms of the temporal bone show typical clinical features. Otorrhagia can be due to other pathological conditions (acute otitis media, chronic otitis media, cancer, glomus tumour), but history of trauma to the head helps to confirm the diagnosis.

In cases of otorrhagia and trauma to the auricle:
- Blood can come from a wound of the auricle and flow secondarily in the external auditory canal.
- Blasting the ear (slap) can lead to a tympanic membrane perforation, a bleeding without temporal bone trauma.

1.5.3.9   Prognosis

Spontaneous healing is the rule. Nevertheless, total functional recovery is not often observed, since some long-term sequelae can be observed. From the simplest to the most severe:
- Chronic ear pain
- Ipsilateral tinnitus
- Ear canal stenosis
- Chronic dizziness and unsteadiness
- Sensorineural hearing loss, from high-frequency hearing loss to dead ear
- Tympanic membrane perforation and cholesteatoma
- Late perilymphatic fistula (see Sect. 1.6.5)
- Meningoceles and encephalomeningoceles of the mastoid and epitympanum (iterative meningitis)

1.5.3.10   Surgical Principles

Closure of CSF Fistulas of the Petrous Bone Roof
See Fig. 1.5.9. The surgical principle is as follows:
- General anaesthesia with the patient in the supine position.
- Supra-auricular vertical pretragal or inferiorly based U-shaped incision.

- Preservation of an inferiorly pedicled temporalis muscle flap including the medial half of the muscle and the pericranium, pushed downwards or harvesting of a free temporalis muscle flap or a simple piece of temporalis fascia.
- Square-limited craniotomy as close to the floor of the middle fossa as possible.
- Cautious elevation of the dura and localization of the bony and meningeal loss of substance. If present, encephalomeningocele is disengaged off the roof of the petrous bone. Engaged piece of brain can be coagulated and sacrificed.
- Bony roof hiatus is reconstructed with a piece of bone or a mixture of bone dust and fibrin glue. The muscle flap is draped on the roof.
- Suspension of the dura and repositioning of the craniotomy bone.
- Suture of the rest of the temporalis muscle on a suction drain.
- Closure of the skin incision.

Middle Ear Exclusion
- General anaesthesia with the patient in the supine position. Antibioprophilaxis with cephalosporins.
- Infiltration of the external auditory canal with lidocaine and epinephrine.
- Postauricular incision.
- Transection of the external auditory canal. Dissection of the lateral part of the meatus and cleavage of the skin from the cartilage of the meatus. Blind sac closure of the skin with Vicryl sutures. The suture is covered medially by a muscular and aponeurotic layer.
- Mastoidectomy and canal wall down technique is carried out, taking care to remove the least piece of

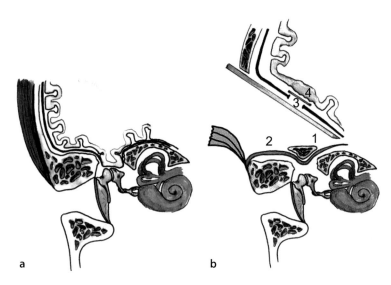

Fig. 1.5.9 a,b A middle fossa approach designed to treat a meningoencephalocele of the petrous bone roof. **a** Preoperative view. Dehiscence of the tegmen leaving access to a meningoencephalocele. The ossicular chain is not dislocated. **b** The tegmen is reconstructed using a bone chip (*1*), engaged in the bone hiatus. A temporalis muscle periosteal flap (*2*) is pushed into the middle fossa to be draped over the roof. The dura is repaired with a periosteal free flap (*3*). The herniated brain is coagulated and sacrificed (*4*)

a   b

epidermal epithelium. The CSF is seen leaking in the middle ear and/or the mastoid.

- The Eustachian tube is filled up and tightly closed with bone wax and little pieces of aponeurosis, muscle, bone chips and bone dust eventually mixed with fibrin glue.
- The middle ear cleft is closed with pieces of muscle or aponeurosis, and eventually with strips of abdominal fat.
- Closure of the skin without drain. A compressive dressing can be used.

Facial Nerve Decompression and Exploration
See Sect. 1.7.2.

Suggested Reading

1. Schuknecht HF (1993) Trauma. In: Pathology of the ear. Lea & Febiger, Philadelphia, pp 279–289

1.5.4 Tumours

1.5.4.1 Squamous Cell Carcinoma of the Temporal Bone

CHRISTIAN MARTIN, OLIVIER STERKERS AND SALVATORE IURATO

Synonyms
Epidermoid carcinoma, spinocellular carcinoma, primary malignant tumour of the temporal bone, malignancy of the temporal bone and ear canal.

Definition
Most frequent primary malignant tumour of the temporal bone arising from the skin of the external auditory canal or from the middle ear cleft. It tends to be locally invasive.

Aetiology/Epidemiology
Squamous cell carcinoma is the most frequent primary malignant tumour of the temporal bone, accounting for 60–80% of all malignancies arising from the skin of the external auditory canal or the middle ear cleft. The incidence is about 1:1,000,000. There are several suspected aetiological factors: local and chronic trauma, ultraviolet radiation, ionizing radiation and chemical exposure, chronic ear discharge, chronic eczema, psoriasis, lupus.

Macroscopically it appears as an ulcerated papillomatous lesion of the skin in the external auditory canal, bleeding to touch. Microscopically there are six histologic types (well differentiated, moderately differentiated, poorly differentiated, clear cell, spindle cell, verrucous). They tend to be locally invasive and only rarely spread to the regional lymph nodes. Distant metastasis to lung, long bones, and liver is rare.

Symptoms
- Otorrhoea, pain and bleeding are the most common presenting symptoms. Note that in most cases of chronic otitis media, pain is not a prominent feature and therefore if a patient has a chronically draining ear with pain, the suspicion of a possible malignancy should be kept in mind.
- Facial palsy due to invasion of the Fallopian canal within the temporal bone.
- Hearing loss.
- Other symptoms will result from tumour spread: trismus and impairment of mouth opening; lower cranial nerves palsy; imbalance or vertigo, headache.

Complications
- Cervical lymph nodes invasion, metastasis
- Intracranial extension

Diagnosis
- Otoscopy: presence of a swelling, polyp or papillomatous and ulcerated tumour that tends to be necrotic and bleeding to touch.
- Biopsy of the lesion under microscope: *any lesion of the external ear or external auditory canal that appears to be inflammatory but does not respond in an appropriate timeframe to standard medications may be malignant and should be biopsied.*
- Palpation of the parotid gland and of the cervical nodes areas.
- Imaging: CT scan using a bone algorithm and MRI with gadolinium localize the tumour (invasion of the tumour from the external auditory canal into the middle ear at the level of the tympanic annulus?) and evidence its intra and extracranial extension.

Additional/Useful Diagnostic Procedures
- Audiovestibular tests
- Arteriography if involvement of the carotid artery in the petrous bone is suspected
- Assessment of lung and liver metastasis

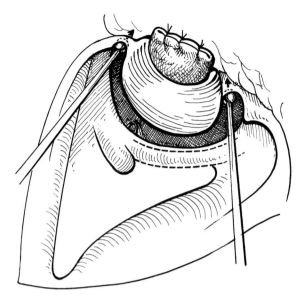

Fig. 1.5.10 Lateral temporal bone resection. An intact wall mastoidectomy is performed by opening the facial recess. The facial nerve is skeletonized (*dotted lines*) and the facial recess is extended anteriorly. The root of the zygoma is drilled away (upper burr) and the bone between the inferior aspect of the external auditory canal and the stylomastoid foramen is removed (inferior burr). Finally, the external auditory canal is removed en bloc (360°) with the tympanic membrane and malleus. Parotidectomy and neck dissection is carried out when needed

Therapy

Conservative Therapy

Radiotherapy may be used in palliative care of patients with extended and aggressive tumours. In most cases radiotherapy is used postoperatively.

Surgery

- Lateral temporal bone resection (Fig. 1.5.10) where the external auditory canal is removed "en bloc" with the tympanic membrane and ossicular chain and tissue lateral to the facial nerve may be adopted in T1 tumours of the external auditory canal and perhaps T2 tumours in the elderly.
- Extended temporal bone resection with a parotidectomy and a supraomohyoid neck dissection and either free flap or local rotation flap repair with a full course of postoperative radiotherapy is the recommended treatment for squamous cell carcinoma of the temporal bone. An excision of the pinna and a wide oval of skin around it should be included in the resection. This is indicated for the management of T2 to T4 external auditory canal tumours and T1 to T4 middle ear cleft tumours.
- Local excision and postoperative radiotherapy have been proposed by some surgeons.

Differential Diagnosis

- *Basal cell carcinoma* which arises from the skin of the auricle or of the external portion of the external auditory canal and comprises 20% of the malignancies of the ear. Usually its appearance is a pigmented nodular lesion, but ulcerative lesions are also common and difficult to differentiate from squamous cell carcinoma.
- *Adenocarcinoma* of the middle ear. The presenting symptoms are hearing loss, tinnitus and vertigo and in advanced cases facial weakness and palsy of the lower cranial nerves. There are two subtype tumours: low-grade primary adenocarcinoma, which is difficult to differentiate from adenomas of the middle ear, but the presence of bony erosion and facial nerve infiltration makes the diagnosis; high-grade or adenoid cystic carcinoma of the temporal bone, which is very difficult to differentiate from an adenoid cystic carcinoma of the parotid gland that invades the temporal bone secondarily.
- *Rabdomyosarcomas* are rare and are seen in children. They are very aggressive tumours.
- *Other tumours*: malignant melanoma, Ewing's sarcoma, lymphoma and secondary metastatic tumours.

Prognosis

Radical surgery associated with postoperative radiotherapy has improved the prognosis in these aggressive tumours. Malignancies limited to the external ear compartment have cure rates from 70 to 90%. Extended temporal bone surgery associated with radiotherapy yields about 50% 5-year survival in patients with large tumours.

Suggested Reading

1. Clark LJ, Narula AQ, Morgan DA et al. (1991) Squamous carcinoma of the temporal bone: a revised staging. J Laryngol Otol 105:346–348
2. Kinney SE (1991) Malignancies of the temporal bone and ear canal. In: Jackson CG (ed) Surgery of skull base tumors. Churchill Livingstone, New York, pp 197–210
3. Moffat DA, Chissonne-Kerdel JA, Da Cruz M (2000) Squamous cell carcinoma. In: Jackler RK, Driscoll CLW (eds) Tumor of the ear and temporal bone. Lippincott Williams and Wilkins, Philadelphia, pp 67–83

1.5.4.2   Vestibular Schwannoma

OLIVIER STERKERS,

CHRISTIAN MARTIN AND WOLFGANG ARNOLD

Synonyms

Acoustic neuroma, cerebellopontine angle tumour.

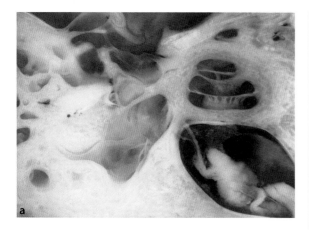

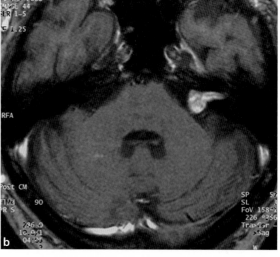

Fig. 1.5.11 a Celloidin embedded section showing a vestibular schwannoma within the internal auditory canal. Vestibular schwannoma before (b) and after (c) fractionated stereotactic radiotherapy

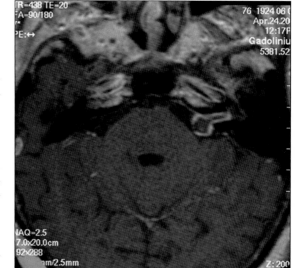

Definition

Slowly growing solid or cystic benign tumour which arises from the Schwann-cells of the vestibular nerve within the internal auditory canal (Fig. 1.5.11a). It can extend into the cerebellopontine angle.

Aetiology/Epidemiology

Vestibular schwannomas account for approximately 7% of all intracranial tumours and 80% of cerebellopontine angle tumours. The number of newly diagnosed cases per year is around 13 per one million individuals. Occult tumours have been identified during autopsies and incidentally discovered on MRI with a prevalence of 0.8%.

The tumours are usually solid but may be partially or mainly cystic. They generally arise from the Schwann cell in the vestibular ganglion within the internal auditory canal and are histologically composed of alternating regions of Antony type A and B areas. Vestibular schwannomas typically grow slowly at a rate of 0–3 mm per year. Vestibular schwannomas are either part of the familial disorder neurofibromatosis type 2 (NF-2) (5%) or sporadic tumours (95%). The gene responsible for the development of vestibular schwannomas has been isolated to chromosome 22q12, which codes for the tumour-suppressor merlin (or schwannomin).

Symptoms

About 90% of patients present with unilateral progressive haring loss; however, 5% will present with a sudden hearing loss. In 80% of patients tinnitus is the first clinical symptom. Five percent of patients with vestibular schwannomas have normal hearing at the first presenta-

tion. Patients, especially when asked, will often report quite mild balance disturbance.

Rare presentations include facial numbness or pain, earache or facial weakness, cerebellar ataxia or symptoms of hydrocephalus (headache, visual disturbance, mental status change, nausea, and vomiting).

Complications

Early diagnosis and management of vestibular schwannomas should prevent subsequent complications by compression of the brainstem such as central vestibular disorders, hydrocephalus (headache, vomiting, visual disturbances), and facial (tic, palsy) and lower cranial nerve irritations (n. trigeminus, pain hypoanaesthesia).

Diagnostic Procedures

Recommended European Standard

- *Otoscopy*: normal findings. Present or previous middle ear disease does not exclude the diagnosis.
- *Pure tone audiometry*: Most patients have a high-frequency sensorineural hearing loss at presentation (Fig. 1.1.17) but any pattern of hearing loss (or normal hearing) may be encountered.
- *Speech discrimination testing*: Discrimination usually is worse than expected from the audiogram, but a normal speech discrimination does not eliminate the diagnosis. The test is of great value to access the usefulness of hearing in the neuroma ear, especially when hearing conservation surgery is being considered.
- *Stapedius reflexes*: decay (Fig. 1.1.17) or missing in up to 70% of patients.
- *Electric response audiometry*: This is the most sensitive audiological test in vestibular schwannoma diagnosis (Fig. 1.1.17). It indicates a retrocochlear abnormality in more than 90% of vestibular schwannoma patients: nevertheless a normal response is observed in 5% of vestibular schwannoma patients (mainly in small tumours).
- *Vestibular caloric testing*: hyporeflexia or areflexia is commonly observed but a normal test finding does not eliminate the diagnosis.
- *MRI*: MRI with gadolinium enhancement is the most accurate diagnostic tool for identifying vestibular schwannoma (Fig. 1.1.27).

Additional/Useful Diagnostic Procedures

- *Hitselberger sign*: reduced sensitivity of the skin of the posterior wall of outer ear canal of the affected side.
- *Otoacoustic emissions*: In many cases otoacoustic emissions are present, indicating undisturbed cochlear blood flow.
- Electronystagmography or videonystagmography (to disclose central vestibular abnormalities).
- Clinical and electrical examination of the facial nerve.

- Clinical examination of the trigeminal and lower cranial nerves.
- Neurologic and ophthalmologic examinations.
- CT: When a patient cannot be examined by MRI (claustrophobia, cardiac pacemaker, etc.), CT with contrast provides visualization of medium or large vestibular schwannomas. Its sensitivity is moderate for intracanalicular and very small vestibular schwannomas.

Therapy

Recommended European Standard

Conservative Treatment

- Since especially in the elderly vestibular schwannomas are slowly growing tumours, a *wait and see strategy* should be considered at least in the short term (6–12 months) for patients with a small vestibular schwannoma (in older patients and individuals in poor health).
- *Radiotherapy*: Stereotactic radiosurgery (gamma knife) or fractionated stereotactic radiotherapy (55–60 Gy) may stop vestibular schwannoma growth mainly in small intracanalicular and extracanalicular lesions (Fig. 1.5.11b, c). Fractionated stereotactic radiotherapy or radiosurgery as the first therapeutic option is recommended in bilateral vestibular schwannomas (e.g. morbus Recklinghausen) (Fig. 1.5.12) but only when the tumours are small.
- Annual imaging is recommended for all patients being managed conservatively for the rest of their life or until vestibular schwannoma growth is seen to a certain limit.

Surgical Treatment

- *Translabyrinthine approach* in patients with medium-sized and large tumours and in patients with small tumours with poor hearing

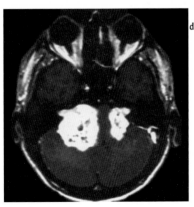
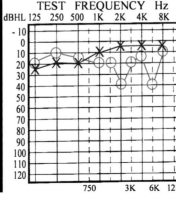

Fig. 1.5.12 Bilateral acoustic schwannoma in m. Recklinghausen with the audiogram of the same patient. The hearing threshold is very good considering the size of the tumours. Often NF2 patients have tumours that infiltrate the cochlear nerve without interrupting the nerve fibres, whereas unilateral sporadic tumours damage the hearing by compression of the cochlear nerve fibres (From Arnold et al. [1])

Table 1.5.1 MRI characteristics of selected cerebellopontine angle masses

Abnormality	T1	T2	T1 + gadolinium
Vestibular schwannoma	Hypointense	Isohypointense	Enhancing
Meningeoma	Hypointense	Isohypointense	Enhancing
Lipoma	Hypointense	Isointense	Variable
Haemangioma	Hypointense	Isohypointense	Enhancing
Facial neuroma	Hypointense	Isohypointense	Enhancing
Epidermoid	Hypointense	Isohypointense	Non-enhancing
Arachnoid cyst	Hypointense	Hyperintense	Non-enhancing

- *Middle fossa approach* in patients with intracanalicular or small tumours with good hearing as an attempt to preserve residual hearing
- *Retrolabyrinthine or retrosigmoidal approaches* in patients with large extracanalicular vestibular schwannomas

Additional Useful Surgical Procedures
- Intraoperative facial nerve monitoring.
- Intraoperative hearing monitoring: may be useful in hearing preservation surgery.

Differential Diagnosis
- *Meningioma* is, in most cases, recognized on radiologic features (tumour usually extrinsic to internal auditory canal, sessile with peritumoral dural enhancement and intratumoral calcifications). MRI characteristics are similar of those of vestibular schwannoma. An enhanced "dural tail" is a distinguishing feature. Meningioma is usually a positive finding on a somatostatin scintigram. The strategy of meningioma treatment does not differ from that of vestibular schwannoma.
- Other cerebellopontine angle lesions (cholesteatoma, arachnoid cyst, lipoma, haemangioma, glomus tumour, facial neuroma) can in most cases be recognized by their radiologic aspects and MRI characteristics (Table 1.5.1).
Note that most tumour types can exhibit considerable variability in imaging characteristics. If the radiologist is aware of the differential diagnosis, special sequences (fat suppression, fluid-attenuated inversion recovery) can be performed to help sort out lesions that appear similarly on standard images.

Prognosis

Conservative Therapy (see Fig. 1.5.11 b and c)
With radiotherapy tumour control is around 96%, tumour regression 35%, lesion of the trigeminal nerve less than 5.6%, facial weakness 2%, and hearing loss 32%. There is no CSF leak and no mortality.

If irradiation cannot stop tumour growth (in about 4% of cases), surgery is technically sometimes extremely difficult. Malignant transformation after radiotherapy is also valid for neuromas.

Surgery
Complete vestibular schwannoma resection and preservation of facial and/or cochlear function depends on the experience of the surgeon. In experienced hands, complete tumour removal is possible in 95% of cases. According to international statistics, deafness occurs in 80% of patients, facial palsy in 20–40%, long-lasting dizziness in 50–60%, CSF leak in 5–10%, meningitis in 2% and mortality in approximately 1%.

Translabyrinthine Approach
See Fig. 1.5.13. The procedure is as follows:
- General anaesthesia with the patient in the supine position.
- Postauricular incision.
- Mastoidectomy.
- Closure of the middle ear cleft with pieces of fat or muscle.
- Extended exposure of the dura of the posterior fossa and middle fossa. Complete labyrinthectomy and complete exposure of the internal auditory canal.
- Opening of the dura.
- Section of the vestibular nerves and identification of the facial nerve in the internal auditory canal.
- Debulking the tumour in the cerebellopontine angle.
- Tumour resection with preservation of the facial nerve.
- Careful haemostasis.
- Closure of the translabyrinthine approach with pieces of fat.
- Closure of the skin incision with no drain.

Retrosigmoid Approach
See Fig. 1.5.14. The procedure is a follows:

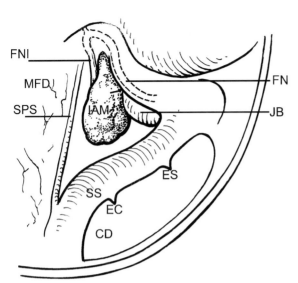

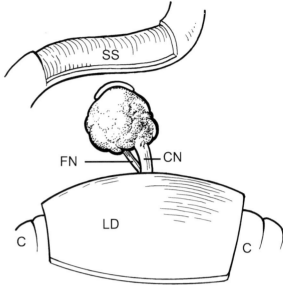

Fig. 1.5.13 Extended translabyrinthine approach (Sanna). Notice the extended exposure of the middle fossa dura (*MFD*) and of the cerebellar dura (*CD*) behind the sigmoid sinus (*SS*). *EC* emissary vein (Citelli), *ES* emissary vein (Santorini), *SPS* superior petrosal sinus, *FN* facial nerve protected by bone, *FNI* facial nerve identified at the fundus of the internal auditory canal, *JB* jugular bulb, *IAM* dura mater of the internal acoustic meatus distended by the tumour, *arrow* cochlear aqueduct

Fig. 1.5.14 Retrosigmoid approach. No retractor is used in this procedure. *SS* sigmoid sinus, *FN* facial nerve, *CN* cochlear nerve, *LD* lyophilized dura protecting the cerebellum (*C*) (From Sterkers [2], with permission)

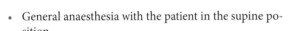

- General anaesthesia with the patient in the supine position
- Skin incision along the posterior margin of the mastoid process
- Limited craniotomy behind and close to the sigmoid sinus
- Incision of the dura and exposure of the cerebellopontine angle without retractor
- Drilling of the medial posterior wall of the internal auditory canal
- Section of vestibular nerves and identification of the facial nerve in the cerebellopontine angle
- Dissection of the tumour in the cerebellopontine angle and then in the internal auditory canal
- Section of the vestibular nerves and removal of the tumour in the fundus
- Verification of the fundus with an endoscope
- Careful haemostasis
- Closure of the internal auditory canal with a piece of fat
- Suture of the dura and closure of the retrosigmoid approach with pieces of fat
- Closure of the skin incision with no drain

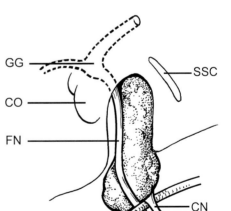

Fig. 1.5.15 Middle fossa approach. The middle fossa retractor is not shown. *GG* geniculate ganglion; *SSC* blue line of the superior semicircular canal, *FN* facial nerve, *CN* cochlear nerve, *CO* cochlea, *CIA* inferior cerebellar artery (From Sterkers [2], with permission)

Middle Fossa Approach

See Fig. 1.5.15. The procedure is as follows:

- General anaesthesia with the patient in the supine position
- Supra-auricular vertical pretragal or inferiorly based U-shaped incision
- Limited craniotomy as close to the floor of the middle fossa as possible
- Elevation of the middle fossa dura and insertion of the middle fossa retractor
- Drilling of the superior wall of the internal auditory canal after exposure of the geniculate ganglion and the facial nerve labyrinthine portion and/or exposure of the blue line of the superior semicircular canal
- Incision of the dura of the internal auditory canal
- Identification of the facial nerve in the anterior portion of the internal auditory canal
- Section of the superior vestibular nerve at its lateral end
- Separation of the tumour from the facial and cochlear nerves
- Removal of the tumour after division of the inferior vestibular nerve
- Closure of the internal auditory canal with abdominal fat
- Suspension of the dura and reposition of the craniotomy bone
- Suture of temporalis muscle on a suction drain
- Closure of the skin incision

References

1. Arnold W, Ganzer U, Iurato S (2007) Checklist otorinolaringoiatria CIC, Rome
2. Sterkers JM (1991) Chirurgie du neurinome de l'acoustique. Arnette, Paris

Suggested Reading

1. Haseqawa T, Fujitani S, Katsumatu S et al. (2005) Stereotactic radiosurgery of vestibular schwannomas; analysis of 317 patients followed for more than 5 years. Neurosurgery 57:257–265
2. Kaylie DM, Horgan MJ, Delashaw JB et al. (2000) A meta-analysis comparing outcomes of microsurgery and gamma knife radiosurgery. Laryngoscope 110:1850–1856
3. Kondziolka D. Lunsford LD, McLaughlin MR et al. (1998) Long term outcomes after radiosurgery for acoustic neuromas. N Engl J Med 339:1426–1433
4. Jackler RK, Driscoll CLW (2000) Tumors of the ear and temporal bone. Lippincott Williams and Wilkins, Philadelphia. Clinical effectiveness guidelines: Acoustic Neuroma (Vestibular Schwannoma). BAO-HNS (London) Document 5, Spring 2002
5. Lunsford LD, Niranjan A. Flickinger JC et al. (2005) Radiosurgery of vestibular schwannomas; summary of experience in 829 cases. J Neurosurg 102:195–199
6. Maire JP, Huchet A, Milbeo Y et al. (2006) Twenty years experience in the treatment of acoustic neuromas with fractionated radiotherapy: a review of 45 cases. Int J Radiat Oncol Biol Phys 66:170–178
7. Ramsden RT, Saeed SR (2006) Surgical management of vestibular schwannoma. In: Scott-Brown's otolaryngology, 7th edn. In press.
8. Shin M, Ueki K, Kurita H, Kirino T (2002) Malignant transformation of a vestibular schwannoma after gamma knife radiosurgery. Lancet 360:309–310
9. Sterkers O, Bebear JP, Fraysse B et al. (2001) Le neurinome de l'acoustique: diagnostic, traitement et suivi. Soc Fr Otorhinolaryngol Chir Face 113–116
10. Wilkinson JS, Reid H, Armstrong GR (2004) Malignant transformation of a recurrent vestibular schwannoma. J Clin Pathol 57:109–110

1.5.4.3 Paragangliomas of the Temporal Bone

OLIVIER STERKERS AND CHRISTIAN MARTIN

Synonyms

Glomus tumours, chemodectomas, nonchromaffin paragangliomas.

Definition

Glomus tumours are vascular neoplasms developed in the temporal bone from the branchiomeric paraganglia. These tumours form a clinical spectrum from small limited lesions confined to the promontory of the middle ear (tympanic paraganglioma) to extensive lesions developed in the jugulotympanic region with skull base involvement (jugulotympanic paraganglioma). Paragangliomas demonstrate a slow and insidious pattern of growth.

Aetiology/Epidemiology

Paragangliomas of the temporal bone are the most common tumour of the middle ear and the second most common tumour of the temporal bone. Most occur in Caucasian adults with a female-to-male preponderance. Usually, there is a solitary paraganglioma of the temporal bone. Multicentric lesions can occur in 10% of cases, mostly combined with a ipsilateral carotid body tumour. In the familial tumours, the tendency for multicentricity is higher (up to 50%). Linkage analysis has identified the long arm of chromosome 11 as one site of familial tumours. Because the chief cells of glomus tumours are cells of the diffuse neuroendocrine system, glomus tumours are associated with secondary malignancy of cells

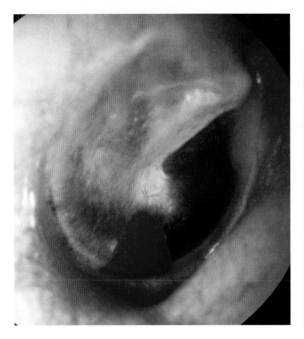

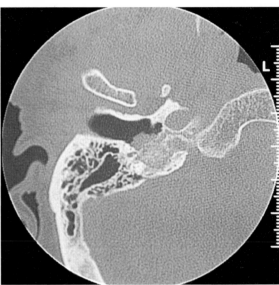

Fig. 1.5.16 The pulsating red mass behind the inferior quadrants of this right tympanic membrane is a glomus tumour (chemodectoma) limited to the middle ear (class A tumour)

Fig. 1.5.17 Glomus tumour, CT scan, axial view. Enlarged jugular foramen with irregular bony erosion. The carotid foramen and canal are intact (class B tumour)

with similar derivation in up to 7% (thyroid carcinoma, pheochromocytoma and multiple endocrine neoplasias). Although glomus tumours are histologically benign, up to 4% can develop metastases. Approximately 1–3% of paragangliomas demonstrate secretory activity (mostly norepinephrine).

Symptoms

Pulsatile tinnitus is the most common presenting symptom followed by hearing loss.

When the glomus is limited to the tympanic region, patients can complain of otalgia, ear fullness, otorrhoea and aural bleeding. When the glomus arises from the jugular foramen, neurologic deficit is the second major group of symptoms: facial and lower cranial nerve paralysis (hoarseness, dysphagia). Horner's syndrome can be observed.

Complications

Paragangliomas rarely metastasize and most often spread along paths of least resistance. Complications may result from the invasion of the cochleovestibular apparatus (sensorineural hearing loss, vertigo), the foramen jugulare with lower cranial nerve paralysis (pulmonary infections, etc.), the petrous apex (abducens and trigeminal palsy), and the cerebellopontine angle (see Sect. 1.5.4.2).

Diagnosis

- Inspection and palpation of the neck (cervical mass and trapezius weakness in extensive jugulotympanic glomus).
- Inspection of the oral cavity and pharyngolarynx (tongue deviation, decreased gag reflex, vocal cord paresis in extensive jugulotympanic glomus).
- Otoscopy (ear microscopy): pulsating retrotympanic vascular mass (Fig. 1.5.16). In larger lesions a polypoid vascular mass may be seen in the external auditory canal. Cessation of pulsation can be obtained with positive pressure on pneumatic otoscopy (**Brown's sign**).
- Audiovestibular testing: Pure tone and speech audiometry are performed to assess the degree of conductive and sensorineural impairment. Vestibular studies are limited to patients who describe dizziness or vertigo.
- Imaging: High-resolution CT and MRI are mandatory for the diagnosis of glomus tumours and for the evaluation of their extension. CT helps to define the extent of involvement of the temporal bone by the tumour (Fig. 1.5.17). MRI helps to characterize the vascular nature of the tumour, which is often heterogeneous ("salt and pepper" aspect in T2 images). MRI obviates the need for angiography. CT and MRI allow one to classify the tumour (Table 1.5.2).
- Catecholamine secretion : measure of cathecholamine levels and 24-h urinary metanephrines and vanillylmandelic acid.

Table 1.5.2 Classification of Fisch

Class A	Tumour limited to middle ear (glomus tympanicum)
Class B	Tumour limited to the tympanomastoid area with no infralabyrinthine involvement (glomus hypotympanicum)
Class C	Tumours involving the infralabyrinthine compartment of the temporal bone and extending into the petrous apex
Class De	Tumours with intracranial extradural extension
Class Di	Tumours with intracranial intradural extension

Additional/Useful Diagnostic Procedure

Radionuclide scintigraphy (with indium-111 octreotide) is used for detection of multicentric or metastatic lesions in familiar tumours or when several tumour were found on head and neck imaging.

Therapy

Conservative Therapy

- No treatment: proposed in asymptomatic patients
- Radiotherapy: proposed to slow or stop growth of large lesions when the expected morbidity and mortality of the surgical tumour resection would exceed the risk of the tumour itself, especially in the elderly and individuals in poor health

Surgery

- Transcanal approach: indicated for class A.
- Mastoid-extended facial recess approach: indicated for class B.
- Infratemporal fossa approach with rerouting the facial nerve: proposed for classes C and D (Fig. 1.5.18).
- Two-stage operation is proposed for large intracranial extension.

Additional Useful Procedures

- Embolization: Preoperative arteriography provides information on vascular pedicules filling the tumour, collateral circulation, and permits embolization of the tumour. This procedure is not necessary in class A tumours.
- Peroperative cranial nerve monitoring: Facial nerve monitoring as well as hypoglossal and vagal monitoring allow a safer dissection of the nerves.

Differential Diagnosis

- Vascular retrotympanic abnormalities: high jugular bulb, ectopic or aneurysm of the intrapetrous carotid artery.
- Middle ear lesions: facial neuroma, meningioma, adenoma, cholesteatoma, cholesterol granuloma, etc.
- Jugular foramen tumours: schwannoma, meningioma, plasmocytoma, endolymphatic sac tumour, Langerhans cell histiocytosis, metastatic diseases, etc.

Prognosis

- The outcome of patients with glomus tympanicum (type A) is generally excellent.
- For the others tumours the results of surgery depend on the volume and extension of the tumour. Depending upon the extent of disease, the vascular structures at risk include the extratemporal and the intratemporal carotid artery, the external carotid artery, and the internal jugular vein. Larger tumours involving the cavernous sinus place the more distal carotid artery and its branches at risk. The incidence of lower cranial nerve deficit is higher in class C and D tumour resection. Facial paresis and hearing loss are frequent sequelae of therapy.
- Long-term imaging follow-up is necessary except for class A tumour.

Surgical Procedure: Infratemporal Fossa Approach (Type A according to Fisch)

- General anaesthesia with the patient in the supine position.
- Sweeping C postauricular and upper-neck incision.
- Blind sac closure of the external auditory canal.
- Neck dissection with identification of the common, internal and external carotid, internal jugular vein and lower cranial nerves. The external carotid is ligated.
- Subtotal petrosectomy exposing the Fallopian canal from the oval window to the stylomastoid foremen (Fig. 1.5.18a).
- Transposition of the facial nerve to the first genu (Fig. 1.5.18b). The periosteum of the stylomastoid foramen is sutured anteriorly to support the nerve without tension.

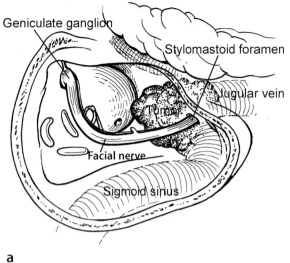

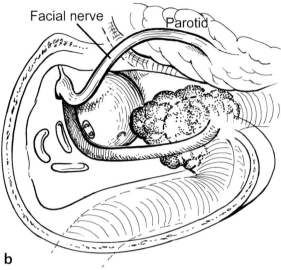

a   b

Fig. 1.5.18 a,b Infratemporal fossa approach type A (Fisch). After exposure of the facial nerve in the parotid and identification of the great vessels and nerves in the neck, the skin of the external auditory canal is cut and removed. **a** An extended mastoidectomy is then carried out and the Fallopian canal is exposed. **b** The facial nerve is mobilized and transposed anteriorly in a new Fallopian canal and groove in the parotid. After ligation of the sigmoid sinus and identification of the carotid artery, the infratemporal fossa will be exposed, the caroticotympanic artery is coagulated and cut and the tumour is mobilized and removed

- Obliteration of the Eustachian tube and exposure of the intrapetrous portion of the carotid.
- Ligation of the sigmoid sinus.
- Dissection of the tumour with progressive coagulation in the middle ear and mastoid cavity and then from the intrapetrous carotid.
- Exposure of the jugular bulb, which is frequently involved, and obliteration of the inferior petrous sinus and ligation of the internal jugular vein.
- Resection of the foramen jugulare remnant with, when possible, lower cranial nerves preservation.
- Removal of the intradural extension when necessary and closure of the dural defect with abdominal fat.
- Closure of the petrous cavity with abdominal fat with reposition of the facial nerve.
- Suture in two layers without drain.

Suggested Reading

1. Fisch U, Mattox DE (1988) Microsurgery of the skull base. Thieme, New York
2. Jackler RK, Driscoll CLW (2000) Tumors of the ear and temporal bone. Lippincott Williams and Wilkins, Philadelphia
3. Jackson CG (1991) Surgery of skull base tumors. Churchill Livingstone, New York

1.5.5 Petrous Bone Cholesteatoma

SALVATORE IURATO

1.5.5.1 Synonyms

Medial cholesteatoma of the temporal bone, petrosal cholesteatoma.

1.5.5.2 Definition

Epidermoid cyst of the petrous portion of the temporal bone.

1.5.5.3 Aetiology/Epidemiology

Epidermoids account for 1.5% of all intracranial tumours (the temporal bone being the most frequent site in the base of the skull). They may be congenital or acquired:
- *Congenital*: from aberrant epithelial remnants
- *Acquired*: from deep ingrowths of an epitympanic cholesteatoma in patients who have not been operated on or in patients who have already been operated on (residual disease)

1.5.5.4   Types (Sanna's Classification)

- Supralabyrinthine cholesteatoma
- Infralabyrinthine cholesteatoma
- Cholesteatoma of the petrous apex (apical cholesteatoma)
- Infralabyrinthine cholesteatoma invading the pyramid apex
- Massive labyrinthine cholesteatoma

1.5.5.5   Symptoms

There is very slow growth, with the individual being symptom-free for years.
- Hearing loss (conductive or sensorineural).
- Progressive facial paralysis.
- Other symptoms are vertigo and tinnitus.
- In acquired petrous bone cholesteatoma, otorrhoea may be present.

1.5.5.6   Complications

- Involvement of the facial nerve, otic capsule, carotid artery, dura, sigmoid sinus and jugular bulb.
- CSF leak.
- Recurrence if complete exenteration has not been achieved.

1.5.5.7   Diagnostic Procedures

- Otoscopy (ear microscopy), hearing examination.
- CT: key examination to demonstrate bone erosion (Fig. 1.5.19). Note that CT does not differentiate between congenital cholesteatoma and cholesterol granuloma.
- MRI: key examination to demonstrate dura invasion and to differentiate congenital cholesteatoma (low signal intensity on T1-weighted scans and high signal intensity on T2-weighted scans) from cholesterol granuloma.

1.5.5.8   Surgical Treatment

Total removal of all squamous epithelium: if complete exenteration or adequate exteriorization is not obtained, there will be rapid recurrence of cholesteatoma.
- Marsupialization of the cavity in the case of small infralabyrinthine cholesteatomas.
- Middle fossa approach for small supralabyrinthine cholesteatomas with good hearing.

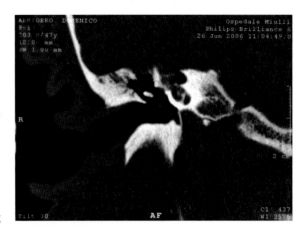

Fig. 1.5.19 Supralabyrinthine cholesteatoma. This coronal CT section shows a large osteolytic lesion in the supralabyrinthine part of the petrous bone with involvement of the superior semicircular canal, cochlea and the first portion of facial nerve. The middle ear is free of disease

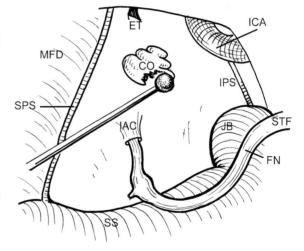

Fig. 1.5.20 Transcochlear approach (Sanna): The procedure implies transection of the external auditory canal, with posterior rerouting of the facial nerve (*FN*) from the geniculate ganglion (*GG*) to the stylomastoid foramen (*STF*). *ICA* internal carotid artery, *SPS* superior petrosal sinus, *IPS* inferior petrosal sinus, *JB* jugular bulb, *IAC* content of the internal auditory canal, *MFD* middle fossa dura, *SS* sigmoid sinus, *ET* Eustachian tube, *CO* cochlea

- Modified transcochlear approach (Sanna) in most cases (Fig. 1.5.20): wide petrosectomy with posterior rerouting of the facial nerve, closure of the Eustachian tube, obliteration of the defect with abdominal fat and closure of the external auditory canal. Hearing function is sacrificed.

1.5.5.9   Differential Diagnosis

Note that the CT and MRI techniques have revolutionized the diagnosis (and management) of petrous apex lesions.

- *Cholesterol granuloma*: see Sect. 1.5.6.
- *Mucocele*: mucous effusion in a well-pneumatized petrous apex. Bony architecture is well preserved on CT. Low intensity on T1-weighted images and high signal intensity on T2-weighted images.
- Tumours.

1.5.5.10   Prognosis

Annual follow-up with MRI is mandatory especially if the defect has been obliterated.

Suggested Reading

1. Ferlito A, Devaney K O, Rinaldo A et al. (1997) Ear cholesteatoma versus cholesterol granuloma. Ann Otol Rhinol Laryngol 106:79–85
2. Fisch U, Mattox D (1988) Microsurgery of the skull base. Thieme, New York
3. Muckle RP, De la Cruz A, Lo WM (1998) Petrous apex lesions. Am J Otol 19:219–225
4. Sanna M et al. (1993) Petrous bone cholesteatoma. Skull Base Surg 3:201–213
5. Thedinger BA, Jackler R K (1994) Lesions of the petrous apex. In: RK Jackler, DE Brackmann (eds) Neurotology. Mosby, St Louis, pp 1169–1187

1.5.6   Petrous Apex Cholesterol Granuloma

OLIVIER STERKERS AND CHRISTIAN MARTIN

1.5.6.1   Synonym

Cholesterol cyst.

1.5.6.2   Definition

Cholesterol granuloma is probably the most common cystic lesion of the petrous apex and represents the end result of complete obstruction of an air cell tract to the petrous apex early in life.

1.5.6.3   Aetiology/Epidemiology

Cholesterol granuloma has not been so uncommon since the development of MRI imaging. Obliteration of a well-developed cell tract in the petrous bone leads to mucoid fluid retention and breakdown products of blood from the capillary network of the mucoperiosteal lining (haemosiderin). This produces a foreign-body reaction with macrophage accumulation, giant cells and the distribution of cholesterol crystals within the soft tissue lining of the cyst. The continued accumulation of fluid is responsible for breakdown of bony walls of the space and compression of the adjacent soft tissue structures. Evolution of the lesion is highly variable and many of them remain asymptomatic.

1.5.6.4   Symptoms

The usual presenting symptoms of an expanding lesion in the petrous apex are a conductive hearing loss from a serous effusion caused by Eustachian tube obstruction, headache, from pressure on the dural covering, diplopia related to involvement of cranial nerve VI, facial hypoaesthesia caused by compression of cranial nerve V (*Gradenigo syndrome*), sensorineural hearing loss and vestibular abnormalities by a compression of the internal auditory canal. The facial nerve is relatively resistant to paresis from this slowly expansive lesion.

1.5.6.5   Diagnosis

- **Otoscopy** (ear microscopy): normal or presence of serous otitis.
- Clinical evaluation of cranial nerve function (V,VI,VII).
- **Audiovestibular testing**: Pure tone and speech audiometry are performed to assess the degree of conductive and sensorineural impairments. Tympanometry is performed to assess the presence of a middle ear effusion. Auditory brainstem response is performed in the case of sensorineural hearing loss. Vestibular studies are limited to patients who describe dizziness or vertigo.
- **Electrical facial nerve testing**: electromyography and electroneuronography to evaluate facial nerve function (see Sect. 1.7.1).
- **Imaging**: High-resolution CT and MRI are mandatory for the diagnosis of petrous apex lesions. CT scanning visualizes a well-shaped enlargement of the apical cell, the bony destruction and its relationship to vital structures, including the internal auditory canal, cochlea, vestibular labyrinth, carotid artery and jugu-

lar bulb. MRI is highly suggestive with hyperintense signals on T1 and T2 sequences, and no gadolinium enhancement.

1.5.6.6   Therapy

Conservative Therapy
There is no treatment in asymptomatic patients with a periodic imaging follow-up.

Surgery
- Drainage procedures of the petrous apex (infralabyrinthine or infracochlear) depending on the location of the cholesterol granuloma and the anatomy of the petrous bone.
- Transotic approach: in extensive petrous bone cholesterol granuloma with dead ear.

Peroperative facial nerve monitoring is an additional useful surgical procedure

1.5.6.7   Differential Diagnosis

- **Congenital or acquired cholesteatoma**: Facial nerve palsy is frequent. Only MRI differentiates the lesion from cholesterol granuloma with hypointense T1, hyperintense T2 and no gadolinium enhancement.
- **Vascular lesion**: internal carotid aneurysm.
- **Benign solid lesions**: schwannoma, chondroma, meningioma, paraganglioma.
- **Malignant lesions**: chondrosarcoma, lymphoma, eosinophilic granuloma, metastatic lesions.

1.5.6.8   Prognosis

- Drainage procedures allow pain relief and the recovery of some cranial nerve dysfunction.
- Potential long-term recurrence implicates serial clinical and imaging follow-up.

Suggested Reading

1. Brackmann DE, Shelton C, Arriaga MA (1994) Otologic surgery. Saunders, Philadelphia

1.6 Inner Ear

ANDREAS ARNOLD, WOLFGANG ARNOLD, ROBERTO BOVO, UWE GANZER, KARL-FRIEDRICH HAMANN, SALVATORE IURATO, JAN KIEFER, KERSTIN LAMM, WALTER LIVI, ALESSANDRO MARTINI AND GERARD M.O'DONOGHUE

1.6.1 Zoster Oticus

SALVATORE IURATO AND WOLFGANG ARNOLD

1.6.1.1 Synonyms

Herpes zoster oticus, herpes zoster cephalicus, Ramsay Hunt syndrome.

1.6.1.2 Definition

Disease characterized by the rapid onset of peripheral facial paralysis associated with severe otalgia and ipsilateral varicelliform vesicles involving the auricle and the external auditory canal.

1.6.1.3 Aetiology/Epidemiology

Caused by reactivation of the varicella zoster virus at the level of the ganglion cells of cranial nerves VII and VIII, herpes zoster oticus accounts for approximately 10–15% of acute facial palsy cases.

1.6.1.4 Symptoms

- One or 2 days of general malaise with fever.
- Burning earache followed by a vesicular eruption involving the aperture of the external auditory canal and the auricle. The bluish-red vesicles eventually form crusts within a few days.
- Facial palsy.
- Sensorineural hearing loss and vertigo (lesion of cranial nerve VIII).
- Pain in the pharynx (lesion of cranial nerves IX and X).
- Facial pain due to involvement of cranial nerve V.
- Headache, neck stiffness, photophobia.

1.6.1.5 Complications

Persistent complete hearing loss, persistent vertigo, postherpetic pain, persistent facial paralysis.

1.6.1.6 Diagnostic Procedures

- Inspection: varicella zoster vesicles on the lateral surface of the auricle, concha and entrance of the auditory canal (Fig. 1.6.1). Vesicles may occur over the face and neck and may involve the buccal mucosa. **Warning**: the vesicles may be small or may resolve before the patient is evaluated (pay attention to encrusted areas).
- Otomicroscopy: vesicles or vesicle remnants in the external auditory canal and on the tympanic membrane.
- Audiometric evaluation: sensorineural hearing loss.
- Vestibular tests: spontaneous nystagmus towards the affected side (at the beginning), later towards the opposite direction.
- Serological confirmation: rarely utilized.

1.6.1.7 Therapy

Conservative Treatment
- Local treatment of the vesicles with drying agents (e.g. 70% alcohol) and acyclovir cream.
- Antiviral treatment with acyclovir (800 mg five times a day orally). Alternatively, brivudin or famciclovir may be given.
- Prednisolone, 100 mg/day for 3–5 days together with proton pumps blockers. Alternatively, prednisone, 1 mg/kg of body weight daily orally for 7–10 days with tapering to zero over the following 10 days.

Surgical Treatment
In cases of persistent facial paralysis, gold weight implant in the upper eyelid, hypoglossal-facial anastomosis.

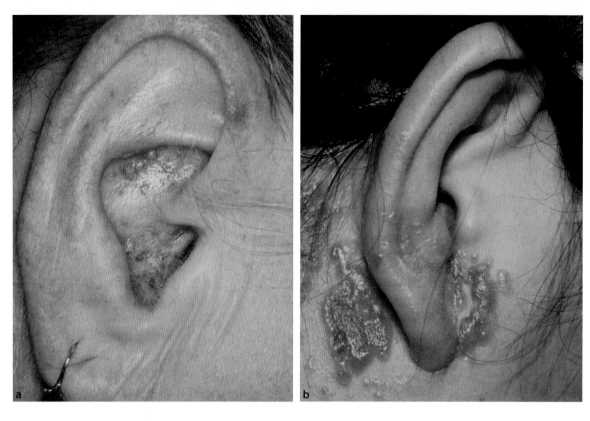

Fig. 1.6.1a,b Herpes zoster oticus. **a** Numerous vesicles (some of them crusted) are seen scattered throughout the concha. **b** Numerous vesicles in the concha, in front and behind the auricle

1.6.1.8   Differential Diagnosis

- Bell's palsy (idiopathic facial palsy): the characteristic cutaneous lesions and the high incidence of cochlear and vestibular symptoms differentiate zoster oticus from Bell's palsy.
- External otitis, perichondritis, erysipelas, neoplasm, labyrinthitis, Melkersson–Rosenthal syndrome.

1.6.1.9   Prognosis

- The prognosis for recovery of the facial function is less favourable than that of Bell's palsy. Incomplete recovery is frequent (only less than 50% of the patients recover satisfactorily). Prognosis is worse in elderly patients.
- Often persistent neuralgia (years).
- Complete hearing loss and complete vestibular areflexia are irreversible.

Suggested Reading

1. Niparko JK (1994) The acute facial palsies. In: Jackler RK, Brackmann DE (eds) Neurotology. Mosby, St Louis, pp 1291–1319
2. Gross G, Doerr H-W (2006) Herpes zoster. Recent aspects of diagnosis and control. Karger, Basel
3. Schaitkin BM et al. (2000) Idiopathic (Bell's) palsy, herpes zoster cephalicus, and other facial nerve disorders of viral origin. In: May M, Schaitkin BM (eds) The facial nerve. Thieme, New York, pp 319–338

1.6.2   Labyrinthitis

WOLFGANG ARNOLD

1.6.2.1   Synonym

Acute or chronic inflammation of the labyrinth.

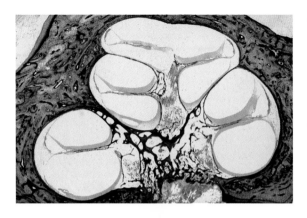

Fig. 1.6.2 Mild serous labyrinthitis in the course of lethal viral meningitis. Protein deposits can be seen in the perilymphatic spaces

1.6.2.2 Definition

Acute or chronic serous (Fig. 1.6.2) or purulent (Fig. 1.6.3) inflammatory reaction within the fluid spaces and membranes of the vestibulocochlear labyrinth caused by bacteria, viruses, spirochetes or fungi.

The route of infection may be *otogenic, meningogenic* or *haematogenic.*

1.6.2.3 Viral Labyrinthitis

The symptoms are:

- **Otogenic:** during the course of a viral infection of the upper respiratory tract including the middle ear (picornavirus, influenza virus, parainfluenza virus, respiratory syncytial virus, coronavirus, adenovirus). Serous effusion of the middle ear, vestibular disturbances, combined or pure sensorineural hearing loss, tinnitus. No earache.
- **Meningogenic:** during the course of mumps, measles or parainfluenza meningitis. Route of infection are the internal auditory canal and the cochlear aqueduct. Protein deposits can be seen in the perilymphatic spaces (Fig. 1.6.2). Clinical signs of meningitis are fatigue, vomiting, headache, stiff neck, fever, and unilateral or bilateral deafness.

1.6.2.4 Bacterial or Purulent Labyrinthitis

Aetiology/Epidemiology

Purulent (suppurative) bacterial labyrinthitis may be secondary to acute otitis media or purulent meningitis. In acute otitis media, bacteria may enter the inner ear through the oval and round windows (Fig. 1.6.3).

Purulent labyrinthitis is frequently followed by meningitis as the microorganisms gain access to the subarachnoid space through the cochlea aqueduct or internal auditory canal. Bacterial labyrinthitis can be a complication of cholesteatoma, spontaneous or acquired labyrinth fistula or may occur in malformations of the cochlea with enlarged perilymphatic spaces (Mondini dysplasia).

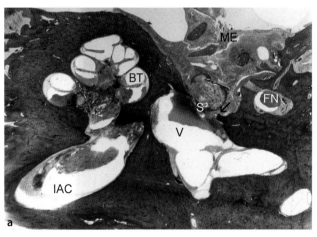
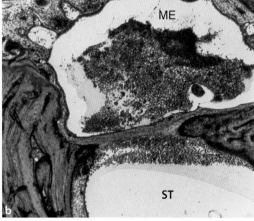

Fig. 1.6.3 a Purulent otogenic labyrinthitis and meningitis in a 4-year-old child, who died from the disease. The route of penetration is the oval window (*arrow*). **b** Acute otogenic labyrinthitis. The route of penetration is the thickened round window membrane. On both sides of the round window membrane purulent exudates can be seen. *IAC* internal auditory canal, *S* stapes, *FN* facial nerve, *ME* middle ear cavity, *BT* basal cochlear turn, *V* vestibule, *ST* scala tympani, basal turn

The most frequent bacteria causing otogenic labyrinthitis are pneumococci, *Haemophilus influenzae*, *Streptococcus* (A), *Escherichia coli* and *Klebsiella pneumoniae*.

The most frequent bacteria causing meningogenic labyrinthitis are meningococci, pneumococci and *Hemophilus influenzae* type B.

Symptoms
- **Otogenic labyrinthitis**: severe vertigo with nystagmus, vomiting, high fever. It invariably results in complete hearing loss and is often followed by facial paralysis.
- **Meningogenic labyrinthitis:** classic symptoms of meningitis, severe vertigo with nystagmus, vomiting, unilateral or bilateral, often fluctuating hearing loss or complete deafness. Postinflammatory rapid ossification of the cochlear fluid spaces.

Complications of Otogenic Bacterial Labyrinthitis
Meningitis, encephalitis, brain abscess, complete deafness, lethal outcome.

1.6.2.5   Haematogenic Labyrinthitis

- *Treponema pallidum*: congenital or acquired syphilis (third stage). Fluctuating hearing loss, endolymphatic hydrops, dizziness. Hennebert sign positive. If untreated, it results in complete hearing loss.
- *Mycobacterium tuberculosis*: formation of tuberculous granuloma along vascular spaces which spread into the labyrinth spaces. Progressive sensorineural hearing loss. In most cases it is associated with a systemic haematogenic spreading of tuberculosis.
- **Mucormycosis:** systemic, in many cases fatal mycotic sepsis (caused by, e.g., *Rhizopus*, *Absidia*) in immunodepressed patients (AIDS, leukaemia, diabetes): high temperature, meningitis, deafness, facial palsy, vertigo, purulent sinusitis.

1.6.2.6   Diagnostic Procedures

Recommended European Standard
- Otoscopy or ear microscopy: serous or purulent otitis media, pulsating tympanic membrane, cholesteatoma, bone fracture
- Hearing examination: tuning fork, audiogram (mixed or pure sensorineural hearing loss, deafness)
- Frenzel glasses: at the beginning nystagmus in the direction of the affected ear, later in the opposite direction
- High-resolution "emergency CT"

Microbiology
- Culture taken from the purulent ear secretion or from the nasopharynx
- Blood cell differentiation, blood sedimentation rate
- CSF diagnostic: cell count, protein and sugar elevation, culture taken from the CSF

Additional/Useful Diagnostic Procedures
- Serology: rubella virus, paramyxovirus, influenza virus, adenovirus, syphilis
- Bone scintigraphy (single photon emission scintigraphy)
- Counselling: neurology, neuropaediatrics, dermatology

1.6.2.7   Therapy

Conservative Treatment for Viral Labyrinthitis
- Glucocorticoids, initially 500 mg intravenously for 3 days followed by oral administration of prednisolone starting with 120 mg per day, then reducing the dosage by 10 mg per day
- Treatment of the rhinogenic infection (nasal spray, mucolytica)
- Vestibular suppressant medications and antiemetics
- Antibiotics intravenously to avoid bacterial superinfection (cephalosporine, aminopenicillin with or without a β-lactamase-inhibitor)

Conservative Treatment for Bacterial Labyrinthitis
- High doses of antibiotics, e.g. cephalosporines (third generation), chloramphenicole and aminoglycosides, according to the smear culture results
- Vestibular suppressant medications and antiemetics
- In lues III, penicillin G or tetracycline
- In tuberculosis, tuberculostatic therapy
- In mucormycosis, amphotericine B, control of diabetes
- Infusions with electrolytes; antipyretica

Surgical Therapy
Each otogenic labyrinthitis caused by bacteria needs surgical intervention.

Surgical Principles
- Myringotomy, insertion of ventilating tubes (Fig. 1.4.5)
- Mastoidectomy, radical ear surgery, labyrinthectomy

1.6.2.8   Prognosis

- Early onset of therapy (antibiotics, antimycotics) is obligatory in this life-threatening infection of the temporal bone.
- Deafness and long-lasting dizziness. Lethal outcome in most cases of generalized mucormycosis.
- In cases of bilateral complete deafness following bacterial meningitis, early cochlear implantation is recommended before ossification of the cochlea occurs (see Sect 1.6.12).

Suggested Reading

1. Arnold W, Bredberg G, Gstöttner W et al. (2002) Meningitis following cochlear implantation: pathomechanisms, clinical symptoms, conservative and surgical treatment. ORL J Otorhinolaryngol Relat Spec 64:382–289
2. Gulya AJ (1998) Infections of the labyrinth. In: Bailey BJ (1998) Head & neck surgery—otolaryngology, 2nd edn. Lippincott-Raven, chap 145
3. Schachern PA, Paparella MM, Hybertson R et al. (1922) Bacterial tympanogenic labyrinthitis, meningitis and sensorineural damage. Arch Otolaryngol Head Neck Surg 118:53–57
4. Schuknecht HF (1993) Infections of the ear. In: Pathology of the ear, 2nd edn. Lea and Febiger, Philadelphia

1.6.3   Contusio Labyrinthi

WOLFGANG ARNOLD

1.6.3.1   Synonym

Concussion of the labyrinth.

1.6.3.2   Definition

Microinjuries of the vestibulocochlear organ (bleeding, membrane ruptures, microfractures) caused by a blunt concussion of the skull, with or without fracture of the skull base or contusio cerebri.

1.6.3.3   Symptoms

Sensorineural hearing loss affecting all frequencies or mainly the frequencies above 3 kHz. In lateral (parietal) trauma, mainly the opposite ear is affected (contrecoup); when the blunt forces act from behind (occipital trauma) then both labyrinths can be damaged. Vertigo and tinnitus are accompanying symptoms.

1.6.3.4   Complications

- Luxation of the ossicles (e.g. incus), perilymphatic fistula, slowly progressive sensorineural hearing loss, deafness, long-lasting vertigo, subdural bleeding, posttraumatic endolymphatic hydrops.
- Postconcussion disequilibrium syndrome: pathomechanisms and symtoms are identical with those of benign paroxysmal vertigo (see Sect. 1.6.15) and cupolithiasis [1].

1.6.3.5   Diagnostic Procedures

Recommended European Standard
- Detailed history (of forensic importance)
- Inspection of the skull, searching for skin injuries, haematoma
- Inspection of the oral, nasal and nasopharyngeal cavities
- Otoscopy or ear microscopy, searching for fracture signs, haemotympanum, rupture of the tympanic membrane
- Hearing examination: tuning forks, audiogram, tympanogram, stapedius reflexes
- Frenzel glasses: to exclude vestibular irritation or loss of function of one vestibular organ

Additional/Useful Diagnostic Procedures
- Schüller-X-ray, high-resolution CT: to exclude fractures
- Examination of the vestibular function (electronystagmography, video-oculography)
- Examination of the sense of smell to exclude rupture of the fila olfactoria

1.6.3.6   Therapy

Conservative Treatment
The recommended European standard is use of antioedematous principles (see Sect. 1.6.5).

Surgical Treatment
If there is an additional conductive hearing loss caused by trauma of the middle ear structures, reconstruction of the ossicular chain is recommended some weeks following the injury.

1.6.3.7   Prognosis

The prognosis is uncertain: in many cases complete restoration of the cochleovestibular deficit is possible; in some cases progressive hearing loss and/or long-lasting vertigo are possible.

References

1. Schuknecht HF, Davison RC (1956) Deafness and vertigo from head injury. Arch Otolaryngol 63:513–528

Suggested Reading

1. Schuknecht HF (1969) Mechanism of inner ear injury from blows to the head. Ann Otol Rhinol Laryngol 78:253–262
2. Von Schulthess G (1961) Innenohr und Trauma mit besonderer Berücksichtigung des Krankheitsverlaufes. Fortschr Hals-Nase-Ohrenheilk 7:1–102
3. Tuohimaa P (1978) Vestibular disturbances after acute mild head injury. Acta Otolaryngol Suppl 359:3–67

1.6.4   Otoliquorrhoea/Otorhinoliquorrhoea

SALVATORE IURATO

1.6.4.1   Definition

An abnormal communication between the subarachnoid space and the middle ear is a precondition:
- **Otoliquorrhoea**: outflow of CSF into the external auditory canal through a rupture of the tympanic membrane.
- **Otorhinoliquorrhoea**: if the tympanic membrane is intact, CSF drains from the middle ear into the nose through the Eustachian tube.

1.6.4.2   Aetiology/Epidemiology

- *Congenital (labyrinthine and perilabyrinthine abnormalities)*: bone and meningeal defects in the tegmen tympani and tegmen antri areas, cochlear dysplasia, arachnoid granulations, defects in the Fallopian canals, enlarged and patent cochlear aqueduct (labyrinthine abnormalities), fissula ante fenestram, stapes malformations, cerebral herniations (meningoencephaloceles) in the middle ear and mastoid
- *Acquired* (more common): head trauma specially in cases of temporal bone fractures (see Sect. 1.5.3); in 29% of longitudinal fractures and in 44% of transverse fractures

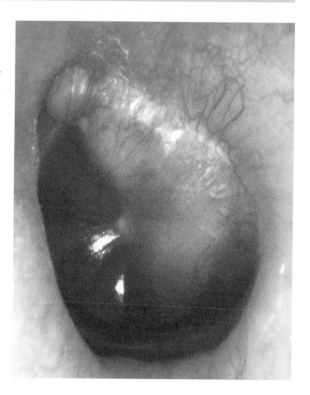

Fig. 1.6.4 This patient was operated on to remove a vestibular schwannoma with a leak along the posterior wall of the pharynx and a watery rhinorrhoea on bending her head forwards. The tympanic picture mimics a serotympanum

- *Postoperative* CSF leak: e.g. complication of vestibular schwannoma surgery, middle and posterior fossa surgery, surgery for chronic ear disease (less frequently)

1.6.4.3   Symptoms

A watery pulsating secretion when there is a tympanic membrane perforation or rupture. When the tympanic membrane is intact, there is clear fluid behind the tympanic membrane simulating a serous otitis media (Fig. 1.6.4). Outflow of watery fluid from the nose (otorhinoliquorrhoea). Coughing at night. A sensation of salty fluid in the mouth.

1.6.4.4   Complications

Recurrent meningitis, meningoencephalitis.

1.6.4.5 Diagnostic Procedures

- Clinical history
- Otoscopy/ear microscopy (Waterlike fluid behind the tympanic membrane? Clear secretion through a perforation?)
- Inspection of the oral cavity (Any leak along the posterior wall of the pharynx?)
- Queckenstedt's sign (a rise in the CSF pressure compressing the veins in the neck)
- Hearing examination: tuning fork, audiogram, tympanometry
- High-resolution CT scan (axial and coronal scan)
- MRI to prove herniated brain tissue within the temporal bone
- Laboratory tests: glucose content examination (50% of blood sugar), protein content (maximum 2 g/l), β_2 transferrin
- In some cases, intrathecal fluoroscein (attention to complications such as seizures and transverse myelitis with paralysis!), CSF scintigraphy

1.6.4.6 Therapy

Conservative Treatment

- Rest in bed, with the head elevated. Avoid straining at stool.
- Never occlude the external auditory canal!
- Diuretics (acetazolamide).
- Antibiotic treatment to prevent ascending infections: cephalosporins, ciprofloxacin.
- Continuous lumbar CSF drainage (attention to the sterility and the volume and rate of flow!) if the above-mentioned measures do not work.

In vestibular schwannoma surgery careful sealing during surgical closure and a compressive bandage are necessary to prevent postauricular CSF leak.

Surgical Treatment

Surgical treatment is necessary when CSF fistulas do not heal spontaneously. The best approach for spontaneous and post-traumatic leaks is through the middle fossa (Fig. 1.5.9). For CSF fistulas following vestibular schwannoma surgery, revision of the surgical wound and insertion of plugs of periostium and abdominal fat should be performed.

1.6.4.7 Differential Diagnosis

- Serotympanum (Fig. 1.4.6a)
- Monolateral serous rhinitis
- Rhinorrhoea

Suggested Reading

1. Hoffman RA (1994) Cerebrospinal fluid leak of temporal bone origin. In: Jackler RK, Brackmann DE (eds) Neurotology. Mosby, St Louis, pp 919–928

1.6.5 Sudden Sensorineural Hearing Loss (Including Perilymphatic Fistula)

KERSTIN LAMM

1.6.5.1 Synonyms

Sudden deafness, sudden idiopathic sensorineural hearing loss.

1.6.5.2 Definition

Sudden sensorineural hearing loss is characterized by an *acute* in the majority of cases *unilateral hearing loss originating in the inner ear* of *unknown pathogenesis and origin*. Hearing loss may be slight, moderate, profound or complete and concerns the high, middle, deep or all frequencies. The disease is accompanied by tinnitus in about 85% of cases and dizziness in about 30% of cases.

1.6.5.3 Epidemiology

The incidence ranges between 20 cases per 100,000 residents per year in Austria and Germany, eight to 13 cases per 100,000 residents per year in Japan and about 11 cases per 100,000 residents per year in the USA.

Women are equally affected as men, most frequently at the age of 50 ± 5 years. However, there is an increasing incidence in younger people, whereas children are rarely concerned.

1.6.5.4 Aetiology/Classification

The cause is still unknown. The following pathomechanisms are currently discussed:
- Impairment of cochlear blood flow due to vasomotor paralysis or vasospasm, endothelial oedema or other endothelial disorders resulting in microcirculatory rheological disturbances
- Impairment of cochlear blood flow due to systemic rheological disorders
- Malfunction of ion channels in hair cells resulting in cellular dysfunction
- Synaptic dysfunction due to insufficiency or toxicity of afferent neurotransmitters

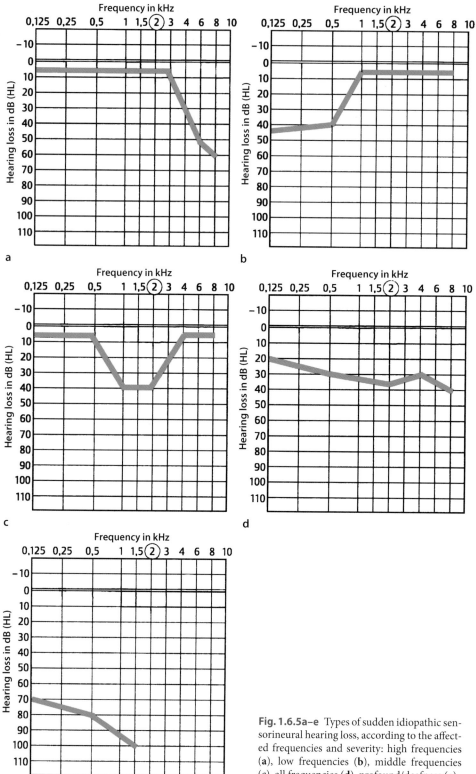

Fig. 1.6.5a–e Types of sudden idiopathic sensorineural hearing loss, according to the affected frequencies and severity: high frequencies (**a**), low frequencies (**b**), middle frequencies (**c**), all frequencies (**d**), profound/deafness (**e**)

- Malfunction of the cochlear efferent pathways
- Malfunction of ion channels in strial cells resulting in endolymphatic water–electrolyte imbalance, potentially even in endolymphatic hydrops
- Inflammatory tissue alterations, e.g. within the endolymphatic sac
- Alteration of other biochemical and physiological mechanisms involved in cochlear homeostasis

According to the affected frequencies and severity the following types of sudden idiopathic sensorineural hearing loss can be distinguished (Fig. 1.6.5):

- **High-frequency idiopathic sensorineural hearing loss**, which may be due to cellular malfunction of outer (below 50 dB HL) and inner (beyond 60 dB HL) hair cells (Fig. 1.6.5a).
- **Low-frequency idiopathic sensorineural hearing loss**, which may be due to endolymphatic water–electrolyte imbalance or even endolymphatic hydrops as a possible result of impaired blood flow within the vascular stria and subsequent hypoxic cellular damage (Fig. 1.6.5b).
- **Middle-frequency idiopathic sensorineural hearing loss**, which may be due to impaired blood flow within the spiral lamina and subsequent hypoxic cellular damage of the organ of Corti or, alternatively may be due to genetic defects (Fig. 1.6.5c).
- **All-frequency idiopathic sensorineural hearing loss**, which may be due to blood flow impairment in the spiral modiolar artery and/or upstream arteries resulting in hypoxic damage of cochlear tissues (Fig. 1.6.5d).
- **Profound idiopathic sensorineural hearing loss and deafness**, which may be due to thrombotic or embolic blood flow obstruction in the arteria cochlearis communis or spiral modiolar artery resulting in hypoxic damage of cochlear tissues. Perilymphatic fistula due to rupture of the round window membrane or lesion of the oval window which may result in acute profound hearing loss or even deafness is a disorder of a distinct origin and, therefore, cannot be referred to as idiopathic sensorineural hearing loss by definition (Fig. 1.6.5e).
- **Other types**, such as fluctuating hearing thresholds, progressive hearing loss in spite of current therapy etc.

1.6.5.5   Symptoms

Patients complain about symptoms in the following descending order of incidence:

- *Acute unilateral subjective hearing loss*, although this symptom may be not perceived in cases of slight hearing loss restricted to a few frequencies

- *Tinnitus* (in about 85% of cases)
- *Feeling of pressure in the ear*
- *Dizziness* (in about 30% of cases)
- *Distorted hearing, diplacusis, hyperacusis*
- *Periaural dysaesthesia*
- *Secondary psychoemotional ailments* such as anxiety, fear, distress, restlessness, agitation, resignation and sense of guilt

1.6.5.6   Complications

Complications such as fluctuating hearing threshold or progressive hearing loss in spite of current therapeutic intervention raise the question of a distinct cause such as beginning Ménière's disease, pressure variations of CSF, vestibular schwannoma and (auto)immune-mediated disease.

Another complication may concern psychoemotional and psychosocial problems in cases of persistent hearing loss and/or tinnitus (see Sect. 1.6.8).

1.6.5.7   Diagnosis

Recommended European Standard

1. Detailed case history
   - Side, onset and duration of hearing loss
   - Associated symptoms such as tinnitus, dizziness, feeling of pressure in the ear, periaural dysaesthesia, secondary psychoemotional ailments
   - Previous idiopathic sudden sensorineural hearing loss or previous hearing loss due to noise exposure or other diseases, previous pure tone audiograms
   - History of otorhinolaryngological diseases and surgery
   - History of head trauma and/or other accidents
   - History of internal, neurological, psychiatric or psychosomatic or orthopaedic diseases
   - Family status, profession, still working, claim for early retirement, retired
   - Recreational activities
2. Microscopy of the ear canal and ear drum
3. Rhinoscopy using 0°/30° endoscopes
4. Posterior rhinoscopy using a 70° endoscope
5. Sonography of the maxillary and frontal paranasal sinus
6. Pharyngoscopy
7. Hypopharyngoscopy and laryngoscopy using a 90° endoscope
8. Tympanometry and stapedial reflex measurements (ipsilateral and contralateral evoked reflex responses at 0.5, 1, 2 and 4 kHz)
9. Pure tone audiogram (0.125, 0.25, 0.5, 0.75, 1, 1.5, 2, 3, 4, 6 and 8 kHz)

10. Transitory evoked otoacoustic emissions
11. Vestibular tests using video-oculography
12. Auditory evoked brainstem responses (ABRs) or cerebral MRI in the case of equivocal ABR measurement results or pathological ABRs and/or video-oculography findings and/or in the case of a previous or suspected intracranial disease
13. Blood pressure measurement

Useful Additional Diagnostic Procedures

- Audiometric tinnitus measurement (frequency-matching, intensity, minimal masking level using broadband or narrowband noise or pure tones, residual inhibition) (Fig. 1.6.7)
- Speech audiometry
- Distortion products of otoacoustic emissions
- Auditory evoked cortical responses
- Electrocochleography
- Glycerol test according to Klockhoff
- Tympanoscopy in cases of profound hearing loss or deafness
- Blood cell count, haemoglobin, fibrinogen, lipids, creatinine, C-reactive protein
- Serologic tests on borrelia, lues, herpesvirus type 1, herpes zoster virus, HIV
- Doppler duplex sonography of extracranial vessels
- Depending on case history internal, neurological, psychosomatic, orthopaedic, genetic examination

1.6.5.8   Therapy

Sudden idiopathic sensorineural hearing loss must be managed with care and as soon as possible concerning the diagnostic procedures and the mode and beginning of therapy. According to the categories of the Oxford Centre for Evidence-Based Medicine (http://www.cebm.net), the evidence level of most clinical trials on therapy of sudden deafness is relatively low. In addition, the clinical trials considered in the Cochrane International Register of Controlled Clinical Trials, e.g. prospective, randomized, placebo-controlled and double-blind conducted studies, are of relatively high level of evidence; however, the underlying study protocols vary tremendously. Therefore, universally valid therapeutic options based on reproducible results are not available. Instead, therapeutic recommendations are merely formed empirically.

Spontaneous recovery rates range from 31 to 68%; however, these data were revealed from retrospective, non-randomized and mostly non-controlled trials on a few patients only. Furthermore, the term "recovery" was not exactly defined, e.g. partial remission was not distinguished from complete remission, and a persistent tinnitus was not taken into consideration. Patients would not regard themselves as fully recovered when their tinnitus is still persistent.

However, in well-informed patients presenting with a slight hearing loss without previous ipsilateral or contralateral hearing loss and without tinnitus and/or dizziness, one may await spontaneous recovery for a few days.

Conservative Therapy

Basic therapeutic interventions comprise normalization of systemic blood pressure, heart rate and haematocrit level (below 45). For patients complaining of moderate to severe psychoemotional ailments such as anxiety, fear, distress, restlessness, agitation, resignation and sense of guilt, a psychotherapist should be included.

Recommended European Standard

According to the aforementioned cause and pathogenesis possibly involved, therapeutic recommendations differentiate between the various types of sudden idiopathic sensorineural hearing loss.

- **High-frequency idiopathic sensorineural hearing loss.** A daily dose of 250–500 mg *prednisolone* intravenously on three consecutive days is recommended.

In the case of partial or no remission, prednisolone treatment should be continued orally for 16 days, starting with 100, 80, 60, 40, 20, 10, 5 and 2.5 mg each dosage for two days.

Prednisolone therapy should be accompanied by gastric proton pump inhibitors (40 mg omeprazole per day or 150 mg ranitidine per day or others).

Prednisolone is a synthetic analogue of endogenous corticosteroid hormones classified as glucocorticoids. Besides anti-inflammatory effects, prednisolone possesses multiple other cellular effects. The rationale for administration of prednisolone is based on the consideration that inflammatory tissue alterations are also elicited by tissue ischaemia and hypoxia. In addition, prednisolone mobilizes amino acids for gluconeogenesis, alters glucose utilization and influences protein metabolism. Finally, prednisolone binds with equal affinity to both glucocorticoid and mineralocorticoid receptors widely distributed in cochlear tissues, thereby contributing to restoration of cellular osmolarity, electrochemical gradients, transmembrane ion flux and neuronal conduction.

In patients presenting with *contraindications* (e.g. diabetes, severe chronic gastritis, gastric or duodenal ulcera) *for the treatment with prednisolone*, intravenous infusion of a hyperoncotic hydrophilic haemodilutive plasma-expanding agent, such as *hydroxyethyl starch or others* (250–500 ml/day for 5–10 days) is a good alternative option.

However, contraindications (e.g. arterial hypertension) should be noted, and potential side effects (e.g. temporary pruritus) should be considered. *In the case of contraindications for haemodilution*, another haemorheological active drug such as *pentoxifylline* (100 mg, equivalent to 5 ml/day dissolved in 100 ml 0.9% isotonic saline) may be intravenously infused for 5–10 days.

Additional administration of scavangers of toxic free oxygen radicals such as *α-lipoic acid* (600 mg/day orally) during haemodilutive or haemorheological infusion therapy may be reasonable to prevent reperfusion injury within the cochlea.

- **Low-frequency and middle-frequency idiopathic sensorineural hearing loss**. A daily dose of 250–500 mg *prednisolone* intravenously on three consecutive days is recommended. In the case of partial or no remission, prednisolone treatment should be continued orally for 16 days together with gastric proton pump inhibitors as described above. Additional *osmotic infusion therapy* using *mannitol* (15 g in 100 ml solution) and *acetazolamide* (500 mg) intravenously on three consecutive days may be administered. Acetazolamide (250 mg/day) may be continued orally for 10 days.

  In patients presenting with *contraindications* (e.g. diabetes, severe chronic gastritis, gastric or duodenal ulcer) *for the treatment with prednisolone,* initial osmotic therapy is recommended.

- **All-frequency idiopathic sensorineural hearing loss**. A daily dose of 250–500 mg *prednisolone* intravenously on three consecutive days is recommended. In the case of partial or no remission, prednisolone treatment should be continued orally for 16 days together with gastric proton pump inhibitors and additional *haemodilutive/haemorheological infusion therapy* together with *α-lipoic acid* should be administered as described for high-frequency idiopathic sensorineural hearing loss.

  In patients suffering from an elevated fibrinogen level (above 300 mg/dl) *fibrinogen and low density lipoprotein apheresis* may be a good alternative to haemodilutive or haemorheological infusion therapy. However, the expense is relatively high and the long-term outcome on hearing gain was proved to be equally effective as with conventional therapy as described above.

- **Profound idiopathic sensorineural hearing loss and deafness**. A daily dose of 500 mg *prednisolone* intravenously on three consecutive days together with *haemodilutive/haemorheological infusion therapy* and *α-lipoic acid* should be administered as described for high-frequency idiopathic sensorineural hearing loss. Prednisolone treatment should be continued orally for 16 days together with gastric proton pump inhibitors

as described, and haemodilutive/haemorheological infusion therapy and α-lipoic acid should be continued for another seven consecutive days.

In patients suffering from an elevated fibrinogen level (above 300 mg/dl) *fibrinogen and low density lipoprotein apheresis* may be additionally tried (but see the comments for all-frequency idiopathic sensorineural hearing loss).

In the case of minor or no remission at all, perilymphatic fistula due to rupture of the round window membrane or lesion of the oval window may be considered and *tympanoscopy* should be performed preferably within 5–10 days after onset of hearing loss.

Useful Additional Therapeutic Strategies

If initial therapy with prednisolone and/or haemodilutive or alternative haemorheological agents is only partially or not effective at all, and this is the case in over 25% of patients, *hyperbaric oxygenation therapy* (ten to 15 sessions on ten to 15 consecutive days) should be started as soon as possible, preferably within 3–6 weeks after the onset of idiopathic sensorineural hearing loss.

Obsolete Therapeutic Options

- Isobaric oxygenation therapy, e.g. breathing of oxygen under normal atmospheric pressure
- Ozone therapy
- Ultraviolet light irradiation
- Ultrasonic therapy
- Laser irradiation of any type or mode
- Electromagnetic stimulation
- Suggestive psychotherapy, hypnosis
- Acupuncture
- Autohaemotherapy, autologous blood transfusion
- Monotherapy with vasodilative agents which may induce intracochlear vascular steal effects resulting in an impaired cochlear blood flow

Surgery

In the case of progressive hearing loss in spite of current therapeutic intervention or in the case of minor or no remission of profound hearing loss, *tympanoscopy* should be performed to exclude or seal a rupture of the round window membrane or a lesion of the oval window (see Sect. 1.6.5.9).

1.6.5.9 Differential Diagnosis

Sudden sensorineural hearing loss may also be attributable to the following diseases:

- **Perilymphatic fistula**. Perilymphatic fistulae of the oval or round window are rare clinical findings. They may occur during skull trauma, following stapes surgery, middle ear surgery, after lifting heavy weights or spontaneously.

Perilymphatic fistulae in the area of the annular ligament of the stapes footplate cause sensorineural hearing loss and dizziness of different extent. They can occur after stapes surgery with insufficient sealing of the prosthesis. Congenital perilymphatic fistulae of the stapes footplate occur in cases of malformation of the stapes and cause recurrent meningitis. They are usually detected during exploration of the oval window.

Perilymphatic fistulae of the round window membrane are rare findings in cases of sudden hearing loss. There are no clear clinical symptoms characteristic for round window membrane rupture. In some cases the history reveals strong physical exertion (explosion trauma after Goodhill).

All diagnosed perilymphatic fistulae should be completely sealed with connective tissue and fibrin glue to avoid labyrinthitis and/or meningitis. Surgical sealing of the ruptured round window membrane or annular ligament with connective tissue sometimes results in partial or complete, but not predictable, restoration of hearing.

- Haematological diseases (e. g. polycythaemia, polyglobulia, leukaemia, exsicosis).
- Cardiovascular diseases.
- Bacterial labyrinthitis (due to otitis media, borrelia, lues). See Sect. 1.6.2.
- Meningitis.
- Virus infection (adenovirus, herpesvirus type 1, herpes zoster virus, mumps virus, HIV).
- Encephalitis disseminata (multiple sclerosis).
- Autoimmune vasculitis (e. g. Cogan's syndrome).
- Intoxication (drugs, industrial pollution).
- Renal failure, dialysis.
- Intracerebral tumours (e. g. vestibular schwannoma).
- Barotrauma or decompression trauma of the inner ear. See Sect. 1.5.1.
- Acute noise induced hearing loss, acoustic trauma. See Sect. 1.6.9.3.
- Head trauma with labyrinthine contusion. See Sect. 1.6.3.
- Severe distortion trauma of the cervical spine.
- Pressure variations of CSF (e. g. after CSF puncture).
- Cochlear malformation.
- Genetic defects, hereditary sensorineural hearing loss.
- Genetic syndrome (e. g. Usher, Pendred).
- Psychogenic hearing loss.

1.6.5.10   Prognosis

The prognosis is most favourable in low-frequency and middle-frequency idiopathic sensorineural hearing loss without previous hearing loss. However, recurrence rates of such hearing losses range up to 30%.

Patients with slight to moderate threshold shifts recover better than patients presenting with moderate to profound hearing loss.

A relatively worse prognosis is expected in profound hearing loss or even sudden deafness.

Suggested Reading

1. Gulya AJ (1993) Perilymphatic fistulas. In: Nadol JB, Schuknecht HS (eds) Surgery of the ear and temporal bone, Raven, New York
2. Albegger KW, Arnold W, Biesinger E, Brusis T, Ganzer U, Jahnke K, Jaumann MP, Klemm E, Koch U, Lamm K, Lenarz T, Michel O, Mösges R, Probst R, Strutz J, Suckfüll M, Vassuer M, Westhofen M, Zenner HP (2003) Sudden deafness. Revised Guidelines. Consensus commission of the Association of the Scientific Medical Societies in Germany. http://www.uni-duesseldorf.de/awmf
3. Lamm K (2003) Hyperbaric oxygen therapy (HBO) for the treatment of acute cochlear disorders and tinnitus. Editorial. ORL Otorhinolaryngol Relat Spec 65: 315–316.
4. Lamm K, Arnold W (1999) How useful is corticosteroid treatment in cochlear disorders? Otolaryngol Nova 9:203–216

1.6.6   Ménière's Disease

SALVATORE IURATO AND WOLFGANG ARNOLD

1.6.6.1   Synonyms

Ménière's syndrome, idiopathic endolymphatic hydrops, morbus Ménière.

1.6.6.2   Definition

The syndrome is characterized by: recurrent spontenous attacks of vertigo, fluctuating hearing loss (at the early beginning mainly affecting low frequencies) tinnitus and aural fullness.

According to the American Academy of Otolaryngology—Head and Neck Surgery at least two attacks of objective rotational vertigo, each of 20-min duration or longer must occur to confirm the diagnosis of Ménière's disease. Unilateral sensorineural hearing loss must be documented audiometrically on at least one occasion.

The diagnosis "Ménière's disease" always is a diagnosis "per exclusionem" since other diseases of the cochleovestibular system can mimic Ménière's symptoms.

1.6.6.3 Aetiology/Epidemiology

Temporal bone histopathology from Ménière's patients are usually showing dilatations (hydrops), distortions and/or ruptures (Fig. 1.6.6) of the delicate membranes separating the endolymphatic from the perilymphatic fluid compartements. Hydrops can develop simultaneously as well in the cochlear as in the vestibular compartments, but also isolated in only one of the compartments (this may explain why in Ménière the symptoms can only consist of attacks of vertigo or hearing loss with tinnitus). A malfunctioning spiral ligament and /or endolymphatic sac (disturbed resorption of the endolymph, immunologic factors causing "saccitis") seem to be involved in the pathophysiology of endolymphatic hydrops. Recently the homing of Herpes Type I viruses has been demonstrated as well within the endolymphatic sac as in ganglion cells of Scarpa's ganglion. Reactivation of these viruses seems to be triggered by (immunologic) stress factors clinically causing the typical symptoms of the disease.

There are many known causes of endolymphatic hydrops: viral labyrinthitis, autoimmune inner ear disease (e.g. Cogan's syndrome), otosclerosis, leukaemia, otosyphilis, surgical trauma to the inner ear, temporal bone trauma, etc. When the cause cannot be identified, the term "Ménière's disease" is used. The incidence is one in 8,000 individuals per year in Europe. Approximately 30% of patients will develop contralateral involvement over time (25% at 10-year follow-up).

1.6.6.4 Symptoms

Classic symptoms are:
- Recurrent attacks of rotational vertigo (the most disabling symptom for the patients) which last from several minutes to hours. Vertigo is often associated with nausea and vomiting.
- Fluctuating, unilateral low-frequency hearing loss of the sensorineural type (upsloping audiometric pattern). In the late stages of the disease, there is flat or downsloping non-fluctuating sensorineural hearing loss (hearing threshold of 50–60 dB, speech discrimination of 50–60%).
- During the attacks, subjective tinnitus and aural fullness/pressure are present. Between attacks patients are not dizzy but aural fullness and tinnitus may persist. Vertigo attacks can vary in frequency, intensity and

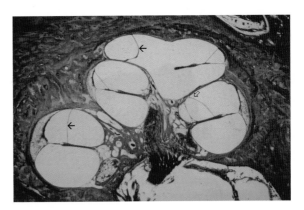

Fig. 1.6.6 Severe endolymphatic hydrops ($\leftarrow$) with distension of Reissner's membrane, ruptures and adhesions ($\hookleftarrow$) in a patient, age 58 who suffered from bilateral Ménière's disease

duration. Generally the attacks increase in severity and frequency with progression of the disease. The frequency and intensity of the vertigo attacks decrease after approximately 5–10 years.

1.6.6.5 Diagnostic Procedures

- Clinical history: extremely important.
- Physical examination: normal findings. Between the attacks patients usually display horizontal, spontaneous nystagmus beating away from the affected ear (paretic nystagmus).
- Electrocochleography: a significant enhancement of the summating potential to action potential amplitude ratio (more than 30%) occurs in 60% of patients with Ménière's disease.
- Auditory brainstem response.
- MRI with contrast medium plays an important role in excluding a retrocochlear lesion (vestibular schwannoma) in *any patient* with unilateral neurotologic symptoms!

1.6.6.6 Additional/Useful Diagnostic Procedures

- Blood sedimentation rate, antinuclear antibody test for autoimmune ear disorders (see Sect. 1.6.7); fluorescent treponemal antibody absorption test to rule out syphilis.
- Glucose tolerance and thyroid function tests are recommended as hypothyroidism and diabetes may be associated with the disease. Lipid profile.
- Caloric tests (with electronystagmography): reduced caloric response on the affected side.

- Glycerol test (1.2–1.5 ml/kg body weight of glycerol mixed with lemon juice): frequently used in the past, but much less nowadays because of its side effects (headache, nausea, vomiting).

Note: *the diagnosis is often by exclusion.*

1.6.6.7   Differential Diagnosis

- Vestibular schwannoma
- Sudden sensorineural hearing loss
- Autoimmune hearing loss
- Migraine

1.6.6.8   Therapy

Recommended European Standard

Conservative Treatment

1. In acute attacks bed rest, vestibular suppressant medication (diazepam) and antiemetics (transdermal scopolamine, thiethylperazine, prochlorperazine) are recommended
2. To prevent attacks, decrease the amount of fluid in the inner ear by diet and diuretics
   - Diet: low salt intake (less than 3 g per day) and reduced water intake
   - Diuretics: acetazolamide, chlortalidone, hydrochlorothiazide, furosemide. Replace potassium if needed
3. In addition
   - Vasoactive drugs (betahistidine) to improve blood flow in the inner ear
   - Steroids to suppress inflammatory and/or allergic tissue reactions within the inner ear (endolymphatic sac)
4. Avoidance of caffeine, alcohol, tobacco
5. Antiviral approach [1]: oral acyclovir (800 mg 3 times a day) for 3 weeks; if the patient feels better, reduce the dose to 800 mg 2 times a day for 1 month and then to 800 mg daily for another month before ending the treatment.

Semiconservative Treatment

- Insertion of a *transtympanic ventilating tube* (Montandon) (Fig. 1.4.5)
- Transtympanic unilateral *chemical labyrinthectomy with gentamicin*: good results on vertigo control, low to moderate risk of hearing deterioration
- For bilateral cases, intramuscular *streptomycin*
- Following insertion of a transtympanic ventilating tube (Fig. 1.4.5), self-administered treatment with the

Meniett device (intermittent low-pressure pulses to stimulate the flow of the endolymph)

- Intratympanic dexamethasone injections (0.4–1.0 ml)
- Intratympanic application of ganciclovir 50 mg/ml per 10 days through a ventilating tube or a microwick inserted into the tympanic membrane [2].

Surgical Treatment

- Endolymphatic sac decompression: Sham operation or first-line procedure? Control of vertigo attacks in approximately 70% of patients.
- Vestibular neurectomy (middle fossa or retrosigmoid approach). This procedure has a 98% success rate in relieving vertigo, which is the most distressing symptom, but does not improve hearing.
- Labyrinthectomy, which implies the complete loss of hearing; high success rate in eliminating major vertigo attacks.
- Vestibulotomy: high success rate (control of vertigo 90%, reduction of tinnitus loudness 60%, risk of hearing loss).
- Tenotomy (section of the tensor tympani and stapedius muscle tendons): a new entry.

Note: *Ménière's disease does not have a currently known cause and this may explain the variety of therapeutic options and some geographical differences.*

References

1. Gacek RP (2008) Evidence for a viral neuropathy in recurrent vertigo. ORL 70:6–15
2. Guyot JP, Maire R, Delaspre O (2008) Intratympanic application of an antiviral agent for the treatment of Ménière's disease. ORL 70:21–26

Suggested Reading

1. Arnold W, Ganzer U (2006) Checkliste: Hals-Nasen-Ohren-Heilkunde. Thieme, Stuttgart, pp 190–193, 531–533
2. Arnold W, Niedermeyer HP (1997) Herpes simplex virus antibodies in the perilymph of patients with Ménière's disease. Arch Otolaryngol Head Neck Surg 123:53–56
3. Bojrab DI, Bhansali SA, Battista RA (1994) Peripheral vestibular disorders. In: Jackler RK, Brackmann DE (eds) Neurotology. Mosby, St Louis, pp 629–650
4. Committee on Hearing and Equilibrium (1995) Guidelines for the diagnosis and evaluation of therapy in Menière's disease. Otolaryngol Head Neck Surg 113:181–185
5. Hamann K, Arnold W (1999) Ménière's disease: a review. Adv Otorhinolaryngol 55:137–168
6. Vrabec JT (2003) Herpes simplex virus and Ménière's disease. Laryngoscope 11:1431–1438

1.6.7 Autoimmune Inner Ear Disease

ROBERTO BOVO AND ALESSANDRO MARTINI

1.6.7.1 Synonyms

Autoimmune hearing loss, immune-mediated inner ear disease.

1.6.7.2 Aetiology/Epidemiology

- An underlying genetic predisposition results in autoimmune disease expression following immunoregulatory defects in immune response to unknown environmental pathogens.
- Today there is substantial evidence of autoimmune mechanisms in relapsing polychondritis (Fig. 1.3.2c), cochlear vasculitis (e.g. Cogan's syndrome), progressive sensorineural hearing loss of both sides and some types of sudden deafness.
- With regards to Ménière's disease, around 16% of bilateral cases and 6% of monolateral cases may be due to immune dysfunction.
- Autoimmune inner ear disease represents less than 1% of all cases of hearing impairment or dizziness; nevertheless, the diagnosis might be overlooked because of the lack of a specific diagnostic test. The disease seems to be more common in females than in males; the first onset of symptoms generally occurs between 20 and 50 years of age.
- Sympathetic cochleopathy: sudden sensorineural hearing loss in the last hearing ear (similar to sympathetic ophthalmopathy).

1.6.7.3 Symptoms

- Hearing loss: a rapidly progressive, often fluctuating, *bilateral* sensorineural hearing loss over a period of weeks to months. The progression of hearing loss is too rapid to be diagnosed as idiopathic progressive sensorineural *hearing loss* or presbyacusis and too slow to conclude a diagnosis of sudden sensorineural hearing loss.
- Tinnitus: 25–50% of patients also have tinnitus (ringing, hissing, roaring) and aural fullness, which can fluctuate.
- Vertigo and/or imbalance: generalized imbalance, ataxia, motion intolerance, positional vertigo and episodic vertigo may be present in up to 50% of patients.
- Occasionally only one ear is affected initially, but bilateral hearing loss occurs in most patients (80%), with symmetric or asymmetric audiometric thresholds.

- Systemic autoimmune disease coexists in up to 20% of patients (systemic lupus erythematosus, rheumatoid arthritis, disseminated vasculitis, Sjögren's syndrome, myasthenia gravis, Hashimoto's thyroiditis, Cogan's syndrome, Behçet's disease, sarcoidosis, Wegener's granulomatosis, colitis ulcerosa, relapsing polychondritis; Fig. 1.3.2c).

1.6.7.4 Diagnostic Procedure

- Currently, the diagnosis of autoimmune inner ear disease is based either on clinical criteria or on a positive response to steroids. There is seldom convincing evidence from broader laboratory tests indicating autoimmunity.
- Detailed history: Endocrine diseases? Recurrent fever?

Physical Examination

Otoscopy findings are usually normal; nevertheless external ear skin and/or cartilage inflammation and/or facial palsy may rarely occur (e.g. relapsing polychondritis), as well as tissue destruction at the level of the tympanic membrane, middle ear and mastoid (e.g. Wegener's granulomatosis).

Laboratory Studies

There are no antigen-specific tests (migration inhibition test, lymphocyte transformation test and western blot analysis) that are commercially available and proven to be useful for the diagnosis of systemic autoimmune diseases.

In clinical practice next to the indispensable blood sedimentation rate (BSR) a non-specific antigen screening test may be useful for evidence of systemic immunologic dysfunction; yet it does not strictly correlate with a diagnosis of immune-mediated inner ear disease.

Recommended tests are:

- Blood tests for autoimmune disorders: levels of circulating immune complexes, BSR, antinuclear antibodies, rheumatoid factor, complement C1Q, smooth muscle antibody, TSH and antimicrosomal antibodies, antigliadin antibodies (for celiac disease), HLA testing.
- Blood tests for conditions that resemble autoimmune disorders: fluorescent treponemal antibody absorption test (for syphilis), Lyme titre, HbA1c (for diabetes, which is often also autoimmune-mediated), HIV (HIV is associated with auditory neuropathy).

Note that a commercially available test, called "anti-68 kD (hsp-70) western blot" (OTOblot™) was reported to detect a local autoimmune inner ear process in the absence of any systemic autoimmune process and to be correlated with steroid responsiveness. The test uses purified hsp-70 kDa antigen from a bovine kidney cell line and is based on the assumption that the 68-kDa protein is heat shock protein 70 (hsp-70). Unfortunately, this assumption has now been refuted: in fact, there is mounting evidence that the target antigen of the 68-kDa antibody is not hsp-70 (as was believed over the last 15 years), but the human choline transporter-like protein 2 (CTL2). Furthermore, the sensitivity and specificity of this test are very low.

1.6.7.5   Differential Diagnosis

- Bilateral Ménière's disease
- Luetic inner ear disease
- Lyme disease
- Toxoplasmosis
- Treatment with ototoxic drugs (gentamicin, cisplatin)
- Charcot–Marie–Tooth disease (hereditary neuropathy)
- Large vestibular aqueduct syndrome
- Endocranic hypertension

1.6.7.6   Therapy

- Prednisolone, 1 mg/kg per day for 4 weeks followed by a gradual tapering over several weeks to a maintenance dose of 10–20 mg per day or every other day. Shorter-term or lower-dose long-term therapy either has been ineffective or appears to increase the risk of relapse. Patients often learn the necessary maintenance dose to preserve their hearing, as the disease activity often waxes and vanishes. If hearing suddenly worsens or tinnitus reappears in one or both ears during the tapering period, repetition of the initial high-dose treatment is indicated.
- Oral as well as systemic steroid treatment over long period of time should always be accompanied by proton pump inhibitors to avoid a gastric ulcer.
- In patients with no response to steroids within 6–8 weeks, methotrexate and cyclophosphamide have been used over the long term. These agents are associated with considerable toxicity and the decision regarding when and how to use them should always be multidisciplinary. The normal oral dose of methotrexate is 7.5–20 mg weekly with folic acid. Cyclophosphamide in addition to steroids has been used with the following regimen: cyclophosphamide 5mg/kg per day intravenously for 2 weeks, followed by a rest period of 2 weeks, and then a final period of infusions for 2 weeks.

1.6.7.7   Prognosis

Autoimmune inner ear disease is analogous to rapidly progressive glomerulonephritis. If not treated, the inner ear inflammation progresses to severe irreversible damage within 3 months of onset (and often much more quickly). On the other hand, steroid responsiveness is high and with prompt treatment the hearing loss may be reversible. Nevertheless, several patients become steroid-dependent.

Suggested Reading

1. Arnold W (1977) Systemic autoimmune diseases associated with hearing loss. Ann N Y Acad Sci 29:187–202
2. Disher MJ et al. (1997) Human autoantibodies and monoclonal antibody KHRI-3 bind to a phylogenetically conserved inner-ear-supporting cell antigen. Ann N Y Acad Sci 830:253–265
3. Bovo R, Aimoni C, Martini A (2006) Immune-mediated inner ear disease. Acta Otolaryngol 126:1012–1021
4. McCabe B (1979) Autoimmune sensorineural hearing loss. Ann Otol 88:585–589
5. Yoo TJ, Yazawa Y (2003) Immunology of cochlear and vestibular disorders. In: Luxon L (ed) Audiological medicine—clinical aspects of hearing and balance. Taylor & Francis, London, pp 61–87

1.6.8   Tinnitus

KERSTIN LAMM

1.6.8.1   Synonym

Ringing in the ears (from Latin *tinnire* meaning "ringing").

1.6.8.2   Definition/Symptoms

It is important to distinguish between objective and subjective tinnitus:
- Patients affected by an **objective tinnitus** notice a *real existent endogenous acoustic source* originating in the middle ear, Eustachian tube, soft palate or extracranial or intracranial vessels. Such acoustic phenomena may also be perceived by the non-affected fellow human being using a stethoscope; however, the incidence of this kind of tinnitus is relatively seldom. Depending on the underlying disease, the patients notice intermittent clicks or crackles due to spasm of the middle

ear muscles or myoclonus of soft palate muscles, respiratory noise and breath, respectively, due to an abnormally wide Eustachian tube, or a pulsatile noise due to intracranial hypertension, glomus tumour, angioma, aneurysm, arteriovenous fistula, stenosis or thrombosis of extracranial or intracranial vessels as well as due to systemic rheological diseases such as hyperglobulinaemia or anaemia.

- In contrast, a **subjective tinnitus** is exclusively perceived by the affected patient. In most cases it consists in an intermittent or continuous whistling or fizzling, in broadband or narrowband noise, hum, ping or ringing, or even in pure tones of various frequency, intensity and duration. Such auditory perceptions emerge from deficient neuronal plasticity within the central auditory system triggered by an auditory input failure. In this respect, a subjective tinnitus is *a symptom of any disease of the peripheral and/or central auditory system* associated with malfunction of hearing. In this particular context it should be emphasized that *tinnitus is not* a symptom of an organic or functional disease of the cervical spine, temporomandibular joint or any other orthopaedic or dental distress; likewise tinnitus is not caused by emotional, mental or physical distress, although the intensity and annoyance of tinnitus may be amplified by such problems.

1.6.8.3   Epidemiology

There are no epidemiological data available concerning the incidence and prevalence of an **objective tinnitus.**

A transient **subjective tinnitus** is perceived by about 35–45% of the population of industrial nations at least once in their life; 13–17% have perceived tinnitus over a longer period in their life, with an annual incidence of 0.33% in Germany.

The point-prevalence of a constant chronic tinnitus (perceived as longer than 6 months up to years) averages about 4% of the population of industrial nations, of which about 0.5–1% regard themselves as severely psychoemotionally affected.

Of those patients who perceive tinnitus over a longer period in their life, 35–37% *notice the tinnitus in a silent environment only (grade I)*; 44–51% perceive their tinnitus permanently, however it *may be masked by moderate environmental noise (grade II)*. In only 14–17% of cases is tinnitus *perceived even in a relatively loud environment (grade III)*.

According to a recent evaluation of about 12,000 members of the German Tinnitus Support Group (Deutsche Tinnitus-Liga, http://www.tinnitus-liga.de) who perceived tinnitus for more than 6 months up to years, 45% localized their tinnitus in both ears, while a further 24% localized their tinnitus perception in the middle of the head. Of the unilaterally affected, 29% perceived tinnitus in the left ear and 20% in the right ear.

The high incidence of bilateral tinnitus averaging about 46% and the slight preference of the left ear is also known from former evaluations among non-selected populations.

The prevalence of tinnitus is only somewhat higher (by 1–5%) in females than in males.

Respecting the age distribution, manifestation of tinnitus is most common between 40 and 60 years of age; however, there is an increasing incidence of noise-induced tinnitus in younger people owing to exposure to leisure noise such as noisy toys, amplified music, motorcycling and other loud recreational activities. Data from long-term studies concerning the incidence and prevalence of a chronic tinnitus (for more than 6 months up to years) in this population are not available so far.

1.6.8.4   Aetiology

Concerning an **objective tinnitus**, there are no data available regarding the incidence of the underlying diseases, as mentioned already in Sect. 1.6.8.2.

The **subjective tinnitus** is a symptom of any diseases of the peripheral and/or central auditory system associated with malfunction of hearing in the following descending order of incidence: in **32%** tinnitus is being caused by **noise-induced damage of the inner ear** due to single or repetitive exposure to industrial or leisure noise; in **12%** by **acute acoustic trauma of the inner ear** due to single or repetitive sound impulses from pistols, revolvers, military rifles, sport guns, firecrackers, fireworks and others; in **8–10%** by **idiopathic sensorineural hearing loss** (sudden deafness); in **8%** by **Ménière's disease** (morbus Ménière); in **7%** by **age-related sensorineural hearing loss** (presbyacusis); in **6%** by **toxic labyrinthitis** due to an acute serous or purulent otitis media; in **4%** by **chronic otitis media** inclusive of cholesteatoma; in **2–3%** by **otosclerosis**; and in **1%** by a **vestibular schwannoma** (acoustic neurinoma).

In the **remaining 20–23%** tinnitus may be caused by obliteration of the outer ear canal with wax, exostosis or others; myringitis, rupture or perforation of the ear drum; dysfunction of the Eustachian tube due to acute or chronic infections of the upper respiratory tract; barotrauma of the middle ear; tympanosclerosis; luxation of the incudomalleal or incudostapedial articulation; rupture of the round window membrane; perilymphatic fistula of the round or oval window; labyrinthine contusion or fracture of the temporal bone due to head trauma; meningitis or encephalitis; ototoxic medication (aminoglycosides, cisplatin, etc.); intoxication by alcohol or drugs; peridural anaesthesia; lumbar puncture; multiple sclerosis; neurofibromatosis; neurolues; polyneuropathia; varicella zoster infection; systemic viral infections (rubella, measles, mumps, etc.); borreliosis; inner ear hearing loss associated with various syndromes (Alport, Addison, Cogan, Usher, etc.) or other autoimmune diseases (sympathic cochleopathia similar to sympathic ophtalmopathy, periarteritis nodosa, granulomatosis Wegener, lupus erythematodes, etc.); inner ear hearing loss associated with diabetes, arterial hypertension, renal failure etc.; and congenital inner ear hearing loss.

In summary, *there are almost 100 diseases of the peripheral and/or central auditory system which may cause tinnitus.* In this respect, an accurate otoneurological diagnostic procedure is of prime importance.

1.6.8.5   Diagnostic Procedures

Recommended European Standard
1. Detailed case history in the style of standardized tinnitus questionnaires, e. g. according to Goebel and Hiller (1998)
    – Type/character of tinnitus: unilateral, bilateral, in the head; intermittent or continuous; frequency; masking level by environmental noise—grade I–III (see Sect. 1.6.8.3); fluctuant or constant loudness
    – Visual analogue scale (range from 1 to 10) concerning loudness and annoyance
    – Onset and duration
    – Potential causal relationship and trigger mechanisms (exposure to noise of any kind, etc.)
    – Associated hearing problems, hyperacusis or phonophobia
    – Vestibular complaints
    – History of otorhinolaryngological diseases and surgery
    – History of head trauma and/or other accidents, actions under civil law
    – History of internal, neurological, psychiatric or psychosomatic or orthopaedic diseases
    – Alleviating or amplifying circumstances
    – Tinnitus-associated and/or other complaints (sleep disturbance, concentration and attention problems, psychoemotional and psychosocial problems, etc.)
    – Family status
    – Profession, still working, claim for early retirement, retired
    – Recreational activities
2. Microscopy of the ear canal and ear drum
3. Compression–decompression test using the Politzer balloon
4. Tympanometry and stapedial reflex measurements (ipsilateral and contralateral evoked reflex responses at 0.5, 1, 2 and 4 kHz)

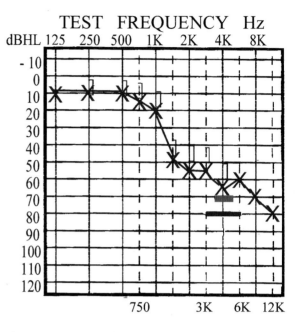

Fig. 1.6.7 Tinnitus analysis: the patient described his tinnitus as similar to a 4-kHz tone with an intensity of 70 dB. A broadband 80-dB noise masked the tinnitus which was heard again by the patient after 1 min, which means that a residual inhibition was not present. *Red line* tinnitus, *blue line* broadband noise

5. Pure tone audiogram (0.125, 0.25, 0.5, 0.75, 1, 1.5, 2, 3, 4, 6 and 8 kHz)
6. Audiometric tinnitus measurement [frequency-matching, intensity (Fig. 1.6.7), minimal masking level using broadband or narrowband noise or pure tones, residual inhibition]
7. Auditory evoked brainstem responses

Useful Additional Diagnostic Procedures
• Transitory evoked otoacoustic emissions
• Distortion products of otoacoustic emissions
• Auditory evoked cortical responses
• Speech audiometry
• Vestibular tests using video-oculography
• Electrocochleography
• Cerebral MRI in the case of pathological auditory evoked brainstem responses and/or video-oculography findings and/or in the case of a suspected intracranial disease
• CT scan of the temporal bone in the case of chronic otitis media, mastoiditis, cholesteatoma, head trauma, etc.
• Doppler duplex sonography of extracranial and intracranial vessels, if necessary angio-MRI
• Rhinoscopy using 0°/30° endoscopes

- Posterior rhinoscopy using a 70° endoscope
- Sonography of the maxillary and frontal paranasal sinuses
- Pharyngoscopy
- Hypopharyngoscopy and laryngoscopy using a 90° endoscope
- Exploratory vestibular tests using Frenzel glasses
- Depending on the case history, internal, neurological, psychosomatic or orthopaedic examination

1.6.8.6 Therapy

Objective Tinnitus

Treatment is directed to the underlying disease:

- In the case of spasms of the middle ear muscles, myringotomy and insertion of a grommet or transection of the tensor tympanic muscle or stapedial tendon may be helpful.
- In the case of a myoclonus of soft palate muscles, injection of botulinum toxin achieves relatively good results.
- If the patient perceives respiratory noise and breath owing to an abnormally wide Eustachian tube, an attempt to treat the tinnitus by application of an inert ointment onto the ear drum or myringotomy and insertion of a grommet may be worthwhile.
- A pulsatile tinnitus due to intracranial hypertension may require neurosurgery in selected cases. A pulsatile tinnitus due to angioma, aneurysm, arteriovenous fistula, stenosis, thrombosis of extracranial or intracranial vessels as well as due to systemic rheological diseases such as hyperglobulinaemia or anaemia should be treated by the angiologist and vascular surgeon, respectively.
- For surgical and/or radiation therapy of a glomus tumour, see Sect. 1.5.4.3.

Subjective Tinnitus

Subjective tinnitus cannot be treated directly. In fact, treatment is targeted to the underlying disease of the peripheral and/or central auditory system to achieve elimination of auditory input failure, thereby correcting pathological neuronal plasticity within the central auditory system. It is important to explain these issues to the patient in the acute stage, e.g. **first tinnitus counselling**.

1. **Acute stage (less than 3 months' duration)**. Acute tinnitus due to noise-induced damage or acoustic trauma of the inner ear, idiopathic sensorineural hearing loss (sudden deafness), acute attack of Ménière's disease, toxic labyrinthitis, rupture of the round window, perilymphatic fistula of the round or oval window, labyrinthine contusion or fractures of the temporal bone

due to head trauma should be treated with a daily dose of 250–500 mg **prednisolone** intravenously on three consecutive days. In the case of partial or no remission, prednisolone treatment should be continued orally for 16 days, starting with 100, 80, 60, 40, 20, 10, 5 and 2.5 mg each on two consecutive days. Prednisolone therapy should be accompanied by gastric proton pump inhibitors (40 mg omeprazole per day or 150 mg ranitidine per day or others).

In patients presenting with contraindications (e.g. diabetes, severe chronic gastritis, gastric or duodenal ulcer) for the treatment with corticosteroids classified as glucocorticoids such as prednisolone, infusion therapy as described below may be a good alternative option.

In cases of severe hearing loss, *additional* intravenous infusion therapy using a hyperosmotic hydrophilic haemodilutive plasma-expanding agent, such as *hydroxyethyl starch* or others (250–500 ml/day for 5–10 days), would be reasonable to improve microcirculation. However, contraindications (e.g. arterial hypertension) should be noted, and potential side effects (e.g. temporary pruritus) should be considered. *In the case of contraindications for haemodilution*, another haemorheological active drug such as *pentoxiphylline* (100 mg, equivalent to 5 ml/day dissolved in 100 ml 0.9% isotonic saline) may be intravenously infused for 5–10 days.

If this initial therapy with prednisolone and/or haemodilutive or alternative haemorheological agents is only partially effective or not effective at all, and this is the case in over 25% of patients, *hyperbaric oxygenation therapy* should be started as soon as possible (ten to 15 sessions on ten to 15 consecutive days). However, according to clinical trials therapeutic results on tinnitus are only available from patients suffering from acoustic trauma, noise-induced hearing loss and idiopathic sensory-neural hearing loss (sudden deafness); therefore, hyperbaric oxygenation therapy should be restricted to these three indications.

For additional treatment of tinnitus due to an acute attack of Ménière's disease, toxic labyrinthitis, rupture of the round window, perilymphatic fistula of the round or oval window, labyrinthine contusion or fractures of the temporal bone due to head trauma, see the specific sections.

Likewise, for treatment of all other diseases of the peripheral and/or central auditory system which may cause a subjective tinnitus, such as chronic otitis media, cholesteatoma, mastoiditis, otosclerosis and vestibular schwannoma (acoustic neurinoma), see the specific sections.

2. **Subacute stage (duration of more than 3 months up to 1 year) and chronic stage (duration of more than 1 year)**. In both, the subacute and the chronic stage a

second tinnitus counselling should be performed as follows:

– Tinnitus is an auditory phantom perception which emerges from deficient neuronal plasticity within the central auditory system triggered by an auditory input failure due to any disease of the peripheral and/or central auditory system.
– It is ensured that all aforementioned initial therapies and/or other causal treatment of the underlying disease of the peripheral and/or central auditory system have failed to ameliorate or eliminate tinnitus at the latest by the end of the subacute stage.
– The patient should be briefed that *the following* pharmaceuticals, natural remedies and other therapeutic strategies have been *proven to have no persistent effect on subacute and/or chronic tinnitus in placebo-controlled clinical trials:* intratympanal application of glucocorticoids, lidocaine, glutamate-receptor agonists or antagonists; systemic administration of antiarrhythmics such as lidocaine, anticonvulsive drugs such as lamotrigine or carbamazepine, antidepressives such as trimipramine, nortriptyline or amitriptyline, benzodiazepines such as diazepam or alprazolam, vasodilative drugs such as pentoxifylline, cyclandelate, prostaglandin E1, analogues of histamine such as betahistine, antagonists of histamine receptors such as cinnarizine, calcium antagonists such as flunarizine or trimetazidine, GABA agonists such as baclofen, antiphlogistic drugs such as azapropazone, diuretics such as dyazide, melatonin, zinc, vitamins, *Ginkgo biloba*, laser therapy of any kind with or without *Ginkgo biloba*, acupuncture of any kind, ultrasonic therapy and electromagnetic stimulation of any kind.
– Therefore, in the chronic stage correction of pathological neuronal plasticity within the central auditory system cannot be achieved directly by pharmaceuticals, natural remedies or other treatment strategies already mentioned, but can be achieved indirectly by compensation of the remaining hearing loss using hearing aids as soon as possible. However, in cases where hearing loss is less than 30 dB HL at three or fewer frequencies (2 kHz included), a broadband noise generator (formerly tinnitus masking device) may be helpful to defocus on tinnitus.
– In addition, active listening to music of someone's own choice and/or to audiobooks are reasonable therapeutic auditory training strategies which may be helpful to direct the patient's attention to external auditory stimuli again.

– Patients presenting with tinnitus-associated and/or other complaints, such as sleep disturbance, concentration and attention problems, psychoemotional and psychosocial problems, should be admitted to a cognitive tinnitus coping therapy including a multimodal behavioural treatment in a specialized psychotherapeutic–psychosomatic outpatient department, or in selected cases to a psychotherapeutic–psychosomatic inpatient clinic.
– A promising novel therapeutic innovation is neurofeedback training, which has been shown to effectively relieve stress-associated symptoms and thereby annoyance of tinnitus.

1.6.8.7   Prognosis

The outcome is dependent on the quality of the initial and the following medical attendance, e.g.:

- Briefing of the patient that tinnitus perceptions emerge from deficient neuronal plasticity within the central auditory system triggered by an auditory input failure.
- An accurate case history and otoneurological examination to diagnose the disease of the peripheral and/or central auditory system which has caused the tinnitus.
- Briefing of the patient that pharmaceutical and/or surgical treatment can be only targeted on the tinnitus-underlying disease of the peripheral and/or central auditory system to achieve elimination or at least reduction of the auditory input failure and malfunction of hearing, respectively.
- Including technical devices if necessary.
- Including psychotherapeutic–psychosomatic treatment strategies if necessary.

Suggested Reading

1. Bartels H, Staal MJ, Albers FW (2007) Tinnitus and neural plasticity of the brain. Otol Neurotol 28:178–184
2. Dohrmann K, Elbert T, Schlee W, Weisz N (2007) Tuning the tinnitus percept by modification of synchronous brain activity. Restor Neurol Neurosci 25:371–378
3. Dohrmann K, Weisz N, Schlee W, Hartmann T, Elbert T (2007) Neurofeedback for treating tinnitus. Prog Brain Res 166:473–485
4. Møller AR (2006) Neural plasticity in tinnitus. Prog Brain Res 157:365–372
5. Schenk S, Lamm K, Gündel H, Ladwig KH (2005) Neurofeedback-based EEG alpha and EEG beta training. Effectiveness in patients with chronically decompensated tinnitus. HNO 53:29–37

1.6.9 Noise-induced Hearing Loss

UWE GANZER AND ANDREAS ARNOLD

The disorder is defined as hearing loss caused by acute or chronic exposure to high-intensity sound.

1.6.9.1 Explosions

Definition
Impulse sound exposure with an intensity above 150 dB(A) SPL peak equivalent with a peak sound pressure duration greater than 3 ms.

Aetiology/Epidemiology
Explosion traumas are seen in explosives fabrication and the processing industry, in the military, in the gas, tyre and chemical industry as well as in motor vehicle accidents. Additionally, they can occur from a physical injury to the ear, such as a blow to the side of the head, diving head first into water or deployment of an airbag.

Symptoms/Findings
An explosion trauma of the ear generally leads to inner ear damage concomitant with a rupture of the eardrum and, most often, a disruption of the ossicular chain (Fig. 1.4.1b). This leads to a unilateral or bilateral, moderate to severe combined (conductive and sensorineural) hearing loss with otalgia, tinnitus and, frequently, vestibular symptoms. At the time of examination, a serous otitis media has commonly developed.

Complications
Complete hearing loss and tinnitus are feared. Further complications are long-lasting vertigo and rupture of the round window membrane.

Diagnostic Procedures
- Detailed patient history—important in the case of a later lawsuit and for expert reports.
- Complete ENT examination.
- Otomicroscopy, with special attention to perforations of the tympanic membrane, haemotympanum and pathologic secretion.
- Hearing test battery: tuning fork, audiogram, speech audiogram, testing of recruitment. Mostly, the findings are a single-sided or unilateral pronounced high-frequency hearing loss or a pancochlear sensorineural hearing loss up to deafness. Recruitment is positive. In the case of rupture of the ear drum and/or luxation of ossicles, an additional conductive hearing loss is present.
- Vestibular testing: exclusion of spontaneous and provoked nystagmus with Frenzel glasses. Positional and positioning tests and examination of vestibulospinal reflexes. Assessment of vibration nystagmus can be helpful.

Additional/Useful Diagnostic Procedures
- Video-oculography (VOG) or electronystagmography (ENG). An eventual caloric testing must be performed with cold and warm air insufflation in the case of ear drum injury.
- Tinnitus analysis with subjective loudness assessment and testing of masking possibility (Fig. 1.6.7).

Therapy

Conservative Treatment
- As in sudden hearing loss (see Sect. 1.6.5)
- Initiate hyperbaric oxygen therapy as soon as possible!

Surgical Treatment
- In the case of complete hearing loss and suspicion of rupture of a cochlear window: tympanotomy and covering of a perilymphatic fistula
- In case of ear drum rupture: myringoplasty, tympanoplasty
- The surgical treatment is no replacement for conservative therapy. If needed, it is carried out additionally

Differential Diagnosis
The circumstances surrounding the patient's accident and the clinical findings derived from the patient's medical history should allow consideration of other possible diagnoses:
- Cochlear window rupture
- Sudden hearing loss (see Sect. 1.6.5)
- Toxic inner ear damage
- Craniocerebral injury, distortion of the cervical spine (whiplash injury)

Prognosis
- If high-dose glucocorticoid and rheologic therapy, perhaps combined with a hyperbaric oxygen therapy, is administered within 12 h after an acute incident, recovery of hearing is expected in up to 75% of cases. A

minor high-frequency sensorineural hearing loss and a more or less disturbing tinnitus can persist in spite of rapid and correct therapy.
- The chances of spontaneous recovery without therapy is low. Sometimes untreated post-traumatic hearing loss is progressive.

Surgical Principles
- Myringoplasty (see Sect. 1.4.6)
- Tympanoplasty (see Sect. 1.4.6)

Special Remarks
With occupational explosion trauma, special compensation insurance must be addressed (Berufsgenossenschaft in Germany, SUVA in Switzerland, INAIL in Italy).

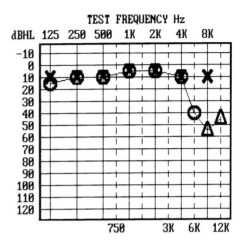

Fig. 1.6.8 Acoustic trauma at the right ear following airbag (full-size) explosion

1.6.9.2   Impulsive Noise Trauma

Synonyms
Shooting trauma, muzzle blast trauma.

Definition
Impulse sound exposure with an intensity above 150 dB(A) SPL peak equivalent with a peak sound pressure duration shorter than 3 ms (normally 0.4–1.5 ms).

Aetiology/Epidemiology
The main cause of shooting trauma is inappropriate use of a handgun, e.g. in the military, by police or by hunters. However, also guns firing blanks and toy guns produce sound pressures greater 100 dB(A)! Additionally, fireworks and airbags (Fig. 1.6.8) can cause muzzle blast trauma.

Symptoms/Findings
Otomicroscopy shows no abnormalities. In audiometric testing, there is an acute, most often unilateral mild to moderate sensorineural hearing loss of around 4 kHz (c^5 notch) and a positive recruitment. Tinnitus in the damaged ear is common. Sometimes otalgia or vestibular disturbance is present. In the case of repeated muzzle blast trauma in a short period of time (toy gun), a steep high-frequency hearing loss above 2 kHz develops.

Complications
Persistent tinnitus. Complete deafness or persistent vestibular vertigo is very rare.

Diagnostic Procedures
- Detailed patient history—important in the case of a later lawsuit and for expert reports
- Complete ENT examination
- Otomicroscopy, with special attention to perforations of the tympanic membrane
- Hearing test battery: tuning forks, audiogram (typical c^5 notch), speech audiogram, testing of recruitment
- Tinnitus-analysis with subjective loudness-assessment and testing of masking possibility

Additional/Useful Diagnostic Procedures
- Distortion products of otoacoustic emissions (DPOAE), otoacoustic emissions (OAE).
- Vestibular testing: exclusion of spontaneous and provoked nystagmus with Frenzel glasses. Positional and positioning tests and examination of vestibulospinal reflexes.
- Caloric vestibular testing with or without VOG/ENG.
- Brainstem evoked response audiometry (BERA): at the earliest 1 week after the incident, because of the additional noise exposure.

Therapy

Conservative Treatment
- As in sudden hearing loss (see Sect. 1.6.5).
- With more severe inner ear damage, initiate additional hyperbaric oxygen therapy as soon as possible.

Surgical Treatment
- In the case of complete hearing loss and suspicion of rupture of a cochlear window: tympanotomy and closure of a perilymphatic fistula (see Sect. 1.6.5).

- The surgical treatment is no replacement for conservative therapy. If needed, it is carried out additionally.

Differential Diagnosis

Derived from patient history, the event of accident and clinical findings any of the following other possible diagnoses should be considered:
- Cochlear window rupture
- Contusio labyrinthi
- Distortion of the cervical spine (whiplash injury)

Prognosis

- An initial good recovery of the high-frequency hearing loss occurs in approximately half of the cases. After some weeks, a remaining hearing loss or a persisting tinnitus must be considered as permanent damage. A post-traumatic increase of hearing loss above 2 kHz is possible. A spontaneous recovery of a high-frequency tinnitus is rare.
- If high-dose glucocorticoid, rheologic therapy and hyperbaric oxygen therapy is administered as soon as possible, recovery to normal hearing is frequently achievable.

Special Remarks

With occupational blast trauma any special compensation insurance must be addressed (Berufsgenossenschaft in Germany, SUVA in Switzerland, INAIL in Italy).

1.6.9.3 Acute Acoustic Trauma

Definition

Broadband sound exposure with an intensity above 100 dB(A) SPL peak equivalent for minutes to hours.

Aetiopathology

Exposure to non-impulse permanent sound causes metabolic as well as mechanical ultrastructurally visible damage at the level of the organ of Corti (outer hair cells, stereocilia). Excessive demand for oxygen and subsequent progressive ischaemia of the cochlea lead to production of free radicals, depletion of endogenous cellular antioxidants and, finally, apoptotic cell death.

Epidemiology

- Discotheques: averaged over 15 min, a music sound pressure level of 100–110 dB(A) with sound pressure peaks of up to 125–130 dB(A) SPL can be measured.

- Concerts: heavy metal, punk, hard rock reach sound pressure peaks of up to 120 dB(A), rock and pop up to 110 dB(A).
- Walkman: averaged music sound pressure level of 85–89 dB(A). In 3% of Walkman-users sound pressure levels reach up to 110 dB(A).
- Musical instruments: drums, percussion and wind instruments played indoors quickly reach sound intensities loud enough to cause hearing loss. Infants are most endangered (music school!).
- Toys: tool imitations, toy ambulances, military imitations, etc. produce an average sound pressure level of up to 100 dB(A) at a distance of 10 cm from the ear or 130–140 dB(A) directly at the ear.
- Motor sports, airplanes, do-it-yourself hobbies can reach sound intensities of up to 100 dB(A).
- Low-level flights: 50% have peak levels around 85–119 dB(A) and 2% even peak levels of around 120–125 dB(A) with impulselike, steep peak attacks. Such sounds can be encountered at or near airports.

Symptoms

Acute, most often bilateral, mild to moderate high-frequency sensorineural hearing loss (c^5 notch) with positive recruitment. Tinnitus is frequent, as is a temporary threshold shift. Otalgias or vestibular symptoms occur rarely.

Complications

Permanent hearing loss and/or tinnitus.

Diagnostic Procedures

- Detailed patient history—important in the case of a later lawsuit and for expert reports.
- Complete ENT examination.
- Otomicroscopy: without pathological findings.
- Hearing test battery: tuning fork, audiogram (typical c^5 notch), speech audiogram, testing of recruitment. Findings are most often a unilateral or more severe on one side c^5 notch or a pantonal sensorineural hearing loss of varying degree. The recruitment is always positive.
- Tinnitus analysis with subjective loudness assessment and testing of masking possibility.

Additional/Useful Diagnostic Procedures

- Vestibular testing: exclusion of spontaneous and provoked nystagmus with Frenzel glasses. Testing of vibration nystagmus. Positional and positioning tests and examination of vestibulospinal reflexes
- VOG/ENG with caloric vestibular testing

- DPOAE, OAE
- BERA: at the earliest 1 week after the incident, because of the additional noise exposure

Therapy

Conservative Treatment

As in sudden hearing loss (see Sect. 1.6.5).

Differential Diagnosis

Derived from patient history and examination:

- Explosion trauma (see Sect. 1.6.9.1)
- Shooting trauma (see Sect. 1.6.9.2)
- Sudden idiopathic hearing loss (see Sect. 1.6.5)
- Contusio labyrinthi (see Sect. 1.6.3)

Prognosis

The prognosis is unfavourable despite correct therapy; progress is possible.

1.6.9.4   Occupational Hearing Loss

Definition

Bilateral, mostly symmetric sensorineural hearing loss following intermittent exposure to broadband and/or impulse sound with an intensity above 80–85 dB(A) and a daily exposure of 6–8 h (work shift) over many years. Therefore, it is a matter of chronic noise damage.

Aetiopathology

Chronic noise exposure causes metabolic as well as mechanic ultrastructural visible damage at the level of the organ of Corti, initially causing a loss of outer hair cells, leading finally to neuronal degeneration. Typically, hearing loss initially occurs as a sensorineural high-frequency notch, normally at 4 kHz (c^5 notch). The middle frequencies, e.g. the main speech frequencies, are affected considerably later. The recruitment is always positive. In approximately 70% of cases, a bilateral tonal tinnitus exists. The extent and the progress of the hearing loss depend on the intensity, duration of exposure and frequency composition of the sound as well as the duration of recovery phases and the *individual noise susceptibility*. An individual noise susceptibility is suspected in genetically predamaged inner ears, after sudden hearing loss, after treatment with ototoxic medication and trauma. Moreover, humans with blond hair, fair complexion and lightly coloured eyes seem to be especially endangered owing to a lack of melanin.

Aetiology/Epidemiology

By definition, noise-induced hearing loss is an effect of working in noise and therefore occurs most frequently in metalworkers, mineworkers, airport workers, radio operators, disc jockeys and military personnel as well as construction workers and orchestra musicians, etc.

Symptoms

Because of extensive recruitment, this progressive binaural hearing loss leads to an important communication problem in noisy environments (conversation of multiple persons, theatre, restaurant). A pronounced hyperacusis is common. Tinnitus is found in 70% of patients.

Complications

Social isolation following hearing loss, psychiatric impairment secondary to the tinnitus.

Diagnostic Procedures

- Detailed patient history, including professional and recreational sound exposure. If necessary, inquire regarding professional sound exposure at employment or special insurance organizations (Berufsgenossenschaft in Germany, SUVA in Switzerland, INAIL in Italy).
- Complete ENT examination.
- Otomicroscopy: without pathological findings.
- Hearing test battery: tuning fork, audiogram, speech audiogram, tympanometry, stapedial reflexes, testing of recruitment.
- Tinnitus analysis (Fig. 1.6.7) with subjective loudness assessment and testing of masking possibility.

Additional/Useful Diagnostic Procedures

- OAE, DPOAE, transitory evoked otoacoustic emissions.
- BERA, auditory evoked cortical responses.
- VOG/ENG.
- Vestibular testing: exclusion of spontaneous and provoked nystagmus with Frenzel glasses. Positional and positioning tests and examination of vestibulospinal reflexes.

Therapy

Conservative Treatment

- A pharmacological therapy of the chronic noise-induced hearing loss is not possible. Glucocorticoids and rheologics (see Sect. 1.6.5) can be used in an attempt to treat the tinnitus.

- In most cases, the hearing loss can be compensated for with hearing aids. In selected cases, a tinnitus masker can be helpful.

Additional Useful Therapeutic Strategies

By avoidance of noise or use of effective ear protection when working in a noisy environment, the progress of the chronic noise induced hearing loss can be prevented.

Differential Diagnosis

- Presbyacusis (see Sect. 1.6.11), progressive idiopathic hearing loss, hereditary sensorineural hearing loss.
- Drug-induced or toxic sensorineural hearing loss.
- Post-traumatic sensorineural hearing loss following contusio or commotio labyrinthi, craniocerebral injury, distortion of cervical spine (whiplash injury).
- If evident asymmetry of hearing thresholds and/or pathologic findings in vestibular testing or BERA are present, the diagnosis of noise-induced hearing loss is unlikely and a search for a retrocochlear cause of hearing loss (tumour of the cerebellopontine angle, multiple sclerosis, etc.) is necessary.

Prognosis

- After cessation of activity in a noisy environment, noise-induced hearing loss is not progressive anymore. This is the reason why routine use of noise protectors or a change to a less noisy work environment can stop the progression of hearing loss.
- If a sensorineural hearing loss shows progression despite cessation of noise exposure, other or additional causes must be sought.

Special Remarks

1. To reliably distinguish professional noise-induced hearing loss from other types of hearing losses, the following requirements must be fulfilled:
   - An adequate noise exposure has to be confirmed.
   - The hearing loss must have developed during the time of noise exposure.
   - The hearing loss must be more or less symmetric.
2. The patient history must cover questions regarding earlier ear diseases and head injuries.
3. If a noise-induced hearing loss is suspected, any special compensation insurance (Berufsgenossenschaft in Germany, SUVA in Switzerland, INAIL in Italy) must be addressed.
4. For an assessment of noise-induced hearing loss, the recommendations of special insurance organizations (e.g. Berufsgenossenschaft in Germany, SUVA in Switzerland, INAIL in Italy) are important guidelines, which must be obeyed.

Suggested Reading

1. Dobie RA (2001) Noise-induced hearing loss. In: Bailey BJ (ed) Head neck surgery-otolaryngology. 3nd edn. Lippincott-Raven, Philadelphia
2. Sataloff J, Sataloff RT, Menduke H, et al. (1983) Intermittent exposure to noise: effects on hearing. Ann Otol Rhinol Laryngol, 92:623–628
3. Spoendlin H (1971) Primary structural changes in the organ of Corti after acoustic overstimulation. Acta Otolaryngol, 71:166–176

1.6.10 Ototoxicity

SALVATORE IURATO

1.6.10.1 Definition

Adverse effect to the cochlear or vestibular portion of the inner ear caused by pharmaceutical agents.

1.6.10.2 Aetiology/Epidemiology

The most ototoxic compounds in clinical practice are aminoglycoside antibiotics (streptomycin, dihydrostreptomycin, neomycin—all routes of administration, kanamycin, gentamicin), loop diuretics, quinines and chemotherapy agents (cisplatin) (Table 1.6.1).

The incidence of ototoxicity has not been accurately determined. Risk factors are a decreased renal function, increased daily doses, extended duration, concomitant administration with more than one ototoxic drug and prematurity.

1.6.10.3 Symptoms

The following symptoms may be temporary or permanent: high-pitched tinnitus (earliest sign of cochlear damage), hearing loss (with or without vertigo), nausea, dizziness. Initially the loss of hearing affects the high frequencies. As damage progresses, the lower frequencies become involved.

1.6.10.4 Audiometric Monitoring of Risk Patients on Ototoxic Drug Therapy

- Establish "baseline" hearing level (air-conduction thresholds at 0.5, 1, 2, 4, 6 and 8 kHz).
- Repeat the test during therapy (every 2 days, every week). Ototoxicity is defined as a shift from the

Table 1.6.1 Ototoxic compounds in clinical practice

Drugs	Main damage	
	Primarily ototoxic	Primarily vestibulotoxic
Streptomycin	+	+++
Dihydrostreptomycin	+++	+
Neomycin	+++	+
Kanamycin	+++	+
Gentamicin	+	+++
Ethacrynic acid	+	+
Salicylate	+	
Cisplatin	++	

baseline of 15 dB or more at both 6 and 8 kHz, either unilaterally or bilaterally as assessed 5–7 weeks after beginning of the treatment.

- Monitoring of the status of the cochlea with the acoustic emissions and high-frequency audiometry.

1.6.10.5 Prevention

- Discontinue or change the medication (if it is possible).
- Antioxidant therapy (iron chelators, vitamin E, ascorbic acid).
- Prophylactic treatment (aspirin).
- In a patient who has decreased renal function, dose schedules should be adjusted.

1.6.10.6 Rehabilitation

If the hearing is still serviceable, amplification with a hearing aid may be used.

1.6.10.7 Potential Ototoxicity of Topical Otic Preparations

Through a perforation of the tympanic membrane otic drops may enter into the round window niche, diffuse across the round window membrane and reach the membranous labyrinth. Ototoxic preparations include alcohol, povidone iodide, gentamicin, neomycin, polymixin B, chloramphenicol and hydrocortisone. Non-ototoxic preparations include amphotericin B, sulphacetamide, ciprofloxacin, triamcinolone and dexamethasone.

Suggested Reading

1. Bergstrom LV, Thompson PL (1984) Ototoxicity. In: Northern JL (ed) Hearing disorders. Little, Brown. Boston, pp 119–134
2. Riggs LC, Matz GJ, Rybak LP (1998) Ototoxicity. In: Bailey BJ (ed) Head neck surgery–otolaryngology, 2nd edn. Lippincott-Raven, Philadelphia
3. Slattery W, Brownlee R (1955) Otic preparations. In: Swarbick J, Boylan J (eds) Encyclopaedia of pharmaceutical technology, vol 11. Dekker, New York

1.6.11 Presbyacusis

UWE GANZER AND ANDREAS ARNOLD

1.6.11.1 Synonym

Age-related hearing loss.

1.6.11.2 Definition

Presbyacusis describes the progressive sensorineural hearing loss nearly every human experiences starting in the fifth decade of life. It is more or less symmetric and begins in the higher-frequency range with or without tinnitus.

1.6.11.3 Aetiopathology

Degeneration of hair cells, cochlear neurons, stria vascularis, cochlear nerve and components of the central auditory pathway, e.g. cochlear nuclei.

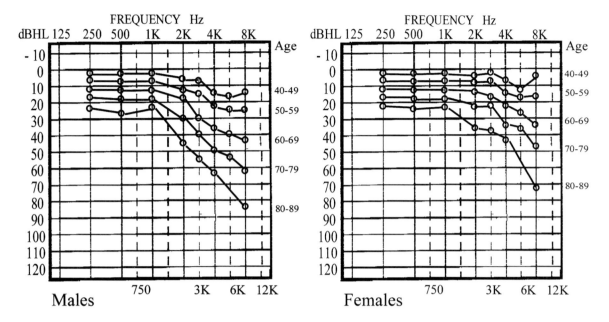

Fig. 1.6.9 Presbyacusis: average hearing loss in industrialized countries correlated with the age

1.6.11.4 Aetiology/Epidemiology

- The hearing loss is caused, on one hand, by the physiologic processes of aging based on individual genetic predisposition and, on the other hand, by exogenous degeneration of parts of the inner ear (supporting cells, basilar membrane, outer hair cells) and central auditory pathway components. The exogenous degeneration is essentially the consequence of environmental influences, nutritional habits, toxicity of legal drugs, professional and recreational noise exposure, ototoxic medications, medical and neurological problems, etc. A hereditary component of presbyacusis has been demonstrated.
- Worldwide, 400 million humans are affected. In the UK 92% of persons older than 60 years show a hearing loss of more than 25 dB. In Denmark, the percentage of hearing loss per decade is 3 dB up to the age of 55 years and 9 dB for persons older than 55 years.

1.6.11.5 Symptoms

Progressive hearing loss with the greatest threshold shift in the high frequencies (Fig. 1.6.9). Speech comprehension is reduced, mainly in ambient noise (party effect), loss of discrimination. Discomfort in noisy environments, during phone calls. Decline of directional hearing. Tinnitus is common.

1.6.11.6 Complications

Psychosocial isolation und suspiciousness of the environment are caused by the loss of ability to communicate, secondary to the hearing loss. Depressive crisis can be triggered by the tinnitus.

1.6.11.7 Diagnostic Procedures

- Detailed patient history, including professional and recreational sound exposure as well as family history.
- Complete ENT examination.
- Otomicroscopy: without pathological findings.
- Hearing test battery: tuning fork, audiogram, speech audiogram, tympanogram and stapedial reflex audiometry. Symmetric sensorineural hearing loss limited to the higher frequencies, pantonal or gently declining from 1 kHz. Poor discrimination in the speech audiogram. Mostly, a positive recruitment is seen. With pancochlear sensorineural hearing loss, recruitment can also be negative.
- Tinnitus analysis with subjective loudness assessment and testing of masking possibility (Fig. 1.6.6).

1.6.11.8 Additional/Useful Diagnostic Procedures

- Basic vestibular testing with Frenzel glasses: exclusion of spontaneous and provoked nystagmus, positional

and positioning tests and examination of vestibulospinal reflexes.
- Brainstem evoked response audiometry: in the case of a clear asymmetry of the hearing loss.
- Vestibular testing with video-oculography/electronystagmography including a caloric test.
- MRI, if the results of vestibular and/or brainstem evoked response audiometry examinations are pathologic.

1.6.11.9 Therapy

Conservative treatment includes the following:
- Binaural hearing aids should be prescribed as soon as possible, with additional hearing training and lip reading training in the case of severe hearing loss.
- Phone amplifier. Optical signal devices to help at home.
- Resocialization, possibly with concomitant psychotherapy.
- Medical therapy only in the case of rapid progress of presbyacusis or disturbing tinnitus. In such cases rheologic drugs, α-lipoic acid or antioxidants such as vitamin C or E can be used. In most cases, these measures remain unsuccessful.

1.6.11.10 Differential Diagnosis

- Hereditary sensorineural hearing loss, otosclerosis
- Symptomatic sensorineural hearing loss with medical or neurological disease or systemic autoimmune disease
- Noise-induced hearing loss, ototoxic medication, etc.
- Traumatic sensorineural hearing loss secondary to contusio or commotio labyrinthi, craniocerebral injury, whiplash injuries

1.6.11.11 Prognosis

Normally, unavoidably slowly progressive hearing loss.

1.6.11.12 Special Remarks

The diagnosis of "presbyacusis" requires the exclusion of all other possible causes. Not every hearing loss in the elderly is a presbyacusis!

Suggested Reading

1. Nadol JB (1996). Schuknecht: presbyacusis. Laryngoscope, 106:1327–1329
2. Roland PS, Eaton D, Meyerhoff WL (2001) Aging in the auditory and vestibular system. In: Bailey BJ (ed) Head neck surgery-otolaryngology, 3rd edn. Lippincott-Raven, Philadelphia
3. Schuknecht HF (1993) Presbyacusis. In: Pathology of the Ear. Lea & Febinger, PA
4. Van Eyken E, Van Camp G, Van Laer L (2007) The complexity of age-related hearing impairment: contributing environmental and genetic factors. Audiol Neurotol, 12:345–358

1.6.12 Hearing Impairment in Childhood

JAN KIEFER AND GERARD M. O'DONOGHUE

1.6.12.1 Synonym

Childhood deafness.

1.6.12.2 Definition

- **Hearing impairment in childhood** refers to any hearing loss, occurring from birth to late childhood, e. g. around the age of 16 years. It may be unilateral or bilateral.
- It may be present at birth, e. g. **congenital**, or **acquired** after birth, either during the perinatal period of life or later during lifetime. As hearing impairment affects the acquisition of speech, its occurrence is also classified in relation to the stages of speech development as *prelingual* (0–2 years of age), *perilingual* (2–4 years) and *postlingual* (more than 4 years).
- It can be classified into four categories of severity: **mild** (average hearing levels ranging from 10 to 39 dB), **moderate** (average hearing levels from 40 to 69 dB), **severe** (average levels ranging from 70 to 94 dB) and **profound** (hearing loss that has average hearing levels greater than 95 dB).
- In principle, hearing loss can be **conductive** (due to malfunction of the outer ear or the middle ear) or **sensorineural** (due to malfunction of the inner ear or the auditory nerve), or **mixed**.
- Its course may be temporarily, fluctuating, progressive or permanent (**permanent childhood hearing impairment, or PCHI**).

1.6.12.3 Aetiology/Epidemiology

1. By far the commonest cause of hearing loss during childhood is a **conductive hearing loss** caused by **otitis media with effusion** (OME) following episodes of acute otitis media (see Sect. 1.4.4). Fortunately, for most children, the hearing loss is only transient and, if

not, is readily correctible by myringotomy, placement of ventilation tubes and adenoidectomy if conservative treatment fails (see Sect. 1.4.4).

2. Other causes for **conductive hearing loss** may be chronic inflammatory middle ear disease such as chronic mesotympanic otitis media (see Sect. 1.4.6), cholesteatoma (see Sect. 1.4.7), or congenital malformations of the outer ear canal and middle ear (see Sect. 1.2).

3. **Sensorineural hearing loss** is primarily caused by malfunction of the organ of Corti (sensory hearing loss), rarely by malfunction of the auditory nerve (neural hearing loss) or the interface between sensory hair cells and spiral ganglion cells (auditory neuropathy).

4. **PCHI** has a prevalence of approximately one to two per 1,000 children in Europe; literature values range from one to 4.2 per 1,000 children in selected populations.

5. **Congenital hearing impairment:** a genetic cause may account for more than 50% of these cases. Approximately three quarters of these are non-syndromic; one quarter are associated with hereditary syndromes carrying other specific hereditary features in addition to deafness. Most frequently, the hereditary course is autosomal recessive. The commonest findings are mutations in the gene *GJB2*, coding for connexin 26, a gap junction protein in the inner ear that is necessary for the maintenance of the endocochlear potential. Other hereditary causes are autosomal dominant with various phenotypes or X-linked.

Further causes of congenital hearing loss are:
   – Infections during pregnancy (rubella, cytomegalovirus, toxoplasmosis).
   – Inner ear malformations due to developmental arrest in embryonic stages such as Mondini malformation or common cavity malformation. They may be related to syndromes that are associated with other symptoms or occur in isolated forms.

6. **Acquired hearing impairment:** hearing loss may be acquired in the perinatal period owing to hypoxaemia, severe infections, prolonged newborn icterus and others. Following the perinatal period, the commonest cause of acquired inner ear hearing loss in early childhood is bacterial meningitis, with permanent hearing loss complicating up to 30% of affected children, mostly mild or unilateral. However, about 2% of children affected by meningitis develop a bilateral permanent and profound hearing loss. Vaccination against *Haemophilus influenzae* type B and early vaccination against *Streptococcus pneumoniae* reduce the risk of developing meningitis as well as the risk for acquired deafness due to meningitis. Other causes include infections (e.g. measles, mumps, varicella), trauma, middle ear diseases and administration of ototoxic drugs.

7. **Progressive hearing impairment:** progressive inner ear hearing loss during childhood can be associated with genetic mutations causing syndromes such as Pendred syndrome (Fig. 1.1.16) and the genetically associated syndrome of a large vestibular aqueduct (Fig. 1.1.26), Usher syndrome (retinitis pigmentosa and progressive hearing loss) and Alport syndrome. Other forms of genetically caused hearing loss occur as progressive hearing loss starting during adolescence. Frequently, the cause of progressive hearing loss remains unknown.

1.6.12.4 Symptoms

The most important symptoms of PCHI are the absence of adequate reactions to environmental sounds and speech as well as the delay or absence of normal speech development, depending on the severity of the hearing impairment. Additional symptoms may be poor general communication skills and behavioural difficulties out of frustration in communicational attempts.

However, it is important to understand that these symptoms are not easy to recognize, even for professional child carers, and that diagnosis even of severe hearing impairments is often considerably delayed, even up to the age of 2–4 years, if based only on the recognition of these symptoms. In many cases, the parents' concern precedes professional diagnosis and should therefore be taken for serious and prompt further hearing assessments for the child.

Risk factors that are associated with PCHI such as a family history of hearing impairment, infections during pregnancy (e.g. rubella, toxoplasmosis, cytomegalovirus), prematurity, low birth weight, necessity of admission to intensive care unit, prolonged newborn icterus, administration of ototoxic drugs (e.g. aminoglycosides), craniofacial abnormalities and hereditary syndromes should draw attention to possible hearing impairment.

Deficits in speech development include receptive skills of speech understanding as well as speech production. Affected areas range from basic skills such as segmentation and analysis of phonemic structure, short-term auditory memory as well as vocabulary to higher levels of speech such as syntax and grammar.

It is important to monitor the speech development of children, since some children may have progressive hearing loss occurring during childhood.

1.6.12.5 Complications

• The early auditory system is particularly receptive to sounds and speech. Sufficient auditory input is necessary to induce the maturation of the auditory system. Failure to stimulate the auditory system during this period (referred to as the critical period) can have lifelong detrimental effects on the acquisition of spoken language. Untreated hearing loss can also compromise a child's reading ability and educational attainment. This may limit access to further education, may restrict employment opportunity and lead to greater dependence on social services later in life. Thus, permanent untreated hearing impairment can have far-reaching consequences for the child, its family and for the wider community. Evidence suggests that early identification and treatment may significantly reduce the impact of PCHI. Fitting of hearing aids or cochlear implantation after the critical period of language development (from 0 to 4–6 years) will not be able to fully recover these effects.

- After meningitis, labyrinthitis may develop to fibrosis and/or neo-ossification of the cochlear duct, making cochlear implantation difficult and less successful. Early diagnosis via MRI or CT after meningitis (Fig. 1.1.25) is recommended to detect possible early signs and proceed to implantation.

1.6.12.6   Diagnostic Procedures

Recommended European Standard: Diagnostic Steps or Investigations in Neonatal Screening for Hearing Impairment

1. General neonatal screening for hearing impairment is recommended (European consensus conference 1998) since diagnosis of hearing impairment is often delayed and early intervention is of great importance. All newborns should be screened during their first days of life. Screening methods should have high sensitivity and specificity, and should be objective as well as time- and cost-efficient. The following methods are available:
   - Automated measurements of otoacoustic emissions (OAE), such as transitory evoked OAE (TEOAE) and distortion products of OAE (DPOAE)
   - Automated brainstem evoked response audiometry (BERA)
   - Automated measurements of amplitude modulation following response (AMFR)
2. If the child fails to pass the screening for hearing impairment, follow-up with eventual rescreening and more extensive auditory testing to confirm or exclude hearing loss is necessary.

History

1. Risk factors that are associated with PCHI such as a family history of hearing impairment, infections during pregnancy, prematurity, low birth weight, necessity of admission to an intensive care unit, prolonged newborn icterus and administration of ototoxic drugs should be investigated.
2. Ask about:

   - Reactions to sound and speech: Does the child startle at loud sounds, does it react to voice when the speaker is not visible, e. g. calming or smiling?
   - Language development: Does the child vocalize, does it imitate (mama, papa), what is the range of vocabulary, are there articulation problems, are there problems with syntax or grammar?
   - Behavioural abnormalities: e. g. aggression, low tolerance to frustration, communicative strategies.

Physical Examination

1. Inspection
   - General physical examination should pay attention to any signs of hereditary syndromes.
   - Look at the facial features of the child and its parents: craniofacial abnormalities, e. g. outer canthi of the eyelid slant downwards in Treacher Collins syndrome or upwards in the branchio-oculo-facial syndrome.
   - Ear anomalies such as hypoplasia or aplasia of the pinna, preauricular appendages and atresic ear canal draw attention to possible conductive hearing loss or associated inner ear malformations.
   - The neck should be evaluated for any branchial remnants (found in the branchio-oto-renal syndrome) or an enlarged thyroid gland (Pendred syndrome and associated enlarged vestibular aqueduct).
   - Blue sclerae are associated with osteogenesis imperfecta.
   - A white forelock and pigmental anomalies of the iris may indicate Waardenburg syndrome.
2. **Otoscopy**: Note anomalies of the pinna and external auditory ear canal, check for the presence of a normal tympanic membrane, possible anomalies of the handle of the malleus, signs of OME (retraction, fluid behind the eardrum) or chronic otitis media. Rarely, a whitish mass behind the eardrum may indicate congenital cholesteatoma (Fig. 1.4.14). Note that in sensorineural hearing losses, the tympanic membrane is normal.
3. Rhinoscopy: to exclude nasal stenosis, choanal atresia, nasal infections.
4. Pharyngoscopy: to exclude hyperplastic or infected adenoids or tonsils.

Audiological Testing

We distinguish between **subjective** and **objective** auditory tests. Subjective tests require some form of reaction of the subjects tested, whereas objective tests can be carried out without active feedback. Even in small children and babies, age-adequate subjective tests are possible (e. g. behavioural response audiometry, conditioned response audiometry); however, they require special expertise. Objective tests such as OAE and BERA can be performed at any age, sometimes requiring sedation. Diagnosis should only be based on the combination of subjective and objective tests, and should be reevaluated at subsequent developmental stages of the child to reach a higher degree of exactitude, to distinguish between transitory, permanent or progressive problems and to account for maturation and developmental processes.

Subjective tests are:

- **Behavioural response audiometry** (age range 0–2 years): Spontaneous responses to sounds such as calming, blinking and startling are watched for by experienced examiners. In visual reinforcement audiometry, reactions of the child such as head turning are reinforced by attractive visual stimuli. Bilateral freefield testing is possible; thresholds found are generally 20–30 dB above real auditory thresholds.
- **Performance test and play audiometry** (age range 2–5 years): This test requires that a child can be actively involved in a task. It uses a conditioned response (e. g. stacking cubes) to evaluate auditory thresholds in bilateral free-field conditions.
- **Pure tone audiometry** (age range from 3.5–4 years upwards): testing side specific pure tone thresholds (see Sect. 1.1.5.2). The child must be able to wear headphones and cooperate in the task.
- **Speech audiometry**: Various speech tests with ageappropriate language material are available. Results are influenced by auditory thresholds, capacity of auditory speech analysis as well as general speech development.
- Tests for **central auditory processing disorders**: Special tests such as the dichotic listening test or hearing in noise are used to diagnose central auditory processing disorders such as in auditory attention deficit syndrome.

Objective tests are:

- **Screening tests**: They are designed to detect hearing losses greater than 30–40 dB, in general without giving detailed thresholds.
- **Tympanometry**: to detect middle ear problems (e. g. OME). Stapedial reflex measurements are useful to estimate thresholds (see Sect. 1.1.5.2).
- **OAE**: OAE reflect the normal activity of outer hair cells. They are generally present when hearing loss does not exceed 30–40 dB. However, they do not reflect the function of inner hair cells and the auditory nerve; therefore, they might be present in cases of auditory neuropathy or neural hearing loss. TEOAE are click-evoked and have a broad response spectrum over the whole frequency range. DPOAE are evoked by continuous two tones and are frequency-specific. By determining growth functions of DPOAE, one can obtain an approximation of auditory thresholds.

- **Auditory brainstem response**: The synchronized neural activity of the auditory pathway (spiral ganglion and cochlear nerve, cochlear nucleus, lateral lemniscus, superior olive and inferior colliculus) is recorded in response to click stimuli (broad frequency response) or tone bursts (limited frequency specificity). Auditory thresholds can be approximated. The method may require sedation in children.
- **AMFR**: Like for auditory brainstem response, the synchronized neural activity is measured but is elicited by sine waves that are amplitude-modulated. Higher frequency specificity can be achieved.

Assessment of Speech and Language Development

As one of the main symptom of PCHI is delayed speech and language development, it is important to include assessment of speech and language development by psychologists, speech and language therapists or teachers of the deaf in a multidisciplinary approach.

Neurological and Ophthalmological Examination

Many children with PCHI have additional neurological and vision deficits. Neurological examination and vision screening should be carried out if indicated.

Diagnostic Imaging

- High-resolution, thin-section CT is the modality of choice to visualize the bony structures of the outer ear, the middle ear, the mastoid, the inner ear and the internal acoustic meatus (Figs. 1.1.23, 1.1.24). Soft tissue masses or fluid in the middle ear or mastoid can also be detected. Special attention has to be paid to detect possible malformations of the ossicles, of the inner ear, e. g. Mondini malformation (Fig. 1.2.2), common cavity, labyrinthine malformations, enlarged vestibular aqueduct (Fig. 1.1.26), or in postmeningitis cases, neo-ossifications of the scala tympani, media or the labyrinth (Fig. 1.1.25).
- MRI is indicated to visualize the fluid content of the inner ear, the auditory and vestibular and facial nerves in the inner acoustic meatus, and to detect central nervous system abnormalities. It is of special importance to detect early signs of fibrosis and neo-ossification of the cochlea after meningitis.

Genetic Testing and Counselling

Genetic testing may be useful in syndromic as well as non-syndromic hearing loss for diagnostic purposes and counselling of patients and parents. Specific genes associated with syndromes such as Waardenburg, Pendred and Usher have been identified. In non-syndromic hearing loss, the *GJB2* gene encodes for the connexin 26 molecule. It can be tested in many centres and may account for approximately 50% of cases of presumed non-syndromic genetic deafness. However, the number of gene mutations associated with deafness continues to increase; more then 100 mutations have been described. Therefore, negative findings in genetic testing do not preclude the genetic origin of a hearing loss.

1.6.12.7 Therapy

Conservative Therapy
- **Early intervention** is a key factor to prevent sequelae of hearing impairment. Even children as young as 3–6 months can be fitted with hearing aids; however, special expertise is needed to fit very small children.
- **Fitting of hearing aids**: The first step in therapy of PCHI is providing adequate amplification by means of hearing aids. They should be fitted on the basis of subjective and objective measures, and bilaterally, if the hearing loss is bilateral. Hearing aids have to be maintained and ear moulds have to be adjusted regularly to fit the ear canals, which typically enlarge with age. In conductive hearing loss, e. g. in ear malformations, that is not ready to be corrected surgically, bone-conduction hearing aids are the treatment of choice (Fig. 1.2.4).
- **Monitor the children's development:** Reactions to sound and speech as well as speech and language development of children fitted with hearing aids have to be monitored by the children's parents, paedaudiologists, teachers and therapists to make sure that amplification is adequate and optimal benefits are obtained. Training of communicative skills and counselling of parents is of great importance and should start as soon as possible.
- **Consider cochlear implantation**: If hearing capacities as well as speech and language development remain insufficient in patients with severe or profound hearing impairment, despite optimally fitted hearing aids, a cochlear implantation has to be considered.

Surgical Treatment

Conductive Hearing Loss
- **OME**: If conservative treatment fails, myringotomy and placement of ventilation tubes should be performed (see Sect. 1.4.4).
- **Chronic mesotympanic otitis media and cholesteatoma**: Surgical treatment is indicated (see Sects. 1.4.6, 1.4.7).
- **Malformations of the ear**: Reconstruction of the outer ear canal and ossicular chain, implantation of active middle ear implants and placement of bone-anchored

hearing aids are possible surgical options (see Sect. 1.2).

Sensorineural Hearing Loss
Function of Cochlear Implants
Cochlear implants replace the function of the inner ear in transferring acoustic sounds into neural excitation patterns. Unlike hearing aids, which amplify sounds acoustically, cochlear implants convert the sounds into electrical stimulation patterns, which electrically stimulate fibres of the cochlear nerve and thus elicit hearing sensations (Fig. 1.6.10). A cochlear implant system consists of two parts: the external speech processor and the implant itself (Fig. 1.6.11). The speech processor picks up external sounds, analyses them for frequency and time content and generates instructions for stimulation. Together with the necessary energy, the information is sent to the implant via a short high-frequency radio connection. The sender is centred over the implant with a magnetic link. The implant receives the instructions and generates electric pulses. These are delivered by the intracochlear electrodes (currently between 12 and 22) that follow the tonotopic organization of the cochlea. Electrodes at the base (near the round window) elicit high-pitched auditory sensations; electrodes near the apex elicit low pitches.

Indications for Cochlear Implantation
- For profoundly deaf children (typically those with hearing losses greater than 100 dB) and those chil-

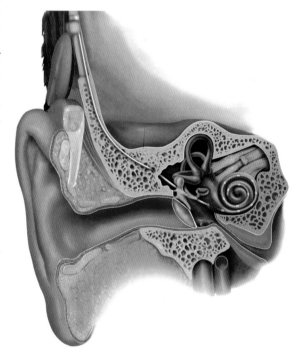

Fig. 1.6.10 Cochlear implant

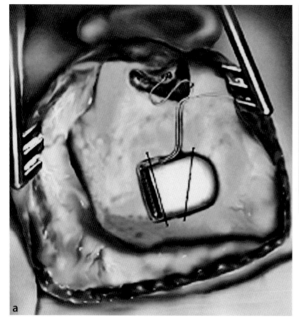

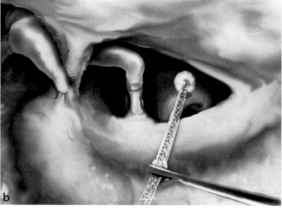

Fig. 1.6.11 a Cochlear implant fixed in the bony recess. **b** Cochlear implant electrode, inserted into the scala tympani of the cochlea through the facial recess and cochleostomy

dren with severe to profound hearing loss, who do not obtain sufficient benefit from powerful hearing aids to develop their speech and language skills, cochlear implants are extremely valuable in providing access to speech signal and sounds.

- Cochlear implantation can be performed as early as 8–12 months if indicated. Early intervention, e. g. implantation before the age of 2 years, is best to make use of critical periods in hearing as well as speech and language development. Therefore, early diagnosis and hearing aid trial periods are of importance.
- Bilateral implantation is possible and beneficial in adults and in children, allowing for better speech understanding under difficult listening conditions and partial development of spatial and directional hearing.
- Children with multiple handicaps in addition to profound hearing loss will obtain significant profit from cochlear implantation in most cases, even if receptive and expressive language development may not be expected owing to, e. g., intellectual handicaps.
- For malformations of the inner ear or neo-ossifications after meningitis, special surgical techniques have been developed.

Contraindications for Cochlear Implantation

- Cochlear implantation is not possible if the auditory nerve is absent. In these cases, brainstem implants may be an alternative approach.
- Cochlear implantation is contraindicated if sufficient rehabilitational and/or technical support for maintenance of the device function cannot be ensured.

Additional Therapeutic Strategies

- Additional speech and language therapy is necessary in most patients with severe and profound hearing impairment.
- General support, careful choice of educational settings and counselling of parents is of importance.
- Children with a cochlear implant require regular programming and control of the speech processor, which is best ensured in multidisciplinary cochlear implant rehabilitation programmes.

1.6.12.8 Differential Diagnosis

- Differential diagnosis between conductive and sensorineural hearing loss is an essential prerequisite.
- PCHI has to be differentiated from central auditory processing disorders that may be mistaken for peripheral hearing loss.
- Non-organic hearing loss (psychogenic) should not be missed, occurring most often in teenage children.
- Unilateral hearing loss is often overlooked in childhood.
- Progressive loss may pass unrecognized; the same is true for hearing loss affecting only part of the frequency range as the findings of the initial objective hearing screening can be normal.

1.6.12.9 Prognosis

Evidence confirms that early identification and treatment, coupled with sustained, appropriate habilitation and educational support can achieve excellent outcomes. Development of spoken language can proceed at rates similar to that for normal-hearing children even in profoundly deaf children, provided that early identification and cochlear implantation are achieved. They can achieve impressive competence with oral communication, and can often attend mainstream schools (with varying degrees of assistance), achieving their full educational potential.

Negative prognostic factors include late age at diagnosis, the presence of other cognitive disabilities, inappropriate communication strategies, inadequate educational and rehabilitational support and poor socioeconomic status.

1.6.12.10 Surgical Procedure: Cochlear Implantation

See Fig. 1.6.10.

The procedure involves the following:
- Monitoring of facial nerve function is recommended to avoid injury to the facial nerve.
- Extended retroauricular incision.
- Cortical mastoidectomy.
- Posterior tympanotomy with identification of chorda tympani, facial nerve, stapedial tendon, stapes and round window niche. The round window membrane may be identified for better localization of the scala tympani.
- Drilling of the bed for the implant housing and preparation of tie-down sutures (Fig. 1.6.11a).
- Cochleostomy of the scala tympani in front of the anterior/inferior aspect of the round window membrane, alternatively incision of the round window membrane (Fig. 1.6.11b).
- Insertion of the cochlear implant electrode until the point of first resistance, no forceful manoeuvres to avoid cochlear trauma, sealing of the cochleostomy (Fig. 1.6.11b).
- Fixation of implant housing with tie-down sutures or tightly sutured periosteum, depending on the type of implant and incision (Fig. 1.6.11a).
- Intraoperative tests to ensure correct function and placement (electrode impedance, implant function, neural responses to electric stimulation and measurement of electrically evoked stapedial reflexes).
- Fixation of the electrode, wound closure, sterile dressing.
- Postoperative radiological control of electrode placement and depth of insertion (transorbital or Stenvers view, Fig. 1.1.21).

Suggested Reading

1. Delaroche M (2001) Audiométrie comportementale du très jeune enfant. De Boeck Université, Louvain-la-Neuve
2. Anonymous (1988) European Consensus statement on neonatal hearing screening finalized at the European Consensus. Development Conference on Neonatal Hearing Screening 15–16 May 1998, Milan, Italy. Scand Audiol 27:259–260
3. Mondain M, Sillon M, Vieu A et al. (1997) Speech perception skills and speech intelligibility in prelingually deafened French children. Arch Otolaryngol Head Neck Surg 123:181–184
4. O'Donoghue GM, Nikolopoulos TP, Archbold SM (2000) Determinants of speech perception in children following cochlear implantation. Lancet 356(9228):466–468

1.6.13 Hearing Aids

WALTER LIVI

1.6.13.1 Definition and Components

A hearing aid is a miniature electronic instrument that detects, amplifies, elaborates and transmits sound to the hearing impaired patient's ear. Its basic components are the *microphone* (input), the *amplifier* (elaborator) and the *receiver* (output).

1.6.13.2 Classification

Hearing aids can be classified into three groups depending on the technology used:
1. **Analogue**: The microphone converts sound waves to a continuous electrical signal that is similar to the stimulus in intensity, frequency and time. The amplifier then amplifies the electrical signal, which can be modified by manual controls (trimmers), and then transmitted to the receiver that reconverts the elaborated electrical signal to a sound wave.
2. **Digitally programmable analogue**: They represent an evolution of analogue hearing aids that differ only in the phase of amplification. The amplified electrical signal is not modified by a manual trimmer but is amplified electronically by the computer. The elaboration of the signal remains an analogue process.
3. **Fully digital**: The microphone converts sound waves into an analogue electrical signal. The analogue-to-digital converter transforms the continuous electrical signal into a series of binary numbers (0–1). The digital sound processor digitally elaborates the numerical signal according to algorithms contained in the program. The analogue-to-digital converter transforms

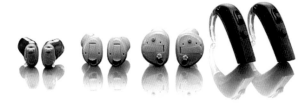

Fig. 1.6.12 From *left to right*, examples of completely inside the canal (CIC), in the concha (ITC), mainly in the external auditory canal (ITE) and behind the ear (BTE) hearing aids

the series of numbers into an electrical signal. The receiver then reconverts the electrical signal into sound waves.

Types of hearing aids are shown in Fig. 1.6.12. Depending on the place in which they are worn, hearing aids can be classified in the following way: *behind the ear* (BTE), *in the ear* (ITE), *body aid*, and *eyeglass aid* (*spectacles*). The choice is influenced by the type and entity of the hearing impairment and by the needs of each patient:

1. **BTE hearing aids**
   - Can be used for all types of hearing impairments.
   - Are composed of a plastic shell that contains the microphone, amplifier, receiver, volume control (or other manual controls or switches) and battery.
   - They are quite small and are placed BTE (pinna).
   - They are connected to the flexible tube of the ear mould by a plastic hook or by a fine wire to a receiver positioned directly in the ear canal (receiver in the ear, RITE) (Fig. 1.6.13). The ear mould is composed of biocompatible material that is made to measure for the ear canal of the patient.

2. **ITE hearing aids**
   - They can be placed completely inside the canal (CIC) or mainly in the external ear canal (ITE) or in the concha of the external ear canal (ITC) (Fig. 1.6.12).
   - They are made of biocompatible material and are well accepted by patients because they are small and practical.

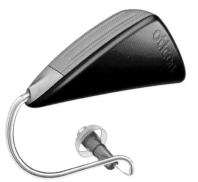

Fig. 1.6.13 The application of modern design to advanced electronic technology. A hearing aid that implements the receiver in the ear (RITE) solution

- They are not a good choice in cases of severe to profound hearing loss because they do not provide sufficient amplification.
- They are not often prescribed to children, because of the limited size of the child's ear canal and its continuous change in size.

3. **Body worn pocket aids**: The plastic case of the aid contains all components except for the receiver, which is placed in the ear canal. They are no longer in use because they are not very practical.

4. **Eyeglasses/spectacles**: All components of the hearing aid are in the arm of the glasses. They can transmit sounds by:
   - **Air conduction**: Air-conduction spectacles are practically obsolete.
   - **Bone conduction**: Bone-conduction spectacles contain the vibrator at the end of the arm and transmit the vibrations to the mastoid. They may be prescribed in cases of mild to moderate conductive loss and of mixed loss up to 35 dB. Note that a much better type of bone-conduction aid is the bone-anchored-hearing aid.

5. **Implantable hearing devices**: A conventional hearing aid takes sound and makes it louder. The amplified sound is conducted to the ear canal either via an ear mould or directly via the hearing aid.
   - A device that is semi-implantable (RetroX) has been classified by the FDA as a transcutaneous air-conduction hearing aid system (TACHAS). This is a conventional hearing aid, where the sound-transmitting silicon tube is placed from behind through the skin and cartilage of the auricle to direct the sound into the outer ear canal.
   - In the Vibrant Soundbridge implantable hearing system a tiny magnet (floating mass transducer, FMT) is directly attached to the ossicular chain (during surgery) and amplifies the natural vibrations of the ossicles. Many patients report that "direct" coupling leads to improved hearing quality and improved speech understanding. The system consists of external and internal parts. The external part, called the audio processor, is worn underneath the hair and held in place with a magnet. It contains a microphone, a battery and electronics. The audio processor converts environmental sounds into signals that are transmitted to the implanted internal coil of the Soundbridge. The implanted part consists of the internal coil, magnet, conductor link and the FMT. The signal from the audio processor is transmitted across the skin to the internal coil, which relays the signal down the conductor link to the FMT. The FMT is attached either to the incus or to the round window membrane (Fig. 1.2.5). The FMT converts the signal into vibrations that directly drive and move the ossicles or via the round window the peri-

lymph and amplify their natural movement. These vibrations then conduct the sound to the basilar membrane and the organ of Corti. This system is designed for mild to severe sensorineural hearing loss (FMT attached to the incus) or for moderate or severe mixed hearing loss (FMT attached to the round window), e. g. cochlear otosclerosis, malformations of the ear. Another middle ear implant is the middle ear transducer, an implantable hearing device where the sound is transmitted by a similar vibrating driving system attached to the head of the malleus.

– A bone-anchored-hearing aid is a hearing aid fixed to a bone-anchored titanium screw, in which bone conduction is used to transmit sound directly via the skull into the cochlea (Fig. 1.2.4).

– In deaf patients cochlear implants are used (see Sect. 1.6.12). Sound is transformed by the so-called speech processor to electric signals which are sent to a retroauricular subcutaneously implanted receiver. The receiver is connected with a stimulating electrode which is inserted into the cochlea.

1.6.13.3 Recommendations

It is well known that hearing impairment can negatively influence interpersonal relations and create difficulties in everyday tasks. The fitting of a hearing aid is necessary for patients who cannot benefit from pharmacological therapy and/or surgical procedures, and in some cases may be of support to the latter.

Criteria

Patients with a bilateral hearing loss with a loss in the better ear of at least 30 dB for at least one of the frequencies examined (from 0.5–3.0 kHz) and when the speech discrimination for monosyllabic words in the better ear is 80%. In cases of monolateral hearing loss, the loss should be 30 dB or more at 2.0 kHz or at two frequencies between 0.5 and 3.0 kHz. Make certain that the patient can properly use the hearing aids after a period of training with the hearing healthcare professional. The patient must also be motivated to use the hearing aid all the time. When deciding on hearing aids, the professional and the patient must evaluate subjective, social, cognitive and lifestyle aspects.

Recommendations for Binaural Fittings in Cases of Bilateral Hearing Loss

Stereophonic hearing is necessary for good speech discrimination, especially in noisy surroundings. If both ears can benefit from amplification, the rule today is to fit binaurally to guarantee the best result for speech discrimination (interpersonal communication). The patient must be motivated to correctly use both hearing aids.

Procedures for Fitting Hearing Aids

Three phases should be respected for an optimal result in fitting a hearing aid:

1. *Prescription*: In this phase the medical specialist is involved and he/she must carry out the testing necessary and an otomicroscopic objective examination. The testing includes subjective and objective tests; that is pure tone audiometry using earphones and free field. Impedance testing with particular attention to the stapedial reflex and in some cases, especially with children, the study of evoked potentials (auditory evoked brainstem responses).

2. *Fitting*: This is carried out by the audiologist/dispenser on the basis of the results from the testing and diagnosis. In this phase the hearing aid is chosen along with any assistive listening devices (if necessary) to satisfy the individual needs of the patient.

3. *Follow-up*: To obtain the maximum benefit from hearing aids it is necessary that the patient and audiologist/dispenser work together closely. After approximately 2 months, the plastic processes are completed. In this phase the medical and paramedical competences (audiologist/dispenser, ENT specialist, speech therapist, psychologist) converge to obtain the best result.

Choosing a Hearing Aid

Although hearing aids from a technological point of view rely on extremely sophisticated technologies, they are "obsolete" from the cosmetic point of view and this is usually the reason why many patients refuse hearing aids. For this reason hearing aids today have been restyled and special attention is given to their "design". If a hearing aid is to be accepted it should be perceived as a modern assistive device for communication, an extension of the patient's body, eliminating the sense of shame that the patient feels by wearing a hearing aid. There is a kind of tabu that is linked to dentures, hearing aids, cosmetics for men and in the past to eyeglasses. But today these negative connotations are decreasing and that changes the perception of the abovementioned items. They are no longer disturbing; they may become a part of fashion trends!

According to the audiological classification of hearing loss there is a distinction on the basis of the average tone threshold into *mild* (threshold between 20 and 40 dB), *moderate* (40–70 dB), *severe* (70–90 dB) and *profound* (90–120 dB) hearing loss. The choice of the hearing aid with respect to the above classification takes into account the audiometric curve (flat, symmetrical, asymmetrical, downward slope, upward slope) and can be categorized as follows:

1. *Sensorineural hearing loss moderate (40–70 dB) to severe (70–90 dB)*
   - *Moderate hearing loss:* (1) digital CIC or ITC; (2) digital BTE with made-to-measure ear mould.
   - *Mild and moderate hearing loss downward slope:* digital BTE with open fitting, traditional (with tube), or RITE.
   - *Severe hearing loss:* digital BTE with custom ear mould.
2. *Postlingual profound hearing loss (above 90 dB) with normal linguistic ability*
   - Digital BTE aids with made-to-measure ear mould.
   - Alternatively, cochlear implant.
3. *Conductive and mixed hearing loss with normal tympanic membrane and external auditory canal*
   - Digital air-conduction hearing aid if the bone-conduction threshold is above 40 dB for the middle to high frequencies (in some cases).
   - Bone-conduction spectacles or better bone-anchored hearing aid if the bone-conduction threshold is more than 35 dB for middle to high frequencies, including 2.0 kHz.
4. *Conductive and mixed hearing loss, with problems related to application to the ear canal: bilateral agenesis of the external auditory canal; chronic bilateral otitis media; after tympanoplasty open or closed, radical cavity*
   - Implantable bone-conduction aids (bone-anchored hearing aids) in adults in some cases and in children (over the age of 6 years).
   - Bone-conduction vibrators mounted on a headband for a child.
   - Bone-conduction spectacles for adults.
5. *Prelingual profound hearing loss in adults who have never used hearing aids.* All hearing aids, including cochlear implants give unsatisfactory results.
6. *Prelingual profound hearing loss in adults who have always used analogue hearing aids.* In many cases digital hearing aids with custom-made ear moulds can be recommended and when possible cochlear implants.

The most frequent complaints that arise from patients using traditional hearing aids are the hearing aid whistles (feedback), loud sounds are uncomfortable, unsatisfactory speech discrimination in noisy surroundings and the perception of the person's own voice altered owing to the occlusion effect of the external auditory canal. To solve these problems today there are digital ITE and BTE hearing aids with artificial intelligence that use technologies capable of improving speech discrimination in noise, eliminating feedback and with the "open fitting" system the problems connected to the occlusion effect are resolved.

Hearing Aid Fitting in Children

Fitting hearing aids in children is difficult both for the diagnosis and in the actual fitting. It is essential that children are fitted with hearing aids at a very early stage (within 6–12 months). To obtain the best results, the family must be actively involved in the process, the child must be placed in an adequate scholastic and social environment and followed closely by a speech therapist. To evaluate the results of the fitting, objective audiometric testing (impedance testing, auditory evoked brainstem response, electrocochleography, otoacoustic emissions) is essential. The testing and the evaluation of the hearing aid fitting must be carried out in a medical environment with the cooperation of the audiologist/dispenser. When the child is in Kindergarten it is important to use a personal FM system to eliminate any interference from background noise present in classrooms. Most hearing-impaired children suffer from moderate hearing loss and in those cases a hearing aid is an adequate solution. In cases of profound hearing impairment, after approximately 6 months of hearing aid use and an accurate evaluation of the entity of the hearing loss and after a careful psychological evaluation and speech evaluation, the possibility of a cochlear implant may be considered and must be carried out before the child is 18 months old.

Suggested Reading

1. Algaba J (2004) A new semiimplantable hearing system device—RetroX. Abstract book, II. Meeting consensus on auditory implants, Valencia, pp 19–21
2. Cotrona U, Livi W (2006) L'adattamento degli apparecchi acustici. Oticon, 3rd edn. Arti grafiche Reggiani, Ozzano dell'Emilia
3. Deddens AE, Wilson EP, Lesser TH, Fredrickson JM (1990) Totally implantable hearing aids: the effects of skin thickness on microphone function. Am J Otolaryngol 11:1–4
4. Dillon H (2001) Hearing aids. Boomerang, New York
5. Fredrickson JM, Coticchia JM, Khosla S (1996) Current status in the development of implantable middle ear hearing aids. Adv Otolaryngol Head Neck Surg 10:33–53

1.6.14 Vestibular Neuritis

KARL-FRIEDRICH HAMANN

1.6.14.1 Synonyms

Vestibular neuropathy, "vestibular neuronitis" (wrong term, because one neuron cannot be inflamed).

1.6.14.2   Definition

Acute unilateral, partial or complete loss of peripheral vestibular function, caused probably by a viral inflammation.

1.6.14.3   Aetiology/Epidemiology

Current findings point to a viral origin (herpes simplex virus) similar to facial palsy. Owing to immunologic deficiencies, herpes simplex viruses, which were already present in the patient as a result of an earlier infection, are reactivated and destroy vestibular sensory fibres. Vestibular neuritis is one of the most frequent peripheral vestibular disorders (about 25% of vertigo patients seen in an ENT vertigo unit suffer from this disease).

1.6.14.4   Symptoms

The symptoms are marked by the acute appearance of severe vertigo, mostly purely rotatory, sometimes accompanied by vomiting, nausea and ataxia. In the acute state a violent horizontal-rotatory nystagmus, beating towards the intact side, is always present. Hearing impairment or tinnitus do not belong to vestibular neuritis.

1.6.14.5   Complications

In the acute state a tendency to fall is obvious, so a prevention against falls is necessary, to avoid orthopaedic sequelae. Not seldom benign paroxysmal positioning vertigo follows a vestibular neuritis within a short delay, this is named "*Lindsay–Hemenway syndrome*".

1.6.14.6   Diagnostic Procedures

A careful questionnaire reveals the sudden onset of the vertiginous complaints, which decrease within a period of some days. The only objective sign is a strong horizontal-rotatory nystagmus, beating to the intact side. The caloric test proves the hypofunction of the lesioned side, which is in the beginning not compensated in the rotatory test. Vestibular spinal tests show a marked deviation and a tendency to falls directed to the lesioned side.

1.6.14.7   Additional Useful Diagnostic Procedures

A lesion in the auditory system, which does not belong to the vestibular neuritis, can be excluded by audiological tests. A vestibular schwannoma, which in very rare cases is mimicked by the same symptoms, can be excluded by MRI.

1.6.14.8   Therapy

Conservative Treatment
Treatment is exclusively conservative. In the early stage of the disease sedating drugs such as H1 antagonists (50 mg dimenhydrinate 2–3 times a day) are recommended, but only for a short time, not longer than 2 days. As soon as possible vestibular habituation training should be started to induce a rapid vestibular compensation.

Corticosteroid treatment is recommended during the first 14 days (start with 500 mg intravenously with decreasing doses to 0 mg within 10 days).

Additional Useful Therapeutic Options
To accelerate vestibular compensation active movements (sports), stimulating agents such as caffeine and avoidance of calming procedures such as bed rest seem useful therapeutic options.

1.6.14.9   Differential Diagnosis

Differential diagnosis of vestibular neuritis is simple, because the duration of vertigo for some days is very characteristic; therefore, benign paroxysmal positioning vertigo, vestibular paroxysmia, Ménière's disease or vestibular migraine can be excluded by a careful questionnaire. The fact that vestibular neuritis is monosymptomatic facilitates the differential diagnosis in patients with additional hearing problems. Although vestibular schwannoma only very seldom becomes apparent by vertigo complaints, MRI allows a clear differential diagnosis.

1.6.14.10 Prognosis

The prognosis is generally favourable. If there are additional factors which can inhibit vestibular compensation, such as sedating drugs, old age or additional abnormalities in the CNS, the complaints can continue for a long time.

Suggested Reading

1.   Arbusow V, Schulz P, Strupp M et al. (1999) Distribution of herpes simplex virus type I in human geniculate and vestibular ganglia: implications for vestibular neuritis. Ann Neurol 456:416–419

2. Brandt T (1999) Vertigo—its multisensory syndromes, 2nd edn. Springer, London
3. Hamann KF (1987) Training gegen Schwindel. Springer
4. Strupp M, Arbusov V, Maag KP et al. (1998) Vestibular exercises improve central vestibulo-spinal compensation after vestibular neuritis. Neurology 51:838–844

1.6.15 Benign Paroxysmal Positioning Vertigo

KARL-FRIEDRICH HAMANN

1.6.15.1 Synonym

Benign paroxysmal positional vertigo.

1.6.15.2 Definition

Benign paroxysmal positioning vertigo (BPPV) is a mechanically induced vertigo caused by a canalolithiasis or a cupulolithiasis.

1.6.15.3 Aetiology/Epidemiology

Normally otoliths are fixed in the otolithic membrane. By head traumatism, in old age or idiopathically, otoliths can be loosened and travel in one or some of the semicircular canals. BPPV is one of the most frequent kinds of vertigo, mainly in the elderly. The different semicircular canals are not affected equally. In 96% of cases the posterior vertical canal is concerned, the horizontal canal in 3% of cases and the anterior vertical semicircular canal only in 1% of cases.

1.6.15.4 Symptoms

The vertigo attacks have a short duration, only a few seconds, typically triggered by certain head movements, for example by head turning in the morning for a look at the alarm clock. BPPV never occurs when the head is not moved.

1.6.15.5 Complications

Complications in the real sense of the word do not exist. As for all forms of vertigo, falls can occur.

1.6.15.6 Diagnostic Procedures

The questionnaire reveals that vertigo appears only during head movements and lasts only for some seconds. Apart from the characteristic complaints, the diagnosis is made by nystagmus observation under Frenzel's glasses. By specific positioning of the head in the plane of one of the semicircular canals (Hallpike manoeuvre), one can prove a BPPV if a typical nystagmus appears. The involved semicircular canal can be identified by analysis of the nystagmus, because the pattern of eye movements for each semicircular canal is known. Other neurotological tests such as caloric or rotatory tests do not show pathological findings; the auditory system is not involved as well.

1.6.15.7 Additional Useful Diagnostic Procedures

Additional diagnostic procedures are not necessary. Imaging techniques are only suitable for exclusion of possible central abnormalities.

1.6.15.8 Therapy

Conservative Treatment
Owing to the mechanical pathophysiologic nature of BPPV only a mechanical treatment is reasonable. The goal of a rational treatment of BPPV is to liberate the semicircular canals from the dislocated otoliths. This can be carried out by liberatory manoeuvres of Semont [2] (Fig. 1.6.14) or Epley [1] (Fig. 1.6.15). Both have principally the same intention, namely to bring the dislocated otoliths by specific movements of the head to a "neutral point" in the vestibular apparatus nearby the utriculus. For the treatment of a canalolithiasis or a cupulolithiasis of the horizontal canal, a barbecue rotation or Brandt–Daroff exercises can be recommended as for a prophylaxis of BPPV.

Surgical Treatment
Only in extremely rare cases (less than 1%) surgical treatment can be indicated. Two procedures exist: (1) neurectomy of the posterior canal nerve, (2) plugging of the affected canal.

1.6.15.9 Differential Diagnosis

Because of the typical clinical signs (vertigo only in combination with head movements, duration of vertigo never more than 60 s, provocation of typical nystagmus by specific positioning), normally the differential diagnosis does not present a problem. One of the rare differential-

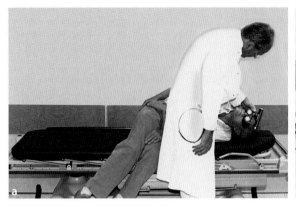 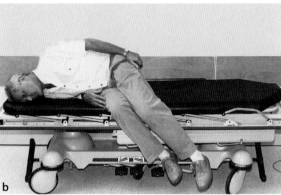

Fig. 1.6.14 a First movement of a liberatory manoeuvre (Semont) for treatment of a canalolithiasis of the left posterior canal: starting from a sitting position the patient is positioned to the left side, the head turned 45° to the unaffected right side.

b Second movement of the liberatory manoeuvre (Semont): the head and trunk of the patient were thrown from the left side to the right side without changing the position of the head relative to the body

diagnostic possibilities is the vestibular paroxysmia, which is characterized by vertigo attacks of a few seconds. But these attacks are not correlated typically with certain head movements which trigger the BPPV.

Another differential diagnosis, but less frequent, is the possibility of a vestibular migraine, which, in contrast to BPPV, should be accompanied by headaches.

1.6.15.10 Prognosis

The prognosis of BPPV is very favourable. After one liberatory manoeuvre about 70% of patients no longer have complaints. In the remaining 30%, repetitive liberatory manoeuvres lead to a complete cure. If necessary, Brandt–Daroff exercises must be continued. The rate of recurrences is relatively high. In a period of 2 years after a liberatory manoeuvre, about 20% of patients complain about vertigo again; in a period of 8 years, the rate of recurrences reaches 55%. Only in extremely rare cases does a surgical treatment become necessary (see Sect. 1.6.15.8).

References

1. Epley JM (1992) The canalith repositioning procedure: for treatment of benign paroxysmal positioning vertigo. Otolaryngol Head Neck Surg 10:299–304
2. Semont A, Freyss G, Vitte E (1988) Curing the BPPV with a liberatory manoeuvre. Adv Otorhinolaryngol 42:290–293

Suggested Reading

1. Baloh RW, Honrubia V, Jacobson K (1987) Benign positional vertigo. Clinical and oculographic features in 240 cases. Neurology 37:371–378
2. Brandt T (1999) Vertigo—its multisensory syndromes, 2nd edn. Springer, London
3. Lempert T, Tiel-Wilck K (1996) A positional manoeuvre for treatment of horizontal canal benign positional vertigo. Laryngoscope 106:476–478
4. Suzuki JI, Tokumasu K, Goto K (1969) Eye movements from single utricular nerve stimulation in the cat. Acta Otolaryngol 68:350–362

1.6.16 Motion Sickness

KARL-FRIEDRICH HAMANN

1.6.16.1 Synonyms

Corresponding to the environment: car sickness, sea sickness, space sickness.

1.6.16.2 Definition

Motion sickness is a special kind of physiological vertigo, induced by an unusual stimulation of the multisensory system, which normally guarantees adequate orientation in space.

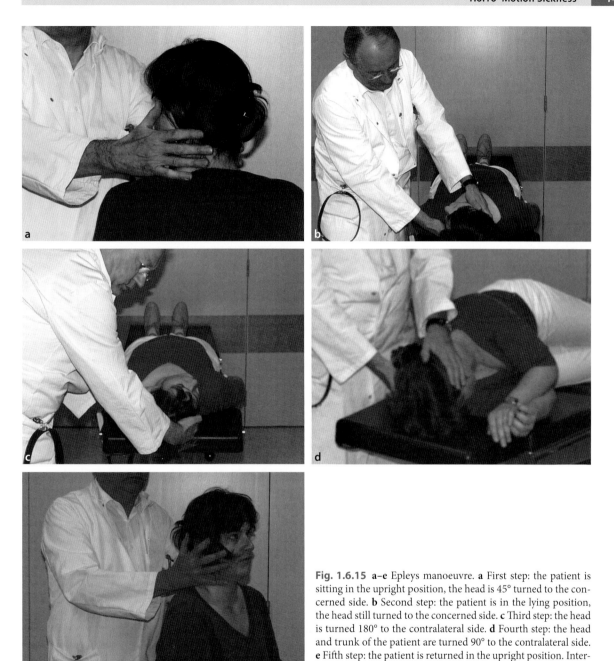

Fig. 1.6.15 a–e Epleys manoeuvre. **a** First step: the patient is sitting in the upright position, the head is 45° turned to the concerned side. **b** Second step: the patient is in the lying position, the head still turned to the concerned side. **c** Third step: the head is turned 180° to the contralateral side. **d** Fourth step: the head and trunk of the patient are turned 90° to the contralateral side. **e** Fifth step: the patient is returned in the upright position. Intervals between each step of 3–5 min

1.6.16.3 Aetiology/Epidemiology

It is generally accepted that motion sickness develops when a sensory conflict between the different sensory systems, responsible for the orientation in space, occurs. Both intrasensory mismatch (within the vestibular system) and intersensory mismatch (between the vestibular and visual system for example) can trigger the symptoms of motion sickness. The crucial condition is that different sensory receptors give different signals about the passive motion of an individual in space. So the perceived pieces of information do not correspond amongst themselves nor to the expected perception pattern, previously adapted by experience. Principally in all people with an intact sensory system motion, sickness can be induced, if certain conditions which can create a sensory conflict are fulfilled.

1.6.16.4 Symptoms

Motion sickness is clinically characterized by nausea, pallor, yawing, vomiting and mainly by a feeling of severe discomfort. These symptoms last not only for the time of conflict stimulation but also for a certain period afterwards, when motion stimulation had stopped.

1.6.16.5 Complications

Complications in the real sense of the word do not exist. Falls and aspiration caused by vomiting are sequelae of the symptoms themselves.

1.6.16.6 Diagnosis

Motion sickness is diagnosed very simply, because the coincidence of the inducing motion and the typical symptoms is pathognomonic. Further diagnostic procedures are not necessary.

1.6.16.7 Therapy

A prophylactic therapy can be useful if it is predictable that a motion sickness inducing sensory conflict will occur. The best prevention consists in a vestibular habituation training with the intention to prepare the orientation system for a conflict stimulation. As a medical prophylactic treatment, scopolamine used in the form of a transdermal skin patch can be recommended. When the symptoms of motion sickness appear, one can try to break free from the sensory conflict situation. In the case of seasickness the suffering person has to leave the cabin and should go on the ship's deck. Then he/she should fixate on an object not too far away. In this way there the correspondence between visual and vestibular information increases. The medical treatment consists in the uptake of an H1 histamine antagonist such as dimenhydrate or meclozine. It must be pointed out that all H1 antagonists have sedative side effects. Interestingly, ginger root, given in a pulverized form, has significantly favourable effects on motion sickness symptoms.

1.6.16.8 Differential Diagnosis

A differential diagnosis of motion sickness does not exist. The only exception is that a real vestibular disease can be triggered also by a specific movement or a sensory conflict.

1.6.16.9 Prognosis

The prognosis of motion sickness is very favourable. At the latest in the moment when the inducing motion ceases, a rapid decrease of the uncomfortable symptoms begins. After some hours, the symptoms of motion sickness disappear.

Suggested Reading

1. Brandt T, Dichgans J, Wagner W (1974) Drug effectiveness on experimental optokinetic and vestibular motion sickness. Aerosp Med 45:1291–1297
2. Brandt T (1999) Vertigo—its multisensory syndromes, 2nd edn. Springer, London
3. Fukuda T (1975) Postural behaviour in motion sickness. Acta Otolaryngol 330:9–14
4. Gay LN, Carliner PE (1949) The prevention and treatment of motion sickness. Science 109:359–360
5. Mowrey DB, Clayson DE (1982) Motion sickness, ginger, and psychophysics. Lancet 20:655–657

1.7 Facial Nerve

ANDREAS ARNOLD AND VINCENT DARROUZET

1.7.1 Idiopathic Facial Palsy

ANDREAS ARNOLD AND VINCENT DARROUZET

1.7.1.1 Synonyms

Bell's palsy, *a frigore* facial palsy.

1.7.1.2 Definition

Bell's palsy is characterized by a sudden onset of incomplete or complete paralysis of facial nerve function without detectable cause. It is usually unilateral.

1.7.1.3 Aetiology/Epidemiology

Bell's palsy affects about two in 10,000 people. The cause remains unclear. The most probable cause is a mononeuritis triggered by reactivation of herpes simplex virus type 1 in the geniculate ganglion. This increases the nerve diameter and leads to compression in its bony channel as it courses through the temporal bone. Other infections known to be associated with facial palsy are *early-summer meningoencephalitis* virus, *Borellia burgdorferi*, herpes zoster, influenza virus, HIV and HTLV-1. Conditions with a higher susceptibility are sarcoidosis, diabetes mellitus, pregnancy, autoimmune-disorders and AIDS. Bell's palsy remains a diagnosis of exclusion.

1.7.1.4 Symptoms

The palsy usually starts suddenly and ranges from weakness of facial movements to a "lifeless" facial drooping on one side. It may also include difficulty in eye closure on the affected side, face twitching, saliva drooling due to the droopy corner of mouth, dry eye or mouth, loss or alteration of sense of taste and sometimes hyperacousis and dysaesthesia on the affected side.

1.7.1.5 Complications

Possible complications are disfigurement from loss of facial movement, difficulty with eating, drinking and speaking, dry eye with corneal ulcers and keratitis due to lagophthalmus, chronic spasm of face muscles or eyelids, chronic taste abnormalities and synkinesis (abnormal reinnervation of facial muscles resulting in tears when laughing or inappropriate salivation).

1.7.1.6 Diagnostic Evaluation

Recommended European Standard

- *History*: time and type of onset (slow, rapid), first time or recurrent, additional symptoms (neurological, hearing, vertigo, taste, pain).
- *Inspection* (see the decision algorithm in Fig. 1.7.1): usually unilateral facial weakness [classification according to House and Brackmann (HB); see Table 1.7.1]. Vesicles in or around the auricle (Fig. 1.6.1) and external auditory canal (Ramsay Hunt syndrome similar to herpes zoster oticus?). Note that peripheral facial palsy includes palsy of the forehead of the affected side; central palsy shows both side movements. Bell's phenomenon (physiological elevation of the globes when lids are closed) becomes visible owing to incomplete lid closure. Complete cranial nerve examination. Other neurological signs?
- *Palpation*: parotid gland (tumour?), dysaesthesia auricle (Ramsay Hunt syndrome similar to herpes zoster oticus?).
- *Complete ENT examination.*
- *Micro-otoscopy*: effusions? cholesteatoma? blisters of herpes zoster? Normal auditory canal and tympanic membrane in Bell's palsy.
- *Hearing tests*: tuning fork, audiogram, tympanogram, stapedial reflexes (see topognostic of facial nerve palsy in the next section).

Additional/Useful Diagnostic Procedures

1. *Sonography of parotid gland*: to exclude a parotid gland tumour.

Decision algorithm

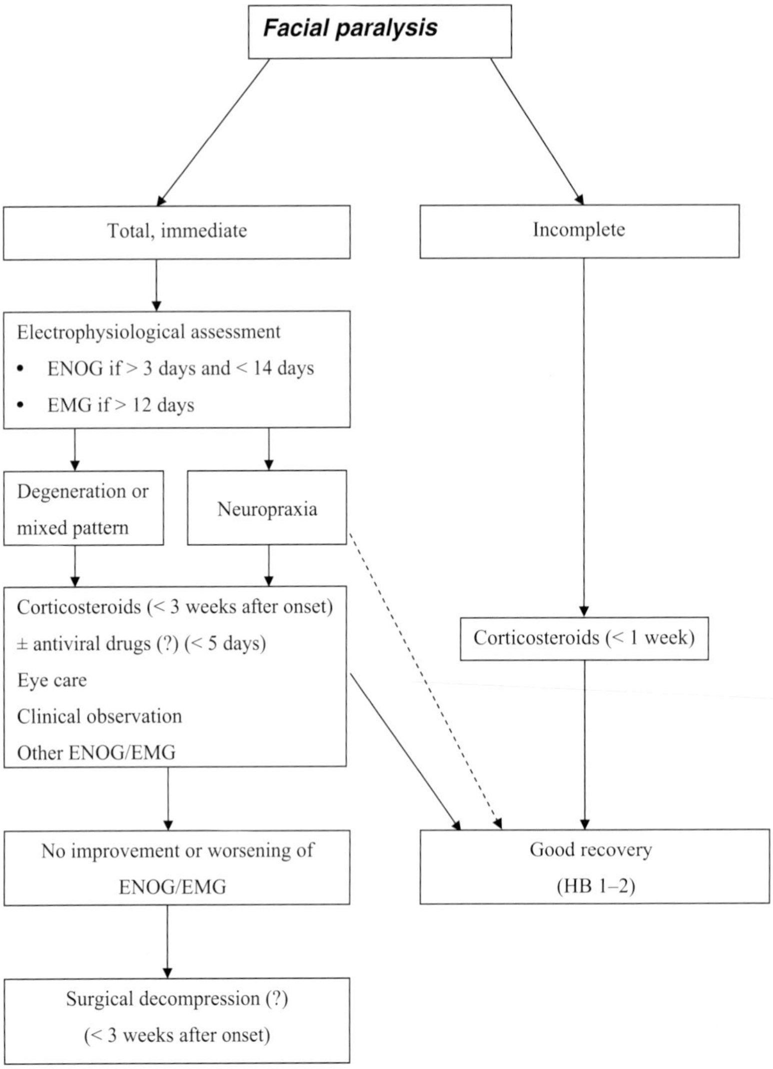

Fig. 1.7.1 Decision algorithm. *EMG* electromyography, *ENOG* electroneuronography, *HB* House and Brackmann

2. *Liquor diagnostics*: always with synchronous or metachronous bilateral facial palsy (borreliosis? multiple sclerosis?).
3. *Topognostic of facial nerve palsy*
   - Tear test (Schirmer test): reduced tear production if palsy is at or proximal to the geniculate ganglion (greater petrosal nerve).
   - Stapedial reflexes: elevated threshold or absence if the site of the lesion is located in or proximal to the tympanic segment of the facial nerve.
   - Evaluation of the taste sense: loss of taste of the anterior two thirds of the lateral tongue shows a loss of function of the chorda tympani and indicates damage proximal to the second genu.

Note that if all of these tests result in normal findings, the lesion must be distal to the tympanic segment of the facial nerve (e. g. mastoid or extracranial segment).

4. *Electrophysiological evaluation* [e. g. nerve-excitability test, electroneuronography (ENOG), electromyography (EMG); see Table 1.7.2]: important for quantification of innervation and reinnervation, prognosis and decision making for surgical intervention. EMG results have prognostic value 10–12 days after the onset of facial palsy.
5. *Differential blood count, glucose and HbA1c, C-reactive protein, erythrocyte sedimentation rate.*
6. *Serologic tests* for herpes simplex virus type 1, *early-summer meningoencephalitis* virus, influenza virus, *Borrelia burgdorferi* and HIV.

Table 1.7.1 House–Brackmann grading system

Grade 1 (*normal*): normal function in all areas

Grade 2 (*mild dysfunction*): slight weakness noticeable only on close inspection. At rest: normal symmetry of forehead. Motion: ability to close eye with minimal effort and slight asymmetry, ability to move corners of mouth with maximal effort and slight asymmetry. No synkinesis, contracture or hemifacial spasm.

Grade 3 (*moderate dysfunction*): obvious but not disfiguring difference between two sides, no functional impairment; noticeable but not severe synkinesis, contracture, and/or hemifacial spasm. At rest: normal symmetry and tone. Motion: slight to no movement of forehead, ability to close eye with maximal effort and obvious asymmetry, ability to move corners of mouth with maximal effort and obvious asymmetry. Patients who have obvious but not disfiguring synkinesis, contracture and/or hemifacial spasm are grade 3, regardless of the degree of motor activity.

Grade 4 (*moderately severe dysfunction*): obvious weakness and/or disfiguring asymmetry. At rest: normal symmetry and tone. Motion: no movement of forehead; inability to close eye completely with maximal effort. Patients with synkinesis, mass action and/or hemifacial spasm severe enough to interfere with function are grade 4, regardless of motor activity.

Grade 5 (*severe dysfunction*): only barely perceptible motion. At rest: possible asymmetry with drop of corner of mouth and decreased or absent nasal labial fold. Motion: no movement of forehead, incomplete closure of eye and only slight movement of lid with maximal effort, slight movement of corner of mouth. Synkinesis, contracture and hemifacial spasm are usually absent.

Grade 6 (*total paralysis*): loss of tone; asymmetry; no motion; no synkinesis, contracture or hemifacial spasm.

7. *Balance tests*: electronystagmography.
8. *Brainstem evoked response audiometry*: vestibular schwannoma?
9. *High-resolution CT* (recommended after trauma): fracture, destructive process, mastoiditis, cholesteatoma?
10. *Magnetic resonance tomography*, enhanced with gadolinium (recommended if neurotological symptoms are present): shows disease of temporal bone, cerebellopontine angle, brain and parotid gland. An inflamed geniculate ganglion can be seen with gadolinium enhancement (Fig. 1.7.2).
11. *Consultation with other disciplines*: neurology, ophthalmology, internal medicine.

Table 1.7.2 Electrophysiological examination

Electroneuronography: A compound action potential is recorded and measured peak to peak by skin electrodes after supramaximal stimulation of the nerve at the stylomastoid foramen. The nerve degeneration can be expressed as a percentage by comparing the compound action potential with that for the normal side. An amount of more than 90% indicates a severe denervation pattern. Repetition and comparison of results obtained day after day are significant. The main advantage of this test is that it can be applied early (from the third day after onset) and is carried out by the otologist. It is not reliable after the 14th day. This test is to be preferred over the Hilger test, or the nerve excitability test: the current necessary to provoke just visible facial muscular contraction is considered as the threshold and is measured bilaterally. A decrease in excitability of 3.5 mA or more indicates nerve degeneration.

Electromyography and **evoked electromyography**: Concentric needle or skin electrodes are used to measure electrical activity of the facial musculature. The first measurement is done at rest. Then the patient is asked to move his/her face, and action potentials are recorded. The third part consists of nerve stimulation at the stylomastoid foramen: evoked action potentials are characterized by their morphology and latency. This test is very reliable and reproducible from the tenth day to elicit a denervation pattern (fibrillation potential but no voluntary or evoked action potential). These tests enable one to distinguish three types of nerve lesions that can be associated in a single nerve:

1. Neuropraxia: Axons are partially demyelinated. Voluntary electrical activity is poor or absent but action potentials are evoked by supraliminar electrical stimuli. There is no need for axonal regrowth and recovery is complete and fast.

2. Axonotmesis: Axons are degenerated. However, neurotubules are intact and axonal regrowth through these tubules can lead to total recovery after some weeks or months.

3. Neurotmesis: No action potentials are detected even after stimulation. Fibrillation potentials are characteristic of this denervation pattern. Neurotubules are compromised. Axonal regrowth is associated with wrong routing, leading to synkinesia, spasm and mass movements

1.7.1.7 Therapy

If the patient is referred early, during the first week, medical treatment is the initial form of therapy (see the decision algorithms in Figs. 1.7.1, 1.7.3). The HB (House and Bruckmann) grading system (Table 1.7.1) is used to assess clinical outcome. Three different situations are to be differentiated:

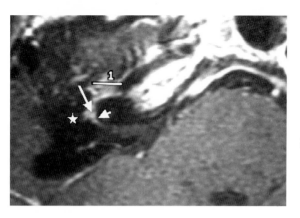

Fig. 1.7.2 Bell's palsy. Contrast-enhanced MRI of the right petrous bone: strong enhancement of the facial nerve at the level of the geniculate ganglion (*arrow*), petrous nerve, initial part of the tympanic portion (*star*) and labyrinthine portion (*arrowhead*)

1. If the palsy is incomplete and not worsening, appearing benign, medical treatment is facultative and the patient is clinically observed until total recovery (HB 1).

2. If the palsy is complete but the EMG pattern is favourable (advocating neuropraxia), or if daily electroneuronograms elicit less than an 85% denervation rate, medical treatment is applied and the patient is closely followed up clinically and, if possible, electrophysiologically. The natural evolution of the disease leads four out of five patients to total or near total recovery (HB 1–2) within some weeks.

3. If the palsy is complete and the ENOG pattern is unfavourable (90% denervation rate) or if the survey of an initially benign looking Bell's palsy demonstrates a clear clinical and electrical deterioration, a surgical decompression of the nerve can be discussed during the first 3 weeks after onset. Confirmation of the poor prognosis with EMG, more reliable than with ENOG alone, and realization of a MRI scan are two prerequisites. The aim of the surgery is to decompress the probably swollen nerve by opening the Fallopian canal at the level of the geniculate ganglion and labyrinthine portion to the meatal foramen, thus avoiding total denervation and its unavoidable associated sequelae (synkinesis, hemifacial spasm; HB 3–4).

Decision algorithm

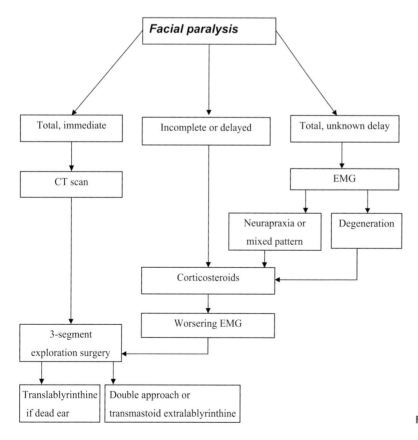

Fig. 1.7.3 Decision algorithm

If the patient is referred late (after 3 weeks), the usefulness of any medication is to be discussed. Great attention must be paid to those patients by watching carefully their outcome. If no recovery at all is observed 6 months after onset, going against the natural evolution of the disease, the diagnosis of Bell's palsy must be reconsidered. A full MRI and CT scan workup, searching for intrinsic tumours of the nerve, must be performed and surgical exploration of the nerve could be considered.

Conservative Therapy

Recommended European Standard Therapeutic Steps

Corticosteroids: 500 mg/day intravenously for 3 days. Can be continued orally for several days.

Antiviral drug (e.g. acyclovir, 3×10 mg/kg per day intravenously or 5×800 mg/day orally).

In the treatment of idiopathic facial paralysis, a combined therapy of antiviral drugs and corticosteroids seems to have a better outcome than therapy with corticoids alone. Other investigators have postulated that in facial palsy corticosteroids are more important than antiviral drugs. Corticosteroids may reduce swelling and relieve pressure on the facial nerve. *To be most effective, they should be given as early as possible.*

Lubricating eye drops or eye ointments protect the eye if it cannot be closed completely. An eye patch (moist chamber) is recommended during sleep.

Additional Useful Therapeutic Options

- Rheologic infusions, e.g. pentoxiphylline, 6% hydroxyethyl starch
- Myofacial training, electrotherapy
- If Lyme disease is suspected, tetracycline, macrolides or third-generation cephalosporins (e.g. ceftriaxon) for 14–21days

Surgery

Recommended European Standard Therapeutic Steps

Normally, no surgical treatment is recommended. However, in some units surgery is offered when EMG assessment has clearly demonstrated irremediable nerve lesion severeness (electrical silence) (Fig. 1.7.3). It must be performed within 3 weeks to be effective.

Additional Useful Surgical Procedures in Selected Cases

Persistent extensive palsy with signs of severe denervation in the EMG and imminent ocular complication may need surgical eye protection (tarsorrhaphia, eyelid gold or titanium inlay).

Facial reanimation after total palsy can be performed by anastomosis of hypoglossal and facial nerves or with regional muscle transposition (e.g. temporalis transposition).

With recurrent paresis, total nerve decompression is a treatment option. If done, it should be performed within 3 weeks to be effective. However, decompression surgery is controversial and has not been shown to routinely benefit patients with Bell's palsy.

1.7.1.8   Differential Diagnosis

- *Complications* of acute otitis media, cholesteatoma, middle ear tuberculosis.
- *Post-traumatic facial palsy* (temporal bone fracture, stab or gunshot wound), iatrogenic after middle ear or parotid surgery.
- *Tumour of parotid gland, vestibular schwannoma, cerebral tumour, facial schwannoma.* All patients with Bell's palsy lasting more than 4 weeks and all patients with recurrent facial palsy should be investigated for the presence of a tumour.
- *Central facial palsy* (e.g. following ischaemic stroke): frontal branch of facial nerve functional!
- *Ramsay Hunt syndrome* (zoster oticus): vesicles?
- *Lyme disease*: recent tick bite or erythema chronicum migrans?
- *Melkersson–Rosenthal syndrome*: recurrent bilateral or alternating facial palsy with cheilitis, fissured tongue and facial oedema (familial, sometimes with rheumatologic symptoms).
- *Congenital hemifacial dysplasias.*
- *Dissection of internal carotid artery*: subintimal or adventitial bleeding occurring secondary to sports, chiropractic manipulations, trauma (distortion of cervical spine) or spontaneously. A partial perfusion stop of the internal carotid artery leads to a compression of the cranial nerves. Functional deficits can also be caused by ischaemia of the cranial nerve nuclei (VI, VII, IX, X, XI). Similar spontaneous or post-traumatic conditions are also possible along the vertebral artery.
- *Bilateral simultaneous or recurrent alternating facial palsy.* Congenital: Möbius syndrome (congenital atrophy or agenesis of ganglion cells of cranial nerves III, VI and VII). Infections: borreliosis, syphilis, leprosy, tuberculous or bacterial meningitis, mononucleosis, HIV, herpes simplex virus, mycoplasma pneumoniae (CSF diagnosis!).
- *Neoplastic*: leukaemia, pontine gliomas, brain metastasis, carcinomatous meningitis.
- *Neurologic*: multiple sclerosis, polyneuropathies, Guillain–Barré syndrome, bulbar paralysis, Parkinson's disease, pons bleeding, bulbospinal neuropathy, Bannwarth's syndrome (neurologic symptoms in bor-

reliosis with meningitis, radiculitis, facial palsy and myocarditis).
- *Autoimmune diseases:* systemic lupus erythematosus, Wegener's granulomatosis.

1.7.1.9   Prognosis

Approximately 60–80% of patients recover completely within a few weeks to months. The outcome depends on the extent of denervation. Incomplete palsy has an excellent prognosis. The sooner partial function returns, the better the chance for complete recovery.

Poor prognostic factors include total palsy, palsy rapidly induced, additional pain or neurotological symptoms, and delayed treatment.

Suggested Reading

1. Adour KK (2002) Decompression for Bell's palsy: why I don't do it. Eur Arch Otorhinolaryngol 259:40
2. Alberton DL, Zed PJ (2006) Bell's palsy: a review of treatment using antiviral agents. Ann Pharmacother 40:1838
3. Bell C (1821) On the nerves; giving an account of some experiments on their structure and functions, which lead to a new arrangement of the system. Philos Trans R Soc Lond 111:398
4. May M, Schaitkin BM (2000) The facial nerve, 2nd edn. Thieme, New York
5. Peitersen E (2002) Bell's palsy: the spontaneous course of 2,500 peripheral facial nerve palsies of different etiologies. Acta Otolaryngol Suppl 549:4–30
6. Rowlands S, Hooper R, Hughes R, Burney P (2002) The epidemiology and treatment of Bell's palsy in the UK. Eur J Neurol 9:63

1.7.2   Traumatic Facial Palsy

VINCENT DARROUZET

1.7.2.1   Definition

Facial paralysis resulting from trauma to the nerve in the temporal bone, internal auditory canal or cerebellopontine angle.

1.7.2.2   Aetiology/Epidemiology

Facial paralysis can result from either a blunt trauma, an open trauma (association of a wound) or a ballistic trauma to the temporal bone or a direct iatrogenic insult to the nerve during otological or otoneurological surgical procedures. Facial paralysis arises in 10–30% of temporal bone fractures. The overall incidence is decreasing like temporal bone fracture incidence, mainly owing to the decrease in the number of road traffic accidents. Iatrogenic lesions are common situations in surgery of tumours in the cerebellopontine angle (acoustic neuroma). Surgery of cholesteatoma is the main cause of iatrogenic lesions in otological surgery, followed by surgery of external and middle ear dysgenesis.

Facial paralysis can be of immediate or delayed onset, depending on the direct or indirect mechanism of the nerve insult. A delayed onset of 1–12 days may be due to a secondary nerve oedema or to viral reactivation (herpesvirus or varicella zoster virus).

1.7.2.3   Symptoms

Traumatic facial paralysis is of a peripheral type. It can be partial or total, immediate or delayed with regard to the trauma. Motor nerve fibre malfunction is evoked by some degree of hemiface paralysis. Depending on the level of the nerve trauma, other symptoms can be observed owing to facial nerve sensitivity or parasympathic fibre malfunction: hypoaesthesia of the Ramsay Hunt area, dry eye due to lachrymal flow defect and ipsilateral hemitongue taste sensation deficit.

1.7.2.4   Complications

Traumatic facial paralysis must be managed with care as for any facial paralysis to prevent subsequent complications such as conjunctivitis, keratitis, eyeball infections and visual sequelae. In contrast to Bell's palsy, an absence of recovery can be observed in the case of nerve trunk disruption or burn, leading to severe aesthetic and functional sequelae.

1.7.2.5   Diagnostic Procedures

Clinical examination and workup are as follows:
- History of the palsy with regard to the trauma: Ask the patient, his/her family or the emergency ward team about the onset mode of the palsy: **immediate** or clearly **delayed**. This is of paramount importance.
- At first examination, facial nerve motor function is evaluated using a quantitative method: A score is given to each of the main movements of the face (forehead wrinkling, eye closure, open mouth smiling, snarling, lip puckering and finally chin wrinkling) and to the facial tone. Patients are scored daily during the first 2 weeks. Other mid- and long-term forthcoming eval-

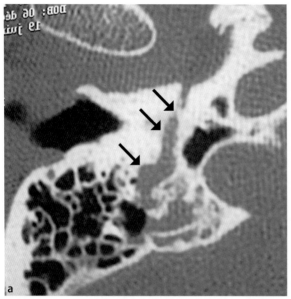

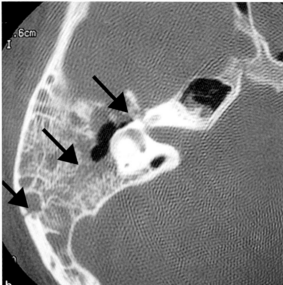

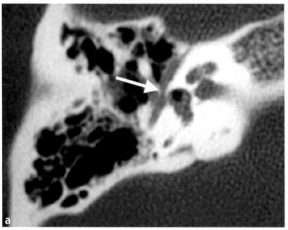

Fig. 1.7.4 a Right petrous bone extralabyrinthine fracture (high-resolution CT, axial view, bone algorithm). The fracture line (*arrows*) crosses the tympanic bone and divides the mastoid segment of the Fallopian canal. **b** Right petrous bone extralabyrinthine fracture (high-resolution CT, axial view, bone algorithm). The longitudinal fracture line is directed towards the geniculate ganglion area. **c** Right petrous bone extralabyrinthine fracture (high-resolution CT, axial view, bone algorithm). The dislocated incus splits the facial nerve at the level of its tympanic portion (*arrow*)

uations are done using the **House and Brackmann (HB) grading system** (see Sect. 1.7.1) designed for the evaluation of functional recovery.

- A complete otological and neurological workup is done as in any temporal bone trauma (see Sect. 1.5.3). A standard audiogram with stapedial reflex measurement is obtained as early as possible.
- Cranial nerves are also checked.
- Eye examination: look for dry eye.

A radiological workup of the temporal bone is to be done. A high-resolution CT scan using a bone algorithm and less than 1 mm slices is the standard examination. Native axial and coronal scan planes are optimal to look at the three parts of the Fallopian canal. It is possible to differentiate *transverse translabyrinthine fractures* (20%), mainly responsible for lesions to the tympanic portion of the nerve (Fig. 1.5.8b) or mainly *extralabyrinthine fractures* (80%), longitudinal or complex, responsible for lesions in the geniculate ganglion area (Fig. 1.7.4). In acute

traumatized patients it is not always possible to obtain coronal scan planes.

An electrophysiological assessment is useful and must be carried out in cases of a complete motor deficit.

Two different electrical examinations are routinely used:

1. **Electroneuronography (ENOG):** see Table 1.7.2
2. **Electromyography (EMG)** and **evoked EMG:** see Table 1.7.2

1.7.2.6 Additional/Useful Diagnostic Procedures

- Complete assessment of main extrafacial branches of the facial nerve: see the discussion of topognostic of facial nerve palsy in Sect. 1.7.1
- Contrast-enhanced MRI in cases of no fracture line
- Ophthalmologist counselling

1.7.2.7   Therapy

The patient is handled in one of two different ways:
1. If the palsy is incomplete, delayed or both, medical treatment is prescribed. The HB grading system is used to assess clinical outcome. If the palsy is complete but the EMG pattern is favourable (advocating neuropraxia), or if ENOG elicits less than 85% of denervation rate, medical treatment is first given and the patient is closely followed up. If during this survey palsy worsens, the ENOG pattern increases or the EMG pattern favours a severe denervation, a surgical exploration of the nerve is proposed after confirmation of the bad prognosis with EMG, which is more reliable than ENOG alone. Demonstration of a clear-cut fracture line crossing the path of the facial nerve on high-resolution CT can help to indicate surgery.
2. Surgery is chosen every time a total and immediate facial paralysis is demonstrated.

Conservative Medical Treatment

Recommended European Standard
- Corticosteroids: 1–2 mg/kg per day for 2 weeks if no contraindication is noticed
- Eye care (closure and eye drops)

Useful Additional Procedures
- Physiotherapy and rehabilitation technique without electrical stimulation.
- Vasodilators, pentoxyphilline, dextran (Stennert's protocol).
- Antiviral drug (acyclovir) use is discussed in the case of a secondarily induced facial paralysis (suspicion of herpesvirus reactivation).

Surgical Treatment
Recommended European Standard
1. Timing: surgery is performed as soon as possible on account of the associated shock and neurological trauma, allowing the patient to recover from his/her trauma and any haematoma can resolve itself.
2. Approaches
   - In the case of a labyrinthine fracture and/or a dead ear, a three-segment decompression technique is performed through a transmastoid translabyrinthine pathway.
   - When bone-conduction hearing is preserved, even partially, nerve decompression is done using a double approach: middle fossa and transmastoid.
   - The labyrinthine portion of the nerve can be reached by a simple transmastoid route through

the attic (so-called transmastoid extralabyrinthine approach) in selected cases when pneumatization is consistent and/or ossicles (incus) are displaced by the trauma. Surgical dislocation of the ossicular chain (section of the head of the malleus and removal of the incus) is otherwise mandatory. But the room is narrow to perform a graft or a decompression at the meatal foramen.
3. Nerve management
   - In the case of preservation of the nerve continuity only a decompression is realized uncovering the nerve in a minimum of half its circumference. Nerve sheath slitting routinely performed by some authors is debatable since some prefer not to add to nerve lesions.
   - In cases of a nerve gap, nerve repair is done according to the usual neurotologic procedures: decompression, rerouting and end-to-end suture and sural or great auricular nerve autograft in cases of a nerve gap larger than 3 mm. Nerve stumps are either sutured using nylon 9/0 or 10/0 stitches or only sealed using fibrin glue. The functional results seem to be the same. When the proximal stump is not available, one can choose between a crossfacial nerve graft, difficult to achieve, and a hypoglossal-facial crossover, easier to perform and leading to more constant results.
   - In case of late management (more than 3 months), great difficulties are faced to assess nerve lesions and even more to locate available nerve stumps in cases of nerve transection because of traumatic neuroma masking the proximal viable stump.
   - After a delay of 2 years after trauma, nerve repair is questionable. EMG can help to check muscle electrical spontaneous activity. If it is absent, it can be better to prefer static procedures such as face-lifting or muscle transposition (pediculized or free muscle transfer).

1.7.2.8   Differential Diagnosis

Post-traumatic peripheral facial paralysis is not difficult to distinguish from central palsies due to brain traumas.

Gunshot Traumas
In cases of gunshot traumas, lesions are usually situated in the tympanic or vertical portion of the nerve. Facial paralysis is usually associated with a dead ear and a CSF fistula. Surgery frequently necessitates a middle ear exclusion to treat the leakage and protect the meninges. Nerve lesions are very difficult to assess. A graft is usually necessary to bridge the nerve loss. A bad outcome can be antic-

ipated because of nerve burning and tearing and because of foreign bodies polluting the operative field.

Iatrogenic Lesions

Iatrogenic lesions are not so common as those following temporal bone traumas. They are to be differentiated:

1. Lesions in the cerebellopontine angle or the internal auditory canal consecutive to tumour resections (vestibular schwannomas, meningiomas). Two situations are to be considered:

   (a) An anatomically-preserved nerve does not respond to electrical stimuli: nerve degeneration will necessitate a total regrowth. If no recovery is observed after 18 months a XII–VII crossover is proposed to the patient using either the classic end-to-end or the side-to-end technique allowing one to preserve the lingual function.

   (b) There is a nerve gap: an immediate repair is necessary. This repair is particularly difficult to achieve in this area. Rerouting and suture is not always sufficient to bridge the nerve gap. Use of a cable graft either sutured or sealed with fibrin glue is the rule when the proximal stump of the nerve is available. The graft is harvested at the expense of the sural nerve or the great auricular nerve, nearer to the ear. Grafting leads to results as good those achieved with nerve rerouting and suturing. More often than not HB 3 or 4 (4>3) is obtained. When the proximal stump is not available, a XII–VII crossover is proposed.

2. Lesions in the middle ear due to iatrogenic injury during middle ear surgery (otosclerosis, cholesteatoma, dysgenesias). Those injuries can be consecutive to wrong use either of sharp instruments (blades, pick or hook) or of more compromising ones such as lasers, electrocauteries or drills. Prognosis is dramatically better in the former than in the latter. Burning (laser, electrocautery) actually leads to severe sequelae even if the nerve is decompressed, owing to degeneration process scarring and loss of tubules. Accidents due to drilling may also be severe because of associated tearing and heat traumas to the nerve.

A golden rule is to be followed: in the case of an immediate and complete facial paralysis following middle ear surgery, not due to lidocaine infiltration, one must reoperate as soon as possible to explore the nerve.

- In the case of nerve herniation through a sheath wound, decompression and wide opening of the sheath is to be done up and down the lesion site.
- In cases of a nerve gap, rerouting and suture or interpositional grafting are chosen depending on the situation of the lesion and the gap length.

1.7.2.9 Prognosis

Recovery depends on the initial severity of the nerve lesions at the time of handling and on the surgical management:

- In the case of neuropraxia (incomplete or delayed palsies), the outcome is good leading to HB 1 (or 2) in all cases.
- In the case of partial or total nerve degeneration (neurotmesis), the result cannot be better than HB 2 (partial degeneration, mixed EMG pattern). More often than not HB 3 is obtained, with synkinesia and mass movements.
- In the case of nerve suture or graft, a HB 3 or 4 is obtained at the best: no frontal movement is observed and synkinesia are constant features.
- In the case of late management (after 3 months), the results seems to be less favourable (HB 4 or less) because of difficulties to locate nerve stumps.

1.7.2.10 Surgical Principles: Double Approach to the Intratemporal Facial Nerve

General anaesthesia with the patient in the supine position, head turned on the contralateral side and fixed.

1. Middle fossa approach
   - Supra-auricular vertical pretragal or inferiorly based U-shaped incision.
   - Square 5 cm × 5 cm limited craniotomy as close to the floor of the middle fossa as possible, above the root of the zygomatic process.
   - Extradural exposure of the roof of the temporal bone enabling the location of the middle meningeal artery and petrous nerve nearby.
   - From there, drilling enables exposure of the geniculate ganglion, labyrinthine and proximal part of the tympanic portion of the nerve.
   - Suspension of the dura and repositioning of the craniotomy bone.
   - Suture of the rest of the temporalis muscle on a suction drain.
   - Closure of the skin incision.

2. Transmastoid approach
   - Patient's head is not fixed.
   - Postauricular incision.
   - Removal of large air cells Opening of the mastoid aditus and epitympanum. Location of the incus.
   - Location of the vertical portion of the nerve at the second genu below the lateral semicircular canal.
   - Wide posterior tympanotomy preserving the incus, exposing the stapes and the tympanic segment of the facial nerve.
   - Closure of the skin.

Suggested Reading

1. Darrouzet V, Guerin J, Bebear JP (1999) New technique of side-to-end hypoglossal nerve attachment with translocation of the intratemporal facial nerve. J Neurosurg 90:27–34

1.7.3   Facial Nerve Schwannoma

OLIVIER STERKERS, CHRISTIAN MARTIN
AND WOLFGANG ARNOLD

1.7.3.1   Synonyms

Facial nerve neuroma, facial nerve neurilemoma, facial nerve neurinoma.

1.7.3.2   Definition

Facial nerve schwannomas may arise throughout the course of the facial nerve from the cerebellopontine angle to the parotid gland. These primary tumours of the facial nerve are uncommon, generally benign and exhibit a slow growth rate.

1.7.3.3   Aetiology/Epidemiology

Facial nerve schwannomas are encountered at around 40 years of age with an equal sex and side distribution. The perigeniculate area and the horizontal and vertical portions of the facial nerve are most often affected (Fig. 1.7.5). Many patients have two or three contiguous areas affected. Tumours are also found along branches of the nerve including the chorda tympani and the nerve of the stapedius muscle. Facial nerve schwannomas that have developed in the cerebellopontine angle and the internal auditory canal can be misdiagnosed as acoustic tumours preoperatively. Neurofibromatous type 2 tumours affecting both sides may be observed in some cases. Malignant schwannoma is an exceedingly rare entity.

1.7.3.4   Symptoms

Symptoms depend upon the location of the lesion. The most common presenting complaint is a slowly progressive facial nerve weakness and/or conductive hearing loss. It begins generally with facial twitching (hyperkinesis). However, a sudden facial paralysis is not uncommon as well as recurrent ipsilateral paralysis. Progressive mainly conductive hearing loss is frequent. Other symptoms include tinnitus, pain, ear canal mass, vestibular symptoms and otorrhoea.

1.7.3.5   Complications

Complete facial paralysis, total deafness and consequences of cerebellopontine angle extension are complications (see Sect. 1.5.4.2).

1.7.3.6   Diagnosis

- Grading of the facial nerve function according to the *House–Brackmann (HB) scale* (see Sect. 1.7.1).
- *Palpation of the neck*: mass in the parotid region when the tumour is extended to the parotid gland.
- *Otoscopy (ear microscopy)*: non-pulsating, grey or reddish retrotympanic mass when the tumour invades the middle ear cavities. Tumours that begin in the vertical portion may sometimes be seen through the external auditory canal.
- *Audiovestibular testing*: pure tone and speech audiometry are performed to assess the degree of conductive and sensorineural impairments. Auditory brainstem response is performed in the case of sensorineural hearing loss. Vestibular studies are limited to patients who describe dizziness or vertigo.
- *Electrical facial nerve testing*: electromyography and electroneuronography to evaluate facial nerve function (see Sect. 1.7.1).

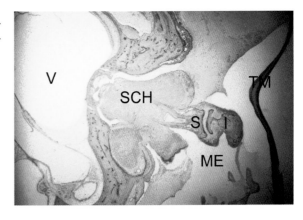

Fig. 1.7.5 Histology section through the oval window niche showing a facial nerve schwannoma which has partly destroyed the stapes suprastructure causing a severe conductive hearing loss. V = vestibule; SCH = facial nerve schwannoma; I = incus; S = stapes; ME = middle ear cavity; TM = tympanic membrane

- *Imaging*: high-resolution CT and MRI are mandatory for the diagnosis of facial nerve schwannomas and for the evaluation of the extension along the facial nerve course. MRI characteristics are isointense or slightly hypointense signals in T1 sequences with homogeneous gadolinium enhancement. Proximal facial nerve tumours simulate acoustic tumours in their MRI aspects.

1.7.3.7 Therapy

Conservative Therapy

No treatment is proposed in patients with no alteration of the facial function, especially in elderly patients. Radiotherapy is used in selected cases (see Sect. 1.5.4.2)

Surgery

- *Middle fossa approach*: proposed for geniculate lesions and internal auditory canal and moderate cerebellopontine angle extension with serviceable hearing.
- *Translabyrinthine or transotic approaches*: proposed for the cerebellopontine angle and internal auditory canal lesions without serviceable hearing.
- *Transmastoid approach*: proposed for tympanic and vertical lesions. It can be associated with a middle fossa approach in cases of geniculate invasion or with parotid gland dissection in cases of extratemporal extension.
- *Facial nerve grafting*: in most cases the facial nerve is interrupted after tumour removal. Immediate cable grafting with the great auricular or sural nerve is the procedure of choice.

1.7.3.8 Differential Diagnosis

- *Geniculate haemangioma*: extrinsic benign facial nerve tumour presenting in all cases with facial palsy. Imaging characteristics differentiate haemangiomas from schwannomas: on CT, enlargement of geniculate ganglion with adjacent bony irregular and unsharp erosion; on MRI, heterogeneous aspect with intense gadolinium enhancement and sometimes intratumoral calcifications. Surgical treatment is similar to that for geniculate schwannomas.
- *Other benign and malignant lesions of the temporal bone*: meningioma, vestibular schwannoma, primary epidermoid tumours, glomus jugulare, parotid malignancies and metastatic lesions.

1.7.3.9 Prognosis

- Facial nerve recovery can at best achieve HB 3 (see Sect. 1.7.1) at 1-year follow-up. Rehabilitation of the facial function is greatly improved by facial exercises.
- Complications arising from translabyrinthine and middle fossa approaches (see Sect. 1.5.4.2).
- If no treatment, serial clinical and imaging follow-up is necessary.

Suggested Reading

1. Jackler RK, Driscoll CLW (2000) Tumors of the ear and temporal bone. Lippincott Williams and Wilkins, Philadelphia
2. O'Donoghue GM (1994) Tumors of the facial nerve. In: Jackler RJ, Brackmann DE (eds) Neurotology. Mosby, St Louis
3. Saleh E, Achilli V, Naguib M et al. (1995) Facial nerve neuromas: diagnosis and management. Am J Otol 16:521–526

Diseases of the Nose and Paranasal Sinuses

Edited by Manuel Bernal-Sprekelsen

2.1 Anatomy of the Nasal Cavity and Paranasal Sinuses

HUMBERTO MASSEGUR AND JACINTO GARCIA

2.1.1 Introduction

Since nasal endoscopy and CT were first introduced into general ENT practice, controversy has arisen over the terminology of the anatomical landmarks in the nasal cavities.

Useful terminology for the rhinologist is sparse in the anatomical nomenclature, and the introduction of different terms by English and French authors has contributed to further confusion.

The Anatomic Terminology Group's (formed in 1993 at the International Conference on Sinus Disease: Terminology, Staging, and Therapy, Princeton, N.J.) first attempt at standardisation has not achieved consensus throughout the world, due either to problems of diffusion or to difficulties in the acceptance of new terminology. This chapter aims to contribute to the unification of anatomical terminology of the nasal cavity and paranasal sinuses, serving as a guide for rhinologists, anatomists and radiologists.

The nasal cavity and the paranasal sinuses are complex structures, made up of an intricate jigsaw of bones. Vascular and neural elements find their way to the mucosa through the tight sutures among them. The bones are first described separately and then as a whole.

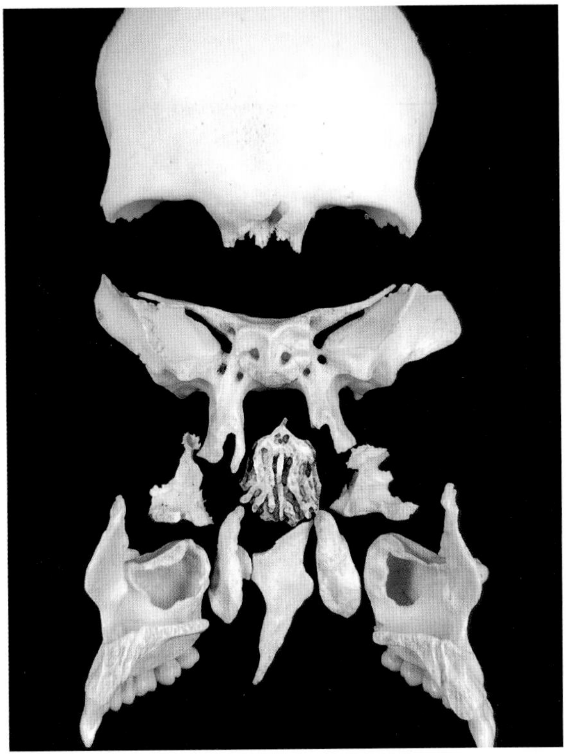

Fig. 2.1.1 The ethmoid bone sits in the middle of all sinonasal bony structures

2.1.2 Ethmoid Bone

The ethmoid bone (os ethmoidal) sits in the middle of the sinonasal structures (Fig. 2.1.1). For the purpose of this text, it is taken as a reference around which all the other bones are situated.

The ethmoid is a middle bone situated under the ethmoidal recess of the frontal bone (Fig. 2.1.2). On its superior face, the lamina cribrosa separates the anterior cranial fossa from the nasal cavity (Fig. 2.1.3). The crista galli stands perpendicularly to the lamina cribrosa, serving as an attachment for the falx cerebri. On the same sagittal plane hangs the perpendicular plate, the lamina perpendicularis: a thin bony sheet that forms the upper part of the nasal septum. Laterally, the ethmoidal cells (cellulae ethmoidales) grow inside the lateral masses of the ethmoid (labyrinthus ethmoidalis). The middle turbinate

basal lamella divides the ethmoidal cells into two complexes, anterior and posterior. All cells draining anteriorly into the basal lamella belong to the anterior complex, and all cells draining posteriorly, except those from the sphenoid, belong to the posterior complex. The "middle ethmoid complex" is, however, an erroneous concept, as it has no anatomical or physiological basis.

The external wall of the lateral mass is a paper-thin plate called the lamina papyracea (lamina orbitalis). It forms a large part of the medial wall of the orbit, together with the lacrimal bone (os lacrimale) and the lateral wall of the sphenoid bone. In its superior border two small grooves (foramina ethmoidale) house the anterior and posterior ethmoidal arteries, nerves and veins coming out of the orbit.

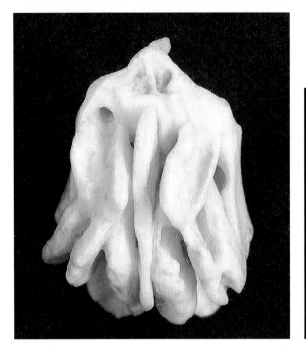

Fig. 2.1.2 The ethmoid bone (anterior view)

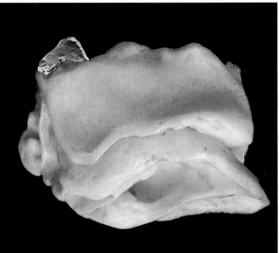

Fig. 2.1.3 The ethmoid bone, lateral view of the crista galli (*silver*)

The medial surface of the lateral mass forms part of the lateral wall of the corresponding nasal cavity. There are three main structures, the middle turbinate (concha nasalis media), the superior turbinate (concha nasalis superior) and the supreme turbinate (concha nasalis suprema).

Each of them has three segments. The first is vertical and inserts into the horizontal part of the nasal bone or in the union between the lamina cribrosa and the lateral mass of the ethmoid (Fig. 2.1.4). The second segment is horizontal and attaches to the lamina papyracea in a frontal plane (Figs. 2.1.5, 2.1.6). The third segment corresponds to the visible part of the turbinate and inserts longitudinally in the lamina papyracea. The horizontal segments are also called basal lamellae. That of the middle turbinate divides the ethmoid cells in two segments, anterior and posterior, as stated previously.

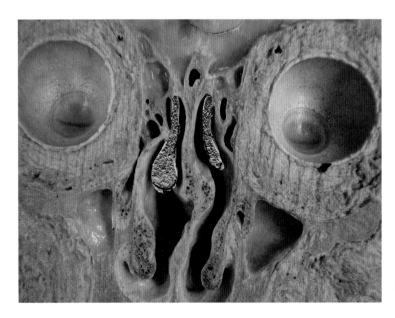

Fig. 2.1.4 Coronal view with the skull base insertion of the middle turbinates (*silver*)

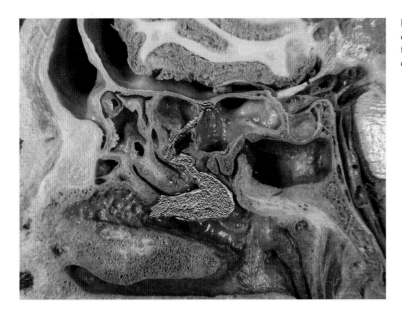

Fig. 2.1.5 Sagittal view of the ethmoid cells with the basal lamella of the middle turbinate, dividing the anterior ethmoid cells from the posterior ethmoid cells

Each turbinate limits its corresponding meatus. The middle meatus contains several well-defined structures that represent significant surgical landmarks.

The uncinate process (processus uncinatus) is a thin, sickle-shaped lamella, a remnant of the first ethmotur-

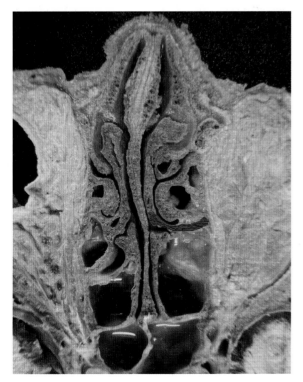

Fig. 2.1.6 Axial view of the ethmoid labyrinths. The right basal lamella of the middle turbinate (*in red*) dividing the anterior and posterior ethmoid cells

binal (Fig. 2.1.7). It is oriented sagittally and inserts, with many variations, into the cranial base, lamina papyracea or anterosuperior part of the lacrimal bone, lamina perpendicularis of the palatine bone and processus ethmoidalis of the inferior turbinate (concha nasalis inferior).

It is curved posteriorly, parallel to the ethmoidal bulla (bulla ethmoidalis), and represents the anterior border of the inferior semilunar hiatus (hiatus semilunaris inferior) and the ethmoidal infundibulum (infundibulum ethmoidale) (Fig. 2.1.8).

The ethmoidal bulla (bulla ethmoidalis) is the anterior ethmoidal cell most constant. It is a semicircular bony bulge, which inserts laterally on the lamina papyracea. In some cases, the superior insertion does not reach the roof of the ethmoid, leaving a space called the suprabullar recess. In the same way, a space between the posterior wall of the ethmoidal bulla and the middle turbinate basal lamella is called retrobullar recess (Fig 2.1.8). The two structures together form the sinus lateralis (sinus ethmoidalis) of Grünwald. However, the term *recess* is usually preferred, considering the limited utility of the term *sinus* in this context and the possible mislead concerning the lateral sinuses of the brain.

Inferior semilunar hiatus (hiatus semilunaris inferior) designates the 2D plane that goes from the posterior border of the uncinate process to the anterior face of the ethmoidal bulla. It is crescent-shaped and serves as the entrance to the ethmoidal infundibulum. The superior semilunar hiatus (hiatus semilunaris superior) is the space between the ethmoidal bulla and the middle turbinate. It allows access to retrobullar and suprabullar recesses.

The ethmoidal infundibulum (infundibulum ethmoidale) is the most important infundibulum of the nose, as the other two infundibula, frontal and maxillary, flow

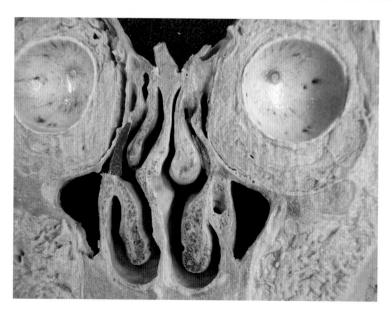

Fig. 2.1.7 Coronal view of the ostiomeatal complex. *Red* the unciform process

into it. It is a funnel-shaped, 3D space limited by the uncinate process medially, the lamina papyracea laterally and the ethmoidal bulla posteriorly. It can lead directly to the frontal recess or end in a pouch (recessus terminalis), depending on the anterosuperior attachment of the uncinate process.

The frontal recess is the most anterior and superior part of the middle meatus, leading to the frontal sinus. It is an inverted funnel, reminiscent of the pneumatisation of the frontal sinus by the ethmoidal cells. It is limited medially and superiorly by the middle turbinate, laterally by the lamina papyracea and posteriorly by the basal lamella of the ethmoidal bulla. All three limits are very variable, depending on the pneumatisation and insertions of the bulla and the capricious situation of the anterosuperior insertion of the uncinate process. The resulting septa of these anatomical variations graphically illustrate the misnomer *frontonasal duct.* Even though the CT images can lead to confusion, the existence of this duct cannot be demonstrated anatomically. The term *frontal recess* should be used instead (Fig. 2.1.9).

Anterior ethmoidal cells are numerous (9 or 10) and variable. They can be categorised into three cell types: uncinate, bullar and meatal. They tend to invade neighbouring structures such as the supraorbital, lacrimal or frontal cells.

The posterior ethmoidal cells are situated behind the basal lamella of the middle turbinate. They are fewer in number (2 to 4) but bigger than the anterior cells. In some cases a single posterior cell, named the sphenoethmoidal cell, or the Onodi cell, invades the body and small wings of the sphenoid bone. The bony dehiscence of the optic canal can be seen within these cells, depending on the extent of pneumatisation (Fig. 2.1.10).

The ostiomeatal complex cannot be considered an anatomical structure. It is a physiological unit of the anterior ethmoidal sinus, where ethmoidal, frontal and maxillary sinuses drain.

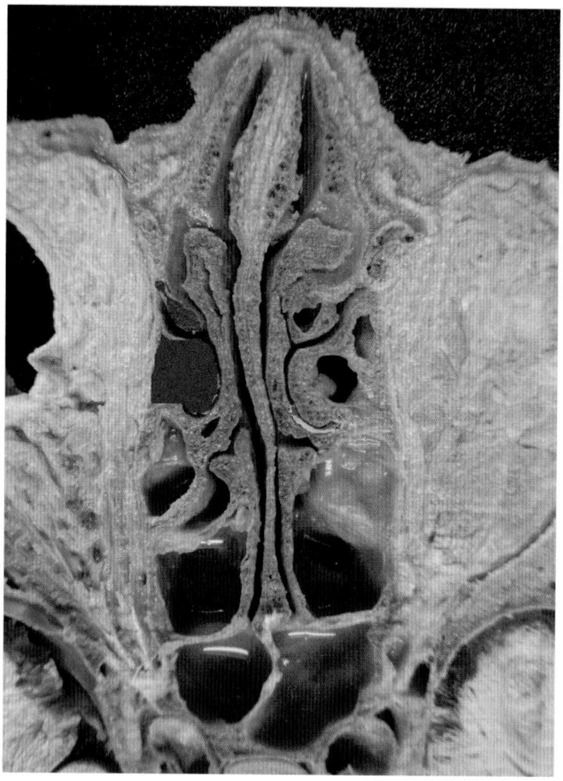

Fig. 2.1.8 Axial view of the ethmoid cells. *Red* unciform process, *blue* bulla ethmoidalis, *yellow* retrobullar recess

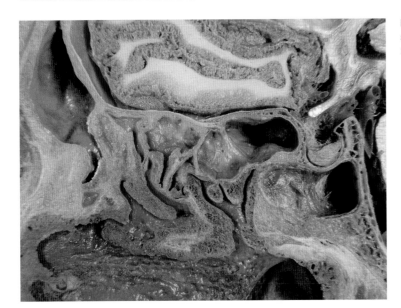

Fig. 2.1.9 Sagittal view of the frontal sinus, frontal infundibulum and frontal recess (*silver*)

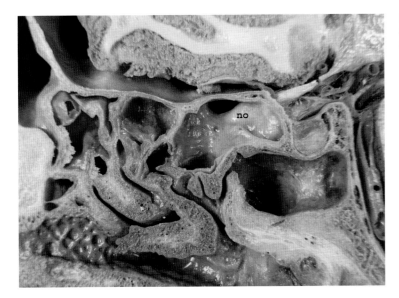

Fig. 2.1.10 Sphenoethmoidal cell or Onodi cell, with the optic canal (*no*) protruding on the lateral wall

2.1.3 Frontal Bone

The lateral masses of the ethmoid bone are very thin in their superior part, as the ethmoidal cells invade the horizontal part of the frontal bone (os frontale) at both sides of the ethmoidal notch (incisura ethmoidalis). Therefore, the roof of the ethmoid consists of the medial portion of the orbital face of the frontal bone (facies orbitalis) (Fig. 2.1.11). The impressions of the ethmoidal cells on the frontal bone are called foveae, and they can vary considerably in depth. This can lead to a significant difference in the height of the roof of the ethmoid compared with the lamina cribrosa. Keros classified these variations into three types: Keros I, when the difference is 1–3 mm,

that is, the roof of the ethmoid and the lamina cribrosa are almost the same height; Keros II, 4–7 mm; and Keros III, 8–16 mm. The latter means that the medial wall of the ethmoid can be extremely thin, posing a significant risk of anterior cranial fossa damage during surgery.

Air cell invasion of the frontal bone is maximal in the frontal sinuses (sinus frontalis). It starts in the frontal ostium (aperture sinus frontalis) and continues along the frontal infundibulum to end in the frontal sinus itself. Altogether, the infundibulum, ostium and sinus take the shape of an hourglass in the sagittal view.

All but the inferior wall of the frontal sinus are formed by diploe. The posterior wall is usually thin and in close contact with the anterior cranial fossa. The inferior wall is part of the roof of the orbit. Both frontal sinuses are

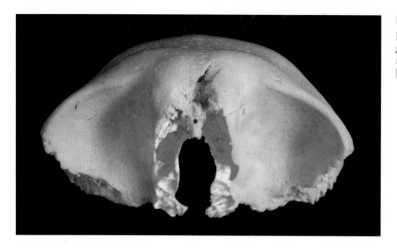

Fig. 2.1.11 Frontal bone with the medial portion of the orbital face *highlighted in grey*, showing the foveae left by the ethmoid cells and the ethmoidal notch for the lamina cribrosa

separated by a thin, oblique, bony wall, responsible for their characteristic asymmetry.

The ethmoidal notch (incisura ethmoidalis) is filled by the lamina cribrosa. The anterior ethmoidal foramen (foramina ethmoidalis anterior) opens in the cribriform plate, right behind the crista galli, allowing the passage of the anterior ethmoidal nerve and vessels in a canal along its lateral edge. The relief of this canal protrudes into the roof of the ethmoid, behind the anterior wall of the ethmoidal bulla, and indicates the posterior limit of the frontal recess (Fig. 2.1.12). This should not be confused with a prebullar cell, commonly found as a fovea between the canal relief and the frontal recess itself.

The posterior ethmoidal foramen (foramina ethmoidalis posterior) can be found in the posterior part of the frontoethmoidal suture. It contains the posterior ethmoidal nerve and vessels. The canal relief can be seen just in front of the sphenoidal sinus or sphenoethmoidal angle.

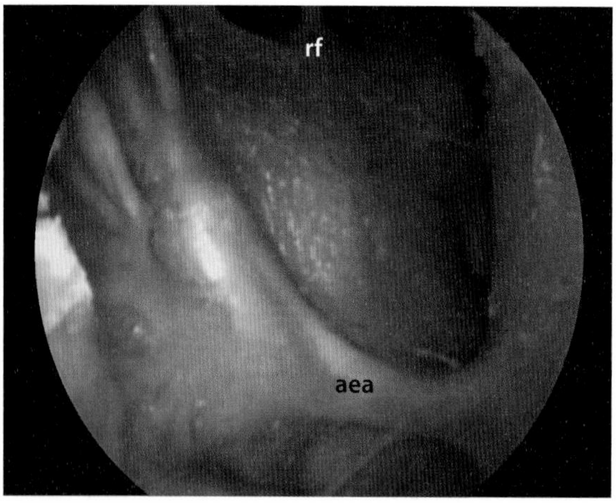

The posterior border (margo sphenoidalis) of the frontal bone articulates with the small (ala minor) and greater wings (ala major) of the sphenoid bone.

The nasal part (pars nasalis) of the frontal bone lies between the orbital parts (pars orbitalis). This portion presents a rough, uneven interval, the nasal notch (margo nasalis), which articulates on either side of the middle line with the nasal bone (os nasale), and laterally with the frontal process of the maxilla (processus frontalis) and with the lacrimal (os lacrimale).

The nasal spine (spina nasalis) is a midline prolongation. The spine forms part of the septum of the nose, articulating in the front with the crest of the nasal bones and behind with the perpendicular plate of the ethmoid (lamina perpendicularis).

2.1.4 Maxilla

The body of the maxilla (corpus maxillae) surrounds the cavity of the maxillary sinus (Fig. 2.1.13). In its anterior and medial part stands the frontal process, which articulates with the frontal bone superiorly, with the lacrimal posteriorly (margo lacrimalis), with the middle turbinate in the ethmoidal crest (crista ethmoidalis) and with the inferior turbinate in the conchal crest (crista conchalis) in the medial face.

Right behind the frontal process is a deep groove, the lacrimal groove (sulcus lacrimalis), which is converted into the nasolacrimal canal, by the lacrimal bone and the lacrimal process (processus lacrimalis) of the inferior nasal concha. This canal opens into the inferior meatus of the nose and transmits the nasolacrimal duct.

Fig. 2.1.12 Endoscopic view of the frontal recess with the relief of the anterior ethmoid artery as a posterior limit. *rf* frontal recess, *aea* anterior ethmoid artery

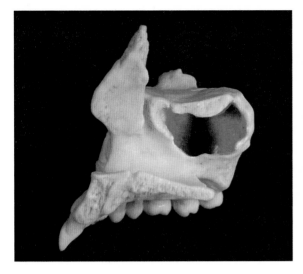

Fig. 2.1.13 Maxillary bone. The maxillary sinus (*silver*)

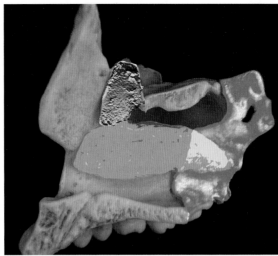

Fig. 2.1.14 Maxillary bone. The lacrimal bone, palatine bone and inferior turbinate attached, leaving a reduced hiatus maxillaries

The maxillary sinus (sinus maxillaris) has a pyramidal shape, whose base corresponds to the medial face and whose vertex points to the zygomatic process of the maxilla (processus zygomaticus). The posterior limit is the infratemporal wall of the maxilla, the inferior limit is closed by the palatine process of the maxilla (processus palatinus) and the alveolar process (processus alveolaris), the anterior wall is the anterior face of the maxilla (facies anterior) and the roof is the floor of the orbit (facies orbitalis).

The maxillary ostium (hiatus maxillaris) is very wide in the disarticulated maxilla. However, in the articulated skull this aperture is greatly reduced in size by several bones. The uncinate process of the ethmoid crosses diagonally to articulate with the ethmoidal process (processus ethmoidalis) of the inferior nasal concha, whose maxillary process (processus maxillaris) covers the inferior margin. The vertical part (lamina perpendicularis) of the palatine hides the posterior notch, and a small portion of the lacrimal bone covers the anterosuperior angle (Figs. 2.1.14, 2.1.15). The remaining gap in the maxillary ostium is closed by connective tissue and mucosa, forming the fontanelle. The uncinate process divides the fontanelle into the anterior and posterior fontanelle. The natural ostium of the maxillary sinus is located in the anteroinferior angle of the fontanelle, and constitutes the connection of the maxillary infundibulum with the ethmoidal infundibulum. It is hidden medially by the concave portion of the uncinate process. It is not unusual to find accessory ostia, seen as round holes in the fontanelle; this should not be confused with the oval-shaped natural ostium, which cannot be seen with a 0° endoscope (Figs. 2.1.16, 2.1.17).

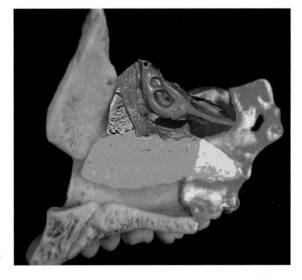

Fig. 2.1.15 Maxillary bone. The unciform process and ethmoid bulla superimposed, leaving the fontanelle gaps

The palatine process (processus palatinus) is a horizontal plate that projects medially towards its contralateral counterpart to form the floor of the nose and the hard palate. The nasal crest (crista nasalis) arises in the suture between these two processes and articulates with the vomer. Anteriorly, the septal cartilage attaches to a thick protrusion called the anterior nasal spine (spina nasalis anterior) (Fig. 2.1.18). Behind the palatine process lies the horizontal process of the palatine bone (lamina horizontalis), completing the floor of the nasal cavity.

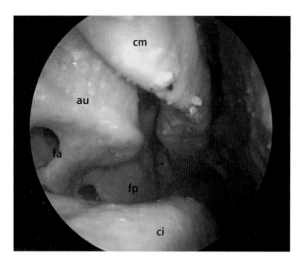

Fig. 2.1.16 Endoscopic view of a right nasal fossa, middle meatus, with several accessory ostia on the anterior and posterior fontanelle

contains an air cell. The sphenoidal process (processus sphenoidalis) attaches to the medial lamina of the pterygoid process. The orbital and sphenoidal processes are separated from one another by the sphenopalatine notch (incisura sphenoidalis), part of the sphenopalatine foramen. The medial wall of the vertical plate has an ethmoidal crest (crista ethmoidalis) for the middle turbinate and a conchal crest (crista conchalis) for the inferior turbinate. The latter separates an inferior concavity belonging to the inferior meatus from a superior concavity in the middle meatus (Fig. 2.1.19). The pyramidal process (processus pyramidalis) projects backwards and laterally from the junction of the horizontal and vertical parts, and is received into the angular interval between the lower extremities of the pterygoid plates (incisura pterygoidea) On its posterior face lies the palatine groove (sulcus pterygopalatinus). Together with the greater palatine groove of the maxilla, they form a canal for the descending palatine vessels and the palatine major nerve.

2.1.5 Palatine Bone

The palatine bone (os palatinum) consists of:
1. The *horizontal plate* (lamina horizontalis)
   This articulates with the palatine process of the maxilla, and forms the posterior prolongation of the nasal crest ending up to the posterior nasal spine (spina nasalis posterior)
2. The *vertical plate* (lamina perpendicularis), with three outstanding processes
   The orbital process (processus orbitalis) projects upwards to the floor of the orbit and articulates with the maxilla, the ethmoid and the sphenoid. It usually

2.1.6 Inferior Turbinate

The inferior turbinate (concha nasalis inferior) is an independent bone situated in the lateral wall of the nasal cavity, with three major reliefs. The lacrimal process (processus lacrimalis) closes the nasolacrimal duct by articulation with the descending process of the lacrimal bone. The maxillary process attaches to the maxilla in the inferior part of the maxillary ostium and with the conchal crest of the palatine bone. The ethmoidal process (processus ethmoidalis) articulates with the inferior end of the uncinate process (Fig. 2.1.20).

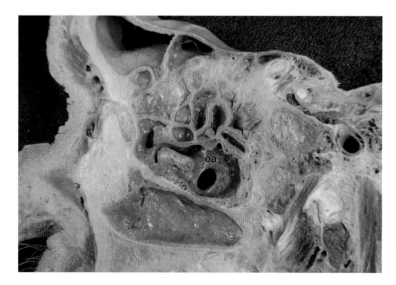

Fig. 2.1.17 Sagittal view of the fontanelle area with an accessory ostium

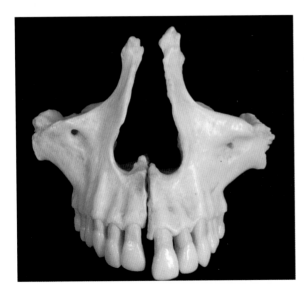

Fig. 2.1.18 Both maxillary bones articulate, forming the nasal framework

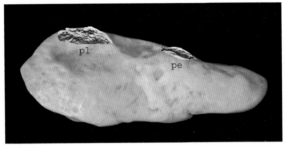

Fig. 2.1.20 Right inferior turbinate. *pl* lacrimal process, *pe* ethmoid process

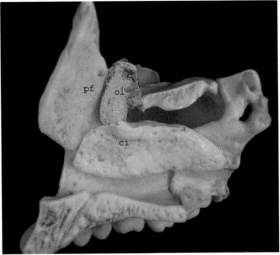

Fig. 2.1.21 The lacrimal bone (*ol*) articulated with the frontal process of the maxillary bone (*pf*) and the lacrimal process of the inferior turbinate (*ci*)

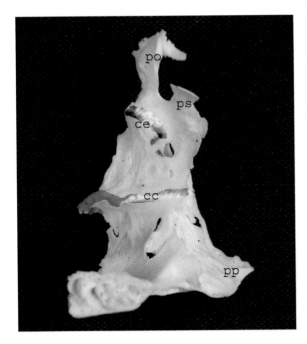

Fig. 2.1.19 Right palatine bone, medial view. *po* orbital process, *pe* sphenoid process, *pp* pyramidal process, *ce* ethmoidal crest, *cc* conchal crest

segment and the ethmoidal cells–lamina papyracea posteriorly.

It articulates with the frontal process of the maxilla and with the lacrimal process of the inferior turbinate to form a canal containing the nasolacrimal duct and sac (Fig. 2.1.21).

2.1.7 Lacrimal Bone

The lacrimal bone (os lacrimale) is a rectangular lamella that completes the middle meatus, with its anteroinferior

2.1.8 Sphenoid Bone

The sphenoid (os sphenoidale) is the posterior bone of the nasal cavity. It articulates with the ethmoid, palatine, vomer, maxilla and frontal bones, forming canals and spaces of outmost importance (Fig. 2.1.22).

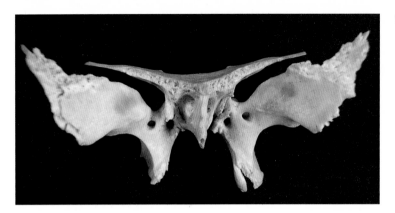

Fig. 2.1.22 Sphenoid bone, coronal view

The body of the sphenoid (corpus sphenoidalis) has a central situation and contains the sphenoidal sinuses. These are variable in shape and size and asymmetrically divided by a bony septum. Pneumatisation may develop in the clinoid and pterygoid processes. Larger air cavities imply weaker protection of the adjacent structures: internal carotid artery, cavernous sinus, optic and maxillary nerves in the lateral wall; hypophysis cerebri, basilar artery and pons in the posterior wall; optic chiasma and anterior cerebral arteries in the upper wall (planum sphenoidale) and lastly, the Vidian nerve in the inferior wall.

The ostia of the sphenoid sinus (apertura sinus sphenoidalis) open in the anterior face of the body. The sinus communicates with the nose via the sphenoethmoidal recess (recessus sphenoethmoidalis). This space is limited by the bony septum (perpendicular plate of the ethmoid and vomer) medially, the upper and supreme turbinates laterally, and the roof of the nasal cavity (rima olfactoria) superiorly.

Medially, the body of the sphenoid has two crests, the sphenoid crest (crista sphenoidalis), which articulates with the perpendicular plate of the ethmoid, and the sphenoidal rostrum (rostrum sphenoidale), which attaches to the vomer (Fig. 2.1.23).

The great wings articulate with the frontal bone (margo frontalis). They have an orbital facet that partially inserts to the maxilla to form the inferior orbital fissure (fissura orbitalis inferior). This is the entrance to the orbit of the infraorbital and zygomatic nerves and the infraorbital artery. The gap between the great and the small wings is called the superior orbital fissure (fissura orbitalis superior). It transmits the ophthalmic, oculomotor, trochlear, and abducens nerves, the three branches of the ophthalmic division of the trigeminal nerve, the orbital branch of the middle meningeal artery and the ophthalmic vein. The small wings attach to the frontal bone closing the ethmoidal notch from behind.

The pterygoid processes of the sphenoid consist of two plates, the medial and lateral (lamina medialis and lamina lateralis), the upper parts of which are fused anteriorly.

The plates are separated below by an angular cleft, the pterygoid fissure (incisura pterygoidea), which shelters the pyramidal process of the palatine bone (Fig. 2.1.24). In this 3D space lies the pterygomaxillary fossa, contained by the posterior wall of the maxillary sinus anteriorly. It contains the pterygopalatine ganglion and the maxillary vessels with all their branches.

The medial plate fuses with the sphenoid process of the palatine bone in a small furrow located in the joint of the pterygoid process and the body of the sphenoid. In

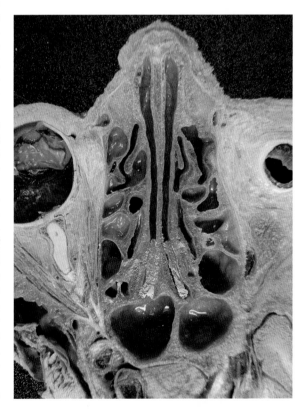

Fig. 2.1.23 Axial view of the sphenoethmoidal recesses (*red*)

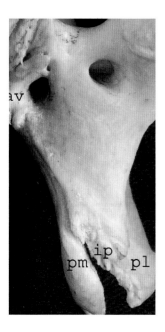

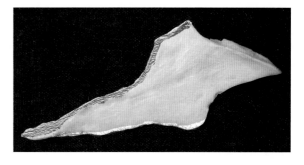

Fig. 2.1.24 Left pterygoid process of the sphenoid bone. *pl* lateral process, *ip* incisura pterygoidea, *pm* medial process

Fig. 2.1.25 The vomer articulates with sphenoid bone (*light silver*), perpendicular plate of the ethmoid (*dark silver*), the septal cartilage (*red*) and the maxillary and palatine crest (*white*)

The anterior border fuses with the perpendicular plate of the ethmoid and the septal cartilage. The inferior border articulates with the crest formed by the maxillae and palatine bones (Fig. 2.1.25).

the medial border of this furrow, a crest articulates with the wings of the vomer (processus vaginalis). A small orifice allows the entrance of the sphenopalatine artery and nerve into the nasal cavity.

2.1.10 Conclusion

The complex anatomy of the nasal cavity and paranasal sinuses is made up of the articulation of all the structures described (Figs. 2.1.26, 2.1.27). This chapter aimed to "deconstruct" the jigsaw and give a detailed description of each of the separate pieces, to understand better the anatomical landmarks and relationships and to provide a 3D view of the anatomy of the nose. Although the perspective differs depending on the instrument of examination (microscope, endoscope, among others), anatomy has not changed significantly over the last centuries.

2.1.9 Vomer

The vomer is situated in the median plane, and it forms the hindmost and lower part of the nasal septum. The uppermost and posterior part presents a groove for the articulation with the rostrum, and two little wings for the processus vaginalis of the sphenoid and palatine bones.

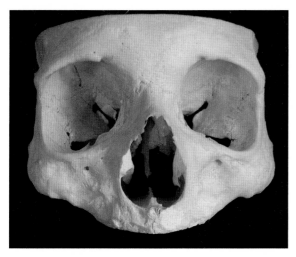

Fig. 2.1.26 Anterior view of the nasal fossae

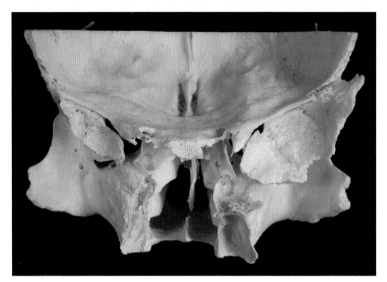

Fig. 2.1.27 Posterior view of the nasal fossae

References

1. Lang J (1988) Klinische Anatomie der Nase, Nasenhöhle, und Nebenhöhlen: Grundlagen für Diagnostik u. Operation. Thieme, Stuttgart
2. Stammberger HR, Kennedy DW et al. (1995) Paranasal sinuses: anatomic terminology and nomenclature. Ann Otol Rhinol Laryngol 104:S7–S16
3. Klossek JM, Serrano E, Desmonds C, Percodani J (1997) Anatomie des cavitées nasosinusiennes. Encycl Med Chir Otorhinolaringol 265:A10
4. Agrifolio A, Terrier G, Duvoisin B (1990) Étude anatomique de l'ethmoide anterieur. Ann Otolaryngol 107:249–258
5. Stammberger H (1991) Functional endoscopic sinus surgery: the Messerklinger technique. Decker, Philadelphia, Pa.
6. Wigand ME, Hosemann W (1990) Endoscopic surgery of the paranasal sinuses and anterior skull base. Thieme, Stuttgart
7. Klossek JM, Serrano E, Dessi P, Fontanel JP (2004) Chirurgie Endonasale sous guidage endoscopique. Masson, Paris

2.2 Physiology of the Nose

JEAN-FRANÇOIS PAPON AND ANDRÉ COSTE

As the initial upper part of the conductive respiratory system, the nose actively participates in airflow dynamics and conditioning of the 10,000 litres of air inhaled every day by an adult. As a specific organ, the nose contains the olfactory organ.

2.2.1 Airflow Dynamics

Air enters the nose through the nostrils. It takes a sharp turn and follows a curved course through the main nasal passage to exit the nasopharynx by the vertical choana; it then takes another sharp turn to the oropharynx. Inspiratory air is directed medially to course along the septum, where the main stream splits into different flows, arching between the inferior and superior turbinates. By comparison with the nasal cavities, airflow through the paranasal sinuses is inconsequential. The nose is responsible for 40–70% of the total airway resistance. The major portion of nasal resistance is confined to the nasal valve, e. g. the few millimetres posterior to the anterior edge of the upper lateral cartilage. The lumen of the nasal valve is regulated by lateral (head of the inferior turbinate) and medial (septum) erectile mucosa, and modulated by the tone of alar muscles and stabilised by bone and cartilage. At the entrance of the nasal cavity, airspeed is between 2 and 3 m s^{-1}, at the nasal valve it reaches 12–18 m s^{-1} and beyond the nasal valve, due to the decrease of nasal resistance, it decelerates to 2–3 m s^{-1}, promoting a disturbed pattern of respiratory airflow favourable for effective exchanges between air and mucosa.

The parameter most sensitive to change in nasal airway resistance is the size of the nasal cavities, which is proportional to the size of the turbinate mucosa. Several factors can affect the turbinate volume and thus the nasal resistance:

- Exercise usually decreases nasal resistance.
- Dust, smoke and alcohol usually increase nasal resistance.
- Pressure on one side of the body induces reflex nasal congestion on that side.

The nasal cycle is another factor affecting the volume of nasal turbinates: in healthy adults, each side of the nose alternatively congests and decongests every 3–7 h, leading to a spontaneous, resistive cycle phenomenon called the nasal cycle. The reason for the existence of this cycle remains unclear, but it occurs in approximately 80% of healthy adults. Although unilateral resistances can fluctuate between severe obstruction and optimum patency, the reciprocity between sides (as one side congests, the opposite side decongests) results in stable, combined resistance.

Sensory receptors of airflow have not been yet identified in nasal mucosa, but sensation of airflow could depend on thermal and/or sensitive stimulation of inhaled air. Moreover, several aromatic substances, notably L-menthol, enhance the sensations of chill, airflow and nasal patency, without modification of objective airflow indices. Thus, sensory interpretations of nasal airflow are influenced not only by ambient and pathophysiological conditions, but also by psychological factors.

The airflow distribution pattern through the nasal cavities and its characteristics are crucial to effective air conditioning.

2.2.2 Air Conditioning

In patients with tracheostomies, absence of nasal respiration induces squamous metaplasia of the respiratory epithelium. Moreover, in asthmatic subjects, oral breathing induces a higher degree of bronchoconstriction after exercise than nasal breathing does. Therefore, nose conditioning of inhaled air is essential to the lower airways, limiting aggression of the fragile structures of the alveoli. Essential in assuring the delicate function of air conditioning are the efficacy of the vascular network in the lamina propria, the contribution of watery secretion, the quantity of seromucous glands, the surface contact between inspired air and mucosa and the beating quality of the cilia.

The nose is responsible for thermal and hygrometric regulation of inhaled air, maintaining a 30°C mean temperature and 98% relative humidity, regardless of the variation of ambient humidity and temperature. The nose also participates in body thermoregulation via adjustment of the nasal mucosa blood flow. Arteriovenous shunts within nasal mucosa allow elevation or decrease of blood flow when heat needs to be lost or retained, respectively. Moreover, in normal conditions, inhaled air is supplemented with nitric oxide (NO) synthesised in the paranasal sinuses. NO-induced broncho- and vasodilatation contribute to improve oxygenation as well as blood perfusion in ventilated alveolar areas, resulting in better function in the entire respiratory system.

During normal breathing, nasal air filtration is facilitated by the disturbed airflow pattern, allowing particles (microorganisms and noxious materials) to attach to the mucosa. The number of particles that will attach to the mucosal surface depends on several factors such as physical size, shape, density and hygroscopicity. Mucus film covering nasal epithelium is responsible for trapping particulates greater than 10 μm, which will be transported to the oropharynx and then swallowed and destroyed by gastric enzymes. Transport of particles depends on the mucociliary clearance, which is determined by the motion of the blanket of mucus from the front of the nose to the nasopharynx by the coordinated waves of cilia. The cilia are 0.3 μm in diameter and 7–10 μm long; there are about 100 cilia per cell. The rate of mucociliary transport is 1–2 mm h^{-1} just behind the anterior portion of the inferior turbinate, and increases to 8–10 mm h^{-1} on the posterior portion of the inferior turbinate. Factors affecting nasal mucociliary clearance are either primary abnormality of cilia (Kartagener's syndrome, primary ciliary dyskinesia) and mucus (cystic fibrosis) or secondary to viruses, bacteria, chronic nasal inflammation (allergic rhinitis) and inhaled pollutants (tobacco smoke).

In addition to physical removal of particles by mucociliary clearance, the nose actively participates in immunological defence of the airways. Immunocompetent cells such as mast cells and lymphocytes T and B are found to migrate in nasal epithelium. These cells participate in antigenic-particle removal, immunological memory and release of preformed and granule-derived mediators of inflammation. Moreover, via HLA-DR and ICAM-1 expression, nasal epithelial cells could act as antigen-presenting cells to infiltrating lymphocytes. In addition, nasal NO and several nasal secretion constituents (peroxidases, interferon, lysozymes, lactoferrin, complement and immunoglobulins [A, G, M and E]) have immunological properties that may act nonspecifically to maintain the sterility of the lower airways. However, in patients with tracheostomies, despite colonisation of the lower airways with pathogenic bacteria, there is no increase in severe pulmonary infections.

2.2.3 Olfaction

Olfaction has a primary role in the regulation of food intake and in the perception of flavour. Olfaction has also an important protective function in the detection of irritating and toxic substances. During normal respiration, olfactory mucosa is sheltered from the inspiratory mainstream and, when sniffing, airflow is redistributed to the upper part of the nasal cavities to the olfactory organ. Humans can detect more than 10,000 different odours and discriminate between 5,000 of them. Age-related olfactory loss appears to begin at 60 years of age, and it becoming significantly worse after age 70. However, women consistently perform better than men do in smelling. The olfactory organ is functional at birth and is unique in the central nervous system, being the only part in direct contact with the environment and in its ability to regenerate damaged or lost neurons. In order to interact with the olfactory sensory neurons, hydrophilic odorants are dissolved in the olfactory mucus, and hydrophobic odorant molecules are bound and solubilised by odorant-binding proteins present in the nasal mucus. After interaction between the odorant molecules and receptor proteins, olfactory transduction (transformation of mechanical stimulation into electrical activity) probably involves an olfactory epithelium G$_{olf}$ protein–coupled cascade, with cAMP and/or inositol-phosphatidyl-3 as an intracellular second messenger, exciting an ion channel in the cilia, which depolarises the olfactory neuron. Depolarisation follows the olfactory axons that synapse in the olfactory bulbs, and then projections go to the amygdala, the prepyriform cortex, the anterior olfactory nucleus and the entorhinal cortex, as well as the hippocampus, hypothalamus and thalamus. The precise mechanism by which the vast number of smells is recognised and discriminated is unknown, but possible theories include specific odorants exciting specific receptors; differing solubilities of odorants, allowing a temporospatial distribution of the odorant across the olfactory mucosa or a response to the molecules' vibration spectra. As three quarters of flavour is contributed to by olfaction, complaints of loss of taste are usually related to olfactory loss. There are three major classifications of olfactory disorders: transport (conductive), sensory and neural. Transport disorders interfere with the access of an odorant molecule to the olfactory receptor, sensory losses result from damage to the olfactory receptor, and neural losses result from interruptions in the peripheral or central nervous olfactory pathways.

Suggested Reading

1. Van Cauwenberge P, Sys L, De Belder T, Watelet JB. Anatomy and physiology of the nose and the paranasal sinuses. Immunol Allergy Clin North Am 2004;24:1–17
2. Ohki M, Naito K, Cole P. Dimensions and resistances of the human nose: racial differences. Laryngoscope 1991;101:276–278
3. Cole P. The respiratory role of the upper airways. St Louis, MO, 1993:1–59

4. Nishino T, Tagaito Y, Sakurai Y. Nasal inhalation of l-menthol reduces respiratory discomfort associated with loaded breathing. Am J Respir Crit Care Med 1997;156:309–313

5. Mangla PK, Menon MP. Effect of nasal and oral breathing on exercise-induced asthma. Clin Allergy 1981;11:433–439

6. Bjermer L. The nose as an air conditioner for the lower airways. Allergy 1999;54 Suppl 57:26–30

7. Ferguson JL, McCaffrey TV, Kern EB, Martin WJ, 2nd. The effects of sinus bacteria on human ciliated nasal epithelium in vitro. Otolaryngol Head Neck Surg 1988;98:299–304

8. Maurizi M, Paludetti G, Todisco T, Almadori G, Ottaviani F, Zappone C. Ciliary ultrastructure and nasal mucociliary clearance in chronic and allergic rhinitis. Rhinology 1984;22:233–240

9. Papon JF, Coste A, Gendron MCet al. HLA-DR and ICAM-1 expression and modulation in epithelial cells from nasal polyps. Laryngoscope 2002;112:2067–2075

10. Jones N, Rog D. Olfaction: a review. J Laryngol Otol 1998;112:11–24

2.3 Examination of the Nasal Cavity and Paranasal Sinuses

JACINTO GARCIA AND HUMBERT MASSEGUR

2.3.1 Examination of the Nasal Cavity

Prior to instrumental examination, the nasal pyramid and maxillae should be inspected and palpated. Nasal deformities of the dorsum, tip or columellae may indicate internal alterations. Crepitation or pain on palpation will disclose fractures of nasal bones. Skin colour and texture and scars or wounds should be assessed. Nasal flapping and alar collapse should also be examined.

Inspection of the face in children can provide useful information about the course and degree of nasal obstruction (adenoid facies, allergic salute). Unilateral rhinorrhea would indicate a choanal atresia or a foreign body in the nostril.

2.3.1.1 Anterior Rhinoscopy

Anterior rhinoscopy is a simple, inexpensive technique that allows visualisation of the anterior third of the nasal cavity. Requirements are a light source (Clar mirror) and a nasal speculum (Killian, Vienna.) The use of an otoscope is recommended for small children.

The examiner stands in front of the seated patient, focusing the light beam on the tip of the nose. One hand holds the patient's head while the other gently opens the nostril with the speculum. Care should be taken not to damage the septum or the nostril by excessive opening of the instrument. The anatomy of the vestibulum can be distorted by the insertion of the speculum. This region is best examined by lifting the nasal tip with the finger. This gives a clear view of the alterations in this area and distortion is minimal.

Rhinoscopy allows examination of the nasal vestibulum, septum, inferior turbinate and meatus and the floor of the nasal cavity. In some cases the rhinopharynx can be directly visualised. Tilting the patient's head backwards gives a consecutive view of the middle turbinate and middle meatus, superior turbinate and roof of the nasal cavity. Vasoconstrictor sprays or topical anaesthetics with epinephrine can be used in selected patients. Structures and deformities such as polyps or septal deviations can be palpated with a cotton swab.

Small children are better examined in the supine position, with the examiner holding the head with one hand while an assistant immobilises the child.

Summarising, the following aspects should be taken into consideration when performing anterior rhinoscopy:

1. The appearance of the mucosa (e. g. colour, humidity)
2. The situation and deformities of the nasal septum
3. Characteristics of nasal secretions (e. g. type, appearance, localisation)
4. Turbinate congestion and meatal patency
5. Presence of tumours, foreign bodies or nasal polyps
6. Bleeding points

2.3.1.2 Posterior Rhinoscopy

This technique is used to examine the posterior part of the nasal cavity, namely the choanae, tail of the turbinates, posterior end of the septum, rhinopharynx and torus tubarius.

It requires the patient's collaboration and the physician's expertise. It may be difficult or even impossible to perform in children. These problems have been largely resolved by nasal endoscopy, and posterior rhinoscopy has become less frequent in everyday practice.

Required instruments include a headlight, a small laryngeal mirror and a tongue depressor. The patient's tongue is depressed while the laryngeal mirror is introduced, facing upwards, in the oropharynx behind the uvula. Contact of the mirror with the lateral or posterior walls of the oropharynx will likely provoke a nausea reflex and topical anaesthetics may be required.

The soft palate is sometimes large or inserts posteriorly, considerably reducing the field of vision. A palate retractor or two feeding tubes should be used to draw the palate forward and allow better exposure of the nasopharynx.

When correctly performed, this technique allows visualisation of:
• The size and shape of the choanae
• Blockage of the nasopharynx, e. g. tumours, adenoid hypertrophy, polyps, cysts, angiofibromas, etc.
• Nasal secretions: type, appearance

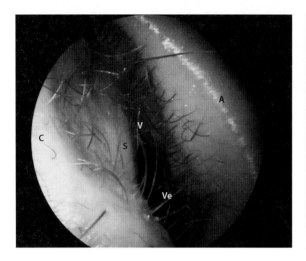

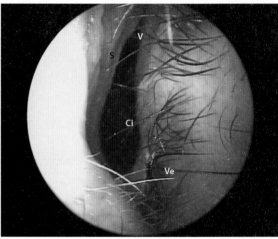

Fig. 2.3.1 Nasal vestibulum *C* columellae, *A* nasal alae, *S* septum, *Ve* vestibulum

Fig. 2.3.2 The endoscope is slightly introduced in the vestibulum. *S* septum, *V* nasal valve, *Ci* inferior turbinate, *Ve* vestibulum

- Size and shape of the tails of inferior and middle turbinates
- Morphology of the torus tubarius and Rossenmüller's fossae

2.3.1.3   Nasal Endoscopy

Nasal endoscopy has become the gold standard in nasal examination, for it provides precise and reliable information on the entire nasal cavity. Even traditionally inaccessible spots such as the sphenoethmoidal recess or the ostiomeatal complex can be thoroughly assessed.

The required equipment consists of a light source, a fibre optic cable and the endoscope itself. The latter can be one of three different types:

1. Rigid telescopes
   They may have different lengths and calibres. For adults, telescopes of 25-cm length and 4-mm diameter are most commonly used. Smaller endoscopes such as the 2.7-mm diameter model are often needed in children. Angulations used for examination are 0 or 30°. More recently, 45 and 70° optics have been developed, being most useful in surgery of the frontal recess.
2. Fiberoptic endoscopes
   These are made of a flexible fibre optic, ranging from 2.2 to 4 mm in diameter. The tip can be bent 130–180° upwards and 80–100° downwards.
3. Laryngo-epipharyngoscopes
   They can be used for posterior rhinoscopy, but they pose the same problems as the classic technique. They are 90° angled, providing a wide field of vision. Posterior rhinoscopy can also be performed with a 70° endoscope introduced through the mouth.

Endoscopic examination should be performed systematically to achieve a complete exploration of the complex anatomy of the nasal cavity.

The procedure should be carefully explained to the patient, especially to children, to obtain cooperation. An anterior rhinoscopy is performed, placing cotton pads soaked in anaesthetic solution with or without vasoconstrictor for 10 min (2% tetracaine in water solution with or without epinephrine 0.1 mg ml^{-1}). Topical anaesthesia may not be needed in all patients but is mandatory in children. Children younger than 3 years of age may need sedation.

The endoscope should be held with one hand while the other holds the patient's head, as for anterior rhinoscopy. The tip of the instrument is soaked in antifog solution. The nasal cavity is entered, and the vestibulum (Fig. 2.3.1), anterior septum (Fig. 2.3.2), valvular region (Fig. 2.3.3) and head of the inferior turbinate (Fig. 2.3.4) can be visualised. The entrance of the inferior meatus is examined, progressing over the floor of the nasal cavity (Fig. 2.3.5). Heading up and backwards, the agger nasi and middle turbinate are reached (Figs. 2.3.6, 2.3.7). Examination of the middle meatus is the main step in the endoscopy procedure, as this area drains all the anterior cavities. The uncinate process and bulla ethmoidalis can often be seen lateral to the middle turbinate (Fig. 2.3.8). The presence of swelling or secretions should be assessed at this point (Fig. 2.3.9). The endoscope is carefully advanced up to the tails of the turbinates and nasopharynx (Fig. 2.3.10). Mobility of the palate and torus tubarius is now assessed as well as the presence of adenoid hypertrophy, cysts or masses in the area (Figs. 2.3.11, 2.3.12). The superior turbinate and sphenoethmoidal recess should also be assessed. The 70°-angled optic can be very useful at this point, even though it is more difficult to handle.

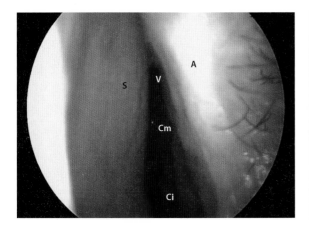

Fig. 2.3.3 Nasal valve. *V* valve, *Cm* middle turbinate, *Ci* inferior turbinate, *S* septum, *A* nasal alae

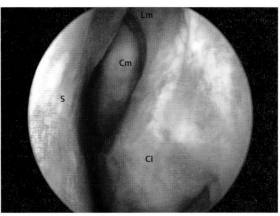

Fig. 2.3.4 Endoscopic view of the middle and inferior turbinates. *Cm* middle turbinate, *Ci* inferior turbinate, *Lm* linea maxillaris, *S* septum

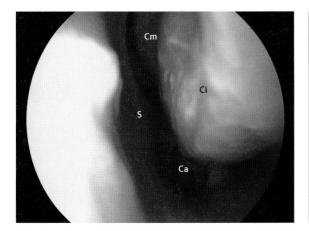

Fig. 2.3.5 Endoscopic view oft the middle and inferior turbinates and choanae. *Cm* middle turbinate, *Ci* inferior turbinate, *Ca* choana, *S* Septum

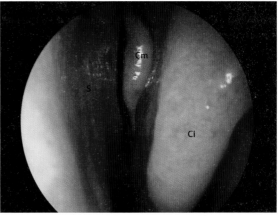

Fig. 2.3.6 Endoscopic overview of the inferior turbinate middle turbinate and septum in a left nasal fossa. *Ci* inferior turbinate, *Cm* middle turbinate, *S* septum

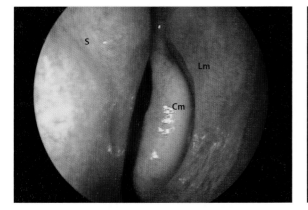

Fig. 2.3.7 Endoscopic view of the agger nasi region in a left nasal fossa. *Cm* middle turbinate, *Lm* linea maxillaries, *S* septum

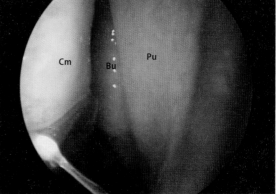

Fig. 2.3.8 The middle turbinate has been medialized and allows the endoscopic view of the middle meatus. *Cm* middle turbinate, *Bu* bulla ethmoidalis, *Pu* uncinate process

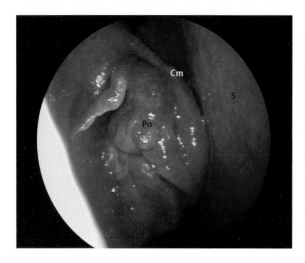

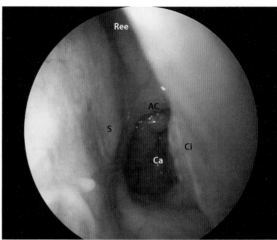

Fig. 2.3.9 Polyposis in a middle meatus. Right nasal fossa. *Po* polyp, *Cm* middle turbinate, *S* septum

Fig. 2.3.10 Endoscopic view of the choanae and the tails of turbinates. Left nasal fossa. *Ree* sphenoethmoidal recess, *AC* choanal arch, *S* septum, *Ca* rhinopharynx, *Ci* inferior turbinate

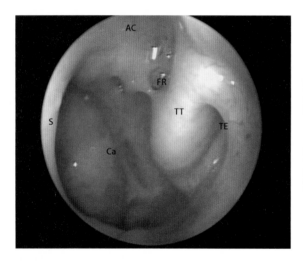

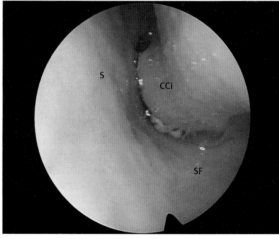

Fig. 2.3.11 Endoscopic view of the rhinopharynx from the left nasal fossa, with a Thornwald cyst on the right side. *AC* choanal arch, *S* septum, *Ca* rhinopharynx with a Thornwald cyst, *Fr* Rosenmüller fossa, *TT* torus tubarius, *TE* Eustachian tube

Fig. 2.3.12 Left nasal choana obstructed by inferior turbinate hypertrophy. *S* septum, *CCI* inferior turbinate, *SF* floor of the nasal fossa

The ostium of the sphenoid sinus can be found 1 cm above the choanal arch and the tail of the middle turbinate (Fig. 2.3.13). With the 70° telescope or the fiberoptic endoscope in the inferior meatus, the ostium of the nasolacrimal duct can be observed. In the middle meatus, a slight luxation of the middle turbinate allows visualisation of the confluence of the ethmoidal ostia.

Septal deviations and other anatomical variations may hinder the examination (Fig. 2.3.14). The use of fiberoptic

endoscopes is highly advisable, even though their image quality is slightly poorer.

2.3.1.4   Nasopharyngoscopy

The nasopharynx can also be examined through the mouth with a 70° nasal endoscope or a 90° rigid laryngoscope. The procedure is similar to that used for posterior

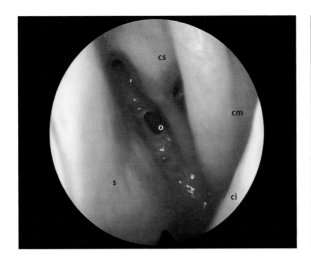

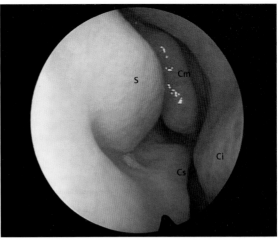

Fig. 2.3.13 Left sphenoethmoidal recess. *O* sphenoid ostium, *Cs* superior turbinate, *Cm* middle turbinate, *Ci* inferior turbinate, *S* septum

Fig. 2.3.14 Deviated nasal septum. Left nasal fossa. *S* septum, *Cs* septal deviation, *Cm* middle turbinate, *Ci* inferior turbinate

rhinoscopy, allowing direct control of the posterior third of the nasal cavity.

2.3.2 Examination of the Paranasal Sinuses

Inspection of the soft tissues and skin above the sinuses can provide very useful information. Swelling, inflammatory signs or painful palpation of the sinusal points often indicate sinus disease. These points of palpation should be the infraorbital region for the maxillary sinus, the frontal and supraorbital region for the frontal sinus and the medial commissure of the eye (Ewing's point) for the ethmoidal sinus.

Diaphanoscopy, or transillumination, consists of illumination of the sinusal cavities from the outside. With correct ventilation of the sinus, the light spread illuminates the cheek or the frontal region. Occupation of the sinusal cavity, on the other hand, results in opacification. However, sinusal transillumination has shown little reliability in clinical practice, and it is therefore scarcely used.

Endoscopic examination of the nasal cavity provides indirect signs of sinusal diseases; such signs may include a purulent discharge in the middle meatus or inferior turbinate.

The sinusal cavities cannot be directly seen unless a puncture is made or a surgical approach has left a wide opening of the sinus into the nasal cavity. In the past, transmeatal puncture was widely used to access the max-

illary sinus when draining or lavage was needed. It is still used occasionally today to introduce an endoscope for direct examination of the sinusal mucosa. The sphenoid sinus can also be accessed through its natural ostium.

2.3.2.1 Transmeatal Puncture

The nasal cavity, specifically the inferior meatus, must be anaesthetised. Cotton pads soaked in an anaesthetic solution with a vasoconstrictor should be placed in the inferior meatus for 10 min. After they are removed the trocar is introduced in the inferior meatus placing the tip in the uppermost part, turning it to face the maxillary sinus. Constant pressure is applied with slight rotating movements, pointing the trocar to the external commissure of the eye until the sinus is entered.

Possible complications of the procedure are posterior wall perforation and orbital penetration, both related with difficulties in trocar insertion due to a foremost anterior perforation.

Once the sinus cavity is reached, it can be either aspirated or irrigated. If the trocar sheath is wide enough to allow the entrance of the telescope, then direct visualisation of the sinus mucosa will be achieved. Biopsy taking is possible by facing the lesion with the trocar while introducing the forceps. The drawback with this technique is the lack of visual control the moment the biopsy it taken. This can be solved by making a puncture through the canine fossa that can be used as a second access to introduce either the forceps or the endoscope inside the sinus.

2.4 Functional Investigations of the Nose

JOSIANE PERCODANI

2.4.1 Introduction

Epidemiological and clinical studies have clearly highlighted the relationships between upper and lower airway dysfunctions. Chronic inflammatory processes that affect upper airways interact with the lower respiratory tract by several mechanisms [1, 2]. At the clinical level, they may participate in the worsening of bronchopulmonary diseases and impair quality of life. However, in many instances, patients with both upper and lower airway pathologies have predominant symptoms at one site and may neglect to report symptoms that concern another site. Physicians involved in respiratory disease management need to know how to evaluate common rhinological problems in order to offer patients a global therapeutic approach.

The physical examination of a patient with a nasal pathology is only considered after meticulous, "detective-style" questioning. This will often orient the diagnosis accurately and guide the choice of any complementary examinations. Although nasal endoscopy is the key step to diagnosis, a complete clinical examination of the nasal pyramid, orbital region, occlusion and buccal cavity should not be neglected, and should be performed with a thorough examination of the ear, nose and throat. Development of the light source and miniaturisation of optical systems have facilitated better exploration of nasal cavities. The differential diagnosis of inflammatory, infectious, architectural and tumoral pathologies is now possible. Nasal endoscopy is not only visual, but it also allows palpation of the mucosa, and can be combined with bacteriological, cytological and histopathological sampling to refine further the diagnosis. Other explorations depend on the data obtained during the patient questioning and the nasal endoscopy.

2.4.2 Rhinomanometry

This set of techniques allows simultaneous measurement of the flow and pressure variations to which an air current is subjected as it passes through the nasal cavities. These data are used to calculate the nasal resistance, based on Poiseuille's law. Two methods satisfy the recommended requirements of the International Committee for the Standardisation of Rhinomanometry [4]: active anterior rhinomanometry, which is the most widespread, and active posterior rhinomanometry. Both are based on the same principle in which the airflow and nostril pressure are measured inside a mask covering the nose and mouth. The choanal pressure is measured in the contralateral nostril, during active anterior rhinomanometry, and in the buccal cavity during active posterior rhinomanometry. Due to the obstruction of one nostril, anterior rhinomanometry cannot be used to study both nasal cavities simultaneously. Active anterior rhinomanometry is simple and rapid to carry out, reproducible, and feasible in all patients, including children. Active posterior rhinomanometry, in contrast, is difficult to carry out in certain patients due to the introduction of a buccal probe. It has the advantage of measuring the overall resistance and provides a better picture of the nasal valve by eliminating the nostril rims.

The total nasal resistance is normally below 0.3 Pascal (Pa) ml^{-1} s^{-1}, and the normal unilateral resistance below 0.6 Pa ml^{-1} s^{-1}.

The examination is carried out after the nose is blown, in a quiet, well-aired room, and out of the direct sun. The examination is over if the resulting values are normal. In cases of supine nasal obstruction, a second measurement should be made after the patient has lain supine for 30 min. When the nasal resistances are high, different manoeuvres are performed to determine which anatomical structures are involved. Cottle's test (opening of the nasogenian fold to increase the valve angle) and Bachmann's test (insertion of a swab into the top of the nasal valve) are considered positive if the resistances return to normal when they are applied. A positive value implies that the valve is involved. When a vasoconstrictor test brings the nasal resistances back to normal, this indicates that the nasal obstruction is due to turbinal hypertrophy.

Rhinomanometry cannot be used to quantify precisely the nasal obstruction. There is in fact no correlation between the magnitude of the increase in nasal resistance and the severity of the obstruction felt by the patient. Certain studies show, however, that the correlation is better in the case of unilateral rather bilateral nasal obstruction.

Nasal challenges are used to measure the specific reactivity of the nasal mucosa to different allergens. They have benefited from the progress and standardisation of rhinomanometry. Nasal challenges consist of measuring the variations in nasal resistance before and after introduction of the allergen. The allergen may be introduced in different ways (direct application to the nasal mucosa, nasal sprays of allergen solutions, aerosols). A strict protocol is required to prevent contamination of the bronchi with the allergenic solutions. Positive criteria are doubling of the nasal resistance and dose-dependent clinical effects. Local treatments and antihistamines should be stopped for at least 48 h before the test, and no acute infection should be present. These tests are time-consuming; only a single allergen can be tested per session. They must therefore be reserved for complex clinical situations in which the clinical history and skin tests do not permit formal identification of the allergen(s) involved. They can therefore be used, for example, in the case of polysensitisation to determine the respective roles of different allergens or, inversely, where there is strong clinical presumption of sensitisation to an allergen that cannot be confirmed by the usual methods. This latter situation is particularly frequent in occupational allergy.

2.4.3 Acoustic Rhinometry

This recently developed technique is based on acoustic scanning and provides an objective geometric study of the nasal cavities [7]. Computerised analysis of the reflexion of sound waves in the nasal cavities is used to deduce a "section area" for each point in time. Using the speed of sound, the distance to the site of this section area within the nasal cavity can be calculated. Jackson in 1977, then Hilberg in 1989 described the principle:

- A pressure wave, emitted by a generator, is directed into the nasal cavity through a tube of constant calibre.
- A microphone placed at the end records the reflexion of the wave after its passage through the nasal cavity. This signal is then amplified, filtered and analysed by computer.

Acoustic rhinometry enables an obstacle within the nose to be quantified and situated on a curve with three undulations in the form of negative waves:

- The first peak is fixed and corresponds to the end of the nasal tube. It is situated approximately 0.5 cm beyond the nostril orifice.
- The second peak is situated approximately 2 cm from the nostril orifice and corresponds to the valve region and the head of the inferior turbinate.

- The third peak is located approximately 6 cm from the nostril orifice and corresponds to the tail of the inferior turbinate.

In patients with turbinal hypertrophy, the smallest section area is situated at the head of the inferior turbinate.

Large variations are apparent, especially beyond the first 3 cm into the nasal cavity, for which the method remains imperfect.

The advantages of this technique are its rapidity, reproducibility, noninvasive character and the minimal cooperation required of the patient [7]. Nevertheless this method still requires validation, and numerous technical problems remain unresolved.

2.4.4 Exploration of Mucociliary Function

Examination of the mucociliary function is not carried out in daily clinical practice. However it should be systematic in cases of chronic purulent or bilateral recurrent nasosinusal infection. Several methods of exploration can be used. The best clinical indication of mucociliary clearance is the saccharin transit time test [8]. It consists on placing some saccharin powder on the inferior turbinate. The time needed by the patient to taste the saccharin is usually less than 20 min. The techniques used to study ciliary beat rate and electron microscopic analysis of ciliary structure are more specific. The investigation of ciliary structure is long and costly [3] and only undertaken in patients selected based on the ciliary beat study. It is in fact unlikely for an abnormality to be found if the beat is normal. The study of nasal mucus quality is still in its experimental stages at present and is not dealt with in this chapter.

These various methods are useful for the diagnosis of primitive or secondary ciliary dyskinesia, and Young's syndrome (which combines chronic rhinosinobronchitis and obstructive azoospermia due to poor mucus viscosity).

2.4.5 Cellular Exploration: Nasal Cytology

Nasal cytology can involve taking a smear or nasal brushing. The nasal smear is obtained under visual control, with a Dacron swab inserted up as far as the middle turbinate. This swab is wiped over the outer surface of the middle turbinate in the non-anaesthetised nasal cavity, with care taken not to cause bleeding. It is then smeared (but not squashed) onto glass slides and air fixed or fixed cytologically. The different epithelial cells and the percentages of each leukocyte type are measured semiquantitatively by May–Grünwald–Giemsa staining. The smear must be performed in the absence of any superinfection, and 15 to 21 days after any corticotherapy.

The normal nasal mucosa does not contain polynuclear neutrophils or eosinophils. Free cells exist in the nasal mucus, and most of these are polynuclear neutrophils. A nasal cytology examination is appropriate in the context of chronic diseases of the nasal mucosa. In allergic patients undergoing allergen exposure, mucosal and secretory eosinophils become dominant. However, an infiltration of polynuclear eosinophils is not synonymous with allergy. Nonallergic rhinitis with eosinophilic syndrome (NARES) is an inflammatory rhinitis characterised by secretory eosinophilia. The existence of eosinophilia exceeding 20% in two successive samples coupled with negative allergological tests will imply a diagnosis of suspected NARES. This examination can only be interpreted validly if strict sampling and interpretation criteria are respected. It therefore requires certain experience both on the part of the operator and on the part of the laboratory. In practice they are mainly useful for eliminating NARES in cases of chronic rhinitis. The indication of nasal cytology in the context of polyposis is relative. In fact neither the diagnosis nor treatment of polyposis is dependent on cytology.

Brushing consists of inserting a fine nylon brush into contact with the middle turbinate and collecting samples of nasal epithelial cells by rotation of the brush during its removal. The advantages of brushing include the possibility of a quantitative cell population study, electron microscopy, immunocytochemical and biochemical analyses [6]. A large number of epithelial cells can be obtained with this method and the ciliary motion examined in vivo by light microscopy. The beats of the cilia are screened and quantified by phase-contrast microscopy or by stroboscopy.

2.4.6 Olfactory Exploration

The exploration of the sense of smell is poorly accessible in daily clinical practice, although impairment of smell or taste may have a substantial impact on quality of life and is not uncommon even in allergic rhinitis. Devices most often proposed for patients to identify different smells are rigid "sniff bottles", perfume testers or microcapsules that release odorant molecules when scratched. The olfactory test developed by the University of Pennsylvania and commercialised as the Smell Identification Test (UPSIT) permits a qualitative identification of different smells. It consists of a booklet of four pages, each containing 10 microencapsulated "smell" molecules. The patient must choose between four possible answers for each stimulus. The score is calculated by comparing the number of correctly identified smells out of 40 [5].

2.4.7 Conclusion

In daily practice, examination of the nose mainly relies on meticulous questioning, and this is followed by complete clinical examination of the upper respiratory tract. Any practitioner can perform anterior rhinoscopy, using a frontal lamp and a speculum or an otoscope with a nasal adapter before and after vaporisation of a topical vasoconstrictor. It is a first step that may be completed, if necessary, by nasal flexible or rigid endoscopy, which requires special instruments and medical experience. Indications of other explorations like rhinomanometry, nasal cytology, mucociliary function or olfactory explorations are less frequent and depend on data obtained during patient questioning and examination.

Suggested Reading

1. Bousquet J, Van Cauwenberge P et al. (2002) Allergic rhinitis and its impact on asthma. Allergy 57:841–855
2. Bousquet J, Vignola AM, Demoly P (2003) Links between rhinitis and asthma. Allergy 58:691–706
3. Chapelin C, Coste A, Reinert P et al. (1997) Incidence of ciliary dyskinesia in children with recurrent respiratory tract infections. Ann Otol Rhinol Laryngol 106:854–858
4. Clement P (1984) Committee report on standardization of rhinomanometry. Rhinology 22:151–155
5. Doty RL, Shaman P, Dann M (1984) Development of the University of Pennsylvania Smell Identification Test: a standardized microencapsulated test of olfactory function. Physiol Behav 32:489–502
6. Maru YK, Munjal S, Gupta Y (1999) Brush cytology and its comparison with histopathological examination in cases of diseases of the nose. J Laryngol Otol 113:983–987
7. Roithmann R, Cole P, Chapnik J, Shpirer I, Hoffstein W, Zamel N (1995) Acoustic rhinometry in the evaluation of nasal obstruction. Laryngoscope 105:275–281
8. Stanley P, MacWilliam L, Greenstone M et al. (1984) Efficacy of a saccharine test for screening to detect abnormal mucociliary clearance. Br J Dis Chest 78:62–71

2.5 Imaging of the Nasal Cavity and Paranasal Sinuses: Anatomy and Anatomic Variations

NAFI AYGUN AND S. JAMES ZINREICH

2.5.1 Anatomy

To correctly interpret imaging studies, it is essential to understand the anatomy of the lateral nasal wall and its relationship to adjacent structures. The lateral nasal wall contains three bulbous projections: the superior, middle and inferior turbinates (conchae). The turbinates divide the nasal cavity into three distinct air passages: the superior, middle and inferior meati. The superior meatus drains the posterior ethmoid air cells and, more posteriorly, the sphenoid sinus (via the sphenoethmoidal recess). The middle meatus receives drainage from the frontal sinus (via the frontal recess), the maxillary sinus (via the maxillary ostium and subsequently the ethmoidal infundibulum) and the anterior ethmoid air cells (via the

ethmoid cell ostia). The inferior meatus receives drainage from the nasolacrimal duct [1–15].

The radiographic evaluation of this morphologic area should focus on the anatomic structures surrounding three specific "tight spots". Anteriorly, the first area comprises the structures surrounding the frontal recess. The second tight-spot area consists of the structures surrounding the infundibulum/middle meatus. The third, posterior-most tight spot includes the anatomic structures surrounding the sphenoethmoidal recess.

On CT scanning, the first coronal images display the outline of the frontal sinuses. The frontal sinuses are funnel shaped. Their aeration varies from patient to patient. They can be small and occupy only the diploic space of the medial frontal bone, or they can be large enough to extend through the floor of the entire anterior cranial fossa. In general, a central septation separates the left and right sides; however, often there may be several septations. The floor of the frontal sinus slopes inferiorly towards the midline.

Close to the midline the primary ostium is located in a depression in the floor. The frontal recess is an hourglass-like narrowing between the frontal sinus and the anterior middle meatus through which the frontal sinus drains (Fig. 2.5.1). It is not a tubular structure, as the term na-

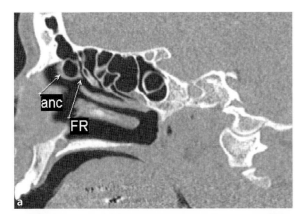

Fig. 2.5.1a–c The frontal recess (*fr*) and surrounding structures are demonstrated in sagittal (**a**),coronal (**b**), and transverse (**c**) sections of CT. The frontal recess drains to the anterior aspect of the middle meatus and surrounded by the agger nasi cell (*anc*) anteroinferiorly, and the ethmoid bulla (*eb*) posterolaterally

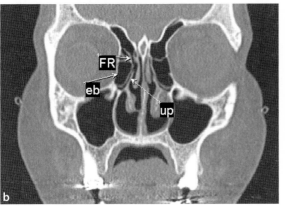

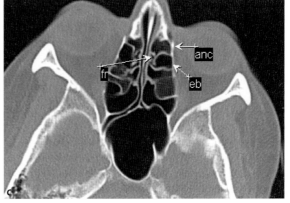

sofrontal duct might imply, and therefore the term *recess* is preferred.

Anterior, lateral and inferior to the frontal recess is the agger nasi cell. The agger nasi cell is a remnant of the first ethmoturbinal, which is present in nearly all patients. It is aerated and represents the anterior-most ethmoid air cell. It usually borders the primary ostium or floor of the frontal sinus, and thus its size may directly influence the patency of the frontal recess and the anterior middle meatus. The frontal recesses are the narrowest anterior air channels and are common sites of inflammation. Their obstruction results in loss of ventilation and mucociliary clearance of the frontal sinus.

2.5.1.1   Frontal Cells

Frontal cells are invariably found in relationship with the anterior ethmoid air cells and the agger nasi cell. The recognition and subsequent definition of the appearance and aetiology of frontal cells was initiated by J. Parson Schaeffer. During the course of his observations of the embryonic development of the sinuses, he discovered that it was possible, although infrequent, for one cell to aerate each half of the frontal bone, each with a separate communication to the frontal recess. Schaeffer coined the term *frontal cell* to describe this phenomenon. Van Alyea subsequently defined the frontal cell as a cell encroaching upon the frontal recess or frontal sinus. He considered supraorbital ethmoid, agger nasi, and intersinus septal cells as well as cells limited to the frontal recess as frontal cells. Bent et al. have defined frontal cells more specifically as belonging to one of four categories. They also state that all frontal cells derive from the anterior ethmoid sinus behind the agger nasi cell and pneumatise the frontal recess above the agger nasi cell. Each type of frontal cell

may obstruct the nasofrontal communication or the frontal sinus itself.

The uncinate process is a superior extension of the lateral nasal wall (medial wall of the maxillary sinus). Anteriorly, the uncinate process fuses with the posteromedial wall of the agger nasi cell and the posteromedial wall of the nasolacrimal duct. The uncinate process has a "free" (unattached) superoposterior edge. Laterally this free edge delimits the infundibulum. The infundibulum is the air passage that connects the maxillary sinus ostium to the middle meatus (Fig. 2.5.2). Posterior to the uncinate is the ethmoid bulla, usually the largest of the anterior ethmoid cells. The uncinate process usually courses medially and inferiorly to the ethmoid bulla. The ethmoid bulla is enclosed laterally by the lamina papyracea.

The gap between the ethmoid bulla and the free edge of the uncinate process defines the hiatus semilunaris. Medially, the hiatus semilunaris communicates with the middle meatus, the air space lateral to the middle turbinate. Laterally and inferiorly the hiatus semilunaris communicates with the infundibulum, the air channel between the uncinate process (caudal border) and the inferomedial margin of the orbit (cranial border). The infundibulum serves as the primary drainage pathway from the maxillary sinus.

The structure medial to the ethmoid bulla and uncinate process is the middle turbinate. Anteriorly it attaches to the medial wall of the agger nasi cell and the superior edge of the uncinate process. Superiorly the middle turbinate adheres to the cribriform plate. As it extends posteriorly, the middle turbinate emits a number of posterolaterally coursing bony structures. The first such "laterally fanning" attachment to the lamina papyracea and posterior to the ethmoid bulla is the basal lamella. This bony structure separates the anterior from the posterior ethmoid sinus.

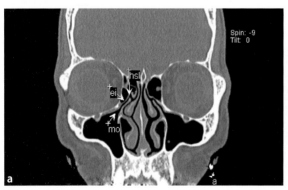

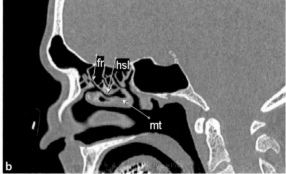

Fig. 2.5.2 a,b The anatomy of the ostiomeatal unit in coronal (**a**) and sagittal (**b**) CT images. The ethmoid infundibulum (*ei*) connects the maxillary ostium (*mo*) to the hiatus semilunaris

(*hsl*), the air space between the uncinate process (*up*) and ethmoid bulla. HSL in turn opens to the more medially positioned middle meatus, which surrounds the middle turbinate (*mt*)

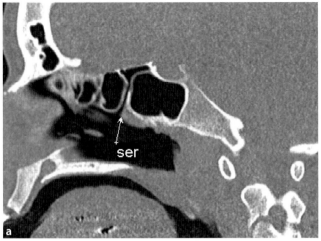
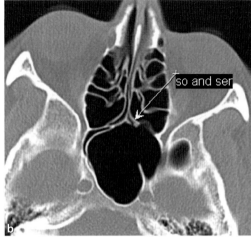

Fig. 2.5.3 a,b The sphenoethmoidal recess anatomy is demonstrated in sagittal (**a**) and transverse (**b**) CT images. The sphenoid ostium (*so*) is usually located along the superior medial and anterior wall of the sphenoid sinus and opens to the sphenoethmoidal recess (*ser*), which is just lateral to the nasal septum

In most patients, the posterior wall of the ethmoid bulla is intact, and an air space is usually found between the basal lamella and the posterior ethmoid bulla. This air space, the sinus lateralis, may extend superiorly to the ethmoid bulla and communicate with the frontal recess. Recently, the sinus lateralis has been renamed by an international surgeon's group and is now called the retrobullar recess cell. If it extends above the ethmoidal bulla, then this extension would be called the suprabullar recess cell. A dehiscence or total absence of the posterior wall of the ethmoid bulla is common and may provide communication between these two usually separated air spaces.

The posterior ethmoid sinus consists of air cells between the basal lamella and the sphenoid sinus. The number, shape and size of these air cells vary significantly from person to person.

The sphenoid sinus is the posterior-most sinus. It is usually embedded in the clivus and is bordered superoposteriorly by the sella turcica. Its ostium is located medially in the anterosuperior portion of the anterior sinus wall and communicates with the sphenoethmoidal recess and posterior aspect of the superior meatus (Fig. 2.5.3). The sphenoethmoidal recess lies just lateral to the nasal septum and can sometimes be seen on coronal images, but it is best displayed in the sagittal and axial planes.

The relationship between the aerated portion of the sphenoid sinus and the posterior ethmoid sinus must be accurately represented so the surgeon can avoid surgical complications. Usually, in the paramedian sagittal plane the sphenoid sinus is the most superior and posterior airspace. When dealing with this relationship, a horizontal, septation-like structure will be present in the sphenoid si-

nus; however, all of these horizontally oriented structures within the sphenoid sinus are separations in the posterior ethmoid sinus, the space above the more inferiorly placed sphenoid sinus. All sphenoid sinus septations are vertically oriented. This relationship is well demonstrated on axial and sagittal images. The number and position of the septations in the sphenoid sinus are variable. Of particular importance are septations that adhere to the bony canal wall, covering the internal carotid artery, which often projects into the posterolateral sphenoid sinus. Less often the canal of the Vidian nerve (pterygoid canal) and the canal of the second division of the trigeminal nerve (foramen rotundum) can project into the floor of the sphenoid sinus.

Anatomically, the paranasal sinuses are in close proximity to the anterior cranial fossa, the cribriform plate, the internal carotid arteries, the cavernous sinuses, the orbits and their contents, and the optic nerves as they exit the orbits (Fig. 2.5.4). The surgeon must be especially cautious when manoeuvring instruments directed cranially and dorsally, to avoid inadvertent penetration and damage to these structures.

2.5.2 Anatomic Variations and Congenital Abnormalities

Even though nasal anatomy varies significantly from patient to patient, some specific variations occur repeatedly within the population. Certain anatomic variations are thought to be predisposing factors for the development

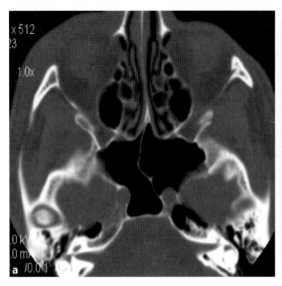
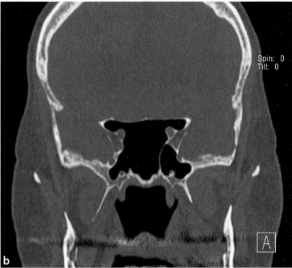

Fig. 2.5.4 a,b Transverse (**a**) CT shows bilateral bulging of the carotid arteries into the sphenoid sinus with probable dehiscence of the bony canal. In a different patient, coronal CT (**b**) demonstrates bulging of the bilateral optic nerves, Vidian nerves and left maxillary nerve into the sphenoid sinus

of sinus disease or surgical complications. Thus, it is necessary for the radiologist and surgeon to be cognizant of these variations, especially if the patient is a candidate for functional endoscopic sinus surgery (FESS).

2.5.2.1 Variations of the Middle Turbinate

2.5.2.1.1 Paradoxical Curvature
Normally, the convexity of the middle turbinate bone is directed medially, towards the nasal septum. When paradoxically curved, the convexity of the bone is directed laterally towards the lateral sinus wall. The inferior edge of the middle meatus may assume various shapes with excessive curvature, which in turn may narrow and/or obstruct the nasal cavity, infundibulum, and middle meatus. Because of this potential narrowing or obstruction, most authors agree that paradoxical middle turbinates can be a contributing factor to sinusitis; however, some report finding no significant relationship between paradoxically curved middle turbinates and recurrent sinusitis.

2.5.2.1.2 Concha Bullosa
A concha bullosa refers to an aerated middle turbinate. It may be unilateral or bilateral (Fig. 2.5.5). Less frequently, aeration of the superior turbinate may occur; however, an aerated inferior turbinate is uncommon. Concha bullosae are classified according to the degree and portion of turbinate pneumatization. When the pneumatization involves the bulbous segment of the middle turbinate, then the term *concha bullosa* applies. Should only the attachment portion of the middle turbinate be pneumatized without the pneumatization extending into the bulbous segment, it is known as a *lamellar concha*.

Although middle turbinate pneumatization has been suspected as a potential cause of middle meatal obstruc-

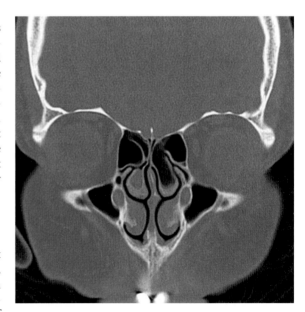

Fig. 2.5.5 Bilateral middle turbinate concha bullosa with opacification of the right one

tion and resultant sinusitis, the definitive relationship between concha bullosa and sinusitis continues to be debated. A concha bullosa involving the middle turbinate may enlarge the turbinate so that it obstructs the middle meatus or the infundibulum, and extensively pneumatized middle turbinates are associated with a higher prevalence of ipsilateral sinus disease. This is especially true when the concha bullosa exists in conjunction with another anatomical configuration that may obstruct the ostiomeatal complex, such as extensively pneumatized ethmoid bulla. The air cavity in a concha bullosa is lined with the same epithelium as the rest of the sinonasal cavities, and thus these concha bullosa cells can experience the same inflammatory disorders that affect the paranasal sinuses. Obstruction of the drainage of a concha may also lead to mucocele formation. Isolated, or smaller conchae bullosae, or those in which pneumatization is confined to the anterior or inferior aspect of the middle turbinate (further from the ethmoid infundibulum), are less frequently associated with sinusitis symptoms.

2.5.2.1.3 Other Variations

The other variations of the middle turbinate are medial displacement, lateral displacement, lateral bending, L-shaped middle turbinate and sagittal transverse clefts. Medial displacement of the middle turbinate is the result of other middle meatal structures (polypoid disease, pneumatized uncinate process) encroaching upon the middle turbinate. Lateral displacement of the middle turbinate is usually due to the compression of the turbinate towards the lateral nasal wall by a septal spur or septal deviation. Either or these two variants may predispose for sinus disease. L-shaped and lateral bending of the middle turbinate, as well as sagittal or transverse clefting may also be observed; however, these variants do not appear to cause sinusitis.

2.5.2.1.4 Nasal Septal Deviation

The nasal septum is fundamental in the development of the nose and paranasal sinuses. Nasal septal deviation is usually congenital but may be posttraumatic in some patients. Misalignment of the facial skeletal components of the adult nasal septum (septal cartilage, perpendicular ethmoidal lamina and vomer) may cause deviation of the nasal septum, deformity of the chondrovomerine articulation, or a septal spur. Asymptomatic septal deviation is observed in 20–31% of the population; however, more significant deviation, especially at the level of the chondrovomerine articulation, may contribute to sinusitis symptoms. Severe asymmetric bowing of the nasal septum may compress the middle turbinate laterally, narrowing the middle meatus, and the presence of associated bony spurs may further compromise the ostiomeatal unit.

Obstruction, secondary inflammation, swollen membranes and infection of the middle meatus have all been observed because of severe nasal septal deviation.

2.5.2.2 Uncinate Process Variations

2.5.2.2.1 Deviation

The uncinate process is one of the crucial bony structures of the wall of the lateral nasal cavity. Together with the ethmoid bulla, it forms the boundaries of the hiatus semilunaris and ethmoid infundibulum, the structures through which the frontal and maxillary sinuses drain. The course of the free edge of the uncinate process may be configured in a variety of ways. In most cases, either it extends slightly obliquely towards the nasal septum with the free edge surrounding the inferoanterior surface of the ethmoid bulla, or it extends more medially to the medial surface of the ethmoid bulla. If the free edge of the uncinate is deviated in a more lateral direction, then it may cause narrowing or obstruction of the hiatus semilunaris and infundibulum. Less frequently, a medial deviation or "curling" of the uncinate is encountered, which may result in the structure's contact and subsequent obstruction of the middle meatus.

2.5.2.2.2 Attachment

In normal anatomy, the upper tip of the uncinate process attaches to the lateral nasal wall in the location where agger nasi cells are commonly found. Anatomic variations of this attachment include attachment to the lamina papyracea, the lateral surface of the middle turbinate, or the cranial bone. It is necessary for the surgeon to be cognizant of any of these variations in the patient undergoing FESS, especially when an uncinatectomy is contemplated. If a variation of uncinate process attachment is present (ethmoidal roof, middle turbinate), then special care should be taken in order to avoid aggressive traction and torque on the upper tip of the structure during uncinatectomy, which may inadvertently damage the ethmoid roof.

Sometimes the free edge of the uncinate adheres to the orbital floor, or inferior aspect, of the lamina papyracea. This is referred to as an atelectatic uncinate process (Fig. 2.5.6). This variant is usually associated with a hypoplastic, and often-opacified, ipsilateral maxillary sinus due to closure of the infundibulum. It is important to note this variant for surgical planning because the ipsilateral orbital floor will be low-lying because of the hypoplastic maxillary sinus. This increases the risk of inadvertent penetration of the orbit during surgery. An additional variation of the uncinate is its extension superiorly to the roof of the anterior ethmoid sinus, causing the superior infundibulum to end as a blind pouch. This is referred to

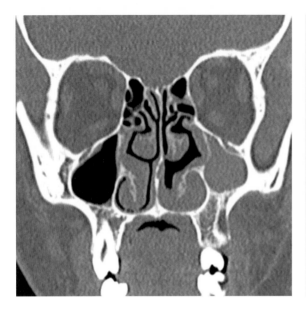

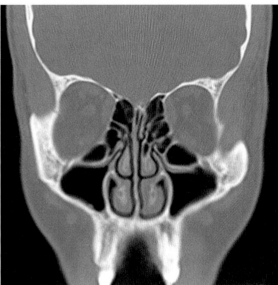

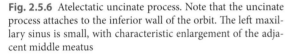

Fig. 2.5.6 Atelectatic uncinate process. Note that the uncinate process attaches to the inferior wall of the orbit. The left maxillary sinus is small, with characteristic enlargement of the adjacent middle meatus

Fig. 2.5.7 Haller cells in coronal CT. Note the proximity of these cells to the ethmoid infundibulum and maxillary ostium

as the lamina terminalis. Here, the infundibulum drains via the posterior aspect of the middle meatus.

2.5.2.2.3   Pneumatization

Pneumatization of the uncinate process, also referred to as an uncinate bulla, has been suggested as a predisposing factor for impaired sinus ventilation, especially in the anterior ethmoid, frontal recess and infundibular regions. Functionally, the pneumatized uncinate process resembles a concha bullosa or an enlarged ethmoid bulla. Pneumatization of the uncinate process is believed to be due to extension of the agger nasi cell within the anterosuperior portion of the uncinate process. Reported incidences of this variation are relatively low, ranging from 0.4–2.5 to 18%.

2.5.2.3   Infraorbital Ethmoid Cells (Haller's Cells)

Infraorbital ethmoid cells are pneumatized ethmoid air cells that project along the medial roof of the maxillary sinus and inferior-most portion of the lamina papyracea, below the ethmoid bulla and lateral to the uncinate process (Fig. 2.5.7). These cells were first identified by Haller in 1765 and subsequently named after him; recently, however, the preferred term for these air cells has been changed to reflect both a growing trend that discourages the naming of structures after anatomists who first de-

scribe them, as well as the need for international standardisation and descriptive nomenclature for anatomical terms. Most often, infraorbital ethmoid cells arise from the anterior ethmoid cells and are closely related to the infundibulum. These cells contribute to the narrowing of the infundibulum and may compromise the adjacent ostium of the maxillary sinuses. Consequently, many authors cite infraorbital ethmoid cells as a factor in recurrent maxillary sinusitis.

2.5.2.4   Onodi Cells

Two primary definitions of Onodi cells have been presented in the literature. The first defines them as the posterior-most ethmoid cells superolateral to the sphenoid sinus that are closely associated with the optic nerve (Fig. 2.5.8). Another, more general description of Onodi cells is a posterior ethmoid cell extending into the sphenoid bone, situated either adjacent to or impinging upon the optic nerve. The reported incidence of Onodi cells ranges from 3.4 to 51%. This discrepancy is most likely due to the use of different criteria to define the variation. Onodi cells abut or may even surround the optic nerve, risking the nerve when surgical excision of the cells is performed.

Onodi cells are also a potential cause for incomplete sphenoidectomy. If a surgeon is operating in an Onodi cell, he or she may recognise landmarks traditionally associated with the sphenoid sinus (internal carotid artery, optic nerve) and therefore may mistakenly conclude that the sphenoid sinus has been entered and consider the operation completed, when in fact it is not.

2.5.2.5 Ethmoid Bulla Variations

The ethmoid bulla is usually the largest and constant anterior-most ethmoid air cell. Its appearance varies considerably, based on the extent of pneumatization. Extensive pneumatization may obstruct the ostiomeatal complex. Elongated ethmoid bullae are usually the result of pneumatization that extends in a superior–inferior direction, rather than in an anterior–posterior direction. Because they do not extend in an anterior or posterior direction, elongated ethmoid bullae are relatively unlikely to obstruct the ostiomeatal complex.

2.5.2.6 Medial Deviation or Dehiscence of the Lamina Papyracea

Medial deviation or dehiscence of the lamina papyracea may be either congenital or the result of prior facial trauma. In either case, this variation puts the orbital contents at risk during surgery because of the dehiscence in the medial orbital wall, as well as the ease of surgically con-

fusing this "medial bulge" with the ethmoid bulla. Both excessive medial deviation and bony dehiscence occur most often at the site of the insertion of the basal lamella into the lamina papyracea, thus rendering this portion of the lamina papyracea most delicate.

2.5.2.7 Aerated Crista Galli

When aeration of the normally bony crista galli occurs, the aerated cells may communicate with the frontal recess. Obstruction of this ostium can lead to chronic sinusitis and mucocele formation within the crista galli. To avoid unnecessary surgical extension into the anterior cranial vault, it is important to recognise an aerated crista galli and to differentiate it from an ethmoid air cell prior to surgery.

2.5.2.8 Cephalocele

Cephaloceles may be congenital, spontaneously occurring, or the result of previous ethmoid or sphenoid sinus surgery. Preoperative coronal CT scanning is useful in the detection of cephaloceles, and is especially suited in displaying the extent of any bony erosion. When diagnosing an isolated soft tissue mass adjacent to the ethmoid or sphenoid roof, a radiologist must consider a cephalocele, especially if there is adjacent bone erosion. The differential diagnosis includes mucocele, neoplasm, and less likely, a polyp associated with an adjacent bony dehiscence. Sagittal and coronal MRI may be employed to narrow the differential diagnosis.

2.5.2.9 Posterior Nasal Septal Air Cell

Air cells are commonly found within the posterosuperior portion of the nasal septum. When present, they communicate with the sphenoid sinus. Any inflammatory disease that occurs within the paranasal sinuses may also affect these cells. Such disease may obliterate this cell, causing it to resemble a cephalocele. CT and MRI usually define the involved pathology and resolve any differential diagnostic problems.

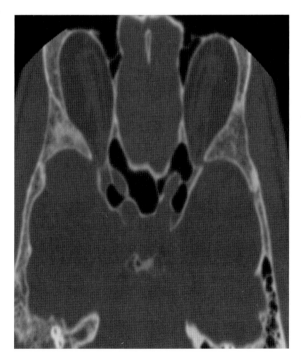

Fig. 2.5.8 Transverse CT shows bilateral Onodi cells that surround the medial and superior aspects of the optic canal. Note the pneumatized anterior clinoid processes

References

1. Babbel R et al. (1991) Optimization of techniques in screening CT of the sinuses. Am J Roentgenol 157:1093
2. Benson ML, Oliverio PJ, Zinreich SJ (2001) Techniques of imaging of the nose and paranasal sinuses. In: Meyers E (ed) Advances in otolaryngology–head and neck surgery, vol 10. Mosby, St Louis

3. Bolger W, Butzin C, Parsons D (1991) Paranasal sinus bony anatomic variations and mucosal abnormalities: CT analysis for endoscopic sinus surgery. Laryngoscope 101:56–64

4. Delano M, Fun FY, Zinreich SJ (1996) Optic nerve relationship to the posterior paranasal sinuses: a CT anatomic study. AJNR Am J Neuroradiol 17:669–775

5. Hosemann W (1990) Dissection of the lateral nasal wall in eight steps. In, Wigand ME (ed) Endoscopic surgery of the paranasal sinuses and anterior skull base. Thieme, Stuttgart

6. Kennedy DW, Zinreich SJ (1988) The functional endoscopic approach to inflammatory sinus disease: current perspectives and technique modifications. Am J Rhinol 2:89

7. Kennedy DW, Zinreich SJ, Hassab MH (1990) The internal carotid artery as it related to endonasal sphenoethmoidectomy, Am J Roentgenol 4:7–10

8. Laine FJ, Kuta AJ (1993) Imaging the sphenoid bone and basiocciput: pathologic considerations. Semin Ultrasound CT MR 14:160–167

9. Melhem ER et al. (1996) Optimal CT screening for functional endoscopic sinus surgery. AJNR Am J Neuroradiol 17:181–187

10. Messerklinger W (1978) Endoscopy of the nose. Urban and Schwartzenberg, Baltimore

11. Stammberger H (1991) Functional sinus surgery. Mosby, St. Louis

12. Stammberger H, Wolf G (1988) Headaches and sinus disease: the endoscopic approach. Ann Otol Rhinol Laryngol 134:3–23

13. Wigand ME, Steiner W, Jaumann MP (1978) Endonasal sinus surgery with endoscopic control: from radical operation to rehabilitation of the mucosa. Endoscopy 10:255–260

14. Zinreich SJ et al. (1988) MR imaging of normal nasal cycle: comparison with sinus pathology. J Comput Assist Tomogr 12:1014–1019

15. Zinreich S et al. (1987) Paranasal sinuses: CT imaging requirements for endoscopic surgery. Radiology 163:769–775

2.6 Diseases of the Outer and Inner Nose

B. MARTINEZ-VIDAL, MICHALINA RUSIECKA, AND MANUEL BERNAL-SPREKELSEN

2.6.1 Erysipela

- Definition of the disease
  - Erysipela is a skin infection that affects the superficial dermis and is caused by *Streptococcus pyogenes* (group A). It usually develops in the extremities and the face, and less commonly on the scalp and genitals.
- Epidemiology/aetiology
  - Erysipelas are more often seen in elderly, infants and children, patients with compromised immunology and diabetes. Predisposing factors are alcoholism, skin ulceration, puncture wounds, fungal infections, chronic lymphatic or venous obstruction, malnutrition and burns. Some authors report higher incidences during the summer.
- Symptoms
  - It usually presents with a sudden onset of fever with chills and general fatigue. The skin lesion is a red, indurated and elevated plaque with well-defined borders that expand rapidly. It is painful, warm and accompanied by variable oedema. On the second or third day, a flaccid bulla may develop, and desquamation of the involved skin occurs within 10 days. Presence of regional lymph nodes is common.
- Complications
  - The most common complication is recurrence, which is seen in 18–30% of the cases, even after proper antibiotic therapy. Recurrence is seen more often in females than in males. Very rarely, in older patients a rapid spread into the deeper layers of the skin, producing necrotising fasciitis, may also occur. A skin infection with *S. pyogenes* could lead to glomerulonephritis.
- Diagnosis
  - Diagnosis is based on the patient's personal history and physical examination, particularly on inspection of the skin. If a blister or purulent secretion is present, a culture and sensitivity should be obtained. Biopsy specimen cultures or fine-needle aspirates are usually negative, and thus are not recommended. Blood cultures are positive in less than 5% of cases.

- Therapy
  - Conservative therapy
    - The preferred antibiotic is penicillin. In mild cases with minor systemic symptoms, penicillin V, 500 mg orally every 6 h for 10 days, or penicillin G benzathine, 1.2 mil U intramuscularly once. Other possibilities are amoxicillin, 500 mg orally twice a day for 10 days, or cephalexin 500 mg orally every 6 h for 10 days.
    - In patients with a known penicillin allergy, azithromycin, 500 mg orally daily, then 250 mg orally daily for 4 days; clarithromycin, 250 mg orally twice a day for 7–10 days; or clindamycin, 300 mg orally three times a day for 7–10 days is recommended.
    - In moderate and severe cases with significant systemic symptoms, hospitalization and intravenous treatment is required: penicillin G, 2–4 mil U intravenously every 4–6 h; Cefazolin, 0.5–1.5 gm intravenously every 8 h; cefotaxime, 1–2 gm intravenously every 8 h; or ceftriaxone 1–2 gm intravenously once a day should be administered. In patients with a penicillin allergy, clindamycin, 600 mg intravenously every 8 h or vancomycin, 15 mg/kg intravenously twice a day may be given.
  - Additional useful therapeutic options
    - Prednisone 30 mg over 8 days might be considered, as well as elevation of the affected site. Moist heat compresses may be useful.
- Surgery
  - Debridement and drainage are indicated when bullae, abscesses or necroses are present.
- Differential diagnosis
  - Contact dermatitis
  - Asteatotic eczema
  - Herpes zoster
  - Angioneurotic oedema
  - Osteomyelitis

2.6.2 Furuncle/Carbuncle

- Definition of the disease
    - A furuncle or carbuncle is an infection that begins at the hair follicle and spreads deeper into the dermis and subcutaneous tissue, forming a seated, firm, tender nodule. After several days, it develops into an abscess with a red, painful, and fluctuant, pus-filled compilation.
    - When several neighbouring hair follicles are infected, the carbuncle swells. It is deeper and wider, often with interconnecting subcutaneous abscesses.
- Epidemiology/aetiology
    - The causative agent is *Staphylococcus aureus*. Cutaneous abscesses are often polymicrobial.
- Symptoms
    - In most cases, symptoms are local and limited to the site of infection. Furuncles usually arise in warm and moist areas such as the neck, axillae, groin, buttocks and thighs, but may occur anywhere where hair follicles are present. Carbuncles are common on the back of the neck. From time to time, systemic symptoms (fever and malaise) and surrounding cellulitis may accompany the presentation.
- Complication
    - One complication is furunculosis: multiple draining sinuses that might develop into ulcers that heal with a visible scar.
- Diagnosis
    - The diagnosis is based on clinical inspection. Culture and sensitivity testing are not necessary when there is no systemic involvement, but should be considered if systemic therapy (in case of fever, significant cellulitis or hospitalization) or when community-acquired methicillin-resistant *Staphylococcus aureus* (MRSA) is considered.
- Therapy
    - When the furuncle is small, application of moist heat seems to promote drainage. Larger furuncles and all carbuncles should be drained by surgical incision. After drainage, the area should be cleaned with an antiseptic (i.e. with chlorhexidine), and mupirocin 2% ointment should be applied twice a day.
    - If no systemic symptoms or extensive cellulitis are present, simple topical care is usually curative, and oral antibiotics are not necessary. Otherwise, systemic treatment is indicated and should cover any possible MRSA.
    - Recommended antibiotics are trimethoprim-sulfamethoxazole, 1–2 tablets orally twice daily; doxycycline or minocycline, 100 mg orally twice daily; or clindamycin, 300–450 mg orally every 8 h. In severe cases, vancomycin, 15 mg/kg intravenously every 12 h; linezolid 600 mg intravenously or orally every 12 h; tigecycline, 100-mg intravenous loading dose, which is followed by 50 mg intravenously every 12 h; or clindamycin, 600 mg intravenously every 8 h.

2.6.3 Atrophic Rhinitis

Atrophic rhinitis is also known as ozaenae, dry rhinitis, and open-nose syndrome.
- Definition of the disease
    - Atrophic rhinitis is a rare, chronic disease of the nasal mucosa and subjacent bones, leading to abnormally wide nasal cavities, dryness, crusting, atrophy, fetor and a paradoxical subjective sensation of nasal obstruction.
- Epidemiology/aetiology
    - The aetiology of atrophic rhinitis is still not clear. Originally it was attributed to colonization by *Klebsiella ozaenae*, and now this form is considered primarily. It is seen mostly in young people in developing countries with warm climates. Although no significant scientific support exists, it is assumed associated with developmental, endocrine, vascular, nutritional, autoimmune and genetic factors.
    - Nowadays, secondary ozaenae can be caused by aggressive surgery for nasal obstruction (excessive turbinate surgery), trauma, granulomatous diseases (Wegener's granulomatosis), and cocaine abuse or radiation therapy.
- Symptoms
    - The predominant symptoms are foul-smelling nasal discharge, crusting and a paradoxical subjective sensation of nasal obstruction. The sensation of nasal obstruction might be produced either by an abnormal airflow pattern or by dysfunctional neurological regulation, both conditions being caused by atrophy. Because of possible septal perforation, a saddle-nose deformity may develop.
- Diagnosis
    - The patient's history and physical examination with rhinoscopy are the main keys to diagnosis. Culture of any discharge serves to confirm the diagnosis as well as to provide an antibiogram. A CAT scan or NMR is useful to evaluate paranasal sinuses.
- Therapy
    - Conservative therapy
        - The first line of treatment should be local antibiotics and nasal irrigation with crust removal. In the later stages nasal drops – glucose 50% and glycerine – may help to reduce the odour and crusting.

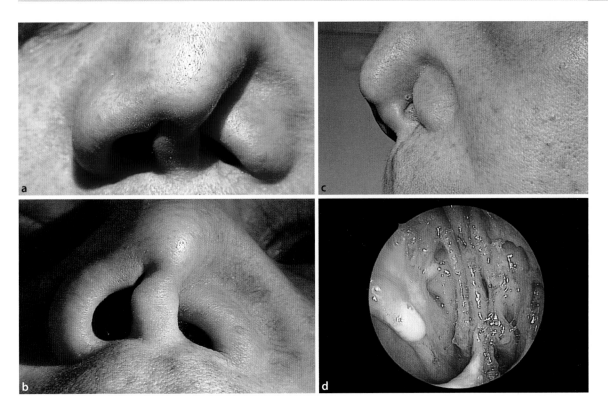

Fig. 2.6.1a–d Alar collapse (**a–c**) and septal necrosis secondary to cocain abuse

- Some authors report utility of systemic streptomycin or riphampicin.
- Surgery
  - Surgical treatment involves closure of the nostrils
  by using a circumferential flap of vestibular skin
  (Young's procedure). Recovery of the nasal mucosa
  may occur after a period of prolonged closure, and
  the nose can be reopened.
- Prognosis
  - In some cases, the disease disappears spontaneously when patients reach middle age.

2.6.4 Midline Granuloma

A midline granuloma is also known as an angiocentric
lymphoma. Formerly, it was referred to as polymorphic
reticulosis, lethal midline granuloma and midline malignant reticulosis.

- Definition of the disease
  - This rare disease is a lymphoma of extranodal presentation, usually of an immature natural killer
  cell strain, and in almost all cases is positive for
  the Epstein-Barr virus. This lymphoma most commonly appears in the midface region, hence its
  name.
- Epidemiology/aetiology
  - This form of lymphoma is rare in Europe and the
  United States, with a higher prevalence in Asia and
  among the native population of Peru. It affects all
  age groups and is more frequent in males.
- Symptoms
  - The most common presentation is nasal obstruction with a destructive mass occupying the nose,
  sinuses and palate. Involvement of extranodal sites
  including the upper airway, gastrointestinal tract,
  skin or testis may be present. Fever, night sweats
  and weight loss seen usually in Hodgkin's lymphoma and other non-Hodgkin's lymphomas (known
  as "B symptoms") are uncommon.
- Diagnosis
  - The diagnosis is based on anatomopathological
  study. The malignancy of the tumour manifested by
  extensive necrosis makes the histological diagnosis
  difficult, and often more biopsies are required for
  confirmation.
- Therapy
  - Therapy consists of radiotherapy with or without
  chemotherapy.

- Prognosis
  - Depending on the stage, patients may either achieve long-term remission or experience a worsening prognosis with relapses, which may include other extranodal sites.

2.6.5 Wegener's Granulomatosis

- Definition of the disease
  - Wegener's granulomatosis is a systemic chronic vasculitis of small- and medium-sized blood vessels, with an autoimmune component. It affects particular organs, with variable predilection.
- Epidemiology/aetiology
  - Wegener's granulomatosis is a rare disease. It affects about 1 in 20,000–30,000 people. It is more prevalent in middle-aged Caucasian patients, although it may appear at any age. No difference between genders has been found, nor is there any evidence for a hereditary element.
- Symptoms
  - The disease may present with pulmonary, upper respiratory tract or renal involvement in a localised or disseminated form. The localised form – confined to the upper respiratory region – is present in 25% of the patients. It consists of nonspecific manifestations such as nasal obstruction, crusting, purulent or bloody rhinorrhea, and painful or painless ulcers in oral or nasal cavities, which are unresponsive to standard medical treatment.
  - In some patients, the nasal septum is perforated, which leads to saddle-nose deformity. Less common symptoms are hoarseness, stridor due to subglottic stenosis, otalgia, otorrhea, and conductive and sensorineural hearing loss. Also, ocular symptoms such as scleritis, conjunctivitis, uveitis and episcleritis may be present.
  - In the disseminated form, pulmonary involvement is manifested by cough, dyspnoea, haemoptysis (due to an alveolar capillaritis, necrotic lesions or endobronchial disease) and pleuritic pain. Systemic symptoms such as weakness, fever, lack of energy, fatigue, loss of appetite, weight loss, night sweats and migratory arthralgias may be present.
  - Ninety per cent of patients have nasal symptoms, and these symptoms are usually the first manifestation of the disease. Pulmonary symptoms without upper respiratory tract symptoms or signs are unusual. Most patients have also renal involvement, even if it is subclinical.
- Diagnosis
  - Diagnosis of Wegener's granulomatosis is based on clinical findings that demonstrate lung (chest x-ray), kidney (urine analysis) or upper respira-

tory tract involvement (oral or nasal ulcers or discharge), along with positive blood analysis for cytoplasmic-staining antineutrophil cytoplasmic antibodies (c-ANCA) and confirming proteinase 3 (PR3) ANCA or myeloperoxidase (MPO) ANCA.
  - Biopsy is essential for diagnosis and often demonstrates no more than nonspecific chronic inflammation and necrosis. The biopsy should be taken from the involved organ, usually meaning nasal mucosa (multiple turbinate and septum specimens). In the absence of nasal involvement, skin, kidney or lung biopsy may be obtained.
  - Bacterial and fungal infections should also be ruled out.
- Therapy
  - Conservative therapy
    - In the induction of disease remission high-dose steroids (e. g. prednisone, 1 mg/kg/day) for 1 month, with tapering over several months are given. In addition, cyclophosphamide (2 mg/kg/day) should be administered for 6–12 months until symptoms disappear. In the maintenance of remission, cyclophosphamide should be replaced, if possible, with less toxic agents such as methotrexate, azathioprine, or mycophenolate mofetil. Antibiotics, mainly trimethoprim-sulfamethoxazole, are given for prophylaxis against *Pneumocystis jiroveci* (formerly *Pneumocystis carinii*) pneumonia (PCP), which may develop during immunosuppression and have a role in preventing recurrences.
    - Sinonasal manifestations may be treated with topical nasal steroids and nasal irrigations, low-dose systemic steroids and antibiotics when bacterial infection (typically *Staphylococcus* species) is suspected.
- Differential diagnosis
  - Microscopic polyangiitis and other vasculitis should also be considered when diagnosis is being made. ANCAs can be positive after use of certain drugs.
- Prognosis
  - Most of the patients respond well to treatment, achieving symptom-free intervals of 5–20 years or more. Anatomical problems (sinusitis, tracheal stenosis) may require surgery (in a small proportion of patients). Relapses can be long and troublesome. Long-term complications are mainly chronic renal failure, hearing loss and deafness.

2.6.6 Nasal Fractures

- Definition
  - A nasal fracture is a disruption of the nasal bone structure, due to trauma. It is the most frequently

fractured facial bone, due to its prominence and delicate structure.

- Epidemiology/aetiology
  - Sports, falls and assaults are the usual mechanisms of fracture. Males are affected twice as often as are females in both adult and paediatric populations, with a peak incidences during the second and third decades of life. Variables such as force, impact direction, nature of the striking object, age and other host factors will influence the pattern of injury to the components of the nose. Young adults often suffer dislocations of major segments, and older patients have comminution of osteopenic nasal bones. Children usually have cartilaginous injuries and greenstick fractures.
- Symptoms
  - Deformity, swelling, epistaxis and periorbital ecchymosis are signs that are suggestive of nasal fracture, whereas bony crepitus and nasal segment mobility are diagnostic.
  - Epiphora occurs in 0.2%. Injuries to the structures that surround the nose occur in cases of high-velocity impacts such as motor vehicle accidents. Severe bilateral injuries to the lachrymal bones are associated with depressed nasal fractures. Hard palate instability and open-bite deformity are signs of Le Fort's fracture, whereas unilateral malar deformity and facial asymmetry suggest a zygomaticomaxillary complex fracture (see Chap. 2.19, Sect. 2.19.1).
- Complications
  - Septal haematoma is one of the most severe early complications of nasal trauma, and without drainage, it results in abscess formation 6–7 days after trauma, producing necrosis of the septal cartilage. Long-term problems such as saddle-nose deformity, perforation, columellar retraction and nasal-base widening may appear. Contiguous spread of septal infection could lead to osteomyelitis, orbital and intracranial abscesses, meningitis and cavernous sinus thrombosis. Cerebrospinal fluid leakage is a common complication of severe nasal and frontal fractures. Surrounding orbital wall fractures could lead to fat or muscle herniation and/or retrobulbar haematoma. Delayed nasal complications include worsening of septum deviation, spurs, internal nasal valve collapse and synechiae, all causing nasal airflow obstruction.
- Diagnostic procedures
  - Inspection
    - Changes of appearance such as deviation and asymmetry, bleeding, watery drainage, changes in nasal breathing and smell. It is useful to compare the current presentation with old photographs (up to 40% of normal individuals have significant nose malformations).
- Physical examination
  - The diagnosis of a nasal fracture is made primarily by physical examination: epistaxis, nasal swelling, and periorbital ecchymosis. Nasal shape, in the lateral and frontal inspection, should be assessed. Grasping the dorsum between two fingers and rocking the pyramid back and forth aids in assessing the mobility of nasal bones. Internal structures should be evaluated by using a headlight and nasal speculum. Clotted blood is removed by suction, and assessment of haematoma, mucosal tears and active bleeding is performed. Bimanual palpation of the septum helps to differentiate septal swelling from haematoma.
- Radiography
  - There is no clear evidence of the role of radiography in the management of nasal fractures. Plain films have up to a 66% false-positive rate as a result of misinterpretation of normal suture lines. In addition, old fractures are difficult to distinguish.
  - Three-dimensional CT is recommended for extensive injuries involving the nasal-orbital-ethmoidal complex.
- Additional/useful diagnostic procedures
  - Using a 0 or 30° 4-mm endoscope is helpful in the assessment of posterior abnormalities. If the patient is heavily sedated, Brown-Gruss provocation manoeuvres may be performed to determine deformities in upper, middle or lower segments by compressing each compartment.
- Conservative treatment
  - Treatment of bleeding
    - For localised bleeding, anterior sources may be cauterised by silver nitrate or sealed with topical materials such as thrombin combined with gelatin foam, fibrin glue, FloSeal® or other procoagulant materials. If conservative measures fail, a formal anterior packing is placed.
    - Bleeding from branches of sphenopalatine or ethmoid vessels requires anterior-posterior packing.
    - Surgical methods such as direct endoscopic vessel cauterization or ligation have been shown to offer better haemostasis and patient comfort. Angiography with embolization can also be considered in cases refractory to more conservative approaches.
  - Timing of reduction
    - Fibrous connective tissue within the fracture line develops around 10 days to 2 weeks after injury. Manipulation should be performed before this point. A short delay period of 2–3 days is also recommended to allow for diminishment of swelling.

– Type of reduction
  • Nondisplaced fractures should be treated with observation alone. Closed nasal reduction is the best choice for simple injuries (isolated, unilateral with medial displacement).
  • An open approach should be considered in severe trauma (bilateral, depressed fractures).
• Prognosis
  – Seventy to 90% of patients are satisfied after closed reduction of the nasal fracture. Three per cent require secondary corrective treatment.
• Surgical principles
  – Topical anaesthesia with cotton pledgets soaked with 4% cocaine or 0.05% oxymethazoline, combined with 4% topical lidocaine should be applied for 5–10 min. Local anaesthesia should also be injected (1% lidocaine and 1:100,000 epinephrine) along the septum, lateral walls and floor of the nasal cavity.
    • Closed reduction
      – The nasal bones are grasped between two fingers, and pressure is applied laterally in the opposite direction of the deviation. A blunt elevator may be used from within the nose in cases of significant medial collapse. Walsham forceps can be of help. Reduction of the septum should be performed with the use of Asch forceps.
      – To prevent collapse of the postreduction framework, nasal packing should be placed for 3–5 days. Septum splints are recommended in comminuted septal fractures with severe mucosal lesions. External nasal splinting for 10 days (Aquaplast®, Thermoplast®) provides nasal protection. Nasal saline sprays prevent crusting, and oral antibiotics should

be prescribed for 1 week if nasal packing or septal splints are placed.
    • Open reduction
      – Immediate repair of fractures by using wide surgical exposure, reduction, fixation and reconstruction of severely damaged structures should be considered.
      – The second option is delayed correction (6 months or more) of persistent deformities, using standard techniques of rhinoplasty.

2.6.7 Deviated Nasal Septum

• Definition of the disease
  – Deviation of the nasal septum is a common cause of unilateral nasal airway obstruction, in which the nasal septum is displaced.
• Epidemiology/aetiology
  – Developmental septal abnormalities may occur. Septal cartilage damage in the neonatal period and during birth can cause severe septal deviation in the absence of a history of nasal trauma. Microfractures sustained during late intrauterine life and during birth may cause weakness in the damaged side of the cartilage. The result is asymmetric bending of the cartilage towards the side of the injury, while the contralateral side achieves dominance over time. In addition, septal deviation from traumatic nose or midface impacts can occur in childhood or adult life.
• Symptoms
  – Patients may present with a history of sinusitis, allergic rhinitis, obstructive sleep apnoea, previous nasal surgery or recent nasal trauma. Unilateral or

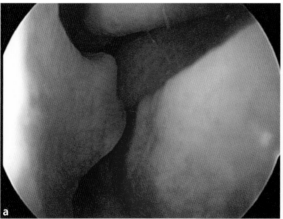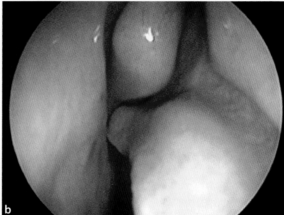

Fig. 2.6.2a,b Septal spur on the left (**a**) and the right (**b**) nasal fossa

bilateral nasal airway obstruction that is unrelieved with decongestants or nasal steroid sprays is often seen.

- Diagnosis
  - On initial examination, external dorsal deviation may be evident, or the columella and caudal septum may be deflected off the midline (caudal subluxation).
  - Inspections of the nasal cavity and anterior-posterior rhinoscopy are helpful in diagnosing the location, type and severity of septal deformity. Both the anterior and posterior septum should be evaluated. The endoscope is also useful in identifying polyps, assessing the severity and extent of posterior septal deviations and bony spurs, and locating areas of septal perforation or mucosal injury. The size of the inferior turbinate should be noted before and after a decongestant spray.
  - Allergic rhinitis can present with pale, boggy mucosa and watery discharge. Vasomotor rhinitis, rhinitis medicamentosa or cocaine abuse usually presents with thickened, hyperaemic mucosa. Lateralising the nasal sidewall with lateral digital pressure on the patient's cheek can assess a narrow internal nasal valve.
- Therapy
  - Septoplasty is a tissue-sparing procedure. The area of deviation is corrected or resected in order to leave behind as much cartilage and bone as possible. Cartilage resection is minimised and can be repositioned, reshaped, or recontoured, using a variety of methods.
  - Indications of septoplasty before the growth period of the nose is finished should be very limited. In these cases, surgery must preserve all the cartilage in order to prevent external changes of the shape of the nose.
  - Submucosal resection, unless for isolated septal spurs, is an obsolete technique.
- Complications
  - Frequent complications include haematoma and infection. Cerebrospinal fluid leak is a rare, but potentially serious complication. It is usually the result of avulsion or damage to the cribriform plate when handling the perpendicular plate of the ethmoid. Bed rest with elevated thorax to reduce intracranial pressure, nasal packing and oral antibiotics usually manage it, as spontaneous resolution usually occurs.
  - Other complications include epistaxis, nasal obstruction due to residual deviation, synechiae, return of the cartilaginous deviation, septal perforation, anosmia and cosmetic nasal deformities such as widened alar rim margins, drooping nasal tip, columella retraction, and a sunken dorsum with a supratip saddle formation.

2.6.8 Septal Haematoma

A septal haematoma is a blood collection under the perichondrium of the septum, which separates the vascular supply from the underlying cartilage. It can result in cartilage necrosis within 3 days.

- Epidemiology/aetiology
  - A septal haematoma is one of the most severe early complications of nasal trauma.
- Diagnosis
  - Signs and symptoms include intense pain, swelling, haematoma of the upper lip and philtrum area, and complete nasal airway obstruction.
- Therapy
  - Management consists of drainage through a mucoperichondrial incision. Immediate treatment is necessary to prevent long-term problems such as a saddle-nose deformity, perforation, columellar retraction and nasal-base widening. In children, septal destruction can lead to devastating nasal and midfacial growth abnormalities.
- Surgery
  - Incision and evacuation of the collection is performed. Drainage of a septal haematoma should provide closure of the incision. Splints or trans-

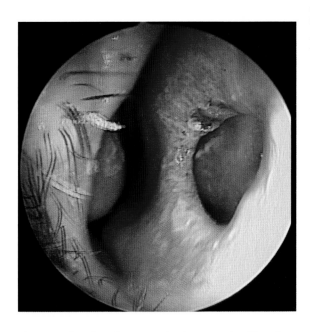

Fig. 2.6.3 Septal perforation with minor crusting. View from the right nasal fossa

septal dissolving sutures are placed to obliterate the potential space and prevent collection. Positioning of a Penrose-like drainage can eventually lead to superinfection. Infection involving the septal cartilage requires surgical treatment by means of resection of the cartilage, which is replaced by a septum-like silicon stent. Reconstruction with autologous cartilage is then performed in a second stage. Oral antibiotics should be given.

2.6.9   Nasal Deformity

- Saddle-nose deformity
  - A saddle-nose deformity is characterised by a loss of nasal dorsal height and compromised nasal support structures. Other features observed are depression of the middle vault and dorsum, loss of nasal tip support and definition, shortened (vertical) nasal length, over rotation of the nasal tip and retrusion of the nasal spine and caudal septum. It is also known as a "Pug nose" or "boxer's nose", both of which refer to various degrees of nasal dorsal depression.
- Epidemiology/aetiology
  - Prevalence is higher in population groups prone to facial trauma (i.e. boxers, athletes), those with histories of intranasal cocaine use, nasal surgery (e. g., radical submucosal septal resection, reductive rhinoplasty) and certain familial and ethnic groups.
  - A saddle-nose deformity can be congenital or acquired. It can be noticed as a part of individual, familial, syndromic, and ethnic characteristics. Most deformities are acquired due to traumatic and iatrogenic causes. Other medical causes are Wegener's granulomatosis, relapsing polychondritis, leprosy (Hansen's disease), syphilis, ectodermal dysplasia and intranasal cocaine use.
- Symptoms
  - Saddle-nose deformities with septal perforations can present with nasal crusting, nasal obstruction and a whistling sound heard during nasal airflow.
- Diagnosis
  - Complete history taking and physical examination are important in diagnosis. The use of intranasal cocaine or heroin should be investigated in patients with nasoseptal perforations. Endoscopic nasal examination of all end nasal structures and a standard series of photographs should be obtained prior to surgical planning for rhinoplasty.
- Therapy
  - Nasal reconstruction indications depend on patient selection, surgeon experience and aetiology of the deformity. Indications for surgery can be functional, aesthetic or, most commonly, both. In individu-

als with a compromised nasal airway, a nasoseptal reconstruction is indicated.
  - Contraindications include patients with malignant, chronic or autoimmune disease conditions, drug abuse, poor perioperative risk profile and unrealistic expectations.
  - Multiple previous rhinoplasties and certain professions (mixed martial artists, boxers, and other contact sports) are relative contraindications.
- Septoplasty
  - Septoplasty is performed to correct nasal obstruction caused by septal deformity.
  - Usually septoplasty is performed under general anaesthesia, with the patient in the supine position with the head elevated by approximately 30%. (Right-handed surgeons approach from the right side.)
  - Local vasoconstrictive anaesthesia is applied not only to reduce postoperative pain, but also more importantly to achieve vasoconstriction of the mucosa and less intraoperative haemorrhage. Lidocaine with adrenaline or epinephrine is used, although in patients with cardiac hypersensitivity, oxymetazoline might be preferred.
  - Septoplasty begins with the incision of septal mucosa. Most operative techniques utilise a hemitransfixion incision at the caudal end of septum, so that deviation at this point might be reached, as well as a transfixion incision that is easily obtained if needed. (Right-handed surgeons normally choose the left side, but that may vary when deviation is convex towards the right.)
  - A columella retractor is placed over the columella, and by pulling it laterally, the caudal border of the septum is exposed. Ala can be protected by an ala protector. A vertical incision with a no. 15 blade over the caudal end of septum is performed, until reaching the plane of the septal cartilage. It is essential to correctly identify the perichondrium and by using the Cottle elevator, dissect and lift it, creating a flap. As the dissection proceeds along the septal cartilage, a longer speculum (no. 5) is introduced so that elevation of the mucoperichondrium is done under constant visual control.
  - The next step is to dissect the mucoperiostium from the nasal floor along the maxillary crest, creating a second (inferior) tunnel, which afterwards should be connected with the pocket previously prepared over the septum.
  - Dissecting over the bony-cartilaginous junction when joining both tunnels might be difficult and is especially prone to membrane perforation.
  - If needed, the same tunnels are to be created on the other side of the septum. Then, deviated parts of septum are identified and removed either with a knife or a Freer chisel. If deviation is due to a shift of

septum from the maxillary crest, the septum must be separated from the perpendicular plate, trimmed along the inferior border, placed back onto the crest and sutured to the periosteum. If the deformity involves the vomer, an osteotome is used. Care must be taken not to break the cribriform plate, because it could cause a cerebrospinal fistula.

- Once the septal deviation is corrected, the flaps and hemitransfixion incision are mattressed with absorbable sutures. Nasal packing to prevent synechiae and postoperative septal haematoma might be advised but should be removed within 72 h.

Suggested Reading

1. Bailey B (2006) Head and neck surgery – otolaryngology, 4th edn. Lippincott Williams & Wilkins, Philadelphia, Pa.

2. Cummings C (2005) Otolaryngology: head and neck surgery, 4th edn. Mosby, New York

3. Isobe, K, Uno, T, Tamaru, J et al. (2006) Extranodal natural killer/T-cell lymphoma, nasal type: the significance of radiotherapeutic parameters. Cancer 106:609–615

4. Jaswal A, Jana AK, Sikder B, Nandi TK, Sadhukhan SK, Das A (2008) Novel treatment of atrophic rhinitis: early results. Eur Arch Otorhinolaryngol 265:1211–1217

5. Leavitt, RY, Fauci, AS, Bloch, DA et al. (1990) The American College of Rheumatology 1990 criteria for the classification of Wegener's granulomatosis. Arthritis Rheum 33:1101–1102

6. Li, CC, Tien, HF, Tang, JL et al. (2004) Treatment outcome and pattern of failure in 77 patients with sinonasal natural killer/T-cell or T-cell lymphoma. Cancer 100:366–375

7. Stevens DL, Bisno AL, Chambers HF et al. (2005) Practice guidelines for the diagnosis and management of skin and soft-tissue infections. Clin Infect Dis 41:1373–1406

2.7 Epistaxis

PAOLO CASTELNUOVO, ANDREA PISTOCHINI AND PIETRO PALMA

2.7.1 Nose: Pertinent Vascular Anatomy

Nasal cavities are supplied by terminal branches of the external (ECA) and internal (ICA) carotid arteries. The vessels originiating from ECA are branches of the facial artery and the internal maxillary artery (IMA). The superior labial artery, from the facial artery, enters the nose laterally to the anterior nasal spine and supplies the anterior nasal septum. The sphenopalatine artery (SPA) and the descending palatine artery (DPA), originating from the IMA, enter the nasal cavities, respectively, through the sphenopalatine foramen and the incisive foramen. The SPA supplies the nasal septum with the septal branch and the middle and inferior turbinates with its nasal branches. The DPA supplies the anterior nasal septum.

The 3 branches of the ICA that supply the nasal cavities are (1) the Vidian artery, coming from the petrous segment of ICA, crossing the basisphenoid in the Vidian canal and reaching the IMA and its first endocranial branch, the ophthalmic artery, with its two ethmoidal branches, (2) the posterior (PEA) and (3) the anterior (AEA) ethmoidal arteries. After passing through the posterior and anterior ethmoid canals (exiting from the orbit through the lamina papyracea), they enter the nasal cavities and cross the ethmoid sinus on the ethmoidal roof. Then they enter the anterior cranial fossa in the olfactory cleft and divide into their meningeal branches.

Anteriorly, the nasal septum presents a vascular plexus (Kiesselbach area or locus Valsalva), which is supplied by both carotid systems (ECA and ICA). Another septal anastomotic plexus can be also found in the Woodroof area, which is another common site of bleeding.

2.7.2 Epistaxis

Epistaxis (synonymous with nasal bleeding, nosebleed and nasal haemorrhage) is a loss of blood from the nasal fossae. It originates from a disruption of the nasal mucosa and vessels and is commonly divided into anterior and posterior epistaxis, depending on the site of origin.

2.7.2.1 Aetiology/Epidemiology

Causes of epistaxis can be divided in local and systemic causes (Table 2.7.1). The most frequent local causes of epistaxis are traumas, including nose picking and inflammatory disease involving nasal mucosa. Endonasal surgery is an obvious cause of bleeding. Nose bleeding is typically recurrent also when it is due to a tumour. Patient medical history has to be investigated accurately, and patients should be systematically asked about hypertension and use of anticoagulants.

Males are slightly more affected than females are until the age of 50, but after 50 no difference between sexes is reported. After the age of 50, severe epistaxis is more frequent.

2.7.2.2 Symptoms

Patients may report nasal obstruction due to clots, or emesis due to blood ingestion. Some accompanying symptoms, like syncopal episodes, are suggestive of underlying cardiovascular problems.

2.7.2.3 Complications

Severe bleeding coming from the oral cavity and hypopharynx may flow back in the nasal cavities. Cardiovas-

Table 2.7.1 Aetiology of epistaxis

Local causes	Systemic causes
Trauma (including surgical trauma)	Coagulation deficits
Inflammatory diseases and infections	Anticoagulant drugs
Tumours	Vascular/cardiovascular diseases, vasculitis
Vascular malformations	HHT, Rendu-Osler-Weber disease

cular complications may occur when the patient looses a large amount of blood, especially when blood pressure is not monitored. Amaurosis may occur as a consequence of intraorbital bleeding of ethmoidal arteries. Ethmoidal artery ligation may lead to external deformities like enophthalmos, diplopia and even blindness.

2.7.2.4   Diagnostic Procedures

2.7.2.4.1   Recommended European Standard
- Nasal endoscopy
- Inspection of the oral cavity, nasal cavity and nasopharynx
- ECG
- Blood tests (blood count, coagulation tests)

2.7.2.4.2   Additional/Useful Diagnostic Procedures
- Blood pressure monitoring
- Microbiology: nasal secretions culture
- CT scan/MRI
- Computerised digital subtraction angiography

2.7.2.5   Therapy

2.7.2.5.1   Conservative Treatment

Recommended European Standard
- As a first remedy, particularly in younger patients with minimal anterior epistaxis, the nostrils should be firmly pinched between fingers and thumb, continuously for 10 min, with the patient seated and the head tilted forward. In many cases digital pressure stops haemorrhage and helps to reduce blood ingestion. More severe epistaxis, when nasal endoscopy is feasible, has to be treated with endoscopic bipolar electrocautery. Chemical cautery with silver nitrate-tipped sticks generally is not quite effective, especially with active bleeding.
- When nasal endoscopy is not feasible, nasal packing is necessary. Traditional anterior and posterior packings are obsolete. Many different resorbable (Surgicel, Gelfoam) and nonresorbable (Merocel, Lyofoam) materials are available. Packing should be coated in antibiotic ointment. Results are similar with the different materials. If the bleeding originates posteriorly, nasal balloons (Epistat) can also be used. Nasal packing has to be removed after 24 h, and nasal endoscopy after decongesting the mucosa has to be performed to identify the site of bleeding. If the Epistat is not slightly deflated or removed after 24 h, then injury of nasal mucosa can occur. If the balloon is kept in place inflated for 48 h,

then tissue necrosis may take place, with consequent septal perforation.
- Once bleeding has stopped, nasal irrigation and the use of antibiotic ointment for some days are recommended.

Useful Additional Therapeutic Strategies
- Avoidance of NSAIDs
- Vitamin C
- Vascular protective drugs
- Topical haemostatic agents
- Nasal washing
- A Foley balloon, which is easily available, can be used instead of Epistat.

2.7.2.5.2   Surgical Treatment

Recommended European Standard
- The treatment of choice is represented by bipolar cauterisation under endoscopic control of the bleeding vessel. Use of nasal packing should be limited as much as possible. Attention should be paid not to simultaneously cauterise nasal septum at the same place bilaterally, to avoid iatrogenic septal perforations.
- In most cases endoscopic bipolar electrocautery of the SPA (especially the septal and nasal branches), AEA or PEA are effective in haemostasis. The procedures can be done under local or general anaesthesia, depending on the patient's general conditions.
- Selective embolisation with polyvinyl alcohol spheres, under general anaesthesia, is needed only in special cases. In a few cases, arterial ligation has to performed, and the IMA is generally closed under endoscopic control by a vascular clip after removal of the posterior wall of the maxillary sinus. The AEA and PEA can also be clipped by way of an external approach (the Howard-Lynch incision); in these cases endoscopic control is also highly recommended.
- ECA ligation has to be considered when other procedures fail to end the bleeding.

2.7.2.6   Differential Diagnosis

Epistaxis shows typical clinical features, and it is difficult to misdiagnose.

2.7.2.7   Prognosis

The prognosis depends on the underlying disease causing epistaxis. The prognosis is good for nose bleeding due to local causes (except for tumours). When epistaxis represents a symptom of a systemic disease, treatment of the primary disease is the main concern. The treatment may be that of long-term therapy, or no effective therapy may be available, e.g. in cases of hereditary hemorrhagic telangiectasia (HHT).

When blood loss reduces the patient's haemoglobin value to $\leq 7 \pm 1$ g/dl, then transfusion should be considered.

2.7.2.8 Surgical Principles

2.7.2.8.1 Endoscopic Nasal Bipolar Electrocautery

- SPA electrocautery is the most effective procedure. A mucosal incision of the lateral wall is made 1 cm anterior to the tail of the middle turbinate. Then, a subperiosteal dissection is initiated and continued until the sphenopalatine foramen is reached, immediately dorsal to the tail of the middle turbinate. The ASP lies just behind the bony point of the foramen. The same area can be easily cauterised also without performing submucosal dissection, especially when the procedure is performed under local anesthesia.
- The septal branch of the SPA can be cauterised over the superior choanal margin, above the tail of the superior turbinate.
- When bleeding from an ethmoidal artery occurs intraoperatively, e.g. during transnasal transethmoidal surgery, then endoscopically assisted electrocautery

is performed after having identified the AEA or PEA on the ethmoidal roof. Ethmoidectomy is necessary to visualise the ethmoidal roof.

Technique

- Zero and 45° rigid endoscopes and suction units are necessary.
- Bipolar cautery improves efficacy and ease of the procedure.
- Ethmoidectomies have to be performed with cutting instruments to avoid mucosa stripping and consequent vagaries of scarring.

2.7.2.8.2 IMA Ligation

A vascular clip may be positioned either endoscopically or via an external approach. The pterygomaxillary fossa has to be exposed through the posterior wall of the maxillary sinus. The posterior wall of the maxillary antrum may be accessed endoscopically after removal of the medial wall of the maxillary sinus, or externally using the Caldwell-Luc approach.

2.7.2.8.3 AEA and PEA Ligation

A full-thickness Howard-Lynch incision is followed by an endoscopically assisted dissection under the orbital periosteum. The AEA is identified 1–2 cm posterior to the

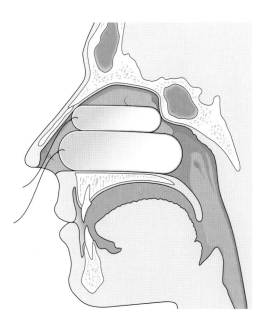

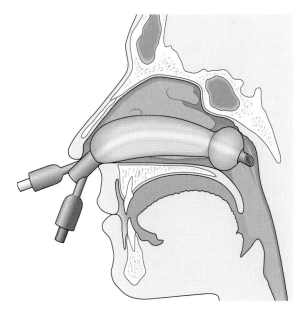

Fig. 2.7.1 Nasal packs (Merocel, Medtronic Xomed, Jacksonville, FL) are inserted parallel to the nasal floor to obtain useful haemostasis

Fig. 2.7.2 Nasal catheter (Epistat, Medtronic Xomed, Jacksonville, FL) is fully inserted and then inflated when also a posterior packing is needed

anterior lacrimal crest. The PEA is located about 1.5 cm behind the AEA. Once identified, arteries are clipped or cauterised with bipolar cautery.

2.7.2.8.4 ECA Ligation

During ECA ligation accurate identification of the ICA is necessary. Injuries to the vagus, superior laryngeal and hypoglossal nerves must be avoided.

2.7.3   Special Remarks

- It is of utmost importance to diagnose coagulation deficits, HHT and vascular tumours (e.g. juvenile nasal angiofibroma) before performing any interventional procedures.
- Major nasal packing should be avoided, as modern devices allow a more effective control of haemostasis while minimising the patient's discomfort.

2.7.3.1   Surface Anaesthesia of the Nasal Mucosa

Every endoscopic procedure should be carried out after having decongested the nasal mucosa with cotton sponges soaked with topical oxybuprocaine hydrochloride and naphazoline.

Suggested Reading

1. Cummings C (2005) Otolaryngology: head and neck surgery, 4th edn. Mosby, New York
2. Douglas R, Wormald PJ (2007) Update on epistaxis. Curr Opin Otolaryngol Head Neck Surg 15:180–183
3. Harvey RJ, Kanagalingam J, Lund VJ (2008) The impact of septodermoplasty and potassium–titanyl–phosphate (KTP) laser therapy in the treatment of hereditary hemorrhagic telangiectasia-related epistaxis. Am J Rhinol 22:182–187
4. Miller TR, Stevens ES, Orlandi RR (2005) Economic analysis of the treatment of posterior epistaxis. Am Rhinol 19:79–82
5. Padua F, Voegels RL (2008) Severe posterior epistaxis–endoscopic surgical anatomy. Laryngoscope 118:156–161
6. Snyderman CH, Goldman SA, Carrau RL, Ferguson BJ, Grandis JR (1999) Endoscopic sphenopalatine artery ligation is an effective method of treatment for posterior epistaxis. Am J Rhinol 13:137–140
7. Srouji I, Lund V, Andrews P, Edwards C (2008) Rhinologic symptoms and quality-of-life in patients with Churg-Strauss syndrome vasculitis. Am J Rhinol 22:406–409
8. Wormald PJ, Wee DT, van Hasselt CA (2000) Endoscopic ligation of the sphenopalatine artery for refractory posterior epistaxis. Am J Rhinol 14:261–264

2.8 Congenital Malformation: Choanal Atresia

PIETRO PALMA, PAOLO BOSSOLESI, CRISTIAN CAMBRIA
AND PAOLO CASTELNUOVO

2.8.1 Rhinopharynx

2.8.1.1 Basics

The choana is the posterior nasal aperture. It is the opening between the nasal cavity and the nasopharynx. It is not actually a structure but rather a space bounded anteriorly and inferiorly by the horizontal plate of palatine bone, superiorly and posteriorly by the sphenoid bone, medially by the nasal septum and laterally by the medial pterygoid plates.

2.8.1.2 Choanal Atresia

2.8.1.2.1 Definition

Choanal atresia is a developmental defect in which a failure occurs of one or both nares to canalise as consequence of a congenital malformation of the posterior portion of the nasal cavity; conspicuous unilateral or bilateral narrowing up to complete coarctation of the opening between the nasal cavity and the nasopharynx represent the relevant clinical features. The atretic plate contains bone in 80–90% of cases, whereas it is constituted by mucosa and fibrous tissue in about 10% of cases. In cases of bilateral involvement, suffocation may occur before the child learns to breathe through the mouth, and severe feeding difficulties are present.

2.8.1.2.2 Aetiology/Epidemiology

A number of theories have been proposed to explain the occurrence of choanal atresia, but not one has gained universal acceptance. The persistence of the buccopharyngeal membrane seems to be the most widely accepted theory, but failure of the bucconasal membrane of Hochstetter to rupture, abnormal mesodermal adhesions forming in the choanal area and misdirection of mesodermal flow due to local factors are also reported in the literature.

Associated malformations occur in 47% of infants without chromosome anomalies. Nonrandom association of malformations can be demonstrated using the (mnemonic) CHARGE association (*c*oloboma, *h*eart abnormalities, *a*tresia of choanae, *r*etarded growth and development of central nervous system, *g*enitourinary anomalies, *e*ar defects).

The unilateral form is more frequent, but a bilateral presentation occurs in 30–40% of the cases, and the incidence of this disorder is estimated to be 1 in 5,000–8,000 live births. There is female-to-male-predominance of 5 to 1 in Caucasians.

2.8.1.2.3 Symptoms

The diagnosis of congenital bilateral choanal atresia is suspected soon after birth when the newborn presents with asphyxia and cyanosis. In unilateral choanal atresia, the picture resembles unilateral nasal obstruction with rhinorrhea and can be confused with other lesions, eluding definitive diagnosis for several years. Respiratory distress in newborns with unilateral atresia is less dramatic, but impaired breast-feeding should raise suspicion.

2.8.1.2.4 Complications

In cases of bilateral choanal atresia, severe hypoxia with suffocation after birth may occur. Suckling difficulties are always present, leading to severe weight loss if appropriate measures are not taken.

2.8.1.2.5 Diagnostic Procedures: Recommended European Standard

When unilateral or bilateral atresia is suspected, nasopharyngoscopy by flexible endoscope is mandatory. Endoscopic examination with rigid endoscopes, when feasible, is helpful to get a clearer picture.

CT scan in axial and coronal projections provides a thorough evaluation of choanal atresia and adjacent structures. The axial views supply fundamental information including site of obstruction, composition of the atretic plate, and unilateral or bilateral involvement. Imaging allows also identification of other congenital malformations such as meningoencephalocele, septal deviation and anatomical sinus variations.

Historical/Useful Diagnostic Procedures

Literature-mentioned diagnostic procedures include visual evaluation of nasal patency with the use of a glass steaming up in front of the nostril(s) opening and plain conventional radiography with contrast solution injected into the nasal fossa. Introduction of a probe through the nose or injection of coloured solution enables the operator to check the patency of the passageway by inspection of the oropharynx.

The aforementioned diagnostic tools are only of historical interest as nasopharyngoscopy represents the current gold standard.

2.8.1.2.6 Therapy

- Conservative Treatment
  - Recommended European standard:
    - None
  - Useful additional therapeutic strategies:
    - None
- Surgical Treatment
  - Recommended European Standard:
    - Choanal atresia is surgically treated through an endonasal endoscopic approach.

2.8.1.2.7 Differential Diagnosis

Complete nasal obstruction in the newborn is undoubtedly suggestive, but there are other conditions to be taken into account to establish the correct diagnosis:

- Hypertrophic pharyngeal tonsil
- Turbinate hypertrophy
- Sinonasal neoplasms
- Nasal polyps
- Septum deformity
- Skull base malformations

2.8.1.2.8 Prognosis

Both bilateral and unilateral choanal atresias need to be treated surgically. According to the literature data, the endoscopic endonasal approach, with or without postoperative stenting, shows good results for a persistent opening of the neochoana and the nasal fossa in 84–100% of the cases.

The transpalatal technique, even if it permits good exposure of the lesion, carries considerable risks such as damage of the palatine vessels. Other possible complications are represented by functional damage of the palatal muscles and palatal leaks.

The manoeuvre of perforation of the atresic plate may lead to injury of the Eustachian tube and skull base.

The most common long-term complication is represented by restenosis of the neochoana due to scar formation around the border of the neo-ostium, developing after bone exposure during surgery.

2.8.1.2.9 Surgical Principles

Problems of feeding and breathing soon after birth are present in bilateral cases and always demand urgent attention. To establish sufficient breathing in an emergent situation orotracheal intubation is mandatory until skilled surgical help is available. The operation can be performed few days after birth. In unilateral cases treatment is not urgent, and it is generally diagnosed later.

Endoscopic endonasal approach represents the first choice approach. Surgery is addressed not only to remove the atretic plate, but also must include removal of the posterior part of the septum as well as development of suitable mucoperiosteal flaps in order to prevent restenosis. The technique is aimed at creating a new opening between the posterior nasal cavity and nasopharynx.

Technique

The technique to be used depends mainly on the type of choanal atresia, unilateral or bilateral, and on the available "surgical space".

In unilateral cases when the surgical space is generally adequate, the technique is as follows.

The first step consists of a vertical incision of the nasal mucosa at the level of the posterior third of the vomer in order to raise two mucoperiosteal flaps. The first flap is developed from the surface of the atretic plate and displaced laterally, whereas the second septal flap is harvested in a posterior–anterior direction from the part of the vomer that has to be removed. The bone is then pierced in the middle and drilled away, up to complete ablation of the inferior portion of the sphenoidal rostrum. The inferoposterior part of the vomer is resected with the use of a back-bite forceps. The mucoperiosteal flap detached from the anterior surface of the atretic plate is used to cover the raw area of the lateral aspect of the neochoana, while the mucosa detached from the posterior aspect of the vomer is employed to cover the medial edge of the neochoana and septum.

At the end of the procedure a Silastic sheet is positioned along the nasal septum and fixed with a transseptal stitch (Vicryl 2-0). Sheeting will allow maintaining sufficient patency of the nasal airway while nasal passageways are irrigated daily with saline solution. The Silastic sheets are kept in place for about 20 days.

In the newborn with bilateral choanal atresia, the surgical procedure differs greatly due to the lack of spaces. The first step is always represented by the vertical incision of the posterior septal mucosa. Then the central part of the atretic plate is pierced bilaterally by a 1-mm osteotome and then widened centripetally by a circular punch while care is taken to avoid leaving bare bony areas. These manoeuvres create a wider operative space, so a flap over the posterior septum can be raised. Bony septum and part of the sphenoid rostrum are then removed. The previously raised septal flap is used to cover the bony areas.

Alternative Technique

The approach can be transpalatal, using microsurgical techniques and an operating microscope.

2.8.1.3 Special Remarks

Keys to avoid postoperative stenosis are represented by:
1. Accurate removal of the posterior edge of the vomer and inferior portion of sphenoid rostrum.
2. Complete covering of bare bone by mucoperiosteal flaps.

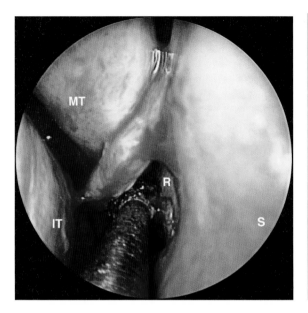

Fig. 2.8.1 Unilateral right choanal atresia. Right nasal fossa, 0° endoscope view. After elevation of the mucosal flaps, the inferior portion of the sphenoidal rostrum is drilled away to perforate the atretic plate. (MT: middle turbinate; IT: inferior turbinate; R: rostrum; NS: nasal septum)

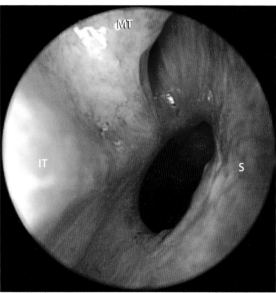

Fig. 2.8.3 Right nasal fossa, 0° endoscope view. Post-operative control after 6 months. The neochoana shows an adequate opening. (IT: inferior turbinate; S: nasal septum)

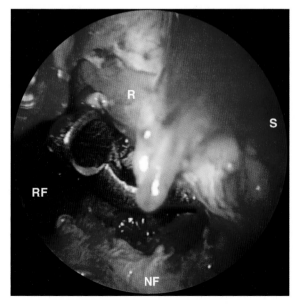

Fig. 2.8.2 Right nasal fossa, 45° endoscope view. The infero-posterior portion of the vomer removal is carved by a back-bite forceps, introduced through the controlateral nasal fossa (R: rostrum; S: nasal septum; NF: nasal floor; RF: rhino-pharynx)

2.9 Nasal Obstruction

JACINTO GARCÍA AND HUMBERT MASSEGUR

2.9.1 Introduction

The "stuffy" nose (also known as nasal blockage or nasal congestion) is the sensation of having difficulty breathing through the nose. It may be unilateral or bilateral, transient or permanent, usually caused by anatomic variations, tumours or changes in the function of the nasal mucosa, which narrow the nasal cavity and increase resistance to the air flow. Therefore, there exist conditions such as atrophic rhinitis or viscosity changes of mucus, which elicit the same sensation despite the wide patency of the nasal cavities.

2.9.2 Aetiology/Epidemiology

The causes that obstruct the nasal airflow can be divided in two main groups:
1. Mechanic or structural causes
   a. Alar collapse caused by insufficient rigidity of the alar cartilages
   b. Vestibular synechiae or scars
   c. Septal deviations
   d. Septal perforations, haematoma, perforation
   e. Nasal polyposis, antrochoanal polyp
   f. Benign tumours: angiofibroma, inverted papilloma
   g. Malignant tumours: squamous cell carcinoma, adenocarcinoma, melanoma
   h. Turbinate hypertrophy
   i. Malformations of the nasal framework
   j. Choanal atresia
2. Functional causes
   a. Allergic rhinosinusitis
   b. Acute or chronic rhinosinusitis
   c. Rhinitis medicamentosa or drug side effects
   d. Rhinitis of pregnancy
   e. Atrophic rhinitis
   f. Chemical injury of nasal mucosa (inhaled drugs, occupational)
   g. Wegener granulomatosis

2.9.3 Diagnostic Procedures

2.9.3.1 Recommended European Standard

- Inspection
  - Are there deformities of the nasal framework?
  - Does the nasal valve collapse at forced inspiration?
  - Is the skin of the nasal vestibule swollen?
- Palpation
  - Are there deformities of the nasal framework?
  - Projecting the nasal tip upwards is a good technique.
  - Is the caudal septum deviated?
  - Is there narrowing of the nasal valve?
- Rhinoscopy before and after vasoconstriction
  - Are there deformities, hematomas or perforation of the nasal septum?
  - Is there turbinate hypertrophy?
  - Is the mucosa red or pale?
  - Are there polyps?
  - Is there purulent secretion?
  - Is a tumour visible?
- Endoscopy of the nose/nasopharynx, before and after vasoconstriction
  - Are there posterior septal spurs?
  - Are the turbinates swollen?
  - Does the middle meatus have purulent discharge?
  - Are there bleeding or pulsating polyps?
  - Are there synechiae?
  - Is choanal atresia evident?
  - Is there adenoid hypertrophy?
  - Are there polyps?
  - Is a tumour visible?

2.9.3.2 Additional/Useful Diagnostic Procedures

- Nasal inspiratory peak flow
- Rhinomanometry (active anterior and posterior)
- Acoustic rhinometry

- Nasomucociliary clearance (dye or reactive particles)
- CT scan (tumours, complications of sinusitis)
- Eosinophils in nasal discharge
- Nitric oxide (presence of inflammation and ciliary dysfunction)
- Biopsy (always after CT scan)

2.9.3.3   Therapy

- Conservative treatment
- Recommended European standard
  - Topic nasal corticosteroids
- Useful additional therapeutic strategies
- Surgical treatment

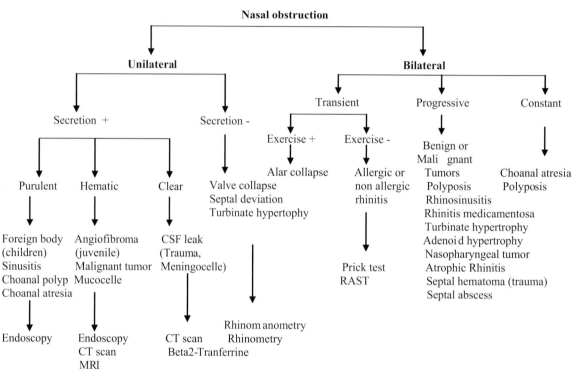

Fig. 2.9.1 Algorithm on nasal obstruction

2.10 Nonallergic Rhinitis and Primary Ciliary Dyskinesia

MIGUEL MALDONADO-FERNÁNDEZ AND JOAQUIM MULLOL

2.10.1 Introduction

Rhinitis is defined by the presence of nasal symptoms such as obstruction, itching, discharge and sneezing [1]. According to its skin test and serum immunoglobulin (Ig)E pattern, chronic rhinitis has been traditionally classified into "allergic" and "nonallergic". Nonallergic rhinitis is therefore defined as chronic rhinitis with negative testing for IgE-mediated sensitivity to aeroallergens. At first blush, conditions such as infectious rhinitis or nasal polyposis would fall into this category. However, for most authors these diseases must be excluded, with the focus only on nonallergic, noninfectious rhinitis.

tion suffers from chronic nasal disease with daily symptoms and the need for medication. According to the Joint Task Force on Practice Parameters in Allergy, Asthma and Immunology, approximately 50% of patients with rhinitis do not have an allergic rhinitis [4]. Nonallergic rhinitis usually develops in the middle-aged population, whereas allergic rhinitis tends to develop predominantly in children. Ageing might therefore be responsible for changes in the nasal mucosa that could affect the course of disease.

2.10.2 Diagnosis

Clinical features including obstruction, itching, discharge and sneezing (at least two of them for more than 1 h most days) [2], with negative allergic background (history, skin-prick test, serum-specific IgE) are the basic criteria for nonallergic rhinitis (Fig. 2.10.1). However there is no specific test for nonallergic rhinitis, so diagnosis is made by exclusion of allergy, sinus disease, and structural or immune alterations.

However, not every rhinitis with a positive skin test is an allergic rhinitis. There is a group of rhinitises without a clear association between their positive skin tests and their symptoms (e.g. a positive test for a seasonal allergen and a clearly persistent behaviour of the specific rhinitis). Furthermore, in a broad group of patients, mixed pathophysiology (both allergic and nonallergic) can be suspected [3]. Therefore, nonallergic rhinitis actually is a group of syndromes without generally accepted diagnostic criteria, sometimes overlapping when comparing different classifications.

2.10.3 Epidemiology

Although uneven definition standards have made figures variable, it is estimated that 2–4% of the general popula-

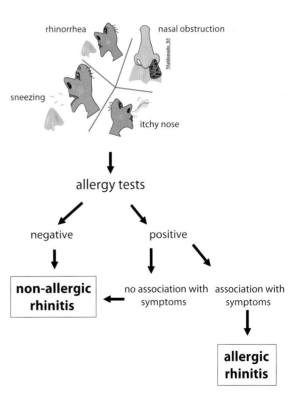

Fig. 2.10.1 Flow chart for chronic rhinitis. Allergic tests in nonallergic rhinitis are either negative or not related to nasal symptoms

2.10.4 Occupational Rhinitis

Occupational rhinitis is an episodic, working-related nasal syndrome characterised by sneezing, nasal obstruction and nasal discharge. It may be due to an IgE-mediated mechanism, which would be a form of allergic rhinitis, or related to nonspecific inflammation of the nose, e.g. exposure to high concentrations of irritating substances, which would be included in the nonallergic rhinitis category. There are many causes of occupational rhinitis, which include grains, laboratory animals, wood dust and latex, and chemicals like platinum salts, acid anhydrides, glues and solvents. Occupational rhinitis may be associated with occupational asthma, a condition that should be further investigated.

Treatment of occupational rhinitis is based on prevention, which can be carried out screening applicants for sensitising work environments. However, in a study performed on laboratory workers, this measure proved inefficient. Environmental control measures like adequate ventilation or the use of masks is another form of prevention. Pharmacologic treatment for occupational rhinitis is similar to treatment for other types of rhinitis, and is based on intranasal and systemic antihistamines, anticholinergic agents, decongestants and intranasal steroids.

2.10.5 Drug-induced Rhinitis

Rhinitis medicamentosa is a term reserved for the worsening of nasal obstruction in patients who use nasal decongestants chronically. This condition is of special concern in neonates because rebound nasal obstruction can lead to difficulty in feeding and to respiratory distress. Signs include erythematous nasal mucosa and swollen turbinates. Its pathologic hallmark is interstitial oedema [5], although hyperplastic goblet cells and increased immunoreactivity for EGFR have been discovered recently. Intranasal steroids have proved to be useful in the management of rhinitis medicamentosa in animal models and in vivo.

A number of drugs are known to cause rhinitis. Among these are:
- Aspirin and other nonsteroidal anti-inflammatory drugs (NSAIDs)
  - In about 10% of adult patients with asthma, NSAIDs are able to trigger an asthmatic crisis by means of cyclo-oxygenase inhibition. This may shift the arachidonic acid metabolism to the lipo-oxygenase pathway, increasing leukotriene synthesis.
- Alpha-blockers
- Angiotensin-converting enzyme (ACE) inhibitors
- Beta-blockers
- Chlorpromazine
- Cocaine
- Guanethidine
- Methyldopa
- Oral contraceptives
- Reserpine
- Phentolamine.

2.10.6 Rhinitis and Pregnancy

Pregnancy rhinitis is defined as nasal congestion in the last 6 weeks or so of pregnancy, excluding an allergic or infectious cause, and with complete resolution of the symptoms within 2 weeks after delivery. It affects roughly one out of five pregnancies. An impairment of nasal patency documented by anterior rhinomanometry and an augmented mucociliary clearance has been observed during pregnancy. In addition, there is an increase of nasal obstruction in women during their peri-ovulatory stage of the menstrual cycle, in conjunction with the rise in serum estrogens. The ultimate treatment for this condition is yet to be found. Nasal decongestants, although useful, tend to be overused by patients with pregnancy rhinitis, which carries the risk of developing rhinitis medicamentosa. Corticosteroids have not been found to be effective.

2.10.7 Rhinitis Associated with Physical and Chemical Factors

Chemical and physical factors may be responsible for nonallergic nasal symptoms, although limits between physiological and pathological influence of these factors are difficult to determine. Immersion in cold water has been found to produce nasal obstruction in a side-specific way. Cold, dry air may cause nasal obstruction and increase of secretions, known as "skier's nose". (However, total nasal patency [e.g. both nasal cavities] has been found kept at a constant level in skiers performing under cold and dry conditions). Ipratropium bromide can be a useful treatment for this condition.

2.10.8 Food-induced Rhinitis

Spicy foods cause watery rhinorrhea, a phenomenon called "gustatory rhinitis". This is caused by stimulation of atropine-inhibitable muscarinic receptors, so the syndrome can be treated with intranasal atropine [6].

2.10.9 Atrophic Rhinitis

Atrophic rhinitis is characterised by progressive nasal mucosal atrophy, which in its late stage (ozena) evolves to crusting, fetor, hyposmia, and enlargement of the nasal space, although with paradoxical nasal congestion. It has been attributed to infection with *Klebsiella pneumoniae* subsp. *ozenae*. Likely due to the use of antibiotics for chronic nasal infection, the incidence of primary atrophic rhinitis has decreased markedly in incidence in the last century. The most frequent type nowadays is secondary atrophic rhinitis resulting from trauma, surgery (e.g. aggressive resection of the turbinates), infection, granulomatous diseases or radiation exposure [7].

2.10.10 Nonallergic Rhinitis Eosinophilic Syndrome

Nonallergic rhinitis can be classified according to the inflammatory type found in the mucosa. *Nonallergic rhinitis eosinophilic syndrome* (NARES) is characterised by nasal perennial symptoms and nasal eosinophilia (more than 20%) with a negative allergy test. Clinical symptoms are usually more intense than in allergic or vasomotor rhinitis, and anosmia is common. The mechanism of eosinophilic infiltration is not known.

Although NARES is usually an isolated syndrome, it may be accompanied by asthma, aspirin intolerance and nasal polyps. For this reason it is sometimes considered an early stage of the Widal (or Samter) triad. Up to 45% of patients with NARES but without a history of respiratory symptoms show bronchial responsiveness. A subgroup of NARES is *blood eosinophilia nonallergic rhinitis syndrome* (BENARS), in which a rise in blood eosinophils is associated with NARES syndrome (Fig. 2.10.2).

It has been found that a proportion of patients with negative skin-prick test show nasal eosinophilia and are positive on nasal challenge. As well, local IgE production has been demonstrated. Therefore exclusion of an allergic basis should include intranasal provocation tests for a proper adscription of patients to the NARES group. Although treatment of NARES may be difficult at times, even requiring systemic steroids [8], intranasal fluticasone, either alone [9] or in combination with oral loratadine [10], may be useful in its management.

2.10.11 Vasomotor/Idiopathic Rhinitis

Vasomotor/idiopathic rhinitis is a classic term that refers to upper respiratory hyper-responsiveness to nonspe-

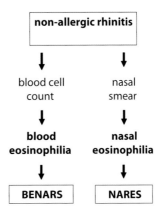

Fig. 2.10.2 Flow chart for diagnosis of nonallergic rhinitis eosinophilic syndrome (*NARES*) and blood eosinophilia nonallergic rhinitis syndrome (*BENARS*)

cific triggers like exposure to strong smells, changes in air temperature or humidity, alcohol ingestion or tobacco smoke. Its diagnosis is based on exclusion of allergy, structural lesions, drug abuse or systemic disease. Infection is usually ruled out if nasal secretion is watery and clear instead of purulent. The term *vasomotor rhinitis* implies a neurovascular dysfunction of the mucosa, which has not been thoroughly documented. Thus, the term *idiopathic* is more appropriate. Sympathetic innervation of the nose increases nasal patency and reduces nasal secretion, whereas parasympathetic innervation of the nose enhances hypersecretion and nasal congestion. Equilibrium between both systems is disturbed towards a hypofunction of the sympathetic innervation and hyperactive parasympathetic innervation. C fibres are nonmyelinated portions of sensory neurons, and might also play a role in vasomotor rhinitis, although no direct proof has been found. It has also been referred to as idiopathic rhinitis, and has been considered a part of the group of *nonallergic noninfectious perennial rhinitis* (NANIPER) [1, 2].

2.10.12 Other Possible Causes of Nonallergic, Noninfectious Rhinitis

2.10.12.1 Emotions

Psychological stress and sexual arousal are known to worsen rhinitis, supposedly by autonomic stimulation [1]. Postclimax rhinitis and/or asthma was confirmed in a four-case series in which physical exercise was ruled out to be the cause, leaving sexual excitement as the most logical trigger.

2.10.12.2 Gastroesophageal Reflux

Vasomotor rhinitis, chronic sinusitis and impaired recovery from sinus surgery have been frequently related to gastroesophageal reflux, but no evidence-based medical studies have been published.

2.10.12.3 Metabolic Conditions

Hypothyroidism and acromegaly have been both connected to rhinitis. However, evidence linking hypothyroidism with nasal disorders is limited. Resolution of rhinitis symptoms with a treatment for hypothyroidism alone has not been documented. In addition, administration of low-dose recombinant human growth hormone over 8 weeks was not found to cause nasal congestion, although higher doses have not been tested.

2.10.13 Primary Ciliary Dyskinesia

2.10.13.1 Introduction

The term *primary ciliary dyskinesia* (PCD) refers to all congenital abnormalities of ciliary function. In 1933 Kartagener published a series of four cases with sinusitis, bronchiectasis and dextrocardia. After the ultrastructural description of cilia in sperm tails, the association of chronic respiratory infections with absence of mucociliary clearance with immobile spermatozoa was observed. Male infertility was added to the syndrome described by Kartagener. Defects in the dynein arms of cilia were described, and the name *immotile cilia syndrome* was proposed. There exists a group of patients with ciliary activity but without effective mucous clearance, in whom cilia are oriented randomly and therefore mucous cannot be propelled effectively. Thus PCD includes the entire family of syndromes.

Normal ciliary beating, responsible for much of the mucous clearance, consists of three phases: an effective propelling stroke, a recovery phase and a recovery stroke. In this last phase, the cilia return to the original position, but without effective retrograde mucous transport.

A normal cilium consists of long microtubules that extend from the cytoplasm to the tip of the cilium. Microtubules can be found in singlets, doublets and triplets, formed by 13, 23 and 33 protofilaments of tubulin, respectively. The microtubule with a complete ring of 13 protofilaments is named "A", and the attached microtubules with incomplete rings of 10 protofilaments each are named "B" and "C". The cilium is anchored to a basal body located in the cytoplasm, and is composed by a central pair of singlets and nine pairs of triplets, which become doublets at a certain point in the length of the cilium. Four groups of proteins hold the structure together. The central singlets are united by connecting bridges, and surrounded by a sheath. Protein spikes radiate from the central singlets to the A microtubule of each doublet. Finally each doublet is fixed to the adjacent by a nexin link. An inner and an outer dynein arm is attached to every A microtubule of the outer doublets. The activity of the cilia is due to the ATPase activity of the dynein. Most of the motility disorders are related to mutations one or more of the proteins involved in the structure of the cilia.

2.10.13.2 Diagnosis

After the exclusion of other sinopulmonary syndromes such as cystic fibrosis, common variable immunodeficiency and Wegener's granulomatosis, an initial screening carrying out a ciliary motility and mucociliary transport analysis is recommended. Ciliary motility analysis requires high-speed film, laser, stroboscopic or photoelectric systems to capture the usual 12-Hz frequency beats of the cilia. Mucociliary transport in the nose can be studied with the saccharin test. If screening is positive, then electron microscopy should be performed to investigate ultrastructure alterations of the cilia.

2.10.13.3 Treatment

As for bronchiectasis from other causes, treatment of PCD consists of antibiotics, physiotherapy and vaccination against influenza virus, *Streptococcus pneumoniae* and *Haemophilus influenzae*. Lung lobectomy is nowadays an infrequent therapeutic tool. Lung transplantation has been performed in final stages of the disease, although there is additional difficulty in adapting a normal lung to a situs inversus patient.

References

1. Bousquet J, Van Cauwenberge P, Khaltaev N, Aria Workshop Group, World Health Organization (2001) Allergic rhinitis and its impact on asthma. J Allergy Clin Immunol 108:S147–S334
2. Lund VJ, Aaronson A, Bousquet J et al. (1994) International Consensus Report on the diagnosis and management of rhinitis. International Rhinitis Management Working Group. Allergy 19:5–34
3. Bachert C (2002) Persistent rhinitis—allergic or nonallergic? Allergy 59:11–15
4. Dykewicz MS, Fineman S (eds) (1998) Diagnosis and management of rhinitis: complete guidelines of the Joint Task Force on Practice Parameters in Allergy, Asthma and Immunology. Ann Allergy Asthma Immunol 81:478–518
5. Graf P, Hallen H, Juto JE (1995) The pathophysiology and treatment of rhinitis medicamentosa. Clin Otolaryngol 20:224–229

6. Raphael G, Raphael MH, Kaliner M (1989) Gustatory rhinitis: a syndrome of food-induced rhinorrhea. J Allergy Clin Immunol 83:110–115

7. Moore EJ, Kern EB (2001) Atrophic rhinitis: a review of 242 cases. Am J Rhinol 15:355–361

8. Moneret-Vautrin DA, Jankowski R, Bene MC, Kanny G, Hsieh V, Faure G, Wayoff M (1992) NARES: a model of inflammation caused by activated eosinophils? Rhinology 30:161–168

9. Webb DR, Meltzer EO, Finn AF, Richard KA, Pepsin PJ, Westlund R, Cook CK (2002) Intranasal fluticasone propionate is effective for perennial nonallergic rhinitis with or without eosinophilia. Ann Allergy Asthma Immunol 88:385–390

10. Purello-D'Ambrosio F, Isola S, Ricciardi L, Gangemi S, Barresi L, Bagnato GF (1999) A controlled study on the effectiveness of loratadine in combination with flunisolide in the treatment of nonallergic rhinitis with eosinophilia (NARES). Clin Exp Allergy 29:1143–1147

2.11 Allergic Rhinitis

JOAQUIM MULLOL AND ANTONIO VALERO

2.11.1 Introduction

Allergic rhinitis is a symptomatic disorder of the nose induced, after allergen exposure, by an immunoglobulin (Ig)E-mediated inflammation of the nasal mucosa. Allergic rhinitis is a global health problem, affecting at least 10–25% of the population [1], and an increase in is its prevalence has been observed in the past 40 years. In European countries, the prevalence of allergic rhinitis has been rated from 17 to 29% [2]. Allergic rhinitis is not a severe disease, but it alters a patient's social life, affecting school performance and work productivity, the costs incurred by rhinitis being substantial. Asthma and rhinitis are common comorbidities, suggesting a concept of "one airway, one disease".

Guidelines for the diagnosis and treatment of allergic rhinitis have already been published [3], but some were not founded on evidence-based medicine and few, if any, considered the patient globally in terms of comorbidities. The Allergic Rhinitis and Its Impact on Asthma (ARIA) Initiative [4] has developed a document that is the state-of-the-art for the specialist as well as for the general practitioner to:

- Update their knowledge of allergic rhinitis
- Highlight the impact of allergic rhinitis on asthma
- Provide an evidence-based documented revision on the diagnosis methods and on the treatments available
- Propose a stepwise approach to the management of the disease

2.11.2 Definition and Classification

Symptoms of allergic rhinitis include rhinorrhea, nasal obstruction, nasal itching and sneezing, which are reversible spontaneously or with treatment. Allergic rhinitis was previously classified as "seasonal" and "perennial".

The new ARIA classification of allergic rhinitis is based on symptoms and quality-of-life parameters. Duration of symptoms is subdivided into "intermittent" or "persistent" disease, while severity is subdivided into "mild" or "moderate-severe", depending on symptoms and quality

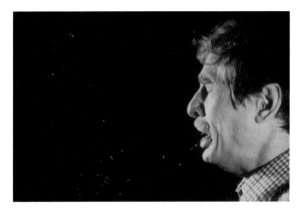

Fig. 2.11.1 Classification of allergic rhinitis (ARIA)

of life (Fig. 2.11.1). This classification has been recently validated [5].

2.11.3 Aetiology and Triggers

2.11.3.1 Allergens

Aeroallergens are very often involved in allergic rhinitis. The increase in domestic allergens is responsible in part for the increase in the prevalence of rhinitis, asthma and allergic respiratory diseases. In the home, the main allergens are mites, domestic animals, insects or plants. Outdoor allergens include pollens and moulds.

Occupational rhinitis is less well documented than occupational asthma is, but is often associated with asthma. Latex allergy, which can manifest with rhinitis-like symptoms, has become an increasing concern to patients and health professionals, who should be aware of the problem and develop strategies for prevention and treatment.

2.11.3.2 Pollutants

Pollutants are involved in the aggravation of nasal symptoms in patients with allergic and non-allergic rhinitis. The interaction between pollutants and rhinitis is suggested by epidemiological evidence, although the mechanism is not well understood. Indoor pollution, including domestic allergens and indoor aerosol pollutants (tobacco smoke), is of great importance, since in industrialised countries, subjects spend over 80% of their time indoors.

Urban-type pollution is in many countries primarily of automobile origin, and the principal atmospheric oxidant pollutants include ozone, nitric oxides and sulphur dioxide. Diesel exhaust fumes may also enhance IgE formation and allergic inflammation.

2.11.3.3   Aspirin and Non-Steroidal Anti-Inflammatory Drugs

Aspirin and non-steroidal anti-inflammatory drugs (NSAIDs) commonly induce rhinitis and asthma.

2.11.4   Mechanisms of Action

In allergic rhinitis, the understanding of the mechanisms of the disease provides a framework for its rational therapy, based on the complex inflammatory reaction rather than on the symptoms alone. Allergy is classically considered to result from an IgE-mediated allergy associated with nasal inflammation of variable intensity. Allergic rhinitis is characterised by an inflammatory infiltrate made up of different cells, including the following:

- Chemotaxis, activation, differentiation and survival prolongation of various cell types including eosinophils, T cells, mast cells and epithelial cells
- Release of mediators by these activated cells, with cytokines, chemokines, histamine and cysteinyl-leukotrienes as the major mediators
- Communication with the immune system and the bone marrow

Nonspecific nasal hyperreactivity is an important feature of allergic rhinitis, and it is defined as an increased nasal response to normal stimuli, resulting in sneezing, nasal congestion and/or secretion. Intermittent rhinitis can be mimicked by nasal challenge with pollen allergens, and an inflammatory reaction occurs during the late-phase reaction. In persistent allergic rhinitis, allergic triggers interact with an ongoing inflammatory reaction, and symptoms are due to this complex interaction.

The concept of "minimal persistent inflammation" [6] has been confirmed in perennial allergic rhinitis. In patients with persistent allergic rhinitis, allergen exposure varies throughout the year, and there are periods in which there is little exposure. Although symptom free, these patients still present with nasal inflammation.

2.11.5   Comorbidities

Allergic inflammation does not limit itself to the nasal airway. Multiple comorbidities have been associated with rhinitis such as asthma, rhinosinusitis and conjunctivitis.

2.11.5.1   Asthma

Nasal and bronchial mucosa share many similarities. Epidemiological studies have shown that asthma and rhinitis often coexist in the same patients. Most patients with allergic (80%) and non-allergic (50%) asthma have rhinitis, and many patients with rhinitis (20–30%) also have asthma. Allergic rhinitis constitutes a risk factor for asthma, and many allergic rhinitis patients have bronchial hyperreactivity.

Pathophysiological studies also suggest that a strong relationship exists between rhinitis and asthma. Although differences exist between rhinitis and asthma, upper and lower airways may be considered a unique entity influenced by a common inflammatory process. Since bronchial challenge leads to nasal inflammation and nasal challenge leads to bronchial inflammation, allergic diseases may be considered systemic. Thus, when considering a diagnosis of rhinitis or asthma, an evaluation of both the lower and upper airways should be made.

2.11.5.2   Other Comorbidities

Other comorbidities include rhinosinusitis and conjunctivitis, while the associations between allergic rhinitis, nasal polyposis and otitis media are poorly understood.

2.11.6   Diagnosis

The diagnosis of allergic rhinitis is based on the coordination between a clinical history (allergic symptoms), nasal examination and diagnostic tests.

2.11.6.1   Clinical History

Clinical history is essential for an accurate diagnosis of rhinitis, assessment of its severity and response to treatment. Although not necessarily of allergic origin, the main nasal symptoms are obstruction, sneezing, itching and rhinorrhea.

2.11.6.2 Nasal Examination

In patients with mild intermittent allergic rhinitis, a nasal examination is optimal, but all patients with persistent allergic rhinitis should have a nasal examination. Anterior rhinoscopy, using a speculum and mirror, reveals limited information. Nasal endoscopy, which can be performed only by specialists, is more useful.

2.11.6.3 Diagnostic Tests

In vivo and in vitro tests used to diagnose allergic diseases are directed towards the detection of free or cell-bound IgE. The diagnosis of "allergy" has been improved by allergen standardisation:

- Routine tests
  - History
    - Clinical
    - Family
  - General ENT examination (rhinoscopy)
  - Nasal airway assessment
    - Peak nasal inspiratory flow (PNIF)
  - Allergy tests
    - Skin tests
    - Serum-specific IgE
- Additional tests
  - Endoscopy
    - Rigid
    - Flexible
  - Radiology: CT scan
- Optional tests
  - Nasal challenge
    - Allergen
    - Lysine aspirin
  - Nasal samples
    - Cytology/nasal secretions
    - Nasal biopsy
    - Nasal swab
  - Radiology: MRI
  - Mucociliary function
    - Nasal mucociliary clearance (NMCC)
    - Ciliary beat frequency (CBF)
    - Electron microscopy
  - Nasal airway assessment
    - Rhinomanometry (anterior, posterior)
    - Acoustic rhinometry
  - Smell test (UPSIT, ZOST, BAST-24)
  - Nitric oxide measurement

2.11.6.3.1 Skin Prick Test

The skin prick test is widely used to demonstrate an IgE-mediated allergic reaction and is a major diagnostic tool in the field of allergy. If properly performed, it gives confirmatory evidence for the diagnosis of a specific allergy. Due to the complexity in performance and interpretation, it is should be carried out by trained health professionals.

2.11.6.3.2 Serum-Specific IgE
The serum-specific IgE test has value similar to that of skin tests.

2.11.6.3.3 Allergen Nasal Challenge
Allergen nasal challenges are mainly used in research and, to a lesser extent, in clinical practice. They are especially useful in the diagnosis of occupational rhinitis.

2.11.6.3.4 Imaging
Imaging is not usually necessary for diagnosis.

2.11.6.3.5 Diagnosis of Asthma
Guidelines for recognising and diagnosing asthma have been published by the Global Initiative for Asthma (GINA) and are recommended. Measurement of lung function and confirmation of the reversibility of airflow obstruction are essential steps in the diagnosis of asthma.

2.11.7 Management and Treatment

The management of allergic rhinitis is based on allergen avoidance, pharmacological treatment, specific immunotherapy and, when possible, the patient education [4, 7].

2.11.7.1 Allergen Avoidance

Most allergen avoidance studies have dealt with asthma symptoms, and very few have studied rhinitis symptoms. A single intervention may be insufficient to control symptoms of rhinitis or asthma. Although more data are needed to appreciate fully the clinical value of allergens, allergen avoidance (including house dust mites) should be an integral part of a management strategy.

2.11.7.2 Pharmacological Treatment

See Figs. 2.11.2 and 2.11.3.

	sneezing	rhinorrhea	nasal obstruction	nasal itch	eye symptoms
H₁-antihistamines					
oral	+++	+++	0 to +	+++	++
intranasal	++	+++	+	++	0
intraocular	0	0	0	0	+++
Corticosteroids					
intranasal	+++	+++	++	++	+
Chromones					
intranasal	+	+	+	+	0
intraocular	0	0	0	0	++
Decongestants					
intranasal	0	0	++	0	0
oral	0	0	+	0	0
Anti-cholinergics	0	++	0	0	0
Anti-leukotrienes	0	+	++	0	++

Fig. 2.11.2 Pharmacological management and drug effects on the symptoms of allergic rhinitis. 0 no effect, + mild, ++ moderate, +++ intense

intervention	SAR		PAR	
	adult	children	adult	children
oral anti-H₁	A	A	A	A
intranasal anti-H₁	A	A	A	A
intranasal CS	A	A	A	A
intranasal chromone	A	A	A	A
subcutaneous SIT	A	A	A	A
sublingual	A	A		
nasal SIT	A	A	A	
allergen avoidance	D	D	D	D

Fig. 2.11.3 Strength of evidence for the treatment of allergic rhinitis. Recommendations are evidence based on randomised controlled trials (*RCT*) carried out on studies performed with the previous classification of rhinitis: seasonal (*SAR*) and perennial (*PAR*) allergic rhinitis. Strength of recommendation: *A* based on RCT or meta-analysis, *D* based on the clinical experience of experts

2.11.7.2.1 H₁ Antihistamines

Drugs

- Old generation: chlorpheniramine, clemastine, diphenhydramine, hydroxyzine, ketotifen, mequitazine, oxatomide
- New generation: acrivastine, azelastine, cetirizine, desloratadine, ebastine, fexofenadine, levocetirizine, loratadine, mizolastine, rupatadine
- Cardiotoxic drugs: astemizole, terfenadine

Mechanism of Action

The mechanism of action of this drug class is blockage of H₁ receptors, and some anti-allergic activity. New-gener-

ation drugs can be used once daily. There should be no development of tachyphylaxis with this drug class.

Side Effects

- Old generation
  - Sedation and/or anticholinergic effect is common.
- New generation
  - There is no sedating effect with most drugs, no anticholinergic effect and no cardiotoxicity.
  - Acrivastine has sedative effects.
  - Mequitazine has anticholinergic effects.
  - Oral azelastine may induce sedation and has a bitter taste.

Comments

New-generation oral H₁-antihistamines should be preferred due to their favourable efficacy/safety ratio and pharmacokinetics. They are rapidly effective (less than 1 h) against nasal and ocular symptoms, but poorly effective against nasal congestion. Cardiotoxic drugs should be avoided [7, 8].

Local Antihistamines

Azelastine and levocabastine are two local antihistamines. They are quickly effective (less than 30 min) against nasal or ocular symptoms. They can produce minor local side effects; azelastine has bitter taste.

2.11.7.2.2 Corticosteroids

Drugs

- Intranasal: beclomethasone, budesonide, flunisolide, fluticasone, momethasone, triamcinolone

- Oral/IM: dexamethasone, hydrocortisone, methyl-prednisolone, prednisolone, prednisone, triamcinolone, betamethasone, deflazacort

Mechanism of Action
Corticosteroids potently reduce nasal inflammation and nasal hyperreactivity.

Side Effects
- Intranasal
  - There are minor local side effects, a wide margin for systemic side effects and there are growth concerns with some molecules only.
  - In young children, consider the combination of intranasal and inhaled drugs.
- Oral
  - Systemic side effects are common in particular for IM drugs.
  - Depot injections may cause local tissue atrophy.

Comments
- Intranasal
  - Corticosteroids are the most effective pharmacological treatment for allergic rhinitis.
  - They are effective against nasal congestion and loss of smell.
  - Effects are observed after 12 h, but maximal effect is usually seen after a few days.
- Oral
  - When possible, intranasal corticosteroids should replace oral or IM drugs.
  - A short course of oral corticosteroids may be needed with severe symptoms [7].

2.11.7.2.3 Chromones (Intranasal, Ocular)
These drugs include cromoglycate and nedocromil, the side effects of which are minor. Their mechanisms of action are not well known.

Intraocular chromones are very effective. Intranasal chromones are less effective, and their effect is short lasting. Overall, they offer excellent safety for therapy.

2.11.7.2.4 Nasal Decongestants

Drugs
- Oral: ephedrine, phenylephrine, phenylpropanolamine, pseudoephedrine
- Intranasal: oxymethazoline, naphazoline, xylometazoline and others

Mechanism of Action
Nasal decongestants are sympathomimetic drugs, which relieve symptoms of nasal congestion.

Side Effects
- Oral: hypertension, palpitations, restlessness, agitation, tremor, insomnia, headache, dry mucous membranes, urinary retention, exacerbation of glaucoma or thyrotoxicosis
- Intranasal: same side effects as oral decongestants but less intense
- Rhinitis medicamentosa is a rebound phenomenon occurring with prolonged use (more than 10 days).

Comments
- Oral
  - Use oral decongestants with caution in patients with heart disease.
  - Oral H_1-antihistamine combined with a decongestant may be more effective than is either product alone, but side effects will also be combined.
- Intranasal
  - This form acts more rapidly and more effectively than do oral decongestants.
  - Limit duration of treatment to less than 10 days to avoid rhinitis medicamentosa.

2.11.7.2.5 Anticholinergics
This class of drugs includes ipratropium. Anticholinergic drugs almost exclusively block rhinorrhea. The side effects of anticholinergics are minor and local, as there is virtually no systemic anticholinergic activity. This drug class is effective in allergic and non-allergic patients with rhinorrhea.

2.11.7.2.6 Leukotriene Receptor Antagonists
The drugs in this class include montelukast, pranlukast and zafirlukast, which block cysteinyl leukotriene type (cysLT) receptors. There are few side effects, and patients demonstrate excellent tolerance with these drugs.

Nasal decongestants are promising drugs used alone or in combination with oral H_1-antihistamines, but more data are needed to pinpoint the effectiveness these drugs.

2.11.7.3 Specific Immunotherapy

Specific immunotherapy is effective when optimally administered. Standardised therapeutic vaccines are favoured when available. Subcutaneous immunotherapy raises contrasting efficacy and safety issues [9]. The use of optimal doses of vaccines labelled either in biological units or in masses of the major allergen has been proposed. Doses of 5–20 μg of the major allergen are optimal doses for most allergen vaccines.

2.11.7.3.1 Subcutaneous Immunotherapy

Subcutaneous immunotherapy (SIT) alters the natural course of allergic diseases. SIT should be performed by trained personnel, and patients should be monitored for 30 min after injection. SIT is indicated in patients:

- Whose symptoms are insufficiently controlled by conventional pharmacotherapy
- In whom oral H_1-antihistamines and intranasal pharmacotherapy insufficiently control symptoms
- Who do not wish to be on pharmacotherapy
- In whom pharmacotherapy produces undesirable side effects
- Who do not want to receive long-term pharmacological treatment

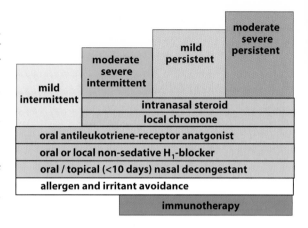

Fig. 2.11.4 Treatment of allergic rhinitis (ARIA)

2.11.7.3.2 Nasal and Sublingual-Swallow Specific Immunotherapy

Nasal and sublingual-swallow specific immunotherapy may be used with doses at least 20–100 times greater than those doses used for SIT, or in patients who had side effects or refused SIT. The indications follow those of subcutaneous injections.

2.11.7.3.3 SIT in Children

Specific immunotherapy is effective. It is not recommended to begin this treatment until the child is older than 5 years of age.

2.11.7.3.4 Education

When possible, patient education is always recommended.

2.11.7.3.5 Surgery

Surgical intervention may be used as an adjunctive intervention in a few and selected patients (e. g. in cases of turbinate hypertrophy or septal deviation).

2.11.7.4 Selection of Medications

Medications have no long-lasting effect when stopped. Therefore, in chronic disease, maintenance treatment is required (Fig. 2.11.4).

- Tachyphylaxis does not usually occur with prolonged treatment.
- Medications used for rhinitis are most commonly administered intranasally or orally.
- Some studies have compared the relative efficacy of these medications, of which intranasal corticosteroids are the most effective. However, the choice of treatment also depends on many other criteria.

- The use of alternative care (e. g. homeopathy, herbalism, acupuncture) for the treatment of rhinitis is increasing. Scientific and clinical support is lacking for these therapies. There is an urgent need for large, randomised and controlled clinical trials for alternative therapies of allergic diseases and rhinitis.
- IM injection of glucocorticosteroids is not usually recommended due to the possible occurrence of systemic side effects.
- Intranasal injection of glucocorticosteroids is not usually recommended due to the possible occurrence of severe side effects.

2.11.7.5 Treatment of Concomitant Rhinitis and Asthma

Treatment of asthma should follow the GINA guidelines. Some drugs are effective in the treatment of both rhinitis and asthma (e. g. glucocorticoids, antileukotrienes), while others are only effective in the treatment of either rhinitis or asthma (e. g. α- or β-adrenergic agonists, respectively). Some drugs are more effective in rhinitis than in asthma (e. g. H_1-antihistamines). Although more studies are needed, optimal management of rhinitis may improve coexisting asthma [10]. Drugs administered by the oral route may affect both nasal and bronchial symptoms. The safety of intranasal glucocorticoids is well established. Large doses of inhaled (intrabronchial) glucocorticoids can induce side effects. One of the problems of dual administration may be the possible additive side effects. Although the addition of intranasal formulations to inhaled formulations does not produce any further significant suppression, more data are needed. It has been proposed that the prevention or early treatment of allergic rhinitis may help to prevent the occurrence of asthma or the severity of bronchial symptoms, but again, more data are needed.

2.11.7.6 Treatment of Conjunctivitis

The options of treatment for conjunctivitis are oral and/or ocular H_1-antihistamines, ocular chromones and saline. Administration of ocular corticosteroids is not recommended.

2.11.8 Special Considerations

2.11.8.1 Pregnancy

Rhinitis is often a problem during pregnancy, since nasal obstruction may be aggravated by pregnancy itself. Caution must be taken when administering any medication during pregnancy, as most medications can cross the placenta. For most drugs, limited studies have been done, and only on small groups, with no long-term analysis.

2.11.8.2 Paediatric Aspects

- Allergic rhinitis is part of the "allergic march" during childhood, but intermittent allergic rhinitis is unusual before 2 years of age. Allergic rhinitis is most prevalent during the school-age years.
- Allergy tests can be done at any age, and they may yield important information. The principles of treatment for children are the same as for adults. Special care has to be taken to avoid the side effects typical in this age group.
- Doses of medication must be adjusted and follow special considerations. Few medications have been tested in children under the age of 2 years.
- In children, symptoms of allergic rhinitis can impair cognitive functioning and school performance, which can be further impaired by the use of (old generation) sedating oral H_1-antihistamines.
- Intranasal glucocorticosteroids are an effective treatment for allergic rhinoconjunctivitis. Their possible effect on growth for some (but not all) intranasal glucocorticoids is of concern. Recommended doses of intranasal momethasone and fluticasone have shown not to affect growth in children with allergic rhinoconjunctivitis.
- Oral and IM glucocorticosteroids should be avoided in the treatment of rhinitis in young children.
- Disodium cromoglycate is commonly used to treat allergic rhinoconjunctivitis in children because of the safety of the drug.

2.11.8.3 Ageing

With ageing, various physiological changes occur in the connective tissue and vasculature of the nose, which may predispose or contribute to chronic rhinitis. Allergy is a less common cause of persistent rhinitis in subjects older than 65 years of age. Atrophic rhinitis is common and difficult to control. Rhinorrhea can be controlled with anticholinergics. Some drugs (reserpine, guanethidine, phentolamine, methyldopa, prazosin, chlorpromazine or angiotensin-converting enzyme [ACE] inhibitors) can cause rhinitis. Some drugs may induce specific side effects in elderly patients. Decongestants and drugs with anticholinergic activity may cause urinary retention in patients with prostatic hypertrophy. Sedative drugs can have even greater side effects.

2.11.9 Key Recommendations [4]

- Allergic rhinitis is a major chronic respiratory disease due to its prevalence, impact on quality of life, impact on work/school performance and productivity, economic burden and links with asthma, rhinosinusitis and conjunctivitis.
- Allergic rhinitis is a risk factor for asthma.
- A new classification of allergic rhinitis has been proposed: "intermittent" and "persistent".
- The severity of allergic rhinitis has been classified as "mild" and "moderate-severe", depending on symptom severity and quality-of-life outcomes.
- Depending on the subdivision and severity of allergic rhinitis, a stepwise therapeutic approach has been proposed.
- The treatment of allergic rhinitis combines allergen avoidance (when possible), pharmacotherapy and immunotherapy.
- Patients with persistent allergic rhinitis should be evaluated for asthma by history, chest examination and assessment of lung function (before and after bronchodilator).
- Environmental and social factors should be optimised to allow the patient to lead a normal life.
- Asthmatic patients should be evaluated (history and physical examination) for rhinitis.
- In terms of efficacy and safety, a combined strategy should be used to treat upper and lower airway diseases.
- In developing countries, a specific strategy may be needed depending on the availability and affordability of interventions.

References

1. Strachan D, Sibbald B, Weiland S, Ait-Khaled N, Anabwani G, Anderson HR, Asher MI et al. (1997) Worldwide variations in prevalence of symptoms of allergic rhinoconjunctivitis in children: the International Study of Asthma and Allergies in Childhood (ISAAC). Pediatr Allergy Immunol 8:161–176
2. Bauchau V, Durham SR (2004) Prevalence and rate of diagnosis of allergic rhinitis in Europe. Eur Respir J 24:758–764
3. Cauwenberge P van, Bachert C, Passalacqua G, Bousquet J, Canonica GW, Durham SR, Fokkens WJ Et al. (2000) Consensus statement on the treatment of allergic rhinitis. European Academy of Allergology and Clinical Immunology. Allergy 55:116–134
4. Bousquet J, van Cauwenberge P, Khaltaev N, ARIA Workshop Group (2001) Allergic rhinitis and its impact on asthma. ARIA Workshop report. J Allergy Clin Immunol 108:S147–S334
5. Bauchau V, Durham SR (2005) Epidemiological characterization of the intermittent and persistent types of allergic rhinitis. Allergy 60:350–353
6. Ciprandi G, Buscaglia S, Pesce G, Pronzato C, Ricca V, Parmiani S, Bagnasco M Et al. (1995) Minimal persistent inflammation is present at mucosal level in patients with asymptomatic rhinitis and mite allergy. J Allergy Clin Immunol 96:971–979
7. Bousquet J, Van Cauwenberge P, Bachert C, Canonica GW, Demoly P, Durham SR, Fokkens WJ Et al. (2003) Requirements for medications commonly used in the treatment of allergic rhinitis. Allergy 58:192–197
8. Simons FE (2004) Advances in H_1-antihistamines. N Engl J Med 351:2203–2217
9. Bousquet J, Lockey R, Malling H (1998) WHO position paper. Allergen immunotherapy: therapeutic vaccines for allergic diseases. J Allergy Clin Immunol 102:558–562
10. Taramarcaz P, Gibson PG (2004) The effectiveness of intranasal corticosteroids in combined allergic rhinitis and asthma syndrome. Clin Exp Allergy 34:1883–1889

2.12 Acute Sinusitis

JEAN MICHEL KLOSSEK, XAVIER DUFOUR AND ELIE SERRANO

2.12.1 Introduction

Sinusitis is (also known as acute bacterial sinusitis [ABS] or acute bacterial rhinosinusitis [ABRS] is an infection and inflammation of at least one of the four paranasal sinuses (frontal, maxillary, ethmoid, or sphenoid). A more global definition would be "Rhinosinusitis is a group of disorders characterised by inflammation of the mucosa of the nose and paranasal sinuses". With acute sinusitis, inflammation is predominantly caused by viral or bacterial microorganisms. Maxillary acute sinusitis is the major localisation addressed in general practice (GP) and studied in the medical literature [1–4]. Only maxillary rhinosinusitis is described below; other forms of sinusitis (description and management) are covered in other sections of this textbook.

2.12.2 Aetiology/Epidemiology

Acute bacterial sinusitis is commonly encountered in clinical practice, affecting between 10 and 15% of the population of central Europe annually [5]. Since adults and children contract an average of two to three, and three to eight viral respiratory tract infections (RTIs) per year, respectively, the number of cases that can progress to ABRS is rather large, although the proportion of viral RTIs that actually progress to ABRS is relatively small (~2%).

Several factors have been suggested to be associated with increased risk of ABRS, including suppression of the immune system, the presence of asthma, allergy, or cystic fibrosis, secondary or environmental smoke exposure, and nasal use of cocaine.

The main causative agents of ABRS are *Streptococcus pneumoniae* and *Haemophilus influenzae*, while *Branhamella catarrhalis*, *Staphylococcus pyogenes*, *Staphylococcus aureus*, and various anaerobes are less frequent pathogens [6, 7]. Complications are rare but can be severe, including intracranial complications, such as meningitis, and orbital complications, such as orbital and preseptal cellulitis or orbital abscess [8].

2.12.3 Symptoms

An accurate and timely diagnosis of ABRS is crucial for an appropriate choice of therapy. Making an unambiguous diagnosis of ABRS is very difficult, especially in maxillary locations and in the primary care setting for at least two reasons: (1) ABRS signs and symptoms (Table 2.12.1) are not specific to bacterial sinusitis and are difficult to differentiate from viral RTIs or other noninfectious causes, and (2) the lack of reliable, convenient, and practical diagnostic tools [2].

In both viral and bacterial infections, symptoms may include nasal congestion, nasal drainage, postnasal drainage, facial pressure/pain, fever, cough, fatigue, maxillary dental pain and ear pressure/fullness. Symptom persisting for over 7 days may be a sign of a bacterial infection. Change in the colour of the nasal discharge, which has been proposed as a potentially useful indicator of ABRS, has not been definitively demonstrated to be a sign of bacterial infection.

2.12.4 Diagnostic Procedures

2.12.4.1 Recommended European Standard

The gold standard for diagnosis of bacterial sinusitis is sinus puncture with aspiration of purulent secretions, but this invasive procedure is seldom performed in primary care [9].

No European guidelines are available for diagnostic procedure; however, for some countries (France, Germany and Spain), national recommendations have been published [2, 3, 10, 11] (Table 2.12.2).

2.12.4.2 Additional/Useful Diagnostic Procedures

- Samples under endoscopic guidance
  - Endoscopic guidance evaluation is ongoing [9], and the technique seems to be a good alternative to sinus puncture even in acute situation.

Table 2.12.1 Symptoms of ABRS and diagnostic guidelines

Country	Diagnosis guidelines

France	Presence of at least 2 of the major factors for >3 days
	• Major factors
	  – Infraorbital sinus pain (despite symptomatic treatment)
	  – Unilateral, pulsating pain (increasing with bowing of the head)
	  – Increase of rhinorrhea and its purulence
	• Minor factors
	  – Fever after the third day
	  – Nasal congestion
	  – Sneezing
	  – Cough

Germany
(Consensus ENT Group)
	Symptoms >4 days and/or severe symptoms
	At least 2 major factors, and 1 minor factor; or 1 major factor and 2 minor factors
	• Major factors
	  – Headache
	  – Sensation of sinus pressure
	  – Obstruction of nasal respiration
	  – Purulent nasal secretion
	  – Impaired sense of smell
	• Minor factors
	  – Cough
	  – Generally not feeling well
	  – Toothache
	  – Irritability
	  – Offensive breath
	  – Earache

Spain	ABRS symptoms usually manifest after the 5th day and persist for ≥10 days • Purulent rhinorrhea • Nasal congestion • Facial pain (especially if unilateral or localised above a sinus) • Postnasal discharge • Hyposmia • Fever • Cough • Fatigue • Maxillary dental pain

- Imaging of the sinuses
  - Standard radiography, CT, MRI or US can reinforce the suspicion of the diagnosis, but have limited value in the routine diagnosis of acute bacterial sinusitis uncomplicated. The main limitation of radiography is the lack of specificity, as this method cannot readily distinguish between an infection and other sinus-related anomalies, such as mucosal thickening, tumours and polyps.
  - Ultrasonography is widely used in northern Europe and The Netherlands, but less so in southern Europe.
  - CT allows for good visualisation of paranasal sinuses and provides high-resolution view of the ostiomeatal anatomy. Although CT can detect a variety of sinus abnormalities, it lacks sufficient specificity, such that viral upper RTIs may produce CT changes identical to those of ABRS. For transillumination, the clinical utility of this method is controversial.

2.12.5 Differential Diagnosis

Difficulties remain in differentiating bacterial rhinosinusitis from viral RTIs or other noninfectious causes, due to

Table 2.12.2 Diagnostic procedures: recommended European standard

Country	Procedure				
	Sinus puncture	Imaging studies	Endoscopy	Physical examination	Nasal swabs
France	No recommendation	X-ray, only in cases of doubt or of treatment failure	No recommendation	No recommendation	No recommendation
Germany	No recommendation	Useful in some cases	Mandatory	Palpation of cheeks and maxillary sinus wall, pain provocation test (fast bowing of the head), and ENT status	Useful in some cases
Spain	No recommendation	CT, only in chronic sinusitis or suspicion of complication	Mostly not necessary	No recommendation	No recommendation

Table 2.12.3 Bacteriology of acute sinusitis in different countries

Country (reference)	Sample collection method	Isolates (n)	Occurrence (%)					
			S. pneumoniae	H. influenzae	M. catarrhalis	S. aureus	S. pyogenes	Other
Europe [7]	Aspirate from punctured sinus	569	20	13	4	12	2	
Finland [7]	Aspirate from punctured sinus	284	13 9–11 14–26	30 43–48 9–11	11 11–14 9–11	4 0–7 2–5	1 0–1 0–1	
Sweden [25]	Aspirate from punctured sinus	200	57 6	24 60	4 2	4 6		7 19

the lack of reliable, convenient, and practical diagnostic tools [4].

2.12.6 Microbiology

Interestingly, there is considerable variation in rates of antibacterial resistance between different countries [6, 7, 12, 13] (Table 2.12.3). For example, in Italy the resistance of *S. pneumoniae* to penicillin is low, but macrolide resistance is high, whereas France has particularly high levels of resistance to both these antibacterial classes. In a comparison between Finland and the rest of Europe (Germany, Belgium, Switzerland, Spain and Austria), *H. influenzae* appeared to be the most frequent cause of bacterial sinusitis in Finland whereas in the rest of Europe *S. pneumoniae* was the most prevalent organism.

The prevalence of antibacterial resistance among the common bacterial pathogens in acute maxillary sinusitis

(AMS)—penicillin, macrolide, and multidrug resistance in *S. pneumoniae,* as well as β-lactamase production in *H. influenzae* and *M. catarrhalis*—is increasing worldwide. The incidence of co-resistance between macrolides and β-lactams is also increasing universally [14]. Bacteria found to be resistant to macrolides are also more likely to be resistant to β-lactams, with the level of co-resistance between the macrolides and the β-lactams currently estimated to be in the order of 50–70%. There have also been reports of penicillin-resistant isolates of *S. pneumoniae* with reduced susceptibility to fluoroquinolones [3].

2.12.7 Complications

ABRS must be managed with care to prevent subsequent complications such as orbital cellulitis, orbital abscess meningitis, brain abscess and subdural-epidural abscess. Maxillary, sphenoid and frontal locations are more common associated with complications than maxillary rhinosinusitis [8].

2.12.8 Therapy

2.12.8.1 Medical Treatment

2.12.8.1.1 Choice of Treatment
Many countries have their own official or unofficial guidelines for the treatment of AMS [10, 11, 15–17] (Table 2.12.4).

Comprehensive treatment of ABRS aims to restore the integrity and function of the ostiomeatal complex by reducing inflammation and restoring sinus drainage, while simultaneously eradicating the bacterial cause of infection and preventing complications. The majority of patients with AMS are treated in the community by primary care physicians [4, 17]. As viruses make a significant contribution to the aetiology of sinusitis and most cases resolve spontaneously, "watchful waiting" combined with symptomatic therapy is the usual initial management strategy.

2.12.8.1.2 Recommended European Standard
Choice of first-line antibacterial therapy is generally considered central in achieving bacterial eradication and clinical success. However, specific treatment recommendations concerning choice of antibacterial agent vary between countries, presumably due to different regulations, aetiology and antibacterial resistance patterns in different countries [2, 18, 19].

- First-line antibacterials
  - Recommended first-line antibacterials are broadly similar across treatment guidelines. An overview of the strengths and limitations of the different classes of antibacterial agents recommended for first-line use in patients with AMS is given in Table 2.12.4 [2, 10, 15–17, 20].
  - Several guidelines include amoxicillin as a first-line treatment option (Belgium, Germany, Finland, Spain, The Netherlands and the United Kingdom), as it is active against the major causative pathogens of AMS and low in cost. However, in France, amoxicillin alone cannot be recommended, with its high prevalence of β-lactam resistance among the most common causative pathogens.
  - Recommendations for alternative first line-treatment options in patients with penicillin allergy vary between countries. Trimethoprim or trimethoprim–sulfamethoxazole is sometimes recommended (United Kingdom, Belgium and The Netherlands). However, trimethoprim–sulfamethoxazole is also associated with high levels of resistance, particularly among *H. influenzae* and *M. catarrhalis*. French guidelines recommend treatment with telithromycin in patients with penicillin allergy, with an additional option of pristinamycin.
  - It therefore appears widely accepted that use of cephalosporins for the treatment of AMS should be limited as far as possible, to minimise the potential for selection of resistance.
- Second-line antibacterials
  - All guidelines recommend treatment with an alternative antibacterial agent in patients who fail to respond to the initial course of therapy. Indeed, US guidelines advocate changing therapy if symptoms have not improved or if they worsen after 3 days of treatment with a recommended first-line regimen.
  - Recommended second-line antibacterials also vary strongly between countries, including second-generation cephalosporins, macrolides, and fluoroquinolones with anti-pneumococcal activity (Table 2.12.4).
  - Telithromycin is recommended as a second-line option in Germany and Spain [21].

Useful Additional Therapeutic Strategies
Analgesics, antipyretics, decongestants, nasal irrigation, steam inhalation and warm packs are generally recommended for symptom relief of AMS. However, some guidelines, including those from the UK-based National Institute for Clinical Excellence, advise against the long-term use of intranasal or oral decongestants. Recently, some countries have considered the use of topical steroids for acute rhinosinusitis in case of moderate symptoms. Additional studies are conducted to confirm such a decision [2].

Table 2.12.4 Summary of treatment guidelines for acute sinusitis

Country	First-line treatment	Second-line treatment	Comments
France	Amoxicillin–clavulanate, 2nd-/3rd-generation cephalosporins (cefuroxime axetil, cefpodoxime proxetil, cefotiam hexetil, but not cefixime) Pristinamycin, telithromycin (especially in patients allergic to penicillin) First-line use of anti-pneumococcal fluoroquinolones (levofloxacin, moxifloxacin) should be restricted to patients at high risk of severe complications	Anti-pneumococcal fluoroquinolones (levofloxacin, moxifloxacin) after bacteriologic and/or radiologic confirmation	Antibacterial treatment recommended if fever persists for 3 days Treatment duration validated: – Amoxicillin–clavulanate 10 days – Cefuroxime axetil, 5 days – Cefpodoxime proxetil, 5 days – Cefotiam hexetil, 5 days – Pristinamycin, 4 days – Telithromycin, 5 days
Spain	Fluoroquinolones (moxifloxacin or levofloxacin) for moderate disease with comorbidity 3rd-generation cephalosporins (intravenous) for severe or complicated disease	Amoxicillin–clavulanate or telithromycin for moderate disease with comorbidity Amoxicillin–clavulanate (intravenous) for severe or complicated disease	
Germany (1)	Aminopenicillin ± β-lactam (e.g. amoxicillin or amoxicillin–clavulanate) 2nd-/3rd-generation cephalosporins	Macrolide Ketolide (telithromycin) 3rd-/4th-generation fluoroquinolone (levofloxacin, gatifloxacin, moxifloxacin)	Macrolides second line because of increasing resistance Ketolides second line because all newer agents are used as such in Germany Treatment for 5 days
Germany (2)	Amoxicillin	Ketolide (telithromycin) If complications: amoxicillin–clavulanate 2nd-generation cephalosporins Macrolides Trimethoprim–sulfamethoxazole Clindamycin Doxycycline	Indicated if symptoms are worsening (fever, pain, purulent rhinorrhea over days) Ketolides second line because all newer agents are used as such in Germany Treatment for 8–10 days
United Kingdom	Amoxicillin Erythromycin, oxytetracycline (adults) Doxycycline (adults) or trimethoprim (children) if penicillin allergic	Amoxicillin, ciprofloxacin	Treatment for 7 days
The Netherlands	Severe or chronic: amoxicillin Trimethoprim if penicillin allergic	Doxycycline Erythromycin	Working Party on Antibiotic Policy (SWAB) and ENT and GP associations do not have specific guidelines for AMS Antibacterials not recommended for acute sinusitis (only if severe or chronic)

Table 2.12.4 *(continued)* Summary of treatment guidelines for acute sinusitis

Country	First-line treatment	Second-line treatment	Comments
Belgium	Amoxicillin Trimethoprim–sulfamethoxazole (adults) and trimethoprim (children) if penicillin allergic	Cephalosporin (cefuroxime axetil) Amoxicillin–clavulanate Tetracyclines Macrolides	First-line treatment for 5–7 days Second-line treatment for 10 days Fluoroquinolones never recommended for upper RTI
Finland	Amoxicillin	Doxycycline (adults) Amoxicillin-clavulanate (adults and children) 2nd-generation cephalosporins and macrolides	In case of treatment failure, choice of second-line therapy should be guided by causative pathogen determined by culture of sinus aspirate Fluoroquinolones to be reserved for infections caused by multidrug resistant pneumococci

2.12.8.2 Surgical Treatment

Antral puncture has become rare since the inception of antibiotics. Samples are recommended specifically to identify the bacterial agent in cases of immunodeficiency, for example.

Surgery (functional endoscopic sinus surgery) may be discussed in cases of recurrent sinusitis after specific investigation (nasal endoscopy, CT).

2.12.9 Prognosis

- Correct high-dose antibiotic therapy over a validated period heals the disease in most cases [2, 18, 22, 23]. In some cases, there may be loss of high-tone sensorineural hearing.
- In cases of recurrence, further investigations are required to eliminate dental infections or local factors (ostiomeatal dysfunction).

2.12.10 Special Remarks

Emerging resistance to antibiotics lead many countries to elaborate guidelines to reduce overuse of antibiotics. European recommendations are not yet available due to the large difference of resistance between countries; nevertheless, an appropriate use of antibiotics in ABRS would be helpful to reduce this increase of bacterial resistance [20, 24].

References

1. Benninger M (2007) Guidelines on the treatment of ABRS in adults. Int J Clin Pract 61:873–876
2. Fokkens W, Lund V, Mullol J (2007) European position paper on rhinosinusitis and nasal polyps 2007. Rhinology 20:S1–S136
3. Klossek J M, Chidiac C et al. (2005) Current position of the management of community-acquired acute maxillary sinusitis or rhinosinusitis in France and literature review. Rhinology 19:S4–S33
4. Thomas M, Yawn BP, Price D, Lund V, Mullol J, Fokkens W (2008) EPOS Primary Care Guidelines: European position paper on the primary care diagnosis and management of rhinosinusitis and nasal polyps 2007—a summary. Prim Care Respir J 17:79–89
5. Grevers G, Klemens A (2002) [Rhinosinusitis. Current diagnostic and therapeutic aspects.] MMW Fortschr Med 144:31–35 (In German)
6. Felmingham D (2004) Comparative antimicrobial susceptibility of respiratory tract pathogens. Chemotherapy 501:3–10
7. Pentillä M, Savolainen S, Kiukaanniemi H, Forsblom B, Jousimies-Somer H (1997) Bacterial findings in acute maxillary sinusitis—European study. Acta Otolaryngol 529:165–168
8. Stoll D, Klossek JM, Barbaza MO (2006) Prospective study of 43 severe complications of acute rhinosinusitis. Rev Laryngol Otol Rhinol (Bord) 127:195–201
9. Benninger MS, Payne SC, Ferguson BJ, Hadley JA, Ahmad N (2006) Endoscopically directed middle meatal cultures versus maxillary sinus taps in acute bacterial maxillary rhinosinusitis: a meta-analysis. Otolaryngol Head Neck Surg 134:3–9

10. Bachert C, Bertrand B, Daele J, Jorissen M, Lefebvre R, Rombaux P et al. (2007) Belgian guidelines for the treatment of acute rhinosinusitis in general practice. B-ENT 3:175–177

11. Blomgren K, Alho OP et al. (2005) Acute sinusitis: Finnish clinical practice guidelines. Scand J Infect Dis 37:245–50

12. Baquero F (1999) Evolving resistance patterns of *Streptococcus pneumoniae*: a link with long-acting macrolide consumption? J Chemother 11:35–43

13. Schito GC, Felmingham D (2005) Susceptibility of Streptococcus pneumoniae to penicillin, azithromycin and telithromycin (PROTEKT 1999–2003). Int J Antimicrob Agents 26:479–485

14. Hoban D, Baquero F, Reed V, Felmingham D (2005) Demographic analysis of antimicrobial resistance among *Streptococcus pneumoniae*: worldwide results from PROTEKT 1999–2000. Int J Infect Dis 9:262–273

15. PRODIGY Guidance. Sinusitis (updated 2002). Available via http://www.prodigy.nhs.uk/home

16. Agence Française de Sécurité Sanitaire des Produits de Santé. Mise au point sur l'antibiothérapie par voie générale en pratique courante (2005). Available via http://agmed.sante.gouv.fr/htm/5/rbp/indrbp.htm (In French)

17. Sociedad Española de Quimioterapia y Sociedad Española de Otorrinolaringología y Patología Cérvico-Facial. Diagnóstico y tratamiento antimicrobiano de las sinusitis. Res Esp Quimioter 16:239–251 (In Spanish)

18. Young J, De Sutter A, Merenstein D, van Essen GA, Kaiser L, Varonen H et al. (2008) Antibiotics for adults with clinically diagnosed acute rhinosinusitis: a meta-analysis of individual patient data. Lancet. 371:908–914

19. Merenstein D, Whittaker C et al. (2005) Are antibiotics beneficial for patients with sinusitis complaints? A randomized double-blind clinical trial. J Fam Pract 54:144–151

20. Williams JW Jr, Aguilar C, Cornell J et al. (2003) Antibiotics for acute maxillary sinusitis. Cochrane Database Syst Rev 2:CD000243

21. Klossek JM, Federspil P (2005) Update on treatment guidelines for acute bacterial sinusitis. Int J Clin Pract 59:230–238

22. Linder JA, Singer DE, Ancker M, Atlas SJ (2003) Measures of health-related quality of life for adults with acute sinusitis. A systematic review. J Gen Intern Med 18:390–401

23. Rosenfeld RM, Singer M, Jones S (2007) Systematic review of antimicrobial therapy in patients with acute rhinosinusitis. Otolaryngol Head Neck Surg 137:S32–S45

24. Molstad S, Erntell M, Hanberger H, Melander E, Norman C, Skoog G et al. (2008) Sustained reduction of antibiotic use and low bacterial resistance: 10-year follow-up of the Swedish Strama programme. Lancet Infect Dis 8:125–132

25. Berg O, Carenfelt C (1988) Analysis of symptoms and clinical signs in the maxillary sinus empyema. Acta Otolaryngol. 105:343–349

2.13 Chronic Rhinosinusitis: Definition, Diagnostics and Physiopathology

J.R. MONTSERRAT, J.M. GUILEMANY, AND J.R. GRAS

2.13.1 Introduction

Until recently rhinosinusitis was usually classified (based on duration) into acute and chronic; the present chapter discusses only adult chronic rhinosinusitis.

To define chronic rhinosinusitis is not easy; data are limited and this entity's definition garners much controversy. Rhinitis and sinusitis usually coexist; thus, the correct term is *rhinosinusitis*. Rhinosinusitis is defined as "…inflammation in the sinuses mucosa associated with inflammation in the nasal mucosa, and often associated with inflammatory changes of the adjacent bony structures" [1].

Although chronic rhinosinusitis has a higher prevalence and morbidity, few epidemiologic studies exist due to the heterogeneity of disease and poor homogeneity in criterion and diagnostic methods. Chronic rhinosinusitis affects to 15–16% of adult population [2].

The factor associated with this aetiology is ciliary impairment, which is divided into primary dyskinesia and secondary dyskinesia. Secondary ciliary dyskinesia is found in patients with chronic rhinosinusitis due to sinonasal epithelium aggression, and is usually reversible with the correction of the sinonasal inflammation and infection. It is clear that in patients with primary ciliary dyskinesia, like Kartagener's syndrome, ciliary impairment is the factor implicated in chronic rhinosinusitis. In cystic fibrosis, the inability of cilia to transport the viscous mucus causes ciliary malfunction and consequently, accumulation and infection in the sinus.

Atopy has been suggested to predispose one to chronic rhinosinusitis. Epidemiologic data reveal an increase of allergic rhinitis in patients with chronic rhinosinusitis [3].

Recent evidence suggests that the lower airway is usually involved in patients with chronic rhinosinusitis, but the interrelationship is poorly understood. Many studies suggest that treatment of the upper airway improves the lower airway, mainly in patients with nasal polyposis and asthma.

Dysfunction of the immune system may cause many pathologies, including chronic rhinosinusitis.

Anatomical variations, such as concha bullosa and nasal septal deviation to the middle meatus, have been suggested as potential risk factors for developing chronic rhinosinusitis. No correlation has been found between chronic rhinosinusitis and anatomic variations.

Currently, there is increasing interest in the concept that chronic rhinosinusitis is induced by fungus that colonise the normal sinus, forming saprophytic crusts. Most of patients with chronic rhinosinusitis exhibit eosinophilic infiltration and presence of fungi by histology or culture. However, presence of bacteria or fungi in sinus cavities does not prove that these pathogens directly create or perpetuate the disease [1, 3].

2.13.2 Clinical Findings

The clinical findings are the signs and symptoms implicated in the clinical assessment of rhinosinusitis. Many studies try to organise the symptomatology; the last consensus document, recently published, constitutes the cornerstone on definition, classification and diagnosis of rhinosinusitis. This consensus is based on clinical symptoms: nasal blockage/congestion, reduction or loss of smell, discharge anterior/postnasal drip and facial pain/pressure. Presence of two or more symptoms one of which should be either nasal blockage / obstruction / congestion or nasal discharge (anterior / posterior nasal drip) +/– facial pain / pressure +/– reduction or loss of smell is mandatory for rhinosinusitis diagnostic associated to endoscopy findings (polyps, rhinorrhea and/or oedema) and/or CT changes [3].

2.13.3 Diagnosis

Although assessment of chronic rhinosinusitis is based on symptoms, there are complementary studies (divided into major and minor tests) that help with diagnosis confirmation. The major tests are endoscopy and CT scan;

the minor tests are mainly represented by nasal cytology, bacteriology and ultrasonography.

Plain sinus X-rays are insensitive for the diagnosis of rhinosinusitis. CT scan is the imaging modality of choice confirming chronic lesions, as it:

- Corroborates the previous clinical diagnostic
- Is a guide to lesions of the different sinuses
- Provides information about anatomical features found in surgery, with the anatomical variations (concha bullosa, paradoxical middle turbinate, Haller cells, prominent agger nasi cell)

The value of radiologic lesions on nasal mucosa is great. In a CT scan, asymptomatic patients present an incidence of sinus occupations, cysts, and mucosal oedema larger than 3 mm, with an incidence of 30 to 60% [1], that percentage being higher in paediatric patients. Viral subclinical infections or physiologic situations on the nasal cycle could be responsible. The nasal cycle might be responsible for oedema in the nasal septum (nasal valve), sphenoethmoidal recess and nasal lateral wall (turbinates, infundibulum), but it is not responsible for frontal, maxillary, and sphenoid occupations [1, 4].

Ultrasonography is an inexpensive screening for sinus pathology, presenting a high sensitivity but a low specificity. Tumours, cysts, polyps and mucosa oedema can generate false-positive results. Sinonasal mucoceles are ultrasonographically clear and are an exception. In conclusion, ultrasonography is useful for differentiating a "supernormal" population, which is irrelevant [1]. No correlation exists between pathologic ultrasonography and clinical evidence of sinusal pathology. Ethmoid and sphenoid evaluation becomes impossible due to technical constraints, but the ethmoid sinus is the key to sinusal inflammatory physiopathology. All these arguments justify the poor application of the ultrasonography. In conclusion, ultrasonography is a rapid, comfortable and innocuous test, but is not diagnostically useful.

Microbiology studies in acute rhinosinusitis have shown a reasonable correlation with germs in the airways, with a prevalence of *Haemophilus influenzae*, *Streptococcus pneumoniae*, *Moraxella catarrhalis* and *Staphylococcus* [1]. In chronic rhinosinusitis, microbiology studies are not conclusive. The technique used to obtain the sample, the cultures themselves and the location of the occupied sinus should be taken into account when interpreting results in the literature. In chronic rhinosinusitis it is accepted that infection is often polymicrobial. The role that anaerobes species play is of question. The anaerobe cultures by sinus puncture (90%) present more positives than do the endoscopically collected cultures from the middle meatus or nasal secretions [1].

Peptostreptococcus spp., *Fusobacterium* spp., *Prevotella* spp., *Streptococcus milleri*, and *Corynebacterium* [1] were the anaerobes species most frequently isolated. *Pseudomonas aeruginosa* and *Proteus mirabilis* could be found in chronic rhinosinusitis of patients with cystic fibrosis or an immunodeficiency [1]. Which of these pathogens is contributory to the disease remains a matter of debate.

2.13.4 Classification

Chronic rhinosinusitis can travel different clinical paths. It can be a consequence of an acute rhinosinusitis, or be an insidious set of symptoms without any recognisable aetiology or prodromal symptoms. Some patients can present with acute exacerbations with chronic rhinosinusitis. Currently, the subacute rhinosinusitis concept is obsolete. In addition, due to the long timeline of 12 weeks in typical chronic rhinosinusitis, it can be difficult to discriminate between recurrent acute rhinosinusitis and chronic rhinosinusitis with or without exacerbations. In recurrent acute rhinosinusitis, the presence of an interval free of disease is mandatory, but currently no criteria of "total recovery" exist. In addition, mucosal radiologic alterations could persist after 2 months of sinusal affection, even if the patient is asymptomatic. These mucosal alterations are difficult to interpret; it could represent normal resolution or a disease persistency. CT scan to confirm the "radiologic healing" in patients without symptoms and normal endoscopy is not viable.

Although previous consensus documents recently have been proposed to be *the* reference document regarding chronic rhinosinusitis [3], the European Position Paper on Rhinosinusitis and Nasal Polyps (EPOS), clearly influenced by the ARIA document [4], tries to quantify the disease severity, dividing it into mild (0–3), moderate (< 3–7) and severe (> 7–10), with a visual analogic scale ranging from 0–10 cm. Very important changes have been done in literature around this topic during 2007.

Based on length of the disease, acute or intermittent rhinosinusitis is defined as duration of symptoms for less than 12 weeks; more than 12 weeks is defined as chronic or persistent [3].

The above emphasises the need to reach a consensus in terms of the classification, the definitions and the diagnostic methods of rhinosinusitis. Only under these circumstances will there exist a useful information interchange on the prognoses, pathologies and treatments of rhinosinusitis.

Due to the variability of symptom intensity and the individual susceptibility on evaluation, varying classifications and definitions of rhinosinusitis persist. In general, the major symptoms of acute rhinosinusitis (nasal blockage, rhinorrhea, facial pain or pressure) are well differentiated, while for the chronic clinical symptoms, only headache and rhinorrhea are emphasised. The partition between acute and chronic disease on duration of symptoms is arbitrary, and no histopathological definition exists defining acute versus chronic disease.

2.13.5 Physiopathology

The key element for nasal health is the maintenance of optimal sinus ventilation and clearance. Obstruction of the ostiomeatal complex contributes to hypoxia inside the sinuses. Intrasinusal lactic acid increases during the middle and long-term stages, which is conducive to bacterial colonisation.

Three key phenomena on sinus mucosa should be delineated: vasodilatation, ciliary dysfunction and glandular impairment. The practise consequence is the presence of oedema, retained secretions and an increased viscosity. This vicious cycle can be difficult to break, and if the conditions persist, they can result in chronic rhinosinusitis. The evidence for chronic rhinosinusitis physiopathology refers to the ostia, ciliary, and glandular functions. The presence of cytokines and adhesive molecules suggests that inflammation holds great importance in chronic rhinosinusitis physiopathology. A highly potent chemoattractant for neutrophils, interleukin (IL)-8 has been demonstrated present in chronic rhinosinusitis tissue [3], together with increased levels of IL-1, IL-4, IL-5, granulocyte macrophage-colony stimulating factor (GM-CSF) and eosinophil cationic protein (ECP) versus control tissue. Cytokines' and adhesion mediators' profiles in chronic rhinosinusitis are similar to those in acute rhinosinusitis and viral rhinosinusitis, except for a significant increase of ECP. This profile is different in nasal polyposis.

Succinctly, cytokines often determine polymorphonuclear adherence to the microcirculation endothelial cells on sinusal mucosa, contributing to attraction, adhesion and migration of the immunocompetent inflammatory cells to the sinusal focus. Adhesion molecules also regulate cytokines. Due to different locations of inflammatory disease, adhesion molecules are also important elements in leukocyte recruitment [1]. The presence of immunoactive substances after curative treatment of the infectious process could be an evocative aspect of rhinosinusitis physiopathology, contributing to persistent feedback inflammation. An important fact is that cytolysis is produced mostly by the presence of inflammatory cells rather than by the presence of microbial pathogens [1, 3, 5].

2.13.6. Therapeutic Principles

Evidence based management for adults with chronic rhinosinusitis should be based on severity of symptoms using a VAS (visual analogical scale). When nasal polyps are not present topical steroids are recommended in a mild illness (VAS: 0–3). After 3 months of treatment when there is a failure of control a long term of macrolides antibiotics is added.

In a moderate /severe (VAS >3–10) chronic rhinosinusitis without nasal polyps topical steroids associated to a long term macrolides antibiotics administration are recommended. Failure after three months of treatment suggest that an endonasal endoscopic surgical procedure should be performed.

In chronic rhinosinusitis with bilateral nasal polys, a very long term of topical steroids are recommended in a mild (VAS: 0–3) and in a moderate illness (VAS >3–7). When there is no improvement after 3 months of therapy surgery should be considered, a postoperative follow-up with topical steroids is mandatory; eventually a short course of oral steroids and a long term of macrolides antibiotics can be necessary.

In a severe chronic rhinosinusitis with nasal polyps (VAS >7–10) a short term of oral steroids associated to topical steroids is recommended. Patient should be evaluated after 1 month of therapy, when improvement is present a very long term of topical steroids is the main treatment, but when there is a failure, surgery is recommended. Follow-up with topical steroids is necessary, a long term of macrolides antibiotics or a short term of oral steroids can be considered.

When signs of complications are present as orbital symptoms like periorbital oedema, displaced globe, double or reduced acuity of vision and ophthalmoplegia or symptoms of severe frontal headache, frontal swelling, meningitis or focal neurological signs is mandatory hospitalisation an urgent investigation and probably a surgical procedure.

References

1. Montserrat JR, Fabra JM, Gras JR, MassegurH, de Juan J, de Juan M (2005) Rinosinusitis aguda y crónica: definición, diagnóstico, clasificación y fisiopatología In: Mullol J, Montserrat JR (eds) Rinitis, Rinosinusitis, Poliposis nasal Ponencia Oficial de la SEORL y PCF Barcelona 2005, II. pp 643–659 (In Spanish)
2. Collins JG (1997) Prevalence of selected chronic conditions: United States, 1990–1992. Vital Health Stat 194:1–89
3. Fokkens W J, Lund V J, Mullol J et al. European Position Paper on Nasal Polyps 2007, Rhinology 45; suppl. 20: 1–139
4. Bousquet J, van Cauwenberge P, Khaltaev N for the ARIA Workshop/World Health Organization (2001) Allergic rhinitis and its impact on asthma. J Allergy Clin Immunol 108:S147–S336
5. Lund VL (1997) Infectious rhinosinusitis in adults: classification, etiology and management. International Rhinosinusitis Advisory Board. Ear Nose Throat J 12:4–22

2.14 Nasal Polyposis

METIN ÖNERCI

2.14.1 Introduction

Although nasal polyps have been identified for a long time, they remain one of medicine's unsolved mysteries. There is no consensus as to the types and formation of polyps; and there are various surgical approaches to their treatment. Nasal polyps are not a single entity; they include different forms, both in growth pattern and response to different medications. Nasal polyposis is varied, encompassing a wide range, from mucosal oedema and solitary polyps to diffuse and massive polyposis

(Fig. 2.14.1). About 5% of the European population suffers from chronic sinusitis. Nasal polyps account for 5% of referrals to ENT clinics and 4% of referrals to allergy clinics. In other studies, the prevalence of nasal polyps was found to be between 1.3 and 5.6%. Davidson found the annual polyp incidence to be 0.43 per 1,000 persons. Nasal polyposis occurs in about 0.6% of adults, but it increases to 15% in patients suffering from bronchial asthma. Up to 95% of patients with the bronchospastic type of analgesic intolerance will develop chronic polypoid sinusitis. Larsen and Tos found polyps in 42% of autopsy specimens. Polyps are more common in male non-asthmatic, atopic patients, whereas in asthmatic patients there is no difference in prevalence between males and females. Eosinophil-dominated diffuse nasal polyposis behaves differently from the non-eosinophil-dominated nasal polyposis. The eosinophil-dominated polyp has a close relationship with asthma and analgesic intolerance. Nasal polyposis exacerbates asthmatic symptoms, and its treatment is known to have a positive effect on asthma. In some cases where only nasal polyposis is present, asthma or aspirin intolerance may develop up to 10 years later. Conversely, nasal polyposis may follow asthma and aspirin intolerance. Fifteen per cent of patients with nasal

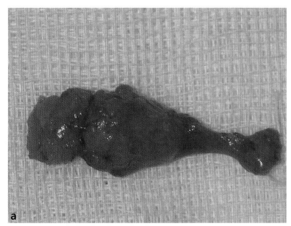

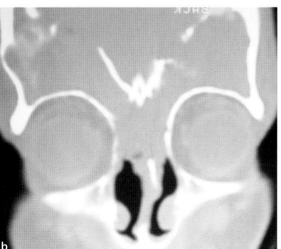

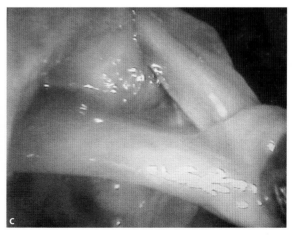

Fig. 2.14.1 a Solitary polyp deriving from the uncinate process, **b** coronal CT, pansinusitis, **c** thick and viscous secretion

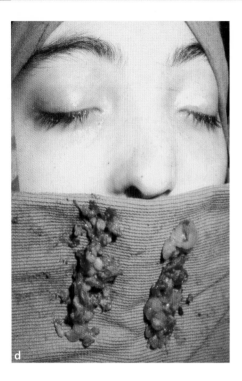

Fig. 2.14.1 *(continued)* **d** diffuse nasal polyposis

2.14.2 Origin of Polyps

The introduction of nasal endoscopy to rhinology has made it possible to detect even small asymptomatic polyps. The site of origin of the polyps is generally identifiable. The majority originate from narrow clefts of the ethmoidal cells. Contact areas may contribute to the formation of polyps. The extent of polyps may be misleading when endoscopically examined. Like the tip of an iceberg, in some patients there appear small polyps behind the middle turbinate, whereas the entire ethmoid sinus may be full of polyps. Radiological studies show the extent of polyposis. However, since CT cannot differentiate between nasal polyps and secretion, the extent of surgery necessary should be decided *during* the surgery, and radical surgery should be avoided whenever possible.

2.14.3 Classification Systems

There are different classification systems according to histology, site of origin and the most common inflammatory cells of the polyps. In recent years, eosinophils are the cells that have drawn the most attention. A distinct eosinophilia in the nasal secretions is characteristic for diffuse eosinophilic nasal polyposis cases. The presence of eosinophils in the tissue and the mucus does not appear to be related to allergy or IgE-mediated hypersensitivity. The eosinophils are upregulated by cytokines, IL-3, GM-CSF and most importantly IL-5. IL-5 appears to have the most dynamic effect on the long-term survival of the eosinophils. In addition to these cytokines in the epithe-

polyps have the bronchospastic type of analgesic intolerance, which increases to 60% in patients who require follow-up surgery for major regrowth of polyps after initial surgery. Nasal polyposis may cause serious complications if not treated (Figs. 2.14.2–2.14.4).

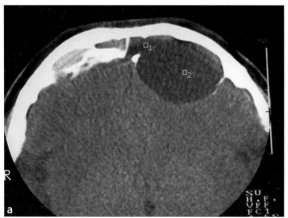
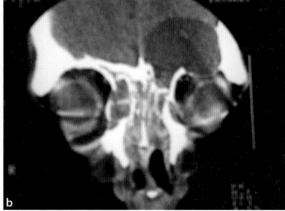

Fig. 2.14.2 a,b Mucocele in a patient with Samter's syndrome with destruction of posterior table of frontal sinus and superior orbital wall

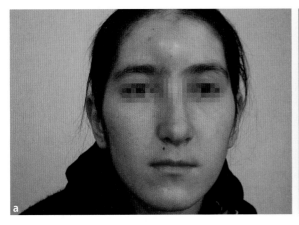
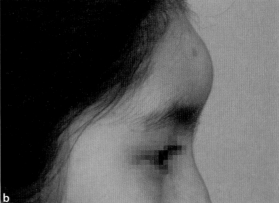

Fig. 2.14.3 a,b Pott's puffy tumour in a patient with diffuse nasal polyposis

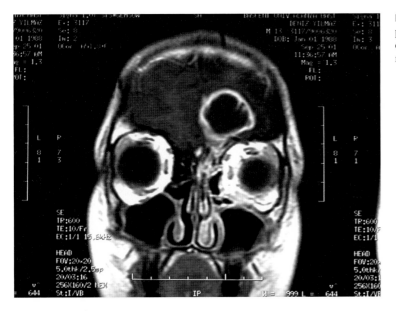

Fig. 2.14.4 Brain abscess in a case of polyps with diabetes mellitus. Histologic exam of the polyps was reported as mucormycosis

lium and endothelium of the nasal polyp, the eosinophil itself can produce similar cytokines. In nasal biopsies, there is an intense infiltration of eosinophils, with ruptured granules dispersed in the tissue. Numerous theories implicating fungi and "superantigens" were suggested to explain the presence of eosinophils. Bachert et al. detected staphylococcal superantigen-specific IgE antibodies to the superantigens SEA and SEB in nasal polyp tissue. Microbial persistence, superantigen production and host T-lymphocyte response are fundamental components of all common chronic eosinophilic-lymphocytic respiratory mucosal disorders. According to the fungi theory, the eosinophils are attracted to a stimulus (fungus) in the mucus in patients who are immunologically sensitive to fungus. Since 40% of the contents of the eosinophils consist of major basic protein (MBP), the secretion of MBP not only kills the microorganism, but also causes epithelial damage from the mucus side, causing secondary bacterial infection. However, some other reports stress the potential role of MBP on the sodium and chloride flux in the epithelium of the polyp epithelial cell.

2.14.4 Treatment

The initial aims of treatment are to relieve nasal blockage, rhinitis symptoms, asthma, and to improve sinus drainage, whereas the final target is to eliminate nasal polyps and sinus pathology and to prevent recurrences. Solitary and non-eosinophilic polyps are not difficult to manage and generally do not recur after surgery. Ostiomeatal unit surgery to remove defined microanatomical narrow passes around this functional key area of the middle nasal meatus, which facilitates drainage and ventilation of the dependent paranasal sinuses, may help recover the circumscribed hyperplastic changes of the remote paranasal sinuses. Even severe changes in the peripheral sinus mucosa may heal subsequently without being specifically treated. The patient with eosinophil-dominated diffuse nasal polyposis presents a challenge to the clinician and the surgeon. Although it is possible to improve nasal breathing, olfaction, rhinitis symptoms and asthma, it is not always possible to eliminate nasal polyps and sinus pathology in these cases. Treatment may help the patient live more comfortably with his or her disease, but in most cases does not eliminate the disease entirely. Therefore, the success of the treatment is dependent on careful evaluation of whether or not there are polyps causing symptoms, obstructing sinus drainage and requiring revision surgery.

2.14.5 Recurrence

Regardless of a medical or surgical approach to treatment, most polyps do recur after treatment. The literature is very scarce regarding comparative studies of medical or surgical treatment of nasal polyposis. These studies generally suggest medical treatment and reserve surgery for patients who respond poorly to medication. The treatment of eosinophil-dominated diffuse nasal polyposis includes topical and systemic corticosteroids (CS), topical diuretics, leukotriene antagonists, immune stimulants and antifungal agents. Aspirin desensitisation and intranasal lysine aspirin have also been suggested for Samter's triad patients. No treatment modality gives a complete cure, and varying success rates have been reported. The best results are with systemic CS. Although the polyps regress with CS therapy, they may recur. Recurrent uses of CS may not be effective due to CS resistance. Some patients cannot use CS because of some medical problems. It is not possible to know in advance which patients will respond favourably to CS therapy and those who will not. Although surgical treatment is an adjunct for medical treatment and should not be considered as the first-line treatment of eosinophil-dominated diffuse nasal polyposis, it is unavoidable in some cases.

2.14.6 Surgery

There are different surgical options described in the literature, ranging from simple polypectomy to nasalisation,

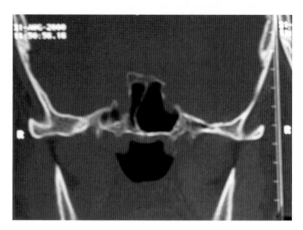

Fig. 2.14.5 A carotid artery bulging into the sphenoid sinus and lacking bony covering

e. g. complete removal of all sinonasal mucosa. Although FESS, which is the standard surgery for sinusitis today, may help patients with primary and limited polyps by improving ventilation, drainage and by opening defined anatomical narrow passages, this surgery does not give satisfactory results in recurrent and advanced diffuse nasal polyposis, since the disease diffusely affects the whole sinus mucosa. The success rates of surgical approaches are variable among reports. Schapowal et al. report 90% recurrence within weeks or months after surgery, whereas Jankovski et al. report a 91% success rate. In diffuse polyposis patients, a more extensive procedure (a "pansinus surgery") is needed. Polypectomy may cause irregular scars that mask anatomical landmarks. Inevitable follow-up procedures are therefore rendered more difficult, and the accompanying risks increase. The surgeon must be aware of the anatomical abnormalities and possible risks (Fig 2.14.5). Wynn and Har-El reviewed 118 patients with asthma (50%) and documented allergy (79%). All patients underwent extensive bilateral nasal polypectomy, complete anterior and posterior ethmoidectomy, and maxillary sinusotomy. One hundred (85%) also had frontal or sphenoid sinusotomy. Follow-up ranged from 12 to 168 (median 40) months. Despite pre- and postoperative nasal and systemic steroid treatment in the majority of patients, 71 (60%) developed recurrent polyposis, 55 (47%) were advised to undergo revision surgery, and 32 (27%) underwent revision surgery. History of previous sinus surgery or asthma predicted higher recurrence and revision surgery rates. History of allergy also predicted recurrence and need for revision.

In recent years, otorhinolaryngologists have realised that recurrent polyp formation in eosinophil-dominated nasal polyposis patients is not a true recurrence, but the result of an ongoing immunological inflammatory reaction. This response may be a reaction to deposits of fungi or staphylococcal superantigens in the nose or sinus cavities. The main pathology lies in the mucus. In other words, the stimulus comes from the mucus, and some patients react differently due to genetic makeup. The secretions are also very thick and viscid, and ciliary activity is not capable of removing this thick mucus (Fig. 2.14.1c). Therefore, the aim of surgery should be to let this thick mucus drain. Any collection or stagnation of the mucus should be prevented, and this extramucosal stimulus burden should be removed.

Mucosa should be preserved as much as possible to avoid scarring, crusting, stenosis and osteitic bone. However, preserving the normal mucosa is not always feasible, because it is sometimes very difficult to differentiate normal mucosa from polypoid mucosa. Moreover, thick mucus may stay in the folds of polypoid mucosa, which in turn starts the vicious circle again. Therefore, all polyps or severe polypoid mucosa that could hide thick mucus should be cleaned as far as access to all the anatomic areas of the nose is permitted. Nasalisation makes sense in that it prevents microbial colonisation and the foci of stimulants such as fungi in the folds of oedematous or polypoid mucosa. However, unnecessary tissue destruction, increased scarring, stenosis, rhinitis sicca, and crusting are the disadvantages of this type of radical surgery. Nasalisation should be reserved mainly for tumours of the nose, and removal of all of the sinonasal mucosal covering should be avoided.

The main cause of recurrence is the areas that have not been opened or drained (see below). If the ethmoidal cells are not opened completely, then the polyps stay in these insufficiently opened cells (Fig 2.14.6). These cells act as a pool for thick mucus. Topical drops cannot reach a sufficient concentration in these cells. Bone inflammation and obliteration of the Haversian system may contribute to the persistence of disease in localised areas, causing irregular bony thickening until such underlying bone is removed. Therefore, all the ethmoid partitions should be opened and removed. A smooth cavity should be created that can be seen, examined and cleaned, and to which medicine can be applied. If there is any pathology in the agger nasi, then these cells should also be addressed. If necessary, the bony prominences should be drilled until no hidden area remains. No free bony spicules should be allowed to remain in the operation field to avoid both granulation tissue and polyp recurrence.

The reasons for failure in surgery of diffuse nasal polyposis are as follows:

- Insufficient ethmoidectomy
- Insufficient removal of septa
  - Insufficient drug concentration behind the septa
  - Insufficient cleaning of the polypoid mucosa behind the septa
  - Pool for collection of secretions
- Insufficient surgery of the frontal sinus
  - Polyps at the frontal recess and frontal ostium area
  - Polyps and mucoceles in the frontal sinus
  - Stenosis of frontal ostium
- Insufficient surgery of the maxillary sinus
  - Insufficient maxillary sinus ostium
  - Reclosure of the ostium
  - Decreased ventilation and drainage
  - Insufficient drainage due to thick secretions
  - Insufficient cleaning
- Insufficient opening of anterior wall of sphenoid sinus
  - Decreased ventilation
  - Decreased drainage
  - Insufficient drug concentration
  - Insufficient cleaning
- Free bony spicules, granulation tissue and polyp recurrence

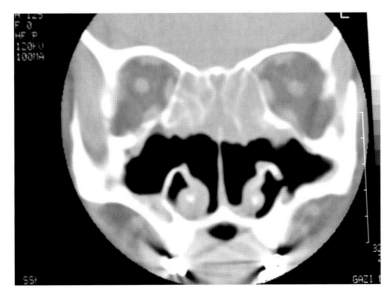

Fig. 2.14.6 A diffuse polyposis case after operation; ethmoid cells were not opened in the previous surgery

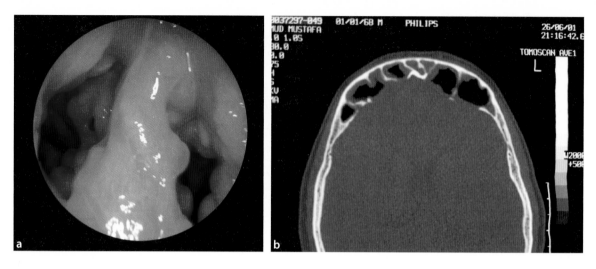

Fig. 2.14.7 a,b Six months after surgery with polypoid mucosa of the frontal sinus. **a** Polyps in the frontal sinus, **b** Axial CT

Regarding the major sinuses, the foremost issue is to have a sufficient opening, which allows the sinus to drain and ventilate sufficiently. Stenosis should be prevented. Normal ostia should remain untouched. If there are polyps in the frontal recess, then they need to be cleaned without damaging the mucosa and without touching the frontal ostium area. However, in recurrent cases it is not sufficient only to drain the sinus, but also to have the possibility of irrigating, cleaning and examining the inside of the sinus, as well as to apply medication. In these cases, the surgeon needs to have a large ostium of the involved sinuses. The maxillary sinus ostium may be connected to the nasoantral window in the inferior meatus. The sphenoid sinus ostium is widened to the extent that the bottom and lateral aspects of the sinus can be seen. If the frontal sinus is opaque and the ostium is blocked, then it may be necessary to widen the frontal ostia, to perform Draf type II or III osteoplasty, and to remove the polyps and mucoceles from the frontal sinus (Figs. 2.14.7, 2.14.8).

Some authors advocate partial resection of the middle turbinate to expand the surgical approach, while others modify it only in cases of abnormalities and leave as much as possible of the middle turbinate intact as a landmark in case revision surgery is needed. In a retrospective evaluation including 100 FESS patients, Giacchi and co-authors preserved the middle turbinate on one side and partially resected it on the other side. The authors observed no side differences in the outcome parameters studied. In a randomised trial, 1,106 matched chronic rhinosinusitis (CRS) patients with and without polyps, who underwent similar functional endonasal sinus surgery with (509 patients) or without (597 patients) partial middle turbinate resection. Partial middle turbinate resection was associated with less synechia formation ($p < 0.05$) and less re-

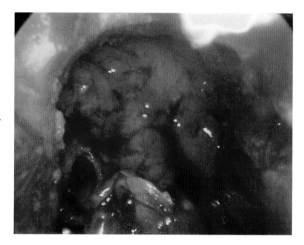

Fig. 2.14.8 Draf type III procedure

vision surgeries ($p < 0.05$) than middle turbinate preservation was. Complications caused particularly by partial middle turbinate resection were not observed. In recurrent cases, the inferior half or two thirds of the middle turbinate can be removed to get better access to the polyps behind the middle turbinate and sphenoid sinus ostium. The possibility that the middle turbinate bone may be osteitic lends support to the removal of the lower half of the middle turbinate. If necessary, septal deviation should be corrected (Fig. 2.14.9). Septal deviation may cause an insufficient exposure of the surgical field in addition to lateralisation of the middle turbinate, resulting in failure of the surgery.

2.14.7 Postoperative Care

Long-term follow-up is crucial. The debris in the nasal cavity should be cleaned by irrigation. Antibiotics and topical steroids (when necessary, systemic steroids) should be continued. The patients must be followed-up closely, and early polypoid tissues, which contain serous fluid, need to be drained. Any persistent disease should be treated prior to becoming symptomatic, since localised persistence of polyp disease eventually leads to diffuse recurrence. However, unnecessary trauma should be avoided, since this may activate granulation of tissue.

2.14.8 Nasal Polyposis in Children

The incidence rate of nasal polyposis in children is quite low. Symptomatic nasal polyps are generally bilateral and associated with systemic disease. Children younger than 16 years of age with bilateral nasal polyposis should be evaluated for cystic fibrosis. Symptomatic diffuse nasal polyps are seen in 20–25% of paediatric patients with cystic fibrosis, in 10% of those with NSAID drug intolerance and in 5% with primary ciliary dyskinesia. They found that 50% of children with nasal polyps have a positive history for polyps, suggesting a genetic role in the development of the disease. The histological structure of the polyps in children is different from that of polyps found in adults. Eosinophilic polyps do not occur as frequently in children as they do in adults. This may be related to frequent upper RTI infections due to systemic diseases such as cystic fibrosis and primary ciliary dyskinesia.

Surgery for nasal polyposis in children should be reserved only for patients with complete nasal obstruction and facial skeletal deformity (broadening of the nasal dorsum; high, arched palate) that negatively affect quality of life. Minimally symptomatic patients should not undergo surgery.

2.14.9 Conclusion

Recovery does not mean complete relief from polyps or polypoid mucosa, but improvement in the symptoms and relief with the help of topical drugs. The mucosa should be preserved as fully as possible. However, in recurrent cases, surgery more extensive is needed. All the ethmoidal cells require opening, and the bony partitions need to be removed. This, in turn, results in access to the entire ethmoidal cavity, allowing topical medication to reach and make contact with the mucosal surfaces. No pooling in the sinuses should be allowed, since stasis and stagnation of the mucus in these areas continues to stimulate the immune reaction. All the entrances of the major sinuses should be cleaned and mucociliary activity restored. If the major sinuses are involved and the lining is completely polypoid, then if possible, the sinus should drain by itself or, if this is not possible, the ostia should be made wide enough ("megaostium") for the sinus to be cleaned. In recurrent cases, Draf type II or III osteoplasty for the frontal sinus may be an option. For the maxillary sinus,

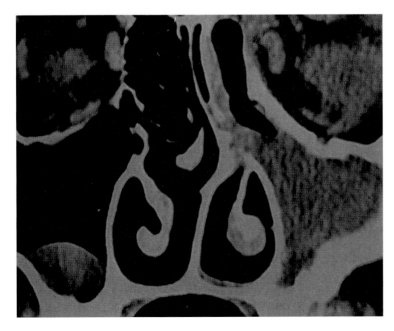

Fig. 2.14.9 Septal deviation with lateralisation of the middle turbinate, resulting in failure of the surgery

the nasoantral window may be opened and the middle meatal antrostomy may be connected to the nasoantral window. The sphenoid sinus deserves close attention due to the critical structures involved, but the ostia can be widened as much as possible. Surgery for eosinophil-dominated diffuse nasal polyposis should be completely radical in terms of opening all the cells, therefore creating an open and smooth cavity, yet it must also be completely functional in terms of preserving the functioning mucosa.

Reading Recommendations

1. Draf W (1991) Endonasal microendoscopic frontal sinus surgery: Fulda concept. Oper Tech Otolaryngol Head Neck Surg 2:234–240

2. Fokkens W, Lund V, Mullol J (2007) European position paper on rhinosinusitis and nasal polyps 2007. Rhinol Suppl:1–136

3. Gordts F, Clement PAR (1997) Epidemiology and prevalence of aspecific chronic sinusitis. Acta Otorhinolaryngol Belg 51:205–208

4. Larsen PL, Tos M (1996) Anatomic site of origin of nasal polyps, endoscopic nasal and paranasal sinus surgery as a screening method for nasal polyps in autopsy material. Am J Rhinol 10:211–216

5. Maran GD, Lund VJ (1990) Clinical rhinology. Stuttgart, Thieme

6. Stammberger H, Hawke M (1993) Essentials of functional endoscopic sinus surgery. Mosby, St. Louis, Mo.

7. Stammberger H (1991) Functional endoscopic sinus surgery. Decker, Philadelphia

8. Wigand ME (1990) Endoscopic surgery of the paranasal sinuses and anterior skull base. Thieme, Stuttgart

2.15 Specific Sinusitis

ANDRÉ COSTE AND JEAN-FRANÇOIS PAPON

2.15.1 Specific Sinusitis (Fungal Rhinosinusitis)

The fungal species involved in rhinosinusitis pathology are typically filamentous organisms and determine two different pathophysiological entities. The fungal element may either act as an allergen or as an infectious agent. In the first case, all types of moulds present in the environment may be involved, while in the second case, only some species have the ability to develop in the human body, especially *Aspergillus*, the commonest being *Aspergillus fumigatus*. Fungi generally have weak invasive power and are opportunist pathogens. Their pathogenicity is expressed only when the host's defences are compromised. It is very important from a prognosis and therapeutic point of view to distinguish between *noninvasive* diseases (*fungus balls* and *allergic fungal rhinosinusitis*) and *invasive* diseases (mainly *acute invasive fungal rhinosinusitis* and exceptionally *indolent or chronic invasive fungal sinusitis*) [3].

2.15.1.1 Fungus balls

2.15.1.1.1 Definition

Fungus balls of the sinuses are localised and poorly aggressive infections without mucosal invasion, encountered in immunocompetent patients. Fungus balls mainly involve the maxillary sinus (89% of cases), but all the sinuses may be involved including the sphenoid.

2.15.1.1.2 Epidemiology

Fungus balls are only encountered in adults and are thought to be more frequent in women.

2.15.1.1.3 Symptoms

Symptoms are nonspecific with a clinical picture of chronic rhinosinusitis responding poorly to medical treatment. They are unilateral and variably associate: chronic pain (especially when the sphenoid is involved), purulent rhinorrhea, obstruction and cacosmia. Fungus balls are frequently incidental findings on imaging.

2.15.1.1.4 Diagnostic Procedure: Recommended European Standard

Inspection produces unremarkable results in most cases, although a swollen cheek may be present.

Rhinoscopy and nasal endoscopy may be normal or show in one of the meatuses:
- Purulent secretions
- Oedema, sometimes with polyps
- Fragments of fungus ball

Sinus CT scan shows different images:
- Unilateral opacity, frequently heterogeneous, involving one or sometimes several sinus cavities, with bone thickening or bone lysis of the nasomaxillary wall
- A pseudometallic foreign body or one or several macrocalcifications
- Microcalcifications
- Sometimes bone lysis more extensive (pseudotumoral forms)

2.15.1.1.5 Surgery

The macroscopic aspect of the fungus balls during surgical removal is often highly suggestive: a solid but crumbly, from brown- to black-coloured mass, with thick creamy secretions.

2.15.1.1.6 Pathology

The pathologic examination of the fungus ball with specific stain (periodic acid–Schiff, Grocott-Gomori) shows the fungal filaments and detects nonspecific inflammation in the mucosa without fungal invasion.

2.15.1.1.7 Mycology

Direct examination reveals fungal filaments in more than 70% of cases. A culture will identify the fungal species in 30–60% of cases but has no diagnostic value, as fungal presence does not necessarily indicate disease. In Europe, *Aspergillus*, especially *A. fumigatus*, is the commonest involved species, but other types of aspergillus or other species may be isolated.

2.15.1.1.8 Additional/Useful Diagnostic Procedures

- Dental examination: looks for devitalised "sinus" teeth
- Standard sinus X-rays: may show unilateral maxillary opacity, with pseudometallic foreign body]
- Dental X-rays: can reveal precise dental status and may show apical material overprojection
- MRI: not practical in cases of fungus ball suspicion, except in cases of pseudotumoral forms in order to distinguish them from tumours, or in cases of immunocompromised patients in whom an invasive fungal rhinosinusitis may be suspected. The fungus ball has a hypodense signal on T_1- and T_2-weighted images [10]. The mucosa has hyperdense signal on T_2- and post-gadolinium T_1-weighted sequences.

2.15.1.1.9 Surgical Treatment: Recommended European Standard

Fungus ball treatment requires a complete surgical removal of the fungus ball. Antifungal therapies are unnecessary.

Surgery consists of creating a large opening of the involved sinuses in order to allow:

- Complete removal of the fungus ball and secretions while preserving the integrity of the mucosa
- Recovery of sinus drainage and ventilation
- Easy endoscopic postoperative follow-up

2.15.1.1.10 Differential Diagnosis

CT scan images are generally highly indicative of the diagnosis and lead to surgery, and then to pathological and mycological examinations. Nevertheless, in cases of pseudotumoral forms, the diagnosis of allergic fungal sinusitis, of fungal invasive rhinosinusitis or even of tumour must be considered, with the knowledge that fungus balls may be associated with tumours.

2.15.1.1.11 Prognosis

Cure should be achieved in all patients after complete removal of the fungus ball and restoration of sinus ventilation and drainage. Long-term endoscopic follow-up is recommended, even though recurrences are exceptional and occur generally when some fungus ball fragments remain after surgery [9].

2.15.1.1.12 Surgical Principles

Endoscopic endonasal surgery is the usual approach [9]:

- A large middle meatal antrostomy, sometimes associated with inferior antrostomy or with an *a minima* trepanning of the canine fossa, is required for maxillary fungus balls; the Caldwell-Luc procedure may be indicated in multiple recurrences or in certain pseudotumoral forms.
- An ethmoidectomy may be associated in cases of ethmoidal extension of the fungus ball.
- A sphenoidotomy is indicated for sphenoidal fungus balls.
- A frontal sinusotomy eventually combined to an external approach if a complete removal of the fungus ball cannot be achieved via the endonasal route.

2.15.1.2 Allergic Fungal Rhinosinusitis

2.15.1.2.1 Definition

The diagnosis of allergic fungal rhinosinusitis (AFS) was developed for patients with recurrent nasal polyps and asthma in mind [5], but there is still not a clear definition and/or panel of criteria. Clearly different from allergic rhinitis with fungus IgE-mediated sensitisation, the AFS concept was inspired by allergic bronchopulmonary aspergillosis, in which the pathogenicity of the fungi could result both from IgE-dependent mechanisms and from immunopathologic mechanisms of infectious origin.

2.15.1.2.2 Epidemiology

AFS is encountered in adults and in children.

2.15.1.2.3 Symptoms

Usual symptoms are those of nasal polyposis (nasal obstruction and congestion, rhinorrhea, sneezing, headache and dysosmia). Nasal polyposis may be unilateral and may be aggressive, with orbital signs (proptosis, diplopia, visual loss). Asthma is frequent.

Diagnostic procedure is the recommended European standard [1, 8]:

- Inspection and clinical examination may show cheek and/or palpebral swelling, proptosis, ophthalmoplegia.
- Nasal endoscopy may be normal or show mucosal oedema, or polyps with or without allergic mucin (thick yellow–green mucus plugs) on one or both sides.
- Sinus CT scan may reveal heterogeneous and serpiginous sinus opacities, with or without pseudocalcifications and bone lysis on one or both sides.
- Pathology consists of allergic mucin with detection of hyphae, eosinophils and Charcot-Leyden crystals.
- Mycology involves identification of various species on mucus fungal culture.
- Serum hypereosinophilia may be present.
- Type I hypersensitivity to fungal species is frequent.
- There may be evidence of asthma.

2.15.1.2.4 Therapy
There is still no consensus as to the treatment modalities of AFS.

Large surgical removal of lesions, mainly via endoscopic sinus surgery, is recommended. Postoperative systemic steroids are recommended by most authors for a duration varying from 2 weeks to several months, but the use of local steroids is not clearly codified.

Antifungal agents (local or systemic) are recommended by some authors.

The indication for specific immunotherapy is not yet clarified.

2.15.1.2.5 Differential Diagnosis
AFS must be distinguished from fungus balls and invasive fungal sinusitis on the basis of clinical features, pathology, allergic investigations and operative findings. Tumours should also be eliminated on the same basis and with the use of imaging.

2.15.1.2.6 Prognosis
Long-term follow-up is recommended based on endoscopic findings, and for some authors, on IgE serum levels. Recurrence is frequently reported.

2.15.1.2.7 Surgical Principles
A large sphenoethmoidectomy on one or both sides is carried out under endoscopic guidance, allowing removal of mucus plugs and mucosal lesions.

2.15.1.3 Invasive Fungal Rhinosinusitis

2.15.1.3.1 Definition
When the fungal spores are not cleared because of immunodeficiency, they may germinate, produce filaments and then invade the surrounding tissues. Invasive fungal rhinosinusitis is therefore defined by the presence of fungal tissue invasion, detected on pathologic examination. This definition may correspond to different clinical forms: acute invasive fungal rhinosinusitis, indolent invasive fungal sinusitis and chronic invasive fungal sinusitis [3].

Acute Invasive Fungal Rhinosinusitis

Epidemiology
Acute invasive fungal rhinosinusitis (AIFRS) is rare and occurs most commonly in immunocompromised patients [3]. Patients affected by leukaemia and lymphoma are especially at risk, in particular in cases of chemotherapy with aplasia and bone marrow transplantation. Neutro-penia is a key factor, especially when neutrophils are below 500/ml. Other main factors are long-term glucocorticosteroid therapy and graft-versus-host disease. AIDS and type I diabetes patients are also at risk. Radiotherapy, long-term antibiotic therapy and malnutrition may also be risk factors for AIFRS.

Symptoms
Palpebral or cheek swelling with fever in an immunocompromised patient is highly suggestive of AIFRS. An unexplained fever in these patients must lead one to suspect AIFRS, especially if nasal congestion, rhinorrhea, epistaxis and/or headaches are reported.

Diagnostic Procedure
Diagnosis criteria have been proposed recently (host factors, clinical and microbiological factors).

Nasal endoscopy may show oedema, ulcerations and/or necrosis with crusts, which are highly suggestive of the diagnosis [2].

Imaging is mandatory (CT scan, MRI), which should show sinus opacities, bone necrosis and orbital and/or intracranial invasion.

A nasal and/or sinus biopsy must be performed each time the diagnosis of AIFRS is suspected, associated with pathologic examination and mycological cultures. Pathology will show fungal elements invading the mucosa, with thrombosis, ischaemia and necrosis [3]. Culture will generally identify the fungus (mainly *A. fumigatus* and *Aspergillus flavus*), and when negative, immunohistochemistry and/or molecular identification techniques may be useful.

Mucormycosis (caused mainly by the genera *Rhizopus* or *Absidia*) represents a distinct entity, as it is generally encountered in type I diabetes patients.

Therapy
The therapeutic strategy must be defined according to a multidisciplinary approach (ENT, haematologist, mycologist, pathologist, ophthalmologist, neurosurgeon and anaesthesiologist).

As soon as the diagnosis of AIFRS is suspected and the biopsies performed, a general antifungal therapy (amphotericin B, 1–1.5 mg/kg/day) is initiated and maintained up to a total dose of at least 1 g. Liposomal amphotericin B or amphotericin B lipid complex may be an interesting alternative, as they possess less renal toxicity and may be used with larger doses (5 mg/kg/day). Itraconazole (400–600 mg/day) is generally recommended after amphotericin therapy. Voriconazole might be a promising alternative to amphotericin therapy [4].

In cases of severe neutropenia, GM-CSF may be used. Diabetes must be kept under control.

A large surgical excision of invaded tissues is recommended.

Differential Diagnosis

Other types of rhinosinusitis, infectious (*Pseudomonas aeruginosa*, tuberculosis, syphilis, rhinoscleroma), inflammatory or granulomatous (sarcoidosis, Wegener's disease) may exhibit vascular or tissue necrosis. Biopsy with pathological examination and mycological culture are the key exams.

Bone erosion is frequently detected in AFS, but the medical background is very different.

Prognosis

The follow-up is monitored by endoscopy and imaging. A long follow-up is necessary even after complete recovery, as recurrences may happen in cases of new occurrences of neutropenia. A mortality rate of 20–80% in immunocompromised patients is reported.

Surgical Principles

Surgical excision of invaded tissues is generally performed via an external approach, or in selected cases via an endoscopic approach. Orbital involvement may lead to larger excisions. In cases of intracranial invasion a combined transcranial approach must be discussed.

Indolent Invasive Fungal Sinusitis and Chronic Invasive Fungal Sinusitis

Indolent invasive fungal sinusitis has been described essentially in immunocompetent African patients but may occur unfrequently in Caucasians, whereas chronic invasive fungal sinusitis is reported in North America. The clinical picture is a nonspecific rhinosinusitis, while imaging shows a pseudotumoral aspect. Treatment is poorly codified and incorporates surgery (which allows biopsies and cultures) with systemic antifungal therapy.

References

1. Bent JP III, Kuhn FA (1994) Diagnosis of allergic fungal sinusitis. Otolaryngol Head Neck Surg 111:580–588
2. de Carpentier JP, Ramamurthy L, Denning DW, Taylor PH (1994) An algorithmic approach to aspergillus sinusitis. J Laryngol Otol 108:314–318
3. deShazo RD, O'Brien M, Chapin K, Soto-Aguilar M, Gardner L, Swain R (1997) A new classification and diagnostic criteria for invasive fungal sinusitis. Arch Otolaryngol Head Neck Surg 123:1181–1188
4. Herbrecht R, Denning DW, Patterson TF et al. (2002) Voriconazole versus amphotericin B for primary therapy of invasive aspergillosis. N Engl J Med 347:408–415
5. Katzenstein AL, Sale SR, Greenberger PA (1983) Allergic Aspergillus sinusitis: a newly recognized form of sinusitis. J Allergy Clin Immunol 72:89–93
6. Klossek JM, Peloquin L, Fourcroy PJ, Ferrie JC, Fontanel JP (1996) Aspergillomas of the sphenoid sinus: a series of 10 cases treated by endoscopic sinus surgery. Rhinology 34:179–183
7. Klossek JM, Serrano E, Peloquin L, Percodani J, Fontanel JP, Pessey JJ (1997) Functional endoscopic sinus surgery and 109 mycetomas of paranasal sinuses. Laryngoscope 107:112–117
8. Serrano E, Percodani J, Uro-Coste E et al. (2001) Value of investigation in the diagnosis of allergic fungal rhinosinusitis: results of a prospective study. J Laryngol Otol 115:184–189
9. Stammberger H (1985) Endoscopic surgery for mycotic and chronic recurring sinusitis. Ann Otorhinolaryngol 119:S1–S11
10. Zinreich SJ, Kennedy DW, Malat J et al. (1988) Fungal sinusitis: diagnosis with CT and MR imaging. Radiology 169:439–444

2.16 Complications of Sinusitis

JOSÉ LUIS LLORENTE PENDÁS AND CARLOS SUAREZ NIETO

2.16.1 Introduction

Although since the pre-antibiotic era the great majority of cases of sinusitis are uncomplicated, sinus infections can readily spread to orbital or intracranial structures, with potential significant morbidity and even mortality. Complicated sinusitis is synonymous with sinus infection, orbital complications and intracranial complications.

Epidemiological data concerning the complications of rhinosinusitis vary widely, and there is no consensus on the exact prevalence of the different types of complications. Orbital complications are more commonly seen in children, and infection arises in most cases because of ethmoid disease.

The bacteria responsible for uncomplicated sinusitis are *Streptococcus pneumoniae*, *Haemophilus influenzae* and *Moraxella catarrhalis*. However, in complicated sinusitis the bacterial spectrum can change depending on the type of complication. The *H. influenzae* cases are commonest in young children. In adults and in orbital complications, *Staphylococcus* and *S. pneumoniae* are most common.

The organisms cultured in intracranial complications may vary but *Staphylococcus aureus* and *S. pneumoniae* are the more frequently isolated. There may be a mixture of organisms, and occasionally no pathogens are identified (20%). Brain abscess are usually due to mixed flora infections, but anaerobes may also be isolated in more than 50% of cases. Cultures of abscess contents or purulent sinusal secretions should always be done in an attempt to establish the aetiological agent. Blood cultures are of little value here.

In a patient presenting with a sinusitis complication, the history and the initial part of the physical examination should aid in ascertaining the source [1]. Complications of rhinosinusitis are classically defined as local, orbital and endocranial. Orbital complications of sinusitis are more commonly seen in children and are more clinically evident. However, intracranial cases in early stages should elicit a high level of suspicion in the examiner.

2.16.2 Diagnostic Procedures

Evaluation of the patient includes a careful history, including that of a recent upper respiratory tract infection, dental/nasal surgery or trauma. A clinical examination, completed if necessary by a nominal laboratory investigation, reveals clues, leading to the diagnosis of complicated sinusitis. An extremely useful test, although not specific, is the white-cell count, which, if elevated in acute rhinosinusitis unresponsive to treatment, is highly suggestive of a complication.

The examination consists of decongesting the nose, anterior rhinoscopy, and nasal endoscopy. In addition, it is recommended that an ophthalmologic examination is also performed by opening the eye (which is generally swollen shut) to examine it for extraocular movements and at the very least, gross visual acuity. Ophthalmologic consultation is obtained, and then the patient is followed closely in order to determine his or her response to treatment.

Radiological evaluation is an indispensable investigational tool for establishing the diagnosis and planning of treatment/management. Conventional plain films of the sinuses are of limited value in complications of sinusitis. The diagnostic modality of choice is CT scan with and without contrast, including axial and coronal high-resolution thin slices, which can reveal any sinus involvement and identify any intracranial or orbital extension (Fig. 2.16.1). CT scan is thought to be the gold standard in the diagnosis of sinusitis. It plays a major role in determining diagnosis and treatment plans. It is crucial to obtain a CT scan of the brain and orbits with contrast whenever a complication is suspected, to determine whether any enhancement is present. If only CT scan without contrast is used, then an abscess could be missed. In meningitis, CT scan of the brain is usually normal. However, low-density mass effect in rim enhancement is usually indicative of an abscess formation. Additionally, MRI has proven to be essential in identifying any intracranial extension. CT is limited in differentiating soft tissue density in acute infection. An appropriate MRI consists of a T_1- and T_2-weighted imaging. In meningitis, patients with a contrast-enhanced MRI show dural enhancement, which is most evident along the falx cerebri tentorium and

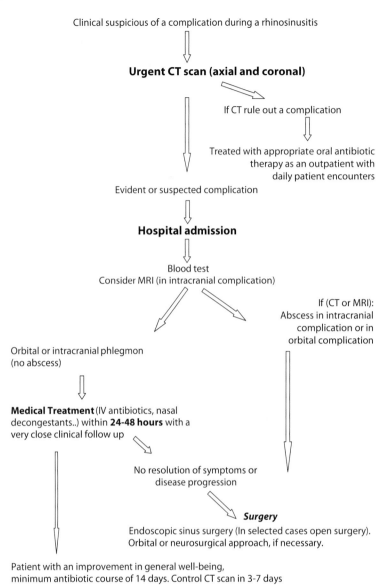

Clinical suspicious of a complication during a rhinosinusitis

Urgent CT scan (axial and coronal)

If CT rule out a complication

Treated with appropriate oral antibiotic therapy as an outpatient with daily patient encounters

Evident or suspected complication

Hospital admission

Blood test
Consider MRI (in intracranial complication)

Orbital or intracranial phlegmon (no abscess)

If (CT or MRI): Abscess in intracranial complication or in orbital complication

Medical Treatment (IV antibiotics, nasal decongestants..) within **24-48 hours** with a very close clinical follow up

No resolution of symptoms or disease progression

Surgery
Endoscopic sinus surgery (In selected cases open surgery). Orbital or neurosurgical approach, if necessary.

Patient with an improvement in general well-being, minimum antibiotic course of 14 days. Control CT scan in 3-7 days

Fig. 2.16.1 Proposed algorithm for selecting diagnosis procedure in complicated sinusitis

convexity dura, but it is not identified by CT scan. Non-contrast T_1- and T_2-weighted images are usually normal. T_1-weighted MRI images are also more sensitive in the diagnosis of cerebritis and/or brain abscesses [2].

2.16.3 Clinical Classification

2.16.3.1 Local Complication: Osteomyelitis

Sinus infection can also extend to the bone, producing osteomyelitis and eventually involving the brain or the orbit. Frontal sinus osteomyelitis with erosion of the anterior sinus wall and subperiosteal abscess produce the classic forehead swelling known as Pott's puffy tumour. Osteomyelitis of the maxilla is rare because of its excellent arterial supply. Sphenoid osteomyelitis is rare as well but when it does occur, it can be disastrous.

Other local complications can be mucoceles or mucopyoceles.

2.16.3.2 Orbital Complications

Periorbital and intraorbital inflammation and infection are the most common complications of acute sinusitis and most often are caused by acute ethmoiditis.

Orbital complications can range from a simple cellulitis to blindness. An awareness of these potential complications, their sequelae, and their management is essential for the ENT health care professional.

These disorders are commonly classified in relation to the orbital septum. The orbital septum is a sheet of connective tissue continuous with the periosteum of the orbital bones, which separates tissues of the eyelid from those of the orbit. Preseptal inflammation involves only the eyelid, whereas postseptal inflammation involves structures of the orbit. Moreover, orbital cellulitis may be a manifestation of a number of systemic diseases such as leukaemia, immunosuppressive disorders or diabetes.

There are some classifications, and they can be staged per the complications as described below: (1) periorbital (or preseptal) cellulitis, (2) subperiosteal abscess, (3) orbital abscess, (4) orbital cellulitis or (5) cavernous sinus thrombosis.

2.16.3.2.1 Periorbital Cellulitis

This type is the most commonly seen in children and is not a true orbital complication. The upper eyelid becomes swollen without evidence of orbital infection. The periorbital swelling is attributable to passive venous congestion, and the infection is confined to the paranasal sinuses. The limitation of spread of infections and oedema is imposed by the septum orbitale. There is no chemosis, limitation of the ocular movement or loss of visual acuity. In the modern era with rapid access to health care and the early use of antibiotics, this complication rarely progresses beyond this point.

2.16.3.2.2 Subperiosteal Abscess

Subperiosteal abscess complication results from the accumulation of pus at the medial aspect of the orbit, between the bone and the periorbita. The commonest origin of the infection is the ethmoid, and the key anatomic barrier preventing the progression of infection is the periorbita. Often, the globe is displaced downwards and laterally, and extraocular movement is impaired. Severe painful proptosis is a common presenting symptom and in later stages, visual acuity may be affected.

2.16.3.2.3 Orbital Abscess

Orbital abscess is a serious complication of the orbital complications. It usually results in severe proptosis and complete ophthalmoplegia. Visual acuity is impaired and may progress to blindness if urgent and proper treatment is not taken.

2.16.3.2.4 Cavernous Sinus Thrombosis

The retrograde spread of the infection to the cavernous sinus throughout the orbital veins causes cavernous sinus thrombophlebitis. This condition is usually bilateral, although of unilateral beginning. The clinical presentation is characterized by sepsis, orbital pain, chemosis, proptosis and ophthalmoplegia. This complication has a poor prognosis, with eventual progression of the infection to coma and death.

2.16.3.3 Intracranial Complications

Inflammatory disease of the frontal, ethmoid and sphenoid paranasal sinuses may extend to the adjacent anterior skull base and then intracranially. Signs of increased intracranial pressure (headache and vomiting), altered mental status or nuchal rigidity require immediate CT scanning (with contrast) or MRI of the brain, orbits and sinuses to exclude intracranial complications. Such complications often demand an interdisciplinary approach for optimal treatment.

Sinus infection may result in epidural or subdural abscess, meningitis or brain abscess. These processes may occur alone or in combination.

2.16.3.3.1 Meningitis

Meningitis is the most common intracranial complication of sinusitis in some series [3]. The most common presenting signs and symptoms were headache, fever and nuchal rigidity. Other symptoms included vomiting, behavioural changes and seizures. Leukocyte count and CSF white cell count were not associated with or indicative of the severity of the condition. Lumbar puncture was done before a CT scan to rule out any intracranial abscess or mass effect.

2.16.3.3.2 Epidural Abscess

Epidural abscess is often clinically indolent, and clinical manifestations only appear when the size of the lesion increases. The dura mater is a natural barrier to infection, and the integrity of this membrane is essential in planning surgical management strategies.

2.16.3.3.3 Subdural Abscess

Subdural empyema often is accompanied by meningitis. It may follow a severe course, with neurologic deficit, seizures and thrombosis.

2.16.3.3.4 Brain Abscess

A brain abscess starts as cerebritis, but as necrosis and liquefaction of brain tissue progresses, a capsule develops, resulting in brain abscess. The clinical presentation depends on the location, size and number of lesions. The most consistent symptom is headache refractory to symptomatic therapy and less commonly, fever, nausea, vomiting or seizures are seen. In other patients, clinical evolution could be indolent, and in the late course of the disease focal signs or altered level of conscientiousness may developed.

2.16.4 Treatment

Spread of infection from paranasal sinuses is uncommon, but when it occurs may lead to serious ocular or intracranial complications. Complicated sinusitis usually requires conservative treatment with parenteral antibiotics and decongestion nose drops. However, if there is no resolution within 48–72 hours or especially if progression of the disease is evident, then surgical intervention should be performed to minimize the sequelae. The treatment of complications of nasosinusal inflammatory processes has seen numerous modifications. Traditionally, cases with purulent collections were treated by external drainage. Currently, the introduction of new optical systems allows such complications to be approached from within the nasal cavity by endoscopic sinonasal surgery.

Treatment of patients with complicated sinusitis demands a teamwork approach consisting of otolaryngologists, neurosurgeons, infectious disease specialists and radiologists. Morbidity and mortality in complicated sinusitis relate directly to the delay in institution of therapy. Both conditions should thus be treated with great urgency [4].

2.16.4.1 Medical Treatment

The mainstay of therapy is an empiric administration of wide-spectrum antibiotics that can cross the blood–brain barrier in cases of intracranial disease. In the presence of orbital or intracranial complications of sinusitis, one must intensify the antibiotic therapy in an effort to achieve therapeutic concentrations against likely pathogens. Parenteral antibiotics are usual administered. Prompt treatment is essential, and antimicrobial drugs should not be withheld until laboratory studies are completed. Table 2.16.1 lists the recommended antibiotics, which must be administered for at least for 14 days. Topical decongestants are essential as adjuvant nasal treatment.

High-dose antibiotics, supportive care, early surgical intervention of sinus disease and early detection and management of central complications are the key elements to improve survival rates [5].

2.16.4.2 Surgical Treatment

Endoscopic sinus surgery should be considered as the gold standard treatment of acute sinusitis and its complications if conservative treatment fails. A mainstay in the treatment of any sinusal complication is eradication of the original source. When sinus disease is the origin, one must adequately treat the sinus infection to avoid the risk of re-inoculation and to facilitate clearance of the intracranial infection.

Table 2.16.1 Antibiotics of choice as empiric treatment in complicated sinusitis

Age group	Orbital complications		Meningitis	Cranial abscess	Osteomyelitis	
	First choice	Alternatives	First choice	First choice	First choice	Alternatives
Adults	Cefuroxime 1.5 g IV/8 h or amoxicillin–clavulanate 1 g/200 mg/IV/8 h	Ceftriaxone 1 g IV/12 h or cefotaxime 2 g/4 h	Ceftazidime 2 g IV/8 h + vancomycin 1 g IV/12 h	Cefotaxime 2 g IV/4 h or ceftriaxone 2 g IV/12 h + metronidazole 15 mg/kg IV/12 h	Cloxacillin 2 g/4 h IV + vancomycin 1 g IV/12 h or rifampicin 600 mg IV/12 h	Ciprofloxacin PO/IV 400 mg/12 h + vancomycin 1 g IV/12 h
Children	Cefuroxime 1.5 g IV/8 h or amoxicillin–clavulanate 40–80 mg daily IV/ divided into 3 doses ± vancomycin 15 mg/kg IV/12 h	Ceftriaxone 100 mg IV/12 h ±vancomycin 15 mg/kg IV/12 h	Cefotaxime 50–70 mg/kg IV/6 h or ceftriaxone 100 mg IV/12 h + vancomycin 15 mg/kg IV/12 h	Cefotaxime 50–70 mg/kg IV/6 or ceftriaxone 100mg IV/12 h + metronidazole 15 mg/kg IV/12 h	Cloxacillin 50–100 mg IV daily, divided into 4 doses	Vancomycin 15 mg/kg IV/12 h

IV intravenous

Surgical drainage of the sinuses is necessary in many patients, but it is planned dependent on the patient's clinical condition and response to medical therapy within the first 48 h. However, the indications for surgical intervention in postseptal infections have become more conservative in recent years.

The major advantage of the endoscopic sinus surgery is the avoidance of an external approach, with less morbidity and superior cosmesis. The endoscopic approach is a safe and convenient procedure, with excellent postoperative recovery of the patients [6].

Endonasal endoscopic surgery facilitates early access to the affected sinuses, enlarging the natural ostia and draining the infection (including the orbit [7]) from the nasal cavity [8].

Occasionally, one needs to complement the endoscopic approach with an additional open sinus approach. In endocranial complications, a craniotomy and surgical drainage are usually required.

In most cases, it is not necessary to be aggressive in the surgery of complicated sinusitis. Endoscopic sinus surgery is a safe procedure with a high success rate in the treatment of such complications. At present, a seldom-traditional approach would be indicated [6].

In osteomyelitis, the treatment of the acute infection consists of drainage and intravenous antibiotic. Once the acute infection is controlled, procedures more definitive such as debridement of devitalized bone or a frontal sinusectomy may be required. The use of long-term intravenous antibiotic has reduced the need for radical bony debridement.

References

1. European Academy of Allergology and Clinical Immunology (2005) European position paper on rhinosinusitis and nasal polyps. Rhinology 18:S1–S87
2. Younis RT, Anand VK, Childress C (2001) Sinusitis complicated by meningitis: current management. Laryngoscope 111:1338–1342
3. Younis RT, Lazar RH, Anand VK (2002) Intracranial complications of sinusitis: a 15-year review of 39 cases. Ear Nose Throat J 81:636–8, 640–2, 644
4. Greenlee JE (2003) Subdural empyema. Curr Treat Options Neurol 5:13–22
5. Donald PJ (1995) Orbital complications of sinusitis. In: Donald PJ, Gluckman JL, Rice DH (eds) The sinuses. Raven, New York, pp 173–189
6. Llorente JL, Del Campo A, Perez P, López A, Rguez N, Sequeiros G, Suárez C (2003) [Complicated sinusitis and endoscopic sinus surgery]. Acta Otorrinolaringol Esp 54:551–556 (In Spanish)
7. Manning SC (1993) Endoscopic management of medial subperiosteal orbital abscess. Arch Otolaryngol Head Neck Surg 119:789–791
8. Bhargava D, Sankhla D, Ganesan A, Chand P (2001) Endoscopic sinus surgery for orbital subperiosteal abscess secondary to sinusitis. Rhinology 39:151–5

2.17 Principles of Functional Endoscopic Sinus Surgery

JACINTO GARCÍA AND HUMBERT MASSEGUR

2.17.1 Introduction

Messerklinger's book *Endoscopy of the Nose*, written in the mid-seventies, explaining the assessment of the physiopathology of sinusitis endoscopic surgery of the nasal sinuses, has remained the standard of care for most inflammatory diseases of the sinuses. The extent of surgery for inflammatory disease has been a matter of controversy. Initially, most surgeons advocated a radical removal of the affected mucosa and the bony walls of the sinuses, whereas in most recent years, the understanding of sinus physiology has led to more conservative approaches. However, wide approaches are used for cranial base surgery, breaking the once-called boundaries of this technique.

In any case, this is an evolving field of surgery, with constant advances in techniques, instrumentation and indications. However, the basic procedures in this section are fully standardised and must be known to any ENT surgeon.

2.17.2 Equipment

The introduction of rigid endoscopes in nasal surgery has changed the way surgeons approach nasal sinuses. Different angulations allow visual control of the intricate anatomy of the paranasal sinuses. Continuous improvement of lenses has increased the field depth and the sharpness of images, allowing greater control of the operating field, without the need for excessive lens movements. In the near future, stereoscopic vision lenses will be available, as well as new instruments to improve spatial position of the surgical tools and anatomical landmarks during the surgery.

The light source must be adequate for the needs of each moment. A simple 250-W light might be enough to work directly through the optic in the office, but xenon light would be compulsory for video recording. Generally, the more elements placed between the light source and the endoscope, namely cameras, beam splitters, etc., the higher the intensity of light needed.

The fibre optic cable should be as thick as possible. It is recommended that its trajectory be the straightest possible, as each bend of the cable produces loss of luminosity.

Surgical instruments for sinus surgery are in continuous evolution, parallel to the evolution of surgical techniques. Most of them were initially designed for rhinological surgery and have been posteriorly refined to adapt to the particular needs of the endoscopic approach.

Following is a list of useful instruments. (Those considered essential are marked in boldface font.)

- Killian nasal speculum
- Bayonet forceps
- **Kuhn-Bolger buttoned probe** for frontal sinus and for maxillary sinus
- **Freer or Cottle elevator**
- **Sickle knife**
- **Blakesley forceps, straight, 45 and 90°**
- **Mackay-Grünwald cutting forceps**
- Struycken cutting forceps
- Curved turbinate scissors
- **Straight and curved suction tubes**
- **Ostrum back cutting forceps**
- **Kuhn-Bolger curette, 55 and 90°**
- **Stammberger punch** for frontal sinus and sphenoid sinus
- Stammberger antrum punch, left and right
- Kuhn-Bolger ("giraffe") forceps for maxillary sinus and frontal sinus
- Smith-Kerrison forceps 2 mm, upward and downward cutting
- Puncture trocar

Suction-irrigation systems may be useful for those who commence this technique.

Microdebriders can help in the removal of large polypoid masses, but they must be used carefully. A good understanding of the cutting settings is needed to avoid accidents. Some of the surgical steps described in this section can be performed with microdebriders (unciformectomy, middle meatal antrostomy enlargement, etc.), but results do not differ significantly, compared with the conventional technique.

Finally, navigation systems allow precise, real-time anatomic orientation during surgery. This could be particularly useful in some cases.

2.17.3 Patient Preparation

Endoscopic exploration of the nasal cavity is mandatory, and other tests like rhinomanometry or allergy test can be useful to assess the patient's status. Prior to surgery, a CT scan with sagittal and coronal views must be obtained. Careful study of the anatomical variations and pathologic conditions must be carried out. When addressing the sphenoid sinus, axial cuts are useful in identifying bulging of the internal carotid artery. Additional sagittal studies are helpful in assessing the anatomy in the frontal infundibulum and frontal recess.

The preoperative and postoperative medical treatment of nasal polyposis and chronic sinusitis is addressed in Chap. 2.13.

In some cases, the application of local anaesthesia can be useful. Surgical patties soaked in adrenaline 1:1,000 are applied to the nasal mucosa 20 min prior to the procedure. After this period, lidocaine 2% with adrenaline 1:100,000 is infiltrated submucosally in the operating area and in the area of the sphenopalatine ganglion. Mild sedation, guaranteeing deglutition reflex and correct ventilation, can be provided with midazolam, propofol or other drugs, under the surveillance of an anaesthesiologist. Nasopharyngeal packing will block the seepage of blood in the pharynx and lower airways, enhancing the comfort of both the surgeon and the patient.

When general anaesthesia is used, surgical patties are inserted into the nasal cavity, but no local anaesthetic is injected.

2.17.4 Surgical Procedures

Surgical treatment of chronic rhinosinusitis comprises "nasalisation" of the sinus cavities, consisting of opening the complex labyrinthine structures of the paranasal sinuses into a single cavity into the nasal fossa. This allows better ventilation and drainage of the affected sinuses as well as an improved distribution of inhaled medications. Nasalisation must sometimes be taken as a radical procedure including complete denuding of the surrounding bone.

The procedure can be divided into different steps
1. Uncinectomy
2. Anterior ethmoidectomy
3. Posterior ethmoidectomy
4. Sphenoidotomy
5. Frontal recess opening
6. Middle meatal antrostomy

Each of them can be performed separately in the case of localised disease, or together in a radical procedure involving all nasal structures.

After removal of the surgical patties, careful exploration of the surgical field must be performed. If the nasal polyps hamper the evaluation of the anatomical landmarks, they must be carefully removed. At regular intervals, the surgeon should stop the dissection to review the CT scan images, which should be available in the operating room during the entire procedure.

2.17.4.1 Uncinectomy

There are two techniques of removing the uncinate process, applicable according to the anatomical characteristics of each case.
1. Classic Messerklinger incision

   After palpation of its free edge to verify its "swing-door" movement, the uncinate process is incised with a Freer or Cottle dissector. The incision line is carried craniocaudally and from an anterior-to-posterior direction, parallel to the lamina papyracea, following the sickle shape of the uncinate process. In most cases, this simple manoeuvre can expose the ethmoidal infundibulum together with the anterior fontanel of the maxillary sinus (Fig. 2.17.1).
2. Uncinate process luxation

   With the angled Kuhn-Bolger probe, the uncinate process is carefully medialized (Fig. 2.17.2a). Then, the paediatric backbiting Ostrum-Stammberger forceps is

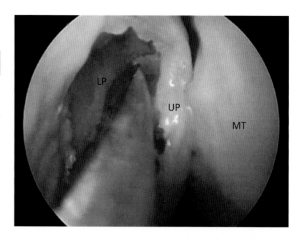

Fig. 2.17.1 Messerklinger incision. Right nasal fossa. The uncinate process is incised craniocaudally and medialized. The ethmoidal infundibulum and lamina papyracea are exposed. *UP* uncinate process, *LP* lamina papyracea, *MT* middle turbinate

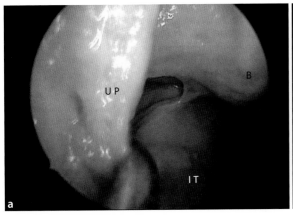 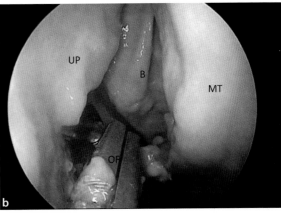

Fig. 2.17.2 a Right nasal fossa. Medial luxation of the uncinate process with a Khun-Bolger probe. *UP* uncinate process, *B* bulla ethmoidalis, *IT* inferior turbinate. **b** Right nasal fossa. Backbiting forceps cutting the uncinate process allow access to the eth- moid infundibulum and maxillary sinus. *UP* uncinate process, *B* bulla ethmoidalis, *MT* middle turbinate, *OF* Ostrum forceps (backbiting)

introduced in the infundibular space to cut transversally the vertical segment of the uncinate process (Fig. 2.17.2b). Care must be taken to remove completely the upper insertions of the uncinate process. This area has many anatomical variations, and incomplete dissections can hamper the approach to the frontal recess.

2.17.4.2 Maxillary Antrostomy

This can be either performed at the beginning of the procedure or at the end of it (Fig. 2.17.3). It is generally easier to do it right after the uncinectomy, because all landmarks are present at this point. The limits of the antrostomy are the inferior wall of the bulla ethmoidalis, superiorly; the inferior turbinate, inferiorly; and the basal lamella of the middle turbinate, posteriorly. Using a 30 or 45° rigid endoscope, the curved aspiration cannula (von Eicken) is propped against the posterior part of the inferior turbinate. Moving the instrument anteriorly will help to locate the fontanelles, through which the sinusal cavity should be entered. The opening is widened with the Kuhn-Bolger curette, Ostrum forceps, Mackay-Grünwald forceps and Stammberger forceps for access to the maxillary sinus. Care should be taken not to strip the sinus mucosa in order to avoid stenosis of the antrostomy. Lesions inside the maxillary sinus can be removed with Kuhn-Bolger angled forceps. If the antrostomy is performed at the end of the surgery, it should be noted that the only landmark present will be the inferior turbinate. This will make the risk of penetrating the orbit slightly higher. Palpation of the fontanelles must be done carefully at the level of the inferior turbinate, in a lateral and caudal direction.

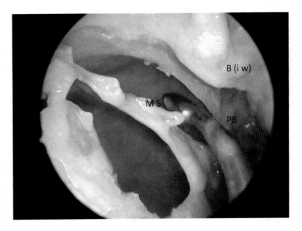

Fig. 2.17.3 Maxillary antrostomy. Right nasal fossa. The posterior limit is the vertical process of the palatine bone and the superior limit the inferior wall of the bulla ethmoidalis. *MS* maxillary sinus, *B(iw)* inferior wall of the bulla ethmoidalis, *PB* palatine bone

2.17.4.3 Anterior Ethmoidectomy

Once the ethmoidal infundibulum is dissected, the bulla ethmoidalis is exposed (Fig. 2.17.4). Anatomical variations depend on the degree of pneumatisation. With a straight aspiration cannula, pressure can be applied to its medial and inferior portion until the anterior wall is perforated. Then, the medial and inferior walls are removed with a Blakesley-Weil forceps. Laterally, the bulla ethmoidalis lies in contact with the lamina papyracea, which must be preserved. The superior wall of the bulla inserts directly into the anterior skull base. In some cases, a su-

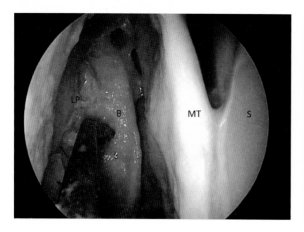

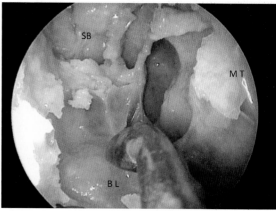

Fig. 2.17.4 Anterior ethmoidectomy. Right nasal fossa. The Khun-Bolger curette is opening the bulla ethmoidalis as the first step to enter the anterior ethmoid cells. *B* bulla ethmoidalis, *LP* lamina papyracea, *MT* middle turbinate, *S* septum

Fig. 2.17.5 Posterior ethmoidectomy. Right nasal fossa. The Khun-Bolger curette is opening the basal lamella of the middle turbinate, to enter the posterior ethmoid cells. *SB* skull base, *BL* basal lamella, *MT* middle turbinate

prabullar space can be found between the bulla and the skull base. The posterior wall of the bulla is sometimes inserted into the lamina papyracea or the basal lamella of the middle turbinate. The rest of the anterior ethmoidal cells must be elevated until the anterior ethmoidal artery relief on the cranial base is located. Dissection is finished when a single cavity limited by the cranial bases superiorly, the middle turbinate, medially, and the lamina papyracea laterally is created.

2.17.4.4 Posterior Ethmoidectomy

Landmarks for this step (Fig. 2.17.5) are the tail of the middle turbinate and the basal lamella inserting in the lamina papyracea. A suction probe or a straight curette is used to open the basal lamella in its most medial and inferior part, penetrating the posterior ethmoid. Blakesley-Weil or Stammberger cutting forceps are used to widen the opening and to excise all the cells until the ethmoidal roof is exposed. Dissection proceeds ventrally to create a cavity between the turbinate wall and the lamina papyracea that connects with the anterior ethmoidectomy.

When radical surgery is planned from the beginning, this step can be done right after opening the bulla ethmoidalis, and then proceeding with the dissection anteriorly to the anterior ethmoidal cells. When additional spatial orientation is needed, a wide maxillary antrostomy can be performed first to identify the maxilloethmoidal angle and the posterior wall of the maxillary sinus. This can be used as a regular landmark to situate the basal lamella of the middle turbinate, which is the limit between the anterior and posterior ethmoidal cells, and to assume the height of the sphenoid sinus.

2.17.4.5 Sphenoidotomy

The sphenoid sinus has a highly variable anatomy, with complex relations with the posterior ethmoidal cells and with many important structures of the cranial base, such as the carotids, the optic nerves and the hypophysis. However, if correctly performed, a sphenoidotomy (Fig. 2.17.6) is neither difficult nor dangerous when approached transnasally or via the sphenoethmoidal recess.

A 0° lens is used to localise the choanal arch, which is the most consistent landmark in finding the sphenoid recess. The straight aspiration cannula is used to enter the sinusal cavity at a point situated 10–12 mm above the choanal arch at the point nearest to the nasal septum. Sometimes the sphenoid foramen can be identified and widened with the Kuhn-Bolger curette or the Stammberger sphenoid sinus punch. Once the sphenoid sinus is opened, the posterior ethmoidectomy can be connected with the sphenoidotomy, in the case of a radical procedure.

The transethmoidal approach has to be performed in a medial direction in order to avoid entering the sphenoid too laterally.

2.17.4.6 Frontal Sinus Surgery

Dissection of the frontal recess (Fig. 2.17.7) is the most difficult step of this surgery, because of its complex anatomy and lack of specific tools to access the uppermost part of the nasal cavity. It is also the procedure with a greater number of potential complications. Identification of the main landmarks is mandatory to avoid them, beginning with identifying the frontal recess during the anterior

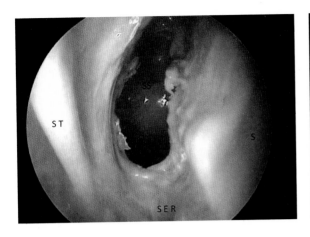

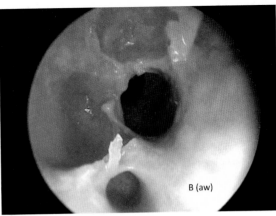

Fig. 2.17.6 Sphenoidotomy. Right nasal fossa. The sphenoid foramen widened through the sphenoethmoidal recess. The posterior wall of the sphenoid sinus can be seen through the opening. *SS* sphenoid sinus, *SER* sphenoethmoidal recess, *S* septum, *ST* superior turbinate

Fig. 2.17.7 Frontal sinus. Right nasal fossa. A 45° view of the frontal recess after removing the uncinate process and the bony walls of the cells that obscure the pathway to the frontal sinus. *FR* frontal recess, *B(aw)* anterior wall of the bulla ethmoidalis

ethmoidectomy. The ethmoidal infundibulum leads to the frontal recess, as it is its natural drainage pathway. When performing the uncinectomy, care should be taken to smoothly excise its upper insertion, for its remaining superior aspect can impede the identification of the frontal recess, thus leading to critical complications. The frontal sinus can be septated or "invaded" by ethmoidal cells, making the identification of the frontal recess even more difficult.

Angled endoscopes, 30, 45 or even 70°, must be used to approach the frontal sinus. The most useful tools are the Kuhn-Bolger probe; 45, 55 and 90° angled curettes; 45 and 90° Blakesley forceps; Kuhn-Bolger giraffe forceps; and Stammberger frontal sinus punch. The head of the patient must be tilted backwards to facilitate exposure.

The main landmarks are the
- Insertion of the middle turbinate at the lateral wall
- Lamina papyracea
- Middle turbinate itself
- Anterior wall of the bulla ethmoidalis
- Relief of the anterior ethmoidal artery

The latter will mark the posterior limit of the frontal recess, once the bulla is removed. The true recess is frequently mistaken for a small recess anterior to the artery, which is only a cul-de-sac.

When all the landmarks are identified, the barriers to the frontal sinus can be removed safely. These will be (as explained earlier) the remnants of the uncinate process and inconstant ethmoidal cells. The goal of the surgery is to provide the frontal sinus with adequate drainage and ventilation. Therefore, exerting too much pressure to enter the sinus must be avoided. Careful dissection of the bony walls obscuring this area should be continued until the recess is fully visible. (Circumferential) mucosal stripping should be avoided as this may enable osteoneogenesis, leading to frontal sinus obstruction. Enlargement of the sinus foramen is rarely necessary. On the contrary, in most cases it is contraindicated because of the risk of stenosis secondary to new bone formation. In the case of a previous stenosis, the enlargement of the frontal ostium (Drafs I, II and III) must be done in an anterior and lateral direction, avoiding the posterior wall of the frontal sinus, where the risk of a CSF leak is more likely to occur.

2.17.5 Postoperative Care

Postoperative care begins in the operating room. Meticulous removal of bone splinters and avoiding mucosal stripping will help to avoid stenosis and synechiae. Controversy arises over total or partial middle turbinate removal. These authors' approach is to consider every case at the end of the surgical procedure. If a lack of support of the turbinate is evident and chances of synechiae to the lateral wall are high, then a turbinectomy is performed. It is important to leave some significant part of the insertion to have a landmark in case a revision surgery is needed. On the other hand, if the turbinate is well preserved, and there is low risk of lateral collapse, then there is no need to remove it. Another option is to induce a synechia between the middle turbinate and the septum, scarring both structures with a curette and bringing them together so the surgical cavity will remain open.

Merocel® or similar dressing is applied at the end of the procedure, and it is left in place for 24–48 h. After this time, the dressing is removed, and debris is aspirated from the cavity. The patient is then instructed to avoid sneezing and to clean the nose with saline and vaporisers several times a day.

The healing process may last 2–6 months, depending on the alterations of the mucociliary transport induced by the surgery. In revision cases, healing takes more time. During that time, weekly visits should be scheduled to remove crusts and fibrin deposits, under endoscopic control and local anaesthesia in the office. Once the crust formation is finished and new oedematous mucosa arises from the surgical field, topical steroids are prescribed to minimise inflammatory response. If purulent discharge is present, oral antibiotics, especially macrolides, are useful to control the infection. Synechia formation must be managed early in the office setting.

Headaches are common in the postoperative period. They are mostly due to obstruction of the frontal recess by thick mucus or oedema. Topic epinephrine can be used as decongestant to help in the cleaning and aspiration of this area.

Postoperative care is one of the cornerstones of the treatment and is of utmost importance in achieving the optimal final results. The involvement of the patient in this care is important to ensure a satisfactory outcome.

Suggested Reading

1. Bernal M, Massegur H,Ademá JM, Sprekelsen C, Moina M, Fabra JM (2001) Cirugía Endoscópica Nasosinusal. Básica y Avanzada. Gràfiques Alzamora. Girona, Spain
2. Hosemann WG, Weber RK, Keerl RE, Lund VJ (2000) Minimally invasive endonasal sinus surgery: principles, techniques, results, complications, revision surgery. Thieme, Stuttgart
3. Klossek JM, Serrano E, Dessi P, Fontanel JP (2004) Chirurgie Endonasale sous guidage endoscopique. Elsevier, Paris
4. Leunig A (2007) Endoscopic surgery of the lateral nasal wall, paranasal sinuses and anterior skull base: principles and clinical examples. Karl Stortz, Tuttlingen, Germany
5. Messerklinger W (1978) Endoscopy of the nose. Urban and Schwarzenberg, Baltimore, Md.
6. Stammberger H (1991) Functional endoscopic sinus surgery: the Messerklinger technique. Decker, Philadelphia, Pa.
7. Terrier G (1991) Rhinosinusal endoscopy: diagnosis and surgery. Zambon Group, Milan
8. Wigand ME, Hosemann W (1990) Endoscopic surgery of the paranasal sinuses and anterior skull base. Thieme, Stuttgart

2.18 Endoscopic Dacryocystorhinostomy: from Diagnosis to Surgery

MANUEL BERNAL-SPREKELSEN, MANUEL TOMÁS-BARBERÁN AND ISAM ALOBID

2.18.1 Introduction

In congenital alterations of the lacrimal pathways, which are manifest from birth, a wait-and-see policy is recommended until the age of 18 to 24 months, at which time tearing usually resolves spontaneously in about 75% of cases.

Eighty percent of the lacrimal pathways belong anatomically to the nose. It is therefore feasible that dacryocystorhinostomy (DCR) may be performed via an endonasal approach. Endoscopic DCR represents a promising approach to obstruction of lacrimal pathways located in the sac and the nasolacrimal duct. Acquired obstruction of the lacrimal pathways is a common problem of elderly female patients, which can be corrected with DCR.

DCR is indicated in patients with chronic obstruction or stenosis of the lacrimal itself (saccal obstruction) or that of the nasolacrimal duct (postsaccal stenosis), when manifestations such as epiphora or repeated infections are severe enough to be bothersome. Unresolved congenital nasolacrimal duct obstruction, congenital dacryocystoceles and other indications for surgery such as punctal agenesis, lacrimal fistula, posttraumatic and postinflammatory canalicular obstruction may need to be drained surgically, as no spontaneous opening can be expected.

Probing, included in the diagnostic rationale, or stenting may avoid surgery by solving the narrowness of the pathways, but must be performed carefully in order to avoid harm.

In 1904 Toti described external DCR, and a transnasal procedure was described by West in 1911. The introduction of rigid nasal endoscopes enabled an endoscopic approach. In a cadaver study, Rice could demonstrate the feasibility of endoscopic intranasal DCR, and the first clinical study was published by McDonogh and Meiring in 1989.

The present section discusses the experience acquired in diagnostic and surgical procedures after more than 800 cases operated endoscopically.

2.18.2 Diagnosis

The key for a correct indication is to exclude presaccal stenosis, which is not suitable for an endoscopic procedure. The best method to assess the site of obstruction consists of probing the lacrimal pathways. If it is possible to pass the proximal canaliculi (superior and inferior) and to enter the superior third of the lacrimal sac through the common canalicus, a presaccal obstruction can be excluded.

Fluorescein dye tests (Jones I and II) or dacryocystographies (of any type) are no longer performed routinely. Since dacryocystographies use a probe to apply the contrast, there is no further need for a radiological evaluation if the probe passes.

CT scan may be indicated to assess dacryocystoceles, the lacrimal sac after prior surgery or after a trauma or to exclude tumours, but it is not routinely employed.

2.18.3 Surgery

Surgery is performed under general anaesthesia. Procedures under local anaesthesia have been done in cases when general anaesthesia was not recommended or when the patient preferred a local anaesthesia. In these cases, infiltration of the supratrochlear and infraorbital nerves (approximately 2 ml of bupivacaine) is added to intranasal anaesthesia. Topical anaesthesia of the lacrimal sac may be difficult when an acute infection is present.

The nasal cavity is vasoconstricted using Cottonoids soaked in topical anaesthesia with epinephrine (1:100,000). Surgery is performed with a 30 or a 45° rigid endoscope. Occasionally, the head of the middle turbinate may need to be trimmed in order to achieve a proper approach to the lacrimal sac.

During the last 6 years, these authors have incorporated a suggestion made by Massegur et al. [3]: an inferior based mucosal flap is created and pushed towards the inferior turbinate. At the end of the DCR this flap is repositioned, partially covering the lateral wall.

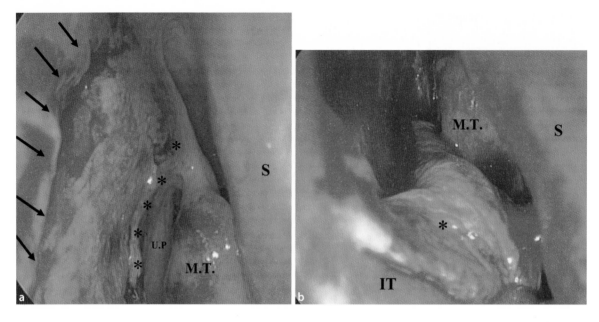

Fig. 2.18.1 a Endoscopic view into a right nasal fossa. The arrows point at the anterior vertical incision of the mucosa on the Agger nasi, the * show the posterior incision on the Agger nasi in front of the uncinate process (U.P.). M.T. = middle turbinate; S = septum. **b** The * identifies the mucosal flap pushed downwards onto the IT = inferior turbinate

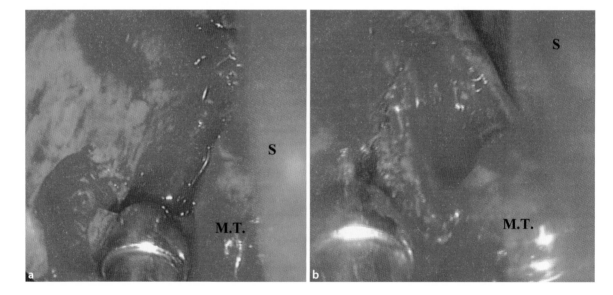

Fig. 2.18.2 a Horizontal bone removal anteriorly by drilling or with the 90° Kerrison rongeur. **b** With the 45° Kerrison rongeur a fracture line is set superiorly, the Agger nasi (frontal process of the maxillary bone) is in-fractured, then removed. The fracture-line is pointed at with the suction probe

This flap is created with the help of a Montserrat knife or a Freer elevator, used to make two vertical incisions through the mucoperiostium down to the bone, in the area of the agger nasi, slightly anterior and superior to the middle turbinate (Fig. 2.18.1a,b). Prior infiltration of this mucosa with local anaesthesia and epinephrine (1:100,000) may be useful, but is not routinely done.

Under irrigation with saline, an ear cutting burr is used to drill the ascending process of the maxilla, exposing a small section of the lacrimal sac surface. (Use of a

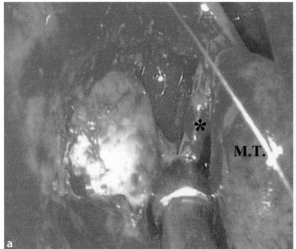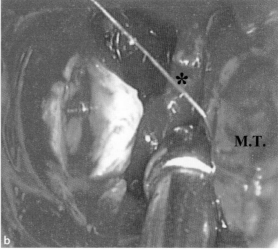

Fig. 2.18.3 a The exposed lacrimal sac (displaying a cholesteatoma-like witish colour) is pushed from outside and fixed with the help of a helper´s finger in order to avoid lateralization during the incision. The * shows remnants of the in-broken frontal process of the maxilla. M.T. = middle turbinate. **b** The sac is open like a book. It remains the surgeon's choice to resect the medial aspect or to create flaps

diamond burr is recommended until the surgeon gains experience with the procedure.) If there is any doubt about the correct identification of the lacrimal sac, the surgeon can introduce a lacrimal probe through the inferior canaliculus and then push gently; the surgeon should be able to identify the lacrimal sac by the resulting bulge. Next, a 90° Kerrison rongeur is used to remove additional bone anteriorly and a 45° Kerrison rongeur to remove the bone superiorly, until the entire medial wall and most of the anterior wall of the lacrimal sac is exposed (Fig. 2.18.2a,b). A vertical incision is then made in the anterior face of the lacrimal sac with the help of a no. 11 or a 45° Phaco knife, and the entire medial wall is removed using a straight Blakesley forceps or a true cutting forceps (Fig. 2.18.3a,b). At this point, pus or mucus usually flows from the sac. The patency of the DCR is checked by a lacrimal probe passed into the nose via the inferior canaliculus, which is seen in the nasal fossa. A silicone probe is used as a stent in each canaliculus for 2–3 weeks after the procedure. Placement of the stents facilitates postoperative care and impedes fibrous closure. Then the mucosal flap is repositioned (Fig. 2.18.2a,b). Intranasal packing, using a reduced Merocel or a foam to fix the mucosal flap, is kept in place for 1 week after surgery. More details of the surgical procedure may be consulted elsewhere [4].

A child's nose is very narrow, therefore, endoscopic DCR, especially in small children, is a technically difficult procedure. Surgery under microscope may provide an enlarged "working space", if a self-retaining speculum is used. The small size of the nostrils makes it difficult to use a drill with an endoscope inside the nose. In children

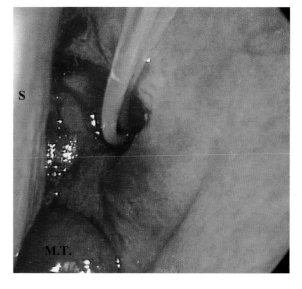

Fig. 2.18.4 Endoscopic view of the situation after reposition of the inferiorly based mucosal flap on a left side. Note that the open sac is not obliterated and the silicone probes are not located below the mucosal flap. The flap may be trimmed superiorly to avoid obliteration of the sac, if needed. M.T. = middle turbinate, S = septum

under the age of 1 year, a 2.7-mm endoscope might better fit into the nose than a 4-mm scope would. Also, handling a hammer and a chisel might be difficult and dangerous in a narrow nose. Ninety and 45° Kerrison rongeurs (Karl Storz, Germany) with a 1-mm bite are more suitable [1, 4].

No other specific instruments are needed compared to surgery in adults, but smaller forceps are recommended.

Technically, the exposure is similar to the one described in adults [1, 3]; however, a more anterior exposure of the lacrimal sac is preferred.

The silicone catheter is fixed on the nasal dorsum with Steri-Strips. In children, fixing a silicone catheter externally on the nasal dorsum is poorly tolerated. It may lead to manipulations and eventually displacements. Putting several knots endonasally prevents manipulations. It is important to allow enough of the eyelid opening before knotting the silicone catheter.

2.18.4 Postoperative Care

Postoperative care after DCR involves removal of the small piece of Merocel after 1 week, and then removal of blood clots and minor crusts once a week for the first 3 weeks.

Patients are allowed to rinse their noses with saline once or twice a day from the second week. Patients are not allowed to blow their noses during the 10 days after surgery, and they are asked to perform gentle massages of the external aspect of the lacrimal sac regularly to facilitate drainage. Eye drops containing steroids and antibiotic are prescribed for 8 weeks to provide continuous flow through the lacrimal system. Use of a lacrimal silicone stent favours the drainage of the eye drops. The silicone probes are removed after 2–3 weeks.

In children, endoscopic removal of fibrin clots and crusts is usually associated with sedation or general anaesthesia. Therefore, the indication for such a procedure should be restricted, as cases with a "second look" do not usually have an improved outcome.

2.18.5 Results

Between January 1990 and December 2007, more than 800 DCRs were performed in more than 550 patients.

The results of 133 patients who underwent DCR between January 1990 and June 1992 were evaluated 1 year after surgery. Our initial results reported DCR as "very good" by 130 patients (85.5%), as "good" by 16 patients (10.5%) and as resulting in "no change" by 6 patients (4%). Postoperative findings included synechiae (34/152 patients, or 22.4%), granulations (10/152 patients, or 6.6%) and obliterative scarring (5 cases, or 3.3%) after a 1-year follow-up. The cases of obliterative scarring relate well with the postoperative failures [1].

The majority of the more than 800 patients who underwent endoscopic DCR were women, with a predominance of 10:1 to men. The mean age was greater than 60 years. More than 120 patients were operated on bilaterally. Some patients had had previous surgery using an external approach.

In more than 60% of the cases, mucous or pus was obtained after lacrimal sac incision. Dacryoliths were seldom encountered. The histologic studies of the medial lacrimal wall showed chronic, unspecific inflammation with different degrees of cellular infiltration. No neoplasia was found. In a third of the cases the nonspecific inflammation may involve the medial lacrimal bone too.

The postoperative evaluation may be done objectively and subjectively.

The best and quickest method to assess the patency objectively is to apply fluorescein drops to the conjunctiva and to observe with the endoscope how it drains towards the nasal cavity. The patients may blink to support the drainage. In an evaluation more passive, the drainage site may be inspected endoscopically while pressing on the external aspect of the lacrimal sac, exactly in the angle of both common canaliculi. Neither fluorescein eye drops testing nor another dye test is performed routinely.

Subjective evaluation includes a "yes" or "no" answer to the question if epiphora or recurrent dacryocystitis has been resolved. Furthermore, female patients are asked if the use of cosmetics has been reinstated.

There were no major intraoperative complications. Orbital fat tissue was exposed in 16 cases (10.5%) in our first series.

Minor cheek ecchymosis (67/152, or 44.1%), subcutaneous emphysema (14/152 cases, or 9.2%) and orbital emphysema (4/152 cases), as observed initially, were no longer seen in those cases when the mucosal flap was repositioned, and since all patients are strictly advised not to blow their noses. There were no episodes of diplopia, important epistaxis, blindness, or soft tissue infection. In some patients, oral antibiotics were prescribed after purulent drainage or middle meatus inflammation was observed during postoperative endoscopy [1]. Local wound care was performed for a mean of 29 days after the DCRs in our first series, with the use of the mucosal flap this period could be reduced to a mean of 20 days.

2.18.6 Discussion

"The search for an alternative to the external approach is motivated by the desire to improve this DCR success rate and to add other advantages, such as a better aesthetic result or better compliance by the patient. The endonasal DCR is a one-stage procedure that permits correction of associated pathology, such as septal deviation or chronic paranasal sinusitis, that may be a causative factor in lacrimal obstruction".

Many newborns suffer from congenital obstruction of the lacrimal pathways. Congenital membranous stenosis of the nasolacrimal duct has been rated between 25 and 50% and incomplete stenosis as high as 50–70%. Fortunately, there is high tendency (of about 85%) of spontaneous relief of epiphora within the first 9 months of life. Thus, indication for endonasal DCR in children younger than 1 year should be studied carefully.

Malformations of the lacrimal pathways or other craniofacial malformations are more frequently manifested in children than in adults. Struck and Weidlich set the age limit for DCR at 1 year. Dilations of the lacrimal sac due to mucous collection, saccal or postsaccal stenosis secondary to trauma or infection and recurrent dacryocystitis are indications to perform DCR before that age, if probing or stenting fail. Figure 2.18.5 offers some recommendations for the stepwise approach to chronic epiphora and dacryocystitis in the paediatric age group.

In the authors' hands, primary DCR achieved a patency rate of 90.3%, and after a revision surgery the rate was 100% [2]. Twenty-four children, with a mean age of 5.6 years (range of 2–14 years) have been operated on by means of an endoscopic approach. A total of 31 sides were operated. Indications for surgery comprised relapsing dacryocystitis (*n* = 22), epiphora (*n* = 7) and two dacryocystoceles. The overall results after more than 1 year of follow-up were good in 28/31 cases. The other three cases needed a revision surgery, which was successful in all three instances. Interestingly, two children had an agenesia of the inferior punctum or canaliculus.

Kominek and Cervenka observed an overall patency rate of 82.3% after a long-term follow-up. The results are poorer when presaccal stenosis exists. Vanderveen studied 22 sides in 17 operated-on children, obtaining a complete resolution of tearing and discharge in 88%.

Technically, the narrowness of the nose is a challenge for an endonasal approach; however, the results are similar to those achieved in adults [2]. It is therefore an excellent alternative to unsuccessful probing or stenting, and clearly indicated in dacryocystoceles or other alterations that do not respond to stenting or probing.

Nasolacrimal intubation may be indicated to avoid the need for DCR for childhood epiphora that fails to resolve spontaneously despite apparently successful probing. Aggarwal et al. achieved complete resolution of symptoms in 28 cases, and only 3 (12%) needed to undergo a DCR.

Presaccal stenosis, or stenosis of the canaliculi, is not a formal contraindication for a DCR procedure, as it prepares the site for subsequent positioning of a Lester-Jones tube. Hakin et al. obtained improved results with a combination of DCR with Lester-Jones tubes in 10/11 cases with canalicular stenosis. In patients who underwent DCR with a canalicular intubation only, the results were also quite good (79%).

Since an external incision is not used, the possibility of pathologic scar formation and/or injury to the medial canthus is avoided. Furthermore, it preserves the pumping mechanism of the orbicularis muscle. Active infection of the lacrimal system is not a contraindication to intranasal DCR, as it drains mucous or pus into a contaminated nasal cavity.

Endoscopic DCR requires special training in the use of endoscopes.

For revision DCR, the endoscopic approach is superior to the external approach. The normal scarring produced after the external incision makes a revision procedure very uncomfortable, and the final aesthetic and functional results are usually poor. In contrast, endoscopic revision DCR is an easy procedure with mainly good results.

The use of the mucosal flap has reduced the cases of "lacrimal sump syndrome", in which the scarring of the opened sac leads to a "kangaroo-like" pouch retaining mucous, which may obstruct the common canaliculus.

The authors have formulated a hypothesis to explain the statistically significant preponderance of lacrimal obstruction in women. The long-term use of cosmetic products, especially on the rim of the lower eyelid, seems to be an important factor. This would explain why lacrimal obstruction most often occurs in elderly women. Arabic women, who use a special, carbon-based cosmetic around the eye (kol), showed particles of that cosmetic within the lacrimal sac, surrounded by an unspecific chronic inflammation.

The low rate of intraoperative and postoperative complications of endoscopic DCR is considered acceptable. Transient periorbital haematomas or ecchmosis, as observed in the past, appear to be due to the fact that the lacrimal sac has a more posterior location in relation to the middle turbinate than has classically been described. The use of the inferiorly based mucosal flap has reduced the incidence completely.

Synechiae occur in some 20% of cases. Most of these adhesions are minor and do not interfere with the functional result.

Treatment Algorithm in children

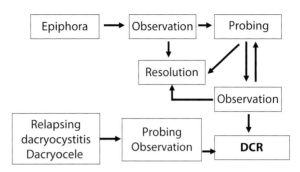

Fig. 2.18.5 Treatment algorithm for children

The classic use of the fluorescein eye drops test to determine the patency of the lacrimal system, and therefore the success or failure of an operation, is controversial. In many cases, the test results will be negative, despite the lack of patient complaints. In the authors' opinion, however, patient satisfaction (*e.g.* lack of epiphora and the ability to use cosmetics again) is the best way to judge the results of endoscopic DCR.

The preponderance of alterations of the lacrimal pathways in women, as seen by others as well, may be related to the long-term use of cosmetics. This is supported by the fact that lacrimal obstruction most commonly affects elderly women, but it does not explain the cases that occur in men.

2.18.7 Conclusion

The intranasal approach has been shown to be a safe alternative to the external approach for endoscopic DCR. The introduction of a mucosal flap to partly cover the lateral wall seems to provide a quicker healing and prevent haematomas or ecchymosis of the cheek. The results of intranasal DCR are comparable to those obtained using the external approach, and the cosmetic advantages are clear. In the near future, more ENT surgeons will be performing this surgery.

References

1. Bernal Sprekelsen M, Tomás Barberán M (1996) Endoscopic dacriocystorhinostomy. Surgical technique and results. Laryngoscope 106:187–189
2. Bernal Sprekelsen M, Massegur H, Tomas M (2003) Endoscopic sinus surgery in children. Rev Laryngol Otol Rhinol 124:145–150
3. Massegur H, Trias E, Adema JM (2004) Endoscopic dacryocystorhinostomy: modified technique. Otolaryngol Head Neck Surg 130:39–46
4. Weber RK, Keerl R, Schaefer SS, Della Rocca RC (eds) (2007) Atlas of lacrimal surgery. Springer, Berlin Heidelberg New York

2.19 Trauma of the Paranasal Sinuses and Orbit

FRANKLIN SANTIAGO MARIÑO SÁNCHEZ, ANDRES OBANDO, MANUEL BERNAL-SPREKELSEN, AND WOLFGANG ARNOLD

2.19.1 Fractures of Frontal Sinus, Midface, Nose-Orbital-Ethmoid, Zygomatic Bone and Orbital Floor

- Definition
  - Isolated or combined fractures of the paranasal bones and sinus system
- Epidemiology/aetiology
  - Common causes of face fractures are motor vehicle accidents, assaults, falls, sports and industrial accidents. Facial trauma is a serious medical and socioeconomic problem, which has fortunately decreased in recent decades in Europe, due to increased use of airbags, belts and helmets. Some reports state that frontal motor vehicle trauma has fallen from a rate of 52 to 26%.
  - Midface fractures represent 10–20% of all facial fractures, while orbital and frontal fractures represent approximately 5%. Predominantly young (20–40 years old) males (male-to-female ratio is 4:1) are injured. Zygomatic fractures are the second most common after nasal bone fractures (again, more frequent in males than in females by a 4:1 ratio). In 80% of cases, the injury is caused by a motor vehicle accident; other causes are trauma from being hit with a fist or a hard object.
- Symptoms
  - The symptoms depend on the paranasal sinus system involved into trauma.
  - In isolated fractures of the frontal, maxillary or ethmoid sinus(es), the only symptom(s) may be pain, swelling and haematoma around the area of the fracture line as well as a bloody nose.
  - In severe fractures of the orbital floor, the patient may spontaneously report diplopia, and during investigation, a deviation of the eye from the horizontal level may be observed.
  - In combined fractures involving the maxilla and zygomatic bone, clenching of the jaw may be disturbed (malocclusion) or painful. Fracture of the sphenoid cavity with disruption of one or both internal carotid arteries results in severe (in many cases), lethal bleeding through the nose.

- Complications
  - Severe bleeding
  - Subcutaneous emphysema
  - Secondary infections
  - Permanent diplopia
  - Alteration of consciousness
  - Mucocele
  - Meningitis
  - CSF leakage
- Diagnostic procedures
  - Inspection (haematoma, emphysema, asymmetry of the face, etc.)
  - Palpation of the bony structures of the nose, maxilla, zygomatic bone, orbital floor, wall of the frontal sinus and hard palate
  - Investigation of skin sensitivity to stimulus to exclude trigeminal nerve lesions
  - CT scan in three levels
  - MRI to exclude intraorbital haematoma, injury of the ocular muscles or brain injury
- Initial management in emergency cases
  - Before treating a fracture in all trauma patients, the fundamental principles of care must be applied (ensuring the patency of the airway, avoid or stop bleeding, ensure circulation and stave off shock).
  - Airway stabilisation in these patients, if necessary, should be achieved either transorally, or via a cricothyroidotomy/tracheotomy. Transnasal intubation should be avoided.
  - Accurate history of the incident
    - Mode
    - Direction
    - Intensity of traumatic force (often difficult or impossible to assess because of associated intracranial, abdominal, or intrathoracic injuries)
  - Wounds should be covered with a sterile dressing, under gentle pressure applied to control bleeding.
  - Tetanus prophylaxis and prophylactic preoperative parental antibiotics for coverage of gram-positive organisms (e.g. Cefazolin, 1 g every 30 min intravenously prior to surgery) is indicated in patients with open fractures. If there is extensive soft tissue damage, additional coverage for gram-negative organisms should be given (e.g. ceftriaxone, 1 g

30 min–2 h intravenously, before surgery); if there is continuity between injuries and the oral cavity or the hypopharynx, anaerobic bacteria should be covered (e.g. Clindamycin, 900 mg administered by intermittent infusion over at least 60 min prior to surgery).

2.19.2 Frontal Sinus Trauma

- Definition
  - Isolated or combined fractures of the anterior or posterior table of the frontal sinus
- Epidemiology/aetiology
  - The force required to fracture the frontal sinus is roughly between 363 and 907 kg. The most common cause is blunt trauma from motor vehicle accidents; the second most common cause is high-impact, sports-related injuries. Frontal sinus fractures compose 5–12% of maxillofacial trauma. The incidence is approximately 9 cases per 100,000 adults. Anterior frontal table fractures alone are a third of the cases, while isolated fractures of the posterior table are rare.
- Complications and sequelae
  - Complications are present in 2–6% of all the cases. In the first 6 months, early complications could appear. These include frontal sinusitis caused by a blocked frontal ostium, retained foreign bodies or bony chips, meningitis or a CSF leak when there is an open posterior table fracture with rupture of the dura mater.
  - Late complications may occur up to a decade after injury. These include mucoceles caused by obstruction in the frontal ostium or trapping of respiratory epithelium, mucopyocele and brain abscesses secondary to a spread of infection through the foramina of Breschet.
- Diagnostic procedures
  - Recommended European standard
    - Inspection
      - The degree of external trauma cannot predict the underlying bony and/or intracranial injury.
      - Patients may present with skin lacerations, asymmetry or depression of the forehead, haematoma and/or ecchymosed over the glabella.
      - Bony fragments or foreign bodies may protrude through an open wound.
    - Palpation
      - Pain with pressure
      - Step-off fractures or crepitus of the bony structures of the forehead and supraorbital ridge

      - Anaesthesia or paraesthesia in the supraorbital nerve distribution
    - Rhinoscopy
      - Epistaxis
      - Clear rhinorrhea, which may suggest CSF leakage
    - CT bone windows in axial and coronal views as well as sagittal reconstruction are recommended.
    - MRI must be performed to exclude brain injuries or intracranial haematoma (Fig. 2.19.1).
    - If watery fluid runs from the nose, the fluid should be tested for CSF. A minimum of 0.5 ml is collect for β-trace protein test or β-2 transferrin test. When the presence of an intermittent CSF leak or an anterior skull base defect is suspected despite a negative lab test, an intrathecal injection of 0.5–1 ml of 5% sodium fluorescein might enhance the dura at the location of the defect under endoscopic view (using UV light).
- Therapy
  - Recommended European standard
    - The goals of the therapy in this type of fracture are to
      - Restore function
      - Prevent complications
- Surgical principles
  - Important issues to consider
    - The degree of fracture displacement and injury of frontal sinus outflow tract (FSOT)
    - The involvement of the walls
    - The association with intracranial injuries
    - Presence of other facial fractures
  - Frontal fracture isolated to the anterior table
    - Nondisplacement and non-obstruction of the FSOT requires conservative treatment.
  - Displaced fracture
    - Endoscopic repair
    - Minimally invasive endoscope-assisted frontal repair is especially useful in minimally displaced fractures. The endoscope also is used to rule out CSF leaks, dura herniation or FSOT obstruction.
    - An open approach is indicated when it is not possible to repair a fracture and/or obstruction of the FSOT by a minimally invasive endoscopic technique (Fig. 2.19.2).
  - Frontal fracture of the posterior table
    - Nondisplaced posterior fracture
      - Patients with linear or nondislocated fractures without evidence of CSF leak and with an intact neurological status can be managed conservatively. Only an anterior table fracture – if dislocated – must be treated.
    - Displacement of the posterior wall

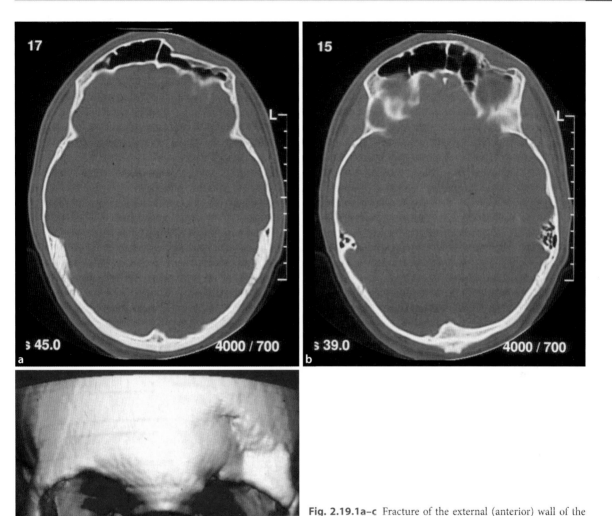

Fig. 2.19.1a–c Fracture of the external (anterior) wall of the frontal sinus. **a,b** Axial CT showing the impression of the anterior wall. **c** Three-dimensional reconstruction showing the impression

– If there is a minor displacement, and it is difficult to determine the status of the dura and underlying brain, a trepanation and transcutaneous rigid or flexible endoscopy are useful options to rule out a dura herniation into the frontal sinus. If there is a significant displacement of the posterior wall with obstruction of the FSOT, an open approach such as a coronal approach is recommended, which permits wide exposure of the frontal sinus and exploration of any dura defects. Frontal sinus obliteration should be carried out in the presence of a total obstruction of the FSOT that cannot be resolved through an endoscopic or external approach. There are different obliteration techniques; one is using abdominal fat after careful obstruction of the FSOT by using fascia or a galea-periost flap.

2.19.3 Midface Fracture

Midface fractures are also known as maxillary fractures and Le Fort fractures.
- Definition/classification
  - Le Fort introduced a classification of midfacial fractures based on cadaver experiments (Fig. 2.19.3).
    - Le Fort I
      - These are low, horizontal fractures that separate the lower alveolar and palatal regions from the upper maxilla, which results in a mobile palate, but a stable upper midface.
      - The fracture extends through the lateral nasal wall and pyriform aperture, across the maxillary alveolus and antral walls to the pterygoid plates.

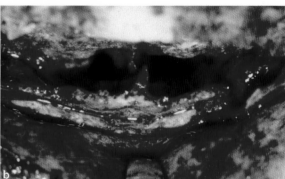

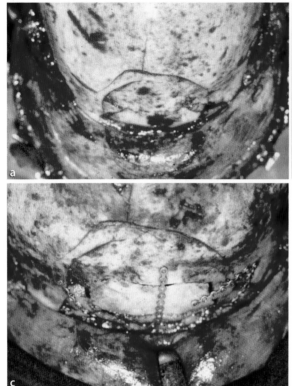

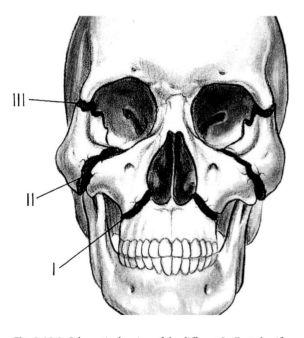

Fig. 2.19.2a–c Surgical repair of a fracture of the anterior wall of the frontal through a coronal approach. **a** Exposure of the fracture. **b** Identification of the frontal infundibulum **c** Fixation with miniplates

Fig. 2.19.3 Schematic drawing of the different Le Fort classification for midfacial fractures

- These injuries generally result from anterior forces directed at the lower midface.
- Le Fort II
  - These are pyramidal, intermediate, horizontal fractures that traverse the orbital floor and nasal bones.
  - Fractures extend through the nasofrontal suture lines, the lacrimal bones, the inferior orbital rims, across the maxillas at or near the zygomatic-maxillary suture lines, and down through the lateral maxillary sinus walls and through the pterygoid plates.
  - They result from forces applied near the level of the nasal bones.
- Le Fort III
  - These represent the most superior fracture pattern and are characterised as complete craniofacial disjunction.
  - Fractures extend through the nasofrontal sutures, the medial orbital walls, through the inferior orbital fissures to the lateral orbital wall at the zygomatic-frontal suture and across the zygomatic-temporal suture.
  - They usually result from anterior forces directed obliquely to the plane of the vertical buttresses.

– In clinical practice, Le Fort fractures are commonly found in combination.
- Symptoms
  – Le Fort I
    • Malocclusion and an anterior open-bite deformity
    • Haematomas and parietal fractures in maxillary sinuses
    • Airway compromise can occur if the palate retrusion is severe.
  – Le Fort II
    • Moderate dislocation
    • Midfacial depression, with participation of sphenoid, orbital content, lacrimal ducts (epiphora) and on some occasions, telecanthus or CSF leakage
  – Le Fort III
    • Immediately after trauma, typical symptoms of facial tumefaction, haematoma, bleeding, eventually shock, commotion or cerebral contusion, loss of vision secondary to intraorbital haemorrhage or to direct optic nerve lesion
    • Complete craniofacial dislocations, often associated with neurosurgical injuries
    • CSF leakage
    • Significant orbital trauma
    • Loss of vision and multiple fractures of the craniofacial skeleton ("dish face")
- Diagnostic procedures
  – Recommended European standard
    • Inspection
      – Asymmetries of midfacial/frontal region
      – Periorbital ecchymosis
      – Massive tissue swelling or subconjunctival haemorrhage
      – Open bite
      – Lingual/buccal region involvement
      – Subcutaneous emphysema
      – Nasal or pharyngeal haemorrhage
    • Palpation
      – Pain with pressure
      – Abnormal mobility of the palate
      – Interruption of normal face structures
      – Steps or tenderness of the underlying bony skeleton
      – Bony crepitation of the midface
      – Immobility of the jaw in all directions, malocclusion and altered state of teeth
    • Pharyngoscopy
      – Teeth avulsion
      – Mucosal injuries
      – Haematomas and ecchymosis (possible evidence of nonvisible fractures)
    • Rhinoscopy
      – Rhinorrhea

– Epistaxis
– Septal luxation
– Septal haematomas
- Visual examination (open-eye injuries and any cause of visual loss must be repaired in the first 6 h after injury)
  – Ocular movement
  – Visual acuity
  – Pupillary function
  – Campimetry
- CT scan in three levels
  – Status of the buttress system
  – Zygomatic arches
  – Orbital volume and herniation of orbital contents
- Additional/useful diagnostic procedures
  – MRI to rule out cerebral trauma or compression of the optic nerve
  – Plain film radiographs are of limited value and should only be reserved for situations in which CT is not available.
- Therapy
  – Recommended European standard
    • Priority rules for treatment (the goals of treatment are to restore function [occlusion], facial height and projection by open reduction and internal fixation)
      – Breathing
      – Severe bleeding
      – Shock
      – Brain
      – Vision
      – Nutrition
      – Fractures (the treatment of fractures should be performed when the patient's situation is stable)
    • General anaesthesia
    • Insertion of a nasogastric nutrition tube
      – In cases with additional injuries of the orohypopharynx, a tracheostomy may be necessary when long-term interdental fixation is planned.
    • In patients with functioning dentition, arch bars and maxillomandibular fixation (MMF) are initially applied. In edentulous patients, a splint or a denture containing an arch bar is fixed to the mandible or maxilla, with circum-mandibular wires or drop wires from the pyriform rim or zygomatic bone.
    • In patients with displaced midfacial fractures, a downward and anterior pull by use of the Rowe-Killey forceps will replace the maxilla and restore its normal position and relationship with the mandible and skull base.
    • Le Fort I: extended sublabial incision

– A two-point stabilisation at the nasomaxillary and zygomatic-facial buttresses is established on each side. Titanium or polyglycolic/polylactic acid, low-profile miniplates, or a combination of both, are placed on the anterior buttresses along with (usually) an L-shaped plate on each zygomatic bone onto the maxilla.

- Le Fort II: transconjunctival-lateral canthotomy or subciliary incision
  – If a greater exposure to the nasoethmoidal complex is required, an external Lynch incision or an extended coronal incision may be used.
  – Fixation at the infraorbital rim and the zygomatic-maxillary buttresses
  – If the nasal bones are comminuted, microplates are used to restore nasal contour.
- Le Fort III: the maxilla must be fixed between two stable platforms
  – The cranium provides the superior stabilisation point, and the mandible the inferior.
  – All displaced fractures of the cranial vault and mandible must be restored to their normal anatomic position. Rigid fixation of all mandibular fractures is vital to ensure this relationship.
  – Displaced subcondylar fractures must be fixed to provide a stable platform, even when only unilateral.
  – Functional elements must be restored, such as the correct orbital volume, including an adequately restored orbital floor with orbital contents free of entrapment, a patent nasal airway bilaterally and maxillary sinuses that will adequately drain.
  – The lateral orbital rims and the buttresses are fixed with miniplates and the nasal dorsum and infraorbital rims with microplates.
- If rigid fixation is considered stable, the MMF may be removed at the end of the operation or within the first 1–2 weeks after the operation. If no stability has yet been achieved, the MMF should be left in place for up to 6–8 weeks.
- Possible complications of the surgical procedure
  – Malunion and resultant malocclusion with temporomandibular joint dysfunction and deformity occur if reduction is not precise, or if loosening of fixation occurs during the postoperative period.
  – Intraoral incisions may develop partial or total dehiscence because of inadequate closure during surgery, poor oral hygiene, local trauma or excessive motion.
  – Injury to tooth roots from misplaced screw holes may result in nonviable teeth.
  – CSF leak
  – Epiphora

- Prognosis
  – Repair of simple maxillary fractures typically restores bony aesthetic contour and function; however, complex fractures often leave the patient with some long-term cosmetic and functional deficits. Early and meticulous surgery is the best way to produce results that restore the patient to the pre-trauma state.

2.19.4 Naso-Orbital-Ethmoid Fracture

A naso-orbital-ethmoid (NOE) fracture is also known as a nasoethmoidal complex fracture or a nasoethmoidal fracture.

- Definition
  – NOE fractures involve injury of the central midface; anatomically they must include the bone to which the medial canthal is attached and may be associated fractures of the frontal bone, nasal bones, lacrimal bones, ethmoid, lesser wings of the sphenoid and maxillary Le Fort fractures.
- Epidemiology/aetiology
  NOE fractures typically result from a forceful blow to the central aspect of the midface. Motor vehicle accidents are the most common cause of injury, which is followed by assault as the second most common cause of injury.
- Symptoms
  – Eye, forehead and nose pain
  – Epistaxis, clear rhinorrhea
  – Epiphora, diplopia
- Complications/sequelae
  – Long-term sequelae of NOE fractures include blindness, telecanthus, enophthalmos, midface retrusion, CSF leak, anosmia, epiphora, recurrent sinusitis, and nasal deformity.
- Classification
  – Markowitz et al. described an accepted classification system. Fractures are classified into three types based on medial the canthal tendon relationship to the central bony fractures fragment.
    - Type 1: there is a single central fragment, with the medial canthal tendon attached
    - Type 2: comminution of the central fragment, with the fracture external to the medial canthal tendon bone insertion
    - Type 3: there is a communication of the central fragment, with the medial canthal tendon disrupted from its bony insertion
- Diagnostic procedures
  – Recommended European standard
    - Inspection
      – Nasal and forehead swelling

- All facial lacerations should be examined, with the aim of ruling out a communication with intracranial structures.
  – Flattened nasal dorsum
  – Assessment of pupillary responses and extraocular muscle mobility
  – Exophthalmos
  – Shortened palpebral fissure
  – Telecanthus
    - Measurement of the intercanthal distance: the normal intercanthal distance is approximately half the width of the interpupillary distance; an intercanthal distance greater than this suggests a NOE fracture as well as a distance of 35 mm; a displaced NOE fracture is considered with a measurement 40 mm or more.
  – Palpation
    - Bimanual palpation by using a Kelly clamp is useful to determine whether a NOE fracture is present and to evaluate the integrity of the canthal tendon. With one hand, the Kelly clamp is placed into the nose under the frontal process, with the index finger of the other hand applying gentle pressure to the medial canthal tendon. A fracture is considered when a canthal or orbital wall motion is felt. Palpation of the nasal pyramid could reveal bone crepitation and retrusion of the nasal bridge.
  – Rhinoscopy
    - One should inspect for septal haematoma and epistaxis. Watery rhinorrhea suggests a CSF leak. If necessary, a sampling of the nasal fluid for laboratory testing should be collected (see Chap. 2, Sect. 2.20.4).
  – High-resolution CT (axial and coronal views) with contrast enhancement of the CSF can assist with the diagnosis of CSF leak. Plain radiographs have limited use.
- Therapy
  – Recommended European standard
    - Goals of surgical therapy include protection of orbital and intracranial contents, prevention of early and late complications, and restoration of aesthetic facial contour.
    - Surgical exposure can be obtained through a coronal incision; a subciliary incision of the lower lid parallel to and 2 mm below the lash line; or a sublabial incision or canthal stab incision, which allows the identification of the severed medial canthal tendon through a 3-mm horizontal stab incision, placed 5 mm to the medial palpebral fissure.
    - Any maxillary or frontal bone fracture should be repaired before reducing the NOE fracture.

  – Type I fracture
    - Nondisplaced, single-fragment fractures do not require surgical repair
    - A displaced fracture usually requires coronal, transconjunctival and sublabial exposure and repair with microplates, one from the frontal bone to the central fragment and one from the maxilla to the central fragment.
  – Type II fracture
    - These fractures require more extensive surgical exposure, e.g. through a sublabial, transconjunctival or coronal incision. A subperiosteal dissection is used to locate – but not to avulse – the medial canthal tendon. Usually, transnasal wiring and microplate repair of the fractures is required.
  – Type III fracture
    - These are associated with more severe trauma, which may require primary bone grafting.
      – Sublabial, transconjunctival and coronal incisions routinely are required. The medial canthal tendon must be identified, and a non-absorbable suture or wire is passed through the stump, and then a bony central fragment is identified and drilled in order to pass transnasal wires.
      – If a central fragment cannot be identified, a piece of ethmoid or maxillary bone is useful. The wire attached to the medial canthal tendon is passed through the central bone, and then continued transnasally. Eventually, the central bone is attached to the stable medial orbital bone with microplates.
      – It is important to rule out a lacrimal duct injury or a significant loss of nasal projection, which may need reconstruction.

2.19.5 Zygomatic-Maxillary Complex Fracture

A zygomatic-maxillary complex (ZMC) fracture is also known simply as a zygomatic fracture.
- Definition
  – The ZMC is a functional and aesthetic unit, constituting the central portion or malar eminence of the zygomatic bone and its attachments to the skull. A ZMC fracture is any isolated or combined fracture of the malar eminence and/or the zygomatic attachments, e.g. an isolated zygomatic arch fracture.

- Epidemiology/aetiology
  - The zygomatic bone is the major buttress of the midface between the maxilla and the skull. The prominent location of the malar eminence makes it prone to fracture. The mechanism of injury involves a blow to the side of the face from a fist, object or from a motor vehicle accident. Minimally or nondisplaced fractures are the result of a moderate force, whereas more severe blows result in displacement of the zygomatic bone or comminuted fractures that involve the inferior orbital rim, the orbital floor, the zygomatic-frontal suture and the zygomatic arch. Zygomatic fractures are the second most common facial fracture after nasal bone fractures. More than 80% occur in men.
- Symptoms
  - Soft tissue swelling in the area of fracture, pain and trismus
  - In some cases, diplopia
  - Unilateral epistaxis
- Complications/sequelae
  - Diplopia
  - Loss of vision
  - Lower eyelid malposition (ectropion, entropion)
  - Enophthalmos
  - Malocclusion
  - Complications related to the material used for reconstruction, which requires its removal
- Diagnostic steps
  - Recommended European standard
    - Inspection
      - The most common findings are swelling and haematoma, malar and periorbital ecchymosis and malar depression or flattening.
      - Trismus is present in 15–27% of the cases, associated with a masseter spasm and/or impingement of the fracture on the movement of the mandible.
      - Ophthalmic findings include inferior displacement of the lateral canthal tendon, subconjunctival haemorrhage and proptosis; acute and severe orbital haematoma may cause loss of vision by compression of the ophthalmic artery or optic nerve.
    - Palpation
      - Pain on palpation and crepitation from subcutaneous emphysema (which in most cases is caused by blowing the nose)
      - Bony step-off when palpating the infraorbital rim, the frontal zygomatic suture line and intraoral in the zygomatic-maxillary buttress
      - Anaesthesia caused by compression of the infraorbital trigeminal branch
    - Rhinoscopy
      - Ipsilateral blood accumulation or epistaxis

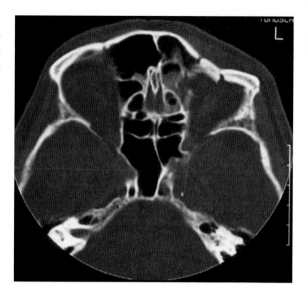

Fig. 2.19.4 Axial CT of the fracture of the zygomatic arch

- High-resolution CT (axial and coronal views) of the orbit and sinuses is the standard imaging method for evaluation and treatment planning. A Waters view radiograph may show evidence of the zygomatic arch fracture and subsequent displacement (Fig. 2.19.4).
- Therapy
  - Recommended European standard
    - Not all ZMC fractures require surgical intervention. In many cases, it is necessary to wait until tissue oedema has resolved, and any deformity can be better appreciated. Patients with nondisplaced or minimally displaced ZMC fractures and a normal ophthalmologic examinations can be treated conservatively. The indications for a surgical treatment include facial contour alteration, persistent difficulties in chewing, visual changes secondary to muscle entrapment, globe displacement and orbital floor disruptions. Medical management includes a soft diet and analgesia.
- Surgical principles
  - The goals of surgical therapy include prevention of early and late complications, and restoration of aesthetic facial contour.
  - An adequate – but not excessive – exposure is necessary to achieve a satisfying functional and aesthetic result. The surgical approach depends on the part of the ZMC unit involved by the fracture.
    - Zygomatic-maxillary buttress
      - A transverse buccal sulcus incision is well hidden and exposes the entire face of the maxilla.

- Frontozygomatic buttress
  - There are three recommended approaches
    - Upper lid blepharoplasty incision, which provides an excellent access to the frontozygomatic suture line
    - Lateral brow incision, which has a higher risk of visible scaring when compared with the upper lid blepharoplasty
    - Hemicoronal incision, which provides wide exposure to the zygomatic and frontal bones
- Infraorbital buttress
  - The orbital rim incision is a faster procedure than the eyelid incisions are, but results in a visible cutaneous scar and may be associated with persistent lower eyelid oedema.
  - The transconjunctival approach provides excellent exposure to the orbital rim and floor and has a low risk of lid ectropion when compared with the subciliary approach.
- Zygomatic arch buttress
  - A direct percutaneous approach could be used in a mild displaced fracture; it is not useful when soft tissue oedema is present, and does not allow a direct observation and bimanual surgical manipulation.
  - The temporal approach, or Gillies approach, is frequently used for isolated fractures that are mild to moderately displaced; it has the advantages of protection of the facial nerve, makes possible a bimanual reduction of the fracture and there is no visible scar.
  - The hemicoronal approach is reserved for severe injures with marked comminution of the zygomatic-maxillary complex.
- When a rigid fixation is necessary, it is done with miniplates, which has some advantages, such as adding stabilisation to the fracture site in three spatial planes, allowing easy fixation and avoiding the possibility of rotating a bone graft or disrupting repaired comminuted fractures.
- Peri- and postoperative antibiotics are administered for 7 days.
- The patient must be evaluated for visual loss during 48 h postoperatively.
- Prognosis
  - Long-term prognoses in ZMC fractures are very good.
    - Three to 4% of the patients have residual facial asymmetry, requiring surgical revision.
    - Persistent diplopia is reported in 7% of the patients, this being the most common ophthalmologic complication and sequela.

2.19.6 Fractures of the Orbital Floor

Fractures of the orbital floor are also known as blowout fractures.

- Definition
  - The true "blowout" is a fracture of the orbital floor, without fracture of the orbital rim, resulting from blunt trauma to the bulbus oculi. However, in many cases of blowout fractures, the orbital rim is involved.
- Epidemiology/aetiology
  - A blowout fracture originates from direct anterior orbital trauma, such as from a fist or a (tennis) ball. The orbital rim remains intact, but the force of the impact is transmitted from the orbital content to the delicate bones of the orbital floor and/or medial wall, causing fractures and displacement into the maxillary and/or ethmoid sinus.
- Symptoms
  - Enophthalmos
  - Diplopia
  - Reduced ocular motility (much more evident when looking upward, because of entrapment of inferior ocular muscles)
  - Periorbital oedema
  - Subconjunctival haemorrhage
  - Reduced sensibility of the infraorbital branch of trigeminal nerve (see Fig. 2.19.2)
  - Periocular air emphysema after nose blowing
- Complications
  - Possible loss of vision is the most ominous complication
  - Permanent diplopia, neuralgia and ocular muscle dysfunction
  - Recurrent sinusitis maxillaris
- Diagnostic procedures
  - Recommended European standard
    - Palpation
      - A search for bony displacement should be done. A bony step can be palpated at the lower rim of the orbit.
      - A check for sensitivity of the infraorbital nerve should be made.
    - Inspection
      - Periorbital haematoma
      - Subconjunctival haemorrhage
      - Enophthalmus
      - CT scanning without contrast provides views of high-density bone. Both axial and direct coronal 1.5- to 2.0-mm cuts to properly evaluate the orbit and its floor should be obtained (see Fig. 2.19.2).
      - MRI enables multiplanar imaging and is excellent for evaluating intraorbital haema-

toma, dislocated soft tissue masses and optic nerve pathology.

- Therapy
  - Recommended European standard
    - Conservative therapy
      - Not all orbital floor fractures require exploration and repair.
      - An afferent pupillary defect is an emergent case, and a lateral canthotomy with cantholysis is indicated if there is any evidence of increased intraorbital pressure or optic nerve lesion.
- Indications for surgery
  - Entrapment of the extraocular muscles, resulting in gaze limitation or diplopia
  - Sagging of orbital fat (hernia), with or without enophthalmos or diplopia
  - Imaging studies revealing a greatly increased relative orbital volume (greater than 5–10% relative increase when compared with the noninjured side) due to the loss of the orbital floor and sagging of the contents into the maxillary sinus.
  - Immediate decompression of the optic nerve is necessary when the lateral orbital wall (orbital plate of the sphenoid bone) impacts the orbital apex or middle cranial fossa.
  - The ideal time for the repair of blowout fractures is either immediately or 7–14 days after the injury, when the oedema/haematoma have been resolved.
- Surgical technique
  - Transconjunctival, subciliary, inferior fornix or mid-lower eyelid incision
  - Orbital contents are then raised out of the fracture line and supported with a titanium plate, thinned cartilage, bone fracture elements to be found in loco, resorbable plate or polydioxanone (PDS) plate
  - Alternatively, a transmaxillary approach with reposition of the fat hernia and stabilisation of the bone fragments by using a balloon catheter is recommended. The catheter is drained through the nose via a bony window drilled through the medial maxillary sinus wall in the direction of the nasal cavity

(anterior part of the lower turbinate). This method has the unique advantage of correcting the level of the orbital floor if necessary postoperatively, by increasing or reducing the fluid pressure in the balloon.

- Prognosis
  - Successful repair of orbital blowout fractures may be complicated by persistent problems. Neuralgia in the distribution of the infraorbital nerve may worsen after surgery. Improvement of this problem, if any, may take 6 months or more. More troubling is persistent diplopia. Enophthalmos can worsen over time. Despite adequately repairing the fracture, atrophy of the orbital fat can occur, resulting in further enophthalmos.

Suggested Reading

1. Chen KT, Chen CT, Mardini S et al. (2006) Frontal sinus fractures: a treatment algorithm and assessment of outcomes based on 78 clinical cases. Plast Reconstr Surg 118:457–468
2. Chowdhury K, Andrews B (2003) Fractures of the midface, naso-orbital-ethmoid complex and frontal sinus. In: Dolan RW (ed) Facial plastic, reconstructive, and trauma surgery. Informa Healthcare, New York, pp 549–595
3. Fraioli ER, Branstetter BF, Deleyiannis FW (2008) Facial fractures: beyond Le Fort. Otolaryngol Clin N Am 41:51–76
4. Larry A (2007) Nasoethmoidal orbital fractures: diagnosis and treatment. Plast Reconstr Surg 120:16–31
5. Linnau KF, Hallam DK, Lomoschitz FM et al. (2003) Orbital apex injury: trauma at the junction between the face and the cranium. Eur J Radiol 48:5–16
6. Manolidis S, Hollier L (2007) Management of frontal sinus fractures. Plast Reconstr Surg 120:32–48
7. Stack BC, Ruggiero FP (2006) Maxillary and periorbital fractures. In: Bailey BJ, Johnson JT, Newlands S (eds) Head and neck surgery, otolaryngology, vol 1, 4th edn. Lippincott Williams and Wilkins, Philadelphia, Pa. pp 975–993
8. Stanley R (1996) Maxillofacial trauma. In: Cummings CW (ed) Otolaryngology head and neck surgery, vol 1, 3rd edn. Mosby, St. Louis, Mo., pp 453–485

2.20 Endoscopic Repair of Anterior Skull Base Defects

MANUEL BERNAL-SPREKELSEN, ISAM ALOBID, JOAQUIM MULLOL
AND ALFONSO GARCIA-PIÑERO

2.20.1 Introduction

Endoscopic repair of defects of the anterior skull base has progressively been introduced in preference to the more aggressive external approach. Different techniques of skull base reconstruction have been proposed, achieving overall results of between 75 and 100% for primary surgery [1, 2].

Ascending bacterial meningitis has been reported as a consequence of these skull base defects and may in fact occur years after trauma or in the absence of active leakage [3]. Endoscopic repair of anterior skull base defects, with or without an active CSF leak, seems to prevent ascending bacterial meningitis in the long term [3]; thus, the endoscopic approach seems to be the technique of choice when approaching anterior skull base defects. One major advantage is that this type of surgery has negligible morbidity.

2.20.2 Diagnosis

The first step in approaching a CSF leak or an anterior skull base defect is to consider if unilateral watery rhinorrhea or bacterial meningitis is present. (The authors have seen some patients who, before the possibility of a skull base defect was explored, were treated for unilateral rhinorrhea with antihistamines for allergic rhinitis], and others for two or more episodes of bacterial meningitis.) In cases with trauma the diagnosis seems obvious, but not as so much in cases with old defects or with spontaneous CSF leaks.

The diagnostic approach is based on biochemical and endoscopic studies, reinforced with imaging, CT scan and/or MRI.

It is not enough to rely on glucose testing of secretions; instead, β_2-transferrin or β-trace verification in samples allows positive and pathognomonic assessment. However, negative tests do not exclude a skull base defect. CSF leaks may appear intermittently or result in a spontaneous closure secondary to brain herniation or to scarring of the arachnoid mater and the nasal mucosa (Fig. 2.20.1). The dura mater itself has little capacity to produce fibroblasts.

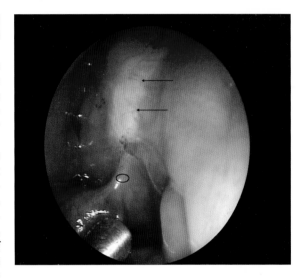

Fig. 2.20.1 Spontaneous closure of a CSF leak after FESS. Note growth of a new mucosa layer upon the dura (*arrows*), which, with scarring of the arachnoid, may stop CSF leakage but not bacterial ascending meningitis, as suffered by this patient before. Fluorescein shines through the dura. The *circle* shows attachment of the middle turbinate to the skull base

Endoscopic assessment of skull defects is useful when there is an active CSF leak, when the dura/brain shows pulsations in cases in which the bone is missing, or when sodium fluorescein has been applied intrathecally, enhancing CSF or the dura. If biochemical testing was positive, intrathecal application of sodium fluorescein should be reserved for the surgical procedure.

During surgery of the skull base, such as for optic nerve decompression or benign or malignant tumours, etc. where a skull base defect with or without a CSF leak is expected, the authors strongly advise applying sodium fluorescein intrathecally. It is very helpful not only in assessing the defect and CSF leak, but also to assess impermeable closure of the leak and the defect performed after, e. g. tumour removal. In other cases, it may be helpful for the differential diagnosis of, e. g. pseudo-rhinorrhea from the Eustachian tube.

Dosage of sodium fluorescein is 0.5–1 ml in a 5% concentration. As sodium fluorescein's specific weight is lower than that of CSF, the patient should be fixed in

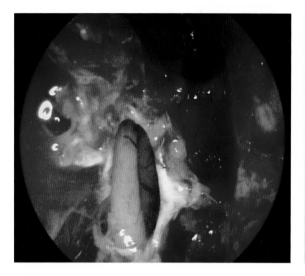

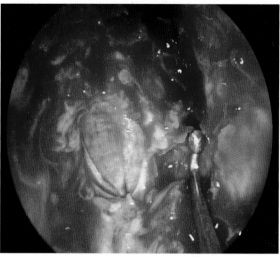

Fig. 2.20.2 Defect of the cribriform plate, with opening of the dura, and the olfactory bulb within the anterior cranial fossa

Fig. 2.20.3 Fascia lata has been positioned upon the dura. Intracranial pressure and pulsations press the fascia towards the dura

the Trendelenburg position, that is, head down and legs up for about 30–45 min before surgery. As this position tends to increase bleeding during surgery, during anterior skull base reconstruction the patients is in a semi-sitting position, and when the moment comes to assess the impermeable closure, the authors revert the patient's position to that of Trendelenburg. Orange light enhancement of fluorescein and Wood's (blue) light to assess fluorescein can be used in cases where the leak is not obvious or active.

Intrathecal sodium fluorescein application is contraindicated in cases of known allergy, recent traumas of the head and in convulsive disease. Complications have been described as being dose dependent, and low if recommended dosages are respected [4].

Imaging of skull base defects is helpful both in large and in small anterior skull base defects. In unclear cases it is important to ask for a 2-mm-slice CT scan. MRI gives additional information when soft tissue is present, e.g. concerning brain herniation, meningoceles or encephaloceles, tumours, etc.

fMRI, unfortunately not available everywhere, may show CSF displacement or circulation. Cisternography is seldom used because active leaks are better diagnosed with a noninvasive method, but it is frequently ordered by other specialists when attempting to diagnose skull base defects.

Ophthalmological fundus exploration may be helpful to exclude or confirm indirect signs of endocranial hypertension.

2.20.3 Surgical Technique

Usually, surgery of defects of the ethmoidal roof and the cribriform plate includes an anterior ethmoidectomy in order to identify the exact entrance of the anterior ethmoidal artery into the endocranium. This prevents its lesion and subsequent intracranial bleeding.

It is of utmost importance to assess the real extension of the defect or leak. After surgery or trauma, the leak might appear smaller than it is. Therefore, bone near the defect or leak has to be palpated to check its potential mobility. Smaller bony fragments should be removed in order to avoid circumscribed osteitis, which may lead to osteal failure. Surrounding mucosa needs to be dissected, leaving bone denuded. Thus, mucosal free flaps are able to adhere to the bone, form a matrix and grow.

Reconstruction of the dural defect depends on its location. A certain type of "underlay" technique is advisable to prevent opening secondary to increased intracranial pressure. Therefore, any material used to reconstruct should be placed either on the dura (from inside) or in between the dura and the bone (Figs. 2.20.2, 2.20.3). This is particularly difficult at the cribriform plate, where no underlay or onlay (on the inner face of the dura) is possible medially. Here it seems to be of help to bend the material towards the crista galli, in an L-shaped fashion. Only in small-millimetre defects do the authors prefer a "bathtub-plug" technique, with autologous fat.

The reconstruction of the lateral wall of the sphenoid sinus requires removal of its anterior bony wall and then drilling laterally. A view within the sphenoid sinus is not difficult to achieve, but to being able to work inside that sinus requires a large opening.

Many autologous tissues have been proposed for use in skull base reconstruction. Interestingly, all seem to work, as the results from the literature show. It is therefore up to the surgeon to decide with which material he/she prefers to work. In the authors' hands lyophilised fascia lata has been shown to adapt quite well. In larger defects it is positioned in a tile-shaped fashion to support intracranial pressure. A trick to measure the size of the defect and trim the corresponding fascia lata is to introduce a 45° Blakesley forceps into the defect; the size of fascia used should double the size of the defect.

A free mucosal graft from the middle or inferior turbinate covers the reconstruction (Fig. 2.20.4) and is adapted by means of the use of Oxycel®. Some authors suggest the use of fibrin glue to fix the mucosa; however, the authors usually find enough blood surrounding the field, which enables fixation of the mucosal graft. Experimental studies have shown mucosa to be fixed after 6 days. This is the period the authors chose for the nasal packing. Another finding of that study was that a mucosal free graft tends to shrink to about 25% of its original surface. Thus, it is recommended to prepare a graft larger than initially estimated.

Lumbar drainage is not used routinely.

2.20.4 Postoperative Handling

Patients receive antibiotics during the period of nasal packing. They are asked not to blow their noses or to

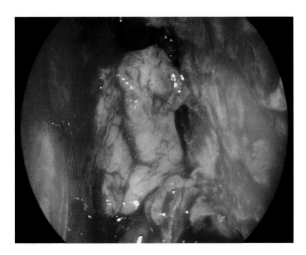

Fig. 2.20.4 A two-layer reconstruction is achieved with a free mucosal graft from the middle or the inferior turbinate. The graft is then fixed by Oxycel®

sneeze open mouthed for about 10 days. They have bed rest for 72 h, with the head elevated 30–40° to reduce intracranial pressure. Subcutaneous heparin treatment should be administered during this time.

Follow-up can be performed once every week to reduce granulation tissue until the defect is covered with mucosal epithelium. Pre- and postoperative assessment of sense of smell is not regularly performed.

It is important to avoid increased abdominal pressure, which would likely result in increased intracranial pressure via venous transmission. Prevention includes prescription of stool softeners with a fibre-rich diet. Patients are also advised not to perform any type of physical exercise for the next 4 weeks (lifting bags or luggage, weights, scuba diving).

2.20.5 Results

Primary surgery of CSF leaks achieves results between 75 and 100%. However, series are difficult to compare because indications, surgical techniques and time of follow-up differ.

Poorer results have been reported in the long term after reconstructions with advancement or rotations flaps coming from the turbinates or the septum [5].

2.20.6 Discussion

Benign intracranial hypertension has been thought to represent a potential cause of idiopathic CSF leaks. Most spontaneous CSF leaks appear in female patients with a tendency towards obesity. Schlosser et al. proposed intrathecal measurements postoperatively; however, invasive diagnostic procedures are accepted with difficulty by asymptomatic patients.

Useful algorithms have been published for the management of CSF leaks [6].

Antibiotic prophylaxis in patients with CSF leaks may be counterproductive. In an extensive review, Rathore et al. found an incidence of 8% of bacterial meningitis in 803 patients treated prophylactically with antibiotics when diagnosed with CSF leaks, compared with only 3% of 389 cases in which no such prophylaxis was prescribed. The explanation may be found in the sub-inhibitory CSF concentration many antibiotics achieve when no infection exists, as they cannot cross the blood–brain barrier in the absence of infection. Thus, pneumococci are reduced, but other microbes such as *Staphylococcus aureus*, gram-negative bacteria or even fungi can grow.

A true indication for prophylactic treatment with antibiotics prevails in the following cases: traumatic leaks or penetrating trauma, iatrogenic leak with infected sinuses, CSF leaks and infected sinus(es), and meningitis. Here, amoxicillin 500 mg/12–24 h or fluoroquinolones (levofloxacin 500 mg/day, or moxifloxacin 400 mg/day) can be used.

It is the recommendation of the Neurosurgery Working Party British Society for Antimicrobial Chemotherapy [7] not to treat prophylactically the following cases: idiopathic CSF leaks, iatrogenic CSF leaks (without infection), CSF leaks secondary to malformation, and CSF leaks secondary to tumour.

β_2-transferrin assessment of active leaks has nowadays been substituted by β-trace determination, which can be performed by nearly any laboratory.

Many different materials have been proposed for the anterior skull base reconstruction: fascia (lyophilised)/(dura), fat (abdominal)/muscle, perichondrium, mucosal grafts, pedicled grafts (septum, middle turbinate) and cartilage/bone [1]. Interestingly, they all seem to work relatively well [2]. The reported overall percentages of closure by means of the endonasal procedure (microscopically and endoscopically) range between 75% and 100% after a first attempt, which rises to 95–100% after a second procedure [3].

Free mucosal grafts seem to be better for closing minor defects than are pedicled grafts or flaps, which may arch or retract during the healing process. Moreover, fistulas treated with local nasal mucosa advancement flaps had a higher rate of failures in the long term [5].

According to Mattox and Kennedy, defects larger than 10 mm must be provided with a bony scaffold to prevent encephaloceles or meningoencephaloceles in the long term. A tile-shaped reconstruction with fascia lata for larger defects provided stable reinforcement for the dura [3].

Lyophilised dura was described to potentially transmit viral disease and thus had to be dismissed as reconstruction material.

Fibrin glue is frequently recommended to improve the attachment of the free mucosal graft. In most cases it is felt that, even with little blood in the operative site, the free mucosal flap adapts well and remains attached to the skull base [3, 8]. This can only be achieved if CSF loss has been terminated, as CSF would certainly detach the mucosa. In cases in which the leakage cannot be halted with only the underlay reconstruction, the use of fibrin glue may be indicated.

No obliteration is recommended after repair of defects in the sphenoid sinus. In these cases, the sinus may be filled with absorbable material, which can be removed 2–3 weeks later. Proceeding as such, mucocele of the sinus can be prevented.

Intrathecally applied sodium fluorescein helps to identify all active leaks; in cases with skull defects, stained CSF can be recognised through the dura or weakened skull base. During surgery it is crucial to assess the impermeable closure of the leak. The complication rate after intrathecal fluorescein application is rather low [4].

Although some authors recommend lumbar drainage, many others have excellent results without it; thus, it may be concluded that there is no need for lumbar drainage if no underlying endocranial hypertension has been found. Moreover, lumbar drainages bear the risk of meningitis, leakage of CSF at the drain site and brain herniation (bed rest is advised).

Collateral measures, some of which have been recommended elsewhere, such as avoiding increased intra-abdominal pressure, reducing intracranial pressure with orthostatic positions, prescribing relaxant medication, prohibiting nose blowing and sneezing with the mouth closed, as well as avoiding physical exercise for a certain period have a positive affect on the final outcome.

The rate of complications after endonasal skull base surgery seems to be low according to the literature, considering the number of procedures that have been performed. Two cases of meningitis, one intracerebral abscess, one case with infection of the thigh, two frontal mucoceles [9] and one intracranial mucocele have been reported. Weber et al. report loss of olfaction disturbances in 17% of cases. This figure seems acceptable, especially considering the risk of bilateral olfaction loss associated with a craniotomy.

Conservative management of dural defects had only a 50% success rate. Moreover, after conservative management of CSF leaks, the rate of ascending bacterial meningitis may be as high as 18.5% [10]. In the light of these findings and the excellent results and low complication rate reported after minimally invasive endonasal surgery, endoscopic skull base revision for patients with CSF leaks is strongly recommend and especially in those with prior ascending bacterial meningitis, even if the CSF leak is not active. Minimally invasive endoscopic reconstruction of the skull base and closure of the CSF leak provides long-term protection against ascending bacterial meningitis in patients who had, and in others who had not, previously suffered such meningitis [3]. Vaccination may be considered as an alternative in cases in which surgery is contraindicated or refused. Nevertheless, vaccination is limited to few microorganisms and has to be repeated.

2.20.7 Conclusion

Intrathecal sodium fluorescein application helps to identify a CSF leak and confirm its impermeable closure. No complications were observed secondary to the use of fluorescein.

Lyophilised transplants in an underlay position together with free mucosal grafts seem to provide excellent long-term results in the reconstruction of defects of the anterior skull base associated with CSF leakage. Furthermore, closure of CSF leaks prevents recurrent episodes of ascending meningitis in the long term, unless new CSF leaks appear. In patients with no previous record of meningitis, reconstruction of anterior skull base defects and/or termination of CSF leaks prevented infection in all cases. Therefore, closure of CSF leaks and repair of skull base defects (even without an active CSF leak) should be considered the standard of care to prevent ascending bacterial meningitis and thus, be included in management algorithms for CSF rhinorrhea/anterior skull base defects. Conservative leak management, even when the active leaks stops, seems to be risky.

References

1. Hosemann WG, Weber RK, Keerl RE, Lund VJ (2000) Minimally invasive endonasal sinus surgery. Thieme, Stuttgart, pp 76–79
2. Hegazy HM, Carrau RL, Snyderman CH, Kassam A, Zweig J (2000) Transnasal endoscopic repair of cerebrospinal fluid rhinorrhea: a meta-analysis. Laryngoscope 110:1166–1172.
3. Bernal-Sprekelsen M, Alobid I, Mullol J, Trobat X, Tomás-Barberán M (2005) Closure of cerebrospinal fluid leaks prevents ascending bacterial meningitis. Rhinology 43:277–281
4. Keerl R, Weber RK, Draf W, Wienke A, Schaefer SD (2004) Use of sodium fluorescein solution for detection of cerebrospinal fluid fistulas: an analysis of 420 administrations and reported complications in Europe and the United States. Laryngoscope 114:266–72
5. Gassner HG, Ponikau JU, Sherris DA, Kern EB (1999) CSF rhinorrhea: 95 consecutive surgical cases with long term follow-up at the Mayo Clinic. Am J Rhinol 13:439–447
6. Lund V (2002) Endoscopic management of cerebrospinal fluid leaks. Am J Rhinol 16:17–23
7. Working Party of the British Society for Antimicrobial Chemotherapy (1994) Antimicrobial prophylaxis in neurosurgery and after head injury. Lancet 344:1547–51
8. Mirza S, Thaper A, McClelland L, Jones NS (2005) Sinonasal cerebrospinal fluid leaks: management of 97 patients over 10 years. Laryngoscope 115:1774–1777
9. Stammberger H, Greistorfer K, Wolf G, Luxenberger W (1997) Operativer Verschluss von Liquorfisteln der vorderen Schädelbasis unter intrathekaler Fluoreszeinanwendung. Laryngorhinootologie 76:595–607
10. Bernal-Sprekelsen M, Bleda C, Carrau R (2000) Ascending meningitis secondary to traumatic cerebrospinal fluid liquid leaks. Am J Rhinology 14:257–259

2.21 Smell Disorders

ISAM ALOBID, JOSEP DE HARO, AND JOAQUIM MULLOL

2.21.1 Introduction

The sense of smell is primal for humans, and one of the important means by which we receive information from our environment. Smell can provide pleasure or warn of danger (e. g. noxious fumes, spoiled food). Smell dysfunctions often produces considerable disability and a poor quality of life. Their aetiology often remains obscure, and physicians will often proceed with a full neuroradiological evaluation, which in most cases is unwarranted and often provides little insight into the underlying pathology.

It is well known that women have greater olfactory sensitivity than men have. Although the exact reason for this difference remains unclear, social, hormonal or genetic factors are thought to be involved [5]. The ability to smell subsides with age, diminishing quality of life and impairing good nutrition. However, the complaint of smell loss should never be attributed solely to age; other causes should be investigated. Smoking leads to a mild but significant decrease of olfactory function, related to the number of cigarettes smoked: however, this decrease can be reversed after smoking cessation is achieved.

The prevalence of chronic smell problems was estimated at 1.42%, or 2.7 million Americans, by the National Health Interview Survey (NHIS). In a recent study of individuals aged 53–97 years, 25% were found to have impaired olfactory function [7]. Two thirds of patients with smell loss not only complained of decreased olfactory function, but also of gustatory loss, and approximately 10% of patients with smell disorders complained of gustatory loss only [2].

2.21.2 Defining Smell Disorders

Numerous terms have been used to describe the manifestations of smell dysfunction:
- *Anosmia* describes the complete loss of detection and recognition of smell.
- *Hyposmia* refers to the general decreased sense of smell.
- *Hyperosmia* is a rare condition that is defined as an increased sensitivity to all odours.

- *Dysosmia* describes a distortion of the sense of smell, and may be the presence (*parosmia*) or absence (*phantosmia*) of a stimulant odour.
- *Cacosmia* occurs when a normally pleasant odour is inappropriately detected as foul or unpleasant.
- *Heterosmia* is the inability to smell one of the few odours in the presence of an otherwise-normal sense of smell.
- *Agnosia* describes the inability to contrast or classify odours, although with the ability to detect them.

2.21.3 Evaluation and Diagnostic Methods

2.21.3.1 History

Having a complete history of the smell dysfunction is the initial and most important step in patient evaluation. The history of the onset and course of the disorder is often paramount in establishing aetiology. This should include demographics, diet, (major) illnesses, medications, hormonal alterations (including questions regarding menstrual status) and nasal symptoms (rhinorrhea, nasal blockage, loss of smell). The patient should be asked about the use of tobacco or cocaine, since these substances can adversely affect the sense of smell. Questions should also be directed to identify any family history of systemic diseases such as diabetes mellitus or hypothyroidism.

2.21.3.2 Physical Examination

The complete physical examination should include the ears, upper respiratory tract, and head and neck. A neurological examination emphasising the cranial nerves and cerebellar and sensorimotor function is essential. The patient's general mood should be assessed, and any sign of depression should be noted. Specific nasal examination should include anterior rhinoscopy and nasal endoscopy. The ears should be examined for serous otitis media, indicating the possibility of a nasopharyngeal mass or inflammation. Palpation for masses in the neck and for thyromegaly is also important.

2.21.3.3 Laboratory Tests

Laboratory tests should be guided by the history and physical examination. Lab tests may include evaluation for allergies (total IgE, specific IgE), infection, diabetes mellitus and thyroid, liver or kidney disease, nutritional deficiencies and malignancy.

2.21.3.4 Imaging Techniques

Imaging studies may be helpful in selected patients, but should be reserved for specific indications. Plain radiographs are generally inadequate for diagnosis. CT is particularly valuable in assessing paranasal sinuses, the skull base and the olfactory cleft. CT scan provides the clearest detail of both bony and soft tissue anatomy and demonstrates the presence of underlying inflammatory diseases. CT is less effective than MRI is in defining soft tissue disease. The use of intravenous contrast media helps to better identify vascular lesions, tumours, abscess cavities and meningeal or parameningeal processes. Functional MRI (fMRI) may be used to measure brain activation in response to olfactory stimuli. Cerebral blood flow in normal subjects during olfactory stimulation was reported to increase in the pyriform cortex and unilaterally in the right orbitofrontal cortex by PET.

2.21.3.5 Olfactory Testing

Olfactory testing usually involves identification of specific odours, an assessment of threshold or both. Quantitative testing of olfactory function is essential to establish the validity of a patient's complaint, characterise the specific nature and severity of the problem, and monitor any change over time. During the lasts decades, standardised general tests of olfactory function have been developed. The quantitative clinical test most widely used is UPSIT [3]. UPSIT consists of a 40-item, forced choice, micro-encapsulated odour, scratch-and-sniff paradigm. The patient's test scores are then compared with norms for the same age and gender.

Other commercially available olfactory tests include the three-item forced-choice microencapsulated Pocket Smell Test [8], the Brief Smell Identification Test [4] and a squeeze-bottle odour threshold test kit.

2.21.3.6 Other Studies

In recent years, event-related potentials to olfactory stimuli have been used in the study of smell processing in healthy and clinical populations. Olfactory biopsy of the olfactory epithelium and ultra-structure study comple-

mented with immunocytochemical analysis may increase the understanding of olfactory function.

2.21.4 Aetiology

Loss of smell is a frequent disorder, but its aetiology remains obscure. Disorders of smell are caused by conditions that interfere with odour contact with the olfactory neuroepithelium (conduction smell loss), injury of the receptor region (sensorial smell loss) or damage of central olfactory pathways (neural smell loss). The history of the disease provides important clues as to the cause. In most instances, loss of smell is caused by nasal and sinus disease, upper respiratory tract infection or head trauma [9]. Major disorders in which smell function is altered or impaired are listed below. Unfortunately, in a fairly substantial number of patients, the precise aetiology remains undetermined. In fact, a number of these patients may well fall into one of the other known diagnostic categories.

Frequent aetiological factors producing smell dysfunction include:

- Nasal and sinus diseases
  - Nasal polyps
  - Allergic rhinitis
  - Rhinitis medicamentosa
  - Rhinitis vasomotora
  - Chronic inflammatory rhinitis (syphilis, tuberculosis, leprosy, Wegener's granulomatosis, sarcoidosis)
  - Nasal septal deformity
  - Foreign body
  - Adenoid hypertrophy
  - Atrophic rhinitis
  - Benign tumour
  - Malignant tumour
- Upper respiratory tract infections
  - Bacterial rhinitis and sinusitis
  - Fungal rhinosinusitis
  - Postviral upper respiratory tract infection
- Trauma
  - Head trauma
  - Postsurgical skull base
  - Postlobotomy (frontal, temporal)
  - Nasal surgery
- Neurodegenerative diseases
  - Alzheimer's disease
  - Parkinsonism

Some *infrequent* aetiological factors producing smell dysfunction include:

- Endocrine–metabolic disorders
  - Diabetes mellitus
  - Hypothyroidism

- Adrenal cortical insufficiency
- Cushing's syndrome
- Chronic renal failure
- Vitamin deficiency (A, B_6, B_{12})
- Zinc deficiency
- Cirrhosis of the liver
- Neurologic diseases
  - CNS tumour
  - AVM
  - Multiple sclerosis
  - Epilepsy
- Drugs
  - Amitriptyline hydrochloride
  - Nifedipine
  - Propranolol hydrochloride
  - Labetalol hydrochloride
  - Chemotherapy
  - Radioactive iodine
- Miscellaneous
  - Kallman's syndrome
  - Radiotherapy
  - Postlaryngectomy
  - Postanaesthesia
  - Schizophrenia
  - Down's and Turner's syndromes
  - Alcoholism
  - Toxic chemical exposure

2.21.5 Treatment

Unfortunately, treatment of smell disorders remains disappointing. A different approach to the treatment is the detection and therapy of underlying causes. Endocrine disturbances should be addressed, and nutritional deficiencies should be corrected. Some drugs may cause smell loss, and these drugs should be discontinued. In addition, early recognition and counselling can help patients to compensate for loss of smell.

Smell disorders are more likely to be treated successfully when the patient has a reversible cause of intranasal interference such as rhinitis, nasal polyps and mechanical obstruction. The use of oral and/or intranasal steroids may be useful. Patients with chronic rhinosinusitis and/or polyps who are resistant to medical treatment can benefit from endoscopic sinus surgery; the surgery can improve conductive defects and reduce local inflammation.

Anosmia subsequent to upper respiratory tract infection may improve over time without specific treatment. Medical treatments are not generally effective in restoring olfactory function in these patients. Recently,

alpha-lipoic acid [6] and the N-methyl-D-aspartic acid (NMDA)-antagonist caroverine have shown promise in improving olfactory loss after upper respiratory tract infection. Controversial results were found after zinc treatment however.

In general, the olfactory system regenerates poorly after head injury. There have been few detailed reports about posttraumatic olfactory dysfunction, especially with regard to improvement of olfaction. Significant recovery of olfactory function has been reported in approximately one third of patients after posttraumatic anosmia, although the mechanism is unclear [1].

References

1. Costanzo R, Becker D (1986) Smell and taste disorders in head injury and neurosurgery patients. In: Meiselman HL, Rivin RS (eds) Clinical measurements of taste and smell. Macmillan, New York, pp 565–578
2. Deems DA, Doty RL, Settle RG, Moore-Gillon V, Shaman P, Mester AF, Kimmelman CP, Brightman VJ, Snow JBj (1991) Smell and taste disorders: a study of 750 patients from the University of Pennsylvania Smell and Taste Center. Arch Otorhinolaryngol Head Neck Surg 117:519–528
3. Doty RL, Shaman P, Dann M (1984) Development of the University of Pennsylvania Smell Identification Test: a standardized microencapsulated test of olfactory function. Physiol Behav 32:489–502
4. Doty RL, Marcus A, Lee WW (1996) Development of the 12-item Cross-Cultural Smell Identification Test (CC-SIT). Laryngoscope 106:353–356
5. Hummel T, Heilmann S, Murphy C (2002) Age-related changes of chemosensory functions. In: Rouby C, Schaal B, Dubois D, Gervais R, Holley A (eds) Olfaction, taste and cognition. Cambridge University Press, Cambridge, pp 441–456
6. Hummel T, Heilmann S, Huttenbriuk KB (2002) Lipoic acid in the treatment of smell dysfunction following viral infection of the upper respiratory tract. Laryngoscope 112:2076–2080
7. Murphy C, Schubert CR, Cruickshanks KJ, Klein BE, Klein R, Nondahl DM (2002) Prevalence of olfactory impairment in older adults. JAMA 288:2307–2312
8. Solomon GS, Petrie WM, Hart JR, Brackin HB Jr (1998) Olfactory dysfunction discriminates Alzheimer's dementia from major depression. J Neuropsychiatry Clin Neurosci 10:64–67
9. Temmel AF, Quint C, Schickinger-Fischer B, Klimek L, Stoller E, Hummel T (2002) Characteristics of olfactory disorders in relation to major causes of olfactory loss. Arch Otolaryngol Head Neck Surg 128:635–641

2.22 Benign Sinonasal Neoplasms

METİN ÖNERCİ

2.22.1 Introduction

There are several benign lesions of the nose and paranasal sinuses, as outlined below. The most common are inverted papillomas, juvenile angiofibromas, pituitary adenomas and fibro-osseous lesions such as fibrous dysplasia. Benign tumours should be differentiated from malignant tumours and other benign structures such as encephaloceles (Figs 2.22.1, 2.22.2).

Benign sinonasal tumours include:

- Sinonasal epithelial tumours
  - Papillomas
    - Sinonasal gland tumours
  - Inverted papillomas
    - Pleomorphic adenoma
    - Myoepithelioma
    - Oncocytoma
- Neuroectodermal tumours
  - Paraganglioma
  - Schwannoma
  - Neurofibroma
- Displaced neural lesions
  - Nasal glioma
  - Pituitary adenoma
- Soft tissue tumours
  - Vascular tumours
    - Juvenile angiofibroma
    - Hemangiopericytoma
  - Fibrous
    - Nasal fibroma
  - Muscle
    - Leiomyoma
    - Rhabdomyoma
  - Bone and cartilaginous
    - Osteoma
    - Ossifying fibroma
    - Fibrous dysplasia
    - Osteoblastoma
    - Aneurysmal bone cyst

One rule to follow for surgery is to completely resect the tumour, with sufficiently safe margins. External approaches have been utilised with success. However, improved visualisation after the introduction of endoscopy and the advancement of imaging technologies and navigation systems have made it possible to remove many benign tumours endonasally. A thorough endoscopic examination after maximal decongestion of the mucosa provides information about the localisation, extent and

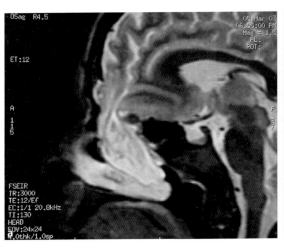
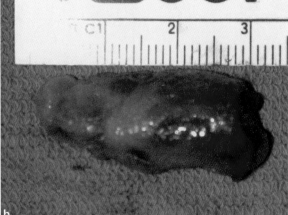

Fig. 2.22.1a,b Nasal encephalocele mimicking a nasal polyp. In unilateral lesions, encephalocele should always be kept in mind. MRI provides adequate information. **a** Lateral MRI image showing the direct continuity of the mass with the intracranial cavity and **b** the lesion after removal

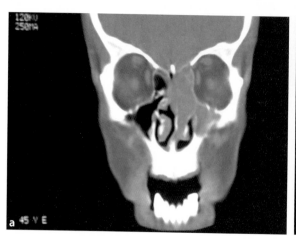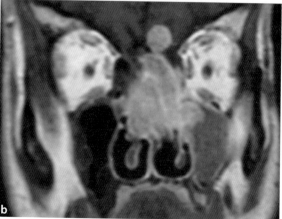

Fig 2.22.2a,b Unilateral mass mimicking a benign tumour, whereas MRI shows it to be esthesioneuroblastoma. **a** Coronal CT, **b** MR image

nature of the tumour. The advantage of the endonasal approach is the avoidance of external scarring and better visualisation during the procedure. If necessary, or, if the surgeon is not experienced enough, external approaches can be utilised. Endonasal tumours such as a schwannoma localised in the nose or a pleomorphic adenoma on the septum present no difficulty for endonasal removal. Radiological examination may show bony involvement, intracranial invasion and spread of the tumour to neighbouring structures. Before surgery, a biopsy should be taken, and the diagnosis for the tumour should be made. The exceptions to preoperative biopsy are juvenile nasopharyngeal angiofibroma (JNA) and nasal encephalocele. Radiological imaging of JNA is generally enough for diagnosis, and biopsy can result in serious bleeding. Encephaloceles should be ruled out if they are suspected, and MRI supplies information that is helpful for diagnostic differentiation (Fig. 2.22.1).

With the increasing use of endoscopes, endonasal surgery is becoming more popular. After the nose has been maximally decongested, the operative field should be exposed to the greatest extent possible. Septoplasty and inferior turbinate surgery should be done if necessary. The middle turbinate can be resected if it prevents exposure of the tumour. The subperiosteal plane is important for dissection, and the tumour is removed under direct vision and with safe margins, if possible. For tumours extending into the frontal sinus and into the lateral and inferior walls of the maxillary sinus, adjunctive external surgery is usually necessary. Improved reconstruction techniques have made it possible to perform surgery more advanced. The medial orbital wall and the skull base should be identified early in the procedure, before significant dissection is performed adjacent to them. The natural barriers of the dura and the orbital periosteum should be maintained whenever possible.

2.22.2 Fibrous Dysplasia

Fibrous dysplasia is a benign, slow-growing tumour. It is more common in the maxilla during the first two decades of life. There is no sex predilection. It is a developmental anomaly of "bone forming mesenchyme", in which normally mineralised bone is replaced by proliferating fibrous tissue and immature woven bone, which has a ground-glass appearance on radiological examination

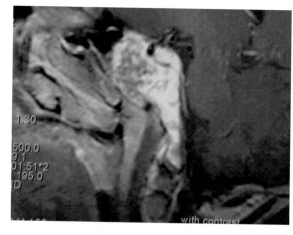

Fig. 2.22.3 Fibrous dysplasia with ground-glass appearance on radiological examination

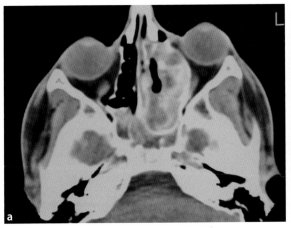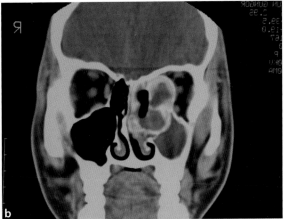

Fig. 2.22.4a,b Ossifying fibroma, with dense capsule. **a** Axial CT, **b** coronal CT

(Fig. 2.22.3). Fibrous dysplasia can be localised in a single bone (monostotic form) or in multiple bones (polyostotic form). The monostotic form is more common, accounting for about 70% of all fibrous dysplasia cases. Ossifying fibromas usually affect women in their second decade of life and is more common in the mandible (90%). The distinction between fibrous dysplasia and ossifying fibromas is difficult to make, although radiological examination may be helpful (Fig. 2.22.4). Histologically there is a peripheral capsule formation in ossifying fibromas but not in fibrous dysplasia. Malignant transformation is not common, occurring in only 0.5% of monostotic and 4% of polyostotic forms. It is widely acknowledged that radiation therapy significantly increases the risk of malignant transformation.

The treatment of fibrous dysplasia is almost always surgical. Treatment is planned according to the age of the patient, growth rate, location and extent of the tumour, cosmetic deformity and functional disturbances. There are some reports in the literature indicating that surgery may activate the tumour and accelerate the growth of the lesion, especially in younger patients, whereas without surgery, the disease would become quiescent after puberty. Therefore, surgery is mainly for patients with cosmetic and functional disturbances. Patients with minimal cosmetic deformity may not require surgery.

On the other hand, surgery should not be delayed until complications appear. The functional deficits may become permanent and irreversible, or the surgery may be more difficult, and the risk of damage to vital structures such as the optic nerve may be more likely. The surgery of choice is the radical excision of all dysplastic bone. However, this procedure may not be possible in all cases, and it may cause further deformities or functional disturbances. If total excision would result in additional deformity and functional disturbance, then conservative surgery is advocated to correct the cosmetic deformity or functional loss.

2.22.3 Endoscopic Pituitary Gland Surgery

Trans-sphenoidal, trans-septal pituitary surgery has traditionally been performed with a sublabial and transfixion incision, and with an operating microscope. However, endoscopic surgery, with its much improved illumination and magnification, in comparison to an operating microscope, has become more popular in the last decade. The most important advantage of the endoscope over the microscope is that angled endoscopes enable surgeons to see the deep and blind areas of the sphenoid sinus and the sella. After tumour removal, the lateral superior and inferior recesses of the sellar cavity can be visualised, and tumour remnants may be detected.

2.22.4 Inverted Papillomas

Inverted papillomas (IP) are the most common neoplasms. They have a unique histological appearance and arise from the membranes lining the nose and paranasal sinuses. IP are named for the histological structure of the tumour that the epithelium inverts into the underlying stroma. A distinct basement membrane that separates the neoplastic squamous epithelium from the underlying tissue stroma can be identified. They do not commonly arise from the nasal floor, septum, nasopharynx, or olfactory groove. The most common site of origin is the lateral nasal wall in the region of the middle meatus and ethmoid cells, and often (in 82% of cases), they secondarily extend into one of the paranasal sinuses. IP, in most cases, commonly involve the maxillary sinus (69%), which is followed by the sphenoid sinus (11–20%) and the frontal sinus (11–16%). Isolated lesions of the sinuses without nasal involvement may occur. In approximately 8% of cases, the tumour may arise from the nasal septum, and in 4% the tumour may be bilateral. IP may also occasionally arise from multiple sites. The histological findings suggest that they evolve from a single lesion from direct extension via metaplasia of the adjacent mucosa. IP are most usually encountered in the fifth through the seventh decades, but the average age of onset is 52 years. It is more commonly seen in males, with ratios ranging between 2/1 and as high as 9/1 according to the literature.

The cause of IP is unknown. Possible theories include proliferation of nasal polyps, allergy, chronic inflammation, environmental carcinogens and virulent infections. An association with allergy, chronic inflammation, nasal polyps, smoking, or other environmental carcinogens is unlikely, since IP are usually unilateral. The rarity of this tumour in children is indirect evidence against viral aetiology. However, Weber et al. found that 16 of 21 IP patients (76%) contained the HPV DNA sequence. All recurrent IP patients in their study were HPV DNA positive, suggesting that the presence of the virus may affect the biological behaviour of these epithelial proliferations, and that there may be a potential etiologic role.

The most common symptom of IP is nasal obstruction. Headache, epistaxis and nasal discharge may also accompany nasal obstruction. Since the symptoms are similar to those of chronic sinusitis, the time of onset of the symptoms to that of patient presentation may be quite long. A high index of suspicion is very important. A unilateral mass requires further investigation with nasal endoscopy, CT scan and biopsy. Coronal-, axial- and sagittal-plane CT scans are very helpful in illuminating the extent of the disease and bone destruction. Bony destruction may be due to the pressure from the tumour and is not always predictive for malignancy, nor does it differentiate benign tumours from nasal polyps. Secondary sinusitis occurs due to obstruction by the IP. MRI scans can help to differentiate retained secretions and chronic sinusitis or mucocele from a sinus neoplasm. In IP, both T_1 and T_2 images are isointense, unlike sinusitis and mucoceles. However it is not possible to determine the foci of SSC from IP.

The aggressive nature of these tumours is well known, and a close association with SSC was reported in several studies, the incidence changing from 2 to 50%, with an average of 10%. Patient age correlates with SCC in IP patients (the mean age of patients with IP/SCC is 9–13 years older than the mean age of those with IP alone). It is also suggested that malignancy tends to be associated with bilateral IP, severe hyperkeratosis, a mitotic index of more than two mitoses per field, absence of inflammatory polyps and the presence of neutrophils. Other variables such as sex, smoking, alcohol use and history of chronic sinusitis were found not to be correlated.

Due to the possibility of IP spread by metaplastic extension to adjacent structures, the treatment of choice is excision with adequate margins. The recommended approach for obtaining such margins is a topic of controversy. Initially, IP were excised transnasally. However, the high rate of recurrence (40–80%) with transnasal excision led to the lateral rhinotomy approach, with a lower rate of recurrence (0–50%). Later, midfacial degloving was developed to avoid external scarring, without compromising the recurrence rate (3–13%). Many studies advocate medial maxillectomy, with reduced recurrence rates. The traditional approach to performing medial maxillectomy is lateral rhinotomy or midfacial degloving. After the introduction of endoscopy, transnasal removal of IP became popular in selected cases, with recurrence rates of 0–17%. Subsequently, transnasal endoscopic medial maxillectomy for IP was reported, with results comparable to those of external approaches.

The advantages of endoscopy are superior magnification, illumination and angled visualisation. An endoscopic approach avoids external scarring, allows inspection of the tumour bed and preserves the superstructure of the nose. An endoscopic medial maxillectomy is possible. Recurrences tend to occur at the buttress between the maxillary antrostomy and the lamina papyracea, which is an area easily visible with endoscopy. Two areas that present difficulty during endoscopic resection are the anterior, anteromedial and lateral walls of the maxillary sinus, and the frontal sinus. In some cases it is also possible to remove an IP located on the posterior wall of the frontal sinus, but if it is not possible, an osteoplastic flap and removal of the frontal sinus mucosa should be performed. For maxillary sinus lesions on the anterior and lateral wall, the canine fossa approach can be utilised.

The key to success of IP surgery is complete visualisation, identifying the attachments of the tumour, removal of the whole mucosa with underlying periosteum and drilling of the bone at these areas. If the tumour is attached to the bony medial orbital wall, then the bone should be removed, leaving the orbital periosteum intact. The cavity must be made wide enough to enable the surgeon to endoscopically inspect during long-term follow-up (Figs 2.22.5, 2.22.6).

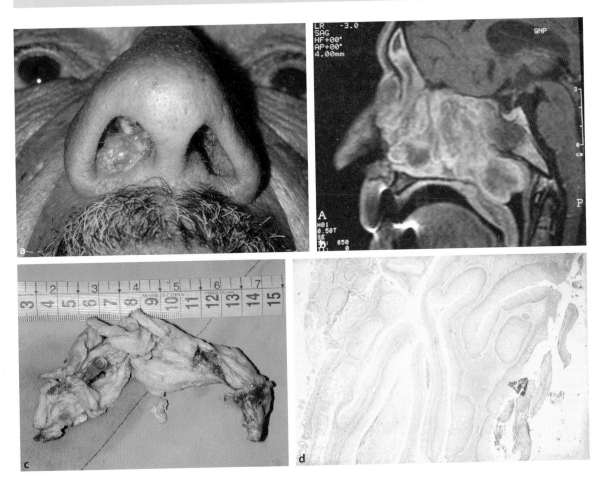

Fig. 2.22.5a–d A very large IP. **a** Nasal view, **b** lateral MRI, **c** IP mass after removal, **d** pathologic section

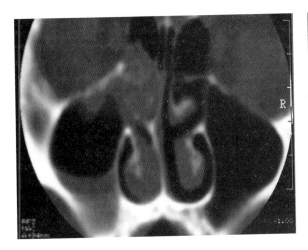

Fig. 2.22.6 Recurrent IP, at the buttress between the maxillary antrostomy and the lamina papyracea

2.22.5 Juvenile Nasopharyngeal Angiofibroma

JNA is a benign, highly vascular tumour that occurs in adolescent males and accounts for 0.05% of all head and neck neoplasms. Although JNA is histologically benign, these tumours may locally behave very aggressively and can cause significant morbidity and, occasionally, mortality. The cause of JNA is unknown. There are varying reports postulating that JNA originates from fibroangiomatous hyperplasia, an ectopic hamartomatous focus or an overgrowth of paraganglionic tissue. The growth of JNA is hormonally influenced. Angiofibromas may have progesterone receptors, androgen receptors and glucocorticoid receptors. While oestrogens can effect angiofibroma growth, the majority of tumours lack oestrogen receptors.

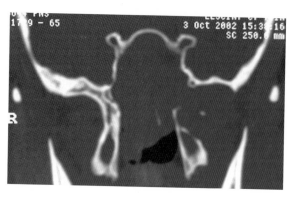

Fig. 2.22.7 A homogeneously enhancing mass in the posterior nasal cavity and nasopharynx, with a widening of the pterygo-palatine fossa

Spontaneous regression is controversial, yet there are multiple reports supporting spontaneous regression. The malignant transformation of JNA is also controversial. However, the reported cases of malignant transformation have been those in which the transformation occurs many years after treatment with radiotherapy, demonstrating the long-term risk of radiation treatment in adolescents.

JNA is thought to originate in the posterolateral nasal cavity, around the sphenopalatine foramen rather than the nasopharynx, as was previously thought. Lloyd et al. found pterygopalatine fossa involvement in all 72 of their patients with JNA. The tumour was present in the ptery-gopalatine fossa and the nasal cavity in 100% of their patients. Therefore they suggested that angiofibroma arises in the pterygopalatine fossa in the recess behind the sphe-nopalatine ganglion, at the exit aperture of the pterygoid canal. This is the area where the sphenoidal process of the palatine bone meets the horizontal ala of the vomer and the root of the pterygoid process of the sphenoid bone.

Nasal obstruction and epistaxis are the most common symptoms of JNA. Headache, Eustachian tube obstruc-tion, nasal speech and mucopurulent rhinorrhea are less common. Ocular symptoms, cranial nerve palsies, and external masses indicate advanced disease. CT and MRI are critical in diagnosis. The characteristic radiographic appearance on CT is that of a homogeneously enhanc-ing mass in the posterior nasal cavity and nasopharynx, with widening of the pterygopalatine fossa and anterior bowing of the posterior maxillary wall (Fig. 2.22.7). On T_1-weighted images, there is low to intermediate signal intensity, and hyperintense signal intensity on T_2-weight-ed images. Biopsy is often unnecessary and can be dan-gerous. However, in atypical patients or in the presence of doubt about the diagnosis, a biopsy should be taken in the operating room under controlled circumstances. JNA are nonencapsulated, and there is a wide-base origin with multiple secondary attachments. On microscopic

examination, there are fibrous stroma and intertwined vascular channels. The vessels are lined with a single layer of endothelial cells, and they lack elastic fibres in their walls. Small-calibre vessels have no smooth muscle, and in large vessels it is incomplete. The absence of a muscular layer in the vessels prevents vasoconstriction. In newer lesions, a vascular pattern predominates. In older lesions, the stroma predominates and may compress the vascular component into narrow slits. Vascular thrombosis can cause further fibrosis and even partial regression.

From its starting point the tumour can extend ante-riorly to the nasal cavity, superiorly to the sphenoid si-nus, posteriorly to the nasopharynx, and laterally into the pterygopalatine fossa and infratemporal fossa. Gener-ally, JNA may show, at least, limited ethmoidal sinus or sphenoid sinus involvement, which does not affect the prognosis or surgical approach. The tumour can enter the orbit via the inferior orbital fissure. It can also enter the cranial cavity by various routes. It can enter the middle fossa through the base of the pterygoids. If it enters the cranial cavity through the superior orbital fissure or the roof of the infratemporal fossa, it lies laterally to the cav-ernous sinus and carotid artery. The tumour may also spread into the cranial cavity through the sphenoid sinus, between the pituitary gland and the carotid artery. If the tumour erodes the fovea ethmoidalis, it enters anterior cranial fossa. There are different classification systems but the most commonly used one is Radkowski classifi-cation:

IA	Limited to nose and/or nasopharyngeal vault
IB	Extension into one or more sinuses
IIA	Minimal extension into pterygomaxillary fossa
IIB	Full occupation of pterygomaxillary fossa, with or without erosion of orbital bones
IIC	Infratemporal fossa with or without cheek involvement or posterior to pterygoid plates
IIIA	Erosion of skull base – minimal intracranial
IIIB	Erosion of skull base – extensive intracranial with or without cavernous sinus

Surgery is widely acknowledged as the main treatment modality for extracranial disease, whereas the manage-ment of intracranial disease remains controversial. The recurrence rate is variable, but on average it is approxi-mately 20%. The high recurrence rate is probably the re-sult of incomplete removal of tumour extensions. There are various surgical approaches, such as:

- Transpalatal
- Sublabial
- Facial translocation
- Lateral infratemporal fossa

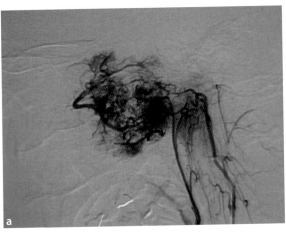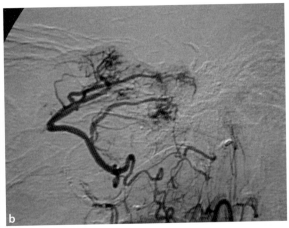

Fig. 2.22.8a,b Embolisation decreases the amount of bleeding during surgery. **a** Before embolisation and **b** after embolisation

- Craniofacial
- Transantral
- Transzygomatic
- Transmandibular
- Lateral rhinotomy
- Combined
- Endonasal

The operative technique is selected according to the location and extent of the tumour, as well as the surgeon's experience. The transpalatal approach is mainly for tumours in the nasopharynx and posterior nasal cavity. For tumours more advanced, lateral rhinotomy and sublabial approaches have been advocated. The facial translocation and lateral infratemporal fossa approaches are used for tumours that extend far laterally into the infratemporal fossa. If intracranial extension exists, craniofacial approaches may be a viable surgical alternative, or radiation therapy may be considered.

After the introduction of endoscopy and improved embolisation techniques into nasal surgery, endoscopic surgery became more popular. (New, revised staging systems were suggested in order to better define the extensions of the tumour and to predict the prognosis.) Embolisation decreases the amount of bleeding considerably (Fig. 2.22.8), although there are some reports on complications related to embolisation. Endoscopic endonasal surgery begins with removal of the lower part of the middle turbinate to create more space and also to enhance visualisation. If the tumour has adhesions to the posterior septum, then an incision is made to the septum, just anterior of where the adhesion starts, and the septal attachment is removed, generally with bipolar cautery. After uncinectomy, the ethmoidectomy is performed until the tumour is reached. The maxillary sinus ostium is identified and widened posteriorly. The posterior maxillary sinus wall, which is thin due to tumour pressure, is removed. The sphenopalatine foramen is exposed and the artery is clipped. All the bony prominences should be drilled or removed with Kerrison forceps until the entire tumour becomes visible. Laterally, the tumour is detached by blunt dissection until fat appears. With angled endoscopes it is easier to identify the border between the tumour and fat. The entire tumour is pushed medially and posteriorly toward the nasopharynx. The nasopharyngeal attachments are then removed and the tumour is removed via the mouth. A problem arises when there is invasion of the cancellous bone at the base of the pterygoids: these tumours may even invade the greater wing of the sphenoid sinus, and this area is generally a site of recurrence. Lloyd et al. found that 93% of their cases of recurrence occurred in patients with invasion and expansion of the cancellous bone at the base of the pterygoid plates. Since this is an area for the tumour to spread to the middle fossa, all patients should be analysed very carefully with detailed imaging studies in relation to the involvement of the middle fossa. When there is extension to the base of the pterygoids, the base of the pterygoids should be drilled and the tumour remnants removed. Endoscopic surgery, with minimised bleeding due to hypotensive anaesthesia and preoperative embolisation in addition to enhanced visualisation, provides the opportunity to work in a less bloody field and, therefore, is becoming more popular. Even some Radkovski stage IIC and IIIA tumours can be removed using endoscopic technique, with results comparable to other surgical modalities (Figs. 2.22.9, 2.22.10).

Full occupation of PMF is not an ominous sign of the tumour, since by drilling the posterior wall of the maxillary sinus and using angled endoscopes, this area can

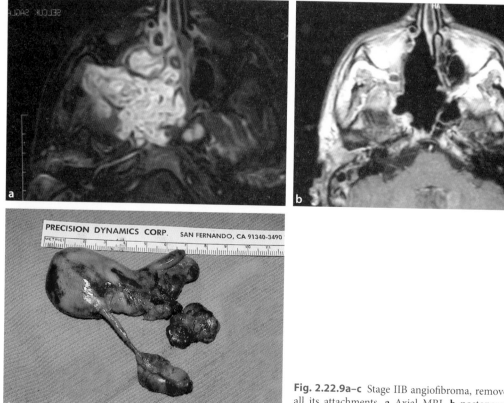

Fig. 2.22.9a–c Stage IIB angiofibroma, removed en bloc with all its attachments. **a** Axial MRI, **b** postoperative axial MRI, **c** specimen after removal

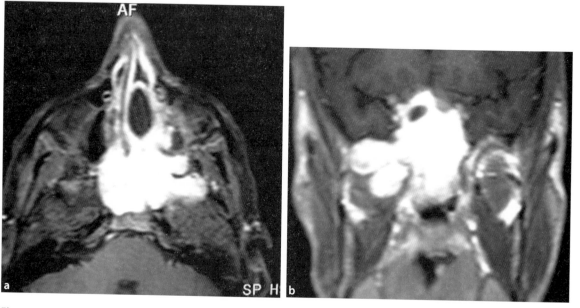

Fig. 2.22.9a–c Stage IIC angiofibroma, removed en bloc with all its attachments. **a,b** Axial and coronal MR images

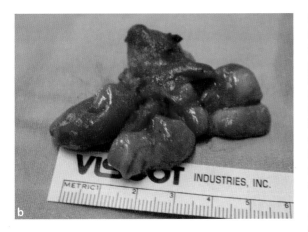

Fig. 2.22.9a–c (*continued*) **c** specimen after removal

be completely cleaned and is not an area for recurrence. Infratemporal fossa extension, though, is a challenge for a surgeon. Infratemporal fossa extension is a route for intracranial extension via the foramen lacerum and foramen ovale. The conventional techniques may be inadequate in removing a tumour, which reaches too far laterally, with cheek fat infiltration. Significant lateral extension into the infratemporal fossa, especially toward the area of the cheek, may not be readily accessible with endoscopes and midline approaches. Even angled endoscopes and angulated instruments will not guarantee sufficient cleaning of the tumour in this area.

Cavernous sinus involvement is not a direct prognostic sign, because the tumour never invades the sinus by cellular infiltration, as do malignant carcinomas. Additionally, penetration is unlikely, and lesions showing cavernous sinus involvement can often be resected through the nose. Furthermore, they generally do not present any problems, except for some venous bleeding after the resection. Even large intracranial extensions that may become adherent to the dura can be dissected. Although the possibility of tumour extension intradurally cannot be denied, to prove intradural extension, either the tumour should be seen intradurally from an initial neurosurgical approach, or the tumour should be shown histopathologically to transgress the dura. There is only one documented case in the literature that fulfilled these criteria. It is often impossible to distinguish radiologically whether the tumour extends intradurally. However, intracranial tumour extension between the pituitary gland and internal carotid artery and intracranial tumour extension posterolateral to the internal carotid artery may present difficulty in surgical resection, possibly resulting in severe haemorrhage if not carefully dissected.

In the management of JNA, a detailed knowledge of cranial base anatomy and a thorough understanding of the natural behaviour of the tumour and of tumour spread patterns are essential. Embolisation, endoscopes, navigation systems and new instruments are very helpful for surgery. All extensions should be removed together with the tumour. If necessary, external approaches should be employed. With the continued advancement of technology, surgery will become easier and safer in the future.

Reading Recommendations

1. Glecih LL (1999) Juvenile angiofibroma: histology and anatomical considerations. Oper Tech ORLHNS 10:95–97
2. Kennedy DW, Keogh B, Senior B, Lanza DC (1996) Endoscopic approach to tumors of the anterior skull base and orbit. Otolaryngol Head Neck Surg 7:257–263
3. Lloyd G, Howard D, Lund VJ, Savy L (2000) Imaging for juvenile angiofibroma. J Laryngol Otol 114:727–730
4. Orten SS, Hana E (1999) Fibrous dysplasia. Otolaryngol Head Neck Surg 10:109–112
5. Sadeghi N, Al-Dahri S, Manoukian JJ (2003) Transnasal endoscopic medial maxillectomy for inverting papilloma. Laryngoscope 113:749–753
6. Schlosser RJ, Mason JC, Gross CW (2001) Aggressive endoscopic resection of inverted papilloma. Otolaryngol Head Neck Surg 125:49–53

2.23 Malignant Tumours of the Paranasal Sinuses and the Anterior Skull Base

ULRIKE BOCKMÜHL

2.23.1 Introduction

Malignant tumours of the nose, the paranasal sinuses and the anterior skull base are rare, accounting for less than 1% of all malignancies and accounting for approximately 3% of those arising in the head and neck. Sinonasal malignancies occur twice as often in males than in females, and are most often diagnosed in patients between 50 and 70 years of age. About 60–70% of the sinonasal cancers develop in the maxillary sinuses, 20–30% in the nasal cavity, 10–15% in the ethmoid sinuses and less than 5% in the frontal or sphenoid sinuses. SCCs (60–70%) and adenocarcinomas (10–20%) make up the majority of these tumours (Table 2.23.1).

Malignant sinonasal tumours may also occur in children, with a different distribution of histological types. In the paediatric age group, they are more likely to be diagnosed as rhabdomyosarcomas.

Industrial exposure to wood dust, nickel, leather, textile dust, chromium, formaldehyde and asbestos has been implicated as causative factors in sinonasal oncogenesis. The influence of several non-occupational risk factors has been discussed controversially. However, it has been shown that there is a two- to threefold excess risk of developing a sinonasal SCC in heavy smokers. As well, HPV types 16 and 18 and EBV have been detected in small subsets of sinonasal carcinomas and are also believed to be etiological agents.

2.23.2 Symptoms

The signs and symptoms of the sinonasal tumours are nonspecific for long periods and depend mostly on their location and size. Nasal obstruction, hyposmia, blood-stained nasal discharge or a vague feeling of pressure or headache may be predominant symptoms. If they occur unilaterally, then this might be the first indication of a tumour. Symptoms such as visual disturbance (e. g. reduction of vision, double vision), meningitis, CSF leak, external swelling of the cheek or forehead, epiphora, and irritation of the first or second branch of the trigeminal nerve (hyperesthesia and pain) are signs of extensive tumour growth beyond the limits of the nose or sinuses.

Table 2.23.1 Most common malignant sinonasal tumour histologies (descending order of frequency) including their reported 5-year disease-specific survival rates after multimodality treatment of surgery and postoperative radiotherapy.

Histologic tumour type	5-year disease specific survival (%)			
	Shah et al. [51]	Suarez et al. [57]	Ganly et al. [18]	Bockmühl et al. [4]
Squamous cell carcinoma	51	65	43.6	57
Adenocarcinoma	57	30	52	65
Adenoidcystic carcinoma	46	100		100
Mucosal melanoma	33	0	0	
Esthesioneuroblastoma	100	70		78
Neuroendocrine carcinoma				
Undifferentiated carcinoma		18	26.3	
Lymphoma				
Sarcoma	58			22
Metastases from other sites				
All	58	71	53.3	60

Most prevalent tumour entities of the authors' patient series are in *italics*

2.23.3 Diagnosis

A complete examination includes assessment of facial asymmetry, visual acuity, pupillary response, extraocular motion and any cranial nerve deficits. Mandibular excursion should be assessed for trismus, which signifies expansion into the pterygoid space. The tympanic cavities should be inspected for effusion related to Eustachian tube dysfunction. Intraoral examination should be directed to the integrity of the palate and upper gingiva. The neck should be assessed for lymph node spread.

The diagnostic workups should always include endoscopy, and CT or MRI. They are important for evaluation of the location and extent of the lesion, surgical planning and postoperative follow-up. To get the optimum information the authors recommend performing *both* CT and MR imaging. The vascularisation of a lesion can be evaluated with digital subtraction angiography. If the tumour has reached or involved the ICA, a balloon occlusion test should be performed along with a perfusion scintigraphy of the brain. It gives information as to whether the ICA can be sacrificed during surgery. In cases with suspected CSF leak a CT or MR cisternography might be a helpful investigative tool.

2.23.4 Classification and Staging

Treatment planning requires meticulous assessment and documentation of the extent of locoregional disease. In 1933 Öhngren was the first to implement a classification system for maxillary sinus tumours, dividing the sinus into halves by an imaginary plane passing through the medial canthus of the eye and the angle of the mandible. This classification system takes into account that *infra*structure tumours present earlier when more amenable to resection and thus have better prognosis, whereas *supra*structure tumours become symptomatic later in the course of disease and are challenging to resect due to proximity to pterygopalatine fossa, infratemporal fossa, orbit and skull base. These principles of the maxillary sinus cancer behaviour were incorporated in the 1977 American Joint Committee on Cancer (AJCC) staging system. Cantu et al. proposed an alternative staging system based on the most commonly accepted unfavourable prognostic factors (intradural extension, involvement of the orbit and particularly of its apex, involvement of the frontal and/or sphenoid sinus, invasion of the infratemporal fossa and the skin). Therefore, and because of the fact that the majority of patients die due to advanced locoregional sinonasal disease, the most recent cancer staging classification of the UICC has included new criteria for the more advanced tumours, as shown in Table 2.23.2.

For international comparison as well as validation and refinement and finally better prediction of the patient's prognosis all sinonasal malignancies should be staged according to the UICC system.

2.23.5 Therapy

2.23.5.1 Treatment Considerations

Management of sinonasal malignancies requires an understanding of the pathology of skull base lesions and the formulation of a treatment plan with a multidisciplinary oncological team.

Treatment decisions should be made on a case-by-case basis with careful consideration of:

- Histology of the tumour
- Tumour stage
- Feasibility of complete resection
- Reconstructive options for restoration of form and function
- Patient's medical condition
- Treatment risks and morbidity
- Surgeon's experience and technical expertise
- Patient's personal preferences

In general, the mainstay of treatment is surgery that is followed by postoperative radiation. When incurable, palliation of symptoms becomes a primary goal, often achieved by adjuvant chemoradiation. The optimum management of sinonasal malignancies is not standardised. Controversy regarding treatment issues is not only fuelled by the general rarity of these tumours, but also by the diversity of histologic types and sites of involvement.

2.23.5.2 Surgical Therapy

2.23.5.2.1 External Approaches

While for the majority of tumours the accepted treatment of choice is complete wide local resection, controversy surrounds the surgical approach that should be used. The type of surgical resection required for tumours of the nasal cavity and paranasal sinuses is dictated by each lesion's anatomical location and sites of expansion. Traditionally, in the last century most sinonasal tumours were removed en bloc via transfacial approaches like lateral rhinotomy or midfacial degloving or as anterior craniofacial resection, which is carried out by a combination of a frontal craniotomy (mainly subcranial approach according to Raveh) and one of the transfacial approaches. All classical external approaches are indicated in the majority of T3 and T4 stage sinonasal malignancies. However, during the last 15 years endonasal procedures have increasingly

Table 2.23.2 UICC system of staging [45, 54]

Stage	Description
Maxillary sinus	
T1	Tumour limited to maxillary sinus mucosa with erosion or destruction of bone
T2	Tumour causing bone erosion or destruction, including extension into the hard palate and/or middle nasal meatus, except extension to posterior wall of maxillary sinus and pterygoid plates
T3	Tumour invades any of the following: bone of the posterior wall of the maxillary sinus, subcutaneous tissues, floor or medial wall of orbit, pterygoid fossa or ethmoid sinus
T4a	Tumour invades anterior orbital contents, skin of cheek, pterygoid plates, infratemporal fossa, cribriform plate, sphenoid or frontal sinuses
T4b	Tumour invades any of the following: orbital apex, dura, brain, middle cranial fossa, cranial nerves other than maxillary division of trigeminal nerve (V_2), nasopharynx or clivus
Nasal cavity and ethmoid sinus	
T1	Tumour restricted to any one subsite, with or without bone invasion
T2	Tumour invading two subsites in a single region or extending to involve an adjacent region within the nasoethmoidal complex, with or without bony invasion
T3	Tumour extends to involve the medial wall or floor of the orbit, maxillary sinus, palate or cribriform plate
T4a	Tumour invades any of the following: anterior orbital contents, skin of nose or cheek, minimal extension to anterior cranial fossa, pterygoid plates, sphenoid or frontal sinuses
T4b	Tumour invades any of the following: orbital apex, dura, brain, middle cranial fossa, cranial nerves other than maxillary division of trigeminal nerve (V_2), nasopharynx or clivus

entered the tumour surgery arena. This section therefore focuses particularly on this progressive surgical technique.

2.23.5.2.2 Endonasal Microendoscopic Surgery

Recent refinements in endoscopic and microscopic techniques along with the development of related surgical instruments have led to expanded endonasal surgery beyond chronic sinusitis to complete resection of sinonasal tumours and lesions at the anterior and central skull base, showing comparable rates of recurrence to an external approach [1, 5]. Moreover, when properly indicated and planned, for malignant tumours endonasal procedures can be superior to the traditional external techniques.

Advantages of the endonasal approach:

- Via the endonasal approach one gets optimal overview over almost the entire paranasal sinus system.
- Dura defects from the lower third of the frontal sinus posterior wall down to the sphenoid roof can be reliably closed exclusively endonasally.
- The bony boundaries of the surgical field can be preserved. This means less danger for cele formation and reduced disturbance for the growing midfacial skeleton in children.

- It is the most minimal invasive way, avoiding visible scars and facial distortion.

General Principles of Endonasal Tumour Surgery

The following preconditions should be realised for successful removal of the pathology and regarding functional and aesthetic aspects:

- The surgeon must have an extensive and reliable knowledge of the anatomy.
- The surgeon must have vast experience in endonasal surgery of inflammatory diseases, traumatology and endonasal duraplasty, and last but not least, must be very familiar with the surgical technique of type III frontal sinus drainage according to Draf.
- The surgeon must be familiar with the prevention and management of possible complications (intraorbital hematoma, damage to the lacrimal system, CSF leaks, major bleeding).
- Since both the microscope and endoscope have advantages and disadvantages, the surgeon should be able to use both in order to optimise his work.
- Navigation is highly recommended.
- The surgeon should also have expertise in head and neck surgery including the different external approaches in this area, e.g. the surgeon must be able to

switch intraoperatively from an endonasal to external approach and to perform an appropriate reconstruction of soft tissue or bone.

- Intracranial extension by itself is not a contraindication for the endonasal approach. Rather, it depends on the degree of extension and the experience of the surgeon. However, those cases should be carefully discussed with the neuroradiologist and the neurosurgeon.
- If the surgeon lacks neurosurgical training, then close cooperation with neurosurgeons not only in major intraextracranial cases is mandatory.
- The surgical procedures should be performed under general anaesthesia.
- In general, the authors achieve vasoconstriction by placing cotton swabs soaked in naphazoline hydrochloride in the nasal cavity for 10 min, which is followed by subsequent injection of lidocaine with 1:200.000 epinephrine at the lateral nasal wall as well as the septum.
- Intraoperatively frozen sections should be obtained to ensure complete tumour removal.

A criticism of the endonasal approach is the impossibility to obtain en bloc resection. Certainly, en bloc removal of tumours is the ideal choice, and it is often achieved in smaller lesions, but radical extirpation of the disease does not depend on it, as shown by the authors' long-term results of inverted papilloma and malignant tumours. Instead, the primary purpose is to identify and widely remove the tumour origin as well as the infiltrated structures, e.g. anterior skull base, dura or lamina papyracea. It is acceptable, therefore, to resect larger tumours segmentally [1]. A typical example of an endonasal microen-doscopic resection of an adenocarcinoma is presented in Fig. 2.23.1.

The authors' philosophy is to dissect around the tumour body from all sides along normal anatomical structures. In many cases this means to start anteriorly with a frontal sinus drainage type III according to Draf, and then resect the upper nasal septum and explore the anterior skull base, dissecting the tumour down to the sphenoid sinus. This includes in many cases the removal of the cribriform plate, the crista galli and the surrounding dura. Laterally, the margin of dissection is the periorbit and medially, usually the nasal septum or the opposite nasal cavity, and in large lesions the opposite periorbit. In a case of periorbital infiltration the periorbit can be removed and reconstructed with Tutoplast Fascia Lata® (Tutogen Medical, Inc., Alachua, Fla.). If the anterior skull base including the dura needs to be removed, the author prefers to dissect laterally to medially, but it is also possible going the other way around. Duraplasty is generally performed as described by Schick et al. If en bloc removal of the tumour is not possible, the author performs a piecemeal resection, since no evidence exists as yet that supports the danger of tumour spread because of debulking. In some circumstances it will be necessary to combine the endonasal approach with an external procedure (e.g. midfacial degloving or a subcranial approach according to Raveh) to achieve clear margins. Then, the surgeon must have the expertise to proceed. Under the circumstances that incomplete tumour removal is expected (tumour abutting the ICA, the optic nerve or the cavernous sinus, e.g. in adenoid cystic carcinoma or chordoma or in metastases) endonasal palliative surgery

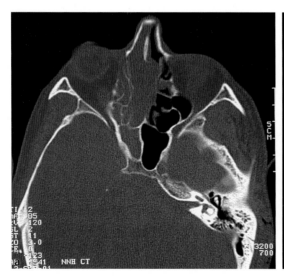
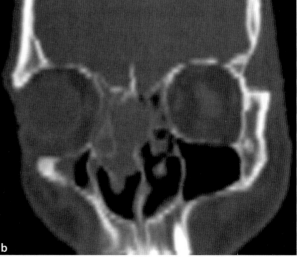

Fig. 2.23.1 a–d Adenocarcinoma (AC) of the right ethmoid sinus extending into the sphenoid sinus and the nasal cavity as well as infiltrating the nasal septum (T4a stage according to the UICC because of the sphenoid sinus involvement). **a,b** Preoperative axial and coronal CT scans showing the space occupying lesion.

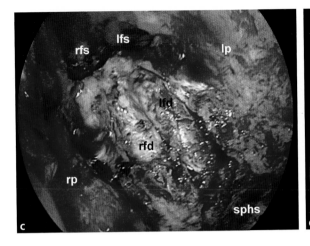

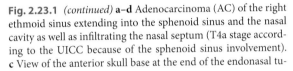

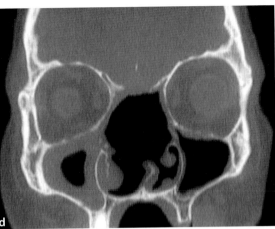

Fig. 2.23.1 *(continued)* **a–d** Adenocarcinoma (AC) of the right ethmoid sinus extending into the sphenoid sinus and the nasal cavity as well as infiltrating the nasal septum (T4a stage according to the UICC because of the sphenoid sinus involvement). **c** View of the anterior skull base at the end of the endonasal tumour resection. *rfs* right frontal sinus, *lfs* left frontal sinus, *lp* left periorbit, *rp* right periorbit, *lfd* left frontal lobe dura, *rfd* right frontal lobe dura, *sphs* sphenoid sinus. **d** Postoperative coronal CT scan without signs of recurrence 4 years after primary endonasal surgery

may be indicated, not for the purpose of cure, but as an attempt to achieve considerable improvement in quality of life. Finally, it is important to recognise when endonasal resection is not in the patient's best interest, e. g. tumour infiltration of the frontal lobe, the cavernous sinus or the orbit. While more recently endonasal endoscopic techniques have extended what can be resected, there is not yet evidence that these increase life expectancy or reduce morbidity, and one who is inexperienced should be very careful adopting advanced procedures. In general, the author recommends endonasal microendoscopic tumour surgery especially for T1 and T2 malignancies.

The tumour locations in which endonasal surgery is indicated are demonstrated in Fig. 2.23.2. In general, T1 and T2 stage malignancies of the nasal cavity and the ethmoid sinus can be safely resected via endonasal procedures. Possibly T3 tumours might also be removable by the endonasal approach if they only superficially infiltrate lamina papyracea and periorbit or the cribriform plate, respectively. This applies to T4a tumours as well if they have grown only marginally into the frontal sinus or have infiltrated the sphenoid sinus without major bony destruction.

In the authors' experience are the following major limitations to the use of the endonasal microendoscopic approach:

- Extensive involvement of the frontal sinus, because it is difficult to remove the diseased mucosa in the supraorbital region and drill the underlying bone (Fig. 2.23.2)
- Extensive intracranial infiltration
- Intraorbital infiltration
- If a tumour originates from the posterolateral, anterior or inferior wall of the maxillary sinus
- Recurrent lesions associated with massive scar tissue

These are limitations that should be managed more properly by external procedures such as the subcranial approach according to Raveh or midfacial degloving.

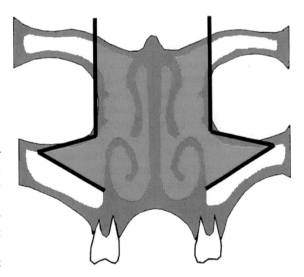

Fig. 2.23.2 Tumour locations in which endonasal surgery is indicated (*orange area*): lesions not exceeding laterally more than a vertical plane through the lamina papyracea (*black line*) and lesions that do not originate from the posterolateral, anterior or inferior wall of the maxillary sinus

2.23.5.2.3 Management of the Orbit

While even 20 years ago the orbit was almost routinely exenterated for any extension of carcinoma towards the orbital floor and the lamina papyracea, now the emerging consensus is that the orbit can often be preserved without compromising overall survival or local control of disease. Carrau et al. examined 58 patients with bony orbital invasion by SCC of the sinonasal tract and found that 3-year survival and local control were not affected by orbital preservation in the absence of orbital soft tissue invasion. A meta-analysis of the literature also supported the sparing of the soft tissue of the orbit when the periorbita has not been transgressed by SCC, because it was not detrimental to the rate of cure or local control. Furthermore, tumour extension into the periorbit does not necessarily condemn the eye to exenteration. Tiwari et al. noted that a thin fascial layer exists around the periorbital fat, which is distinct from the periorbit, and believe that invasion of this layer should determine the need for exenteration. Eye-sparing surgery was associated with local recurrence at the original site of orbital involvement in only 7.8% of cases.

From the author's point of view, involved periorbit can be resected with preservation of orbital contents in cases where there is no invasion of orbital fat, orbital muscles or involvement of the orbital apex. The invasion of any of these structures is an indication for orbital exenteration. The necessity for orbital reconstruction is emphasised for cases with orbital preservation. For orbital floor reconstruction, nonvascularised bone grafts like split calvaria or rib, as well as alloplastic materials like titanium mesh can be used.

2.23.5.2.4 Management of the Neck

Although lymphatic spread to the neck should be suspected as a possible site of metastasis, the overall incidence, regardless of the histological diagnosis, is only 14.3% in the largest available study [7]. The degree of differentiation of sinonasal SCC was observed to be significantly related to the frequency of distant metastases, while there was no association seen in the frequency of lymphatic spread. Generally, in all cases of resectable primary tumours with clinically and radiologically positive metastatic disease in the neck, the lymph nodes should be managed with some form of neck dissection. That applies especially for the histologic tumour types SCC, adenocarcinoma, esthesioneuroblastoma and undifferentiated carcinoma. The management of the clinically N0 neck is debatable. One has to consider that the way of lymphatic spread can be to the prevertebral and retropharyngeal nodes as well as to the cervical nodes, and classical neck dissection may therefore leave residual disease. Thus, the author and others do not advise elective neck dissection in sinonasal malignancy. Since cervical lymph node metastases may become apparent after initial treatment of the primary tumour, thorough neck investigations are mandatory during patient follow-up.

2.23.5.2.5 Postoperative Management

Postoperative Course

In all cases with anterior skull base resection (both cribriform plates and crista galli) and duraplasty or dura strengthening as well as in all cases with large common nasal cavities, the nose should be packed by a continuous ointment tamponade on a silicon sheet that is placed directly on the duraplasty. The silicon film helps re-epithelisation, creating a moistened chamber. If the tumour can be resected by a unilateral paranasal sinus operation, the nose should be packed with rubber finger stalls (Rhinotamp® from the Vostra Co., Aachen, Germany). These should be removed 3–7 days postoperatively. In all expanded endonasal resections the silicon film and the ointment tamponade should be taken out after 7 days. Usually, the patients are hospitalised from 3 days (simple cases) to 10 days (severe cases). During the time of nasal packing the patients are administered antibiotics (usually cephalosporin of the second generation).

After removal of the nasal packing the patients have to nurse their noses, e.g. using greasy ointment several times a day and if necessary, obtain gentle debridement at an outpatient basis. In all cases without duraplasty the author recommends ample douching with a 0.9% saline solution at least twice a day. In this regard, the patients have to be informed that if there was full-thickness mucosal excision, then it may take up to 1 year for normalisation and a possible restart of cilia function. With superficial mucosal damage it may take only several weeks.

Figure 2.23.3 demonstrates the postoperative wound healing after anterior skull base resection.

Follow-Up

Generally, follow-up consists of endoscopic examination of the nasal cavity and MR imaging. In all malignant tumours the author performs regular clinical controls quarterly in the first and second year after surgery, in the third year semiannually and thereafter only annually. Three months after surgery the author usually runs a MRI of the paranasal sinuses and the skull base, respectively, as well as of the neck to exclude lymph node metastases. Afterwards MRI will be repeated yearly. Importantly, preoperative staging includes thoracic CT, which postoperatively will also be repeated yearly, since solitary metastases are resectable.

2.23.5.3 Radiotherapy

Today postoperative adjuvant radiotherapy belongs to the standard combined modality treatment for the majority

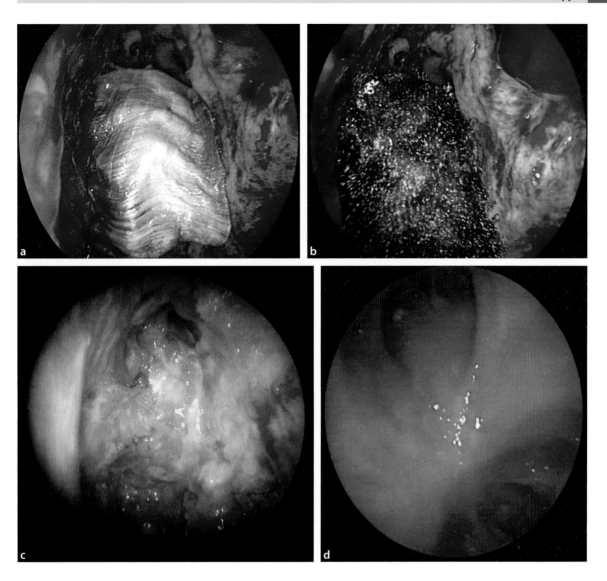

Fig. 2.23.3 a–d Postoperative appearance of the nasal airway and anterior skull base in the same patient (from Fig. 2.23.1) at the end of the operation when the dura was covered with Tutoplast Fascia Lata® (**a**) and with Surgicel on top for stabiliza-tion (**b**). **c** Condition after 6 months, still showing granulation. **d** Condition 1.5 years after primary treatment, presenting normal mucosa

of sinonasal tumours [8, 10]. With the current advent of intensity-modulated radiotherapy (IMRT), treatment can be safely delivered in a spatial, conformal fashion while sparing critical normal surrounding structures, such as the skin, orbit, brain and salivary glands [2, 6]. Radiotherapy alone for larger lesions gives significantly inferior results compared to the combination with surgery. For all T-stage lesions it yields 5-year survival rates less than 20%, in contrast to 5-year survival rates between 35 and 50% for combined surgery and postoperative IMRT [2, 8]. Recently, Waldron et al. found no difference in prognosis of patients who underwent primary IMRT that was followed by salvage surgery for ethmoid sinus cancer and those who received adjuvant IMRT postoperatively. In contrast, Hu et al. reported statistically significant improvements in the 5-year relapse-free and overall survival rates for the preoperative radiotherapy. However, it was apparent from their analysis that preoperative radiotherapy resulted in increased late complications.

To improve local control in advanced tumours and, hence, disease-free survival the use of intraoperative electron beam radiotherapy (IOERT) or intraoperative high-dose-rate (IOHDR) brachytherapy have been successfully introduced.

2.23.5.4 Chemotherapy

Rarity of sinonasal carcinomas, variable tumour histologies, diversity of chemotherapeutic regimens and short treatment follow-up periods have all prevented universal interpretation of the role of chemotherapy in these diseases. However, patients who are deemed inoperable as a result of advanced local disease, distant metastasis or extensive medical comorbidities may nevertheless experience significant palliation with chemoradiotherapy. Both cisplatin and 5-FU act as radiosensitisers by enhancing the effect of radiotherapy on tumour cells.

Moreover, there is sufficient evidence to support chemotherapy as fundamental component of multimodality treatment for sinonasal lymphomas and sarcomas. In other tumour histologies the existing evidence for the beneficial use of systemic chemotherapy outside of the palliative setting awaits a more thorough assessment. Lee et al. [4] reported excellent long-term outcome in locoregionally advanced sinonasal cancer treated with induction chemotherapy, surgery and then followed by concomitant chemoradiotherapy. The 15 patients treated with this regimen had 10-year overall survival, disease-free survival and local control rates of 56, 73 and 79%, respectively [4]. These results are encouraging and appear superior to the survival achieved with surgery and radiotherapy alone. However, further validation is warranted.

2.23.5.5 Outcome

Generally, 5-year disease-specific survival rates of sinonasal malignant tumours that were treated by a combination of surgery (craniofacial resection) and radiotherapy are reported to be between 40 and 70% [3, 8, 9]. Histology, T stage (especially brain, orbital and deep soft tissue involvement, and involvement of the sphenoid sinus), positive surgical margins, previous treatment and lymph node spread have been described to be predictive factors for poor prognosis [8, 9]. Survival rates vary widely, even among tumours of the same histology. Table 2.23.1 presents the results of some selected recently published follow-up studies that evaluated more than 100 patients each. Esthesioneuroblastoma and adenoid cystic carcinoma have the most favourable prognosis, with possible 5-year disease-specific survival rates of up to 100%. However, in the latter, prognosis is determined mainly by distant metastases and slow perineural spread that diminish disease-specific survival to around 40% after 15 years. The two most common histologic types, adenocarcinoma and SCC, are reported to have similar outcomes for overall survival. Looking at disease-specific survival, patients with adenocarcinomas seem to have better prognosis than those with SCCs [1, 3, 8]. Only Suarez et al. [9] have found the reverse proportion in their patient cohort. Ma-

lignant melanomas show, along with undifferentiated carcinomas, the worst prognosis [3, 8, 9]. Although tumour histologic findings play an important role in treatment outcome, the prognostic effect of the histologic type is difficult to establish because of the high number of different pathologic conditions and the small number of most of the histologic types. This is a limitation also of all other predictive factors.

Concerning the outcome of patients whose sinonasal malignancies have been removed exclusively endonasally, the series reported are few and limited so far, and they have not shown an increase in local recurrence rates or poorer prognosis [1]. In particular, the evaluation of our own patients with endonasally resected adenocarcinomas, SCCs and esthesioneuroblastomas ($n = 29$) showed a 5-year disease-specific survival rate of 78.4% compared to 66.4% of the patients ($n = 51$) who underwent conventional external approaches [1]. Thus, especially for the resection of T2-staged squamous cell and adenocarcinomas of the nasal cavity and the ethmoid sinus, the authors advocate the endonasal approach. Possibly T3 tumours might also be removable endonasally if they only superficially infiltrate lamina papyracea and periorbit or the cribriform plate and dura, respectively. That applies to T4a tumours as well if they have grown only marginally into the frontal sinus or have infiltrated the sphenoid sinus, without major bony destruction. In contrast, maxillary sinus tumours should be removed invariably via a transantral approach if necessary, with maxillectomy [8]. In cases of esthesioneuroblastomas the authors recommend endonasal resection for tumours of Morita/Kadish stage A or B (no evidence of intracranial extension). Interestingly, compared to SCCs many esthesioneuroblastomas also infiltrate the dura, but less frequently the brain, resulting in a much higher respectability and finally better outcome.

2.23.5.6 Conclusion

Although sinonasal tumours are rare and form a heterogeneous group in several regards, the last decade has brought important advances in the management of this malignancy. Complete surgical removal of the tumour and postoperative radiotherapy constitute the standard treatment for resectable lesions. Preliminary data of the use of chemotherapy and accelerated radiotherapy appear to indicate substantial benefit for advanced-stage tumours. Significant independent prognostic factors are the histological tumour type, tumour stage, intracranial invasion, involvement of the orbit, nodal stage, surgical margins and previous treatment.

The concept of endonasal microendoscopic surgery is no longer an alternative but a very valid treatment modality in surgery of sinonasal and anterior as well as central skull base tumours. Therefore it is always essential to check whether the endonasal approach is possible. In principle, surgery in this field should be as extensive as necessary, but as minimally traumatic as possible, which requires a lot of experience. In the authors' hands, climbing a stepladder of four surgical techniques has proved to be very efficient:

1. Endonasal
2. Midfacial degloving
3. Osteoplastic frontal sinus approach
4. Subcranial approach according to Raveh

Lateral rhinotomy is generally reserved for conditions under which exenteration of the orbit is needed simultaneously. However, the surgical approach ultimately chosen should provide adequate exposure for safe tumour resection without compromising oncologic principles and while minimising morbidity to the patient. The addition of these modalities may further improve the long-prevailing poor prognosis of these challenging tumours.

Acknowledgement

To Professor Wolfgang Draf for teaching in skull-base surgery.

References

1. Bockmühl U, Minovi A, Kratzsch B, Hendus J, Draf W (2005) Stellenwert der endonasalen mikro-endoskopischen Tumourchirurgie. Laryngol Rhinol Otol 84:884–891

2. Duthoy W, Boterberg T, Claus F, Ost P, Vakaet L, Bral S, Duprez F et al. (2005) Postoperative intensity-modulated radiotherapy in sinonasal carcinoma: clinical results in 39 patients. Cancer 104:71–82

3. Ganly I, Patel SG, Singh B, Kraus DH, Bridger PG, Cantu G, Cheesman A et al. (2005) Craniofacial resection for malignant paranasal sinus tumours: report of an International Collaborative Study. Head Neck 27:575–584

4. Lee MM, Vokes EE, Rosen A, Witt ME, Weichselbaum RR, Haraf DJ (1999) Multimodality therapy in advanced paranasal sinus carcinoma: superior long-term results. Cancer J Sci Am 5:219–223

5. Minovi A, Kollert M, Draf W, Bockmühl U (2006) Inverted papilloma: feasibility of endonasal surgery and long-term results of 87 cases. Rhinology 44:205–210

6. Mock U, Georg D, Bogner J, Auberger T, Potter R (2004) Treatment planning comparison of conventional, 3D conformal, and intensity-modulated photon (IMRT) and proton therapy for paranasal sinus carcinoma. Int J Radiat Oncol Biol Phys 58:147–154

7. Robin PE, Powell DJ (1980) Regional node involvement and distant metastases in carcinoma of the nasal cavity and paranasal sinuses. J Laryngol Otol 94:301–309

8. Shah JP, Kraus DH, Bilsky MH, Gutin PH, Harrison LH, Strong EW (1997) Craniofacial resection for malignant tumours involving the anterior skull base. Arch Otolaryngol Head Neck Surg 123:1312–1317

9. Suarez C, Llorente JL, Fernandez De Leon R, Maseda E, Lopez A (2004) Prognostic factors in sinonasal tumours involving the anterior skull base. Head Neck 26:136–144

10. Tiwari R, Hardillo JA, Tobi H, Mehta D, Karim AB, Snow G (1999) Carcinoma of the ethmoid: results of treatment with conventional surgery and post-operative radiotherapy. Eur J Surg Oncol 25:401–405

2.24 Headache and Facial Ache

PAOLO CASTELNUOVO, FRANCESCA DE BERNARDI AND PIETRO PALMA

2.24.1 Basics

Headache is defined as a pain reported of the head, usually above the eyebrows, which can be a disorder itself or caused by other disorders.

According to the second edition of the International Classification of Headache Disorders [1], all the different headache disorders can be classified into major groups, and each group is then subdivided into types, subtypes and subforms.

The principal groups are:
1. Primary headache
   a. Migraine
   b. Tension-type headache (TTH)
   c. Cluster headache and other trigeminal autonomic cephalalgias (TAC)
   d. Other primary headaches
2. Secondary headache attributed to another disorders, e.g. there is a causal link between an underlying disorder and headache. The headache improves or resolves after relief from the causative disorders. Secondary headache could be attributed to:
   a. Head and/or neck trauma
   b. Cranial or cervical vascular disorders
   c. Nonvascular intracranial disorders
   d. Substances or their withdrawal (nitric oxide [NO], carbon monoxide [CO], alcohol, monosodium glutamate, cocaine, cannabis, histamine, ergotamine, triptan overuse, analgesic overuse, opioid overuse or withdrawal, caffeine withdrawal, oestrogen withdrawal)
   e. Infections (meningitis, encephalitis, brain abscess, subdural empyema, systemic infection)
   f. Disturbance of homeostasis (hypoxia and/or hypercapnia, high altitude, diving, sleep apnoea, dialysis, hypertensive crisis, pheochromocytoma, eclampsia, hypothyroidism)
   g. Disorders of cranium, neck, eyes, ears, nose, sinuses, teeth, mouth or other facial or cranial structures (in this case a facial pain may be present)
   h. Psychiatric disorders
3. Cranial neuralgias or central causes of facial pain (trigeminal neuralgia, glossopharyngeal neuralgia, herpes zoster, Tolosa-Hunt syndrome)

2.24.2 Secondary Headaches Attributed to Sinonasal Disorders

This group of headaches is synonymous with those headaches of sinusitis, rhinosinusitis and dysventilation.

2.24.2.1 Definitions

Diagnostic criteria for secondary headaches are:
1. Headache with one (or more) of the following characteristic and fulfilling criteria 3 and 4
2. Another disorder known being able to cause headache has been demonstrated
3. Headache in close temporal relation with other disorder and/or there is other evidence of a causal relationship
4. Headache is greatly reduced or resolves within 3 months (this interval may be shorter for some disorders) after successful treatment or spontaneous remission of causative disorder

Headache or facial ache can be caused by dysventilation of the paranasal sinuses, infections of the paranasal sinuses (bacterial rhinosinusitis, fungal rhinosinusitis), mucocele and neoplasms.

An alteration of ventilation may be linked to a functional or mechanical cause blocking the sinus prechambers, e.g. the ostiomeatal complex (OMC), the frontal recess (FR) or the sphenoethmoidal recess (SER). The abnormal difference of pressure between the sinusal cavity and the nasal passageway stimulates receptors at the ostium, with consequent headache and facial ache [2–4].

The OMC is a functional entity comprising maxillary sinus ostia, the bulla ethmoidalis, the ethmoidal infundibulum, the uncinate process and the middle meatus. A blockage of the OMC causes dysventilation of maxillary and anterior portions of ethmoidal sinuses.

Typical anatomical variations of the OMC are as follows:
- Pneumatisation of the middle turbinate (concha bullosa)
- Paradoxical curvature of the middle turbinate
- Vomer spurs impinging on the fontanel areas

- Medialisation and pneumatisation of the uncinate process
- Haller's cells
- Pneumatisation of the bulla ethmoidalis ("megabulla")

The FR is a virtual space defined by the cranial thirds of the agger nasi, the uncinate process and the bulla ethmoidalis. Alteration of the reciprocal development of these delimiting structures will narrow the frontal recess, hence causing dysventilation of the frontal sinus.

The SER represents the drainage area for posterior ethmoid and sphenoid sinuses. Anatomical variations, such as pneumatisation of the superior/supreme turbinate, pneumatisation of the sphenoid rostrum, or posterior septal crests may cause dysventilation of the posterior sinusal compartment.

Anatomical "complexity" of the prechambers (OMC, FR and SER) represents typical CT findings of dysventilatory lesions. Opacification of the sinuses may be absent, representing a further stage of the progression of the disease.

Rhinosinusitis is an inflammatory process involving the mucosa of the nose and one or more sinuses. Blockage of the OMC plays an important role in the pathogenesis of rhinosinusitis. Stasis of secretions in the sinus cavity is followed by a bacterial infection, which determines exacerbation of mucosa inflammation, causing decrease aeration of the mucosa and worsening of the ciliary function. Such a vicious cycle is difficult to be break and, if the condition persists over time, it can result in a chronic rhinosinusitis [5].

Fungal rhinosinusitis shows different characteristics of presentation. Invasive forms manifest themselves with an aggressive behaviour and are not discussed in this section. Noninvasive forms include aspergilloma and mediated forms, AFR (allergic fungal rhinosinusitis) and EFR (eosinophilic fungal rhinosinusitis). Sinus aspergilloma is an extramucosal fungal proliferation within one or more paranasal sinuses, filling it/them completely. Eosinophilic forms are triggered by a pathological immunological response [6].

A mucocele is an epithelial-lined mucus-containing sac, completely filling a paranasal sinus and capable of expansion due to erosions of the limiting walls of the involved sinus. It may provoke headache and visible alterations of the craniofacial contour [7].

Trigeminal neuralgia is characterised by paroxysmal attacks of pain, lasting from a fraction of a second to 2 min, affecting one or more branches of the trigeminal nerve. Pain is intense, sharp, superficial or stabbing, and is precipitated by the palpation of the "trigger zone".

Sphenopalatine neuralgia (Sluder's syndrome) is a localised facial pain (the pain involves the eye, nose, palate, maxillary teeth, ear and temple) associated with vasomotor abnormalities such as lacrimation, rhinorrhea, and salivation.

2.24.2.2 Aetiology/Epidemiology

Rhinosinusitis is one of the most common diseases in Europe and the United States, and its incidence and prevalence is increasing cancellare [2].

Rhinosinusitis may be bacterial or fungal. The most common bacterial species isolated from the maxillary sinuses of patients with acute rhinosinusitis are *Streptococcus pneumoniae*, *Haemophilus influenzae* and *Moraxella catarrhalis*. The most frequent microorganisms isolated in chronic rhinosinusitis are *Staphylococcus aureus* (36%), coagulase-negative *Staphylococcus* (20%) and *S. pneumoniae* (17%).

In paranasal aspergilloma, fungal culture is positive between 10 and 75% and *Aspergillus fumigatus* is the commonest isolated fungus, followed by *Aspergillus flavus*. The fungus responsible of EFR belongs more often to the Dematiaceous species.

2.24.2.3 Symptoms

Patients affected by acute rhinosinusitis refer headache whose localisation differs in relation to the involved sinuses, purulent nasal secretions, postnasal drip, nasal obstruction, fever, impairment of olfaction and smell. Some symptoms may be absent, or one complaint may prevail over the others.

Ache is referred in the frontal or maxillary regions when the anterior sinusal compartment is involved, whereas the pain is located in the occipital area, in retro-orbital region or at the vertex when the lesion involves the posterior sinusal compartments.

Chronic rhinosinusitis is characterised by persistence of symptoms for more than 12 weeks. Chronic rhinosinusitis presents episodes of pain, occurring during acute exacerbations that are often precipitated by an upper respiratory tract infection or when sinus ostia are obstructed by polyps. Purulent secretions are typically present.

2.24.2.4 Complications

Complications of rhinosinusitis are classified in "orbital", "osseous" and "endocranial". Orbital complications include periorbital cellulitis (preseptal oedema), orbital cellulitis, subperiosteal abscess, orbital abscess. When the sinus infection extends to the bone, it may provoke an osteomyelitis. Endocranial complications include meningitis, subdural–epidural abscess, and cavernous sinus thrombosis.

2.24.2.5 Diagnostic Procedures

2.24.2.5.1 Recommended European Standard

The Standard includes:

- Nasal endoscopy
  - Swelling of the nasal mucosa, purulent discharge at the ostiomeatal complex and/or sphenoethmoidal recess may be seen
  - Can be negative in mucoceles
- Inspection
  - Can be negative
  - Generally positive in cases of complications: swollen skin over the frontal region, periorbital oedema, proptosis, diplopia are usually revealed
- Palpation
  - Can be negative, but pain may be often evoked by digital pressure at the point of the involved cranial nerve
- Inspection of the oral cavity
  - Can be negative, but purulent secretion on the posterior wall of the oropharynx is a frequent finding

2.24.2.5.2 Additional/Useful Diagnostic Procedures

These procedures include:

- CT scan
  - Imaging is not to be done in acute rhinosinusitis. However, it must be performed in acute, complicated rhinosinusitis as well as in chronic rhinosinusitis.
  - Positive CT findings for headache
    - Anatomical abnormalities conditioning a narrowing of the sinusal prechambers, without opacification of the sinus cavities.
    - Opacification of the involved sinuses. CT scan represents a *sine qua non* if any surgery is to be undertaken.
- MRI
  - MRI is mandatory for the differential diagnosis of unilateral expansive lesions.

2.24.2.6 Therapy

2.24.2.6.1 Conservative Treatment

Recommended European Standard

This Standard includes:

- Antibiotics. The sensitivity report from the laboratory should be used as a guide.
- Steroids. They are commonly used as a topical treatment and are given systemically as a short-term course.
- Antileukotrienes.
- Local decongestants.

Useful Additional Therapeutic Strategies

Some useful strategies are:

- Steam inhalations
- Multidrug cocktails (decongestant, antibiotics, steroid and mucolytics delivered intranasally under pressure)

2.24.2.7 Surgical Treatment

The recommended European Standard includes [2–4, 8–9]:

- FESS (functional endoscopic sinus surgery)
  - Concept: recovery of the diseased sinus is achieved by restoring ventilation and mucociliary clearance through the natural ostia by minimally invasive surgical procedures under endoscopic guidance.
  - FESS procedures are represented by uncinotomy, uncinectomy, anterior and/or posterior ethmoidectomy, opening of the frontal sinus and sphenoidotomy.
  - Paradigmatic indications for FESS are represented by acute complicated, acute recurrent and chronic rhinosinusitis.
  - FESS is also the treatment of choice for aspergilloma. Such a noninvasive form of fungal rhinosinusitis is best treated by opening the natural ostium and then removing all the fungal materials by saline pressure washing. These manoeuvres are in most of cases sufficient to avoid recurrence and use of antifungal drugs.
  - FESS is also the best option for management of mucoceles. Marsupialisation is achieved by opening and enlarging the natural ostium of the involved sinus.
- ESS (endoscopic sinus surgery)
  - ESS is indicated in patients affected by massive polyposis. Surgery is used to widen the endonasal spaces by removing polyps, enlarging the natural ostia and sacrificing the middle turbinate in order to better the efficacy of topical steroids.
  - ESS also represents the best treatment option in cases of eosinophilic fungal rhinosinusitis. In these patients surgery allows clearing of the sinuses from the typical dense and viscous secretion, as well as to remove polyps.

2.24.2.8 Differential Diagnosis

For the specifics of this topic, please refer to Fig. 2.24.1.

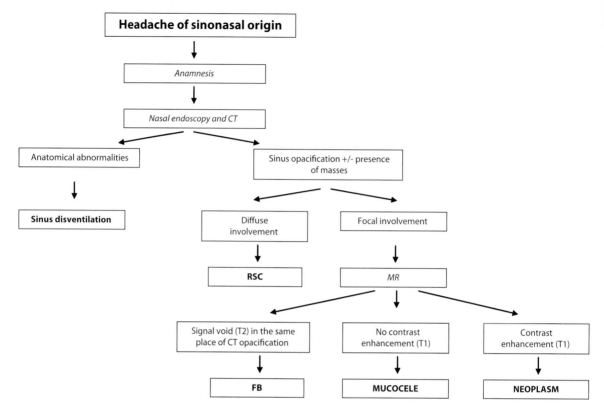

Fig. 2.24.1 Algorithm in the differential diagnosis of headache/facial aches. *RCS*: chronic rhinosinusitis; *FB*: fungus ball

2.24.2.9 Prognosis

In acute rhinosinusitis an adequate course of antibiotics associated with steroids will resolve the disease in most cases.

In chronic rhinosinusitis FESS shows from good to excellent results provided that sinus ventilation and drainage are permanently assured and underlying anatomical abnormalities are corrected.

Aspergilloma cases treated by FESS show high percentage of satisfactory outcome with a low rate of recurrence.

Massive polyposis presents a high rate of recurrence. Multiple-revision-procedure surgeries performed under local anaesthesia are usually inevitable. Enlarged endonasal spaces achieved by ESS makes revision procedures easier for the surgeons, and they are better tolerated by the patients.

Prognosis of EFR is burdened by high risk of recurrence due to the immunological and controversial background of the disease. Improved ventilation, clearing of secretions and reduction of the fungal masses, all of which are achieved by ESS, do help greatly the action of the steroids and/or antileukotrienes that are used to lessen the immunological response.

2.24.2.10 Surgical Principles

2.24.2.10.1 Functional Endoscopic Sinus Surgery

Technique
1. Surface anaesthesia with Cottonoids soaked in oxymetazoline solution
2. Local anaesthesia: 1% lidocaine with 1:200,000 epinephrine
3. Uncinotomy is performed by a backward-biting forceps at Nick's triangle, e. g. the junction area between the vertical and horizontal aspects of the uncinate process
   – When needed, the uncinotomy may be extended to an uncinectomy by removing the vertical and horizontal portions of the uncinate process with a biting forceps
4. Anterior ethmoidotomy
   – The bulla ethmoidalis is opened by a curette at its inferomedial angle, while keeping a safe distance from the laterally located lamina papyracea.
5. Opening of the frontal sinus
   – Cranial portions of uncinate process, bulla and agger nasi are removed by curved instruments under 45° telescope guidance

6. Posterior ethmoidotomy refers to the opening of the basal lamella of the middle turbinate.
7. Sphenoidotomy refers to an enlargement of the natural ostium of the sphenoid sinus either through a transethmoidal approach or a direct route (medially to the middle turbinate)

2.24.2.10.2 Endoscopic Sinus Surgery

Technique

The ESS technique involves the same steps of those of FESS, but their actions are more aggressive. Wider openings are carried out to clear the sinusal cavities by the fungal materials, and removal of the middle turbinate is necessary to reduce the recurrence rate in EFR.

References

1. Headache Classification Subcommittee of the International Headache Society (2004) The International Classification of Headache Disorders: 2nd edn. Cephalalgia 24:S9–S160
2. Stammberger H (1991) Functional endoscopic sinus surgery: the Messerklinger technique. Philadelphia: Decker 283
3. Wigand ME (1990) Endoscopic surgery of the paranasal sinuses and anterior skull base. New York: Thieme Medical Publishers, 1–2
4. Kennedy DW, Zinreich SJ, Rosenbaum AE, Johns ME (1985) 4. Functional endoscopic sinus surgery. Theory and diagnostic evaluation. Arch Otolaryngol 111:576–582
5. Fokkens W, Lund V, Mullol J (2007) On behalf of the European Position Paper on Rhinosinusitis and Nasal Polyps group. European Position Paper on Rhinosinusitis and Nasal Polyps 2007. Rhinology (suppl20):1–139
6. Ebbens FA, Georgalas C, Rinia AB, van Drunen CM, Lund VJ, Fokkens WJ (2007 Sep) The fungal debate: where do we stand today? Rhinology 45(3):178–189
7. Lund VJ (1998 Jan) Endoscopic management of paranasal sinus mucocoeles. J Laryngol Otol 112(1):36–40
8. Kennedy DW (1985) Functional endoscopic sinus surgery. Technique. Arch Otolaryngol 111:643–649
9. Stammberger H, Posawetz W (1990) Functional endoscopic sinus surgery. Concept, indications and results of the Messerklinger technique. Eur Arch Otorhinolaryngol 247:63–76

Diseases of the Nasopharynx

Edited by Uwe Ganzer and Andreas Arnold

3.1 Basics

UWE GANZER AND ANDREAS ARNOLD

3.1.1 Clinical Anatomy

The upper third of the pharyngeal muscle tube (constrictor muscles of the pharynx) is designated as the nasopharynx. This resembles an elongated cavity extending behind the nose from the base of the skull to the lower margin of the soft palate. Cranially and dorsally, the nasopharynx is delimited by the underside of the sphenoid bone and the basilar part of the occipital bone. The posterior wall is in continuity with the deep muscles of the neck and the vertebral fascia in the upper cervical spine. The retropharyngeal space, which contains isolated lymph nodes, is situated between the nasopharyngeal muscle tube and this fascia. Anteriorly the nasopharynx communicates with the nasal cavity through two openings, the choanae, separated by the posterior edge of the nasal septum. Caudally, the nasopharynx passes into the oropharynx. The back surface of the soft palate can be regarded as the „floor". The tensor and levator muscles of the palatine velum constitute the lateral boundary of the nasopharynx in conjunction with the tubal prominence (torus tubarius) and the tube muscles concealed in folds of the mucosa (salpingopharyngeal and salpingopalatine folds).

Immediately below the base of the skull, a deep pharyngeal recess (Rosenmüller's fossa) is situated dorsolaterally on both sides. Below this is the pharyngeal opening of the auditory tube, which is delimited by cartilage. The tube opening is normally closed by mucosal folds; the tube is periodically opened in every deglutition by the interaction of the aforementioned soft palate (pala-tine velum) muscles with the tube muscles, so that air can pass into the middle ear. The pharyngeal tonsil, or adenoid, (a conglomeration of lymphatic tissue) is located at the transition from the posterior wall to the tectum of the nasopharynx (Fig 3.1.1). A smaller accumulation of lymphatic tissue, the tubal tonsil, is likewise to be found in the pharyngeal recesses. At the cranial margin of the pharyngeal tonsil, a depression in the mucosa, the pharyngeal bursa, can often be observed. Occasionally, a cyst (Tornwaldt's cyst) arises here as a result of recurrent inflammations.

3.1.2 Principles of Clinical Examination

- History: blocked nasal ventilation, snoring, predominantly mouth breathing, nose bleeding, headache, recurrent sinusitis, recurrent otitis media, altered character of the voice (rhinolalia clausa or hyponasality)
- Transnasal and transoral endoscopy of the nasopharynx
- Rhinomanometry
- Otoscopy
- Audiogram, tympanometry
- CT scan: coronal, axial, sagittal

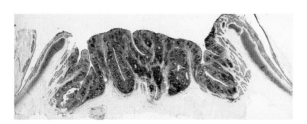

Fig. 3.1.1 Histological section of the pharyngeal tonsil (adenoid). Lateral on both sides, the Eustachian tube orifice with its medially located cartilage is seen

3.2 Adenoiditis

UWE GANZER AND ANDREAS ARNOLD

3.2.1 Synonyms

Nasopharyngitis, coryza.

3.2.2 Definition

Acute manifestation of an initially afebrile catarrhal (predominantly viral) infection of the mucosa of the nasopharynx, adenoids and mostly also of the nose.

3.2.3 Aetiology/Epidemiology

Droplet or smear infection with rhinoviruses, influenza viruses, parainfluenza viruses, respiratory syncytial viruses, adenoviruses, coronaviruses, echovirus and Coxsackie viruses. The prevalence is especially high in the cold months of the year.

3.2.4 Symptoms

Non-purulent watery to viscous nasal secretion, sneezing, nasopharyngeal pain, nasal obstruction owing to swelling of the mucosa, hacking dry cough. Often also hyposmia and hypogeusia.

3.2.5 Complications

Bacterial superinfection with *Haemophilus influenzae*, streptococci, pneumococci, staphylococci, and sometimes meningococci. Transition to purulent secretion, then often fever and nose bleeding. Lateral angina, especially in patients who have already undergone tonsillectomy.

3.2.6 Diagnostic Procedures

3.2.6.1 Recommended European Standard

- Endoscopy: nose, nasopharynx, larynx
- Microscopy of the ear

3.2.6.2 Additional Useful Diagnostic Procedures

- CT scan coronal, axial: paranasal sinuses
- Smear: in therapy-resistant bacterial superinfection

3.2.7 Therapy: Conservative Treatment

- Symptomatic, e.g. sweat-induction treatment. Inhalations with chamomile vapour
- High-dose ascorbic acid, calcium
- Sufficient fluid intake

3.2.8 Prognosis

Recovery without sequelae within a few days.

3.3 Adenoids

UWE GANZER AND ANDREAS ARNOLD

See Figs. 3.3.1 and 3.3.2.

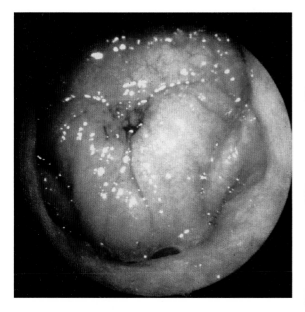

Fig. 3.3.1 Endoscopic view of hyperplastic adenoids

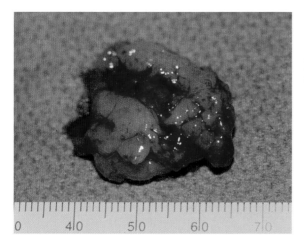

Fig. 3.3.2 Adenoidectomy specimen

3.3.1 Synonyms

Adenoid vegetation, Meyer's disease, adenoid disease, chronic inflammation of the adenoids.

3.3.2 Definition

Hyperplasia of the adenoids owing to chronic inflammation or allergy of the upper airways.

3.3.3 Spectrum of Causative Organisms

Streptococcus pneumoniae, Haemophilus influenzae, Streptococcus A, viruses.

3.3.4 Aetiology/Epidemiology

Hyperplastic adenoids are found almost exclusively in children.

3.3.5 Symptoms

- Impeded nasal breathing
- Chronic mouth breathing
- Hyponasality (rhinophonia clausa)
- Sleep disorders, snoring
- Obstructive sleep apnoea syndrome
- Mucopurulent rhinorrhoea
- Conductive hearing loss
- Lack of appetite owing to reduced ability to smell
- Delay in development

3.3.6 Complications

- Recurrent purulent rhinopharyngitis.
- Congestive sinusitis, sinubronchial syndrome.
- Persistent disorder of tube function followed by otitis media with effusion.
- Recurrent acute otitis media.
- Development of a gothic palate with resulting tooth malalignment and malocclusion because the pressure of the tongue against the maxilla is absent in continuous mouth breathing. Continuous mouth breathing also leads to dryness of the mucosa, so the teeth become susceptible to caries.

3.3.7 Diagnostic Procedures

3.3.7.1 Recommended European Standard

- Inspection: adenoid facies (narrow, pale, dumb facial expression with open mouth and sunken eyes), dried mucus in the nasal orifice (external nares), eczema of the nasal orifice, sometimes halitosis
- Palpation: cervical lymph nodes, also nuchal
- Inspection and if appropriate endoscopy of the inside of the nose, the buccal cavity, the oropharynx and the nasopharynx: tooth malalignment, malocclusion, gothic palate, often also tonsillar hyperplasia, secretion at the dorsal wall of the pharynx
- Microscopy of the ear: retracted tympanic membrane with or without middle ear effusion
- Hearing test: tympanometry, stapedius reflexes (flat tympanogram, reflexes often absent): if appropriate, pure tone audiogram

3.3.7.2 Additional Useful Diagnostic Procedures

- If appropriate, digital examination of the oral cavity and the nasopharynx: ruling out of submucosal cleft palate, juvenile angiofibroma or a cyst.
- Biopsy: if there is suspicion of a neoplasm. If there is suspicion of juvenile angiofibroma, the biopsy must be taken under general anaesthesia and with surgical standby, since severe bleeding may occur and have to be dealt with.
- CT of the cranium: if appropriate angio-MRI or digital subtraction angiography in the case of a putative tumour.

- Clinical laboratory test findings: Epstein-Barr visus (EBV) serology in the case of a putative tumour (see nasopharyngeal carcinoma).
- Consultation with a speech-language pathologist (imperative in the case of a cleft palate) or an orthodontist (in the case of malalignment).

3.3.8 Therapy

3.3.8.1 Conservative Treatment

Conservative treatment is only appropriate preoperatively (e.g. in acute rhinosinusitis) or when surgery is contraindicated (e.g. cleft palate):
- Antibiotics: amoxycillin, macrolides.
- Decongestant nose drops.
- When surgery is contraindicated, there should be long-term treatment with corticoid nasal sprays. Phytoimmunostimulants are often prescribed in German-speaking countries, e.g. Esberitox® N tablets or Lymphozil® Pro tablets. Immunostimulants derived from microorganisms, e.g. Symbioflor® drops or Broncho-Vaxom® for children, are also often administered.

3.3.8.2 Surgical Treatment

The recommended European standard is:
- Surgical removal of the adenoids is the first-line treatment!
- Adenoidectomy: any adenoid hyperplasia with chronically obstructed nasal breathing, recurrent or persistent rhinogenic infections, chronic purulent rhinorrhoea, congestive sinusitis, persistent or recurrent disorder of tube function, otitis media or mucotympanum, chronic bronchitis or in sleep apnoea syndrome.
- Sleep apnoea syndrome: as a rule with simultaneous removal of the palatine tonsils (tonsillectomy).
- Adenoidectomy is only rarely indicated in cleft-palate patients. Simultaneous reconstruction of the velopharynx may be necessary because of the danger of swallowing disturbance and hypernasality.

3.3.9 Additional Useful Surgical Procedure

Myringotomy with or without insertion of grommets.

3.3.10 Differential Diagnosis

- Nasopharyngeal tumour, especially juvenile angiofibroma.
- Tornwaldt's cyst: chronic inflammation of the pharyngeal bursa with cyst formation. Treatment: marsupialization.
- Choanalatresia. See Sect. 2.8.
- Retropharyngeal abscess: owing to a fulminant adenoiditis with transmission of infection into the retropharyngeal lymph nodes ("hot abscess"). Treatment: small abscesses can be incised transorally, larger ones must be opened from an external approach to avoid aspiration.

3.3.11 Prognosis

Recurrences are possible despite correct operation.

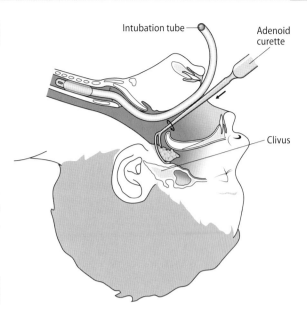

Fig. 3.3.3 Adenoidectomy

3.3.12 Principles of Surgery

1. Myringotomy/grommets (see Sect. 1.4.3.10, Fig. 1.4.5)
2. Tonsillectomy (see Sect. 5.2)
3. Adenoidectomy (Fig. 3.3.3)
   - General anaesthesia.
   - Patient in supine position, reclination of the head.
   - Insertion of the tongue depressor according to Negus or Davis and endoscopy or digital palpation of the nasopharynx.
   - Introduction of the adenoid curette (Beckmann's adenotome) and curettage of the adenoids tangential to the submucosal fascia of the constrictor muscles of the pharynx in the direction of the back edge of the septum.
   - With a smaller adenotome, recurettage of Rosenmüller's fossa, if necessary under visual control with a mirror or an endoscope.
   - Haemostasis with a threaded spherical swab inserted into the nasopharynx for 5 min, which corresponds to the physiological blood clotting period. In some cases the use of bipolar forceps is helpful.
   - Finally, transnasal aspiration of blood, mucus and any dissolved adenoid portions with a thin catheter.

3.3.13 Special Remarks

In physically retarded children or those with recurrent conductive hearing loss and susceptibility to infection, a hyperplastic adenoid must always be considered and speedy adenoidectomy must be aimed for! The risk of surgery is minimal (postoperative haemorrhage less than 1%) compared with the potential advantage for the development of the child!

3.4 Tumours of the Nasopharynx

UWE GANZER AND ANDREAS ARNOLD

All epithelial, mesenchymal and lymphoepithelial neoplasias that occur in the rest of the aerodigestive tract may occur in the nasopharynx, but very much more rarely.

3.4.1 Benign Tumours

Salivary gland tumours (cystadenolymphoma, pleomorphic adenoma). Papilloma, fibroma, lipoma, haemangioma, neurinoma, chondroma, extracranial meningeoma, craniopharyngeoma, juvenile angiofibroma, hypophyseal adenoma.

3.4.1.2 Juvenile Angiofibroma

See also Sect. 2.22.

Synonyms
Nasopharyngeal fibroma.

Definition
Very rare tumour resembling hyperplastic adenoids clinically and a cavernous haemangioma histopathologically. The preferred location is the periosteum of the sphenoid.

Aetiology/Epidemiology
One percent of all head and neck tumours. As a rule, only males aged between 10 and 25 years old are affected. Two thirds of all cases occur between the age of 13 and 17. Hormonal factors seem to play a pathogenetic role in the development of the disease (hormonal disproportion between testosterone and oestrogen) Spontaneous remission can be expected after the age of 25.

Symptoms
- Obstructed nasal breathing
- Recurrent nose bleeding
- Hyposmia

- Unilateral or bilateral disorder of tube function with or without middle ear effusion and conductive hearing loss
- Increasing hyponasality (rhinophonia clausa)
- Sometimes recurrent sinusitis

Complications
Involvement of the adjacent anatomical structures, e.g. infiltration of the base of the skull with invasion of the middle cranial fossa, spreading into the infratemporal fossa and/or the orbit with corresponding symptoms.

Diagnostic Procedures
- Inspection: mouth breathing, protrusion of the eyeball, cranial nerve deficits
- Palpation: cervical lymph nodes, especially nuchal
- Test of cranial nerve function: especially the abducens, oculomotor, trigeminal nerve
- Endoscopy: nose, nasopharynx
- Ear microscopy: retraction of the tympanic membrane, middle ear effusion
- CT: cranium
- Angio-MRI/digital subtraction angiography: identification of blood vessels to the tumour and mostly embolization of the afferent arteries at the same time
- If appropriate, ophthalmological and/or neurological consultation

Additional Useful Diagnostic Procedures
- Biopsy: since there is the danger of haemorrhage, intubation anaesthesia and surgical standby from the start. Alternatively, intraoperative frozen-section histology.
- Donation of the patient's own blood, since this is an *elective* operation.

Treatment

Conservative Treatment
- Primary inoperability: periodic follow-up to detect spontaneous remission.

- Primary inoperability and progressive tumour growth: radiotherapy. Since the patients are relatively young at the time of irradiation, there is danger of a later radiation-induced cancer.
- Long-term oestrogen therapy may also be feasible in occasional cases. The efficacy of this treatment differs greatly from individual to individual; hormone-induced side effects are frequent.

Surgical Treatment

The recommended European standard is:
- Complete resection of the tumour via a transnasal or transmaxillary open or endoscopic access. If necessary, a midfacial degloving is performed.
- Preoperative embolization is appropriate in most cases.

Differential Diagnosis

- Pharyngeal tonsil hyperplasia (*cave* biopsy!).
- Craniopharyngioma (synonym, Erdheim's tumour). This benign, but aggressively growing epithelial tumour originates from remnants of squamous cell epithelium of the hypophyseal duct and/or Rathke's pouch.
- Tornwaldt's cyst (synonym, pharyngeal bursitis) Benign cystic formation from remnants of Rathke's pouch.
- Choanal polyp.
- With the exception of the melanoma, in principle all nasopharyngeal neoplasias.
- Pseudotumours: spondylosis deformans, Forestier's disease (senile ankylosing hyperostosis of the spine).

Prognosis

Tendency for recurrence (up to 30%). Spontaneous remission is possible. After incomplete resection, there is often uncontrolled tumour growth with infiltration of the base of the skull or the orbit.

3.4.2 Malignant Tumours

3.4.2.1   General Remarks

Histological typing: nasopharyngeal carcinoma (70%), malignant lymphoma (20%), adenocarcinoma, adenocystic carcinoma, haemangiopericytoma, osteosarcoma, chondrosarcoma, meningeoma, malignant melanoma, sarcoma, plasmocytoma, chordoma, metastases of other primary tumours (altogether 10%). Very rare metastases from primary malignant tumours located elsewhere (see also CUP syndrome; Sect. 9.7). For TNM classification and staging, see Sect. 9.4.

3.4.2.2   Nasopharyngeal Carcinoma

See also Sects. 9.2, 9.3, and 9.7.

Aetiology/Epidemiology

- Incidence (new cases/inhabitant/year): In central Europe 0.5:100,000–1:100,000, in southern Europe 1:100,000, in southern China, South Asia and in the Middle East and North Africa up to 20:100,000.
- Nasopharyngeal carcinoma shows a predilection for middle-aged patients; however, it is also observed in children.
- Histology: Roughly 50% keratinizing (WHO type 1) and non-keratinizing (WHO type 2) squamous cell carcinomas and 50% undifferentiated (WHO type 3) carcinomas. In the old nomenclature, the latter are also designated as lymphoepithelial carcinomas (Schmincke-Regaud tumour) when containing a greater number of (non-malignant) lymphocytes.
- Infection with EBV is typical for lymphoepithelial carcinoma. EBV is conceivably reactivated by the disorder of T cell function detected in lymphoepithelial carcinoma. Histologically, there is a marked preponderance of B cells in which viral antigens can be demonstrated; they are also found in the submucosal glands. The viral antigens expressed in tumour tissue comprise EBNA 1 (Epstein-Barr nuclear antigen) and LMP 1 (latent membrane protein). High antibody titres against many EBV antigens, including lytic viral antigens, are well recognized and can be clinically used as tumour markers for early diagnosis and control of tumour recurrence after therapy.
- In China, consumption of salted fish containing nitrosamines and smoke from open fires are discussed as additional risk factors.
- A genetic predisposition (HLA class I genotypes) is also discussed as the cause of the disease in view of its raised familial incidence.

Symptoms
- Lymph node metastases, which are often bilateral, are located behind the upper third of the sternocleidomastoid muscle and/or nuchally. They are the first clinical signs of nasopharyngeal carcinoma in about 50% of the cases.
- Obstructed nasal air passage.
- Recurrent nose bleeding.

- Serous middle ear effusion causing conductive hearing loss.
- Hyposmia, anosmia.

Complications
- Infiltration of the base of the skull with involvement of the cranial nerves, abducens nerve palsy being especially frequent.
- Infiltration into the orbit with bulbar protrusion and diplopia or ophthalmoplegia. Infiltration of the infratemporal fossa.
- Severe nose bleeding.
- Therapy-resistant headache.

Diagnostic Procedures
- As in juvenile angiofibroma (see Sect. 3.4.1.1).
- Sonography: neck (imaging of the lymph nodes in front of and behind the sternocleidomastoid muscle as well as nuchally).
- Coronary and axial CT: skull, neck (appraisal of the extent of the tumour and demonstration/exclusion of a retropharyngeal lymph node involvement).
- CT of the thorax to rule out distant metastases.
- Serology: Determination of serum antibodies to Epstein-Barr viruses (virus capside antigen-IgG and antigen-IgA, early antigen, nuclear antigens). Raised titres are definitive tumour markers in undifferentiated or lymphoepithelial carcinomas. The titre is important for diagnosis, whereas the time course of the titre levels during and after treatment is crucial in predicting the prognosis.
- Biopsy of the nasopharyngeal tumour in the absence of putative juvenile angiofibroma. An enlarged lymph node must be totally removed for histological investigation.

Additional/Useful Diagnostic Strategies
- PET-CT: to rule out distant metastases
- Ultrasound: abdomen
- Interdisciplinary consultation with specialists for internal medicine, paediatrics, ophthalmology and/or neurology.

Treatment

Conservative Treatment
The recommended European standard is:
- The treatment of choice in nasopharyngeal carcinoma is primary irradiation of the tumour and lymph node metastases with additional chemotherapy.

- There is no consensus with regard to the different regimes of radiotherapy or chemoradiotherapy. Results from the treatment studies currently being carried out are not to be expected in the near future because of the rarity of the tumour in Europe.
- In primary systemic metastatic spreading (distant metastases), chemotherapy on its own that follows a study protocol may be considered.

Surgical Treatment
- Nasopharyngeal carcinomas are not operated on, since radical resection is not possible. Partial resection does not improve the prognosis.
- Neck dissection (salvage surgery) is indicated in persistent cervical lymph node metastases after radiotherapy/chemoradiotherapy or in recurrences in cervical lymph nodes.
- Otitis media with effusion: myringotomy with or without grommets (see Sect. 1.4.4, Fig. 1.4.6).

Differential Diagnosis
- In principle, all nasopharyngeal tumours, especially craniopharyngeoma and juvenile angiofibroma
- Hyperplasia of the pharyngeal tonsil
- Tornwaldt's cyst

Prognosis
- In undifferentiated (lymphoepithelial) nasopharyngeal carcinoma, the 5-year survival is about 60% for stages I and II, and about 20% for higher stages.
- In keratinizing and non-keratinizing squamous cell carcinomas, the 5-year survival is 20%.

Special Remarks
Since the cervical lymph node metastases are very often the first and for a long time the only early symptom in nasopharyngeal carcinoma, thorough endoscopy and where appropriate biopsy of the nasopharynx are imperative in every case of pathological cervical lymph node enlargement *even when there are no suspicious findings* and also in persistent tympanal effusion in adults.

Suggested Reading

1. Agulnik M, Siu LL (2005) State-of-the-art management of nasopharyngeal carcinoma: current and future directions. Br J Cancer 92:799–806
2. Chang ET, Adami HO (2006) The enigmatic epidemiology of nasopharyngeal carcinoma. Cancer Epidemiol Biomarkers Prev 15:1765–1777

3. Jeyakumar A, Brickman TM, Jeyakumar A, Doerr T (2006) Review of nasopharyngeal carcinoma. Ear Nose Throat J 86:168–170, 172–173, 184

4. Langendijk JA, Leemans CR, Buter J, Berkhof J, Slotman BJ (2004) The additional value of chemotherapy to radiotherapy in locally advanced nasopharyngeal carcinoma: a meta-analysis of the published literature. J Clin Oncol 22:4604–4612

5. Marshall AH, Bradley PJ (2006) Management dilemmas in the treatment and follow-up of advanced juvenile nasopharyngeal angiofibroma. ORL 68:273–278

6. O'Meara WP, Lee N (2005) Advances in nasopharyngeal carcinoma. Curr Opin Oncol 17:225–230

Diseases of the Salivary Glands

Edited by Patrick J. Bradley

4.1 Salivary Gland Anatomy

PATRICK J. BRADLEY

4.1.1 Introduction

In the human, there are three Chief paired salivary glands: the parotid, the submandibular and sublingual, along with several hundred minor salivary glands distributed submucosally throughout all sites of the head and neck (most commonly in the oral cavity).

4.1.2 Parotid Glands

4.1.2.1 Embryology

Each parotid gland develops from a thickening of buccal epithelium. This thickening extends posteriorly towards the ear in a plane superficial to the developing facial nerve. By the third month of embryonic life, the deep aspect of the parotid gland produces bud-like projections between the branches of the facial nerve. These projections merge to form the deep lobe of the gland. By the sixth month, the gland is completely canalised.

4.1.2.2 Anatomy

The parotids are the largest of the major salivary glands. Each is a compound, tubuloacinar, mepocrine, exocrine gland, and it is composed entirely of serous output–producing acini.

Each gland is located in its respective space between the posterior border of the mandibular ramus and the mastoid process of the temporal bone. The external auditory meatus and the temporomandibular joint, with the glenoid fossa and the zygomatic process of the temporal bone, lie posteriorly and superiorly to the gland. Each gland is usually located inferiorly in the neck, sometimes as low as the hyoid. On the deep (medial) surface of each lies the styloid process of the temporal bone. Inferiorly, the parotids frequently overlap the angles of the mandibles, and their deep surfaces overlie the transverse processes of the atlas (C1) vertebra.

Each gland is frequently triangular shaped, with the apex directed inferiorly. On average, the gland is 6 cm in length, with a maximum width of 3.3 cm. In approximately 20% of the population, a smaller accessory lobe arises from the upper border of each parotid duct, approximately 6 mm anterior to the main gland. These accessory lobes overlie the zygomatic arches.

Each gland is surrounded by a fibrous capsule. This fascia passes up from the neck; it was originally thought to separate to enclose the gland. The deep layer is attached to the mandible and the temporal bone at the tympanic plate and the styloid and mastoid processes. This superficial layer is now considered part of the superficial musculoaponeurotic system (SMAS). Anteriorly, the superficial layer of each parotid capsule is thick and fibrous, but more posteriorly, it becomes a thin, translucent membrane. Within this fascia are scant muscle fibres running parallel with those of the platysma muscle. This superficial layer of the parotid capsule appears to be continuous with the fascia overlying the platysma. Anteriorly, it forms a separate layer overlying the masseteric fascia, which is itself an extension of the deep cervical fascia. The peripheral branches of the facial nerve and the parotid duct lie within a loose cellular layer between these two sheets of fascia.

The superior border of each parotid gland is closely attached to the temporomandibular joint, and it encircles the external auditory meatus. An avascular plane exists between the gland capsule, and the cartilaginous and bony acoustic meatus. The inferior border (usually the apex) is at the angle of the mandible, and often extends beyond this to overlap the digastric triangle, where it may lie close to the posterior pole of the submandibular salivary gland. The anterior border just overlaps the posterior border of the masseter muscle, and the posterior border overlaps the anterior border of the sternocleidomastoid muscle.

The superficial surface of each gland is covered by skin and platysma muscle. Some terminal branches of the great auricular nerve also lie superficially to the gland tissue. At the superior border of each parotid lie the superficial temporal vessels, with the artery situated anteriorly to the vein. The auriculotemporal branch of the mandibular nerve runs at a deeper level, just behind the superficial temporal vessels.

The branches of the facial nerve emerge from the anterior border of the gland. The parotid duct also emerges to run horizontally across the masseter muscle, before piercing the buccinators muscle anteriorly, to end at the parotid papilla. The transverse facial artery (a branch of the superficial temporal artery) runs across the area parallel to, and approximately 1 cm above, the parotid duct. The anterior and posterior branches of the facial vein emerge from the inferior border.

The deep (medial) surface of each parotid gland lies on structures collectively called the *parotid bed*. Anteriorly, the gland lies over the masseter muscle and the posterior border of the mandibular ramus, from the angle up to the condyle. Where the gland encircles the ramus, it is related to the medial pterygoid muscle at its insertion onto the deep aspect of the angle. More posteriorly, the parotid is moulded around the styloid process and the styloglossus, stylohyoid and stylopharyngeus muscles from below, upwards. Behind this, the parotid lies on the posterior belly of the digastric muscle and the sternocleidomastoid muscle. The digastric and the styloid muscles separate the gland from the underlying internal jugular vein; the external and internal carotid arteries; and the glossopharyngeal, vagus, accessory and hypoglossal nerves, and the sympathetic chain.

The fascia that covers the muscles in the parotid bed thickens to form two ligaments. The *stylomandibular ligament* passes from the styloid process to the angle of the mandible. The *mandibulo-stylohyloid ligament* (the angular tract) passes between the angle of the mandible and the stylohyoid ligament; inferiorly, it usually extends down to the hyoid bone. These ligaments are all that separate the parotid gland anteriorly from the posterior pole of the submandibular gland superficial lobe.

4.1.2.3   Contents of Parotid Glands

From superficial to deep layers, the facial nerve, the auriculotemporal nerve, the retromandibular vein and the external carotid artery pass through the gland.

4.1.2.3.1   Facial Nerve

Each facial nerve enters the head from the temporal bone, or skull base, at the stylomastoid foramen. The nerve lies about 9 mm from the posterior belly of the digastric muscle, and 11 mm from the bony external meatus. The facial nerve trunk then passes downwards and forwards over the styloid process and associated muscles for about 1.3 cm, before entering the body of the parotid gland. The first part of the facial nerve produces the posterior auricular nerve, supplying the auricular nerve innervating the auricular muscles as well as branches to the posterior belly of the digastrics and stylohyoid muscles.

Inside the parotid gland, the facial nerve separates into two branches, temporofacial and cervicofacial. The division of the nerve is referred to as the *pes anserinus* ("goose foot"). From these two branches, the facial nerve further divides into five further branches: temporal, zygomatic, buccal, mandibular and cervical. The peripheral

branches of the facial nerve form anastomosis between adjacent branches to form the parotid plexus. Davis et al. studied these patterns in 350 cadaveric facial nerves and described six patterns. They demonstrated that in only 6% of cases were there any anastomosis between the mandibular branch and the adjacent branches.

4.1.2.3.2   Auriculotemporal Nerves

Each auriculotemporal nerve arises from the posterior division of the mandibular division of the trigeminal nerve in the infratemporal fossa. It runs backwards, beneath the later pterygoid muscle, between the medial aspect of the condylar neck and the sphenomandibular ligament. It enters the parotid gland on its anteromedial surface, passing upwards and outwards to emerge at the superior border of the gland, between the temporomandibular joint and the external acoustic meatus. This nerve communicates extensively with the temporofacial division of the facial nerve and limits the mobility of the facial nerve during surgery.

4.1.2.3.3   Parotid Lymph Nodes

Lymph nodes are found within the subcutaneous tissues overlying the parotid to form the preauricular nodes, and within the substance of the gland. Typically, most of these nodes within the gland are located laterally to the facial nerve. There are few nodes reported in the deep lobe of the parotid gland. All the parotid nodes drain into the upper deep cervical chain.

4.1.2.3.4   Parotid Ducts

Each parotid duct emerges from the anterior border of the parotid gland and passes horizontally across the masseter muscle. If an invisible line were drawn from the alar base to the commissure, the surface markings of the duct would be delineated by another line running from the tragal cartilage to bisect the alar base–commissure line. The middle third of this line is the surface marking of the parotid duct. Anastomosing branches between the buccal and zygomatic branches of the facial nerve cross the duct. At the anterior border of the masseter, the duct bends sharply to perforate the buccal pad of fat and the buccinators muscle at the level of the second molar teeth. The duct then bends again to pass forwards for a short distance before entering the oral cavity at the parotid papilla.

4.1.2.4   Nerve Supply to the Parotid Glands

The parasympathetic secretomotor nerve supply comes from the inferior salivary nucleus in the brain stem. From there, fibres extend to the tympanic branch of the glossopharyngeal nerve, contributing to the tympanic plexus in the middle ear. The lesser petrosal nerve arises from the tympanic plexus, leaving the middle ear and running in a groove on the petrous temporal bone in the middle cranial fossa. From there, it exits through the foramen ovale to the otic ganglion, which lies on the medial aspect of the mandibular branch of the trigeminal nerve. Postsynaptic postganglionic fibres leave the ganglion to join the auriculotemporal nerve, which distributes the parasympathetic secretomotor fibres throughout the parotid gland.

The sympathetic nerve supply to the parotid gland arises from the superior cervical sympathetic ganglion. The sympathetic fibres reach the gland via a plexus surrounding the middle meningeal artery. They then pass through the otic ganglion, without synapsing, and innervate the gland through the auriculotemporal nerve. There are also sympathetic innervations to the gland arising from the plexuses, which accompany the blood vessels supplying the gland.

Sensory fibres arising from the connective tissue within the parotid gland merge into the auriculotemporal nerve, which passes proximally through the otic ganglion, without synapsing. From there, the fibres join the mandibular division of the trigeminal nerve. The sensory innervation of the parotid gland is via the greater auricular nerve.

4.1.3 Parapharyngeal Space

The parapharyngeal space (PPS) is a potential space located bilaterally in the upper cervical region. The PPS is not readily accessible during routine clinical examination, only becoming clinically relevant when affected by pathological processes such as infections or tumours. The potential wide spectrum of benign and malignant neoplasms encountered in this complex deep anatomic region contributes to the challenge of surgical treatment.

4.1.3.1   Boundaries

The PPS is described as an inverted pyramid, with its base at the skull base and the apex at the greater cornu of the hyoid bone. The *superior boundary* is a small area near the temporal and sphenoid bones, which includes the carotid canal, the jugular foramen and the hypoglossal foramen. The fascia covering the medial pterygoid muscle borders this region of the skull base laterally; medial is the attachment of the pharyngobasilar fascia and posterior the prevertebral fascia. Anteriorly, the medial and lateral borders converge. The *inferior boundary* is formed by the greater horn of the hyoid, and the facial attachments of the posterior belly of the digastric muscle and the sheath of the submandibular gland. The *posterior boundary* is the prevertebral fascia. The *medial boundary* is formed by the pharyngobasilar fascia overlying the superior constrictor

muscle. Medially, the facial layer is the tonsil. The *lateral boundary* is (1) the superior portion of the PPS from above the ramus of the mandible, the fascia of the medial pterygoid muscle and the retromandibular portion of the deep lobe of the parotid gland, and (2) the fascia overlying the posterior belly of the digastric muscle, below the mandible. The *anterior boundary* is the pterygomandibular raphe superiorly and the submandibular space inferiorly.

4.1.3.2   Spaces or Compartments

The previous paragraph described the *prestyloid space* – the anterior space of the PPS – whereas the *retrostyloid space* contains the carotid complex, and thus, this space potentially runs inferiorly into the upper mediastinum. These compartments are separated by the tensor veli palatini muscle and tensor veli palatini fascia, the latter of which arises from the styloid process to cover the tensor veli palatini muscle, and then crosses posteriorly into the parapharyngeal fat.

The prestyloid space extends superiorly into a blind pouch formed by the joining of the medial pterygoid fascia and the tensor veli palatini fascia. Most of the space is occupied by fat. It contains the inferior alveolar, lingual and auriculotemporal nerves and the maxillary artery (resulting in rarely neurogenic neoplasms limited to the salivary glands [neuroma]).

The retrostyloid or poststyloid space contains the carotid artery, with the internal jugular vein related to the posterolateral part of the artery at the skull base. Cranial nerves XI, X, XI and XII, and the sympathetic chain also occupy this space. The vagus nerve lies between the artery and vein, the glossopharyngeal nerve crosses the carotid laterally, and the accessory nerve crosses the internal jugular vein in a direction that is medial to lateral. The hypoglossal nerve ends its vertical course outside the PPS. Lymph nodes and glomus "cells" are also found in this region. A thin, ineffectual membrane separates the retrostyloid part of the PPS from the retropharyngeal space, allowing easy access for the spread of infection and/or tumours from one area to another.

The PPS has numerous lymphatics that drain the paranasal sinuses, the oropharynx, the oral cavity and a portion of the thyroid gland. These nodes have connection with the node of Rouvier in the retropharyngeal space, which drains the nasopharynx, upper oropharynx and sinuses.

4.1.4 Submandibular Glands

4.1.4.1   Embryology

The submandibular glands begin to form at the 13-mm stage, as an epithelial outgrowth into the mesenchyme, forming the floor of the mouth in the linguogingival groove. This proliferates rapidly, sprouting numerous branching processes, which eventually develop lumina. Initially, the gland opens into the floor of the mouth posteriorly; subsequently, the walls of the groove and floor of mouth come together to form the submandibular duct. This process commences posteriorly and moves forward, so that ultimately, the orifice of the duct comes to lie anteriorly, below the tip of the tongue, close to the midline.

4.1.4.2   Anatomy

Each submandibular gland consists of a large, superficial lobe lying within the digastrics triangle in the neck, and a smaller, deep lobe lying within the floor of the mouth posteriorly. The two lobes are continuous with one other around the posterior border of the mylohyoid muscle. The two lobes are not true lobes, as embryologically, the gland – mixed seromucinous – is a single epithelial outpouching.

4.1.4.2.1   Superficial Lobe
Each submandibular superficial lobe lies within the digastrics triangle. Its anterior pole reaches the anterior belly of the digastric muscle, and the posterior pole reaches the stylomandibular ligament. Superiorly, the superficial lobe lies medially to the body of the mandible. Inferiorly, it often overlaps the intermediate tendon of the digastric muscles and the insertion of the stylohyoid. The lobe is partially enclosed between the two layers of the deep cervical facia, which arises from the greater cornu of the hyoid bone and is in close proximity to the facial vein and artery. The superficial layer of the fascia is attached to the lower border of the mandible, and it covers the inferior surface of the superficial lobe. The deep layer of fascia is attached to the mandible, and it covers the medial surface of the lobe. The inferior surface, which is covered by skin, subcutaneous fat, platysma and the deep fascia, is crossed by the facial vein and the cervical branch of the facial nerve, which loops down from the angle of the mandible and subsequently innervates the lower lip. The submandibular lymph nodes lie between the salivary gland and the mandible.

The lateral surface of the superficial lobe is related to the submandibular fossa, a concavity on the medial surface of the mandible and the attachment of the medial pterygoid muscle. The facial artery lies in a groove in its posterior part, at first deep to the lobe, and then emerges between its lateral surface and the mandibular attachment of the medial pterygoid muscle, from which it reaches the lower border of the mandible.

The medial surface is related anteriorly to the mylohyoid, from which it is separated by the mylohyoid nerve and submental vessels. Posteriorly, it is related to the styloglossus, the stylohyoid ligament and the glossopharyngeal nerve, separating it from the pharynx. Between these, the medial aspect of the lobe is related to hyoglossus muscle, from which it is separated by the styloglossus muscle, the lingual nerve and the deep lingual vein. More inferiorly, the medial surface is related to the stylohyoid muscle and the posterior belly of the digastric muscle.

4.1.4.2.2   Deep Lobe
The deep lobe of the each submandibular gland arises from the superficial lobe at the posterior free edge of the mylohyoid muscle and extends forwards to the back of the sublingual gland. It lies between the mylohyoid muscle inferolaterally, the hyoglossus and styloglossus muscles medially, the lingual nerve superiorly and the hypoglossal nerve and the deep lingual vein inferiorly.

4.1.4.2.3   Submandibular Ducts
Each submandibular duct is about 5 cm long in an adult. The wall of the duct is thinner than that of a parotid duct. It arises from numerous tributaries in the superficial lobe, and emerges from the medial surface of this lobe just behind the posterior border of the mylohyoid. It courses the deep lobe, passing upwards and slightly backwards for 5 mm, before running forward between the mylohyoid and the hyoglossus muscles. As it passes forwards, it runs between the sublingual gland and genioglossus, to open into the floor of the mouth on the summit of the sublingual papilla at the side of the lingual frenum, just below the tip of the tongue. It lies between the lingual and hypoglossal nerves on the hyoglossus muscle. At the anterior border of the hyoglossus muscle, it is crossed by the lingual nerve.

4.1.4.2.4   Blood Supply and Lymphatic Drainage
The arterial supply for the submandibular ducts arises from multiple branches of the facial and lingual arteries. Venous blood drains predominantly into the deep lingual veins. The lymphatics drain into the deep cervical group of nodes, mostly the jugulo-omohyoid node via the submandibular nodes.

4.1.4.2.5   Nerve Supply
to the Submandibular Glands
The secretomotor supply of the submandibular glands arises from the submandibular (sublingual) ganglion. This is a small ganglion lying on the upper part of the hyoglossus muscle. There are additional ganglion cells at the hilum of the gland. The submandibular ganglion is suspended from the lingual nerve by anterior and pos-

terior filaments. The parasympathetic secretomotor fibres originate in the superior salivary nucleus and the preganglionic fibres, and then travel via the facial nerve, chorda tympani and lingual nerve to the ganglion via the posterior filaments connecting the ganglion to the lingual nerve. They synapse within the ganglion, and the postganglionic fibres innervate the submandibular and sublingual glands.

The sympathetic root is derived from the plexus on the facial artery. The postganglionic fibres arise from the superior cervical ganglion without synapsing. They are vasomotor to the vessels supplying the submandibular and sublingual glands.

Sensory innervations arise from the submandibular and sublingual glands and pass through the ganglion, without synapsing, and join the lingual nerve, itself a branch of the trigeminal nerve.

4.1.5 Sublingual Glands

When an embryo reaches approximately 20 mm in length, each sublingual gland arises as a number of small epithelial thickenings in the linguogingival groove and on the outer side of the groove. Each thickening forms its own canal, and many of the sublingual ducts open directly onto the summit of the sublingual fold.

4.1.5.1 Anatomy

The sublingual glands are the smallest of the major salivary glands. Each is almond or tadpole shaped. The oval-shaped "head" of the "tadpole" lies in the anterior floor of the mouth, and the wedge-shaped "tail" runs back in the salivary gutter towards the submandibular gland, downwards along the mylohyoid to its attachment on the mandible. It is predominantly a mucous gland. The gland lies on the mylohyoid and is covered by the mucosa of the floor of the mouth, which is raised as it overlies the gland from the sublingual fold. Posteriorly, the sublingual gland is in contact with the deep lobe of the submandibular gland. The sublingual fossa of the mandible is located laterally, and the genioglossus muscle is located medially. The lingual nerve and the submandibular duct lie medially to the sublingual gland between it and the genioglossus. They are un-encapsulated, glandular tissue nests.

4.1.5.2 Blood Supply, Nerve Innervation and Lymphatic Drainage

The arterial supply for the sublingual gland is from the sublingual branch of the lingual artery and the submental branch of the facial artery. Innervation is via the sublingual ganglion, as described above. The lymphatics drain to the submental nodes.

4.1.6 Minor Salivary Glands

The minor salivary glands are distributed widely in the submucosa of the head and neck region, most frequently found in the roof of the oral cavity and oropharynx. They are grouped according to their anatomic location – labial, buccal, palatoglossal, palatal, tonsillar, nasal cavity, nasopharynx, larynx, trachea, etc. They have mixed functional secretions – the labial and buccal are both serous and mucous secreting, whereas the palatoglossal are mucous secreting.

Suggested Reading

1. Bernstein L, Nelson RH (1984) Surgical anatomy of the extraparotid distribution of the facial nerve. Arch Otolaryngol Head Neck 110:177–183
2. Davis RA, Anson BJ, Budinger JM, Kurth LE (1956) Surgical anatomy of the facial nerve and parotid based on 350 cervicofacial halves. Surg Gynaecol Obstet 102:385–412
3. Leppi TJ (1967) Gross anatomical relationships between primate submandibular and sublingual salivary glands. J Dental Res 46:359–365
4. McKean ME, Lee K, McGregor IA (1985) The distribution of lymph nodes in and around the parotid gland. Br J Plast Surg 38:1–5
5. Olsen KD (1994) Tumours and surgery of the parapharyngeal space. Laryngoscope 104:1–28
6. Vidic B, Melloni BJ (1979) Applied anatomy of the oral cavity and related structures. Otolaryngol Clin Nth Am 12:3–14
7. Maheshwar AA, Kim E-Y, Pensak Ml, Keller JT (2004) Roof of the parapharyngeal space: Defining its boundaries and clinical implications. Ann Otol RHinol 113:283–288

4.2 Saliva, Salivation and Functional Testing

PATRICK J. BRADLEY

4.2.1 Saliva

The salivary glands consist of three pairs of large, or major, glands (parotid, submandibular and sublingual) and the smaller, or minor, glands distributed under the mucosa (submucosally) throughout the upper aerodigestive tract. The rate of salivary secretion of individual glands ranges from barely perceptual during sleep, to as high as 4 ml min^{-1} on maximal stimulation. The true volume of saliva per day is unknown, as there is considerable variation both in flow rates among individuals and for the normal volume of mixed saliva.

The specific gravity of saliva varies between 1.000 and 1.010, and increases with increasing flow rate. The osmotic pressure is between half and three quarters that of blood. The viscosity of saliva depends on the distribution of the three glands to the saliva formed. The relative viscosities of the three main glandular secretions after citric acid stimulation were found to be:
- Parotid gland: 1.5 centipoises (cP)
- Submandibular gland: 3.4 cP
- Sublingual gland: 13.4 cP

Thus, viscosity is directly proportional to the percentage of mucus-secreting cells in these individual glands.
- Parotid glands are serous glands, which secrete fluid devoid of mucus
- Submandibular glands are of mixed type, containing serous and mucus cells
- Sublingual glands contain mainly mucus cells.

The majority of saliva is secreted by the major glands, with the smaller glands contributing less than 10% either at rest or when stimulated. Saliva consists of two components that re-secrete by independent mechanisms:
- A fluid component, which includes ions, produced mainly in response to parasympathetic stimulation
- A protein component released mainly in response to sympathetic stimulation

Other factors that can affect salivary composition include:
- Flow rate
  - Flow rate will have marked effect on the concentration of various components of saliva.
- Diurnal variation
  - Unstimulated saliva shows significant circadian rhythms with regard to flow rate and in the concentrations of sodium and chloride, but not in the concentrations of protein, calcium, phosphate and urea. Therefore, the time of the day saliva is secreted has great bearing on the effects of salivary composition and function.
- Age
  - Salivary dysfunction is not a normal consequence of growing older, and is due to systemic diseases, medications, and head and neck irradiation in the majority of cases. Salivary output from the major salivary glands does not undergo clinically significant decrements in healthy individuals. Salivary constituents also appear to be age stable in the absence of major medical problems and medications. It is likely that numerous medical conditions and their treatments contribute significantly to salivary gland dysfunction in the elderly. Another theory suggested is that with ageing, due to the combined effects of atrophy of the acinar cells and progressive replacement of salivary tissue by fat, salivary dysfunction may result.
- Drugs
  - A drug may have no effect on salivary secretion, or it may stimulate or suppress the secretion of saliva. In this way, salivary composition may be altered by virtue of change in concentration of those constituents that are flow-rate dependent. Drugs exert their effects by reflex action, by action on the nervous system, through ganglionic action via the transmitter-releasing drugs, cholinesterase inhibitors, parasympathomimetic or parasympatholytic agents and α- and β-sympathomimetic or sympatholytic agents.
- Source of the saliva
  - Presently, there are at least three types of cells capable of contributing to the composition of saliva, namely the serous and mucus acinar cells and the lining cells of the ducts. Although the compositions of the mucous and serous acinar secretions differ qualitatively and quantitatively, both are concerned with the transportation of electrolytes from serum to saliva, and synthetic amylase and a variety of mucoid substances. Saliva derived from the differ-

ent groups of salivary glands varies in composition, and the relative contribution of each group to the mixed saliva varies considerably.
- Others
  - This category includes hormones, diet, plasma levels, etc.

4.2.1.1   Composition of Saliva

Saliva is composed of a complex mixture of inorganic and organic substances; these can be broadly subdivided into electrolytes, enzymes, other proteins, low-molecular-weight compounds and vitamins. It is estimated that over 200 different proteins and peptides are contained in human saliva. Many of these however may be either isozymes or members of the same protein family. They may range in size from small peptides to large immunoglobulins, and include highly acidic as well as basic proteins. The chemical composition of the secretion of each type of salivary gland differs. The concentration of a given substance in whole saliva varies with species, sex, physical activities, pharmacology state, time of day, etc. No standard state is perfect for comparisons between individuals. Many substances in blood serum are found in saliva. The salivary concentration of some of these is proportional to the serum concentration. Since it is more convenient to obtain a sample of saliva than blood, the former is often used in routine tests to follow changes in disease states and to follow the progress of affected individuals undergoing treatment. With the exception of sialometry (salivary flow rate determination), most salivary function tests must be conducted in special laboratories or clinics. While these tests are helpful, they are invasive, expensive and not always conclusive. Diseases that are considered suitable for such monitoring include:
- Cardiovascular diseases
  - Measurement of serum amylase
- Endocrinology
  - Steroid levels reflect free and true levels of activity
- Infectious diseases
  - HIV testing
  - *Helicobacter pylori*
- Renal diseases
  - Salivary creatinine levels reflect renal function
- Oncology: screening for tumours
  - p53
  - Oral cavity cancer
- Illicit drug monitoring
  - Cocaine
  - Barbiturates
  - Opiates
  - Alcohol
- Psychiatry
  - Monitoring of therapeutic responses to treatment

4.2.1.2   Functions of Saliva

Saliva has the following functions:
- Mechanical cleansing of food and bacteria
- Lubrication of oral surfaces
- Protection of teeth and oral–oesophageal mucosa
- Antimicrobial activity
- Dissolution of taste compounds
- Facilitation of speech, mastication and swallowing
- Formation of food bolus conducive for swallowing
- Initial digestion of starch and lipids
- Oesophageal clearance and gastric acid buffering

4.2.1.3   Salivary Output and Abnormal Functions

Evaluation of salivary output can be determined by measurements of unstimulated and stimulated saliva flow rates. There are a number of different techniques for collecting whole saliva and that of individual gland secretions. However, it is of utmost importance to select a technique that is well defined and has demonstrated high reproducibility. In healthy, nonmedicated adults, the value of unstimulated and chewing-stimulated, whole-saliva flow rates on average range from 0.3 to 1.5 ml min^{-1}, respectively. The salivary flow rate exhibits wide variation in range, and the limits of normalcy for salivary flow in all age groups and both genders are considerable. Salivary gland dysfunction, resulting in inadequate saliva composition and/or reduced salivary flow (hyposalivation), may be temporary or permanent. *Hyposalivation* is a term based on objective measures of the saliva secretion, when the flow rates are significantly lower than are the generally accepted "normal value". Flow rates of unstimulated saliva less than 0.1 ml min^{-1}, and those of chewing-stimulated whole saliva of 0.5–0.7 ml min^{-1}, fulfil the criteria for hyposalivation.

Abnormal function of the salivary glands affects the secretion of the saliva:
- The salivary secretion may be reduced.
- The salivary secretion may be increased.
- The composition of the saliva may be changed at a reduced, increased or normal flow rate.
- The outflow of secretion may be abnormal.

Disorders of salivary secretion and composition can in general be termed *dyschylia*, a term derived from pathologic anatomy.

4.2.1.3.1   Hyposalivation
Inadequate salivary function is often associated with the sensation of a dry mouth, referred to as *xerostomia*. Xerostomia may occur without signs of hyposalivation (in

mouth breathers, xerostomia is related to mucosal dehydration) and hyposalivation may, in turn, occur without the symptoms of xerostomia. Altered salivary composition may occur even when salivary flow is unaffected. Salivary gland dysfunction can be a manifestation of various systemic disorders, or it can be a result of local functional or morphological pathology. Temporary causes of salivary dysfunction include depression, salivary gland infections or side effects of prescribed medications. Medications, especially antidepressants, anti-anxiety agents, anti-hypertensives, diuretics and antihistamines, are the common causes of both hyposecretion and xerostomia.

4.2.1.3.2 Hypersecretion
Increased secretion of saliva is called *hypersalivation*, *ptyalism*, *sialorrhoea* or *hypersialia*. The term sialorrhoea should be restricted to the symptom complex consisting of involuntary flow of saliva from the mouth; this is also known as drooling. This symptom of excess is uncommon, as any excessive saliva is usually swallowed. "False ptyalism" is more common and is either delusional (the patient is alarmed by a sudden awareness of excessive saliva) or due to a faulty neuromuscular control, which leads to drooling despite normal salivary flow, e.g. stroke, parkinsonism, cerebral palsy, etc. Causes are usually local due to increased reflexes, e.g. painful infections, dental procedures or new dentures, or systemic (e.g. nausea) or associated with acid regurgitation. Occasionally hypersalivation may be associated with heavy metal poisoning or iodine toxicity.

4.2.1.3.3 Causes of Salivary Hypofunction
Some causes of hypofunction of the salivary glands include:
- Iatrogenic
  - Medications
  - Radiotherapy
  - Chemotherapy
  - Surgical trauma
- Chronic inflammatory/autoimmune diseases
  - Sjögren's syndrome
- Endocrine disorders
  - Diabetes mellitus
  - Hyper- and hypothyroidism
- Neurological disorders
  - Depression
  - Anxiety
  - Parkinson's disease
- Genetic disorders and congenital abnormalities
  - Cystic fibrosis
- Malnutrition
  - Anorexia
  - Bulimia
  - Anaemia
  - Alcohol abuse
- Infections
  - HIV/AIDS
  - Mumps
  - EBV
  - Tuberculosis
- Others
  - Hypertension
  - Chronic fatigue syndrome
  - Burning mouth syndrome

4.2.2 Functional Testing of Salivary Glands

Functional testing methods include:
- Questionnaires
  - Several scientifically validated questionnaires have been designed specifically for assessing salivary disorders and xerostomia, and may be helpful in clinical practice. The majority of questions relate to xerostomia experienced during mealtime, and therefore these items may be most useful. Salivary hypofunction has been predicted by four additional signs: dryness of lips; dryness of buccal mucosa; absence of saliva produced by gland massage or palpation; and tooth decay, missing teeth and filled teeth (DMFT).
- Sialometry
  - Unfortunately, these tests are complex and difficult to perform. There is substantial variability in flow rates, which make it difficult to define diagnostically useful ranges of glandular fluid production. It has been estimated that unstimulated salivary flow below 45% of normal levels could be defined as salivary hypofunction. In addition, when an individual's glandular fluid production is decreased by about 50%, a person will experience symptoms of oral dryness. The best strategy is to simply monitor a patient's salivary health (both objectively and subjectively) over time.
- The gland itself
  - Anatomy, structure and function can be evaluated by the use of radioisotope scintigraphy, which gives an objective measure of isotope uptake, concentration and excretion – most often used to evaluate the volume of the salivary function tissue of the parotid and submandibular glands.
  - Glandular swellings need to be evaluated by the use of histopathology and imaging techniques, depending on the clinical scenario. The use of sialography, ultrasound, CT and MRI will aid with disease localisation and subsequently, the swelling may need to be biopsied or excised.

- Histopathological evaluation and composition of the glandular structures, as well as differentiating inflammatory from neoplastic disease, should also be performed.
- Drainage of the gland
  - This may be evaluated by the use of sialography: the instillation of a radio-opaque fluid into the major gland ductal system and retrogradely injected will outline the major and minor ductal systems, and also give an outline of the glandular tissue. Sialograms can identify changes in salivary gland architecture, and are useful in the evaluation of major gland swellings. More recently, the use of sialoendoscopy has been advocated, which allows for the most complete exploration of the major ductal systems of the major glands to be examined. Depending on what is found at endoscopy, it is possible to remove stones or debris from the ducts, as well as conduct therapeutic dilatation of stenoses.
- Sialochemistry
  - The composition of saliva changes in disease states, and analysis of the saliva for enzymes, electrolytes, hormones, drugs and immunisation status have been performed, and data are available.
- Microbiology
  - All salivary gland infections should be cultured to identify organisms that may be resistant to commonly used antibiotics.
- Serology/biochemistry/other tests
  - These methods may be required and include the investigation of diseases and conditions such as Sjögren's syndrome, HIV, etc. when auto-antibodies, anti-Sjögren's syndrome A and B (anti-SSA and anti-SSB) and other blood tests are required to aid with making a diagnosis.

4.2.3 Management Options for Symptomatic Hyposecretion

Once a diagnosis of hyposecretion or xerostomia has been established, treatment is designed based on the aetiopathogenesis of the disorder and the prognosis. Methods described and used include:

- Oral hygiene
- Salivary stimulants
- Salivary substitutes
- Treatment with cholinergic agonists
- Acupuncture
- Treatment of the underlying infection
- Symptomatic treatment of Sjögren's syndrome
- Treatment of radiotherapy-induced effects
- Treatment of salivary gland lesions and tumours

Suggested Reading

1. Amerongen AV Nieuw, Veerman ECI (2002) Saliva – the defender of the oral cavity. Oral Diseases 8:12–22
2. Bradley PJ (2006) Salivary disorders: pathology and management. Surgery 24:304–311
3. Mason DK, Chisholm DM (1975) Salivary glands in health and disease. Saunders, Philadelphia, Pa.
4. Ship JA (2002) Diagnosis, managing and preventing salivary gland disorders. Oral Diseases 8:77–89
5. Turner RJ, Sugiya H (2002) Understanding salivary fluid and protein secretion. Oral Diseases 8:3–11

4.3 Clinical Examination and Limited Investigations of Salivary Gland Diseases

JOÃO CARLOS

4.3.1 Clinical Presentation and Evaluation

Symptoms indicative of salivary gland disorders are limited in number and generally nonspecific. Patients usually complain of swelling, pain, xerostomia, foul taste and sometimes sialorrhoea.

Despite the prevalence of modern technology in the identification of salivary gland disorders, a detailed history and thorough physical examination still play significant roles in the clinical diagnosis of the patient.

The most common presenting symptom of benign or malignant neoplasms arising in major salivary glands is an asymptomatic swelling.

The swelling of one or more salivary glands may be a result of duct obstruction, inflammation or neoplasia. A detailed history and physical examination will usually furnish a differential diagnosis as a basis for further testing. Episodic swelling of major salivary glands accompanied by pain and related to salivary stimuli is suggestive of duct obstruction. One study estimates that 80–90% of submandibular gland enlargement is a result of inflammatory disease. Figures 4.3.1 and 4.3.2 display diagnostic algorhythms for acute and chronic swellings.

Pain is reported in 2.5–4% of patients with benign parotid tumours, and 10–29% of patients with parotid cancer. The same symptom is reported in a few patients with benign submandibular neoplasms, and up to 50% of patients with malignant submandibular tumours. Pain is clearly more common with malignant salivary neoplasms, but it is not by itself diagnostic of malignancy.

In general, the duration of symptoms tends to be shorter in those patients with malignant tumours. However, it is possible for patients with salivary cancer to present with an asymptomatic swelling that has been present for several years or even a decade or more. Therefore, the fact that a salivary gland mass has been present for an extended period is no guarantee that it is benign.

For minor salivary sites, the symptoms vary according to the location. They may present with facial pain or swelling in paranasal, epistaxis or nasal obstruction in nasal cavity, painless swelling or ill-fitting dentures in the oral cavity, hoarseness or sore throat.

The age and sex of the patient, in conjunction with knowledge of the demographic features of salivary gland lesions, should also be taken into account in the process of diagnosis. Sjögren's syndrome, for example, is common in menopausal women, while mumps – parotid swelling due to paramyxoviral infection – usually occurs in children between the ages of 4 and 10 years.

A history of systemic disease and of drugs being taken should also be carefully assessed. Dysfunction of these

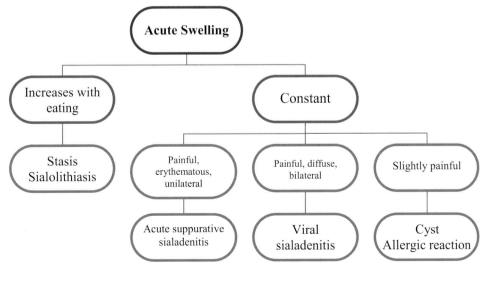

Fig. 4.3.1 Diagnostic algorhythm for acute swelling of the salivary glands

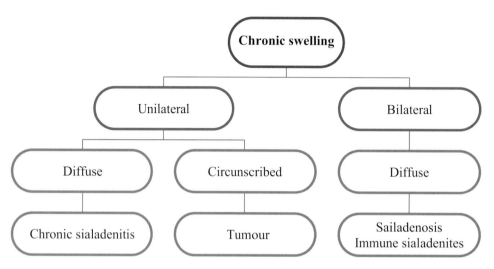

Fig. 4.3.2 Diagnostic algorhythm for chronic swelling of salivary glands

glands is often associated with certain systemic disorders such as diabetes mellitus, arteriosclerosis, hormonal imbalances and neurologic disorders. For example, a salivary gland swelling in a woman of 60 years, with a history of rheumatoid arthritis or other connective tissue disease, has a high chance of being due to Sjögren's syndrome. In such a patient, the possibility of lymphoma needs also to be considered. In a male, particularly if between the ages of 20 and 40 years, a cystic salivary gland swelling should suggest the possibility of HIV infection. Xerostomia or sialorrhoea, for instance, may be due to factors affecting the medullary salivary centre, autonomic outflow pathway, salivary gland function itself, or fluid and electrolyte balance.

Rarely, drugs can give rise to salivary gland swellings, but more often, they are the cause of xerostomia. Xerostomia is often due to the use of psychotherapeutic drugs, diuretics and other antihypertensive drugs.

A careful dietary and nutrition history should be obtained. Patients who are dehydrated chronically from bulimia or anorexia or during chemotherapy are at risk for parotitis. Swelling and pain during meals that is followed by a reduction in symptoms after meals may indicate partial ductal stenosis.

Xerostomia is a debilitating consequence of radiation therapy to the head and neck, and a history of prior radiation should be sought.

4.3.2   Physical Examination

The superficial location of the salivary glands allows thorough inspection and palpation, both extraorally and intraorally, and should be carried out in a systematic way, so as not to miss any crucial signs.

During the initial extraoral inspection, the patient should stand 1–2 metres away, directly facing the examiner. The examiner should inspect symmetry, colour, possible pulsation and discharging of sinuses on both sides of the patient. Enlargement of major or minor salivary glands, most commonly the parotid or submandibular, may occur on one or both sides. Parotitis typically presents as preauricular swelling, but may not be visible if deep in the parotid tail or within the substance of the gland. A masseter hyperplasia can mimic enlargement of the parotid gland, but is easily differentiated by having the patient squeeze the jaws together, which activates the masseter muscle. Submandibular swelling presents just medial and inferior to the angle of the mandible.

During extraoral palpation, the patient's head is inclined forward to maximally expose the parotid and submandibular gland regions. The examiner may stand in front of or behind the patient. A normal parotid gland is barely palpable. The submandibular glands, a swelling of the sublingual glands, and the excretory ducts are palpated bimanually (whenever possible with the palmar aspect of the fingertips), noting the size of any abnormalities and assessing their consistency, surface contours, tenderness, and mobility relative to the skin and underlying tissues. A normal sublingual gland cannot be palpated. It should be noted that observable salivary or lymphatic gland swellings do not rise with swallowing, while swellings associated with the thyroid gland and larynx do elevate. Salivary gland swelling can generally be differentiated from those of lymphatic origin as being single, larger and smoother. The neck should also be carefully examined for lymphadenopathy.

Intraoral inspection should include evaluation of possible asymmetry, discoloration or pulsation, as well as assessment of the duct orifices and possible obstructions. Proper lightning is essential when inspecting within the oral and nasal cavity and pharynx. The openings of Stensen's and Wharton's ducts can be inspected opposite the second upper molar and at the root of the tongue, respectively. A careful survey of minor salivary gland tissue should be performed, especially in the anterior labial, buccal and posterior palatal mucosa. Drying off the mucosa around the ducts with an air blower or tissue, and then pressing on the corresponding glands will allow the examiner to assess the flow of saliva or lack thereof. The flow of saliva, either spontaneous or in response to glandular massage, is an important parameter for differentiating between obstruction, inflammation and normal findings (saliva clear or absent, flocculent, purulent, blood tinged). Dental hygiene and the presence of periodontal disease should also be noted, since deficient oral maintenance is a major predisposing factor to various infectious diseases. The parapharyngeal or tonsillar region may appear prominent due to swelling of deep portions of the parotid gland.

The size and location of a salivary mass are an important consideration. The smaller the salivary gland, the higher the rate of malignancy they boast. Most benign minor salivary gland tumours occur in the oral cavity, while neoplasms arising in other minor salivary sites are usually malignant.

There are certain physical findings that help to distinguish benign from malignant major salivary neoplasms.

Fixation of the tumour either to skin or to deep structures suggests extension of malignant disease outside the gland, with invasion of surrounding tissues.

Facial nerve paralysis in a previously untreated patient usually indicates that a tumour is malignant.

The presence of lymph node enlargement in association with a salivary tumour is another strong indicator of malignancy. Cervical node metastases are noted at presentation in 13–25% of patients with parotid cancer, and 14–33% of patients with submandibular gland cancer.

In patients with malignant submandibular neoplasms, one must be careful to distinguish direct extension to adjacent lymph nodes from actual lymphatic metastases.

Rare clinical entities, such as haemangiomas and other vascular anomalies, may be identified by auscultation.

4.3.3 Limited Investigation

Although a thorough history and complete physical examination are crucial steps in the diagnosis and eventual treatment of any salivary gland disorder, patients occasionally provide little more than vague complaints of pain and/or swelling and no physical signs. In these patients, radiographic diagnostic studies, such as sialography, plain film radiography, CT and MRI, can play an important role in clarifying the aetiology of such nonspecific symptoms (Fig. 4.3.3). For patients with known disease, imaging can assist in treatment selection and planning.

4.3.3.1 Diagnostic Imaging

Careful history and physical examination are often sufficient to establish the diagnosis and the extent of a tumour, and usually furnish a differential diagnosis as a basis for further testing in the major salivary glands. As a general guideline, these studies should only be obtained if they will directly influence the management of the patient. For tumour evaluation, predicting the precise diagnosis is

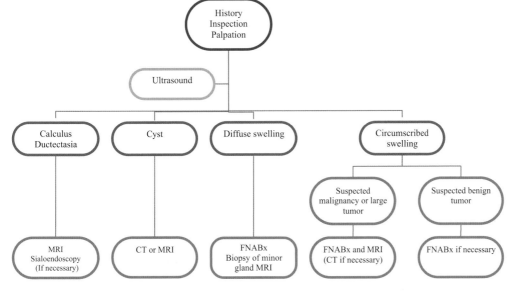

Fig. 4.3.3 Algorhythm for diagnostic investigations in salivary gland diseases

less important than defining the anatomy of the tumour. Particular emphasis is placed on characterisation of the margin and evaluation of possible perineural spread.

In cases of suspected inflammatory disease in the submandibular gland, plain radiographs may demonstrate a calculus in the gland or in Warthin's duct, but their effectiveness is limited by superimposition of bone on the areas of interest and radiolucent calculi.

Sialography relies on the injection of contrast medium into glandular ducts so that the pathway of salivary flow can be visualised by plain film radiographs.

The most common indication for sialography is the presence of a salivary calculus. Often, sialographic examination is unnecessary if the preliminary radiographs detect the calculus beforehand. Other indications for sialography include gradual or chronic glandular enlargement, a clinically palpable mass in one of the glandular regions, recurrent sialadenitis or dryness of the mouth. Sialography can assess perforations or interruption of a duct in trauma cases.

Although conventional sialography can be clinically useful in the diagnosis and the determination of treatment for various salivary disorders, its effectiveness remains arguable, while its rate of usage is highly variable. This method should not be performed if the patient has an acute salivary gland infection, has a known sensitivity to iodine-containing compounds or is anticipating thyroid function tests. Thus, other methods of radiographic diagnosis are currently preferred and have largely replaced sialographic examination.

CT is now more widely used to assess the parotid and submandibular glands. Although stones can be identified, salivary gland inflammation is not generally an indication for CT. Differences between intrinsic and extrinsic parotid gland masses are often difficult to assess, especially when present in the parapharyngeal space. While CT is often utilised as a primary screening tool for the detection of parotid and submandibular gland abnormalities, in difficult cases, a higher-sensitivity approach using both CT and sialography (CT-sialography) can be used.

MRI is preferred for assessment of parapharyngeal space masses, especially in discriminating between deep-lobe parotid tumours and other pathology, such as schwannoma and/or glomus vagale. Some would advocate the use of MRI as the first (and only) technique to evaluate a neoplasm of the major salivary glands. MRI, however, is inferior to CT scanning for the detection of calcifications and early bone erosion. Chronic inflammation of the salivary glands and calculi are not indications for MRI, and pseudomasses may accompany sialolithiasis.

Ultrasound can also evaluate many salivary gland pathologies, providing information about superficial lesions. If the abnormality is accessible to the ultrasound probe, this examination can separate cysts from solids and can identify a dilated duct in calculus obstruction.

Sialoendoscopy is a minimally invasive technique that inspects the salivary glands by using narrow-diameter, rigid, fiberoptic endoscopes. Endoscopic visualisation of ductal and glandular pathology provides an excellent alternative to the indirect diagnostic techniques described above. As such, sialoendoscopy has opened up a new frontier for both evaluation and treatment of salivary gland disease. A lacrimal probe is used to gently dilate the ductal orifice, and then the endoscope is introduced under direct visualisation. During lavage of the glandular duct of interest, direct inspection of the duct and hilum of the gland is performed. Thus, in one setting, at the time of diagnosis, treatment and therapy for benign lesions can be performed. Through a CO_2-laser papillotomy, sialolithectomy can be easily performed. Pharmacotherapy and laser ablation can also be performed. Sialoendoscopy has also been shown to have a significantly low complication rate and is generally well tolerated. This relatively new technique has shown much promise in the diagnosis and treatment of chronic obstructive sialadenitis (COS), sialolithiasis, and other obstructive diseases of the salivary glands.

Nuclear medicine has very specific applications. A technetium-99m pertechnetate scan shows high radionuclide uptake in Warthin's tumours and in oncocytomas.

Fine-needle aspiration (FNA) biopsy provides an opportunity to obtain information about the histology of a salivary tumour prior to the initiation of treatment. FNA biopsy is not essential for every patient. Those who have small, clinically obvious intraparotid tumours will be effectively treated by conventional subtotal parotidectomy, regardless of the histologic diagnosis. Needle biopsy may have its greatest utility in the diagnosis of a submandibular mass, where it can help to distinguish neoplastic from more common inflammatory changes, which may spare the patient unnecessary surgery.

Aspiration cytology may also differentiate a reactive lymph node adjacent to a salivary gland from a tumour within the gland itself. Caution must always be exercised in applying the results if the aspiration cytology is inconsistent with the clinical presentation. FNA biopsy may provide accurate diagnosis in more than 90% of cases.

Many techniques of investigation are research tools and do not, as yet, have an established role in diagnosis. The chief promise of some, such as immunohistochemistry or electron microscopy, is that they may contribute to more precise categorisation of difficult tumour types.

Suggested Reading

1. Ferguson M (1995) Salivary gland dysfunction. In: Norman N, McGurk M (eds) Color atlas and text of the salivary glands: diseases, disorders and surgery. Mosby-Wolf, London, pp 49–55

2. Gayner S, Kane W, McCaffrey T (1998) Infections of the salivary glands. In: Cummings C (ed) Otolaryngology: head and neck surgery. Mosby, St. Louis, Mo., pp 1234–1246

3. Gritzmann N, Rettenbacher T, Hollerweger A et al. (2003) Sonography of the salivary glands. Eur Radiol 13:964–975

4. Loevner L, Battineni M (2006) Imaging of the salivary glands. In: Witt R (ed) Salivary gland diseases surgical and medical management. Thieme, Stuttgart, pp 16–26

5. Nahlieli O (2006) Classic approaches to sailoendoscopy for treatment of sialolithiasis. In: Witt R (ed) Salivary gland diseases: surgical and medical management. Thieme, Stuttgart, pp 79–93

6. Probst R (2006) The salivary glands. In: Probst R, Gerhard G, Iro H (eds) Basic otorhinolaryngology. Thieme, Stuttgart, pp 131–151

7. Rice D (2001) Nonneoplastic diseases of the salivary glands. In: Bailey B (ed) Head and neck surgery: otolaryngology. Lippincott Williams and Wilkins, Philadelphia, Pa., pp 453–461

8. Rosai J (1996) Major and minor salivary glands. In: Rosai J (ed) Ackerman's surgical pathology. Mosby, St. Louis, Mo., pp 815–856

9. Som P, Brandwein M (2003) Salivary glands: anatomy and pathology. In: Som P, Curtin H (eds) Head and neck imaging. Mosby, St. Louis, Mo., pp 2005–2133

10. Ziegler C, Hedemark A, Brevik B et al. (2003) Endoscopy as minimal invasive routine treatment for sialolithiasis. Acta Odontol Scand 61:137–140

4.4 Trauma to the Salivary Glands and their Management

ORLANDO GUNTINAS-LICHIUS

Salivary gland trauma is also referred to as salivary gland injuries.

4.4.1 Definition

Salivary gland trauma is acute trauma of any major salivary gland. It does not include chronic injury to salivary gland tissue resulting from irradiation, chronic infection or chronic obstruction. These salivary gland conditions are sequelae of other diseases or therapy.

4.4.2 Aetiology/Epidemiology

- Salivary gland trauma is uncommon.
- Penetrating trauma: primary reason for acute salivary gland injury, the result of a gunshot or knife wound, or it can be an occupational injury.
- Blunt trauma: mainly caused by acts violence
- Blast injuries: mostly war or occupational injuries
- Often occurs in multiple-trauma victims and can go unnoticed. Typically, these patients are seen months after the trauma, with chronic sequelae.
- In a broader sense, also as iatrogenic trauma: unintentional facial nerve lesion during salivary gland surgery

4.4.3 Symptoms

- Skin laceration and haematoma in the region of a major salivary gland
- Salivary leakage from the wound
- Saliva leakage from scar formation in patients with delayed presentation
- Nerve symptoms: partial or complete, facial palsy or hypoglossal palsy
- Secondary posttraumatic development of a salivary gland swelling due to sialocele formation
- Damage is often overlooked or underestimated, especially when surrounding structures may be injured to the point of being life threatening.

- Damage severe enough to disrupt the submandibular or parotid gland, and have a high probability of being associated with vascular and/or skeletal injury

4.4.4 Diagnostic Procedures

- Recommended European standard
  - History, ascertain nature of the trauma
  - Inspection
    - Localisation of injury site
    - Drainage of injury site
    - Excessive swelling in surrounding tissue
    - Effect of eating on the wound
    - Facial palsy
    - In cases of delayed presentation: saliva drainage in the scar region
  - In cases of open lacerations: direct exploration. Sometimes, a facial nerve lesion can be seen directly in the depths of the wound.
  - Otoscopic examination or ear microscopy
    - Ear canal injury
    - Saliva in the ear canal
  - Inspection of the oral cavity (dental and oral cavity injuries)
  - In cases of submandibular injury: assessment of tongue sensation and mobility
  - Inspection of the salivary ducts and massage of the glands
    - Bloody saliva
    - Blockage
  - Cannulisation of the salivary ducts through the natural ostia, using a lacrimal probe or silastic catheter, gently (not with force) to confirm the integrity of the ducts is important.
  - Inspection and palpation of the facial bones including mandible, zygomatic arch and maxilla
  - Alert patients: detailed evaluation of facial nerve function and mastication
- Additional/useful diagnostic procedures
  - Injection of methylene blue into the natural ostium of salivary duct: helpful in cases with difficult determination of the fistula exit, for instance in a parotid–antral fistula to the maxillary sinus.

– Electrodiagnostics of the facial nerve
  • Electroneurography, and in particular, electromyography in an alert patient. Pathological spontaneous fibrillations (do not usually occur until 14 days after injury) in the mimic musculature during electromyography recording (at rest) are a sign of severe nerve lesion. Initially, only significant decrease of electroneurography response and reduced response of voluntary electromyography should be considered a sign of severe nerve lesion (or lesion of certain nerve branches).
– CT scan in coronal and axial views provides the best evaluation of bone structures, soft tissue delineation and vascular structures.
– MRI is the best tool to evaluate an injured salivary gland.
– To rule out vascular injury: arteriogram, MRA or Doppler studies may be required.
– Sialoendoscopy: optimal to visualise secondary stenosis after injury. It can also be used as interventional sialoendoscopy when the stenosis is dilated endoscopically in the same procedure.
– MR sialography: best imaging tool to visualise the salivary duct system. It is helpful to rule out secondary duct stenosis or to visualise a sialocele.
– Sialography: of limited value, but sometimes necessary in special cases and when MR sialography is not available
– Amylase testing: biochemical analysis of wound or fistula fluid to confirm that it is saliva

4.4.5 Therapy

4.4.5.1 General Aspects

• Acute parotid trauma is usually treated surgically, whereas posttraumatic diseases are often treated conservatively. Due to minimal risk, acute and chronic complications of submandibular trauma are treated in most cases surgically via submandibulectomy.
• Penetrating injury: acute injury should be explored primarily, and injured structure(s) repaired
• Gunshot injuries have a high likelihood of severe tissue damage, infection and tissue necrosis. If the bullet penetrates the salivary gland, a small external wound is commonly associated with a larger intraoral wound. In such cases, wound debridement often needs additional intraoral drainage.
• Posttraumatic secondary sequelae after penetrating injury
  – Chronic salivary fistulas due to parenchymal injuries can be managed conservatively with repeated aspirations and compression, and/or botulinum toxin injection.

– Chronic fistulas due to duct injuries are more resistant to conservative treatment.
• Blunt injury: observation, conservative treatment
• Facial nerve injury: assessment of severity as quickly as possible, because degenerative nerve trauma requires nerve repair immediately for optimal functional recovery

4.4.5.2 Conservative Treatment

The recommended European standard for conservative treatment includes:
• General conservative treatment to reduce saliva flow
  – Pressure dressing
  – Repeated aspiration
  – Parenteral nutrition
  – Antisialogogues
    • Anticholinergic drugs
      – Scopolamine administered via a transdermal patch is effective for 3 days.
    • Atropine sulphate as tablets or drops
      – For adults, 0.4 mg every 4–6 h
      – In children, the suggested dose is 0.01 mg/kg, but generally, 0.4 mg every 4–6 hours should not be exceeded.
    • Cyclophosphamide, adriamycin, vincristine, etoposide (CAVE) chemotherapy: side effects
  – Botulinum toxin injection
    • Botulinum toxin is diluted in a greater amount of normal saline than is used to treat Frey's syndrome:
      – A vial of Botox® is reconstituted with 4 ml normal saline to obtain 2.5 mU/0.1 ml.
      – Alternatively, a vial of Dysport® is reconstituted with 5 ml normal saline to obtain 10 mU/0.1 ml.
      – Between 0.1 and 0.2 ml are injected at each injection point. Four to 10 injections are administered to the parotid gland, depending on the size of the gland, and two to three injections are necessary for the submandibular gland. The injection can be repeated when the effect diminishes, but intervals of 2–3 months between injections should be adhered to minimise the risk of autoantibody development.
    • Radiotherapy
      – To date, low-dose radiation is not offered in any European country, as radiotherapy is reserved mainly for malignant disease. However, it is an alternative in cases in which other conservative therapies fail, and surgery is not possible.
• Development of delayed salivary fistula: confirmation by amylase identification. Conservative treatment is

the treatment of choice, but often, surgical intervention is necessary.

- Development of a sialocele should be confirmed by amylase identification of aspirated fluid. Repeated sterile aspiration and pressure dressings solve many cases. Surgical exploration should be taken into consideration if repeated conservative treatment fails.
- Partial weakness of facial nerve: confirmation by electromyography if available
  - If no nerve lesion is obvious: observation of patient and repeated electromyography. If necessary, a corticosteroid may be used.
  - If there is any doubt, exploration of the region of nerve branches that might have been affected.
    - Secondary/delayed total facial nerve paralysis: confirm by electromyography if available. Observe patient; a corticosteroid may be used.
    - Blunt trauma: observation. Treatment only when symptoms occur. Signs of disruption of salivary tissue by ultrasonography, CT or MRI alone do not justify any intervention.

4.4.5.3 Surgical Treatment

The recommended European standard for surgical treatment encompasses:

- An acute-injury parotid salivary duct should be repaired. In cases of submandibular duct injury, the gland is usually extirpated.
- Injuries to the major salivary gland tissue with duct injury require debridement and closure.
- Complete facial paralysis or evident nerve branch injury must be confirmed by electrophysiological testing, and requires fast surgical repair.
- Delayed development of salivary fistula or of sialocele: if conservative treatment fails, surgical treatment should be considered, in order of invasiveness
  - Fistula closure, proximal duct ligation
  - For parotid gland: tympanic neurectomy, superficial or total parotidectomy
  - For submandibular gland: submandibulectomy
- Tympanic neurectomy: defined as the surgical interruption of anterior and posterior fibres of the tympanic nerve, by drilling into the temporal bone at the hypotympanum. The technique is not described here in detail, as long-term efficiency is doubtful.

4.4.5.4 Prognosis

- Secondary delayed facial palsy: prognosis is as good as that for idiopathic facial palsy. About 85% of patients experience complete recovery within 3–6 months.
- Complete facial palsy or proven dissection of facial nerve or branch and nerve repair: swift repair within

2 months after trauma can result in defective healing, with House-Brackmann grades II–III facial functions at best.

- Salivary fistula and sialocele: utilizing all forms of conservative treatment results in successful treatment of four out of five patients. Only a few require surgical intervention.

4.4.5.5 Surgical Principles

4.4.5.5.1 Parotid Salivary Duct Repair

Salivary duct repair is defined as end-to-end anastomosis of the resected ends of the salivary duct. The repair is done as follows:

1. General anaesthesia is used.
2. Identification of both ends of the duct
   a. The proximal end is identified by massage of the involved gland. The distal end is identified via retrograde cannulisation through the mouth. In unclear situations, a lateral parotidectomy could become necessary.
   b. The ends are debrided and cleaned. If cannulisation is difficult, sialoendoscopy can be used to visualise the end of the distal end of the duct. Diaphanoscopy with the endoscope may help to identify the area in the parotid gland that has to be explored.
3. Mobilisation of both ends to allows tensionless approximation. A microvascular, framed clamp can be helpful.
4. The duct is repaired with a 16- to 20-G silastic stent. The stent should be fixed in the mouth in the oral mucosa. The stent is left in place for 2 weeks.
5. The suturing is performed similarly to that of an anastomosis of small vessels, using 9-0 or 10-0 nonresorbable monofilament suture material, under an operating microscope or by using loops.
6. If primary anastomosis of the duct is not possible, and the duct is injured distally, rerouting of the distal end and oral reimplantation at any point dorsal to the natural ostium is an alternative.
7. In cases of extensive damage, especially in cases of proximal injury, the proximal stump can be ligated, leading to secondary atrophy of the gland. This might be complicated by secondary infection and chronic episodes of pain. In such cases, it might be better to perform a parotidectomy.

4.4.5.5.2 Salivary Gland Wound Debridement

1. General anaesthesia is preferred because the extent of the injury may be greater than was anticipated before surgery.
2. The open parenchyma is explored and facial nerve injury ruled out.

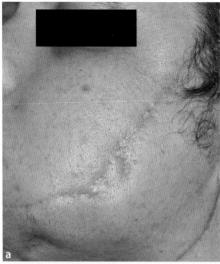

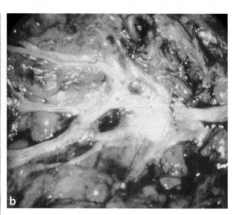

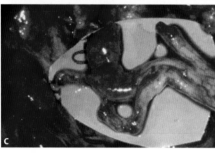

Fig. 4.4.1a–c **a** Patient presented with complete facial palsy 3 months after facial and parotid injury. **b** Exploration shows diffuse scarring of the facial nerve plexus. **c** Complete resection of the scar tissue and reconstruction with nerve grafts is necessary

3. The area is debrided and irrigated. The open parts of the gland are closed with sutures in a layered fashion.
4. Gentle pressure dressing is recommended to prevent saliva accumulation and redrainage through the duct.
5. Antibiotic coverage is indicated, as in any other possibly contaminated wound because of an invasive procedure.

4.4.5.5.3 Facial Nerve Repair
- Primary repair
  - After careful wound cleaning, the cut nerve ends are freshened and re-sutured end to end if the defect is smaller than 1 cm.
  - Mobilisation and rerouting may help to obtain a tensionless situation.
  - For larger defects, reconstruction with (a) nerve graft(s) is necessary; usually the greater auricular or the sural nerve is used.
- Secondary repair (Fig. 4.4.1)
  - The scar tissue has to be resected completely, resulting in clean nerve endings.
  - To obtain a tensionless suture, a reconstruction with (an) interpositional graft(s) is usually necessary.

- If the nerve repair is performed 6 months or more after the trauma, or if it is doubtful/not possible to obtain a freshened proximal facial nerve stump, a hypoglossal-facial-jump-nerve anastomosis is an excellent alternative.

4.4.5.5.4 Submandibulectomy
- In cases of submandibular gland injury, the gland is extirpated.
- In cases of impeded tongue mobility or decreased tongue sensation, exploration of the hypoglossal nerve or of the lingual nerve can be necessary.
- For surgical technique: see Sect. 4.4.5.3 regarding submandibular gland tumours

Additional Reading

1. Van Sickels J E. Management of parotid gland and duct injuries. Oral Maxillofac Surg Nth Am 2009; 21 (2): 243–6
2. Steinberg M J, Hersera AF,. Management of Parotid Duct Injuries. Oral Surg, Oral Med,Oral Path, Oral Radiol Endod 2005; 99(2): 136–41.

4.5 Inflammatory and Non-Inflammatory Affections of the Salivary Glands

FRANCIS MARCHAL

4.5.1 Introduction

In the past, the classic division of salivary gland diseases relied on differential diagnosis. A different concept proposed is to classify these diseases according to their clinical presentation, considering the frequency of episodes and combinations of the associated symptoms. This understanding necessitates separating glands into submandibular and parotid categories because of their different aetiologies and frequencies of these disorders (Figs. 4.5.1, 4.5.2).

Swellings of the parotid, acute and chronic, present in two fashions:

1. Swelling of the entire gland (such as mumps)
2. Partial swelling of the gland (such as tuberculosis, cat scratch disease, benign and/or malignant neoplasms)

In cases of submandibular swelling, the entire gland is considered swollen, and a swelling of part of the gland is difficult to differentiate clinically. In addition, differentiating submandibular gland from adjacent lymph nodes is sometimes difficult and requires the use of radiological imaging. Not infrequently, discrete inflammatory swelling of the parotid or submandibular area is in fact infection of periglandular (submandibular) or intraglandular (parotid) lymph nodes.

Infection of the salivary glands is best defined as an acute and/or a chronic condition that presents as swelling, with or without pain, and with or without systemic unset, which affects the major and minor salivary glands. The most common pathogens identified are viruses and bacteria. The most frequent clinical scenario is that of an adult who presents with swelling of the parotid or submandibular gland, with a diagnosis of obstructive sialad-

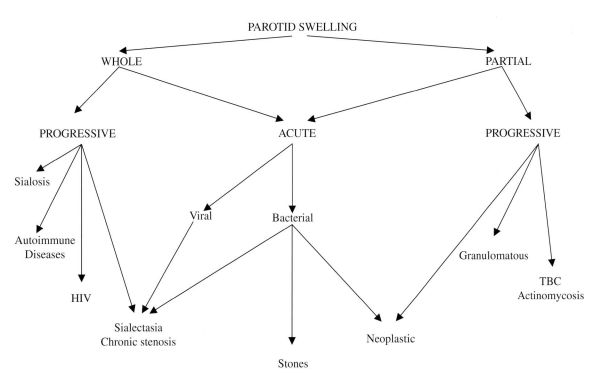

Fig. 4.5.1 Differential diagnosis of parotid swellings

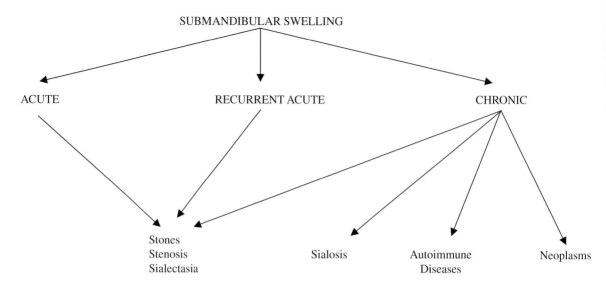

Fig. 4.5.2 Differential diagnosis of submandibular swellings

enitis associated with sialolithiasis, ductal stenosis or sialectasis. Primary obstructive sialadenitis is associated with a bacterial infection. One of the theories proposed for such infective process is the theory of retrograde bacterial infection from the oral cavity.

Infectious salivary swellings have to be differentiated into acute and progressive (chronic). *Acute* is defined as a patient who had a previously normal gland, who experiences a sudden onset of a diffuse, ill-defined swelling of the entire gland or a localised swollen area with indiscrete margins associated with pain, and more rarely erythema, and pus visible at the papilla.

Chronic presentation is a gradual awareness of a diffuse swelling of the entire gland or a discrete, well-defined lump or swelling, usually not associated with pain, sometimes presenting with skin involvement (which might be sign of a neoplasm or tuberculosis).

In the acute phase, patients are treated with anti-inflammatory medications (and antibiotics in cases of pus expression at the papilla). Except for suspicions of abscess, radiologic investigations are usually performed in the resolved acute phase, and include ultrasound, and then by sialendoscopy. In acute, unresolved cases (after approximately 2 weeks of treatment), an MR sialogram or plain CT-MR would be appropriate. In chronic situations, a plain CT-MR, ultrasound-guided fine-needle aspiration cytology (FNAC), or MR sialogram is mandatory.

4.5.2   Viral

4.5.2.1   Mumps

Mumps is the most common viral infection of the salivary glands, presenting with unilateral or bilateral swelling of the parotid glands. In 85% of cases, it affects children under the age of 15 years. It can also affect adults – mainly the elderly or geriatric patients.

Stensen's papilla may be irritated and swollen, but no pus is visible or expressible. Glandular symptoms are often preceded with 1–3 days of a prodromal period, where the patient's complaints might include malaise, discomfort, loss of appetite, chills, headache, fever and sore throat. The swelling lasts usually from a few days to 1 week, and there is no pus at the papilla on examination.

Laboratory findings include leukocytopenia with relative lymphocytosis. Serum amylase can be analysed; it peaks the first week, and normalises at the second or third week. Soluble antibodies directed against the nucleoprotein core of the virus appear within the final week of infection, and disappear within 8 months. Antibodies directed against the outer surface appear several weeks after soluble antibodies do, and can persist for 5 years.

Mumps is due to a paramyxovirus, an RNA virus related to influenza and parainfluenza virus. Mumps is spread by aerosol droplets from the saliva and nasopharyngeal secretions of an infected individual, and spreads easily in highly populated urban areas. Incubation is from 2 to 3 weeks, and the patient is infectious 3 days before the onset of salivary swellings to 7 days afterwards. The peak incidence is at 4–6 years of age, but the incidence has dropped in the last decades because of the systematic introduction of mumps vaccine. Studies have shown that more than 95% of adults have antibodies against mumps. Complications include orchitis (25% in young males), pancreatitis, sensorineural hearing loss (1/20,000 in children, being the first cause of acquired sensorineural hearing loss in children) and meningoencephalitis. Mumps might be a cause of abortion during the first trimester of pregnancy because of the possibility of the mother developing foetal endocardial fibroelastosis.

Classical treatment includes antibiotics, sialagogues and rehydration, the treatment depending on the clinical course and extent of the disease.

It is important to remember that most children who present with an isolated acute, painful parotid swelling do not have mumps; similar symptoms scenarios can be caused by other viruses. These viral infections are not epidemic and are non-infectious, but are sporadic, and are commonly and erroneously labelled mumps. Frequently, parents and general medical practitioners consider that when an acute parotid gland swelling episode arises, it is mumps, but one can only be infected with the mumps virus once, because antibodies are precipitated during the initial infection, and this prevents any secondary infection.

4.5.2.2 Others

Other viruses may mimic clinical mumps, such as influenza and parainfluenza viruses (types 1 and 3), Cocksakie viruses (A and B), echovirus and lymphocytic choriomeningitis virus. Cytomegalovirus and adenoviruses have also been described, mostly in HIV patients. Patients will have the same symptoms as are described for classic mumps.

Parotid HIV manifestations present as enlargements of the gland due to multiple lymphoepithelial cysts. These cysts can be assessed by the use of ultrasound and FNA, which reveal serous fluid with the presence of lymphocytes and macrophages. Their presentation has not been associated with the prognosis of the disease. As the parotid gland contains many lymph nodes at different levels, they might be enlarged, as the HIV virus mainly affects lymphoid tissue. One should not forget a differential diagnosis of solid tumours, which has an increased incidence in the parotids of HIV patients. Infectious causative agents are *Pneumocystis carinii*, adenovirus, *Histoplasma* and cytomegalovirus (CMV), which can be found in the saliva.

Thirty percent of HIV-infected children have proven to have enlargements of their parotid glands.

4.5.3 Acute Bacterial

4.5.3.1 Clinical Course

The disorder is of acute onset, with tender, painful swelling of the salivary gland. Parotids are affected more frequently than are submandibular glands. One of the possible reasons is that the bacteriostatic activity of the parotid saliva is inferior to that of the submandibular saliva. Palpation of the gland elicits pain and purulent discharge at the papilla. Massaging the gland and expressing pus and saliva – although painful – relieves the patient's pain by diminishing the pressure in the ductal system.

Localised infections of the minor salivary glands including sublingual glands can be seen, and have the same causative agents.

Management consists of broad-spectrum antibiotics (after determining the precise bacterial aetiology of the infection) and anti-inflammatories for reducing pain and swelling. In cases of severe infection and associated swelling and tautness of the skin, corticosteroids diminish inflammation and offer quick relief of symptoms. No benefit has been shown thus far with the use of sialagogues for this condition.

The geriatric population is affected by marantic parotitis, caused by dehydration.

Small children can also be affected by this disease in the first 2 weeks of life, in the parotids, and rarely in the submandibular glands, and these episodes most frequently affect premature infants, who are often dehydrated, indicating dehydration as a probable pathogenic factor.

4.5.3.2 Type of Bacteria

The contamination mode of the parotid glands in cases of suppurative parotitis is unknown. Retrograde contamination of the gland by bacteria from the oral cavity, and stasis of salivary flow or reduced salivary flow might be the main causes. Penicillin-resistant, coagulase-positive *Staphylococcus* is commonly encountered, but the flora is usually mixed, containing not only *Streptococcus pneumoniae* and beta-haemolytic *Streptococcus*, but also gram-negative germs, such as *Escherichia coli*. Anaerobic bacteria also play a role, and studies have shown the presence of anaerobic bacteria (*Bacteroides*, *Peptostreptococcus*, and fusobacteria) of up to 30–40%.

Bacteria that affect infants are the same as those that affect adults, such as *Pseudomonas aeruginosa*, *Neisseria catarrhalis* and methicillin-resistant *Staphylococcus aureus* (MRSA). In South-East Asia, *Pseudomonas pseudomallei* has also been reported.

4.5.3.3   Cat Scratch Disease

As this disease involves lymph nodes adjacent to salivary glands, it can involve salivary glands by way of continuous spread. Cats are usually involved, and it is children or young adults contact this disease. *Bartonella henselae*, a gram-negative bacteria, is the pathogen that causes cat scratch disease. Laboratory findings include specific polymerase chain reaction (PCR), or serology. Although generally prescribed, antibiotics seem not to be effective in shortening the course of the disease. The affected lymph node disappears spontaneously with few months.

4.5.3.4   Actinomycosis

Actinomycosis affects lymph nodes adjacent to salivary glands, presenting as salivary gland affection. The pathogen is *Actinomycetes israelii*. Other pathogens include *Actinomyces propionica*, *Actinomyces viscosus* and *Actinomyces odontolyticus*. There are three forms of infection:
1. Acute, associated with suppuration
2. Chronic, slowly progressive, with marked induration
3. Subacute and represented by a slightly tender and tumour-like mass attached to the bone

Treatment of the acute phase is surgical, with eventual drainage of the pus. Broad-spectrum antibiotics are administered.

4.5.4   Recurrent Bacterial or Chronic Parotitis

4.5.4.1   Recurrent Parotitis in Children

Recurrent parotitis in childhood is the most frequent non-viral affection of salivary glands in children, which usually resolves around puberty. Its precise origin remains unclear, and as a result, no specific treatment exists. Sialendoscopy, which is relatively a new technique, seems to be effective in significantly reducing the symptoms.

The disease is characterised by recurrent episodes of acute or subacute, unilateral or bilateral, swelling of the parotid glands, and usually associated with fever and pain. Mucopurulent saliva can be expressed from the papilla, which is often erythematous. Episodes recur every several months, sometimes more often, but the child is usually free of symptoms between episodes. The age of presentation has been reported from 8 months to 16 years, but more frequently from 5 to 7 years, and the symptoms usually decrease or cease at puberty (92% those affected are symptom-free adults of by age 22, in-

dependent of treatment). Histological appearance of the salivary gland reveals massive infiltration with lymphocytes, with lymph follicle formation and cystic ductal formations (sialectasis).

Anti-inflammatory medication is usually prescribed. Antibiotics are given in cases of purulent discharge or persistent swellings despite anti-inflammatory treatment. Among aetiological factors considered are congenital malformations of the parotid ducts, familial history of the disease and impaired rates of secretion (primary or secondary infections, and local manifestations of systemic immunological disease).

Ultrasound is the exam of choice, and is pathognomonic of the disease, revealing typical diffuse oedema and a multiple hypoechogenic, polycystic appearance. Sialendoscopy is the other diagnostic procedure utilised, revealing diffuse reduction of the calibre of Stensen's duct, associated sometimes with multiple localised stenoses, and rarely, salivary stones. Parotid surgery, described previously, as well as ligation of the duct should be absolutely avoided.

4.5.5   Obstructive Ductal Pathologies: Stones, Strictures, and Tumours

See Fig. 4.5.3 for examples of obstructive duct pathologies.

4.5.5.1   Anatomy of the Ductal System

The papilla of Wharton's duct is extremely thin, and difficult to catheterise, whereas Stensen's papilla is wider. The diameter of Wharton's duct is approximately 2–3 mm in a normal gland, and the diameter of Stensen's duct is 1–2 mm. Ductal anatomy, however, differs from one patient to the next.

4.5.5.2   Stones

Sialolithiasis is the main cause of unilateral, diffuse parotid or submandibular gland swelling. It results in a mechanical obstruction of the salivary duct, causing repetitive swelling during meals, which can remain transitory or be complicated by bacterial infections. Traditionally, recurring episodes of infections lead to open surgery. Sialolithiasis still represents the most frequent reason for excision of the submandibular gland, but this attitude has begun to change drastically since the advent of sialendoscopy, which allows glandular preservation. Its incidence varies, according to different authors, from 1/5,000 to 1/30,000.

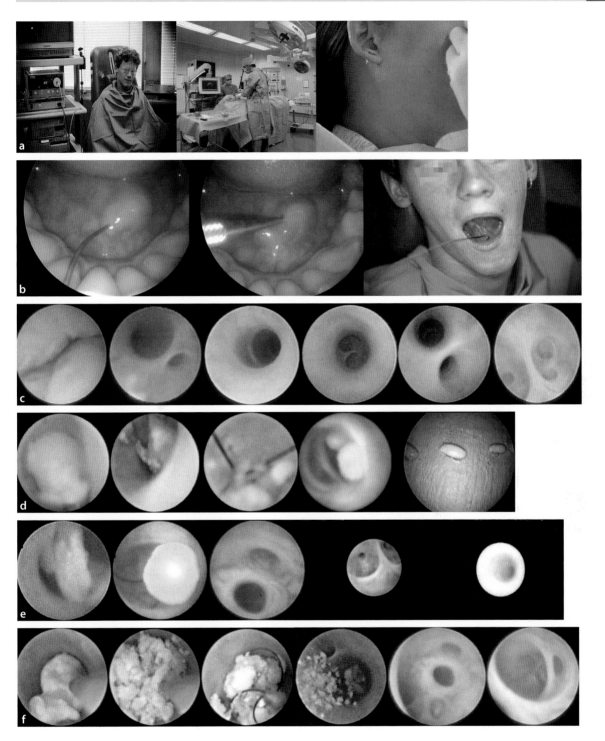

Fig. 4.5.3a–f Sialendoscopic technique and findings. **a** Positioning of the patient and of the scope in parotid, **b** sialendoscopic procedure, **c** normal duct, **d** mucous plugs and multiple stones, **e** stones and strictures, **f** laser fragmentation and stenosis dilatation

Salivary stones are localised in the submandibular gland in 60% of cases, and in the parotid gland in 40% of cases. This difference with previous published data is in part due to the sensitivity of the new detection methods used. Multiple stones are also often present in both the parotid and submandibular glands.

Stones are composed of organic and inorganic substances, in varying ratios. The organic substances are glycoproteins, mucopolysaccharides and cellular debris. The inorganic substances are mainly calcium carbonates and calcium phosphates. The chemical composition consists mainly of microcrystalline apatite $[Ca^5(PO_4)^3OH]$ or whitlockite $[Ca^3(PO_4)^2]$.

The exact pathogenesis of sialolithiasis remains unknown. One hypothesis is that intracellular microcalculi become niduses for further calcification. The other is that aliments, substances or bacteria present within the oral cavity might migrate into the salivary ducts, laying foundation to additional calcification.

Epidemiological studies as well as animal studies have shown that increased calcium intake do not necessarily lead to salivary calculi. Tobacco smoking has been shown to affect saliva in chronic smokers, resulting in increased cytotoxic activity, decreased polymorphonuclear phagocytic ability and reduction of salivary amylase, as well as reduction of salivary protecting proteins, such as peroxidase, and a likely decrease in salivary flow.

A clinical pathological study on submandibular glands removed for sialolithiasis showed the following:
1. No correlation between the degree of gland alteration and the number of infectious episodes
2. No correlation between the degree of gland alteration and the duration of evolution
3. Despite appropriate indications for submandibular gland removal, close to 50% of the removed glands were histopathologically normal or close to normal.

A conservative approach even in long-standing sialolithiasis appears therefore justified.

The Sialendoscopy Working Group of the European Salivary Gland Society (ESTC) has proposed a new classification for stones (lithiasis), strictures and dilatation – the LSD classification (Fig. 4.5.4).

4.5.5.3   Strictures

Strictures of the salivary ducts do cause the same symptoms as salivary stones do. They can be divided in four types:
1. Type I consists of membranous strictures, thin and localised, usually located in second-and higher-generation branches.
2. Type II consists of large (but smaller than 1 cm) strictures usually affecting the main ducts.

3. Type III are diffuse strictures affecting the main duct, with a normal intraglandular ductal system.
4. Type IV are stenotic processes affecting the entire ductal system, which can be divided further into IVa (diffuse reduction of calibre without other strictures) and IVb (diffuse reduction of calibre associated with irregular strictures).

4.5.5.4   Dilatations

Dilatations are mostly associated with strictures, and can be best diagnosed by MR sialography or plain sialography.

4.5.5.5   Tumours

Intraductal tumours (benign or malignant) are a very rare condition, the symptoms of which may mimic that of a salivary stone. Diagnosis is performed by biopsy under endoscopic control, and treatment is planned according to the diagnosis.

4.5.5.6   Radiological Assessment of Salivary Duct Obstruction

Figure 4.5.5 presents several forms of radiologic assessment of salivary duct obstruction.

Ultrasound is the first-line radiological assessment of obstructive pathologies. As it is a dynamic examination, the examiner's experience in the salivary field is crucial. In some European countries, it is performed by an otorhinolaryngology head and neck surgeon who has received proper training. MR sialography, when accessible, is the further exam of choice; it possesses excellent sensitivity and specificity, and also has the advantage of being non-invasive and offers the same images as does classic sialography, but without any injection of contrast medium. Sialography, being in most areas still the gold standard, has some disadvantages: irradiation of the patient, pain often associated with the procedure and potential allergy to contrast medium. Standard x-rays are less indicated, as the sensitivity is poor in case of small stones and parotid stones.

4.5.5.7   Indications and Contraindications of Sialendoscopy

The indications for sialendoscopy in both children and adults are all salivary gland swellings of unclear origin including swellings associated with stones, strictures, inflammatory, or tumour and other processes that might cause obstruction of the duct.

Table III
Endoscopic classification of salivary lithiasis (L).

Score		Endoscopic definition
L0		Duct free of stones
L1		Floating stone
L2	a	Fixed stone, totally visible, inferior than 8 mm
	b	Fixed stone, totally visible, superior than 8 mm
L3	a	Fixed stone, partially visible, palpable
	b	Fixed stone, partially visible, non palpable

Table IV
Endoscopic classification of salivary stenosis (S).

Score	Endoscopic definition
S0	No stenosis
S1	Intraductal Diaphragmatic stenosis (unique or multiple)
S2	Unique ductal stenosis (main duct)
S3	Multiple or diffuse ductal stenosis (main duct)
S4	Generalized ductal

Table V
Endoscopic classification of dilatations (D).

Score	Endoscopic definition
D0	No dilatation
D1	Unique
D2	Multiple
D3	Generalized

Fig. 4.5.4 The LSD classification

Contraindications include acute inflammatory processes. Salivary gland infection and inflammation leads to an increase of fragility of the ductal system, and increases the risk of perforation during sialendoscopy. There are also technical contraindications, related to the material used (if a small-diameter sialendoscope is not available in cases of diffuse stenosis) or to patient anatomy (accessibility of stones and strictures).

4.5.5.8 Tools for Sialendoscopy

The tools needed for sialendoscopy (Fig. 4.5.6) comprises:

- Salivary probes of increasing diameters, ranging from 4.0 to 6.0. They should not be introduced too far, as to minimise duct trauma and prevent perforation.
- A specially designed conic dilator used intermittently between the uses of salivary probes, for gentle dilation of the papilla. As it is a non-invasive procedure, there should be minimal trauma to the papilla, and systematic marsupializations should be avoided.
- Different types of sialendoscopes, the diameter of which should vary from 0.9 to 2.3 mm, including a working channel. A slight angulation at the tip of the endoscope has proven most effective in exploring some parts of the duct that might be difficult to reach with straight endoscopes. In addition, the bevelling of the tip allows for easier catheterisation, and dilatation of the papilla and additional intraductal strictures.
- Different types of interventional instruments that can be introduced in the working channel, such as calculus retrieval baskets, forceps, disposable balloon dilators (low and high pressure), laser fibres and drills.

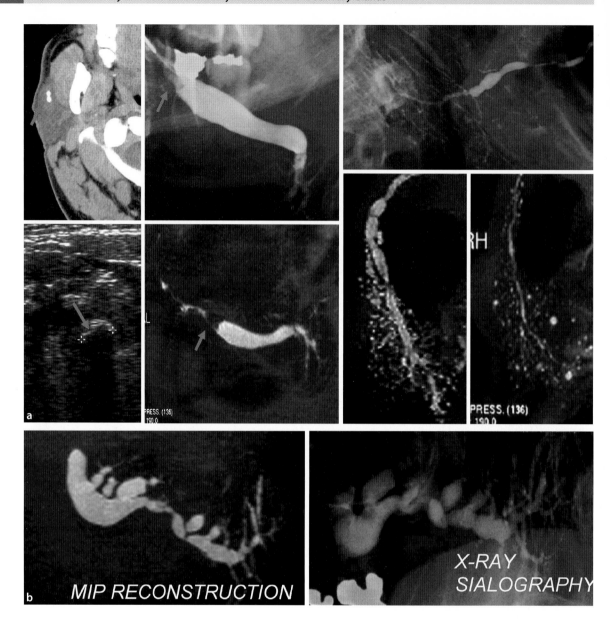

Fig. 4.5.5a,b Radiological assessment of ductal pathologies. **a** *Left* sialolithiasis with CT, sialography, ultrasound and MR sialography. *Right* chronic sialadenitis, and sialodochitis with multiple strictures: sialogram (*top panel*) MR sialography (*bottom panel*). **b** Radiological evaluation of parotid ductal dilatations. MR sialography (*top panel*), sialogram (*bottom panel*). (Schematic courtesy of Dr. Becker)

4.5.5.9 Importance of Restricted Marsupialization

Marsupialization should be completely avoided at the beginning of the procedure. The irrigation liquid has a dilating effect, which provides excellent vision of all ductal branches. Early marsupialization leads to poor visual conditions, and makes the technique more difficult to master because of the irrigation liquid escaping from the opening of the duct system. Furthermore, marsupialization of the ductal papillae, especially in the parotid, should be either completely avoided or kept as small as possible to prevent retrograde passage of air and aliments.

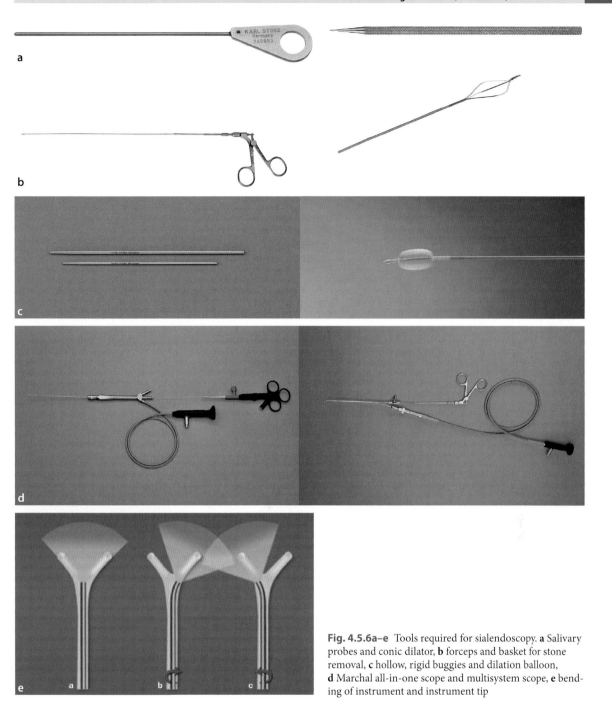

Fig. 4.5.6a–e Tools required for sialendoscopy. **a** Salivary probes and conic dilator, **b** forceps and basket for stone removal, **c** hollow, rigid buggies and dilation balloon, **d** Marchal all-in-one scope and multisystem scope, **e** bending of instrument and instrument tip

4.5.5.10 Anaesthesia

Diagnostic sialendoscopy generally requires local anaesthesia of the papilla and the ductal system. A topical anaesthesia is applied or an injection is given at the papilla at the beginning of the procedure. After introduction of the sialendoscope, anaesthesia of the ductal system is induced with an irrigation solution of Xylocaine.

Taking into account that interventional sialendoscopy is usually performed in the same sitting, sedation or even general anaesthesia can be applied by the anaesthesiologist. This largely depends on the level of difficulty of the individual case.

4.5.5.11   Complications

Sialendoscopy is a technically challenging procedure with a relatively long learning curve. The sialendoscope should only be advanced when distal vision is adequate and non-obstructed. Perforations of the ductal system associated with ductal manipulation could lead to diffuse swellings of the floor of the mouth, and even become life threatening.

4.5.5.12   Interventional Sialendoscopy

Blind retrieval of stones, or treatment of strictures (as described in Subsect. 4.5.5.3) should be avoided, and these procedures should be performed only under direct visualisation.

Calculi are either grasped with the basket or forceps when they float in the lumen or fragmented with a laser beam before the they are retrieved. The laser must be used in tandem with continuous rinsing. Lasers used include the holmium:YAG laser (2,104 nm), the thulium laser (…nm) and the dye laser (350 nm). Potential dangers due to its absorption characteristics in the surrounding tis-

sues and to the heating generated from the fragmentation within the narrow salivary ducts must be considered.

Strictures can be dilated with balloon catheters under endoscopic vision, or with introduction of increasingly sized sialendoscopes.

An algorithm for interventional sialendoscopy is presented in Fig. 4.5.7.

The results of interventional sialendoscopy are directly related to the size of the calculi and the severity of the strictures in both submandibular and parotid glands. According to the literature, overall successful results of interventional sialendoscopy vary from 78 to 93%.

Interventional sialendoscopic procedures might involve antibiotic, anti-inflammatory and corticoid medications, depending on the extension of the surgery. Postoperative, frequent self-massages of the gland are recommended. The diet should be acid free, and no sialagogues should be administered. Clinical controls are performed directly after the intervention. Patients with ruptures of Wharton's duct, or in cases of deliberately extended marsupialization of the latter, must be subjected to careful clinical monitoring because of the risk of oedemic diffusion and/or infection of the floor of the mouth, which might develop into a life-threatening emergency.

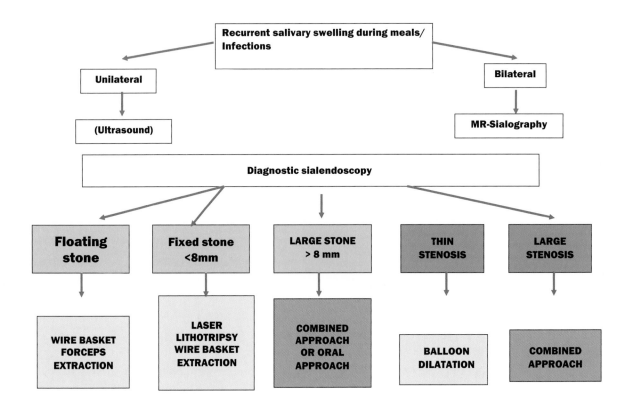

Fig. 4.5.7 Decisional algorithm for interventional sialendoscopy

4.5.5.13 Limitations of Sialendoscopy and Alternative Techniques

In cases of too-large stones, or too-tight strictures, and before considering retrieving the salivary glands when the stone is too large to be fragmented, and/or when the stenosis is too tight to be dilated, the following combined techniques can be applied.

4.5.5.13.1 Parotid Gland

Sialendoscopy is performed classically. Once the stone or stenosis is located endoscopically, the sialendoscope or light source is stabilised (Fig. 4.5.8a).

The patient is then positioned for a classic external parotid approach (with facial nerve monitoring), and 1:200,000 saline and adrenaline solution infiltrated into the planned incision and lateral to the intraparotid illuminated area (Fig. 4.5.8a).

The surgical approach used may be either classic or face-lift type (Fig. 4.5.8b), depending on the age and wishes of the patient. The length of the incision required is calculated on whether the surgical access required is to explore the anterior or posterior part of the parotid duct. The skin is then elevated as is done for the classic facelift approach, and the light source is then activated, in order to localise the stone or the stenosis process. A U-shaped, superficial musculoaponeurotic system (U-SMAS) flap is then prepared and dissected around the lighted area (Fig. 4.5.8b).

When the parotid is exposed, the salivary tissue is dissected very carefully with the use of loops or operating microscope, in order to access Stensen's duct. Since the duct crosses several branches of the facial nerve, one has to be extremely cautious with the dissection. The use of a neurostimulator may help with the identification of the facial nerves and with minimising the possibility of local trauma and subsequent nerve damage. The duct is then incised over the calculus or the stenotic segment with microsurgical instruments (Fig. 4.5.8c). After the calculus has been removed, the distal part of the duct must be examined with the sialendoscope to ensure that a second stenosis or another calculus has not been overlooked. After endoscopic verification that no other pathology is present, the duct is then closed using 7-0 or 8-0 Prolene sutures. In cases of stenosis, the use of a vein graft as a ductoplasty patch will reduce the chance that the stenosis will persist or recur (Fig. 4.5.8c). When large dilatations are present, microsurgical reduction of the resultant enlargement of the duct should be performed. At the end of the procedure, a stent may be introduced either from the external approach or via sialendoscopy forwarded on the guidewire orally. The stent is then attached with a non-absorbable suture close to Stensen's papilla (Fig. 4.5.8c).

The stent's ideal duration of stay should be 2–3 weeks. After completion of the closure, either primary or when a vein graft has been used, it is recommended that the repaired duct is irrigated with the sialendoscope to ensure that a "watertight" closure of the suture line has been achieved to avoid leakage of saliva. The use of fibrin glue may also aid with securing a salivary seal (Fig. 4.5.8d). The U-SMAS patch is then sutured back with interrupted 4-0 or 5-0 Vicryl sutures. The skin is sutured either with intradermal 4-0 or with separate 6-0 Prolene sutures (Fig. 4.5.8d).

The cosmetic results are excellent with this surgical approach: no glandular tissue is removed and the scar is hidden (Fig. 4.5.8d).

The direct approach for removing calculi in the parotid glands through a direct incision in the jaw should be avoided for several reasons: visible scar, and a greater risk of facial palsy and/or salivary fistula.

4.5.5.13.2 Submandibular Gland

Classic sialendoscopy is performed. Once the stone or stenosis is located endoscopically, the sialendoscope or a light source is stabilised.

With the help of an assistant, the floor of the mouth can be pushed upwards by digital pressure from below the patient's mandible, which aids surgical access (Fig. 4.5.9a). Infiltration of the anterior and later, the floor of mouth area, is performed with xylo-adrenalin 1% with 1:200,000 saline (Fig. 4.5.9a). The size and location of the incision is guided by the location of lighted area, and is usually about 2 cm in length (Fig. 4.5.9a). Extreme caution while dissecting in the region of the floor of the mouth needs to be exercised, as the lingual nerve crosses Wharton's duct. After the duct has been clearly identified, it must be dissected from the lingual nerve, which is isolated and preserved. Two coloured Silastic bands are positioned around the duct and the nerve (Fig. 4.5.9b). Traction on the tubing around the duct permits stretching of the duct, and aids with the dissection. Finger palpation allows for precise localisation of the stone, and for the planning of ductal incision with microinstruments (Fig. 4.5.9b). Once the stone has been removed (Fig. 4.5.9b), it is imperative to use the endoscope for completion of the exploration of the remaining distal duct to ensure that residual stones or other pathologies have not been overlooked. The placement and insertion of a 0.45-mm-diameter guidewire should be inserted with the endoscope through the repaired ductotomy, to lie in a position in the posterior portion of the duct (Fig. 4.5.9c). The sialendoscope is removed, and the guidewire left in position, over which the stent is introduced and positioned to ensure stenting of the ductoplasty area (Fig. 4.5.9c). The stent is then sutured with a nonresorbable suture close to Whar-

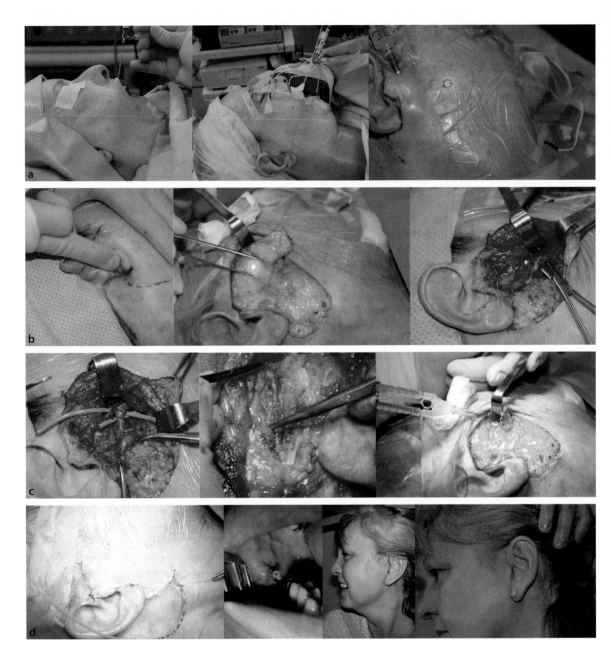

Fig. 4.5.8a–d The parotid combined technique. **a** Positioning of the scope and infiltration, **b** incision, skin and mass dissection and duct preparation, **c** duct incision and reconstruction, **d** skin closure and results

ton's papilla. The stent should stay in position for about 3 weeks, depending on the tolerance of the patient to the foreign body. The stent and suture should be removed as indicated, and the patient needs to be encouraged and supported during the recovery period. The surgical area is closed, one layer onto the duct and the other layer to the submucosal and mucus membrane by using 5-0 or 4-0 Vicryl (Fig. 4.5.9c).

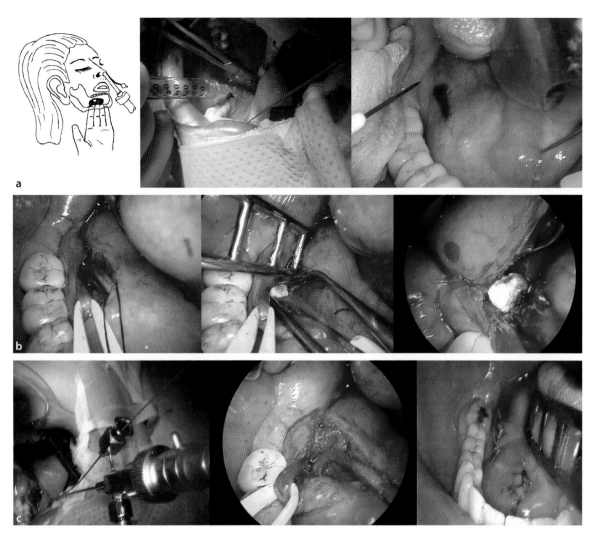

Fig. 4.5.9a–c Submandibular combined technique. **a** Lifting of the gland by assistant, infiltration and posterior incision, **b** after posterior sublingual removal, preparation of Wharton's duct (pulled with suture) and lingual nerve, incision of the duct and stone liberation, **c** reintroduction of the scope, suture of the duct and stent insertion

4.5.5.14 Other Treatment Options

External lithotripsy, developed in the 1990s, requires several sessions at intervals of a few weeks. Once fragmented, calculi are supposed to pass spontaneously, since no stone extraction is described with this technique. The remaining debris can be seen as the ideal nidus for further calcification and sialolithiasis recurrence. Success rates (clearing of the duct) are limited to a maximum of to 75% for the parotid, and 40% for the submandibular gland.

4.5.5.15 Training for Sialendoscopy

The European Sialendoscopy Training Centre (www.sialendoscopy.com), located in Geneva, Switzerland, gathers world experts in the field of sialendoscopy. Under the auspices of the European Salivary Gland Society, it trains clinicians in the indications and procedures associated with diagnostic and therapeutic sialendoscopy, including conferences, live demonstrations and hands-on courses (using animals). Since the first course in January 2002, approximately 500 physicians from 53 countries have received tuition and gained experience in this new field.

4.5.6   Cystic Diseases

4.5.6.1   Hydatid Disease

This diagnosis is suspected in endemic areas, and is extremely rare. Salivary glands are stricken with a cystic condition, and the diagnosis is usually made postoperatively.

4.5.6.2   Ranulas

A ranula is a mucocele of the floor of the mouth, arising from an isolated accessory salivary gland, or from the sublingual gland. It sizes fluctuates, and it might plunge deeper in the floor of mouth and neck, below the mylohyoid muscle. There is no associated pain. The treatment consists of surgical removal of the entire cyst, and it might include in some cases the entire sublingual gland to avoid recurrences.

4.5.6.3   HIV Pseudocysts

For information on HIV pseudocysts, please see Sect. 2.2, "Viral Infections".

4.5.7   Granulomatous Diseases

They are of different types of granulomatous diseases affecting the salivary glands:
- Tuberculosis
- Crohn's disease
- Melkersson-Rosenthal syndrome
    - Cheilitis granulomatosa (Miescher-Melkersson-Rosenthal syndrome)
- Granulomatous giant cell sialadenitis
    - Submandibular or sublingual
- Xanthogranulomatous sialadenitis
- Wegener's granulomatosis
- Churg-Strauss granulomatosis
- Sialadenitis after sialography
- Inflammatory pseudotumours
    - Eosinophilic granuloma
    - Kimura's disease
    - Angiolymphoid hyperplasia with eosinophilia
    - Lymphomatous granulomatosis
    - Rosai-Dorfman disease

Duct obstruction secondary to a stone or (more rarely) to a tumour is the commonly identified cause. The parotid is involved in most cases. Symptoms include painless, firm nodules in the parotid area. Histological confirmation of the disease includes typical noncaseous granulomas.

4.5.7.1   Mycobacteria

Mycobacterium tuberculosis and atypical mycobacteria both affect lymph nodes adjacent to the salivary glands or the intraglandular tissue.

Usually, they are contaminated by local infection affecting the mouth, the pharynx or the lungs. The clinical presentation can be an acute inflammatory lesion or a chronic tumorous lesion.

Diagnosis of mycobacterium tuberculosis is best made by a purified protein derivative (PPD) skin test, which is then followed by FNA, to avoid unnecessary surgery. Treatment relies on medical management using a combination of antibiotics including Isoniazid, Rifampicin and Pyrazinamide.

In cases of atypical mycobacteria, both adults and infants can be infected; it is commonly seen in children between 2 and 5 years, and in adults suffering from immunodeficiency disorders. *Mycobacterium avium*, *Mycobacterium intracellulare* and *Mycobacterium scrofulaceum* are the organisms responsible, and the diagnosis made either by culture performed after therapeutic excisional biopsy of the lymph node, or by a specific PPD test. Its diagnosis is often delayed, as the classic PPD test remains negative. Treatment is surgical excision, but sometime curettage may eradicate the localised infection, depending on its location. Chemotherapy may play a role in suboptimal surgery.

4.5.7.2   Sarcoidosis

Sarcoidosis is a systemic disease affecting multiple organs. Its aetiology remains unclear, but several hypotheses have been made, including auto-antigens and infectious organisms. Salivary glands are usually affected, specifically the parotid glands. Symptoms include swelling and xerostomia. Laboratory findings include diminishing amylase and kallikrein levels during the acute phase of the disease, and the presence of angiotensin-converting enzyme (ACE). Diagnosis is confirmed if there is radiologic and histologic evidence of non-caseous epithelial granulomas. Biopsies can be obtained from minor salivary glands or the parotids, although there is less sensitivity with salivary gland biopsies. Corticosteroids are the best therapeutic option.

Heerfort's disease, also called uveoparotid fever, is associated with parotid enlargement, uveitis and facial palsy. It is a rare form of sarcoidosis occurring patients in their 20s.

Additional Reading

1. Arduino PG, Carrozzo M, et al. (2006) Non-neoplastic salivary gland diseases. Minerva Stomatol 55:249–270
2. Marchal F, (2007) A combined endoscopic and external approach for extraction of large stones with preservation of parotid and submandibular glands. Laryngoscope 117:373–377
3. Marchal F, Dulguerov P et al. (2002) Submandibular diagnostic and interventional sialendoscopy: new prcedure for ductal disorders. Ann Otol Rhinol Laryngol 111:27–35
4. Faure F, Querin S et al. (2007) Pediatric salivary gland obtructive swelling: sialendoscopic approach. Laryngoscope 117:1364–1367
5. Marchal F, Chossegros C et al. (2008) Salivary stones and stenosis. Rev Stomatol Chir Maxillofac 109:233–236

4.6 Sjögrens Syndrome and Sialosis

MIGUEL CABALLERO

4.6.1 Other Salivary Disorders

4.6.1.1 Sjögren's Syndrome

4.6.1.1.1 Definition

Sjögren's syndrome (SS) is a systemic autoimmune disease that presents with sicca symptomatology of the main mucosa surfaces. The spectrum of the disease extends from sicca syndrome to systemic involvement (extraglandular manifestations) and may be complicated by the development of lymphoma. The histological hallmark is focal lymphocytic infiltration of the exocrine glands, determined by a biopsy of the minor labial salivary glands.

4.6.1.1.2 Classification

When sicca symptoms appear in a previously healthy person, the syndrome is classified as primary SS. In association with another systemic autoimmune disease, most commonly rheumatoid arthritis (RA), systemic sclerosis (SSc) or systemic lupus erythematosus (SLE), it is classified as *associated SS*.

4.6.1.1.3 Epidemiology

SS primarily affects perimenopausal Caucasian women, with a female-to-male ratio ranging from 14–24:1 in the largest reported series. The disease may occur at all ages, but typically has its onset in the fourth to sixth decade of life, although some cases are detected in younger female patients.

4.6.1.1.4 Pathogenesis

The aetiopathogenesis of primary SS is a sequential, multistep process that eventually leads to selective damage of the exocrine glands, with consequent target organ dysfunction. The autoimmune process is initiated by a specific combination of intrinsic (individual predisposition) and extrinsic (exogenous agents) factors that generate an abnormal immune response. Thus, the immune system is not capable of discriminating between foreign and self-molecules, and generates an autoimmune response against altered/abnormal self-antigens expressed by the epithelium of the exocrine glands. The abnormal responses of both T and B cells against these molecules contribute the histopathological lesion characteristically observed in primary SS (autoimmune epithelitis) and to alterations in the synthesis of numerous intermediate molecules (cytokines and chemokines), perpetuating the autoimmune lesion. Posterior activation of mechanisms of tissue damage (such as apoptosis) leads to chronic inflammation of the exocrine glands, with fibrosis and loss of physiological function.

4.6.1.1.5 Symptoms

Glandular Manifestations

- Xerostomia, the subjective feeling of oral dryness, is the key feature in the diagnosis of primary SS, occurring in more than 95% of patients.
- Other oral symptoms may include soreness, adherence of food to the mucosa and dysphagia.
- Reduced salivary volume interferes with basic functions such as speaking or eating, and the lack of salivary antimicrobial functions may accelerate local infection (candidiasis), tooth decay, periodontal disease and angular cheilitis.
- Chronic or episodic swelling of the major salivary glands (parotid and submandibular glands) is reported in 10–20% of patients and may commence unilaterally, but often becomes bilateral.

Other Glandular Manifestations

- Xerophthalmia, the subjective feeling of ocular dryness, produces sensations of itching, grittiness, soreness and dryness, although the eyes have a normal appearance. Other ocular complaints include photosensitivity, erythema, eye fatigue or decreased visual acuity.
- Reduction or absence of respiratory tract glandular secretions can lead to dryness of the nose, throat and trachea, resulting in persistent hoarseness and chronic, nonproductive cough.
- Involvement of the exocrine glands of the skin leads to cutaneous dryness. In female patients with SS, dryness of the vagina and vulva may result in dyspareunia and pruritus, affecting quality of life.

Extraglandular Manifestations

- Patients with primary SS often present with general symptomatology, including fever, generalized pain, fatigue, weakness, sleep disturbances, anxiety and depression.
- Joint involvement, mainly generalised arthralgias, is seen in 25–75% of patients. Less frequently, joint disease presents as an intermittent symmetric arthritis primarily affecting small joints.
- Although the main cutaneous manifestation of patients with primary SS is skin dryness, a wide spectrum of cutaneous lesions may be observed, the most frequent of which is vasculitis. Raynaud's phenomenon is probably the most frequent vascular feature observed in primary SS (around a third of patients).
- Involvement of internal organs occurs in 10–20% of patients. Two types of pulmonary involvement are predominant in primary SS, bronchial/bronchiolar involvement and interstitial lung disease. Some patients may present chronic pancreatitis. Liver function tests may be altered in 10–20% of patients with primary SS. The main causes are chronic hepatitis C virus (HCV) infection (especially in geographic areas with high prevalence) and primary biliary cirrhosis (PBC). Renal involvement has been found in only 5% of patients; the main types of renal involvement described are interstitial renal disease and glomerulonephritis.
- Peripheral neuropathy is the most frequent neurological involvement; the most frequent types of neuropathy are mixed polyneuropathy, pure sensory neuropathy and mononeuritis multiplex. Some patients may present an associated myelopathy.
- Psychiatric disorders, including depression and anxiety, have also been described in many patients with SS. Nearly a third of patients with primary SS have thyroid disease.

4.6.1.1.6 Diagnostic Approach

Sicca features are symptoms that usually receive little attention, and may be considered trivial by both doctor and patient. Although often elusive, an early, accurate diagnosis of SS can help prevent, or ensure, timely treatment of many of the complications associated with the disease.

Recommended European Standard

- Inspection (cheilitis, parotid swelling, etc.)
- Palpation of the parotid and submaxillary glands
- Inspection of the oral cavity and nasopharynx

Special Tests

- Oral involvement
  - Several methods to assess have been proposed, such as measurement of the salivary flow rate, sialochemistry, sialography or scintigraphy.
- The main ocular tests are Schirmer's test and rose Bengal staining.
- Minor salivary gland biopsy remains a highly specific test for the diagnosis of SS, although it is an invasive technique that, when not correctly performed, may be accompanied by local side effects. Focal lymphocytic sialadenitis, defined as multiple, dense aggregates of 50 or more lymphocytes in perivascular or periductal areas in the majority of sampled glands, is the characteristic histopathologic feature of SS. The key requirements for a correct histological evaluation are an adequate number of informative lobules (at least four) and the determination of an average focus score (a focus is a cluster of at least 50 lymphocytes). However, nonspecific sialadenitis is quite common in biopsy samples of minor salivary glands in healthy control populations. Although sialadenitis is the key histopathologic feature of SS, its presence in the absence of symptoms and markers suggestive of SS should be interpreted with caution.

Laboratory Findings

- The most frequent analytical features are cytopenia (33%), raised erythrocyte sedimentation rate ([ESR] 22%) and hypergammaglobulinaemia (22%). The most frequent cytopenia detected are normocytic anaemia (20%), leucopoenia (16%) and thrombocytopenia (13%), seen more frequently in patients with positive immunological markers.
- The main immunological markers found in primary SS are
  - Antinuclear antibodies (ANA), are the most-frequently-detected antibodies in primary SS (in more than 80% of cases), and titres >1/80 play a central role in differentiating SS from non-autoimmune causes of sicca syndrome.
  - Anti-Ro/SS-A and La/SS-B antibodies are detected in 30–60% of patients and are closely associated with most extraglandular features.
  - Rheumatoid factor (RF)
    - In nearly 50% of cases, patients with primary SS also present with a positive RF.
  - Hypocomplementaemia and cryoglobulinaemia are two closely related immunological markers that have been linked with more severe SS.
  - Circulating monoclonal immunoglobulins may be detected in nearly 20% of patients with primary SS.

Differential Diagnosis

The proven diagnosis of SS requires not only documentation of sicca symptoms, but also objective evidence of dry eyes and mouth, and analytical evidence of autoimmunity, as sicca syndrome has many causes. The most frequent cause of sicca features is the chronic use of "drying" drugs (mainly antihypertensive, antihistamine and antidepressant agents), especially in the elderly. After this, there are two other main causes of a sicca syndrome. First, some processes may mimic the clinical picture of SS through a nonlymphocytic infiltration of the exocrine glands by granulomas (sarcoidosis, tuberculosis), or amyloid or malignant cells. Secondly, extrinsic factors, mainly chronic viral infections (HCV, HIV) may induce a lymphocytic infiltration of exocrine glands.

A variety of hematopoietic malignancies and carcinomas can cause salivary gland enlargement, as can amyloidosis and certain chronic infections such as tuberculosis or sarcoidosis, HCV, infectious parotitis, metabolic disorders (uraemia, diabetes mellitus), bulimia, Mikulicz's syndrome, and drug-related parotid enlargement (e.g. iodides, phenylbutazone, propylthiouracil).

Test imaging (ecography, NMR) and tissue-sampling fine-needle aspiration (FNA) will help to assess the diagnosis.

Therapy

At present, there is no treatment capable of modifying the evolution of SS, and the therapeutic approach is based on symptomatic replacement or stimulation of glandular secretions, while extraglandular involvement requires an organ-specific therapy with corticosteroids and immunosuppressive agents, similar to that applied in SLE patients.

Recommended European Standard

- Treatment of oral sicca and salivary gland manifestations is mainly symptomatic and is typically intended to limit the damage resulting from chronic involvement.
  - Mouth dryness may be avoided by sipping fluids throughout the day, chewing sugarless gum and using a saliva substitute–containing carboxymethylcellulose as a mouthwash. Moisture replacement products can be effective for patients with mild or moderate symptoms.
  - For patients with SS who have residual salivary gland function, stimulation of saliva flow with a secretagogue is the treatment of choice, and at present is the most efficacious means to prevent long-term oral complications. Two muscarinic agonists (pilocarpine and cevimeline) have been approved for the treatment of sicca symptoms in SS. These agents stimulate the M1 and M3 receptors present on salivary glands, leading to increased secretory function.
  - Oral candidiasis should be treated with nystatin.
  - Use of anticholinergic medications, alcohol and smoking should be avoided whenever possible.
  - Oral hygiene and regular dental visits are essential.
  - Salivary stones must be promptly removed, preserving viable salivary tissue.

  - The pain of suddenly enlarged salivary glands is generally best treated with warm compresses and nonsteroidal anti-inflammatory drugs.
- Treatment of other sicca manifestations
  - Frequent use of tear substitutes will help replace moisture, and preservative-free formulations help avoid the irritation that can occur with frequent use, while lubricating ointments and methylcellulose inserts are usually reserved for nocturnal use.
  - In moderate-to-severe xerophthalmia, frequent use of preservative-free artificial tears – in dosing intervals as often as hourly – is highly recommended.
- Treatment of systemic manifestations
  - As a rule, the management of extraglandular features should be organ specific, with corticosteroids and immunosuppressive agents being limited to severe involvement.
  - Nonsteroidal anti-inflammatory drugs usually provide relief from the minor musculoskeletal symptoms of SS.
  - Hydroxychloroquine may be used in patients with fatigue, arthralgias and myalgias.
  - For patients with moderate extraglandular involvement (mainly arthritis, extensive cutaneous purpura and nonsevere peripheral neuropathy), 0.5 mg/kg/day of corticosteroids may be sufficient, while in patients with internal organ involvement (pulmonary alveolitis, glomerulonephritis or severe neurological features), a combination of prednisone and immunosuppressive agents (cyclophosphamide, azathioprine, mycophenolate mofetil) is suggested.
  - In refractory cases, off-label use of biological agents should be considered. Recent studies have demonstrated the lack of efficacy of anti-tumour necrosis factor (TNF) agents in primary SS. In contrast, a promising treatment is rituximab (anti-CD20), a monoclonal agent approved for the treatment of B-cell lymphoma.

Complications

Primary SS usually progresses very slowly, with no rapid deterioration in salivary function or dramatic changes in sicca symptoms. The main exceptions to this benign course are the development of extraglandular manifestations and the high incidence of lymphoma (Fig. 4.6.1).

Prognosis

With respect to extraglandular involvement, SS patients may be divided into two groups with a different prognosis. A more stable, chronic SS course is usually found in patients with predominantly periepithelial lesions (such as interstitial nephritis, liver or lung disease), while those with predominantly extraepithelial expression (glomerulonephritis, polyneuropathy and vasculitis) present

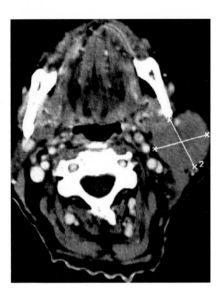

Fig. 4.6.1 CT scan: lymphoma of the parotid in a patient diagnosed with Sjögren's syndrome

a higher morbidity and mortality. Cryoglobulinaemia probably plays a central aetiopathogenic role in this latter group of patients, contributing to the development of the main extraepithelial manifestations.

4.6.1.2 Sialosis

4.6.1.2.1 Definition
Sialosis (sialoadenosis, or sialadenosis) is a form of salivary gland swelling characterized by persistent, asymptomatic, bilateral, diffuse, non-inflammatory, non-neoplastic parotid swelling with occasional involvement of the submandibular salivary gland and, rarely, the minor salivary glands.

4.6.1.2.2 Classification
Sialosis is related to four main conditions:
1. Idiopathic
2. Nutritional
   a. Malnutrition
   b. Bulimia
   c. Gastrointestinal disease
   d. Amylophagia
   e. Vitamin A deficiency
3. Drug induced
   a. Alcohol
   b. Antihypertensives
   c. Naproxen
   d. Valproic acid

4. Endocrine/metabolic
   a. Diabetes insipidus
   b. Diabetes mellitus
   c. Hypothyroidism
   d. Cirrhosis of the liver
   e. Uraemia

4.6.1.2.3 Epidemiology
There is no sex predilection, and the peak age incidence is between 30 and 70 years of age.

4.6.1.2.4 Pathogenesis
An autonomic neuropathy, seen as a demyelinating polyneuropathy, seems to be the common underlying basis for this seemingly disparate group of patients with sialosis. The neural dysregulation results in excessive stimulation of protein synthesis and/or inhibition of its secretion, resulting in cellular hypertrophy. Normal acini measure up to 40 μm in diameter, while in sialosis, measurements achieve 50–70 μm.

4.6.1.2.5 Signs and Symptoms
Generally, signs and symptoms include symmetric, painless parotid gland swellings, with normal in-tone on palpation, and after of years of evolution.

4.6.1.2.6 Diagnostic Approach

Recommended European Standard
- Clinical history
- Physical examination
  - The groove between the mastoid process and the ramus of the mandible becomes obliterated, and there is appreciable swelling that gives a trapezoid appearance.
- Palpation of the parotid and submaxillary glands
- Blood analyses
  - Study of liver enzymes, bilirubin, protein and albumin levels
- CT scan, searching any intraglandular lesions or calcified bodies
- MRI for excluding other diseases (the best image test for salivary glands study)
- FNA biopsy
  - Swelling could be associated with benign acini/acinic cells and adipose tissue but no inflammatory or abnormal cells.
- Sialography
  - There is a lack of arborisation being caused by the separation of secretory ducts from each other and compression of smaller interlobular canaliculi.

- Sialochemistry has virtually no benefit in diagnosis, although raised concentrations of potassium and amylase activity have been reported.
- Sialometry is of little practical value because salivary secretory activity depends of the aetiology.

4.6.1.2.7 Differential Diagnosis

The differential diagnosis must be performed from other pathologic states that cause bilateral parotid swelling.

- Diabetic parotid sialosis can be differentiated with the evaluation of serum glucose levels.
- Epidemic parotitis, or mumps, is a painful viral disease that occurs once and confers immunity.
- Bulimic parotid swellings are associated with chronic emesis and serum electrolyte changes.
- SS with bilateral parotid swellings can be diagnosed by the presence of xerostomia, xerophthalmia, classic serum antibodies and a frequent association with a systemic connective tissue disease.
- Sarcoid-induced bilateral parotid swellings have some hallmarks such as lung infiltrates, hilar lymphadenopathy and microscopic granulomas.
- The bilateral parotid swellings seen in HIV disease reflect the presence of lymphoepithelial cysts and/or a lymphoproliferative infiltrate readily imaged by a CT scan, whose origins can be substantiated by blood studies.
- Non-Hodgkin's lymphoma, causing bilateral parotid swellings, is best diagnosed by the presence of widespread organ involvement, lymphadenopathies and histologic examination.

4.6.1.2.8 Therapy

Recommended European Standard
Treatment of sialosis is unnecessary.

4.6.1.2.9 Complications

There are no important related complications.

4.6.1.2.10 Prognosis

The prognosis of the patients with sialosis depends on the aetiology.

Suggested Reading

1. Fox RI (2005) Sjögren's syndrome. Lancet 366:321–331
2. Ioannidis JP, Vassiliou VA, Moutsopoulos HM (2002) Long-term risk of mortality and lymphoproliferative disease and predictive classification of primary Sjögren's syndrome. Arthritis Rheum 46:741–741
3. Kassan SS, Moutsopoulos HM (2004) Clinical manifestations and early diagnosis of Sjögren's syndrome. Arch Intern Med 164:1275–1284
4. Mandel L, Vakkas J, Saqi A (2005) Alcoholic (beer) sialosis. J Oral Maxillofac Surg 63:402–405
5. Ramos-Casals M, Tzioufas AG, Font J (2005) Primary Sjögren's syndrome: new clinical and therapeutic concepts. Ann Rheum Dis 64:347–354
6. Ramos-Casals M, Solans R, Rosas J, Camps MT, Gil A, Del Pino-Montes J et al. (2008) GEMESS Study Group. Primary Sjögren's syndrome in Spain: clinical and immunologic expression in 1,010 patients. Medicine (Baltimore) 87:210–219
7. Scully C, Bagán JV, Eveson JW, Barnard N, Turner FM (2008) Sialosis: 35 cases of persistent parotid swelling from two countries. Br J Oral Maxillofac Surg 46:468–472
8. Theander E, Manthorpe R, Jacobsson LT (2004) Mortality and causes of death in primary Sjögren's syndrome: a prospective cohort study. Arthritis Rheum 50:1262–1269

4.7 Salivary Glands: Benign Tumours

DAVIDE LOMBARDI

4.7.1 Definition of the Disease

Salivary gland benign tumours encompass a large spectrum of different histologies, mainly those of epithelial origin (Table 4.7.1).

4.7.2 Epidemiology/Aetiology

Salivary gland tumours account for about 2–3% of all neoplasms of the head and neck region, with an annual incidence of 5 new cases per 100,000 inhabitants.

Roughly 70–85% of salivary gland neoplasms originate in the parotid gland, whereas the occurrence in the submandibular and minor salivary glands is much lower (about 10% each). The observation of a sublingual gland neoplasm is a rare event.

The overwhelming majority (80–85%) of parotid gland (PG) tumours is benign, and the rate decreases for the submandibular gland (SMG; 40–55%), minor salivary glands (MSG; 20–50%) and sublingual gland (SLG; 15–30%).

Among benign salivary gland tumours, *pleomorphic adenoma* (PA) is most frequently encountered, accounting for about 60% of all salivary gland tumours. PA originates within the PG in about 80% of cases, whereas the remaining 20% occur in the SMG and MSG.

Its annual incidence is about 2.4–3.05 new cases per 100,000 inhabitants. The age of presentation ranges from 10 to 90 years, with a peak incidence at 46 years. A slight female predominance is reported. PA is composed of epithelial and myoepithelial cells associated with mesenchymal components within a stroma of mucoid, chondroid, myxoid and osteoid origin. Epithelial cells may be of different types, including cuboidal, squamous, spindle and clear cells. According to the proportion between chondromyxoid stroma and the number of cells, three subtypes of PA have been identified: classical, cellular (cell rich) and myxoid (also known as hypocellular, or stroma rich) (Figs. 4.7.1–4.7.3).

The second commonest histotype among benign salivary gland tumours is *Warthin's tumour* (WT), which is almost exclusively localised in the PG, although rare cases involving the periparotid lymph nodes have been

Table 4.7.1 Classification of salivary gland benign tumours according to the WHO Classification [1]

Benign epithelial tumours	Benign soft tissue tumours
Pleomorphic adenoma (also known as benign mixed tumour)	Haemangioma
Myoepithelioma	
Basal cell adenoma	
Warthin's tumour (also known as papillary cystadenoma lymphomatosum)	
Oncocytoma	
Canalicular adenoma	
Sebaceous adenoma	
Lymphadenoma	
Sebaceous	
Non-sebaceous	
Ductal papillomas	
Inverted ductal papilloma	
Intraductal papilloma	
Sialoadenoma papilliferum	
Cystadenoma	

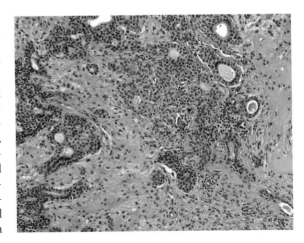

Fig. 4.7.1 Histologic features of PA (classic variant): neoplasm made of myxoid stroma with chondroid metaplasia and aggregates of myoepithelial cells with epithelial ducts covered by cubic and cylindrical cells (haematoxylin and eosin staining [HE])

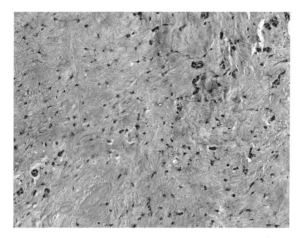

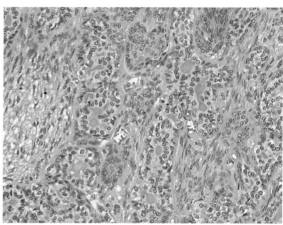

Fig. 4.7.2 Histologic features of PA (myxoid or hypocellular variant): the neoplasm is almost completely composed of myxoid stroma, with rare myoepithelial cells and epithelial ducts (HE)

Fig. 4.7.3 Histologic features of PA (cellular variant): prevalence of myoepithelial cells in solid aggregates; epithelial ducts are visible, whereas the myxoid stroma is scarce (H-E)

reported. WT is a lesion made up of glandular and cystic structures lined by a bilayered epithelium and a stroma where lymphoid tissue with germinative centres is present (Fig. 4.7.4). WT accounts for 3.5–30% of all salivary epithelial tumours, and large variations have been reported in different geographical areas. This discrepancy may be due to smoking, since a substantial proportion of patients with WT are smokers. Another possible factor in the development of WT is radiation exposure. Though the occurrence of WT before 40 years is very rare, age at presentation may range from 12 to 92 years, with a peak incidence at 62 years. Nowadays, the previously reported strong male predominance is no longer observed.

Other epithelial tumours, such as *basal cell adenoma* and *oncocytoma*, are much rarer, since they account for only 1–3 and 1% of all salivary gland tumours, respectively.

Among benign nonepithelial tumours, the most frequently encountered are mesenchymal lesions, which account for about 1.9–4.7% of all salivary gland tumours. The vast majority arise within the PG and SMG (85 and 10%, respectively). *Haemangiomas*, which usually occur in the first decade of life, account for 40% of benign mesenchymal tumours and for 70–80% of all vascular lesions of salivary glands (Fig. 4.7.5). Neural tumours and lipomas are more rarely found, whereas other types of mesenchymal lesions are only occasionally observed.

4.7.3   Symptoms

The clinical presentation of benign tumours of the salivary glands is quite repetitive, with slight differences related to the site of origin.

4.7.3.1   Pleomorphic Adenoma

4.7.3.1.1   Lesions Arising in the Superficial Lobe
The usual feature here is a painless lump in the preauricular or retromandibular areas (Fig. 4.7.6). The tumour mass usually shows well-defined margins; at palpation, it may appear mobile over superficial and deep planes, with firm or hard consistency. Large tumours may appear as polylobulated lesions. Growth is generally slow, and the patient does not report any sudden change in mass size

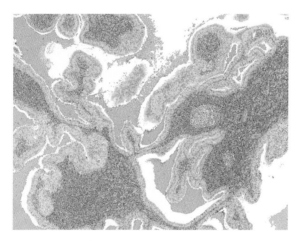

Fig. 4.7.4 Histologic features of WT: neoplasm made of cystic areas and papillary digitations, with double-layered epithelial cells surrounding a central part of lymphatic tissue (HE)

and/or morphology in relation to meals. On occasion, the presenting complaint may be parotid abscess due to superinfection of an otherwise-asymptomatic nodule.

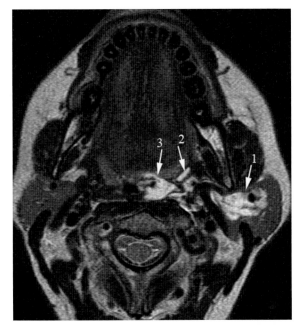

Fig. 4.7.5 Parotid gland haemangioma. MRI shows a hyperintense lesion located in the parotid gland (*1*), parapharyngeal space (*2*) and pharyngeal mucosal space (*3*). Both signal intensity and the trans-spatial pattern of growth are consistent with haemangioma

4.7.3.1.2 Lesions Arising in the Deep Lobe

The lesion presents as swelling that is less well defined in borders and is barely palpable. Medialisation of the lateral oropharyngeal wall and/or the soft palate may be observed. When a remarkable oropharyngeal wall displacement is present, dysphagia and/or dyspnea due to reduced pharyngeal space and/or cranial nerves (IX, X) dysfunction may be referred.

4.7.3.1.3 Lesions Arising in the Accessory Lobe

About 1–8% of all parotid tumours originate in the accessory lobe. When a neoplasm arises in this site, a mid-cheek mass with the same physical features of a lesion of the superficial lobe is evident (Fig. 4.5.7).

4.7.3.2 Submandibular Gland

The most common presentation is a slow-growing, usually painless mass in the submandibular region. No volume changes while eating are observed. The lesion is mobile over superficial and deep planes.

4.7.3.3 Sub-lingual Gland

A submucosal mass in the anterior floor of the mouth, lateral to the lingual caruncle is commonly observed. The lesion is slow growing, usually painless and may cause discomfort in lingual movements and during speech.

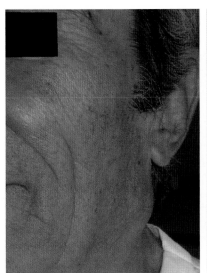
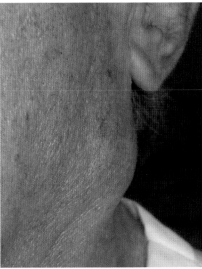
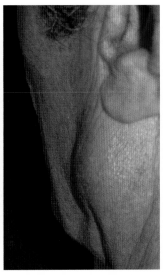

Fig. 4.7.6 Typical clinical presentation of a superficial lobe left parotid gland neoplasm, with a lump clearly visible in the retromandibular region

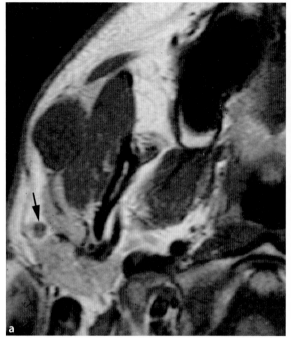
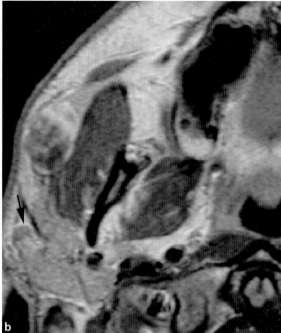

Fig. 4.7.7a,b Accessory lobe PA. On MRI, a nodular lesion is seen in the masseteric lobe of the right parotid gland, exhibiting a hypointense signal on precontrast acquisition (**a**) and bright, nonhomogeneous enhancement after contrast administration (**b**). The lesion shows sharp peripheral borders and does not infiltrate the masseter muscle. An intraparotid lymph node (*arrows*) is also visible

SLG benign tumours are rare, and any lesion in this area should be considered malignant until proven otherwise.

4.7.3.4 Minor Salivary Glands

The more frequent presentation of these tumours is a slow-growing, painless, submucosal mass arising in any head and neck region (sinonasal tract, oral cavity, and pharynx, larynx, trachea and parapharyngeal space), with the oral cavity and oropharynx being the most frequently involved sites. Superficial ulceration is seldom observed in benign tumours of the MSG (Fig. 4.5.8). According to the site of origin, different complaints may be present:
- Sinonasal tract: nasal obstruction, recurrent sinusitis
- Nasopharynx: otitis media due to Eustachian tube compression
- Oropharynx: dysphagia
- Larynx: dyspnea, hoarseness
- Trachea: dyspnea

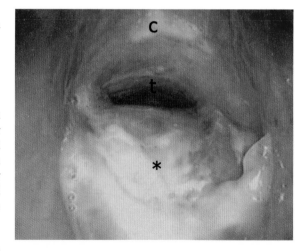

Fig. 4.7.8 Endoscopic appearance of a PA (*asterisk*) arisen from a MSG of the tracheal posterior wall; the neoplasm has an irregular surface and causes a remarkable narrowing of the respiratory space. *c* Cricoid arch, *t* trachea

4.7.4 Diagnosis

In terms of diagnosis, the recommended European standard is as follows:

- Palpation of the gland and ipsilateral neck lymph nodes (levels I–V)
- Inspection of the oral cavity, floor of the mouth and oropharynx
- When a MSG lesion is suspected, endoscopic evaluation of the involved site(s) of onset
- Inspection of scalp and skin of the pre-auricular region
- Evaluation and palpation of major salivary gland excretory ducts (Stensen's and Wharton's), with and without concomitant compression on the relative gland
- Palpation of contralateral gland and neck lymph nodes
- Ultrasonography (US) of the salivary gland and of the ipsilateral neck lymph nodes, better if combined with US-guided fine-needle aspiration cytology (FNAC) or core biopsy as a first step (Figs. 4.7.9, 4.7.10); US study should also include the contralateral gland and lymph nodes, especially when there is risk for bilateral involvement (e.g., WT)
- MRI (or CT with contrast agent when MRI is not feasible) when dealing with lesions with critical extension, deep lobe and/or parapharyngeal space involvement, recurrent disease after previous surgery or clinically suspicious for malignancy (Figs. 4.7.11–4.7.14)
- SL tumours should be evaluated by CT or MRI, due to their limited visibility at US, and to better define their local extension.
- When dealing with MSG tumours, an imaging study (CT and/or MRI) to better evaluate local extension of the lesion should be performed, according to the site of onset of the neoplasm. A biopsy under local anaesthesia should also be carried out.

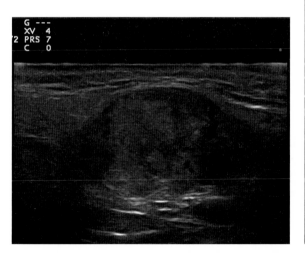

Fig. 4.7.9 Ultrasonography of PA: nodule with oval morphology and hyperechoic structure in superficial lobe of the parotid gland

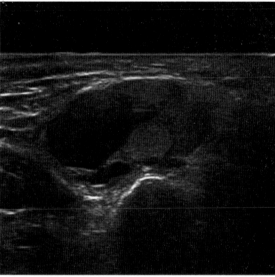

Fig. 4.7.10 Ultrasonography of WT: the parotid gland nodule is well circumscribed with a heterogeneous structure due to presence of solid and cystic areas

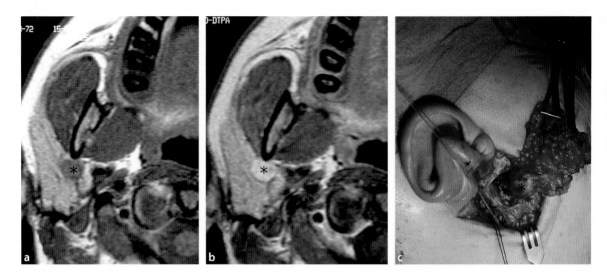

Fig. 4.7.11a–c Parotid gland pleomorphic adenoma (*asterisk*). The nodular lesion shows a typical MRI pattern consisting of a hypointense signal (similar to muscle) on precontrast acquisition (**a**) and bright enhancement after contrast administration (**b**). The same nodule, during surgery, (**c**) appears to belong to the superficial lobe with protrusion or extension between the facial nerve divisions into the deep lobe

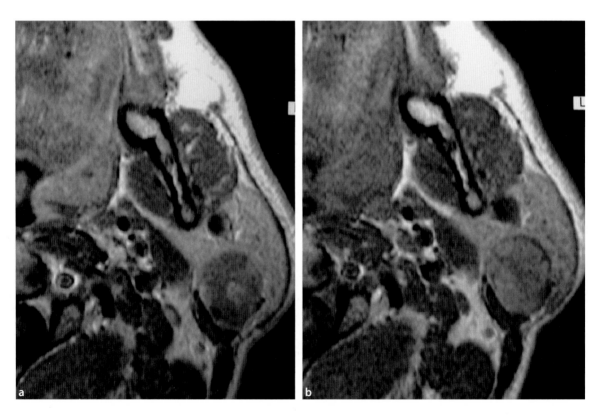

Fig. 4.7.12a,b Parotid gland Warthins Tumour. On MRI, the (**a0**) lesion displays spontaneously hyperintense areas that may account for the accumulation of proteinaceous fluid, cholesterol crystals or hemorrhagic changes (**a**). After contrast, (**b**) the pattern of enhancement is generally nonhomogeneous (**b**)

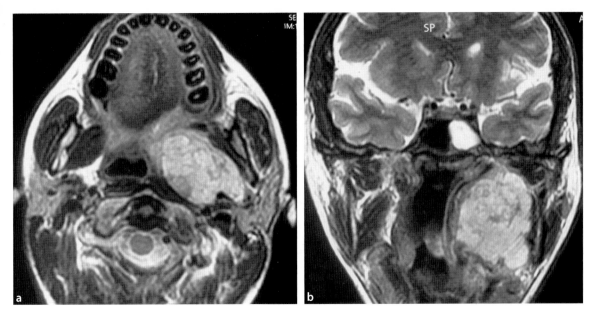

Fig. 4.7.13a,b Parapharyngeal space PA. A huge, nonhomogeneous mass lesion with lobulated contours occupying the prestyloid parapharyngeal space (**a**), compressing both the medial pterygoid and longus capitis muscle. The significant displacement of the pharyngeal wall is better visualised on the coronal plane (**b**)

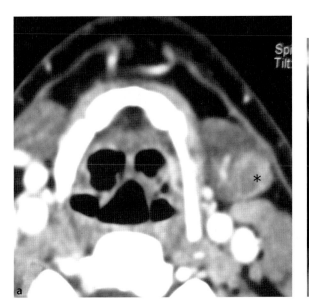
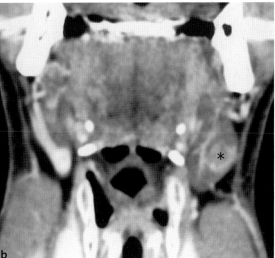

Fig. 4.7.14a,b Multislice CT (MSCT) of submandibular gland pleomorphic adenoma (occasional finding). Axial (**a**) and coronal reconstruction (**b**) detect a small nodular lesion within the submandibular gland (*asterisk*), wich is fairly enhanced after contrast application. The information provided by MSCT is insufficient for characterisation (a diagnosis) of the lesion

4.7.5 Additional/Useful Diagnostic Procedures

PET-CT scan in case of clinical history of malignancy either in the head and neck or in other body districts can be helpful.

4.7.6 Therapy

4.7.6.1 Surgery

The recommended European standard of indications for surgery is:
- Parotid Gland
  - Lesion limited to the superficial lobe: superficial (or lateral) parotidectomy or extracapsular dissection (Fig. 4.7.11)
  - Lesion involving or arising within the accessory lobe: superficial parotidectomy anteriorly extended to involve the accessory lobe
  - Lesion involving the deep lobe: total parotidectomy
- Submandibular Gland
  - Submandibular gland excision
- Sub-lingual Gland
  - Sublingual gland excision
- Minor Salivary Gland
  - Wide excision of the lesion according the site of origin

4.7.7 Differential Diagnosis

Differential diagnosis of the various tumours encompasses the following:
- Parotid gland tumours
  - *Inflammatory*: sialolithiasis, acute suppurative parotitis, chronic non-autoimmune parotitis, subacute necrotising parotitis, necrotising sialometaplasia
  - Parotid enlargement due to granulomatous and/or autoimmune disorders: Wegener's granulomatosis, sarcoidosis, Sjögren's disease
  - *Parotid enlargement due to metabolic–endocrine disorders or toxic agent administration (sialoadenosis):* malnutrition, cirrhosis, endocrine dysfunctions (diabetes), toxic agents (mercury, lead), radio-iodine treatment

  - *Cystic lesions*: obstruction duct cyst, lympho-epithelial cysts (HIV patients), dysgenetic polycystic disease
  - *Infectious*: epidemic parotitis (mumps), mycobacterial parotid lymphadenitis
  - *Congenital, malformative*: I–II branchial cleft cyst, sebaceous cyst
  - *Neoplastic: primary parotid gland malignancy,* parotid *lymph-node metastases from skin cancer* (squamous cell carcinoma, melanoma), parotid *lymph node metastases from head and neck cancer* (conjunctiva and ocular adnexa, lacrimal pathway, nasopharynx, naso-ethmoidal complex, maxillary sinus), *lymphoproliferative disorders* (mucosal-associated lymphoid tissue [MALT] lymphoma, non-Hodgkin's lymphomas), *metastasis from non–head and neck cancer* (kidney, breast, lung)
  - *Facial nerve lesions*: schwannoma, neurinoma
  - *Temporomandibular joint lesions*
  - *Mandibular bone lesions*
  - *Masticatory space and muscle lesions*
- Accessory lobe lesions
  - Cystic lesions: obstruction duct cyst
  - Inflammatory: Stensen's duct stones
  - Neoplastic: accessory lobe malignant lesions, adnexal lesions, neural tumours, lymph node metastases, lymphoproliferative disorders
  - Arteriovenous malformations
- Submandibular gland tumours
  - Inflammatory: sialolithiasis
  - Infectious: acute suppurative sialoadenitis, acute lymphadenitis
  - Cystic lesions: obstruction duct cyst
  - Congenital, malformative: II branchial cleft cyst, sebaceous cyst
  - Neoplastic: level IB lymph node metastases from head and neck cancer (floor of the mouth and oral tongue, cheek, maxillary sinus, lips), primary SMG malignant neoplasms, lymphoproliferative disorders
- Sub-lingual gland tumours
  - Cystic lesions: ranula, obstruction duct cyst, dermoid cyst
  - Neoplastic: malignant SLG and floor of the mouth tumours, neural and vascular lesions
  - Infectious: floor of the mouth abscess, Ludwig's angina
- Minor salivary gland tumours
  - Inflammatory: ranula, mucocele
  - Infectious: submucosal abscess
  - Neoplastic: non-salivary malignant lesion

4.7.8 Prognosis

The main issues in prognosis of benign tumours of salivary glands are the recurrence rate and/or malignant degeneration.

Despite the benign nature, PA has the tendency to recur, mainly due to incomplete excision, multifocality, and/or intraoperative cellular spillage for accidental rupture of the tumour. The recurrence rate is quite variable: when simple enucleation of the tumour is performed, the risk of recurrences ranges from 20 to 45%; conversely, when a complete excision is obtained, the rate drops to 2–7%. Younger patients are the most frequently affected by recurrent PA. The majority of recurrences is multifocal and generally occurs within 10 years of primary surgery (Fig. 4.7.15). Second and further recurrences may occur in about 20–40% and 20% of cases, respectively.

Some histologic characteristics of PA may explain the relative high risk of incomplete excision and therefore of recurrence. In fact, PA often lacks a true complete capsule and is characterised by the presence of a so-called pseudocapsule, which can be incomplete. This incompleteness explains different modalities of merging between the neoplasm and the surrounding healthy parotid tissue, with finger-like tumour projections extending into the parenchyma, or the presence of satellite nodules. Moreover, neoplasms with a high content of stroma (hypocellular or stroma-rich type) tend to recur most frequently, mainly due to the high prevalence of an incomplete pseudocapsule.

Treatment of recurrent PA is one of the most challenging and complex issues in salivary gland tumours, due to the complexity of revision surgery, the high risk of facial nerve lesions and of further recurrences, especially when multiple nodules are found. The wide spectrum of available treatment options includes a "wait-and-see" policy, revision surgery with different approaches and grades of aggressiveness and radiotherapy.

PA has also the potential for malignant degeneration into carcinoma ex pleomorphic adenoma (CEPA) in 5–10% of cases. The most common site for CEPA is the PG, whereas occurrence in the SMG and MSG is much lower; elderly patients (in the sixth to seventh decade) are the most frequently affected. Clinically, a malignant degeneration should be suspected whenever a salivary gland mass, especially if long standing, has a rapid growth and gives rise to complaints like pain, facial nerve palsy and lymph node swelling (Fig. 4.7.16).

Only exceptionally (about 1% of cases) does WT has a malignant degeneration, so that the main concerns in terms of prognosis are the risk of multifocality and bilateral involvement, and the possible association with other salivary gland neoplasms. WT is multicentric (synchronous or metachronous) in up to 20% of cases, with bilateral involvement in up to 15% of patients. Malignant degeneration is exceedingly rare (about 1%) in WT.

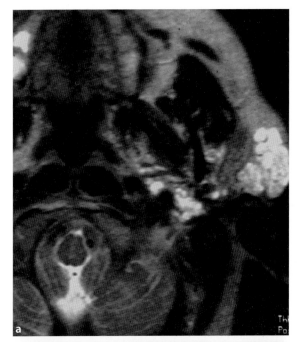

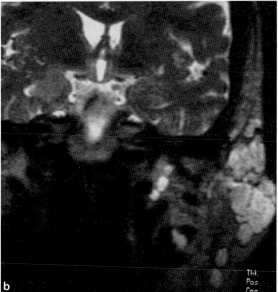

Fig. 4.7.15a,b Recurrent parotid gland PA. A cluster of hyperintense nodules is demonstrated by MRI into the superficial and deep lobe of the parotid gland, within the parapharyngeal space and in the subcutaneous fat

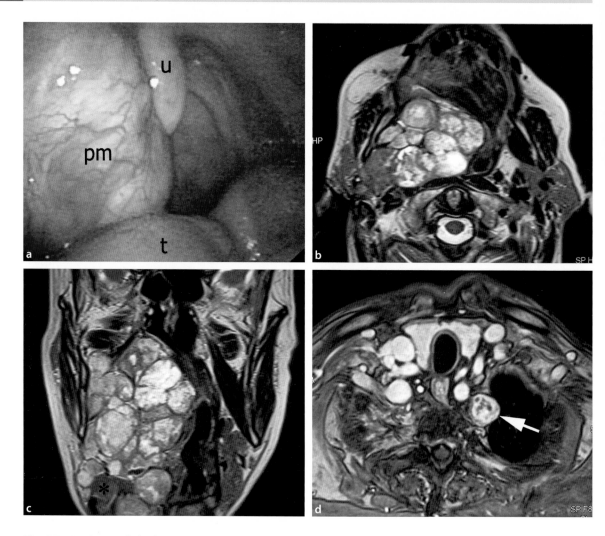

Fig. 4.7.16a–d Parotid gland CEPA. At transoral inspection, the right oropharyngeal wall is medialized by a parapharyngeal mass (*pm*). *t* Tongue, *u* uvula. (**a**). A large, multinodular mass occupies the parapharyngeal space, extending inferiorly to the level of the hyoid bone. The submandibular gland is encircled and displaced by nodules (*asterisk*) (**b,c**). A contralateral nodule is seen in the proximity of the left lung apex (*arrow*) (**d**)

4.7.9   Follow-Up

Since the topic of this chapter is benign lesions of salivary glands, follow-up strategy is focused on lesions with high risk of recurrence:

- *PA of PG superficial lobe or SMG*: clinic and US evaluation once a year for at least 10 years; when a recurrence is observed or suspected, MRI (or CT with contrast agent) is mandatory to define: site, dimension and local extension of the lesion, number of nodules, possible involvement of critical areas (stylomastoid foramen, parapharyngeal space, etc.) (Fig. 4.7.15)

- *PA with high risk for recurrence* (previous incisional biopsy, intraoperative tumour spillage, already treated recurrence, hypocellular variant): clinical evaluation and US every 6 months and MRI once a year for the first 5 years, then clinical evaluation and US for at least 5 years

- *PA involving the deep lobe of the PG or the parapharyngeal space*: this site may be hardly observed by US (deep location, scar); so, whenever US is not fully reliable, MRI is required

- *WT*: the risk of contralateral PG involvement is up to 15%; for this reason a periodic bilateral evaluation by US should be performed

- *MSG*: CT or MRI according to the site of origin

Additional Reading

1. Eveson JW, Auclair P, Gnepp DR, El-Naggar AK (2005) Tumours of the salivary glands. In: Barnes L, Eveson JW, Reichart P, Sidransky D (eds) World Health Organization classification of tumours 9. Pathology and genetics of head and neck tumours. IARC Press, pp. 209–281

2. Myers EN, Ferris RL (eds) (2007) Salivary gland disorders. Springer, Berlin Heidelberg New York

3. Bradley PJ (2001) Recurrent salivary gland pleomorphic adenoma: etiology, management and results. Curr Opin Otolaryngol Head Neck Surg 9:100–109

4. Stennert E, Guntinas-Lichius O et al. (2001) Histopathology of pleomorphic adenoma in the parotid gland: a prospective unselected series of 100 cases. Laryngoscope 111:2195–2200

5. Marshall AH, Qureishi S, Bradley PJ (2003) Outcomes short- and long-term: Patients views following surgery for benign salivary gland surgery. J Laryngol Otol 117:624–629

4.8 Primary and Secondary Malignant Salivary Gland Neoplasms

ORLANDO GUNTINAS-LICHIUS

Salivary gland neoplasms are also known as salivary gland cancer and salivary gland malignomas.

4.8.1 Definition

4.8.1.1 Primary Neoplasm

A primary neoplasm is a malignant tumour of a major salivary gland: parotid, submandibular, sublingual gland or of the minor salivary glands (all mucus-secreting glands in the lining membrane of the upper aerodigestive tract). The most important World Health Organisation (WHO) classified histologic subtypes are listed in Table 4.8.1.

4.8.1.2 Secondary Neoplasm

Lymphatic metastases to lymph nodes within the salivary gland of a tumour of other origin, haematogenous metastases from distant primary tumours or direct invasion from cancers that lie adjacent to the salivary glands are considered secondary neoplasms.

4.8.2 Aetiology/Epidemiology

4.8.2.1 Primary Neoplasm

The aetiology of primary neoplasms is unknown. There are at least two theories of tumorigenesis:
1. In the *multicellular theory*, each type of neoplasm is thought to originate from a different cell type within the salivary gland unit.
2. In the *bicellular reserve cell theory*, the origin of the neoplasms can be traced to the basal cells as reserve cells with potential to differentiate into different salivary gland cells. Recent molecular studies support the reserve cell theory.

There is some evidence that environmental factors such as radiation, viruses, diet or certain occupational exposures may increase the risk of salivary gland cancer. Cancer of the salivary glands accounts for 0.3–0.9% of all cancers. Salivary gland cancers make up 1–3% of all head and neck cancers. The incidence is 1–3 per 100,000 persons in Europe. The mean age is 55–60 years. About 80% of these neoplasms arise from the parotid gland, 10% from

Table 4.8.1 The most important salivary gland neoplasms

Neoplasms – Carcinomas	Relative Percentage (%) Incidence (or comment)
Acinic Cell	5–11%
Mucoepidermoid	35% (80% Located in Parotid)
Adenoid Cystic	15% (10% of all SCCa in Head and Neck Region)
Low-grade Adenocarcinoma	
Epithelial-Myoepithelial	1%
Basal Cell Adenocarcinoma	
Sebaceous	
Papillary Cystadenocarcinoma	
Mucinous Adenocarcinoma	
Oncocytic	
Salivary Duct	
Myoepithelial	
Carcinoma in Pleomorphic Adenoma	3 –12% (75% Located to Parotid)
Small Cell	
Squamous Cell	Rare: Most likely secondary
Undifferentiated	
Others:	
Malignant Lymphomas	5% of all extranodal lymphomas
Non-epithelial Malignancies	
Secondary Malignancies – Metastases	Mainly Skin, Lung, Kidney and Breast

the submandibular gland, up to 5% from the sublingual gland and 5% from the minor salivary glands. Whereas three fourths of all parotid tumours are benign, the majority of other salivary gland tumour localisations are malignant.

4.8.2.2   Secondary Neoplasm

For aetiology, see "Definition" above. In regions with high incidence of skin cancer (such as Australia), secondary neoplasms in the parotid gland represent the majority of malignant parotid tumours (in Australia two of three neoplasms are parotid), chiefly due to metastatic squamous carcinoma.

4.8.3   Symptoms

4.8.3.1   Parotid Glands

In three of four cases, secondary neoplasms are benign tumours for some time: a painless, slowly increasing swelling in the region of a salivary gland. Facial palsy – most probably incomplete or of only a few peripheral nerve branches – is present in only one of four cases of parotid gland malignoma. Pain and skin infiltration are negative prognostic factors, indicating advanced disease. Advanced tumours present with cervical adenopathy.

4.8.3.2   Submandibular Glands

Both benign and malignant tumours usually present as a painless, mobile mass in the submandibular triangle. Again, pain, skin infiltration and fixation to the mandible are signs of local extension. Weakness or numbness of the tongue indicates spreading along the hypoglossal nerve or the lingual nerve, respectively.

4.8.3.3   Minor Salivary Glands

Presentation depends on the site of the tumour and does not differ from other malignant tumours such as squamous cell carcinoma. The palate is the most common site, and the tumour usually manifests as a submucosal mass or ulceration. The second most common site is the sinonasal tract. Symptoms are nasal obstruction, epistaxis or a nasal mass.

4.8.4   Diagnostic Procedures

- Recommended European standard
  - Inspection
    - Red, prominent auricle
    - Swollen skin over the mastoid
    - Facial palsy
  - Palpation
    - Painful, fixed or mobile tumour
    - Skin infiltration
  - Inspection of the oral cavity and the neck
  - Inspection of the skin of head and neck
    - Possible skin cancer
  - Palpation of the neck
    - Possible metastasis
  - Ultrasound of major salivary glands and neck
  - Tumour staging using the tumour–node–metastasis (TNM) system (Tables 4.8.2, 4.8.3)
- Additional/useful diagnostic procedures
  - Fine-needle aspiration cytology (when necessary, ultrasound guided)
  - Otoscopy or ear microscopy in cases of parotid tumours: possible infiltration of the ear canal
  - MRI of the neck: evaluation of the extent of the disease, especially for deep-lobe parotid tumours or those with parapharyngeal extension. Good in early detection of perineural spread.
  - CT of the neck: possible bone infiltration
  - X-ray of the chest: staging procedure
  - MRI of the abdomen: in cases of secondary neoplasm
  - Electrodiagnostics of the facial nerve: in cases of facial palsy or unclear situations
  - [18]FDG-PET: of limited value in comparison to CT and MRI, but superior in distinguishing tumour recurrence from posttreatment fibrosis during follow-up
  - Frozen section: should be reserved for cases where fine-needle aspiration was not possible, or the results were unclear. Note: sensitivity and specificity of frozen sections is less than that of fine-needle aspiration cytology.

4.8.5   Therapy

4.8.5.1   General Aspects

- High-grade tumours (squamous cell carcinoma, carcinoma ex pleomorphic adenoma, undifferentiated carcinoma and salivary duct carcinoma) result in poorer outcomes than do low-grade tumours (acinic cell carcinoma, low-grade adenocarcinoma). Histologic as-

Table 4.8.2 TNM staging of major salivary glands

Component	Definition
T (size or depth of invasion of the primary tumour)	
TX	Primary tumour cannot be assessed
T0	No evidence of primary tumour
T1	Tumour is 2 cm, without extraparenchymal extension[a]
T2	Tumour >2 cm to 4 cm, without extraparenchymal extension[a]
T3	Tumour >4 cm and/or tumour with extraparenchymal extension[a]
T4a	Tumour invades skin, mandible, ear canal or facial nerve
T4b	Tumour invades base of skull, pterygoid plates or encases carotid artery
N (presence or absence of tumour in the regional lymph nodes)	
NX	Regional lymph nodes cannot be assessed
N0	No regional lymph node metastasis
N1	Metastasis in single ipsilateral lymph node ≤3 cm in greatest dimension
N2	Metastasis in a single ipsilateral lymph node >3 cm but not >6 cm; or in multiple ipsilateral lymph nodes, none >6 cm; or in bilateral or contralateral lymph nodes, none >6 cm
N2a	Metastasis in single ipsilateral lymph node >3–6 cm
N2b	Metastasis in multiple ipsilateral lymph nodes ≤6 cm
N2c	Metastasis in bilateral or contralateral lymph nodes ≤6 cm
N3	Metastasis in a lymph node >6 cm
M (presence or absence of distant metastases, including lymph nodes that are not regional)	
MX	Distant metastasis cannot be assessed
M0	No distant metastasis
M1	Distant metastasis

From the American Joint Committee on Cancer, 2002

[a]Clinical or macroscopic evidence of invasion of soft tissues. Microscopic evidence alone does not constitute extraparenchymal extension

signment to high-grade or low-grade tumours may be difficult.

- Other negative prognostic factors are lymph node metastasis (N⁺), advanced stage, cancer of minor salivary glands, positive surgical margins (R⁺), perineural spread, facial palsy and initial pain.
- Conservative treatment, i.e. radiotherapy alone or radiochemotherapy, is reserved for non-resectable tumours. In cases of distant metastases, radiotherapy or chemotherapy may be part of palliative care.
- In resectable cancer, complete surgical excision – and depending on the tumour characteristics, adjuvant radiotherapy or adjuvant radiochemotherapy – is the treatment of choice.

4.8.5.2 Conservative Treatment

- Recommended European standard
  - Adjuvant postoperative radiation therapy
    - Adjuvant postoperative radiation therapy after surgery seems to be superior to surgery alone in the treatment of advanced salivary gland cancer.
      - Selection criteria for adjuvant therapy

Table 4.8.3 Stage grouping of major salivary glands

Stage	T	N	M
I	T1	N0	M0
II	T2	N0	M0
III	T3	N0	M0
	T1	N1	M0
	T2	N1	M0
IVA	T4a	N0	M0
	T4a	N1	M0
	T1	N2	M0
	T2	N2	M0
	T3	N2	M0
IVB	T4b	Any N	M0
	Any T	N3	M0
IVC	Any T	Any N	M1

From the American Joint Committee on Cancer, 2002

- High-grade tumours
- Facial nerve infiltration
- Incomplete resection (R+)
- Extracapsular spread
- Perineural infiltration

- Radiation doses range from 50 to 75 Gy (median of 60 Gy), typically using 2 Gy fractions per day in 30 fractions. Three-dimensional conformal radiotherapy (3DCRT) and intensity-modulated radiotherapy (IMRT) lead to better tumour dosimetry and hence, to less radiation-related complications.
  - Adjuvant postoperative radiochemotherapy or chemotherapy: to date there is no rational basis for adjuvant chemotherapy after surgery in salivary gland cancer. This treatment option should be reserved for clinical studies.
  - Inoperable tumours: in cases of planned radiation for inoperable tumours, tumour-debulking surgery is not warranted by an improvement of locoregional control.
  - Inoperable tumours: fast-neutron radiation therapy may provide higher locoregional control rates than do photon or electron radiation therapy, but it is available only in a few centres in Europe. However, overall survival seems not to be improved by fast-neutron radiation therapy.
  - Chemotherapy as palliative treatment: platinum-based chemotherapy is the only palliative chemotherapy that has shown efficiency in incurable salivary gland neoplasms. Median survival is increased by about 2.5 months by platinum-based chemotherapy.

4.8.5.3   Surgical Treatment

- Recommended European standard
  - Goals: complete tumour resection and avoidance of unnecessary morbidity
  - Parotid tumours: the minimal approach to small tumours (T1/T2) of the superficial lobe is a lateral parotidectomy. Whether a total parotidectomy may result in superior locoregional control is unclear. Larger tumours and all deep-lobe tumours are treated by total parotidectomy (Fig. 4.8.1). Tumour extending beyond the parotid gland may need an extended parotidectomy including skin, soft tissue, masseter muscle resection, infratemporal fossa dissection, mastoidectomy or even petrosectomy. Facial nerve resection in cases without facial nerve infiltration (radical parotidectomy) does not result in increased tumour control. In cases of facial nerve infiltration, the involved branches of the nerve are resected.
  - Submandibular tumours
    - Small tumours are treated by resection of the gland.
    - Advanced tumours need wide en bloc resection of the submandibular triangle, and may need resection of the floor of the mouth, mylohyoid and digastric muscles, or marginal/segmental mandibulectomy. Infiltration and consecutive thickening of the lingual, hypoglossal, mylohyoid or marginal mandibular nerve indicate resection of the involved nerves.
  - Minor salivary gland tumours
    - In the oral cavity, small tumours are treated by wide local excision; advanced tumours require radical excision with segmental/marginal mandibulectomy, or partial maxillectomy.
    - Sinonasal tract tumours are usually high-grade tumours and need partial or total maxillectomy. Infiltration of the second (V2) or third (V3) branch of the trigeminal nerve are managed by nerve resection, as these nerves provide a route to skull base invasion.
  - Treatment of the neck: in cases of clinical evidence of a neck metastasis, a neck dissection is performed as selective, radical–modified or radical neck dissection according to the extent of neck infiltration (Fig. 4.8.1b). It is unclear in which cases of negative neck metastases (N0) do patients profit from elective neck dissection. Recent studies report occult metastasis rates as much as 25–40% independent of the histological subtype. Older reports recommend neck dissection only for high-grade tumours. The highest occult metastasis rate is seen in advanced stages (T3/T4). The type of neck dissection is still

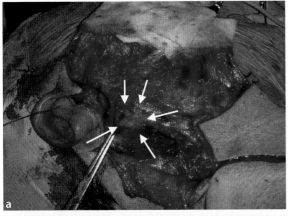

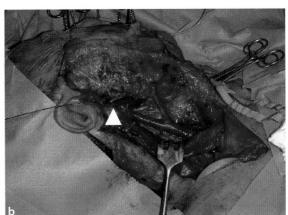

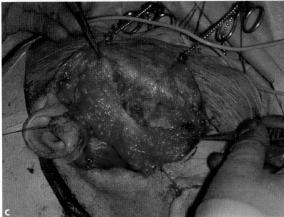

Fig. 4.8.1a–c a Mucoepidermoid carcinoma of the left parotid (*arrows*). **b** Site after total parotidectomy and neck dissection; *arrowhead* delineates facial nerve bifurcation. **c** Defect filling with umbilical fat

controversial. At the very least, selective neck dissection of levels I–III should be performed. A radical–modified neck dissection may lead to better locoregional control.

- Surgery of secondary salivary gland cancer: in general performed in conjunction with resection of the primary tumour, or in cases of secondary metastases, as localised treatment for tumour control. Skin cancer, especially squamous cell cancer of the head, may be an indication for elective parotidectomy, as the occult parotid metastasis rate is reported to be up to 40%; ultrasonography may indicate that a parotidectomy should be performed for any suspicious lesion in the parotid.

4.8.6 Differential Diagnosis

- Benign salivary gland tumour: clinically often not distinguishable. Fine-needle aspiration cytology helpful to differentiate

- Chronic sialadenitis or sialoadenosis: long history. Diffuse involvement of the entire salivary gland, often involvement of several salivary glands
- Sialolithiasis: painful swelling related to eating. Ultrasonography can localise the salivary stone. Massage of the gland leads to secretion of purulent saliva of the related salivary duct, or no saliva can be elicited because of complete blockage of the duct by the stone.

4.8.7 Prognosis

- Five-year overall survival range is from 50 to 70%.
- Ten-year overall survival range is from 45 to 65%.
- Five-year disease-free survival range is from 55 to 65%.
- Ten-year disease-free survival range is from 35 to 55%.
- The most important negative prognostic factors are TNM classification, older age and positive surgical margins. Tumour grading is not a reliable prognostic factor.

4.8.8.1 Lateral Parotidectomy

A lateral parotidectomy is defined as the resection of all parotid tissue lateral to the facial plexus.

4.8.8.1.1 Technique

The surgical technique is as follows:

1) General anaesthesia is used.
2) The patient is placed in the supine position in order to minimise intraoperative bleeding, and with the head hyperextended and rotated to the opposite side. The table is placed in the reverse Trendelenburg position as far as is feasible.
3) In addition to standard surgical coverage, the ipsilateral side of the face may be covered with a transparent sheath to guarantee optical monitoring of the face by the assistant surgeon. By doing this, even slight movements of the face become obvious when anaesthesia is performed without relaxation. In addition, electric monitoring can be performed optionally.
4) A preauricular and submandibular lazy-S incision (modified Blair's incision) is performed. Alternatively, a retroauricular facelift incision can be used. If a neck dissection is planned, the submandibular incision can be modified easily. If the tumour lies laterally to the main trunk of the facial nerve, or if an exposure of its intramastoid segment is necessary, Blair's incision can also be extended retroauricularily.
5) By blunt dissection, the parotid gland is separated from the ear cartilage in the preauricular region and from the sternocleidomastoid muscle until the digastric muscle is exposed. It is often necessary to ligate the greater auricular nerve. Ligation is mandatory to prevent from neuroma formation. Preparation of the anterior buccal skin flap is vital. The flap is lifted in the layer between the parotid pseudocapsule and the deep buccal fascia, combined with a short subplatysmal dissection in the neck. The fascia has to be protected to maintain a barrier in order to decrease the possibility of Frey's syndrome. Of course, any tumour infiltration can lead to a modification of the approach.
6) The primary approach to identify the facial nerve depends on the site and extension of the lesion. The preparation of the entire plexus, i.e. the nerve trunk and all peripheral braches, is performed under microscopic control or by using loops to minimise nerve trauma. There are three surgical approaches:
   a) Anterograde approach: identification of the facial nerve at its exit at the stylomastoid foramen. Then, the bifurcation and the different branches are prepared in a proximal-to-distal direction. Three landmarks help to identify the main trunk:
      i) Conley's pointer is a conchal cartilage extension of the ear canal at the medial end of its anterior–inferior edge. The nerve lies 5–6 mm inferiorly to this pointer.
      ii) The tympanomastoid fissure is more easily felt than seen. The facial nerve lies 6–8 mm caudally to the anterior end of the fissure.
      iii) The posterior belly of the digastric muscle lies in the same plane as does the facial nerve.
   b) Retrograde approach: the best landmark to start with this preparation is the middle third of the zygomatic arch where the frontal branch crosses its periosteum. A zygomatic branch is found about 1 cm inferior to the arch. Alternatively, identification of Stenson's duct might be helpful, which is crossed by a buccal branch.
   c) In many cases, a combination of anterograde and retrograde approach is necessary. In any case, the parotid surgeon has to be trained in all these techniques.
7) The anterograde as well as retrograde preparation, or the combination of both procedures, lead step by step to exposure of the entire peripheral nerve plexus including the trunk and bifurcation. Hereby, the parotid tissue lateral to these nerve structures is progressively dissected free and finally delivered. Touching the tumour should be avoided. If the tumour lies in the lateral lobe, the lateral parotid should be removed with the associated tumour en bloc.
8) Defect filling is a controversial topic in malignant disease, as it could hinder the palpation and detection of recurrent disease. Furthermore, the decision depends on the size of the defect and the patient's wish. There are two options:
   a) Preparation of a muscle flap from the craniolateral aspect of the sternocleidomastoid muscle, lateral to the spinal accessory nerve, which is rotated anteriorly into the defect. The mastoid attachment has to be preserved to assure occipital blood supply to the flap. During ultrasonography (less in CT or MRI) for follow-up, the muscle flap can impede the differentiation between scar tissue and recurrent disease.
   b) For large defects, abdominal fat is primarily used (Fig. 4.8.1c). The fat is harvested via a peri-umbilical incision. Meticulous bleeding control is necessary to avoid abdominal haematoma formation. Some overcorrection is necessary because of postoperative shrinkage. The fat is fixed with several sutures, avoiding any contact with nerve branches. During follow-up, it is easy, especially when using

MRI, to differentiate the fat tissue from recurrent disease.

9) A Redon drain can be placed without contact to nerve structures. The wound is closed in two layers by subcutaneous and cutaneous sutures. A circular head–neck bandage is recommended. If a drain was placed, it should be removed within 24–72 h.

4.8.8.2 Subtotal and Total Parotidectomy

Often a total parotidectomy is declared when only a subtotal parotidectomy was performed. It is important to differentiate both techniques: a *subtotal* parotidectomy includes a lateral parotidectomy, somewhat medial to the facial plexus, but not necessarily including the deep portion, under preservation of the facial nerve. To fulfil the criteria for *total* parotidectomy, a complete resection of the deep portion is mandatory.

4.8.8.2.1 Technique

1. Subtotal/total parotidectomy starts with lateral parotidectomy (see above).
2. The main trunk and the facial nerve branches are dissected from the underlying tissue in atraumatic fashion. Systematically, every branch is gently lifted by using rubber slings to dissect the underlying parotid tissue.
3. Stretch and compression trauma to the nerve must be avoided. Finally, the underlying masseter muscle should be visible within the entire area.
4. To clear the retromandibular space, it is mandatory to resect the retromandibular vein by ligation, distally in the submandibular fossa and proximally next to the zygomatic arch. Finally, the parotid tissue of the deep lobe has to be resected completely along the skull base, up to the stylomastoid process.

4.8.8.3 Facial Nerve Reconstruction

- Sacrifice of the facial nerve should always be limited to the involved nerve branches. Involvement is guided during surgery by frozen sections.
- Reconstruction of the facial nerve is the first choice for facial reinnervation. It results in the best return of nerve function to the face. Dynamic muscleplasty (temporal muscleplasty or masseter muscleplasty) is only the second method of choice, and static slings are the third. An exception is the reinnervation of the eye by an upper eyelid gold weight. This method is first choice for eye reanimation and can be performed in combination with nerve reconstruction surgery.
- If nerve reconstruction is possible and desired by the patient, it should be performed in the same session, the end of the tumour surgery (Fig. 4.8.2). The shorter the delay between facial nerve lesion and reconstruction, the better functional result that can be expected. Postoperative radiotherapy is not a contraindication for nerve suturing.
- All facial nerve repairs employ the epineurium as a suture layer, and the repairs should be done with the aid of a microscope. Typically, nonabsorbable, monofilament 8-0 to 10-0 suture material (depending on the calibre of the nerve branch or trunk) is placed to the nerve stumps and/or grafts.
- A tension-free primary repair is in most cases not possible. Parotid cancer surgery often results in a segmental defect within the facial nerve fan, requiring several nerve grafts (Fig. 4.8.2b). Nearly all grafts can be performed with the greater auricular nerve, which is of-

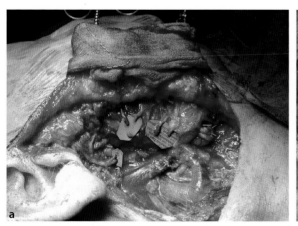 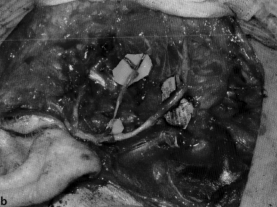

Fig. 4.8.2a, b **a** Situation after radical parotidectomy of an adenoidcystic carcinoma, with partial facial nerve resection. **b** Reconstruction by interpositional nerve grafting with several parts of the greater auricular nerve directly after tumour resection

ten lying within the operation field, or with the sural nerve, which allows longer grafts or double grafts.

- When there has been irreversible damage to the proximal facial nerve in its intracranial or intratemporal portion, or in cases with very long defects not favourable for grafting, reconstruction by a hypoglossal-facial-nerve jump anastomosis is the method of choice.

4.8.8.4   Submandibulectomy

1. Normally done under general anaesthesia, often combined with a neck dissection
2. A curvilinear incision is made in a natural skin crease 3–4 cm below the lower border of the mandible overlying the submandibular gland; the incision is carried down, cutting the platysma in the subcutaneous plane.
3. Care has to be taken to avoid injury of the marginal mandibular nerve. The facial vein is ligated, and upward retraction of the superior vein ligature displaces the nerve superiorly. The facial artery is also ligated and transected.
4. The gland is mobilised bluntly. The digastric muscle, the hypoglossal nerve and the mylohyoid muscle are identified.
5. The mylohyoid muscle is retracted superiorly, and the gland (gently) inferiorly. This manoeuvre exposes the submandibular duct and the lingual nerve. Warthin's duct is doubly ligated and divided. This exposes the deep portion of the submandibular gland. The gland and the tumour are excised en bloc.
6. A Redon drain can be placed without contact to nerve structures. The wound is closed in two layers by subcutaneous and cutaneous sutures. A circular head–neck bandage is recommended. If drainage was placed, it should be removed within 24–72 h.

4.8.8.5   Resection of Minor Salivary Gland Cancer

Surgery depends on the site of minor salivary gland cancer. See above sections on transoral tumour excision, maxillectomy and mandibulectomy.

4.8.8.6   Neck Dissection

Neck dissection is normally performed as a one-step procedure together with a primary tumour resection (Fig. 4.8.1b). For technique, see Sect. 4.8.5.3 on neck dissection for head and neck cancer.

4.8.9   Special Remarks

4.8.9.1   Treatment of Frey's Syndrome (Gustatory Sweating)

- Subclinical manifestation is proven by Minor's iodine–starch test in 85 to 95% of patients. Clinically relevant Frey's syndrome appears in less than 5% of patients after parotidectomy. Treatment of choice is local botulinum toxin injection.
  - Minor's iodine–starch test: the patient's face and the hair region on the affected side is painted with an iodine solution (15 g iodine, 100 ml castor oil and 900 ml ethanol), which is allowed to dry for 1–2 min. Then, the entire area is dusted with starch powder. The patient eats a sialogogue (lemon slice, apple) to evoke gustatory stimulation. Typically, within 5 min, the starch turns blue in the area where saliva is produced.
  - Botulinum toxin injection: either Botox® or Dysport® is used. *A unit of Botox® is not equivalent to a unit of Dysport®.*
    - When using Botox®, the drug is reconstituted with 2 ml preservative-free normal saline, yielding a concentration of 5 mU/0.1 ml Botox®.
    - Using Dysport®, the medicament is reconstituted with 2.5 ml saline, yielding a concentration of 20 mU/0.1 ml Dysport®. After mapping, 0.1 ml of the botulinum toxin solution is injected intradermally at each intersection point, i.e. either 5 mU Botox® or 20 mU Dysport® per intersection point. Local anaesthesia is not necessary. The injections should be begun caudally and end cranially in the outlined area; otherwise, bleeding from the injection points could be disturbing to the patient. To prevent unintentional transient weakness of regional mimic muscles, it is important not to inject botulinum toxin ventrally to the anterior border of the masseter muscle, and to respect the orbicularis oculi muscle.

4.8.9.2   Treatment of Synkinesis Due to Facial Nerve Reconstruction

- Facial synkinesis is the involuntary movement of several mimic muscles at the same time as the result of aberrant nerve regeneration after severe nerve lesion, without or after facial nerve reconstruction. Blepharospasm (involuntary eye closure) can be especially disturbing for patients.
- Treatment of choice is botulinum toxin, with the goal being to weaken involuntary movements. Botulinum

toxin is especially effective for treating blepharospasm.

- Preparation of the drug: see the last paragraph in the previous section. Typically, treatment is begun with administration of 5 mU Botox® or 20 mU Dysport® in the upper and lower lateral portions of the orbicularis oculi muscle, respectively. An optimal effect lasts about 4 months. To reach this duration of effect, it might be necessary to increase the dosage in follow-up sessions. Dose reduction is necessary in cases of overweakening.
- Treatment of synkinesis of the lower face is more difficult, and lower dosages per injections point are needed than in the upper face.

Additional Reading

1. Bibbo M,. Fine Nedle Aspiration of Salivary Glands. Acta Cytol 2009; 53(4): 367–8.
2. Sinha UK, Ng M Surgery of the Salivary Glands. Otolaryngol Clin Nth Am 1999; 32(5): 887–906.
3. Sclanna J M, Petruzzelli G J,. Contemporary Management of Tumours of Salivary Glands. Curr Oncol Rep 2007; 9 (2): 134–8
4. Preuss SF, Klaussman JP Wittwkindt C, Drebbers U, Beutner D, Guntinas-Lichius O,. Submandibular Gland Excision. J Oral Maxillofac. Surg 2007; 65(5): 953–7.
5. Guntinas-Lichius O, Gabriel B, Klussmann JP., Risk of facial palsy and severe Freys Syndrome after conservative parotidectomy for benign disease; analysis of 610 operations. Acta Otolaryngol 2006; 126(10): 1104 9
6. Bradley P J., "Neck Dissection in Salivary Cancer" Chapter in "neck Dissection – Management of regional disease in head and neck cancer. Edited by Ferlito A, Robbins KT, Silver CE, Pleural Publishers. 2009.
7. Munir N, Bradley P J Management of Neoplasms of the submandibular triangle. Oral Oncol 2008; 44: 251–60.
8. Bradley P J, McClelland L, Metha D,. Paediatric Salivary Gland Epithelial Neoplasms. ORL 2007; 89: 137–145.
9. Bradley P J Salivary Disorders: Pathology and Management, Surgery 2006; 24(9): 304–311.
10. Marshall A H,. Quereshi S M., Bradley P J Outcomes – Short and Long-term: Patients views following surgery for Benign Salivary Gland Neoplasms. J Laryngol Otol 2003; 117: 624–629.

4.9 Salivary Gland Surgery: Principles

PATRICK J. BRADLEY

4.9.1 Indications for Surgery

The indications for surgery in salivary gland diseases or disorders are broadly:

1. To establish as precise a diagnosis as is possible to guide the clinician towards an optimal mode of treatment
2. Patients may be cured after surgery; or more frequently after biopsy or excision surgery, and after histopathological evaluation of the surgical specimen, the clinician will be able to evaluate and predict patient's ultimate prognosis.

4.9.2 Biopsy Procedures

The use of fine-needle techniques to aspirate or biopsy (FNA or FNAB) salivary tissue is now widely employed and a well-established diagnostic technique. However, the diversity of salivary gland pathology makes FNA a particularly challenging area for the cytopathologist. In experienced hands, the sensitivity and specificity of FNA is high, but fallible, and occasionally prone to misinterpretation of a benign lesion as malignant, or vice versa. When the preoperative diagnosis is certain, then the information can be invaluable to the surgeon and the patient; but when the diagnosis is in doubt or inconclusive, then the decision to treat still rests on the clinical signs and suspicion. Some clinicians now prefer the use of fine-needle biopsy, which in some hands, leads to higher accuracy of a subsequent correct pathologic diagnosis.

Open biopsy in the presence of skin ulceration is the only clinical scenario in which such biopsy is indicated in the management of major salivary gland swellings. However, when there is suspicion of a minor salivary gland tumour, then incisional or punch biopsy should provide a diagnosis, before embarking on excisional surgery, and usually results in more informed and more appropriate clinical decision making.

The labial gland biopsy has an important role in establishing the investigation of generalised salivary gland swellings, suspected involvement of salivary glands by systemic disease (e.g. Sjögren's syndrome) or when investigating xerostomia.

The procedure of labial gland biopsy involves, after an injection of local anaesthetic, a 1.5- to 2-cm incision made parallel to the vermelion border in the middle of the lower lip, between the midline and the corner of the mouth. At least five lobes of labial glands are obtained by blunt dissection. After routine histological fixation and preparation, the biopsy is evaluated according to a procedure in which an inflammatory focus is defined as an accumulation of at least 50 mononuclear leukocytes per 4 mm². According to the European criteria, a biopsy is positive at a focus score of >1 per 4 mm². The pathognomic histological finding in biopsies is a focal infiltrate of mononuclear lymphoid cells in the salivary glands, replacing glandular epithelium (lymphoepithelial lesion), and which is progressive, as demonstrated by an increase of focus score over time. One differential diagnostic feature of focal sialadenitis is the granulomatous inflammation seen in sarcoidosis. The specificity of a positive labial biopsy is 86.2%, and the sensitivity is 82.4% in patients with primary Sjögren's syndrome diagnosed according to the European criteria. More recently, it has been recommended that biopsy of the sublingual gland may be an alternative to labial gland biopsy, giving better tissue delivery, minimising risk of complication and being better tolerated by patients.

Frozen section and its uses in salivary gland surgery are controversial, but when positive for the information sought, can minimise the consequences of surgery. Indications for its use include:

- Providing the diagnosis and type of tumour
- May indicate the need for further tests – microbiology
- Evaluation of adequacy of surgery – margins
- Involvement of perineural and/or perivascular invasion

Limitations of frozen section include:

- The fact that the diagnosis may remain in doubt – "wait" paraffin section
- Sampling error, leading to inaccurate diagnosis
- Inability to grade aggressiveness of tumour

4.9.3   Excisional Salivary Gland Surgery

When considering surgery, it is important to consider the disease processes that can affect salivary glands. It is best to consider these under broad headings:

- Infections
  - Acute
  - Chronic
  - Recurrent
  - Bacterial
  - Viral
- Non-infectious conditions
  - Sialadenitis
  - Sialolithiasis
  - Sialadenosis
  - Mucoceles
  - Cysts
- Neoplasms
  - Benign
  - Malignant
  - Primary and secondary

Surgery is the treatment of choice for all benign and malignant salivary gland neoplasms, with or without the need for adjuvant radiotherapy with or without chemotherapy. Malignant salivary gland tumours are classified clinically and pathologically as "high grade" and "non–high grade". All salivary glands – major and minor – are at risk of developing benign and malignant neoplasms.

Surgery is also indicated for recurrent chronic sialadenitis, which most frequently affects the parotid and submandibular glands. Sialadenitis frequently coexists with sialolithiasis, or ductal stenosis or stricture. Investigations are warranted prior to recommending gland surgery, and should include sialoendoscopy to separate ductal from parenchymal disease. Since the introduction of sialoendoscopy, it is now possible to treat more conservatively such episodes of gland swellings, recurrent sialadenitis and reverse ductal pathology by the removal of stones, and dilate strictures, if found, thus minimising the likelihood of recurrence.

parotid surgery has been described as surgery of the facial nerve. A classification of parotid surgery may include:

- *Limited excision*: facial nerve identification and mass excision
- *Superficial or lateral parotidectomy*: facial nerve identification and salivary tissue lateral to the nerve removed. This may be partial or complete lateral parotidectomy – known as a "classic parotidectomy"
- *Deep lobe parotidectomy*: Identification of the facial nerve and dissecting the salivary tissue deep to the nerve
- *Total conservative parotidectomy*: identification and preservation of the facial nerve, with removal of all of the salivary tissue
- *Radical parotidectomy*: removal or excision of the facial nerve and all salivary tissue
- *Extended radical parotidectomy*: a more radical parotidectomy to include bone – mandible or temporal – skin, muscle, etc.
- *Neck dissection* may be performed when a malignant tumour is being removed – selective, modified or radical.

The facial nerve should be preserved if it is functioning preoperatively, and should only be sacrificed – branch, division or trunk – if removing part of the nerve will ensure complete removal of a malignant tumour. Should part of the facial nerve be sacrificed, then it should be repaired, primarily by a cable graft – usually the greater auricular nerve. An extended parotidectomy should be considered if there is evidence of bony or cartilaginous invasion by tumour. The use of a facial nerve monitor or a stimulator may help the novice to identify the facial nerve, and is more useful when the facial nerve is being re-explored for recurrent tumours, etc. The nerve stimulator is very useful when surgery has been completed. The facial nerve is stimulated; a twitch or move demonstrates a functioning nerve, and the patient can be reassured that the nerve, even if showing some weakness, can return to its preoperative level of function. Monitors and stimulators will never, however, replace knowledge of anatomy and surgical experience.

4.9.3.1   Parotid Gland Surgery

Surgery of the parotid gland is most frequently indicated for benign and malignant tumours. Secondary indications are for swellings that demonstrate chronicity and in whom FNA remains inconclusive, and thirdly for recurrent chronic inflammatory/cystic sialadenitis.

The extent of surgery performed is dependent on the anticipated or diagnostic pathology and its location relative to the facial nerve, either lateral or medial. Frequently,

4.9.3.2   Submandibular Gland Surgery

The most common indication for surgery is sialadenitis with or without sialolithiasis. The next less frequent indication is a neoplasm, either salivary gland in origin or as part of a neck dissection for cancer. The submandibular gland should be removed in toto, as frequently, recurrence of disease occurs in the remaining gland tissue – infections or neoplasm. When the indication for gland removal is infection, then a subcapsular excision is recommended, as this approach avoids/minimises trauma to the cranial nerves – mandibular branch of the facial nerve, lingual and hypoglossal nerves. Should the indication for surgery be a neoplasm, then the submandibular gland should be excised extracapsularly to reduce the risk of incomplete tumour excision and subsequent local recurrence. It is advocated that because salivary gland neoplasms (both benign and malignant) are at risk for soft tissue extension (with or without lymph node metastasis), a more extensive excision be performed, including selective neck dissection in which levels Ib, IIa, and III are removed.

Surgery for sialorrhoea or drooling may be considered within a treatment plan for some patients whose symptoms do not improve with posture change and physiotherapy. This involves the relocation of the submandibular duct from the anterior floor of mouth to the anterior faucal pillar bilaterally.

4.9.3.3 Surgery of the Sublingual Gland

There are two conditions affecting the sublingual glands that necessitate surgical attention, tumours and ranulae. Removal of a sublingual gland tumour should involve an initial incisional biopsy to confirm the diagnosis prior to recommending a more radical excision; a malignant diagnosis is more likely than benign disease.

4.9.3.4 Minor Salivary Gland Surgery

As there are more than 1,000 minor salivary glands located in the head and neck area, minor salivary gland disease may present in any anatomical site. The most frequent site affected is the oral cavity. Salivary gland tumours – benign and malignant – are the most frequent indication for surgery, but occasionally infection and stones may involve this tissue. As minor salivary glands are located beneath the mucosa, neoplasms present as slow-growing, non-ulcerative swelling, and only tend to present with symptoms when the mass has grown in size, causing organ obstruction. An incision or punch biopsy should be performed to confirm the diagnosis – benign or malignant – prior to recommending an extensive surgical procedure. Tumour surgery for malignant disease requires more extensive surgery if tumour-free margins are to be achieved.

4.9.4 Complications Associated with Salivary Gland Surgery

Surgery is the agreed treatment of choice for salivary neoplasms, both benign and malignant. Because this is facial surgery, patients naturally are reluctant to agree to it unless the procedure is carefully explained, and a minimal risk of sequelae and complications is made by the surgeon. When undertaking such surgery, the objective is the complete removal of disease, with minimal surgical morbidity and no tumour recurrence. Listed in Table 4.9.1 are the recognised morbidities associated with parotid and submandibular gland surgery, divided into early (Immediate – > 4 weeks) and late (after hospital discharge).

The results of a survey concerning the early and late sequelae and complications of 212 patients who underwent parotid surgery for benign salivary neoplasms (of whom 173 patients responded) is presented in Table 4.9.2. Ninety-nine per cent of patients knew the exact date of their respective surgeries. Eighty-five per cent of patients felt the preoperative information helped them prepare for what followed, whereas 10% felt it did not help, and 5% did not respond to the question. No patient reported a recurrence of his or her tumour in the follow-up period.

Table 4.9.1 Early and late complications of salivary gland surgery

Early (Immediate – 4 weeks)	Late (after hospital discharge)
Nerve paralysis: Facial, Lingual, Hypoglossal	Frey's syndrome
Haemorrhage/haematoma	Hypaesthesia of local skin
Infection	Cosmetic deformity: divot defect
Skin-flap necrosis	Hypertrophic scar
Trismus	Recurrence of disease – tumour/infection
Salivary fistula/sialocele	
Seroma	

Table 4.9.2 Early and late sequelae/complications after parotid surgery

Complication	% Short -Term (Within 6 months)	% Long-term (after 6 months)
No problem	16.9	52.5
Sensation around ear/cheek	66.2	30.6
Painful wound	22.5	3.1
Facial sweating while eating	22.5	12.5
Altered shape of face/skin/ear	26.9	3.1
Difficulty with shoulder	9.4	3.1
Facial weakness (partial)	26.3	1.9

4.9.5 Avoidance of or Minimising Complications after Salivary Gland Surgery

Informed consent and considerate explanation are the first step to minimising patients' dissatisfaction of the results of major salivary gland surgery. Results of patient satisfaction surveys (what few are available) can provide the surgeon with a realistic view of patients' perception of the procedure.

To minimise postoperative complications, the following should be borne in mind:

1. The incision employed very much depends on the experience and expertise of the surgeon. In general, benign neoplasms proven on FNAC can be surgically treated by a partial surgery or even extracapsular dissection. However, the facial nerve trunk should be sought initially to determine the location of the tumour proximity to the nerve. This form of surgery is associated with minimal impairment of cosmesis and a lower incidence of gustatory hyperhydrosis. This limited type of surgery should only be undertaken by experienced parotid surgeons. Suggestion as to performing a parotidectomy with endoscopic instruments is said to be associated with minimal morbidity – but results reported in the literature are without prolonged patient follow-up. The submandibular gland may also be removed by transoral methods, also associated with minimal trauma and patients' complaints.

2. All nerves that function preoperatively should be preserved and return to function at some time after surgery. Temporary injury or paresis may occur, reported to be 18–25%, and is frequently the result of traumatic manipulation of the nerve or branches, excessive skeletonization of the nerve, close proximity of electrocautery to the nerve, or occasionally, nerve conduction fatigue from overzealous use of the nerve stimulator. As for recovery of temporary facial nerve weakness, 38% of patients' weaknesses resolved within 1 month, 78% within 3 months and all recovered within 7 months. The incidence of permanent palsy is usually very low in benign neoplasms, and may be higher when a malignant tumour has been encountered; the reported incidence in functioning nerves ranged from 2 to 8%.

3. Sialocele after parotidectomy is uncommon, but not rare. This is the accumulation of saliva without drainage underneath the skin, most usually seen after parotid surgery. Sialoceles have been reported in 30% of lateral parotidectomies (more than near-total parotidectomies), and can generally be treated by observation, with an expectation of resolution within 1 month. When the saliva leaks through the wound or drain site, then the term *salivary fistula* should be used; this complication lasting more than 4–6 weeks is rare. The use of injectable Botox into the remaining or residual gland should be offered, with high expectation of fistula resolution.

4. The development of gustatory hyperhydrosis, facial skin sweating or Frey's syndrome is due to the aberrant regeneration of the parasympathetic cholinergic fibres that normally innervate the parotid gland being redirected to innervate the sweat glands. Typically, such symptoms develop 6–12 months after surgery. Approximately 15% of patients complain bitterly about the symptom and seek relief. The use of local injections of Botox has dramatically improved patients' quality of life, and after injection, the sweating disappears or is suppressed within 14 days, and remains quiescent for a period of 12–18 months. The treatment can be repeated at intervals.

5. First-bite syndrome is occasionally reported by patients after parotid surgery, most usually in the parapharyngeal space. When they commence eating, severe pain

is experienced around the jaw on the first bite, in the side on which was operated. The current theory suggests that this syndrome is due to loss of sympathetic innervation to the parotid gland from the superior cervical ganglion. Treatment for this syndrome, i.e. procedures and injections, so far has had a low success rate.

6. Avoidance of divot and sensory defects can help ensure that a patient's quality of life improves significantly after parotid surgery.

The extent of the facial deformity depends on the volume of the salivary tissue removed. The stigma of a visually prominent facial scar after parotid surgery can be distressing to a young patient. One method to minimise scarring is to use the face-lift incision, hiding the posterior scar within the hairline. Using this incision also allows for the elevation of the superficial musculoaponeurotic system (SMAS) rotation advancement flap, which is associated with decreased incidence of development of divot defect and Frey's syndrome. The use of the sternocleidomastoid muscle (SCM) rotation flap may be used in conjunction with the SMAS flap or alone, when the divot defect after surgery has been more extensive. The use of the SCM flap has been associated to reduce the likelihood of developing Frey's syndrome.

Preservation of the posterior branch of the great auricular nerve (GAN) demonstrates a lesser area of sensory deficit than the deficit of those in whom the trunk of the nerve has been divided. It has been suggested that preservation of the posterior branch of the GAN should be preserved if it does not compromise tumour resection. If this is not possible, the patient and surgeon should be comforted in that only minor, if any, long-term disability will ensue.

Suggested Reading

1. Bradley PJ (2004) Salivary gland neoplasms. Surgery 22:169–172
2. Berquin R (2006) Sublingual gland biopsy. Eur Arch Otorhinolaryngol 263:233–236
3. Bree R de, van der Waal I, Leemans CR (2007) Management of Frey syndrome. Head Neck 29:773–778
4. Curry JM, Fisher KW, Heffelfinger RN, Rosen MR, Keane WM, Pribitkin EA (2008) Superficial musculoaponeurotic system elevation and fat graft reconstruction after superficial parotidectomy. Laryngoscope 118:210–215
5. Henney SE, Brown R, Phillips DE (2008) Parotidectomy: the timing of post-operative complications. Eur Arch ORL DOI 10.1007/s00405-009-0980-1
6. Johnson JT, Ferlito A, Fagan JJ, Bradley PJ, Rinaldo A (2007) Role of limited parotidectomy in management of pleomorphic adenoma. J Laryngol Otol 121:1126–1128
7. Kawashima Y, Sumi T, Sugimoto T, Kishimoto S (2008) First-bite syndrome: a review of 29 patients with parapharyngeal space tumour. Auris Nasus Larynx 35:109–113
8. Marshall A H, Quraishi S M, Bradley PJ (2003) Patients perspective on the short- and long-term outcomes following surgery for benign parotid neoplasms. J Laryngol Otol 117:624–629
9. Munir N, Bradley PJ (2008) Management of neoplasms of the submandibular triangle. Oral Oncol 44:251–260
10. Ryan WR, Fee WE (2009) Long-term great auricular nerve morbidity after sacrifice during parotidectomy. Laryngoscope 119:1140–1146
11. Witt RL (2009) The incidence and management of sialocele after parotidectomy. Otolaryngol Head Neck Surg 1450:871–874

Diseases of the Oral Cavity, Oropharynx, Hypopharynx, Cervical Esophagus

Edited by Viktor Bonkowsky

5.1 Oral Cavity

VIKTOR BONKOWSKY AND PETRA GERDEMANN

5.1.1 Basics

5.1.1.1 Embryology

In the first embryonal weeks an ectodermal depression occurs as the stomodeum, or primitive oral cavity. The buccopharyngeal membrane separates the stomodeum from the primitive foregut. At approximately 3 weeks of gestation the buccopharyngeal membrane tears and the oral cavity becomes contiguous to the foregut. This portion of the foregut is developing into the oropharynx.

The development of the tongue can be divided into two parts. At the end of the fourth week the tuberculum impar in front of the foramen caecum on the floor of the stomodeum occurs. Laterally two oval swellings on either side of the foregut start to grow symmetrically and merge medially and with the tuberculum impar. They form the anterior two thirds of the tongue. The posterior third develops from the primitive copula from the second arch mesoderm and from a mesodermal swelling of the third and fourth arches. The upper and lower lips are formed from the mandibular and maxillary processes. At the same time—between the sixth and seventh weeks—the fusion of the primary and secondary palates occurs.

5.1.1.2 Anatomy

Oral Cavity

The oral cavity is divided into two sections:

1. The **oral vestibule** is the part of the mouth outside the teeth bounded laterally by the mucosa of the lips and the cheeks and the lateral aspect of the mandibular and maxillary alveoli. The main muscles which form the oral vestibule are the orbicularis oris muscle and the buccinator muscle. The *orbicularis oris muscle* encircles the opening of the mouth and helps to close the lips and keeps the mouth closed. The origin and the insertion of the muscle lie into the skin. The orbicularis oris muscle continues laterally into the *buccinator muscle*. It helps to compress the cheeks against the teeth and helps during chewing (Fig. 5.1.1). The blood supply of the oral cavity musculature is the inferior and superior labial arteries, which are branches of the facial artery. The maxillary division of the trigeminal nerve innervates the buccal mucosa and the mucosa of the lips. The motor innervation of all these muscles of facial expression is from the facial nerve.

Multiple minor salivary glands are widely distributed in the mucosa of the lips and the cheeks. The parotid (Stensen's) duct arises from the anterior border of the gland as a termination of various extraglandular ductules. It traverses the masseter muscle, penetrates the buccinator muscle and empties into the oral vestibule opposite the upper second molar.

2. The **oral cavity proper** is the space between the medial surfaces of the maxillary and mandibular alveoli. The cranial border of the oral cavity proper is the hard and the soft palate. It separates the oral and the nasal cavities. The oral cavity opens through the oropharyn-

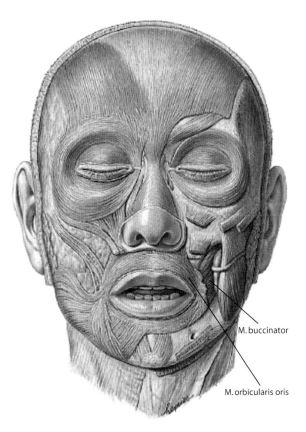

M. buccinator

M. orbicularis oris

Fig. 5.1.1 Muscles of facial expression. (Figure 139 in [1])

geal isthmus into the oropharynx. The anterior two thirds of the tongue belong to the oral cavity proper. The V-shaped row of the circumvallate papillae represents the exact anterior border. The posterior third of the tongue is present in the oropharynx.

The anterior two thirds of the tongue is connected by the frenulum on the floor of the oral cavity. The openings of Wharton's ducts are located on both sides of the frenulum (Fig. 5.1.2). They transport a large amount of saliva which is produced by both submandibular glands. The openings of the submandibular glands are called the "*caruncles*". Adjacent to the ducts are the sublingual glands. They give the floor of the mouth the cobblestoned surface. Multiple minor sublingual ducts open into the mucosa. The anterior part of the sublingual gland has a proper major duct that empties into the caruncle.

The Tongue

The V-shaped row of the circumvallate papillae in front of the foramen caecum separates the tongue into two portions. The base of the tongue is covered by lymphoid tissue, a component of Waldeyer's ring, the lingual tonsil (Fig. 5.1.3).

In addition to the circumvallate papillae, the anterior mobile part of the tongue is covered by different kinds of papillae. The filiform papillae just have mechanical functions; they are distributed all over the dorsum of the tongue. The foliate and the circumvallate papillae are all taste receptors. The foliate papillae lie especially at the lateral borders of the tongue; the fungiform papillae are on the dorsum.

The tongue musculature can be divided into an extrinsic and an intrinsic system (Fig. 5.1.4). The extrinsic mus-

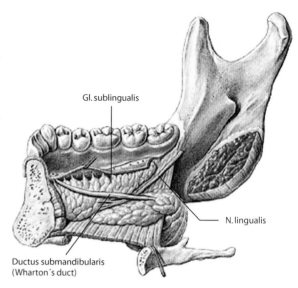

Fig. 5.1.2 Topographic situation of sublingual gland, lingual nerve and Wharton's duct. (Figure 210 in [1])

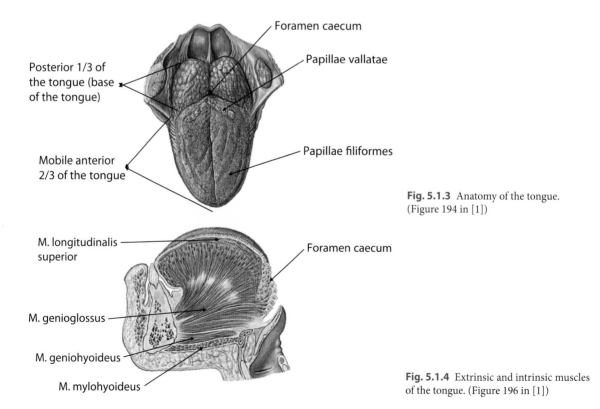

Fig. 5.1.3 Anatomy of the tongue. (Figure 194 in [1])

Fig. 5.1.4 Extrinsic and intrinsic muscles of the tongue. (Figure 196 in [1])

cles include the genioglossus, hyoglossus and styloglossus muscles. They arise from adjacent bony skeletal parts such as the hyoid, the mental spine of the mandible and the styloid process. They help to move the tongue; they cause depression, retraction and elevation. All these extrinsic muscles pass into the intrinsic muscles of the tongue.

The intrinsic musculature is arranged with vertical, transverse and longitudinal muscle fibres. They offer the possibility to change the shape of the tongue.

Innervation

The innervation of the tongue is shown in Fig. 5.1.5.
- Motoric innervation: Hypoglossal nerve (CN XII)
- Sensible innervation: Lingual nerve (CN V)—anterior two thirds of the tongue
- Glossopharyngeal nerve (CN IX)—posterior third of the tongue
- Sensory innervation: Lingual nerve via chorda tympani nerve (CN VII)—anterior two thirds of the tongue
- Glossopharyngeal nerve (CN IX)—posterior third of the tongue

Blood Supply

The blood supply of the tongue is from the lingual branch of the external carotid artery. The lingual artery has multiple branches: the dorsal lingual, the sublingual and the deep lingual arteries. The venous drain is the lingual vein and the facial vein.

Lymphatics

The cheeks, upper lip, a part of the lower lip and the anterior two thirds of the tongue drain into the submandibular nodes and finally into the upper deep jugular digastric nodes (Fig. 5.1.6) (Level I, II and III). The central portion of the lower lip and the tip of the tongue drain into the submental nodes. The lymphatic drain of the tongue is ipsilateral and contralateral, which must be noticed with carcinoma of the tongue and its metastatic processes.

Floor of the Mouth

The floor of the mouth is the caudal border of the oral cavity. It is formed by different muscle layers (Fig. 5.1.7). The *mylohyoid muscle* is the main component. It arises from the inner surface of the mandible and is inserted on the hyoid. It is formed like a triangle diaphragm, supporting the structures of the mouth. It also helps to elevate the hyoid. The submandibular glands lie below the muscle. Upon the mylohyoid muscle lies the *geniohyoid muscle*. On the caudal outer surface of the mylohyoid muscle lies the anterior belly of the *digastric muscle*.

Innervation

The innervation of the floor of the mouth is complex and dependent on the development of the muscles. The mylohyoid muscle and the anterior belly of the digastric

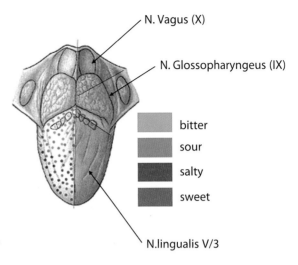

Fig. 5.1.5 Innervation of the tongue. (Figure 195 in [1])

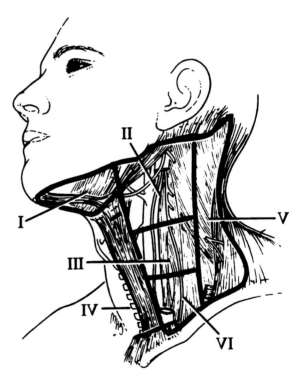

Fig. 5.1.6 Lymph nodes of the oral cavity. (Figure 204 in [1])

muscle are innervated by a branch of the mandibular division of the trigeminal nerve. (The posterior belly of the digastric muscle is reached by the facial nerve!). The geniohyoid muscle is innervated by fibres from the cervical spinal cord which accompany the hypoglossal nerve.

Blood Supply

The blood supply is from the facial artery and the lingual artery.

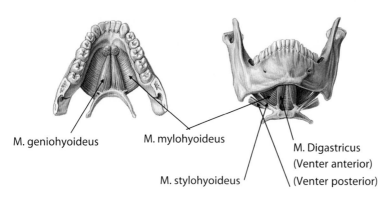

Fig. 5.1.7 Floor of the mouth. (Figure 203 in [1])

M. geniohyoideus   M. mylohyoideus

M. stylohyoideus

M. Digastricus
(Venter anterior)
(Venter posterior)

5.1.1.3   Physiology

The functions of the oral cavity are:
- Food ingestion
- Speech production
- Taste reception
- Accessory respiratory function

Food Ingestion

The lips are the entrance of the aerodigestive tract and help to close the mouth during chewing, so that the food stays in the oral cavity. In the mouth the tongue helps during chewing to chop up the food bolus by various changes of its shape and pressing the bolus against the teeth and the hard palate. The teeth are important during chewing, especially the molars, with a high molar occlusal force. The bolus is mixed with saliva. The salivation starts as a result of smelling the food and it continues when the bolus is placed in the oral cavity. The salivary glands produce 1,500 ml of saliva each day. It is composed of 99% water and 1% enzymes, proteins and salts. Chewing food and mixing it with saliva prepares the bolus for swallowing.

Speech and Articulation

Air expelled from the lungs causes the vocal cords to vibrate and produce sound. It resonates in the upper pharynx, the paranasal sinus and the nose. "Articulation" means to shape the sound into understandable words by the vocal tract; therefore, the coordinated movement of the tongue, teeth, lips and mouth is necessary. Clear and distinct speech needs a competent oral cavity without congenital anomalies or other abnormalities.

Taste Sensation

The tongue tastes four qualities, sweet, salty, bitter and sour, through the taste receptors. The flavour recognition is a combination of olfactory sensations through the nose, gustatory stimuli of the taste buds and mechanical and thermal receptors. Three cranial nerves carry taste sensation of the oral cavity and the oropharynx.

Accessory Respiratory Function

"Mouth breathing" is not the normal respiratory way. It occurs in stress situations, during increased cardiovascular demands and in times of nasal congestion, as in an upper respiratory tract infection. Air respired through the mouth is not humidified and warmed as it is by normal nasal respiration. Oral respiration is not as physiologic as nasal breathing.

5.1.2   Clinical Tests

5.1.2.1   Inspection and Palpation

The most important clinical tests for evaluating disorders of the oral cavity are inspection and palpation. The results have to be considered in combination with the patient's history.

The examination of the salivary secretion is a component of the inspection of the oral cavity. The opening of Stensen's duct can be seen by lateralization of the cheeks. Through smearing of the cheek the saliva is mobilized and its consistence can be evaluated. The submandibular glands are examined in an analogous way.

The cranial nerve functions should be evaluated as well. The movement of the tongue indicates the hypoglossal nerve. It can be tested by putting out the tongue and moving it up and down on both sides. In the case of hypoglossal palsy, the tongue deviates to the paretic side. To examine the motor innervation of the soft palate, the gag reflex needs to be elicited. The soft palate deviates to the healthy side in the case of glossopharyngeal palsy.

The general sensory innervation can be checked with a cotton-tipped swab to evaluate equal sensations on both sides of the tongue and the cheeks.

Any abnormal lesions can be palpated to evaluate consistence and extension. Any subtle surface abnormalities that may be neoplastic warrant biopsy.

5.1.2.2   Taste Testing

Disorders of taste can be verified by the application of test solutions with the four main tasting qualities: sweet, salty, bitter and sour. For the examination, fluid glucose as a sweet stimulus, sodium chloride as a salty stimulus, citric acid as a sour stimulus and quinine sulphate as a bitter stimulus are applied. The solutions are available in different concentrations (Table 5.1.1). The fluids are applied on the lateral tongue with a cotton-tipped swab. Usually all qualities are identified in the lowest concentration. The handling of this kind of subjective testing is easy but has a low degree of reliability and reproducibility. Another possibility of taste testing is the electrical stimulation of the taste buds. The application of synchronized direct current causes metallic and sour taste sensations. By increasing the current, one can verify the exact threshold.

Objective taste testing is possible but very expensive and needs special assumptions. It should be reserved for special centres.

5.1.2.3   Ultrasonography

The tongue and the floor of the mouth may be examined sonographically during reclining of the head. Deep structures are delineated in transverse and longitudinal scans; guiding muscles are the mylohyoid and geniohyoid muscles. In general, B-scans are necessary. Depending on the penetrating and resolving power, probes of 5–10 MHz are used.

5.1.2.4   Radiology

Radiologic evaluations have a role in specific disease entities of the oral cavity. Because of the exposed position of all structures of the oral cavity, most disorders can be detected by clinical inspection. But for extended infectious diseases and for the extension of tumours of the tongue and the floor of the mouth, CT scans and MRI are useful. In general, MRI is preferable because of its ability to distinguish the extent of tumour masses in soft tissue. To visualize the relationship of the tumour to osseous structures, CT scans are more valuable. In addition, CT scans are useful for a suspected abscess in the tongue or the floor of the mouth.

In general, whenever CT or MRI is performed, imaging the neck to visualize cervical lymphatic nodes should complete the examination.

Table 5.1.1 Concentrations of test solutions

Sweet	Glucose	5, 10, 40%
Salty	Sodium chloride	2.5, 7.5, 15%
Sour	Citric acid	1, 5, 10%
Bitter	Quinine	0.075, 0.5, 1%

5.1.3   Congenital Disorders

There exist multiple congenital disorders of the oral cavity. For appropriate treatment an extensive history of the patient and his/her family is necessary as well as a complete physical examination. In the case of congenital syndrome, the patient may have multiple anomalies, so the assistance of a paediatrician as well as a geneticist is useful. Clinical tests, X-rays and swallowing function tests should be performed. The hearing functions needs to be examined too.

5.1.3.1   Congenital Epulis

Aetiology/Epidemiology
This is a formation of granular cell myoblastoma, a benign neoplasm, commonly located on the edge of the oral mucosa on the alveolar and maxillary processes. It is commonly found in female patients.

Symptoms
Epulis is shown as a light-red neoplasm on the oral mucosa and can lead to difficulties during food ingestion. X-rays show arrosion of the bony alveolar processes.

Therapy
Treatment is surgical excision, including the periosteum.

5.1.3.2   Torus Palatinus and Mandibularis

Aetiology/Epidemiology
These are bony exostosis, located on the surface of the hard palate and on the lingual surface of the mandible. They are covered with mucosa.

Therapy
Treatment is only required when the formation is large and the upper and lower dentures do not fit any more, and the exostosis has recurrent infections, ulceration or neoplasm.

5.1.3.3   Ankyloglossia

Aetiology/Epidemiology

The presence of an elongated lingual frenulum, which fixes the whole tongue to the floor of the mouth, limits the mobility of the tongue.

Symptoms

It can result in significant symptoms for the patients. They have difficulties with speech, eating and swallowing.

Therapy

Surgical treatment by the division of the frenulum is required. In severe cases (thick frenulum), a Z-plasty may be necessary.

5.1.3.4   Lingual Thyroid

Aetiology/Epidemiology

Usually, thyroid tissue derives from the foramen caecum in the middle of the tongue base and develops to its anatomic position in front of the trachea at the level of the second and third tracheal rings. The development occurs between the seventh and the 12th weeks of embryogenesis. The normal pathway of the thyroid—the thyroglossal duct—is obliterated. In cases of failure of thyroid descent, the thyroid may persist in the lingual base.

Symptoms

Symptoms are dysphagia, dyspnoea and speech affection. Patients could be hypothyroid.

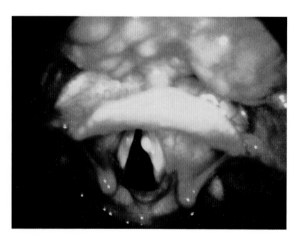

Fig. 5.1.8 Lingual thyroid

Diagnostic Procedures

Physical examination reveals a mass in the lymphoid tissue of the base of the tongue. When lingual thyroid is suspected, normal thyroid tissue should be searched. Thyroid function tests, cervical ultrasound and thyroid scanning should be undertaken (Fig. 5.1.8).

Therapy

Therapy requires the suppression with thyroid hormone to decrease the size of the lingual thyroid. Radioactive iodine ablation as well as surgical excision may also be necessary.

5.1.3.5   Hypoplastic Mandible

This symptom is usually associated with first arch syndromes. A brief description follows.

Pierre Robin Anomaly

The characteristic triad is a combination of cleft palate, micrognathy and glossoptosis. Firstly, the development of the first arch arrests and the triad occurs secondarily. Airway obstruction may occur during childhood and become life-threatening, so tracheotomy in combination with glossopexy could be necessary. In some cases mandibular growth has a normal state by approximately 6 years.

Treacher Collins Syndrome (Franceschetti–Treacher Collins Syndrome, Dysostosis Mandibulofacialis)

This mandibulofacial dysostosis is a syndrome of craniofacial dysmorphia. It typically occurs in the combination of hypoplastic mandible and middle face, low-set ears with congenital aural atresia, hypoplastic mastoid and epitympanum and cleft palate. It has an autosomal-dominant inheritance pattern.

Crouzon's and Apert's Syndromes

The main common factor of both syndromes is the craniofacial dysostosis manifested as abnormal premature synostosis of multiple skull suture lines. Maxillary hypoplasia occurs commonly in Crouzon's syndrome; other common findings are mild mental retardation, congenital aural atresia, hypertelorism and prognathic mandible.

Early fusion of cranial suture lines causes a brachycephalic appearance; in combination with cleft palate, syndactyly of hands and feet and mental retardation it is called "Apert's syndrome".

5.1.4 Infectious and Inflammatory Disorders

The gingiva, the hard palate and the peridontium are covered with keratinized mucosa, which is firmly adherent to underlying structures. The buccal mucosa, the mucosa of the soft palate, the mucosa of the floor of the mouth, the mucosa of the retromolar space and the tongue are nonkeratinized and are easy to deform by the movement of the structures during speech and mastication. In the normal state the mucosa has a moist, smooth and pink appearance. Oral mucosa provides an effective protective barrier against infectious diseases of the oral cavity. The epithelium provides a physical as well as a biochemical barrier. The chemical barrier includes the saliva with all its components, especially salivary immunoglobulins. Multiple causes of inflammatory and infectious diseases include bacteria, viruses, fungi as well as chemical irritants, systemic autoimmune diseases, diabetes mellitus and alcohol and nicotine abuse.

5.1.4.1 Tongue Anomalies

Fissured Tongue

Synonym
Lingua plicata.

Aetiology/Epidemiology
The incidence of a wrinkled tongue is 10%. It follows an autosomal-dominant inheritance pattern.

Symptoms
There are no clinical symptoms. The fissures may occur laterally, medially or are spread all over the tongue (Fig. 5.1.9). A wrinkled tongue can be combined with Melkersson–Rosenthal syndrome, Down's syndrome or acromegaly.

Therapy
No therapy is necessary.

Mappy Tongue

Synonym
Lingua geographica.

Aetiology/Epidemiology
A mappy tongue is caused by a desquamation of filiform papillae in different regions of the tongue. The tongue has characteristic irregular-shaped white and red spots. The

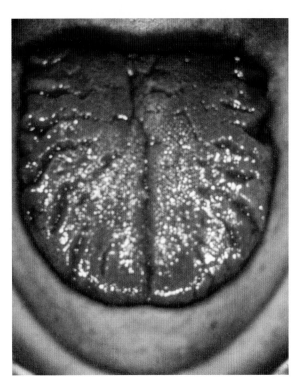

Fig. 5.1.9 Fissured tongue

fields move along the tongue; the different colours and patterns give the surface a "mappy" look.

Symptoms
There are no clinical symptoms, except burning of the tongue and gustatory relay or loss in some cases. Inflammatory signs occur in histologic findings.

Therapy
The treatment can be started by the application of vitamin A and zinc; they should support the epithelization of the mucosa.

Black Hairy Tongue

Aetiology/Epidemiology
Black hairy tongue is caused by a filamentous hyperkeratosis of the filiform papillae, which looks like hairs on the tongue's surface. The elongation of papillae is caused either by a loss of desquamation or by an increased production of keratin. The hyperkeratosis is triggered by antibiotic treatment, nicotine abuse, chronic mucosal irritation and metabolic imbalance.

Symptoms

Patients have a black surface of the tongue, having a hairy appearance caused by the elongation of the filiform papillae. Patients do not complain of pain or burning of the tongue.

Therapy

Hairy tongue does require treatment of the causal disease.

Hunter's Glossitis

Aetiology/Epidemiology

Hunter's glossitis is a nutritional anaemia, caused by pernicious anaemia in the case of malabsorption with a deficit of intrinsic factor.

Symptoms

The tongue shows an atrophic inflammation; associated symptoms are burning of the tongue combined with paraesthesia and dry mouth. The surface of the tongue is atrophic and glazed, sometimes with a flushed appearance (Fig. 5.1.10).

Diagnostic Procedures/Therapy

To diagnose the cause of the glossitis, the serum level of vitamin B_{12} must be measured. In the case of a low concentration, folic acid needs to be substituted.

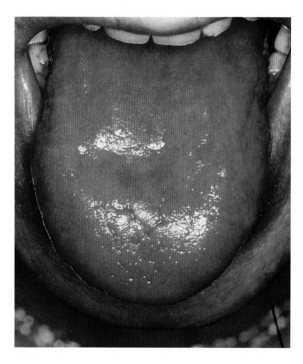

Fig. 5.1.10 Hunter's glossitis

5.1.4.2   Bacterial Infections

Chronic Gingivitis

Aetiology/Epidemiology

This is the most common form of gingivitis; the incidence is up to 90% in middle age. Bacterial factors and food particles in combination with poor dental hygiene cause an irritation of the mucosa. There is an overgrowth of commensal bacteria.

Symptoms

A painless diffuse erythema of the gingival occurs, sometimes with ulcers present on the tooth enamel.

Therapy

Therapy requires appropriate dental hygiene and treatment of carious lesions of the teeth.

Acute Gingivitis

Aetiology/Epidemiology

The most important aetiologic factors are poor dental hygiene as well as immune and nutritional deficiencies. Gingivitis is caused by β-haemolytic streptococci and by staphylococci.

Symptoms

Gingiva is erythematous and inflamed, bleeds easily and hurts during eating. Sometimes an oral fetor exists.

Differential Diagnosis

Acute necrotizing ulcerative gingivitis and herpetic gingivitis need to be considered.

Therapy

Therapy requires management of the acute bacterial infection with oral antibiotics (penicillin or ampicillin) and an improvement of oral hygiene. Local anaesthesia may be helpful.

Acute Necrotizing Ulcerative Gingivitis

Synonyms

Vincent's stomatitis, gangrenous pharyngitis.

Aetiology/Epidemiology

This disease is usually found in older patients and in patients with a lowered resistance to infections. This form of gingivitis leads to a necrosed and sloughed gingiva by an overgrowth of fusiform bacteria and *Borrelia vincentii*. Predisposing factors are poor oral hygiene and immune deficiencies.

Symptoms

The disease initially shows a hyperaemia and swelling of the gingiva. A pseudomembrane covering necrotic epithelium occurs on the gingival margin. Lesions occur craterlike along the alveolar margin and the entire gingiva. Bleeding occurs easily. The disease is very painful; sometimes lymphadenitis is associated with it. Patients complain of a metallic taste.

Diagnostic Procedures

Vincent's stomatitis is diagnosed by the characteristic clinical symptoms and oral swab. Typical organisms in culture and biopsy sections may be found.

Differential Diagnosis

Differentiation of Vincent's angina from acute tonsillitis, herpes infection, agranulocytosis or syphilis is difficult, since all may produce ulceration or membranes.

Therapy

Therapy requires aggressive oral hygiene directed against fusiform bacteria, antibiotic treatment with penicillin or ampicillin and local aseptic treatment such as hydrogen peroxide or sodium perborate.

Syphilis

Synonym

Lues.

Aetiology/Epidemiology

Syphilis is a sexually transmitted disease. In industrialized countries it has a low incidence; during the last few years it has been increasing. The incidence in 2003 in Germany was 3.6 per 100,000 people, which means an increase of 20% in comparison with 2002. In African countries, combined infection of syphilis and HIV often occurs. Primary, secondary and tertiary syphilis may all occur in the oral cavity. Especially primary and secondary syphilis have manifestations in the oral cavity. *Treponema pallidum* causes syphilis.

Symptoms

- In primary syphilis, a solitary painless chancre occurs after an incubation period of 2–3 weeks. Extragenital localizations are the lips, the tongue, buccal mucosa and the hard and the soft palate (Fig. 5.1.11). Sometimes the venereal ulcer is followed by a slight fever, other constitutional symptoms and a painless lymphadenitis.
- In secondary syphilis, a skin eruption of various appearances with mucous patches occurs on the lips and intraorally. There is latency of between 4–6 months. Because of the inflammation which accompanies the

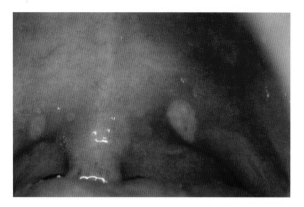

Fig. 5.1.11 Primary affection of syphilis

mucous patches, these lesions are often painful. The patches are highly communicable because of the high bacterial concentration. In secondary syphilis, the local manifestations are often combined with a specific tonsillitis or pharyngitis and more general symptoms.
- In tertiary syphilis, the formation of a gumma starts after 3–10 years. Gummas are painless, well-defined ulcers. Healing with scar formation is possible.

Diagnostic Procedures

Microbial detection is possible in primary syphilis by dark-field microscopy. Serologic tests for syphilis verify the diagnosis (*Treponema pallidum* haemoagglutination test, fluorescent treponemal antibody absorption) and are necessary in cases of secondary and tertiary syphilis.

Differential Diagnosis

The main differential diagnosis is among neoplasm, specific angina-like mononucleosis and Vincent's angina and diphtheria.

Therapy

Therapy is required with 2.4×10^6 units of benzathine penicillin G intramuscularly biweekly or 1.2×10^6 units of procaine penicillin per day intramuscularly for 15 days in primary, secondary and latent syphilis (duration of infection less than 1 year). Alternative therapy with 200 mg doxycycline per day or 2 g erythromycin per day for 2 weeks in penicillin-allergic patients is recommended. In tertiary and latent syphilis (duration of infection more than 1 year) 2.4×10^6 units of benzathine penicillin intramuscularly once a week for 3 weeks is recommended. After therapy a serologic test for syphilis needs to be performed.

Submandibular Space Abscess

Synonym
Ludwig's angina.

Aetiology/Epidemiology
Proliferation of bacteria and bacterial invasion through the enamel organ causes necrosis of bone surrounding the tooth root. Usually, patients undergo tooth treatment and drainage of the root abscess. If the root abscess is not drained and stays unchecked, infection can spread freely into the soft facial compartment of the neck and the mediastinum. Infection mostly spreads from the mandibular teeth, in some cases from injury to oral mucosa. Abscesses can also be caused by trauma, lingual tonsillitis or salivary gland disease. Infection can spread to the deeper neck spaces, to the submandibular, the parapharyngeal and the retropharyngeal spaces. The prevertebral space can also be involved. Deeper neck infections can cause different life-threatening complications such as upper-airway obstruction and mediastinitis. When all three of the primary mandibular spaces are infected (bilateral submandibular and sublingual space) this is known as Ludwig's angina.

Symptoms
Clinical symptoms include high fever, pain in the floor of the mouth, trismus and drooling. Patients cannot speak or swallow because of tongue involvement. Oedema, submandibular induration, tenderness and swelling are evident (Fig. 5.1.12). The skin beneath the chin is erythematous and oedematous; the oedema can be spread down onto the skin of the anterior neck and descend onto the chest wall.

Diagnostic Procedures
Complete blood counts as well as bacterial cultures should be obtained. For estimation of the extension of an abscess formation, accessory CT scans and ultrasound are necessary.

Therapy
Conservative Treatment
Antibiotic therapy should be initialized as soon as possible to prevent the patient from having a progressing infection with life-threatening complications. High-dose penicillin or cephalosporin is recommended. Whenever the therapy starts conservatively with intravenous antibiotics, the general rule is that patients must respond within 18–24 h. If they do not, a surgical exploration is necessary to detect occult abscesses.

Surgical Treatment
Surgical treatment is necessary:
1. If there is obvious abscess formation
2. If anaerobic bacteria are present, seen by gas within the soft tissues in the CT scans, indicating an aggressive anaerobic fasciitis.
3. If there is no improvement after conservative treatment (see above!)

Surgical Procedures
Typically, the submandibular and submental space is opened through horizontal incision paralleling the mandible over the mylohyoid muscle or below the angle of the mandible. During surgery, upon opening the abscess cavity, one should obtain bacterial cultures as well as biopsies in the case of oedema to exclude neoplasm. All loculated areas of the abscess must be opened and drained.

After surgery the number of white blood cells and the fever must decrease. If they persist, another occult abscess cavity exists and the CT scans should be repeated. In the case of a residual abscess, a further surgical drainage is necessary. Sometimes tracheotomy or nasopharyngeal intubation may be necessary to control the airway. Removal of suspected teeth if panoramic X-ray identifies a source needs to be done.

Apparent and unapparent mucosal injuries of the tongue can lead to an abscess of the tongue. Clinical symptoms are obvious. Surgical therapy is also required as well as antibiotic treatment.

Actinomycosis

Aetiology/Epidemiology
Actinomycetes bacteria cause actinomycosis.

Symptoms
Infection starts as a painless nodule, which is located in the mucosal and submucosal tissues. Often the nodule erupts intraorally or to the surface of the skin. Patients present with swelling and erythematous skin or mucosa.

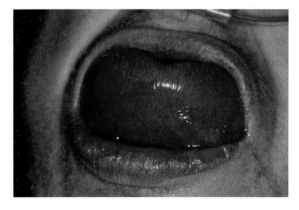

Fig. 5.1.12 Ludwig's angina with oedema of the tongue

Chronic draining fistula persists, especially when the submandibular or the parotid gland are infected.

Therapy
Treatment requires appropriate identification of actinomycetes and penicillin therapy for a long time: 10×10^6–20×10^6 units of penicillin G per day intravenously for 4–6 weeks, after that 2–4 g penicillin V per day or 1.5 g amoxicillin per day orally for 6–12 months.

5.1.4.3 Fungal Infections

Mucosal Candidiasis

Aetiology/Epidemiology
Candida albicans is found in 15–25% of normal mucosa surfaces. It is a normally saprophytic organism. Often patients with immune deficiencies develop mucosal candidiasis. Organ transplants, HIV infection and diabetes mellitus are predisposing factors as are radiation therapy and long-term antibiotic or corticoid therapy.

Patients present with dysphagia, sore throat and painful swallowing.

Diagnostic Procedures
The mucosa of the oral cavity shows red, irregular and flat lesions (Fig. 5.1.13). Sometimes there are white plaques with a red margin, which start bleeding on scraping the plaques. Diagnosis is confirmed by a Gram stain, which demonstrates a mass of mycelia or by a culture.

Therapy
Treatment is the application of topic antifungal medication such as nystatin or clotrimazole five times per day for 7–14 days. In severe cases systemic application of 100–200 mg fluconazole per day for 14–21 days could be necessary.

5.1.4.4 Viral Infections

Herpetic Gingival Stomatitis

Aetiology/Epidemiology
Herpes simplex virus infections of the oral cavity are mainly caused by herpes simplex virus type 1. Infections of herpesvirus type 2 are usually located in genital regions. The route of transmission is usually direct contact or droplet transmission. The incidence in adults is 85–90%. The incubation period is between 5 and 7 days.

In most cases initial infection happens in childhood and has its manifestation in the oral cavity.

Symptoms
In primary manifestation of herpes simplex infection the gingiva and the oral mucosa are erythematous and accompanied by a characteristic low-grade fever, malaise and lymphadenitis. Vesicular lesions occur in the oral cavity, and these erupt within 24 h and are flat, grey ulcers with a halo-sign appearance (Fig. 5.1.14). Young patients present with fetor, hypersalivation and painful food ingestion. Erosions heal after 1 week without scar formation.

Reactivation of the virus occurs as labial herpes, often triggered by pregnancy, stress, sunlight or feverish infections. The virus persists after initial infection in ganglionic cells. Favoured manifestation is at the mucocutaneous border of the lips, sometimes the nasal vestibule, the cheeks or the eyelids. Clinical symptoms are paraesthesia as well as burning skin and mucosa; within a few hours crops of vesicular lesions occur.

Complications
In patients with immune deficiencies, herpes infection can take a progressive course; in such cases it is called "Pospischill–Feyrter disease". Vesicular lesions spread all over the facial skin; life-threatening herpetic meningitis is possible.

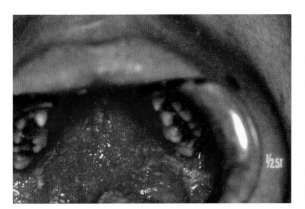

Fig. 5.1.13 Oral candidiasis

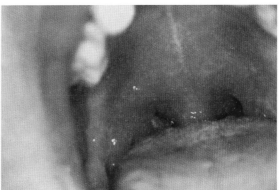

Fig. 5.1.14 Gingivostomatitis herpetica

Diagnostic Procedures

Diagnosis of the infection is by clinical symptoms. Viral infection can be established by assay, but it is very expensive and commonly not necessary.

Therapy

The virus cannot be eliminated; early treatment with antiviral medication is necessary to decrease the viral load. In the case of primary infection, 5×200 mg aciclovir per day orally for 10–14 days is required. In the case of reactivated infection, topical application of penciclovir or aciclovir is necessary. Local aseptic treatment to avoid bacterial infection is required.

Prognosis

The disease is self-limited and does often not recur; however, certain patients suffer from recurring infections. Complications are a bacterial superinfection with staphylococci or streptococci.

Herpes Zoster

Aetiology/Epidemiology

The first contact with varicella zoster virus causes chickenpox, mostly during childhood. Dormant varicella zoster virus persist in ganglionic cells (trigeminal nerve ganglion) and may be reactivated and affect the area of the nerve, in ganglionic cells of which the virus is in a latent state. Predisposing factors are immune deficiencies such as HIV and immune-depressing therapy.

Symptoms

Vesicular lesions similar to chickenpox arise in a dermatomal distribution on one side. The areas innervated by the second and the third division of the trigeminal nerve are affected. When the maxillary branch is affected, lesions occur ipsilaterally on the soft and the hard palate, on the uvula and on maxillary gingiva. When the mandibular nerve is affected, the mucosa of the lower lip, the tongue and the floor of the mouth are affected. Nearly all patients present with neuralgic pain before vesicular lesions can be seen.

Diagnostic Procedures

Clinical symptoms verify the diagnosis.

Therapy

Therapy is just useful if it is started within 3 days after lesions occur! Therapy of herpes zoster requires antiviral medication such as 5×800 mg aciclovir per day orally for 7–10 days to decrease the intensity of the infection and the neuralgic pain. Analgesic agents are useful; in the case of postinfectious neuralgia, amitriptyline and carbamazepine are helpful.

Herpangina

Aetiology/Epidemiology

An infection with Coxsackie A virus causes herpangina. In some cases infection with Coxsackie B virus is possible. Children up to 7 years are mostly affected. The disease starts after an incubation period of 4 days.

Symptoms

Patients present with fever, headache and pharyngitis. Characteristic symptoms include severe sore throat, excessive salivation and nausea. It is a self-limited process in which small vesicles on the soft palate occur later on. They are surrounded by a red margin and erupt early (Fig. 5.1.15). The vesicles are marked by crops of flat lesions on the tonsils, the soft palate and the uvula.

Differential Diagnosis

The main differential diagnosis is the infection with herpesvirus. The affection of the whole gingiva during herpes simplex infection is the main difference; clinical symptoms are more severe. Aphthous stomatitis as well as bacterial pharyngitis and viral enanthema like chickenpox or measles may be confused with herpangina.

Diagnostic Procedures

Clinical symptoms verify the diagnosis.

Therapy

Therapy is symptomatic; oral treatment with local anaesthetics and silver nitrate is useful to accelerate the healing.

Note that no specific treatment for viral pharyngotonsillitis (caused by adenoviruses, Epstein–Barr virus, Coxsackie A virus, rhinoviruses, influenza viruses, parainfluenza viruses) exists, and use of antibiotics for viral tonsillitis should be avoided as much as possible).

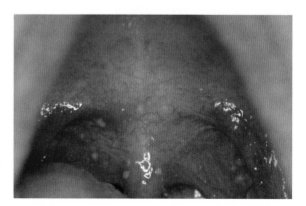

Fig. 5.1.15 Herpangina

HIV-Associated Mucosal Anomalies of the Oral Mucosa

Aetiology/Epidemiology

Infectious changes of the lip and oral mucosa are often associated with HIV-infected patients. The lesions are not caused by HIV itself; they follow from the immune deficiency. Oral candidiasis is usually the first and most frequent opportunistic infection. Viral infections are very common too. Varicella, herpes and cytomegalovirus are the most important.

Symptoms

The course of the infections is more progressive and severe than in patients without HIV. The viral infections define HIV progress.

Therapy

Systemic therapy with aciclovir and ganciclovir—in the case of herpes simplex, varicella or cytomegalovirus—is required; the dose and application form depend on the infection and the immunologic state of the patient. An interdisciplinary approach is necessary to treat this opportunistic infections.

Hairy Leucoplakia

Hairy leucoplakia is found in patients with severe immunocompromised conditions, mostly in the case of HIV infection. It proves HIV is present and counts as a pathognomonic sign; this condition heralds the onset of full-blown acquired immunodeficiency syndrome (AIDS). A shaggy appearance of the tongue is apparent and may vary in colour from white to grey to black. The preferred localization is the lateral surface and the dorsum of the tongue. It is speculated that an infection of the tongue mucosa with Epstein–Barr virus occurs. There is no therapy other than symptomatic treatment.

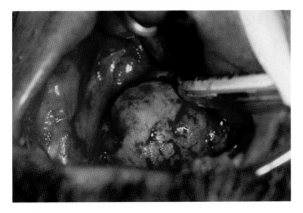

Fig. 5.1.16 Kaposi's sarcoma of the oropharynx

Kaposi's Sarcoma

Since the introduction of antiretroviral therapy, including the protease inhibitors, Kaposi's sarcoma (Fig. 5.1.16) is very rare. In 90% of all HIV-associated Kaposi's sarcomas, human herpesvirus type 8 can be found. Kaposi's sarcoma may occur long before other opportunistic infections.

It can be divided into an early phase, with cutaneous and lymphatic affection, and an advanced stage, with gastrointestinal or/and pulmonal affection, sometimes with extensive oral affection.

Symptoms

Skin and especially oral mucosa show red to livid macules, plaques or nodes; sometimes they are confluent.

Diagnostic Procedures

Examination, palpation (lymph nodes!), blood examination and biopsy with special search for human herpesvirus type 8 verify the diagnosis.

Therapy

It is very important to optimize the antiretroviral therapy. Sarcoma can be regressive or disappear completely.

There are different options depending on the stage:
- Limited cutaneous sarcoma: Radiotherapy, laser therapy or cryotherapy; sometimes excision is necessary.
- Disseminated sarcoma: Systemic therapy with α-interferon is indicated. Success depends on the level of CD4 cells at the beginning.

Aphthous Stomatitis

Aetiology/Epidemiology

The cause of aphthous ulcers is unknown; in some cases viral pieces could be evaluated. The disease may be familiar. The preferred age is between 20 and 30 years. Predisposing factors are times of stress and hormonal imbalance. A chronic inflammatory condition with heavy infiltration of lymphocytes in the submucosa of the ulcers occurs.

Symptoms

Multiple spherical flat craterlike lesions form in the mobile mucosa of the oral cavity. Oral aphthous disease can be distinguished in three clinical variants:
1. Minor type (Mikulicz) (80–90%): This has superficial little (2–5 mm) aphthous ulcers in the anterior part of the oral cavity; healing occurs without scar formation within 1 week.
2. Major type (Sutton) (10%): The painful ulcers are more extended (1–4 cm) and infiltrate the mucosa. The preferred localizations are the tongue and the lips; a pseudomembrane covers the crater. Swab shows fusiform bacteria and borrelia. The defect heals within

2 weeks with scar formation. Mostly, disease is accompanied by lymphadenitis.

3. Herpetiform type (5%): These are very small aphthous lesions, with less general symptoms.

Differential Diagnosis

Differential diagnoses are Behçet's syndrome and herpesvirus infection. Symptoms such as febrile temperatures, eye symptoms, malaise and arthritis accompany Behçet's syndrome.

Therapy

The therapy required is the application of local anaesthetics, local corticoid treatment such as Volon A salve and aseptic agents.

5.1.5   Autoimmune Diseases

5.1.5.1   Behçet's Syndrome

Aetiology/Epidemiology

The cause of this disease is unknown, but it is speculated that it has an autoimmune or viral origin. The syndrome occurs often in male patients in eastern countries such as Turkey.

Symptoms

Major symptoms are aphthous ulcers, genital ulcers and uveitis. Minor symptoms are polyarthritis, gastrointestinal symptoms and anomalies of the vasculature.

Diagnostic Procedures

The general rule to verify the diagnosis of Behçet's syndrome is the appearance of three major symptoms or of two major symptoms and one minor symptom.

Therapy

Therapy includes treatment with immunosuppressants such as cyclophosphamide, colchicines and steroids. Local application of Volon A salve is useful.

5.1.5.2   *Pemphigus vulgaris*

Aetiology/Epidemiology

The origin is unknown; genetic disposition, medication such as ibuprofen and other autoimmune diseases seem to be predisposing factors.

Pemphigus vulgaris is a disease with antibodies targeted against the desmosomes of the epithelium leading to bullous desquamation and supraepithelial split with Tzanck cells. In half of the patients oral manifestation occurs.

Symptoms

The mucosa of the oral cavity is spread with blisters, filled with bloody or serous discharge. Within hours the blisters erupt and flat lesions occur. Primarily the lesions are not painful, but after eruption the pain is severe. Patients complain of odynophagia and throat and tongue pain.

Diagnostic Procedures

Immunofluorescence is used for diagnosis after biopsy to detect the antibodies. Antibodies can be found in the skin and mucosal areas as well as in the serum.

Therapy

High-dose systemic application of corticoids in combination with immunosuppressants (azathioprine, methotrexate) is the most important branch of therapy. The disease may be lethal if it stays unchecked and untreated.

5.1.5.3   Lichen Ruber Planus

Aetiology/Epidemiology

The cause of lichen planus is still unknown; an autoimmune origin is speculated. The use of specific medication (arsenic combinations, malarial medication) and stress seem to trigger the disease. Multiple varieties of lichen planus exist. The most common form in the oral cavity is the reticular form.

Symptoms

The disease often occurs on the mucosa and on the skin at the same time. In 25–70% of cases the oral mucosa is associated with it. On the buccal mucosa, the lips and the tongue, a lacelike reticular pattern of white lines appears (Wickham lines) (Fig. 5.1.17). Patients show no clinical symptoms, except they present with an erosive form, which is very painful.

Diagnostic Procedures

Colloid bodies are detected in the lower epithelial layers and an infiltration of lymphocytes can be found. Histology is used to verify the diagnosis; the detection of colloid bodies proves the diagnosis.

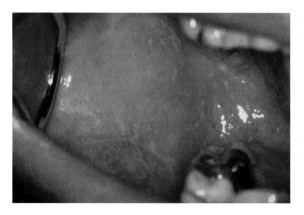

Fig. 5.1.17 Reticular pattern of white lines in buccal mucosa (Wickham lines)

Differential Diagnosis

In the case of erosive lesions, *Pemphigus vulgaris*, syphilis and systemic lupus erythematosus need to be differentiated.

Therapy

The disease is self-limited and requires the use of topical steroids to prevent scarring. Retinoin and isoretinoin are useful in some cases.

Erosive Lichen Planus

Erosive lichen planus, another variety of this autoimmune condition, may ulcerate and is surrounded by a white margin similar in appearance to leucoplakia. The most common localization is the buccal mucosa and the gingiva. Clinical symptoms are more severe than with lichen ruber planus; patients complain of burning of the tongue and pain, especially during eating. With an incidence of 4%, squamous cell carcinoma may occur in erosive lichen planus. Therapy is similar to that for lichen ruber planus; topical anaesthetics seem to be helpful.

5.1.5.4   Systemic Lupus Erythematosus

Aetiology/Epidemiology

This is a chronic systemic disease of the vasculature with involvement of the skin and the possibility of the affection of all other organs. In 40% of cases the oral mucosa is involved.

Symptoms

Intraorally discoid erythematosus lesions occur, sometimes ulcerating. The butterfly rash of the facial skin over the nose and the cheeks is characteristic for systemic lupus erythematosus. At the same time, general symptoms of fever, muscular pain and involvement of the CNS and the kidney often occur.

Diagnostic Procedures

To verify the diagnosis of systemic lupus erythematosus a complex blood and histologic examination is necessary; a dermatologist should be involved. Generally, antinuclear antibodies can be detected.

Therapy

Therapy requires topical and systemic application of steroids and lies in the hand of the dermatologist.

5.1.5.5   Sjögren's Syndrome

Aetiology/Epidemiology

This is an autoimmune condition with antibodies targeted against the epithelium of the ducts of exocrine glands. The disorder occurs most commonly in middle-aged women.

Symptoms

Primary Sjögren's syndrome includes symptoms of the eye and the oral cavity. Major symptoms are a dry mouth—associated with an inability to moisten the food bolus and swallowing—and xerophthalmia. Speech can also be affected. Parotid glands appear hyperplastic, but painless. Often Sjögren's syndrome occurs with a characteristic triad of symptoms:

1. Xerostomia
2. Keratoconjunctivitis sicca
3. Accompanying rheumatoid disease

Secondary Sjögren's syndrome is the destruction of the salivary and lacrimal glands, on the one hand, accompanied by symptoms of another connective tissue disorder, for example rheumatoid arthritis, on the other hand. Patients with Sjögren's syndrome have an increased incidence of the development of lymphoma. Regular inspection and examination of the enlarged parotid glands is necessary.

Diagnostic Procedures

Diagnosis is possible by serologic tests such the measurement of C-reactive protein and antibodies against parotid parenchyma and SS-A and SS-B antibodies. Further, a biopsy of the lip mucosa which includes at least five little glands is useful.

Therapy

Therapy includes a combination of steroids and immunosuppressants to treat the rheumatoid disease. Careful dental management is essential to prevent severe dental disorders, which can occur because of the poor salivary flow. Artificial saliva may be helpful. The application of 3×5 mg pilocarpine per day to activate salivary flow is possible.

5.1.5.6   Wegener's Granulomatosis

Aetiology/Epidemiology

This is an autoimmune disease which leads to necrotizing vasculitis of the upper and lower respiratory tract as well as the renal system. In most cases the first location of manifestation is the nose, but it can also occur in the middle ear, the oral cavity and the oropharynx. It leads to granuloma into the tissues.

Symptoms

In the oral cavity, ulcers or hyperplastic lesions of 1–2 cm occur. Biopsy is necessary to verify the diagnosis, demonstrating necrotizing vasculitis and palisading histiocytes. During the acute onset of Wegener's granulomatosis, titres of antineutrophil cytoplasmic antibodies (C-ANCA) are elevated. During the initial state they are elevated in 50% of patients and during the general state in 95% of patients.

Therapy

Therapy includes trimethoprim/sulphamethoxazole in local cases and cyclophosphamide, methotrexate and oral corticosteroids in severe cases.

5.1.5.7   Lymphomatoid Granulomatosis

Synonym

Lethal midline granuloma.

Aetiology/Epidemiology

This disorder is considered to be a located mucocutaneous T-cell lymphoma.

Symptoms

The main symptom is the ulceration of mucosal surfaces, in both the nose and the sinus. In some cases, the oral cavity is also affected. Erosions of the hard palate occur, generally in the area of the junction.

Therapy

The therapy required is low-dose radiation; in systemic cases chemotherapy may be helpful. The disease has a high mortality rate, between 50 and 70% over a 5-year period.

5.1.5.8   Necrotizing Sialometaplasia

Aetiology/Epidemiology

This is an ulcerative lesion characteristically found on the junctions of the soft and the hard palate.

Symptoms

It occurs as a necrotizing, painful ulcer with deep infiltration, and has the appearance of a carcinoma. The palate and the nose may be perforated and destructed.

Diagnostic Procedures

On histopathologic examination, a metaplastic change to epithelial cells lining small salivary gland ducts is seen. Diagnosis is verified by biopsy.

Therapy

Treatment requires topically applied lidocaine, a self-limited course of the disease is possible.

5.1.5.9   Melkersson–Rosenthal Syndrome

Aetiology/Epidemiology

The cause of this disorder is unknown.

Symptoms

A characteristic triad is the combination of a fissured tongue, cheilitis granulomatosis and recurrent facial palsy. Perioral oedema, paraesthesia, salivation and massive swelling of the upper or lower lips are associated with it.

Diagnostic Procedures

Lip biopsy is helpful, on histopathologic examination granuloma and giant cells are detected.

Therapy

Therapy includes corticosteroid application; sometimes the application of dapsone is possible.

5.1.6 Neoplasms of the Oral Cavity

5.1.6.1 Benign Neoplasms

There are multiple structures within the oral cavity from which benign tumours develop. These include tumours of the epithelium, the mesenchyme, and ectodermal elements, including nerves within the oral cavity. Generally treatment is surgical excision. Clinically important benign tumours are briefly described.

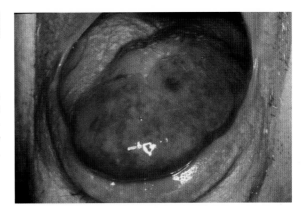

Fig. 5.1.18 Hemangioma of the tongue

Epidermoid Cysts

These occur as firm, well-encapsulated masses. Treatment is excision and recurrence is uncommon. If adnexal structures are found (e.g. hair follicles, sebaceous glands), a dermoid cyst is diagnosed.

Haemangioma

The tumour appear as enlarged blood-filled sinuses under the mucosa of the floor of the mouth, buccal space or lips. Often the intraoral tumour is in contact with an external facial haemangioma and the entire tumour has a significant cosmetic and functional abnormality. The tumour occurs at birth or shortly thereafter. Haemangiomas frequently involve the tongue and then airway obstruction follows (Fig. 5.1.18.).

Note that the real size of haemangiomas is adequately assessed when the patient lies down on a table. Then the blood sinuses will expand, showing the true, and often underestimated, extent of the tumour.

The natural history of haemangioma is that of spontaneous regression over the course of several years. This does not occur in all cases. Cases that may require intervention include haemangiomas of the upper aerodigestive tract with airway obstruction and enlarging haemangiomas.

Lympangiomas

These tumours also occur at birth or shortly thereafter. Unlike the vascular counterpart, haemangioma, spontaneous regression of lymphangioma does not occur. These neoplasms may develop to a significant size and are intimately associated with many vital structures of the neck, making removal very difficult. The natural history of the disease is that of unrelenting recurrences of the tumour after excision. Patients should be informed regarding the inevitable recurrence of this tumour. Attempts at complete removal of the tumour should be performed at the initial operation. The use of steroids is controversial.

Ranula

This is a mucocele of the sublingual glands. The ranula is a bluish mass with a well-mucosalized covering in the floor of the mouth, just lateral to the sublingual frenulum.

When the ranula is confined above the mylohoid muscle in the floor of the mouth, it is best removed through a transoral approach (Fig. 5.1.19).

Tumours may also herniate through the lateral aspect of the mylohoid muscle and occur as a soft mass in the submandibular region. In these cases a combined transoral and external approach is necessary. The sublingual gland should be removed completely for the operation to be adequate and to prevent recurrence.

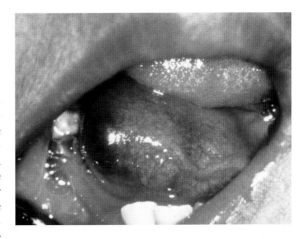

Fig. 5.1.19 Ranula

5.1.6.2 Malignant Neoplasms of the Oral Cavity and the Lips

Epidemiology

More than 95% of cancers in the oral cavity are squamous cell carcinomas. Like in other ENT carcinomas, smoking and alcohol abuse are well-known risk factors, and the incidence is higher in males. An overview of incidence, histopathology and prognosis is shown in Table 1.3.1.

Diagnostic Procedures

The diagnostic procedures are described in Sect. 1.1.4. For all tumours of the oral cavity they include:

- Inspection and palpation
- Endoscopy (essential part of panendoscopy) and biopsy with histologic diagnosis
- Imaging techniques (CT, MRI, ultrasound)

TNM Classification

The detailed TNM classification is described in Sect. 1.1.4.5.

Assessment and Tumour Management

The typical presentation of squamous cell carcinoma of the oral cavity is a persistent sore mouth. Many lesions remain asymptomatic and are found only on careful examination of the oral cavity by a dentist during routine dental care.

Patients with advanced disease (T3 and T4) have involvement of surrounding oral cavity structures, especially the mandible. Mandible invasion is very important for treatment planning and may be best determined by CT scanning with bone windows. The ultimate assessment of mandibular invasion comes at the time of surgical resection, when direct palpation and inspection of the mandibular periosteum and cortical bone is possible.

Once assessment of the primary tumour and examination for regional metastases have been completed, a biopsy is necessary to confirm the diagnosis.

Panendoscopy allows the surgeon to evaluate again the primary tumour and to rule out a second primary tumour.

TNM classification of tumours of the oral cavity is described in Sect. 1.1.4.5.

Therapy

Like in other head and neck cancers, three treatment options prevail:

1. Surgery of the primary tumour and the neck
2. Surgery combined with adjuvant radiation or adjuvant radiochemotherapy
3. Primary radiochemotherapy

These treatment options need to be discussed with the patient in any individual situation. Most would agree, however, that for these tumours the best cure rates can be obtained with combined therapy consisting of surgery followed by radio- (chemo-) therapy. Indications for primary radiochemotherapy and adjuvant radiotherapy are discussed in Sect. 1.3.

Surgical Principles

Floor of the Mouth Carcinoma
See Fig. 5.1.20.

The recommended treatment for early-stage carcinoma (T1 and T2) is transoral excision. Spontaneous healing is possible and demonstrates in many cases good results. Reconstruction can be done either with primary closure or with a skin graft to prevent contracture.

Advanced-stage carcinoma (T3 and T4) often involves the tongue or the mandible, necessitating a wider resection including marginal mandibulectomy or segmental mandibulectomy and partial tongue resection. Marginal mandibulectomy is preferred over segmental mandibulectomy whenever it is oncologically feasible.

Not all lateral segmental resections need to be replaced, and the decision regarding reconstruction of the lateral mandible should be made on a case-by case basis.

All anterior mandibular segmental resections need to be reconstructed to avoid major cosmetic and functional deficits.

Frozen-section analysis of bone margins is not possible, so a generous margin of bone must be taken to avoid positive margins.

Definitions of Mandibulectomy
Mandibulotomy: Osteotomy of the mandible to permit exposure, no bone resected.

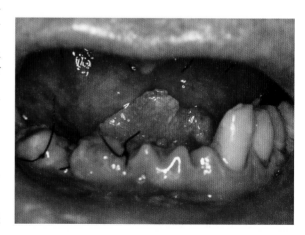

Fig. 5.1.20 Floor of the mouth carcinoma (T2)

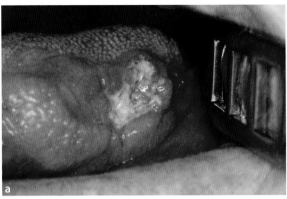
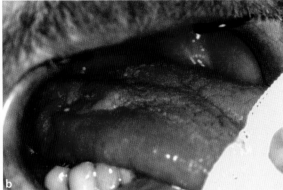

Fig. 5.1.21a,b Tongue cancer. **a** exophytic with little deep infiltration; **b** infiltrative with large submucosal extension

Marginal mandibulectomy: A portion of the mandible, typically the alveolus or lingual plate is resected while leaving the continuity of the mandible intact.

Segmental mandibulectomy: A portion of the mandible is resected, with disruption of condyle-to-condyle continuity (Ramus, angle, body).

Methods of Restoration of the Mandible
- Soft tissue only: Regional pedicled flap, skin graft
- Reconstruction plate: Plate and screw with a pedicled regional flap
- Microvascular free flaps with bone: (preferred option): Fibula, scapula, radius, iliac crest

In advanced stages of oral cavity carcinoma adjuvant radio- or radiochemotherapy is necessary to improve local control and disease-free survival rates.

Tongue Carcinoma

In general, there are two forms of tongue carcinoma: exophytic with little deep infiltration and infiltrative with a large submucosal extension deep into the tongue (Fig. 5.1.21).

The recommended treatment for T1 and T2 tumours is transoral resection and primary closure.

Advanced-stage carcinoma (T3 and T4) is best treated with surgical resection and reconstruction with regional myocutaneous flaps or free tissue transfer combined with adjuvant radiochemotherapy.

If a total glossectomy is necessary to obtain free margins, quality of life after a possible operation needs to be discussed extensively with the patient.

Retromolar Trigone Carcinoma

This area of the oral cavity is often *inadequately examined*, thereby allowing tumours to grow to a large size before diagnosis (Fig. 5.1.22). The thin mucosal covering over the ascending ramus and angle of the mandible with little

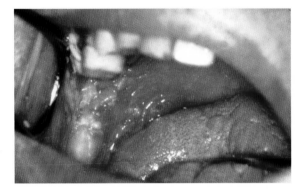

Fig. 5.1.22 Cancer of the retromolar trigone

intervening submucosal tissues is an ineffective barrier to tumour spread. Spread of the tumour along the inferior alveolar nerve may also occur with marrow invasion.

Similarly, extension in the posterior floor of the mouth and tongue may occur, and the true extent of the retromolar trigone tumour may be underestimated on clinical examination.

The surgical principles are not different from those for floor of the mouth and tongue tumours. Not all necessary lateral segmental resections of the mandible must be replaced. The defect may be closed primarily or with a regional flap. The decision regarding reconstruction of the lateral mandible should be made on a case-by-case basis.

Lip Carcinoma

Lip carcinoma is easily identified; therefore, the patient seeks attention sooner than for lesions of other cancers of the oral cavity.

Excision of lip cancers (T1–T4) is the treatment of choice. Multiple methods of lip reconstruction are available after resection of the cancer.

Defects involving one third or less of the width of the lip may be closed primarily without difficulty. The excision is planned in the shape of a V. Defects up to one half to two thirds require larger perioral advancement flap such as the Karapandzic flap or the technique according to Bernard.

5.1.6.3 Nonsquamous Carcinomas of the Oral Cavity

The most common nonsquamous carcinoma of the oral cavity is of minor salivary gland origin. These malignancies typically appear as firm submucosal masses most frequently located on the hard and soft palates. The adenoid cystic carcinoma is the most frequent minor salivary gland malignancy, followed by adenocarcinoma and mucoepidermoid carcinoma.

The natural history of adenoid cystic carcinoma is frequent local recurrence or distant metastases as the patient is followed for prolonged periods of time (10–15 years).

Management of adenoid cystic carcinoma consists of wide surgical excision with an attempt on negative margins. There is inevitable perineural invasion that makes complete resection in the oral cavity difficult. Postoperative radiotherapy is used by many surgeons with both negative and positive margins.

Note that in patients with negative margins, there may be some justification to save radiotherapy for management of the eventual recurrence.

5.1.6.4 Melanoma

Melanoma of the oral cavity is rare, representing less than 1% of all melanomas. However, the oral cavity is the most common location for mucosal melanoma.

Treatment is wide excision and neck dissection in patients with clinically positive adenopathy or sentinel node dissection.

Reference

1. Putz R, Pabst R (eds) (1993) Sobotta: Anatomie des Menschen. Kopf, Hals, obere Extremität. vol 1, 21st edn, version 2.0. Urban und Schwarzenberg, Munich

Suggested Reading

1. Arnold W, Ganzer U (2005) Checkliste Hals-Nasen-Ohren-Heilkunde, 4th edn. Thieme, Stuttgart
2. Boenninghaus HG, Lenarz T (2007) HNO, 13th edn. Springer, Berlin
3. Graham JM, Scadding GK, Bull PD (eds) (2007) Pediatric ENT. Springer, Berlin
4. Lee KJ, Toh EH (2007) Otolaryngology. A surgical notebook. Thieme, New York
5. Myers EN (ed) (2008) Operative otolaryngology: head and neck surgery, 2nd edn. Elsevier Saunders, Philadelphia
6. Seiden AM, Tami TA, Pensak ML, Cotton RT, Gluckman JL (2001) Otolaryngology. The essentials. Thieme, Stuttgart

5.2 Oropharynx and Hypopharynx

VIKTOR BONKOWSKY AND PETRA GERDEMANN

5.2.1 Anatomy of the Oropharynx

The oropharynx extends from the soft palate superiorly to the level of the superior edge of the epiglottis inferiorly. The lingual side of the epiglottis, the back of the tongue and Vallecula's region in front of the epiglottis belong to the oropharynx and are important subdivisions for carcinoma. It is continuous with the mouth through the oropharyngeal isthmus formed by the palatoglossal muscles on each side. The anterior border is the posterior third of the tongue, especially the circumvallate papillae (Figs. 5.2.1, 5.2.2).

The lymphatic drain of the oropharynx reaches the lymph nodes of levels II and III, additionally to the retropharyngeal nodes (Fig. 5.2.3). Most of the time there is a bilateral drain.

5.2.1.1 The Palate

The hard palate is formed by the two palatal processes of the maxilla and the horizontal processes of the palatine bones. The anteriorly positioned incisive fossa and the greater and lesser palatine foramina posteriorly allow the passage of the nasopalatine and palatine arteries and nerves (Fig. 5.2.4). All the bony parts are covered with mucosa.

The soft palate is formed by different muscles (Fig. 5.2.5). The *tensor veli palatine muscle* tenses the palatine velum and opens the Eustachian tube by swallowing. The elevator of the soft palate, the *levator veli palatine muscle*, arises from the temporal bone. It is attached to the palatine aponeurosis at the upper part.

From lateral and caudal, the fibres of the palatoglossus and the palatopharyngeal muscle ascend to the lower part of the palatine aponeurosis. The space between the pharyngeal arches forms the tonsillar fossa.

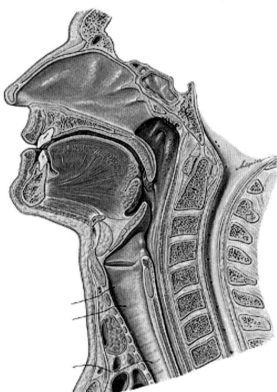

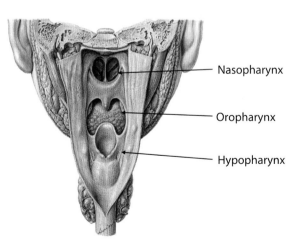

Fig. 5.2.1 Subdivisions of the pharynx I. (Figure 254 in [1])

Fig. 5.2.2 Subdivisions of the pharynx II. (Figure 275 in [1])

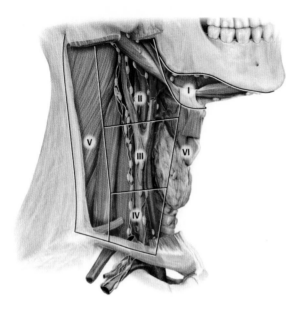

Fig. 5.2.3 Classification of the lymph nodes of the neck

Innervation

The motor innervation of the soft palate muscles is carried by branches of the vagus and glossopharyngeal nerves, except the tensor veli palatine, which is innervated by the mandibular division of the trigeminal nerve.

Sensation reception from the soft palate is carried by the lesser palatine nerve. The hard palate is innervated by branches of the maxillary division of the trigeminal nerve, the greater palatine nerve and the nasopalatine nerve.

Blood Supply

The blood supply of the palate is from ascending branches of the facial artery as well as from the branch of the maxillary artery. The palatine vessels and nerves pass through the palatine canal.

5.2.1.2   The Tonsils

The palatine tonsils are a component of Waldeyer's tonsillar ring. Waldeyer's ring consists of the lymphoid tissue on the base of the tongue (lingual tonsil), two (palatine) tonsils, the adenoids (nasopharyngeal tonsil) and the lymphoid tissue on the posterior pharyngeal wall. This collection of lymphoid tissue is the first to sample and react to antigens in the air and food entering the body, and serves as a defence against infection and plays an important role in the development of the immune system. Waldeyer's ring grows throughout childhood until the age of about 11 years and after that decreases spontaneously.

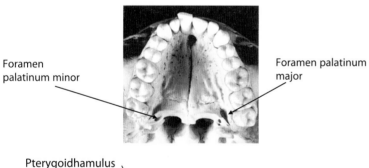

Foramen palatinum minor

Foramen palatinum major

Fig. 5.2.4 The bony palate. (Figure 172 in [1])

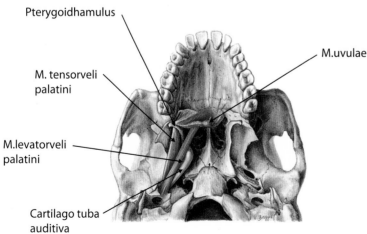

Pterygoidhamulus

M. tensorveli palatini

M.levatorveli palatini

Cartilago tuba auditiva

M.uvulae

Fig. 5.2.5 Muscles of the soft palate. (Figure 682 in [1])

The palatine tonsils are placed in the space between the palatopharyngeal and palatoglossus muscles. The palatine tonsils are the largest component of the ring and have a specialized histologic structure. The matrix is lymphoid tissue with crypts, which shows a deep extension into the tissue. The cells are organized in lymphoid follicles, so they maximize the surface which comes in contact with antigens. The lymphoid tissue is adherent to a capsule, so inflammation of the tonsils is limited.

The location of the tonsils and their design allow direct exposure of the immunologically active cells with the antigens entering the upper aerodigestive tract. The tissue is involved in the production of immunoglobulin and inducing secretory immunity. This tissue is more active during childhood between the ages of 4 and 10 years and maximizes the immunologic memory in this way. Therefore, the tissue increases and sometimes it is so extended that it could lead to breathing and swallowing problems. This is called "hyperplasia of the tonsils" (Fig. 5.2.6). If problems are severe, tonsillectomy is indicated. Tonsillotomy or unilateral tonsillectomy is possible in young children.

After puberty the lymphoid tissue starts to involute.

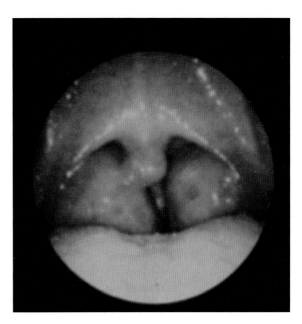

Fig. 5.2.6 Hyperplasia of the tonsils

Innervation

The innervation of the tonsils is from a tonsillar branch of the glossopharyneal nerve.

Blood Supply

The palatine tonsil has a rich blood supply from the external carotid artery branches. The lower pole of the tonsil receives branches from the following arteries:
- The dorsal lingual artery
- The ascending palatine artery from the facial artery
- The tonsillar branch of the facial artery

The upper pole of the tonsil receives branches from the following arteries:
- The ascending pharyngeal artery
- The lesser palatine artery.

In cases of severe secondary haemorrhage after tonsillectomy, detailed knowledge of the arterial blood supply of the tonsils is necessary.

Note that the internal carotid artery lies approximately 2 cm from the palatine tonsils, but contributes no branches.

Venous drainage is more diffuse with a venous peritonsillar plexus about the capsule. The venous blood flows into the lingual and pharyngeal veins, which feed into the internal jugular vein.

The lymphatic drain is to the tonsillar lymph node (behind the angle of the mandible) and to the upper jugular digastric lymph nodes (levels II and III).

5.2.1.3   Tongue Base

The sulcus terminalis, just posterior to the circumvallate papillae, divides the anterior two thirds of the tongue from the posterior oropharyngeal portion. The posterior part of the tongue has no papillae, but is covered with the lymphoid tissue of the lingual tonsils.

The hypoglossal nerve provides motor innervation. The glossopharyngeal nerve mediates taste from the posterior tongue. The lingual artery provides a rich blood supply.

The tongue base develops embryologically as a single structure and therefore has a rich lymphatic communication across the midline. The lymphatic drainage is primarily to the upper deep cervical nodes and retropharyngeal nodes. The tongue lymphatics are plentiful, and tumours therefore occur with early metastases.

5.2.2   Anatomy of the Hypopharynx

The hypopharynx is a mucosalined tube bounded by muscles posteriorly and laterally and by the larynx anteriorly. For classification, it is subdivided into the pyriform sinus, posterior pharyngeal wall and postcricoid region.

The pyriform sinus has the shape of an inverted pyramid:
- It is open superiorly where it is contagious with the glossopharyngeal sulcus of the oropharynx and inferiorly ends in an apex.

- Medially it is limited by the larynx (aryepiglottic fold).
- Laterally it is limited by the thyroid cartilage.

The posterior pharyngeal wall is contagious with the lateral wall of the pyriform sinus. The constrictor muscles are deep to this region.

The postcricoid region extends from the posterior surface of the arytenoids and covers the posterior aspect of the cricoid.

5.2.3   Physiology

The tongue forces the bolus through the oropharyngeal isthmus in the oropharynx. The palatoglossus muscle then contracts to prevent reflux in the oral cavity. The larynx then elevates, and through a combination of tongue thrusts and pharyngeal muscular contractions the food is propelled through the hypopharynx into the oesophagus. Any lack of coordination or sensation can significantly impair swallowing, resulting in aspiration.

5.2.4   Acute Bacterial Infections

5.2.4.1   vAcute Streptococcal Pharyngotonsillitis

Aetiology/Epidemiology
Acute angina is usually a bacterial infection of the tonsils with group A β-haemolytic streptococcus, rarely with staphylococcus and haemophilus. Other pathogens include anaerobic bacteria, viruses and specific bacteria such as gonococci and *Corynebacterium diphtheriae*. Acute angina most commonly occurs in children aged 5–6 years.

Symptoms
This infection is characterized by fever, dry sore throat, odynophagia and cervical lymphadenopathy.

Complications
Complications of bacterial tonsillitis, when it stays unchecked and untreated, may be peritonsillar, retropharyngeal or parapharyngeal abscess including airway obstruction, deep neck infection, septicaemia, meningitis, mediastinitis and thrombophlebitis of the jugular vein.

The major consideration in treating the β-haemolytic streptococcal infection is in preventing possible following diseases, such as poststreptococcal glomerulonephritis and acute rheumatic fever.

Diagnostic Procedures
On examination, the pharyngeal mucosa may appear erythematous; the tonsils may be swollen and red, sometimes with yellow or white spots, often accompanied by malodorous breath (Figs. 5.2.7, 5.2.8). In some cases the tonsils touch each other in the midline ("kissing tonsils").

Inspection as well as high white cell blood counts and high concentration of C-reactive protein verify the diagnosis. Throat culture is only necessary during a rapid or recurrent course.

Therapy
The primary antibiotic treatment of streptococcal pharyngotonsillitis consists of penicillin V for a 10-day course. In the case of patients who are allergic to penicillin, clindamycin or erythromycin may be utilized. Sometimes recurrent acute episodes of tonsillitis occur, sometimes with complete recovery between the episodes. Bacteria stay in the crypts of the tonsils, so aggressive chemical therapy may not reach the focus of the infection. The agreement is that patients with recurrent tonsillar infections (six to seven episodes per year, several episodes for two or more consecutive years) need to undergo tonsillectomy.

5.2.4.2   Lingual Tonsillar Infection

Aetiology/Epidemiology
The disease occurs usually in adults, especially in immunocompromised patients or in patients with diabetes.

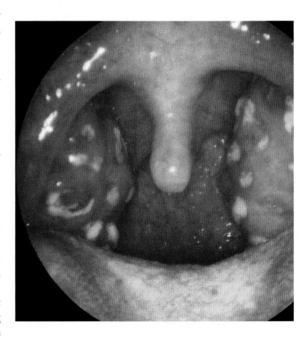

Fig. 5.2.7 Acute angina

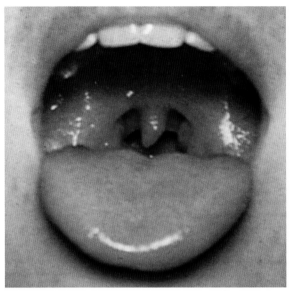 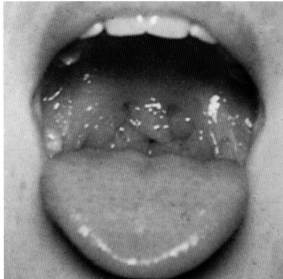

Fig. 5.2.8 Normal tonsills on the *right side*, kissing tonsills on *the left* side

Bacterial pathogens are similar to those of acute pharyngotonsillitis.

Symptoms
Patients present with severe pain, sore throat, dyspnoea and dysphagia. Airway obstruction may occur when the inflammation spreads to the epiglottis; in some cases abscess formation occurs (Fig. 5.2.9).

Diagnostic Procedures
Inspection shows a red and swollen lingual tonsil, sometimes with yellow spots.

Therapy
Antibiotic treatment with macrolides or penicillin V for 10 days is required.

Fig. 5.2.9 Epiglottic abscess

5.2.4.3   Lingual Cysts

Aetiology/Epidemiology
Lingual cysts are usually epithelial cysts. Sometimes they fill up with mucus or pus and extend in the floor of the tongue or into the vallecula (Fig. 5.2.10).

Symptoms
Patients present with dysphagia and sometimes with dyspnoea.

Diagnostic Procedures
Inspection shows a globular tumour, often shiny yellow.

Therapy
Surgical excision is induced. Because of possible swelling of the floor of the tongue, air passage must be guaranteed.

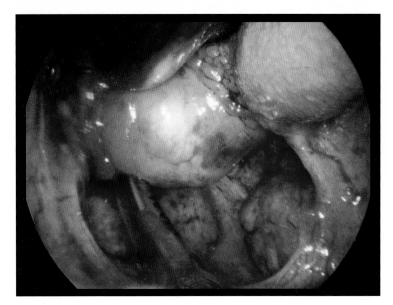

Fig. 5.2.10 Lingual cyst

5.2.4.4   Vincent's Angina

Synonym
Gangrenous pharyngitis.

Aetiology/Epidemiology
Vincent's angina is caused by *Treponema vincentii* and *Spirochaeta denticulata*, which both exist in the normal flora of the mouth. Infection arises in times of overcrowding and it tends to have a slow, sometimes insidious onset. It is an air-contact infection with an incubation period of 1–3 days. It is usually found in patients with poor oral hygiene and lowered resistance.

Symptoms
Patients complain of fever, sore throat, unilateral pain on swallowing and cervical lymphadenopathy.

Diagnostic Procedures
On examination, one tonsil shows a white, necrotizing exudative membrane sometimes combined with an ulcerative lesion (Fig. 5.2.11). Significant is the difference between local symptoms and the relatively stable and good general conditions and feeling of the patient. Laboratory diagnosis depends on typical findings in cultures and biopsy.

Differential Diagnosis
Differential diagnosis is acute tonsillitis, syphilis, diphtheria and neoplasm.

Therapy
Treatment is usually with aggressive oral hygiene and antibiotics, primarily with penicillin.

5.2.4.5   Diphtheria

Aetiology/Epidemiology
Corynebacterium diphtheriae is the pathogen which leads to diphtheria. Despite the widespread immunization in

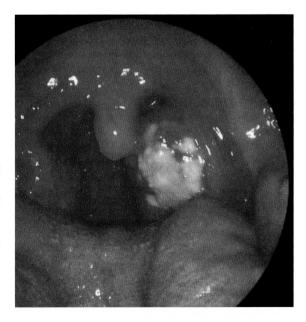

Fig. 5.2.11 Vincent's angina, left side

children, the incidence of diphtheria is increasing, mostly in nonimmunized patients, often from eastern Europe.

Symptoms

Patients complain of severe sore throat, low-grade fever and cervical lymphadenopathy. Sometimes it is accompanied by malaise, headache and nausea. Significant is the sweet fetor ex ore of the patients.

Tonsillar infections with *Corynebacterium diphtheriae* lead to acute pharyngitis characterized by grey, velvety, firm adherent pseudomembranes covering the tonsils (Fig. 5.2.12). Infection may spread over the pillar and the soft palate. When the membranes are wiped, the underlying surface bleeds easily. Toxigenic strains are able to produce lethal diphtheria exotoxin. It may be spread systemically and lead to myocarditis, nephritis and encephalitis.

Diagnostic Procedures

Inspection is the first step to verify the diagnosis. Direct cultures should be obtained for smear and culture (Krebs–Loeffler medium) tests.

Differential Diagnosis

The diphtheritic membrane needs to be differentiated from pseudomembranes of infectious mononucleosis, candidiasis and acute pharyngitis.

Therapy

Treatment of diphtheria has to start immediately; antitoxin should been given within the first 48 h of onset, without confirmation of the result of throat culture, depending on the clinical symptoms. Allergy testing against horse serum needs to be done before application of the antitoxin. Less severe symptoms require 20,000–40,000 IU, nasopharyngeal diphtheria requires 40,000–60,000 IU and severe symptoms require 80,000–100,000 IU.

Antibiotics are required too. Antibiotics are ineffective against the circulating toxin, but symptoms in patients who are treated early with penicillin may be less severe. Penicillin G is required, 50,000 IU/kg per day for 4 days, and penicillin V is required for the following 5 days.

The patient needs to be isolated. Two to 4 days after adequate therapy the patient is not infectious any more. Before discharge, patients need to be pathogen-free, evidenced by the throat culture of the last 3 weeks. In 2% of patients bacteria cannot be eliminated, so they have to undergo tonsillectomy to eradicate the focus.

5.2.4.6 Syphilis

See Sect. 5.1.4.2.

5.2.5 Complications of Oropharyngeal Infections

The widespread use of antibiotics and the rapid diagnosis of acute tonsillitis have decreased the incidence of nonsuppurative complications. Suppurative complications are still commonly encountered.

5.2.5.1 Nonsuppurative Complications

Scarlet Fever

Aetiology/Epidemiology

Scarlet fever is caused by streptococci, which produce a pathognomonic erythrogenic exotoxin.

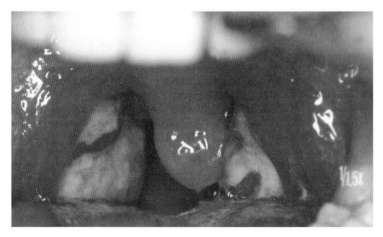

Fig. 5.2.12 Diphtheric pseudomembranes covering the tonsils

Symptoms

It is associated with high fever, dysphagia, a yellow membrane covering the tonsils and an erythematous rash, beginning on the thorax, spreading all over the body and excluding the perioral region (Fig. 5.2.13). The desquamation of the tongue causes the characteristic "strawberry tongue". Facial flush and petechiae occur in body folds and on the soft palate.

Therapy

Traditional treatment is with penicillin for 10 days. Supportive therapy may be required with mild oral desinfection and analgesia.

Acute Rheumatic Fever and Poststreptococcal Glomerulonephritis

Aetiology/Epidemiology

1. Acute rheumatic fever occurs 15–20 days after a pharyngeal infection with group A β-haemolytic streptococci. Streptococcal infection leads to a production of cross-reactive antibodies, which react with heart tissue, and subsequent endocarditis, myocarditis and pericarditis. There are fewer therapy options when heart damage occurs.
2. Poststreptococcal glomerulonephritis occurs 10 days after a pharyngotonsillar infection with group A β-haemolytic streptococcus. The incidence is 10–25%. Immune complexes as well as circulating autoantibodies of the streptococcal antigen damage the glomerulus, and acute nephritic syndrome occurs.

Therapy

Preventing rheumatoid fever and glomerulonephritis means eradicating streptococcal infection. Patients need therapy with penicillin or have to undergo tonsillectomy to eliminate the reservoir of the pathogen. Medical therapy of glomerulonephritis and heart disease depends on the clinical symptoms and the state of the disease.

5.2.5.2 Suppurative Complications

Peritonsillary Abscess

Synonym
Quinsy.

Aetiology/Epidemiology

The abscess usually lies in the space between the tonsillar capsule and the surrounding pharyngeal muscle bed. Typical localizations are the upper pole and along the palatoglossal arch. Usually the process starts with an acute infection of the tonsils and cellulitis of the surrounding tissues and progresses into an abscess beyond the tonsillar capsule. The abscess usually occurs in patients with recurrent acute tonsillar infections and with chronic tonsillitis, which stays untreated. It is more common in young adults.

Symptoms

Patients present with a history of acute tonsillar infection and sometimes with initial improvement, if they received medication. Symptoms intensify during development of the abscess and patients complain of odynophagia, sometimes with dehydration. Generally they complain of unilateral soreness, drooling and trismus; otalgia on the affected side may occur.

Diagnostic Procedures

On examination, patients have a swollen and bulging palate, the tonsil is displaced to the midline and the uvula deviates to the healthy side (Fig. 5.2.14). Cervical lymph

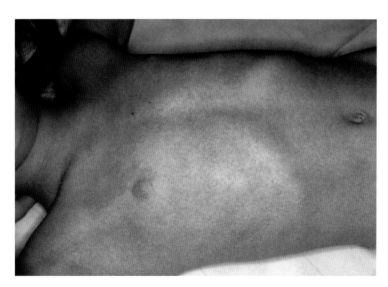

Fig. 5.2.13 Scarlet fever exanthema

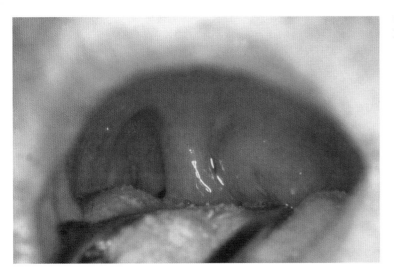

Fig. 5.2.14 Peritonsillary abscess on the left side

nodes become swollen and tender. Needle aspiration may confirm the diagnosis. Microbiologic examination shows a mixed infection with aerobic and anaerobic bacteria. Owing to the swelling, airway obstruction may occur. Ultrasound may verify the diagnosis.

Therapy

Treatment of peritonsillary abscess consists of opening of the abscess by aspiration or incision and intravenous antibiotics as well as careful follow-up. Aminopenicillin or cephalosporin IV may be indicated. After treatment of the acute infection, patients should undergo tonsillectomy because of the high recurrence rate of peritonsillary abscess.

Another possibility of treatment is a "quinsy tonsillectomy", which is a tonsillectomy during acute infection.

Because it can be difficult to differentiate peritonsillar cellulitis from a true abscess, the option to treat the infection initially with intravenous antibiotics and hydration may be favoured. If the patients improve within 24 h, the infection is mostly cellulitis and the patient may improve under the therapy.

Complications

If a peritonsillary abscess stays untreated, the abscess may spread into the deep neck spaces and may lead to septicaemia and mediastinitis.

Parapharyngeal Abscess

Aetiology/Epidemiology

The parapharyngeal space lies laterally to the pharynx and starts superiorly at the skull base and ends inferiorly at the level of the hyoid bone. The medial boundary is the superior constrictor muscle. The lateral margin is the mandible, the parotid and the pterygoid muscle. The posterior boundary is the prevertebral fascia. The parapharyngeal space is divided into an anterior and a posterior division by the styloid process. The carotids and the cranial nerves are located in this space, so an abscess may spread along these structures. Pus from the tonsillar region may go through the superior constrictor muscle along preformed openings of nerves and vessels.

Symptoms

Patients present with severe symptoms of odynophagia, drooling, pain of the throat and neck and tender swelling of the neck, in the region of the angle of the mandible. Trismus may also be present owing to inflammation and oedema around the pterygoid musculature. If only the posterior compartment of the parapharyngeal space is involved, there may be no trismus, but rather swelling of the posterior pharyngeal wall and of the posterior pillar.

Diagnostic Procedures

On examination, patients have tonsillitis, asymmetric pharyngeal swelling and if the abscess extends more inferiorly, airway obstruction may occur. Definitive diagnosis requires a CT scan (Fig. 5.2.15).

Therapy

If an abscess is verified, a surgical drain is necessary. Control of the airway is necessary as well as intravenous antibiotics adapted to the disease.

The safest approach to the parapharyngeal space is through a lateral cervical approach. The great vessels need to be identified; a drainage of the opened abscess is necessary for a period of 24–72 h.

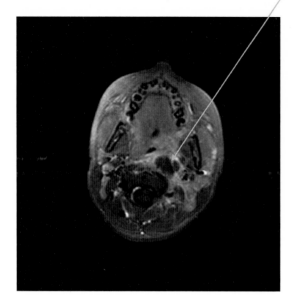
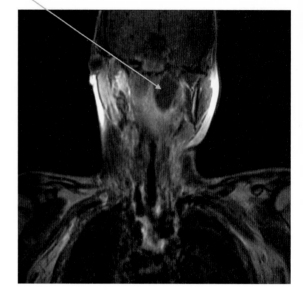

Fig. 5.2.15 Parapharyngeal abscess

Retropharyngeal Space Infection

Aetiology/Epidemiology
The retropharyngeal space lies behind the pharynx, just anterior to the prevertebral fascia. It extends from the skull base to the tracheal bifurcation without an anatomic border; behind the oesophagus the space is called the "retrooesophageal space". In the space there are two layers of lymph nodes. The retropharyngeal abscess often occurs in children, when retropharyngeal lymph nodes start swelling after airway infection and an abscess may occur in the retropharyngeal space. A retropharyngeal abscess rarely occurs in adults; tuberculosis may be the most common diagnosis.

Symptoms
Patients present with trismus, drooling, dyspnoea and dysphagia. Examination shows a fluctuant mass at the posterior wall of the pharynx and oedema of the pharynx and larynx. The anterior longitudinal ligament may be affected, so the head cannot be moved. Patients have fever and malaise.

Diagnostic Procedures
X-ray and ultrasound may be helpful and may show abscess formation. The most important evaluation is through CT scans. They show a hypodense retropharyngeal region with a ring-form enhancement. The presence of air confirms the diagnosis.

Therapy
Once an abscess has been diagnosed, surgical drainage is necessary. A vertical incision followed by blunt dissection is made just off the midline in the posterior pharyngeal wall. Intubation may be difficult, the abscess cavity may be injured and infectious material may be aspirated. Additionally, high-dose intravenous antibiotics may be given.

Abscess of the Base of the Tongue

Aetiology/Epidemiology
Mostly an abscess of the base of the tongue may follow an acute infection of the lingual tonsil.

Symptoms
Patients present with dyspnoea, odynophagia, trismus, drooling and swelling and reduced movement of the tongue. Generally, patients have fever and malaise. On examination, the base of the tongue and the pharyngeal mucosa are oedematous. The swelling may spread into the epiglottis and the larynx and may lead to airway obstruction.

Diagnostic Procedures
Ultrasound shows hypodense regions—the abscess formation—in the base of the tongue. A CT scan is required. If the abscess is identified, a surgical drain is necessary.

Therapy

The abscess cavity needs to be drained into the pharynx. A sufficient airway needs to be ensured; if necessary, the patient must be intubated or undergo tracheotomy. Intravenous antibiotics are necessary.

5.2.6 Chronic Bacterial Infections

5.2.6.1 Chronic Tonsillitis

Aetiology/Epidemiology

Recurrent infections of the tonsils and of the peritonsillar tissue lead to permanent inflammation in the tonsillar crypts and scarring of the tonsillar tissue. Bacteria may grow in the badly drained crypts. The organisms responsible for chronic tonsillitis are similar to those which cause acute infection, with a predominance of β-haemolytic streptococci. Chronic infected tonsils are considered as a "focus" which may activate other chronic inflammatory diseases in the body by spreading bacteria and mediators.

Symptoms

Patients complain of recurrent or persistent sore throats, dysphagia, malaise, malodorous tonsillar concretions as well as fetor ex ore. Cervical adenopathy is present too.

Diagnostic Procedures

On examination, tonsils may be covered with debris or there may be purulent material in the tonsillar crypts. Tonsils appear atrophic and scared, often with surrounding peritonsillar erythematous tissue. In blood counts, the number of white blood cells as well as the concentration of antistreptolysin may increase.

Therapy

Treatment consists of analgesics, and an antibiotic when indicated. Tonsillectomy as a definitive therapy may be indicated; it is generally suggested when the patient complains of recurrent infections of more than five to seven per year or several infections in two or more subsequent years.

5.2.6.2 Chronic Pharyngitis

Aetiology/Epidemiology

Chronic inflammation of the pharynx occurs when the mucosa is irritated over a long period. The structure of the pharyngeal tissue will be changed. Chronic inflammation of the pharynx may occur in two different forms:

1. Chronic hyperplastic pharyngitis, with an erythematous mucosa and lymph follicles
2. Chronic atrophic pharyngitis, with white secretion and a thin layer of mucosa

Chronic inflammation may be caused by extrinsic or intrinsic factors. The most common extrinsic factors are nicotine, alcohol, chemical inhalational irritants and all known allergens. Intrinsic factors may be all acute and chronic infectious diseases such as tonsillitis, rhinosinusitis and bronchitis. Medication such as steroids, antidepressants and psychotropic agents can be causative factors too.

Symptoms

Patients present with a foreign body sensation, rhinorrhea, coughing and hawking.

Diagnostic Procedures

The diagnosis is confirmed by local findings and the history of the patient. It may be completed with a microbiologic examination. In addition, the causative agent should be identified. Gastrooesophageal relux disease needs to be ruled out.

Therapy

Therapy requires the elimination of predisposing factors and mucosal care. Antiallergic and antiphlogistic treatment may be necessary as well as symptomatic therapy with inhalation, fluids, secretory agents and oily emulsions.

5.2.7 Acute Viral Infections of the Oropharynx

5.2.7.1 Acute Pharyngitis

Aetiology/Epidemiology

Adenovirus, rhinovirus, reovirus, respiratory syncytial virus, influenza viruses and parainfluenza viruses have all been shown to be possible pathogens. Secondarily, bacterial superinfection mostly with *Haemophilus influenzae* may occur.

Symptoms

Patients presenting with viral pharyngitis commonly complain of sore throat, difficulty swallowing and often more general symptoms such as fever and headache. Usually oropharyngeal erythema, mostly without tonsillar exudate, as well as rhinorrhoea and sinusitis can be found.

Diagnostic Procedures

Inspection shows dry and erythematous pharyngeal mucosa, sometimes encrusted. Lymphoid follicles on the pharyngeal wall swell and appear as little pink nodes (Fig. 5.2.16). Cervical lymph nodes enlarge and become tender. Oropharyngeal cultures obtained during the infection are not always useful to detect the pathogen. The normal flora of the pharyngeal mucosa includes multiple bacterial organisms, so the affecting species cannot be identified.

Therapy

The treatment for these infections is generally symptomatic; analgesia and warm fluids may be helpful. Only in rare cases of bacterial superinfection are antibiotics necessary. Mostly, pharyngitis is self-limited and resolves within 3–4 days.

5.2.7.2   Infectious Mononucleosis

Aetiology/Epidemiology

Infectious mononucleosis may appear asymptomatic or cause a disease of variable severity. During primary infection the Epstein–Barr virus causes acute pharyngitis as a part of infectious mononucleosis syndrome. It has high incidence rates in children and young adults, it is transmitted by oral contact and is also called "kissing disease".

Symptoms

It manifests itself after an incubation period of up to 4 weeks as a severe attack of acute tonsillitis, cervical marked adenopathy, fever, malaise and hepatosplenomegaly. The tonsils are severely enlarged and are classically covered with extensive grey-white exudates (Fig. 5.2.17). Sometimes tonsillar hypertrophy causes airway obstruction.

Diagnostic Procedures

In the complete blood count, the white blood cell count is—after a period of leucocytopenia—elevated for lymphocytes, which are atypical in structure (activated T cells). The Epstein–Barr virus specific antibody serologic test gives a positive result as does the monospot test, which is more sensitive. To exclude liver affection, liver enzymes should be examined; EKG and ultrasound findings of the liver should also be obtained.

Therapy

The treatment required is supportive with bed rest until the fever has resolved, intravenous fluids, anti-inflammatory drugs and analgesia. To avoid bacterial superinfection at the beginning of the disease, during leucocytopenia antibiotics may be useful, for example with cephalosporins. Bacterial infection may complicate the

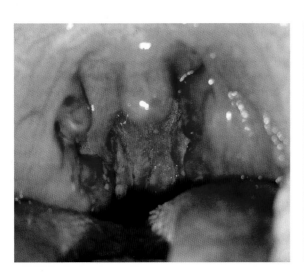

Fig. 5.2.16 Acute pharyngitis

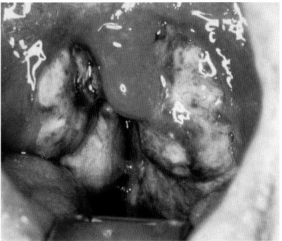

Fig. 5.2.17 Infectious mononucleosis

situation. Treatment with amoxycillin or ampicillin can cause a generalized maculopapular exanthema, mostly on the ninth day of therapy (Fig. 5.2.18). Patients with hepatosplenomegaly should avoid physical activity for almost 3 months. In the case of progressive airway obstruction due to tonsillar swelling, a short course of steroids may be helpful. Sometimes tonsillectomy must be indicated.

5.2.7.3   Herpangina

See Sect. 5.1.4.4.

Aetiology/Epidemiology

Tonsillar infection with Coxsackie virus—mostly group A, rarely group B—results in herpangina; the onset of this infection usually appears during childhood. The incubation period is 1 week.

Symptoms

Herpangina occurs as ulcerative vesicles over the tonsils, the pharynx and the soft palate. Patients present with general symptoms such as headache, malaise, fever, odynophagia and lymphadenitis. Additionally, palmar and plantar vesicles may occur (hand, foot and mouth disease).

Diagnostic Procedures

For diagnosis the increasing concentration of antibodies against Coxsackie virus needs to be measured.

Therapy

Treatment for this viral infection is also symptomatic; antiviral medication with aciclovir may be tried.

5.2.8   Tonsillectomy

5.2.8.1   Indications

Indications for the procedure cover a wide range of illnesses and conditions. The most important indications are:

- Recurrent tonsillitis or peritonsillar abscess
- Obstructive tonsillar hyperplasia with airway obstruction and sleep apnoea
- Suspicion of a malignant tumour (biopsy)

The most frequent indications is recurrent tonsillitis. Different guidelines have been developed to define "recur-

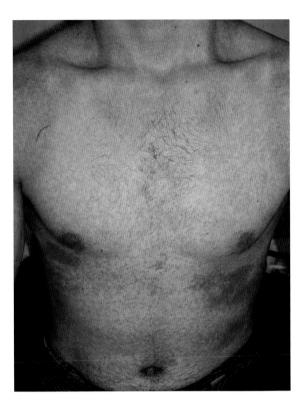

Fig. 5.2.18 Exanthema caused by ampicillin treatment of infectious mononucleosis occurring on the ninth day after beginning ampicillin treatment

rent". The American guidelines suggest that a patient who experiences four or more episodes of acute tonsillitis per year would benefit from a tonsillectomy. These guidelines are helpful, but should not be used rigidly. For example, few, very severe infections may be a better indication for surgical intervention than frequent mild infections.

In children, a watch-and-wait attitude is often useful if the otolaryngologist is the first physician consulted by the parents to evaluate the child. However, if the patient has been seen by a paediatrician who has referred the patient, conservative treatment has usually failed and the patient would usually benefit from tonsillectomy.

The indication for tonsillectomy in children under 5 years should be considered very strictly because post-tonsillectomy haemorrhage in this age group is life-threatening.

5.7.8.2   Surgical Technique

Tonsillectomies are usually performed under general anaesthesia; the patient is usually intubated using a standard orotracheal tube. Various techniques are available to achieve the same goal.

All of the techniques use the principle of careful dissection in the subcapsular plane and meticulous haemostasis at the end of the procedure.

The mouth gag should be inserted (correct length) and the orotracheal tube should be controlled after insertion. The orotracheal tube needs to be centred on the tongue. This is best achieved by positioning the tube in the midline at the tongue base. The thumb of the nondominant hand is placed on the tube against the lower incisors. The middle and the ring finger retract the upper-left molars to open the mouth for gag insertion. In this manner the tube should not move. The gag is inserted in a similar manner, as one would intubate the patient. Once in place, the gag is opened and the lower lips are not caught in the retractor.

Cold Technique

- Retract the tonsil with a blunt instrument (Denis Brown forceps) to avoid unnecessary traumatizations of the tonsils,
- The key to tonsillectomy is getting in the correct plane. This is the potential space between the tonsillar capsule and the constrictor muscle. Failure to dissect in this plane leads to tonsillar remnants as well as a more bloody operation. When retracting the tonsil medially, one can see the lateral aspect of the tonsil submucosally.
- With use of Metzenbaum/tonsillectomy scissors, the mucosa at the upper pole is incised. Using the lower blade of the scissors, one divides the mucosa of the anterior pillar over the tonsil.
- Using the upper blade of the scissors, one divides the posterior pillar in a similar fashion. This frees the tonsil from its mucosal attachments, which makes dissection easier.
- To obtain entry into the correct plane, the scissors are turned perpendicular to the tonsil plane and inserted just lateral to the tonsillar border. The scissors are then opened and a relatively bloodless plane should be seen. With the scissors still open in this space, the forceps are repositioned with one blade in this newly developed space (grasping the upper tonsillar pole).
- The tonsil is then retracted towards the lower pole of the contralateral tonsil; considerable dissection can be done with this move alone. When dissecting, one must regrasp the tonsil occasionally to maintain traction.
- A tonsillectomy dissector is used to reflect the constrictor muscle off the tonsil. Dissection should not proceed to the lingual tonsils because then troublesome bleeding will occur.
- The lower pole can be either divided with a tonsil snare or clamped and the divided pole is secured using a suture.

- Meticulous haemostasis is necessary. Haemostasis can be achieved using bipolar diathermy or 2-0 sutures.
- The gag must be released and reopened to reexamine the tonsillar fossa for bleeders which had been temporarily tamponized by the open gag.

Hot Technique
See Fig.5.2.19.

Monopolar Cautery
The monopolar technique using coagulation is most frequently used. It is necessary to remove smoke with suction aids.

Usually an insulated tip is used for this operation. With the tonsils retracted the cautery is used to incise the tonsil mucosa on the medial aspect of the anterior pillar. Entry in the correct plane can then be achieved using scissors as described for the cold technique. Entry is best performed at the upper pole with retraction of the tonsil inferiorly and medially.

Smooth, purposeful movements using the cautery with the tonsil constantly retracted allow for easier dissection and less char formation. Haemostasis is achieved either with monopolar or bipolar cautery.

Coblation
The coblation technique uses a bipolar current to create a plasma field, which can then split tissue. This occurs at temperatures of only 60–70°C, which is less than those produced with conventional radiofrequency and electrocautery. This decreased temperature required in the coblation technique is thought to diminish surrounding tissue damage. When correctly used, the plasma field slices the peritonsillar connective tissue, while a coexisting low-power current coagulates vessels. Larger vessels are controlled with the coagulation-only pedal without creation of the plasma ion field. The literature indicates that coblation may offer an alternative, safe technique that affords decreased or similar haemorrhage rates, as well as decreased pain. This new technique has been met with initial enthusiasm like many other new techniques in tonsillectomy at the beginning. This enthusiasm often dissipates, however, when these procedures and their complications are compared with those of traditional technique such as electrodissection and cold knife technique.

5.2.8.3   Key Points

- In tonsillectomy in patients with considerable fibrosis, it is more difficult to find the correct plane. In this case, blunt dissection may be the safest way to remove the tonsil. Care must be taken with monopolar cautery, which may create a plane within the fibrotic tis-

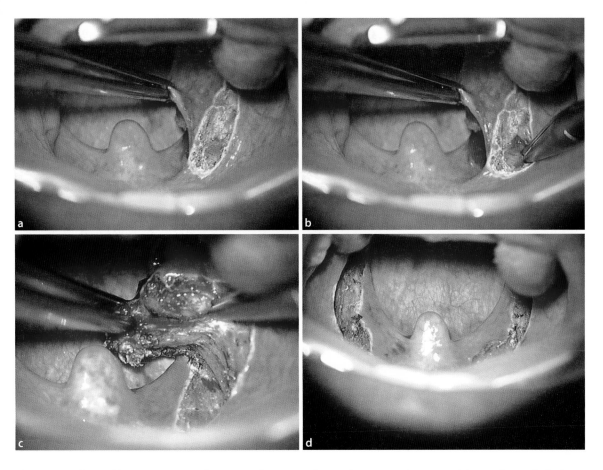

Fig. 5.2.19a–d Tonsillectomy: **a** incision; **b** exposing the correct plane with scissors; **c** dissection of the tonsil towards the lower pole; **d** completion of tonsillectomy on both sides

sue and place at risk major vessels lateral to the constrictor muscle.

- Keep in mind the proximity of the carotid artery to the tonsils.
- Care must be taken to avoid leaving excessive tonsil tissue at the inferior pole as well as to avoid unnecessary excessive dissection into the hypopharynx and the tongue base.

5.2.8.4 Complications

Haemorrhage is the main potential complication and may be either primary or secondary. In minor cases of bleeding, the clot can be removed with suction or forceps and the bleeding area can be cauterized with silver nitrate

In cases of major or life-threatening haemorrhage, the ABC principles must be observed. In children it is wise to prepare the patient for the operating room and con-

trol the bleeding under general anaesthesia sooner rather than later.

Tonsillotomy means partial resection of hyperplastic tonsils. The anterior and posterior pillar and the fibrous capsule of the tonsils are not removed in tonsillotomy. The obstructive part of the tonsils is only resected. Tonsillotomy is indicated in early childhood (under 6 years) when snoring, respiratory obstruction, dysphagia and failure to grow exists and no chronic or acute infection of the tonsils is present. In these cases, tonsillotomy may be a suitable method for treating tonsillar hyperplasia in early childhood.

Complications such as secondary postoperative bleeding are reduced in tonsillotomy according to the literature, because the capsule of the tonsils remains intact and the vessels of the peritonsillar space are not exposed to the saliva. The prerequisite for long-term success is strict limitation of this intervention to the diagnosis of tonsillar hyperplasia.

5.2.9 Neoplasms of the Oropharynx and Hypopharynx

The vast majority of pharyngeal tumours are squamous cell carcinomas. Other malignancies include lymphoma, minor salivary gland tumours, sarcoma and metastatic lesions.

Lymphomas occur most commonly in the tonsil, where they represent 16% of all neoplasms. Lymphomas can occur anywhere in Waldeyer's ring, and are almost always non-Hodgkin's lymphoma. Treatment is primarily nonsurgical.

5.2.9.1 Epidemiology

An overview of the incidence, histopathology and prognosis is shown in Table 1.3.1.

These cancers are strongly associated with tobacco and alcohol use. Minor association occurs with poor oral hygiene, human papilloma virus, syphilis and Epstein–Barr virus.

5.2.9.2 TNM Classification

The detailed TNM classification is shown in Tables 1.1.4.5.2 and 1.1.5.4.1.

5.2.9.3 Symptoms

The most common symptoms are a sore throat, dysphagia, a globus sensation, a neck mass and ear pains. These patients can have significantly advanced cancers, however with a paucity of symptoms.

5.2.9.4 Diagnosis

Documentation of a detected mass in the pharynx should include:
- Multidimensional size of the tumour
- Location in the different regions of the pharynx
- Mobility of the lesion
- Relationship to the prevertebral fascia
- Relationship to the larynx and vocal cords

CT and MRI are useful in evaluating the deep extent of the tumour and the tumour's relationship to surrounding structures.

Endoscopy in the operating room will add to the evaluation of the tumour and biopsies are made.

Following full examination, the tumour should be staged as described next.

5.2.9.5 Staging

Oropharyngeal primary tumours are staged mainly by size, while for hypopharyngeal tumours the location and the relation to the larynx are also important.

The detailed classification is described in Sect. 1.1.5.4.

5.2.9.6 Treatment

Tonsil Carcinoma
See Fig. 5.2.20.

The tonsil is the most common site of cancers of the oropharynx. Like in other head and neck cancers, three treatment options prevail:
1. Surgery of the primary tumour and the neck
2. Surgery combined with adjuvant radiation or adjuvant radiochemotherapy
3. Primary radiochemotherapy

These treatment options need to be discussed with the patient in any individual situation. Most would agree, however, that for these tumours the best cure rates can be obtained with combined therapy consisting of surgery followed by radio- (chemo-) therapy.

Before surgery the tumour's resectability must be assessed. Important areas or structures to evaluate for invasion by cancer are:
- The prevertebral fascia
- Carotid artery
- Skull base

If these areas are involved, the tumour would be judged by most surgeons to be unresectable, and the patient should be treated with radio- (chemo-) therapy.

The surgical principles are as follows:
- *Transoral surgery* is possible in T1, T2 and selected T3 tumours. Transoral surgery can be done with special laser equipment or with monopolar cautery using an insulated tip. Reconstruction procedures are not necessary in most cases. Healing occurs with granulation followed by epithelization like in tonsillectomy procedures. Proper patient selection is the most critical aspect in planning transoral resection. The surgeon must be able to adequately visualize the tumour throughout the procedure.
- *Mandibulotomy*: Osteotomy in the midline allows one to swing the mandible laterally and the tumour is approached through the floor of the mouth and is resected in continuity with the neck dissection specimen. Today this approach is not used very often in European countries, because many of these tumours may be operated on by transoral access.
- *Segmental mandibulectomy* (angle and ascending part of the mandible) is performed when the mandible is invaded by the tumour. Segmental mandibulectomy

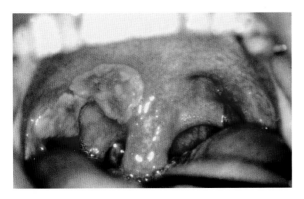

Fig. 5.2.20 Oropharyngeal cancer (soft palate and tonsil)

may be performed in the setting of a composite resection, that is resection of a segment of the mandible in continuity with a cancer of the oropharynx. Reconstruction is necessary and is described briefly in Sect. 5.1.6.2.

Tongue Base Tumours

Tongue base tumours (Fig. 5.2.21) are particularly difficult to manage because of the important function of the tongue base. The tongue base is important to propel food over the larynx and provide sensation and bulk to protect the larynx. The removal of the tongue base even without any removal of the supraglottis can therefore cause severe aspiration. If resection would require removal of large

portions of the tongue base, a laryngectomy must be considered to prevent aspiration. Owing to these concerns, attempts have been made to treat tongue base tumours primarily with chemoradiation. If a surgical therapy is chosen, different approaches are available:

- *Transoral laser resection*: Adequate exposure and visualization of the tumour must be guaranteed, special equipment is necessary.
- *Suprahyoid pharyngotomy approach*: Carefully selected tumours of the tongue base may be resected and reconstructed through a suprahyoid pharyngotomy with good opportunity for tumour clearance, little morbidity and good cure rates.
- *Lateral pharyngotomy approach*: The potential for airway compromise as a result of postoperative pharyngeal oedema and dysphagia necessitates a temporary tracheotomy in most cases of suprahyoid and lateral pharyngectomy.

In most cases of tongue base tumours, a combined therapy with surgery and adjuvant radiochemotherapy is necessary.

Soft Palate and Pharyngeal Walls

Cancers of the soft palate (Fig. 5.2.22) or pharyngeal walls are treated analogously to tonsil and tongue base tumours.

Hypopharyngeal Carcinoma

Hypopharyneal squamous cell carcinomas are typically highly infiltrative with significant submucosal spread. The majority of hypopharyngeal cancers occur in the pyriform sinus (Fig. 5.2.23)

In hypopharyngeal cancer, the tumour's relationship to the oesophagus and larynx must be thoroughly evalu-

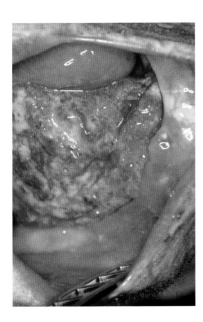

Fig. 5.2.21 Cancer of the tongue base with extension to the floor of the mouth

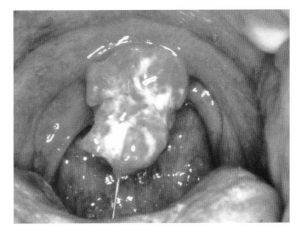

Fig. 5.2.22 Cancer of the soft palate (uvula)

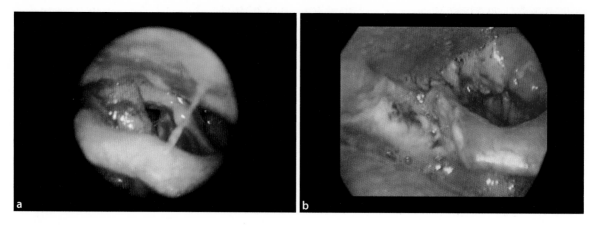

Fig. 5.2.23a,b Cancer of the hypopharynx: **a** before resection; **b** after transoral laser resection

ated. At the upper extent of the tumour, oropharyngeal involvement of the tonsil or tongue base may be detected. At the lower extent, involvement of the oesophagus may influence resectability. Vocal fold mobility must be assessed to detect laryngeal involvement. Fixation against the prevertebral fascia suggests unresectability.

For hypopharyngeal cancer, the same three treatment options exists like for tonsil carcinoma (see earlier)

The surgical principles, however, are different:

1. Transoral laser surgery in T1 and T2 tumours especially of the pyriform sinus (transoral approach) (Fig. 5.2.23).
2. Lateral pharyngectomy and partial hypopharynx resection (external approach) when a transoral approach is not possible because of insufficient transoral exposure of the hypopharynx and the tumour.
3. Total laryngectomy and partial pharyngectomy (T2, T3, selected T4 tumours). Patients with 3 cm of residual mucosa in the transverse dimension can usually undergo primary closure. If less than 3 cm remains, pedicled flap or free flap reconstruction may be required.
4. Total laryngopharyngectomy is required for cancer involving the postcricoid area, advanced cancer of the posterior pharyngeal wall and cancer involving the pyriform sinus with extension across the midline posteriorly. Reconstruction requires free jejunum or tubed free tissue transfer such as the radial forearm flap.

Surgical therapy for advanced hypopharyngeal cancer should only be employed with the patient's complete understanding of what this morbid procedure involves. In all advanced cases, postoperative radio- (chemo-) therapy should be employed.

In all pharyngeal carcinomas (oropharynx and hypopharynx), treatment of the neck is of course very important. The whole pharynx has a rich lymphatic drainage usually to both sides; therefore, in many cases a bilateral treatment of the neck is necessary. Indications and surgical principles of neck dissection are described in Chap.

Reference

1. Putz R, Pabst R (eds) (1993) Sobotta: Anatomie des Menschen. Kopf, Hals, obere Extremität. vol 1, 21st edn, version 2.0. Urban und Schwarzenberg, Munich

Suggested Reading

1. Arnold W, Ganzer U (2005) Checkliste Hals-Nasen-Ohren-Heilkunde, 4th edn. Thieme, Stuttgart
2. Boenninghaus HG, Lenarz T (2007) HNO, 13th edn. Springer, Berlin
3. Graham, JM, Scadding GK, Bull PD (eds) (2007) Pediatric ENT. Springer, Berlin
4. Lee KJ, Toh EH (2007) Otolaryngology. A surgical notebook. Thieme, New York
5. Myers EN (ed) (2008) Operative otolaryngology head and neck surgery, 2nd edn. Elsevier Saunders, Philadelphia
6. Seiden AM, Tami TA, Pensak ML, Cotton RT, Gluckman JL (2001) Otolaryngology. The essentials. Thieme, Stuttgart

5.3 Oesophagus

VIKTOR BONKOWSKY

5.3.1 Clinical Anatomy

The oesophagus begins below the cricoid cartilage at the level of the sixth cervical vertebra. Endoscopically, this is about 16–19 cm from the upper incisor teeth. During its vertical descent, the cervical oesophagus shifts to the left.

Note that surgical access to the cervical oesophagus is best through an incision in the left side of the neck because of its anatomic location.

The thoracic oesophagus is pushed back to the midline by the aorta. The aortic arch lies at the junction of the proximal and middle third of the oesophagus, while the distal third passes just behind the heart. The oesophagus is a conduit 20–25 cm long.

The oesophagus has three areas of anatomic narrowing that become important when confronted with a foreign body or caustic ingestion:

1. Upper oesophageal sphincter (Fig. 5.3.1), which is formed by the cricopharyngeus muscle and is located behind the cricoid cartilage (16–19 cm away from the upper incisors)
2. Anterior compression by the aortic arch and left mainstem bronchus (20–25 cm away from the upper incisors)
3. The gastrooesophageal junction (38–44 cm away from the upper incisors)

The oesophagus is composed of four layers: the mucosa, the submucosa, the muscularis and the adventitia.

The external muscle layer is composed of largely striated muscle within the proximal third of the oesophagus, mixed striated and smooth muscle within the middle third, and smooth muscle in the lower third. The fluid transition that occurs between these segments shows a remarkable coordination, innervated in part by the myenteric plexus of Auerbach, also located within this layer.

The outermost adventitia contains neurovascular structures and elastic fibres that are continuous with fibres interspersed within the inner layers of the oesophagus. This complex network allows the oesophagus to distend in response to bolus feeding and resume its normal shape after deglutition.

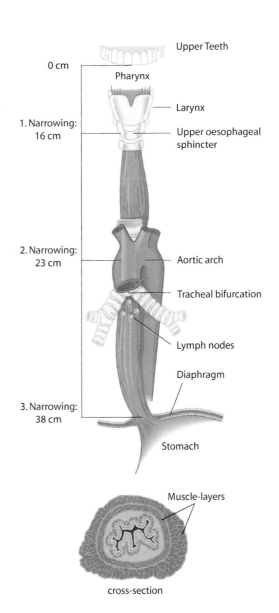

Fig. 5.3.1 Anatomic narrowing of the oesophagus (Figure 15.1a in [1])

5.3.2   Physiology

The oesophagus is capable of propelling different kinds of food, regardless of posture and opposing thoracic and abdominal pressure. In addition it prevents reversal of this flow except when emesis becomes necessary. The adult swallows 50–60 times per hour while awake and six to seven times per hour while asleep. The swallowing can be divided in three phases:

1. Oral phase
2. Pharyngeal phase
3. Oesophageal phase

The oral, or preparatory, phase is under voluntary control. The pharyngeal and oesophageal phases are controlled by reflex.

5.3.3   Clinical Tests

5.3.3.1   Imaging Techniques

Contrast Oesophagram
The best technique to examine the oesophagus is barium swallow. When a contrast swallow is used to confirm an oesophageal perforation, the swallow should be performed with a water-soluble contrast material such as meglumine diatrizoate (Gastrografin). On the other hand, patients suspected of aspiration should be given thin suspensions of barium, because the water-soluble materials are more irritating to the tracheobronchial tree.

CT and MRI
The use of CT and MRI for evaluating oesophageal disease is limited to pretreatment staging of oesophageal carcinoma and for identifying and characterizing disease extrinsic to the oesophagus.

5.3.3.2   Invasive Diagnostic Tests

Manometry
Oesophageal manometry is primarily used to assess peristaltic activity within the body of the oesophagus, and lower oesophageal sphincter pressure and relaxation in achalasia. Oesophageal manometry helps to establish the diagnosis of achalasia and diffuse oesophageal spasm.

Intraluminal pH measurements
Oesophageal pH monitoring is the gold standard for detecting clinically significant gastrooesophageal reflux.

Patients must stop proton pump inhibitors 72 h before pH-metry and histamine receptor antagonists at least 24 h before the study. Then pH monitoring over a 24-h period is performed.

Oesphophagoscopy
Oesophagoscopy is the best method for assessing mucosal integrity, inflammation and malignancy of the oesophagus. Simultaneously, a diagnostic test (biopsy) and therapeutic intervention (foreign body removal) can be done if necessary. Gastroenterologists generally prefer flexible fibre-optic instruments that allow better optics, air insufflation for distension and better access to the distal oesophagus. Otolaryngologists are usually trained in the use of rigid telescopes, which allow easier use of instrumentation and provide a more accurate view of the oesophagus inlet and postcricoid area. The technique of oesophagoscopy is described in Chap. 1.

5.3.4   Congenital Anomalies

5.3.4.1   Oesophageal Atresia

Oesophageal atresia is the most frequent congenital oesophageal disease (1:3,000 to 1:5,000). It is combined in the majority of cases with tracheooesophageal fistula. Oesophageal atresia with a distal tracheooesophageal fistula occurs most often and accounts for 85% of these cases. The most frequent types are summarized in Fig. 5.3.2.

Aetiology and Pathogenesis
In the fourth and fifth weeks of fetal life, an incomplete division of the trachea and digestive portion of the foregut leads to abnormal communication or fistula. As activating causes exogenous factors are discussed.

Symptoms
During or shortly after birth, it results in foamy salivation from the nose and the mouth. Regurgitation of food, cough attacks and cyanosis occur.

A polyhydramnion of the mother can be a sign of an oesophageal atresia since the fetus cannot swallow the amniotic fluid.

Diagnosis
Early diagnosis can be made if a soft 10-Fr catheter cannot be passed to the stomach. Typically one meets resistance after 10–12 cm. On X-ray of the thorax and abdomen, the presence or absence of air in the stomach indicates

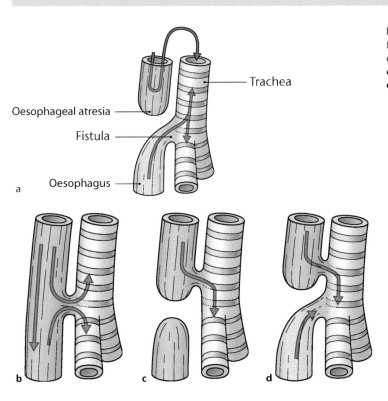

Oesophageal atresia

Fistula

a   Oesophagus

Trachea

b   c   d

Fig. 5.3.2a–d Types of tracheo-oesophageal fistula (TOF). **a** Oesophageal atresia with distal TOF. **b** Isolated, H-shaped TOF. **c** Oesophageal atresia with proximal TOF. **d** Separate proximal and distal TOFs

the presence or absence of a tracheooesophageal fistula. Only small amounts (0.5 ml thin barium) should be used for the radiologic confirmation because of the danger of aspiration.

Note that water-soluble contrast media should be avoided, as they will cause a fulminant pneumonitis if they are aspirated.

Therapy

To avoid pulmonal complications, regular suctioning of the oesophageal pouch is necessary. The feeding occurs parenterally. Surgical correction should be carried out as soon as possible. Definitive repair includes division and closure of the fistula and direct oesophageal anastomosis.

Risks and Complications

Oesophageal stricture is the most common postoperative complication. The sudden appearance of choking or pneumonia after surgery indicates the recurrence of tracheooesophageal fistula.

5.3.4.2   Dysphagia Lusoria

The most frequent underlying vessel anomaly is a left-sided-originating a. subclavia dextra, which in 80% of cases passes behind the oesophagus, in 15% between the trachea and the oesophagus and in 5% ventral to the trachea.

Symptoms

A clinically relevant dysphagia arises rarely. Symptoms usually occur in middle age.

Diagnosis

In the barium swallow, an impression of the oesophagus is proved from outside. MRI shows the vessel anomaly.

Therapy

A functional therapy is only indicated with correspondingly distinct dysphagia.

5.3.5   Functional Disorders

Basically, similar leading symptoms occur in all oesophageal diseases (functional, inflammatory or tumorous disorders):

- Dysphagia
- Retrosternal burning or pain
- Problems at food transportation or regurgitation

Note that a dysphagia that is based on motility disorders of the oesophagus is rather intermittent, progresses very slowly and occurs with liquid and fixed food. For obstructive oesophageal diseases, on the other hand, a constant and increasing dysphagia is typical which affects food, and only with increasing illness are liquids also affected.

First, functional disorders of oesophageal motility are explained. They can be divided into primary and secondary malfunctions.

5.3.5.1   Primary Motility Disorders

Achalasia

Aetiology and Pathogenesis
Achalasia is characterized by an incomplete relaxation of the lower oesophageal sphincter; this leads to a dilatation of the oesophagus. Achalasia is one of the most common primary motor disorders and appears to relate to degenerative changes within the vagal nucleus, vagal trunks and myenteric ganglia of the oesophagus.

The cause of this neuron degeneration is unknown. Infectious, toxic, ischaemic or genetic causes are discussed. The illness manifests itself in middle age (30–50 years).

Symptoms
Leading symptoms are dysphagia, regurgitation and convulsive pains. The patients often point to the xiphoid as the place of the strongest dysphagia.

Diagnosis
A barium swallow shows a typical picture: marked oesophageal dilatation proximal to the lower oesophageal sphincter and narrowing of the lower oesophageal sphincter. Oesophagoscopy with biopsy is obligatory for the exclusion of a carcinoma (frequency of a secondary carcinoma with long-existing achalasia 5–10%). Through the food retention, signs of oesophagitis are found in the oesophagus. Oesophageal manometry shows a clearly increased rest pressure (35 mm Hg higher than the pressure in the stomach) and an absence of relaxation during swallowing.

Therapy
The method of choice with symptomatic patients in stages I and II is the endoscopic balloon dilatation of the lower sphincter or surgical myotomy.

Diffuse Oesophageal Spasm
Tertiary, abnormally strong, simultaneous contractions of the oesophagus with normal function of the lower oesophageal sphincter are referred to as idiopathic diffuse oesophagus spasm. A regular propulsive peristalsis is missing.

Aetiology and Pathogenesis
The cause is unknown. Degenerative changes of the vagal innervation are discussed.

Symptoms
Dysphagia and retrosternal pains are the prevailing symptoms, often simulating cardiogenic pain. However, there should be no exertional pain and an occasional relationship with swallowing along with associated dysphagia help in the diagnosis.

Diagnosis
A barium oesophagram demonstrates segmentation of the barium column in the distal two thirds of the oesophagus owing to simultaneous contractions, producing the so-called corkscrew appearance. Manometry shows prolonged, high-amplitude nonperistaltic or tertiary contractions.

Therapy
A treatment attempt with calcium antagonists and nitrates should be made at the beginning of a therapy. In the case of pain attacks, *N*-butylscopolamine is employed.

5.3.5.2   Secondary Motility Disorders

Motility disorders can also be found within the framework of different basic diseases such as metabolic and endocrine disorders, as well as various neuromuscular diseases (scleroderma, systemic lupus erythematodes, dermatomyositis). Diabetes mellitus and alcoholism lead to a peripheral neuropathy with disordered peristalsis.

Dysphagia due to neighbourhood processes is also included in this group. So are scoliosis, mediastinal tumours and thyroid gland tumours.

5.3.6   Pharyngooesophageal Diverticula (Zenker Diverticulum)

This is the most common of the oesophageal diverticula. It occurs as a protrusion of posterior hypopharyngeal mucosa between the oblique and transverse fibres of the cricopharyngeal muscle in the posterior midline, an inherently weakened area of the oesophagus known as Killian's triangle (Fig. 5.3.3).

5.3.6.1   Symptoms

Dysphagia/odynophagia, regurgitation of undigested food, aspiration (recurring pneumonitis), globe/foreign body feeling, and fetor ex ore.

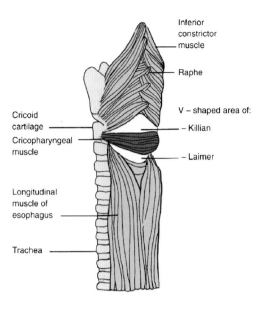

Inferior constrictor muscle

Raphe

V – shaped area of:

– Killian

– Laimer

Cricoid cartilage

Cricopharyngeal muscle

Longitudinal muscle of esophagus

Trachea

Fig. 5.3.3 Killian's triangle

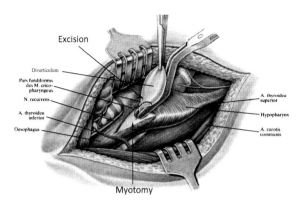

Excision

Diverticulum

Pars fundiformis des M. crico-pharyngeus

N. recurrens

A. thyroidea inferior

Oesophagus

A. thyroidea superior

Hypopharynx

A. carotis communis

Myotomy

Fig. 5.3.4 Conventional excision of a Zenker diverticulum and myotomy

5.3.6.2 Diagnosis

A barium swallow is usually diagnostic, demonstrating a fluid-filled sac.

Note that an endoscopy is generally quite hazardous because the sac has no muscular component and is easily perforated. Malignant degeneration is very seldom (less than 0.5%).

5.3.6.3 Therapy

If the diverticulum is symptomatic, surgical treatment is indicated. Different surgical methods are available:

1. Conventional excision (diverticuloectomy) or diverticulopexy through a left-sided cervicotomy combined with a sufficiently long myotomy of the cricopharyngeal muscle (Fig. 5.3.4).
2. Endoscopic division of the cricopharyngeal bar with the CO_2 laser
3. Endoscopic division of the cricopharyngeal bar with a stapler (Endo-GIA-30) (Fig. 5.3.5)

Conventional Transcervical Diverticuloectomy

- Rigid endoscopy and exposure of the diverticula, placement of a nasogastral tube and packing the sac of the diverticula with a running gauze strip (Fig. 5.3.6).
- Transverse incision in a skinfold near the level of the cricoid cartilage, which marks the cricoid muscle.
- Exposure of the sternocleidomastoid muscle and separation of the sternocleidomastoid muscle and the ca-

rotid sheath from the strap muscles, thyroid gland and laryngotracheal complex.

- Retraction of the sternocleidomastoid muscle and carotid sheath laterally to allow entry into the retropharyngeal prevertebral space and exposure of the prevertebral fascia.
- Placement of a hook in the posterior aspect of the thyroid cartilage and retraction of the laryngotracheal complex and the thyroid gland medially.
- Exposure of the cricopharyngeal muscle and of the packed diverticula in the posterior midline to avoid injury to the recurrent laryngeal nerve.
- Performance of the myotomy (at least 3 cm) of the cricopharyngeal muscle at the level of the cricoid cartilage. The muscle fibres are separated from the hypopharyngeal mucosa in the midline with a haemostat.

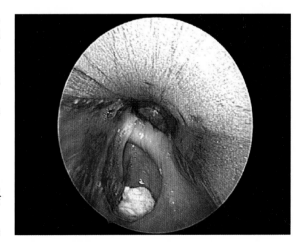

Fig. 5.3.5 Endoscopic view of the cricopharyngeal bar (retention of a pill in the sac of the diverticulum)

- Grasp of the tip of the diverticular sac with a clamp and excision of the sac. Excessive traction on the sac may lead to overresection of hypopharyngeal mucosa and may result in a stricture. In contrast, too much hypopharyngeal mucosa after resection is without sequelae. That means it is much better to preserve more mucosa than too little.
- A 3-0 gastrointestinal suture is used to close the mucosa. Mucosal edges must be inverted or a fistula will develop. Alternatively, a stapler can be used. Diverticulopexy was developed to avoid the risk of entering the pharynx.

Endoscopic Approach

Transorally the diverticular bar is exposed with a special diverticuloscope (Weerdascope, Storz) (Fig. 5.3.5). The diverticular bar (cricopharyngeal bar) is divided with the CO_2 laser or with an Endo-GIA stapler.

The main complications after conventional resection are salivary fistula and recurrent nerve paralysis.

The endoscopic approaches have a higher risk of mediastinitis. The endoscopic approach is not possible in cases of inadequate exposure of the diverticular bar because of anatomic limitations.

Note that it is necessary to select a technique with which the surgeon is experienced and is best suited to the patient's need.

The mucosal surface of the Zenker diverticulum should be examined endoscopically to rule out squamous cell carcinoma

A significant percentage of patients with a Zenker diverticulum will have a second cause of dysphagia. Oesophagogastroscopy and barium oesophagrography will help reveal the correct diagnosis.

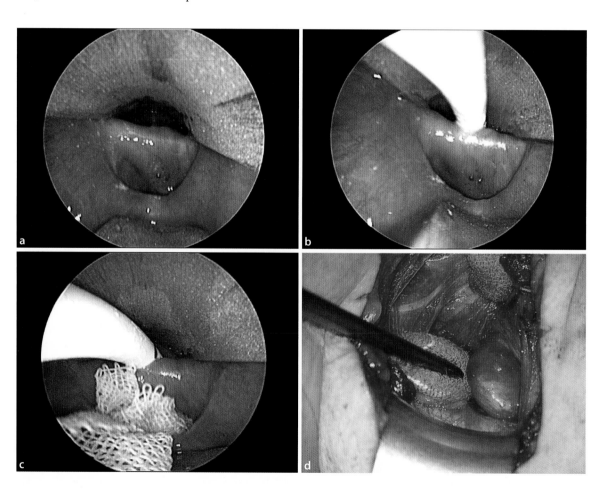

Fig. 5.3.6a–d Endoscopic exposure and packing of the diverticula with a gauze. **a** diverticular bar exposed with the diverticuloscope; **b** nasogastral feeding tube in the cervical oesophagus; **c** diverticulum sac packed with gauze, nasogastral feeding tube placed in the oesophagus; **d** transcervical approach, packed diverticula clearly visible

5.3.7 Infectious and Inflammatory Disorders

Infection or inflammation of the oesophagus typically produces dysphagia and odynophagia, so patients with these disorders may frequently present to the otolaryngolgist.

5.3.7.1 Infectious Oesophagitis

Fungal Infection

The disease is caused most frequently by *Candida albicans*, typically as a result of antibiotic therapy suppressing bacterial commensals, immunosuppression or the development of haematologic malignancies.

Symptoms

Mild dysphagia up to refusing all oral intake because of associated pain.

Diagnosis

Endoscopy reveals raised white plaques with or without ulceration. Brushings or biopsies may be obtained from these lesions.

Therapy

Orally administered flucanozole or ketoconazole provides effective treatment and is preferred over nystatin suspension.

Viral Infection

Second to *Candida albicans*, the most common organism causing oesophagitis is herpes simplex virus type 1 (HSV-1) Although it is more common in immunocompromised patients or those with predisposing factors, it may also occur in otherwise healthy individuals.

HSV-1 oesophagitis starts as a cluster of vesicles within the lower third of the oesophagus. In immunocompromised patients these lesions may progress to a diffuse ulcerative oesophagitis. Patients typically present with extremely severe pain with swallowing. Labial herpes may precede or coincide with the oesophageal lesion. In immunocompetent patients the infection resolves in 2 weeks. In immunocompromised patients the disease may progress to severe haemorrhage, perforation or dissemination.

Endoscopy enables the collection of brushings or biopsy material for culture and characteristically will reveal discrete, punched-out ulcers.

Therapy is with acyclovir.

Bacterial Infection

Bacterial infection accounts for 10–15% of cases of infectious oesophagitis. It seems to largely reflect colonization after oesophageal injury, for example from radiation therapy or gastrooesophageal reflux or nasogastric tubes, and once again tends to occur in immunocompromised patients. Organisms are generally consistent with oral flora; however, therapy should be culture-directed.

5.3.7.2 Noninfectious Oesophagitis

Gastrooesophageal Reflux Disease

Gastrooesophageal reflux disease (GORD) is used to describe any condition in which symptoms or histopathologic change results from refluxed gastric acid. This includes oesophagitis as well as extraoesophageal manifestations. Estimates suggest that GORD affects 7–10% of the population on a daily basis, and 40% on a monthly basis.

A certain amount of acid reflux is considered physiologic and occurs after meals. Whether it becomes pathologic depends on:

- Frequency
- Volume
- Duration of exposure

Defence mechanisms against gastrooesophageal reflux are:

- A competent lower oesophageal sphincter
- Peristaltic clearance of oesophageal acid
- Oesophageal epithelial resistance
- A competent upper oesophageal sphincter

Although the pH of the refluxate is important, it is the pepsin concentration that seems to be responsible for the mucosal injury.

Symptoms

The most common symptom of GORD is heartburn, a retrosternal and epigastric burning pain that may radiate to the back, arm, pharynx and ear when severe. Occasionally it must be distinguished from cardiac pain. However, if it dissipates rapidly with nitroglycerine, it is unlikely to be oesophageal in origin. The severity of pain often does not correlate histologically with the amount of oesophageal inflammation. Pain that is aggravated by hot or cold liquids, citrus juices or alcohol suggests ulcerative oesophagitis.

Oesophageal Symptoms

Common symptoms are heartburn, regurgitation, dysphagia, and chest pain. Less common symptoms are odynophagia water brush (excessive salivation prompted by acid reflux) and subxiphoid pain.

Extraoesophageal Syndromes

Association with gastrooesophageal reflux has been established, but there is good evidence for causation only when it is accompanied by an oesophageal syndrome for:

- Chronic cough
- Laryngitis
- Asthma (reflux as a cofactor)

Proposed association with GORD but neither association nor causation has been established for:

- Pharyngitis
- Sinusitis
- Recurrent otitis media

Diagnosis

When symptoms of gastroesophageal reflux are typical and the patient responds to therapy, no diagnostic tests are necessary to verify the diagnosis. If the patient fails to respond or has atypical symptoms or complications, a number of tests are available:

- The 24-h pH probe is currently the definite test for reflux.
- Endoscopy may show characteristic mucosa changes in the distal oesophagus. However, the presence of normal-appearing mucosa does not rule out the possibility of reflux disease because about 50% of patients with symptomatic reflux have normal findings on endoscopic examination.
- ENT examination (posterior laryngitis, granuloma of the vocal cord) to detect extraoesophageal syndromes.

Treatment

- Dietary changes such as avoiding foods that are acidic (citrus fruits) or foods that can cause gastric reflux (fatty or fried foods, coffee or tea).
- Lifestyle changes (smoking cessation, weight reduction (body-mass index greater than 25), avoidance of eating within 3 h before bedtime.
- Medical therapy: Proton pump inhibitors in a step-down manner (esomeprazole 40 mg daily for 8–12 weeks). After the initial therapy, the patient is advised to titrate the dose to find the lowest dose that provides satisfactory control of heartburn.
- Surgical therapy: Only when medical therapy fails, the so-called antireflux surgery is indicated.

5.3.8   Trauma

5.3.8.1   Caustic Ingestion

In the USA there are 5,000 accidental lye ingestions per year by children under 5 years. Such injury is also seen in adults with mental retardation and in adults trying to commit suicide. The most common agents are alkaline (60%) such as sodium or potassium hydroxides, which are found in many household cleaners, and acid corrosives.

Pathophysiology

Alkalis tend to penetrate faster than acids, causing a liquefaction necrosis that may extend rapidly through the mucosa to the underlying muscle of the oesophagus.

Acids produce a coagulation necrosis with superficial eschar that helps to prevent deeper penetration leading to greater damage within the stomach.

Liquid products are more easily swallowed and produce the most damage at normal narrowings within the oesophagus. Solid substances may attach to the oral mucosa and are more difficult to swallow, thereby more often causing damage to the oral cavity and pharynx.

Classification

Burns are classified as follows (Table 5.3.1):

1. First-degree burn: superficial causing hyperaemia and oedema but no significant scarring.
2. Second-degree burn: additional penetration through the submucosa into the muscle, producing necrosis and deep ulceration. Stenosis may occur over the next week.
3. Third-degree burn: Transmural lesion, eroding into the mediastinum, pleural cavity or peritoneal cavity.

Clinical Findings

The immediate goal in these cases is to accurately access the location and extent of injury and to prevent the development of complications such as stricture or perforation.

Acute patients may complain of burning of the lips, tongue or pharynx and dysphagia. Excessive salivation with drooling is frequently present, wheezing and stridor suggest airway involvement.

Note that 50% of patients complaining of two of the following symptoms—drooling, vomiting and stridor—will have serious oesophageal burns. The presence of only one of these symptoms tends to be associated with very little oesophageal burn.

If oesophageal perforation occurs, severe chest pain, subcutaneous emphysema sepsis and shock may happen.

Haematemesis and abdominal pain suggest gastric injury.

Diagnostic Evaluation

1. Typical history (accidental or suicidal ingestion) and typical clinical findings.

Table 5.3.1 Classification of burns by depth of injury

Grade	Depth	Endoscopy
First degree	Mucosal	Mucosal hyperaemia and oedema
Second degree	Transmucosal, with or without involvement of muscularis. No extension to periesophageal tissue	Haemorrhagic, exudative, ulcerative pseudomembranes
Third degree	Full-thickness injury with extension into perioesophageal tissue. May involve mediastinal or intraperitoneal organs	Complete obliteration of oesophageal lumen by massive oedema; charring and eschar; full-thickness necrosis with perforation

2. Radiographic evaluation (X-ray of the chest and abdomen). A more sensitive study to detect early perforation is CT of the chest.
3. Flexible endoscopy is the most sensitive method for establishing the extent of injury. Endoscopy should be done as soon as possible within the first 48–72 h after the ingestion by an extremely experienced endoscopist. After this time, the risk of perforation during the endoscopy is much higher. The examination is most safely done with a paediatric endoscope with minimal air insufflation. When the first injury is recognized, further endoscopy has to be done with extreme caution to avoid mucosal injury, creating a false lumen and full-thickness perforation. If there is any doubt about the safety of the procedure, the endoscopy has to be stopped. The burns may be classified according to Table 5.3.1. This simple classification is very useful to predict the severity of the injury and the probability of stricture formation.

Therapy

Acute measures such as airway management and volume substitution are used in the initial phase. The greatest concern is to prevent oesophageal stricture or perforation. If second-degree or third-degree burns are found at endoscopy, prompt administration of broad-spectrum antibiotics and steroids is indicated. Use of antifungal agents should also be discussed. There is no doubt about the use of antibiotics because they decrease the bacterial load and the formation of granulation tissue is minimized. Also they help to prevent intramural spread and possibly mediastinitis. Administration of steroids is more controversial. If steroids are used, this should be done within 24–48 h of injury and then stricture formation may be reduced.

Early dilatation is useful and necessary in stricture formation. It should be started in the fifth or sixth week after the injury. The technique is extremely important because perforation could easily occur. Endoscopy and dilatation should only be performed in a endoscopic unit under fluoroscopic guidance. Dilatation is done over a guidewire whose position is radiologically controlled (Savary dilatator). First, a small bougie is used and then the size is increased until a moderate resistance is felt or blood is seen. Repeated dilatations after the appearance of blood indicate the likelihood that the stenosis will be torn, resulting in more severe stricture after this tear heals.

The incidence and interval of repeated dilatations depends on the degree of stenosis. The early placement of a nasogastric tube has been advocated by some groups to prevent stenosis: however, the data are insufficient to universally support this approach.

Late Risks and Complications

Up to 13% of patients with a caustic injury will develop a squamous cell cancer, even years or decades after the injury. Therefore, endoscopic control is necessary.

5.3.8.2 Oesophageal Perforation

Oesophageal perforation may occur from a variety of causes, but the most common cause is iatrogenic, resulting from endoscopic manipulation or dilatation.

Iatrogenic Perforation

The most common sites of iatrogenic oesophageal injury are the cervical oesophagus at the cricopharyngeus and the thoracoabdominal oesophagus at the diaphragmatic hiatus.

Injury at the cricopharyngeus (upper oesophageal sphincter) happens because of:
1. Inadvertent introduction of the oesophagoscope into the pyriform sinus
2. Narrowing of the upper oesophageal sphincter
3. Prominent cervical osteophytes

Injury at the diaphragmatic hiatus tends to occur as the oesophagus angles anteriorly towards the diaphragm, which is often not appreciated by the endoscopist.

An iatrogenic perforation is also possible by placement of a nasogastric tube, traumatic endotracheal intubation or after dilatative tracheotomy.

External Trauma

Penetrating trauma can of course lead to an oesophageal perforation. Also sudden high pressure (blunt trauma) may sometimes cause oesophageal rupture.

Spontaneous Rupture

Spontaneous rupture is known as Boerhaave syndrome and is caused by severe vomiting. The majority of spontaneous oesophageal perforations occur in the distal oesophagus, where it seems to be an inherent weakness within the left posterolateral wall.

Diagnosis

If a perforation happens, it is extremely important to make the diagnosis rapidly. Persistent pain and fever after oesophagoscopy should alert the clinician.

Note that as many as 50% of patients will be asymptomatic for the first 8 h following injury.

Symptoms

Perforation of the cervical oesophagus causes:
- Neck pain (more than 90%)
- Subcutaneous emphysema (more than 50%)
- Dysphagia and odynophagia

Fever and leucocytosis will develop over the first 24 h.
More distal perforation causes:
- Retrosternal chest pain or shoulder pain
- Problems and pain with respiration
- Subcutaneous emphysema

Radiology

A water-soluble contrast medium, such as Gastrografin, is used for the oesophagogram and confirms perforation in about 80% of cases. Gastrografin is preferable because it causes less mediastinal inflammation. However, if the test is negative, a thin-barium swallow may demonstrate the perforation because it remains more sensitive.

Lateral cervical radiographs may demonstrate widening of the retrooesophageal space and streaks of air in the soft tissue planes (prevertebral air) and subcutaneous or cervical emphysema.

Chest radiographs may demonstrate pneumomediastinum, mediastinal widening or pneumothorax

CT with contrast is helpful if an abscess is suspected.

Therapy

It has been clearly shown that delays in diagnosis and treatment are associated with increased mortality. There-

fore, medical therapy should begin even before the perforation has been verified.

For perforation of the cervical oesophagus, medical therapy includes:
- Intravenous high-dose antibiotics (clindamycin, ampicillin, sulbactam).
- Allowing nothing per mouth and intravenous hydration and alimentation.
- Nasogastric suction. This may be helpful and may be used for nutritional support if the tube can be safely passed.

Treatment needs to be individualized and patients need to be closely monitored. Any deterioration in overall status or signs of sepsis will necessitate surgical drainage.

There remains considerable controversy as to whether medical therapy alone is adequate or whether all oesophageal perforations need surgical intervention. In cervical perforation there is a clear trend to medical therapy alone. Generally, appropriate treatment depends on the site and size of the perforation, the time since the injury happened and the health status of the patient.

Surgical therapy includes:
- Incision along the lower third of the anterior border of sternocleidomastoid muscle.
- Retraction of the carotid artery and jugular vein laterally and retraction of the laryngotracheal complex medially.
- Blunt dissection to the retrovisceral space and prevertebral fascia (Fig. 5.3.7).
- The perforation is sought and, if found, is closed with 3-0 absorbable sutures. This step is not a requirement for successful treatment because cervical oesophageal perforations heal with adequate drainage in the absence of a distal obstruction.
- Finger dissection in the posterior mediastinum, irrigation of this area and insertion of a soft suction drain into the mediastinum.

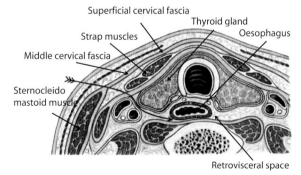

Fig. 5.3.7 Surgical route to the retrovisceral space

For perforation of the middle and lower oesophagus, there is a higher complication rate and a combined surgical and medical therapy is usually favoured.

5.3.9 Foreign Bodies

The oesophagus is the most common site of foreign body impaction within the gastrointestinal tract.

Adults usually describe a history of having eaten fish or chicken and present with dysphagia, odynophagia and sometimes drooling. On the other hand, most foreign body ingestions in children go unnoticed and the history may be very misleading.

Radiographs should be obtained in all patients and include both anteroposterior and lateral neck films as a chest X-ray. It is important to remember that negative X-ray findings do not rule out a foreign body.

In the case of a clinically or radiologically suspected foreign body, endoscopy is necessary. Foreign body endoscopy is an ENT emergency.

Foreign body endoscopy is diagnostic and therapeutic. Endoscopy should be performed within the first 6 h after ingestion. A rigid oesophagoscope, which allows procedures with an open tube, is clearly preferred. The foreign body is carefully removed under direct vision. If a disk battery is ingested and becomes lodged in the oesophagus, it should be emergently removed, as it will release a caustic solution that may cause significant injury to the oesophageal mucosa. After endoscopic removal of a foreign body, the oesophagus is again examined to recognize a lesion or perforation. Postoperatively, patients need to be observed for any signs of perforation. A Gastrografin contrast study is performed before oral food intake is resumed and the patient is discharged.

All of the complications due to foreign bodies are closely related to direct or indirect perforation.

5.3.10 Neoplasms

Oesophageal neoplasms are not very common but are potentially quite lethal. Squamous cell carcinoma is the most common malignancy of the oesophagus and has one of the worst prognoses of any cancer, with an average 5-year survival rate of about 10%.

5.3.10.1 Benign Neoplasms

Leiomyoma is by far the most common benign neoplasm. Because it arises from smooth muscle, it is gener-

ally found within the distal two thirds of the oesophagus. Most patients are asymptomatic, but those who do have symptoms complain of dysphagia.

A barium oesophagram is diagnostic, revealing a smooth, well-circumscribed mass and irregularity of the surrounding mucosa.

During endoscopy, biopsy is contraindicated, because it may lead to bleeding, infection and perforation.

The therapy of choice is surgical enucleation.

The most common benign tumour within the cervical oesophagus is a fibrovascular polyp, which is composed of fibrous and vascular tissue covered by smooth mucosa. It is intraluminal and usually pedunculated. It may occasionally reach a very large size and prolapses into the larynx or even outside the mouth (Fig. 5.3.8). Surgical removal is therefore indicated and this may be done endoscopically.

5.3.10.2 Malignant Neoplasms

Approximately 90–95% are squamous cell carcinoma. Risk factors are excessive alcohol and tobacco use. Increased risk has been noted with caustic injury, long-standing achalasia and chronic oesophagitis of any cause. For cervical oesophagus carcinoma (postcricoid area) a special link to Plummer–Vinson syndrome exists.

Patients presenting with carcinoma elsewhere in the head and neck undergo endoscopy including oesophagoscopy to rule out the possibility of a second primary carcinoma. The incidence of coincidental oesophageal carcinoma varies between 1.0 and 6.5%.

Symptoms
Initially, the symptoms tend to be mild, nonspecific and easily ignored, explaining why most lesions are advanced

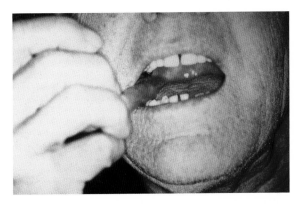

Fig. 5.3.8 Fibrovascular polyp of the cervical oesophagus protruding through the mouth

when they are finally discovered. The leading symptom is progressive dysphagia especially with solid food.

Note that dysphagia in oesophageal cancer means that more than 50% of the lumen has been compromised.

Diagnosis

Endoscopy is essential for direct inspection and histologic confirmation. A barium oesophagram (double-contrast technique) is also helpful in making the diagnosis, but it is not as accurate as endoscopy.

Note that to prevent perforation during endoscopy in oesophageal cancer, it is important never to force the instrument. If the lesion is submucosal and stenotic, biopsy may prove difficult and should be combined with brushings for cytology.

For staging of the oesophageal cancer, CT scanning is the procedure of choice.

Therapy

Surgical resection remains the most effective treatment for cure combined with different neoadjuvant or adjuvant strategies. But many of the patients with oesophageal car-cinoma present with advanced disease, so about 40% of the patients may be inoperable.

For lesions of the cervical oesophagus, in most of the cases a laryngectomy with oesophagectomy is required (Fig. 5.3.9). A safe method for single-stage reconstruction is gastric pull-up. Resection of the cervical oesophagus and preservation of the laryngotracheal complex is difficult and needs a nearly perfect combination of site and extent of the tumour and special surgical expertise.

Palliation therapy is important and includes endoscopic placement of an indwelling stent, laser therapy and bypass procedures.

The prognosis is generally bad (5-year survival rate less than 20%).

References

1. Boenninghaus HG, Lenarz T (2007) HNO, 13th edn. Springer, Berlin
2. Denecke HJ (1980) Die otorhinolaryngologischen Operationen im Mund-Halsbereich. Springer, Berlin
3. Graham JM, Scadding GK, Bull PD (eds) (2007) Pediatric ENT. Springer, Berlin

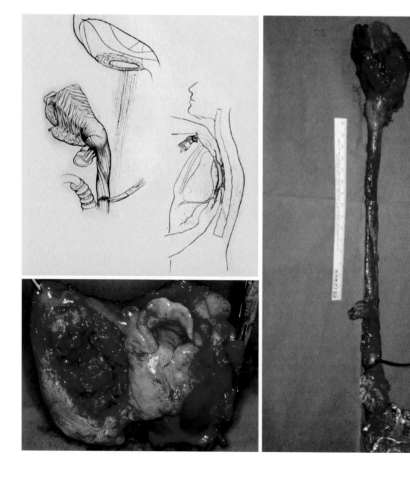

Fig. 5.3.9 Total pharyngolaryngooesophagectomy and reconstruction with gastric pull-up

Suggested Reading

1. Becker W, Buckingham RA, Hedringer PH, Korting GW, Lederer FL (eds) (1969) Atlas der Hals-Nasen-Ohrenkrankheiten einschließlich Bronchien und Ösophagus. Thieme, Stuttgart

2. Becker W, Naumann H, Pfaltz CR (1989) Hals-Nasen-Ohrenheilkunde, 4th edn. Thieme, Stuttgart

3. Benninghoff A; Drenckhahn D, Zenker W (eds) (1994) Anatomie: makroskopische Anatomie, Embryologie und Histologie des Menschen, 15th edn. Urban und Schwarzenberg, Munich

4. Berendes J, Link R, Zöllner F (1978) Hals-Nasen-Ohren-Heilkunde in Praxis und Klinik, vol 3, 2nd edn. Thieme, Stuttgart

5. Braveny I, Maschmeyer G (2002) Infektionskrankheiten Diagnostik—Klinik—Therapie. medco, Munich

6. Lalwani AK (2004) Current diagnosis and treatment in otolaryngology—head and neck surgery. Lange Medical Books/McGraw-Hill, New York

7. Lentze MJ, Schaub J, Schulte FJ, Spranger J (2003) Pädiatrie Grundlagen und Praxis, 2nd edn. Springer, Berlin

8. Myers EN (ed) (2008) Operative otolaryngology head and neck surgery, 2nd edition. Elsevier Saunders, Philadelphia

9. Naumann HH, Helms J, Herberhold C, Kastenbauer E (eds) (1992) Oto-Rhino-Laryngologie in Klinik und Praxis, vol 2, 1st edn. Thieme, Stuttgart

10. Patterson GA, Cooper JD, Deslauriers J, Lerut AEMR, Luketich JD, Rice TW (2008) Pearson's thoracic and esophageal surgery, vol. 2. Elsevier Churchill Livingstone, New York

11. Putz R, Pabst R (eds) (2004) Sobotta: Atlas der Anatomie des Menschen, 21st edn. Elsevier, Munich

12. Probst R, Grevers G, Iro H (2008) Hals-Nasen-Ohren-Heilkunde, 3rd edn. Thieme, Stuttgart

13. Seiden AM, Tami TA, Pensak ML, Cotton RT, Gluckman JL (2001) Otolaryngology. The essentials. Thieme, Stuttgart

14. Strome M, Kelly JH, Fried MP (1985) Manual of otolaryngology diagnosis and therapy. Little, Brown, Boston

15. Strutz J, Mann W (2001) Praxis der HNO—Heilkunde, Kopf - und Halschirurgie. Thieme, Stuttgart

16. Theissing J (2006) HNO—Operationslehre, 4th edn. Thieme, Stuttgart

5.4 Nasopharynx

VIKTOR BONKOWSKY

5.4.1 Evaluation of the Adenoids

The adenoid path in the child's nasopharynx is a normal structure with specific immunologic function. The size may vary from child to child. Respiratory infections affect the size of the adenoids.

Examination of the adenoids in children is generally difficult. In some cases fibre-optic nasoendoscopy may be possible. In a cooperative child, examination of the nasopharynx with a postnasal mirror may be performed.

Clinical symptoms are more important when evaluating the size of the adenoids. Nasal obstruction, snoring, sleep-related disorders, mouth breathing and hyponasal speech are most relevant.

5.4.2 Adenoidectomy

5.4.2.1 Indications

Adenoidectomy remains one of the most commonly performed surgical operations in the paediatric age group. The positive effect of adenoidectomy has been shown in improving the physical condition and quality of life in children with

1. Obstructive adenoid tissue
2. Recurrent and chronic rhinosinusitis
3. Otitis media with effusion

The value of adenoidectomy in recurrent acute otitis media and preventing abnormal craniofacial growth is constantly debated in the literature. It is also uncertain whether a "chronic adenoitis" exists.

5.4.2.2 Surgical Principles

- Traditionally the adenoids have been removed by curettage.
- The mouth gag is inserted to retract the tongue forward and open the mouth.
- The palate is inspected and palpated for evidence of a submucous cleft. The adenoids are inspected with a 70° endoscope or with a mirror.
- With use of a curette adenoid tissue can be removed.
- Haemostasis is achieved with armed swabs, only occasionally with bipolar coagulation.
- Counting of swabs before and after the operation is obligatory.

5.4.2.3 Complications

Postoperative bleeding may occur, although not as often as after tonsillectomy. Regrowth of adenoids is possible, which may require revision surgery. Other complications are nasopharyngeal stenosis, transient or persistent phelpharyngeal insufficiency and Eustachian tube injury

Diseases of the Larynx

Edited by Patrick J. Bradley

6.1 Anatomy and Physiology of the Larynx and Hypopharynx

CESARE PIAZZA, JOÃO CARLOS RIBEIRO, MANUEL BERNAL-SPREKELSEN, ANTÓNIO PAIVA, AND GIORGIO PERETTI

6.1.1 Anatomy of the Larynx

6.1.1.1 Generalities

The larynx is part of the respiratory system and is located at the upper level of the airway (Fig. 6.1.1). Because of its strategic and unique position, in relation to the crossover between the air and food passages, it is often referred to as part of the upper aerodigestive tract. It is also known as the organ of phonation, owing to special modifications of its anatomy during evolution that have rendered it able to produce voice. Indeed, from a physiologic point of view, it is essentially a valve or sphincter with a triple function: (1) that of an open valve in respiration; (2) that of a partially closed valve whose orifice can be modulated in phonation; (3) that of a closed valve, protecting the trachea and bronchial tree during deglutition.

The laryngeal cavity extends from the tip of the epiglottis down to the inferior border of the cricoid cartilage, where it continues into the trachea. It is placed in the visceral compartment of the neck, corresponding to the anterior cervical triangle delimited by the hyoid bone superiorly, the sternal notch inferiorly and the medial borders of each sternocleidomastoid muscle laterally. In the adult, it is located on the ventral side of the bodies of the fourth, the fifth and the sixth cervical vertebra (usually more cranially in women, and more caudally in men), whereas in the child it is usually positioned somewhat cranially, reaching the second cervical vertebra with its superior aspect at birth. In any case, the larynx is separated from the vertebral column by the dorsal wall of the oropharynx and hypopharynx. The position of this organ is influenced by movements of the head and neck and it also moves during deglutition and phonation. It is elevated when the head moves posteriorly (extension) and is depressed when the head is displaced anteriorly (flexion). This fact has profound clinical and surgical implications. The ideal position for every open-neck surgical procedure on the larynx, in fact, is the extended position, with the organ being stretched upward by the suprahyoid muscles, well above the sternal notch. By contrast, during microendoscopic laryngeal surgery, in the case of difficult exposure of the endolarynx (particularly when the anterior commissure must be accurately assessed or manipulated), the

flexed position is of help owing to detension of the prelaryngeal strap muscles and posteroinferior drop of the whole laryngopharyngeal complex. For the passage of the rigid laryngoscope, endotracheal tube or bronchoscope, it is also essential to know the position which brings the axes of the mouth, oropharynx and laryngeal inlet into line; this is achieved by bringing the neck forward (in a flexed position) and at the same time extending the head fully at the atlanto-occipital joint (Boyce–Jackson position).

6.1.1.2 Embryology

The respiratory system arises as an outgrowth of the digestive tract. In particular, the larynx develops from a two-part anlage: the supraglottis from the buccopharyngeal bud (fourth arch of the branchial system), and the glottis and subglottis from the tracheobronchial bud (fifth and sixth arches). This fact has a major impact in oncologic practice, where the glottic plane represents an embryologic barrier between the superior and the inferior lymphatic drainage.

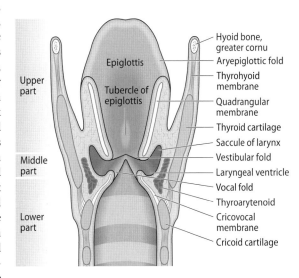

Fig. 6.1.1 Coronal section through the larynx and the cranial end of the trachea: posterior aspect

6.1.1.3   Supraglottis

The clinical term 'supraglottis' refers to that part of the larynx which lies above the glottis. It includes the laryngeal inlet, or aditus (the aperture between the larynx and the pharynx) (Fig. 6.1.2), the laryngeal ventricle (the space between the false and true vocal folds), the false vocal folds, the laryngeal (or posterior) surface of the epiglottis, the arytenoid cartilages and the laryngeal (or medial) aspects of the aryepiglottic folds.

The vestibular or false vocal folds are composed of the thickened lower border of the quadrangular membrane, covered by respiratory mucosa. The ventricle presents a fusiform, cranial recess which is called the 'saccule.' It is a pouch which ascends forwards from the ventricle, between the vestibular fold and the thyroid cartilage, and occasionally reaches the upper border of the cartilage. Laterally, the saccule is separated from the thyroid cartilage by the thyroepiglottic muscle, which compresses the saccule, expressing its secretion onto the vocal cords, which lack glands, to lubricate and protect them against desiccation and infection. Saccules occasionally protrude through the thyrohyoid membrane. Both the laryngeal ventricle and the saccule may on occasion become pathologically enlarged owing to obstruction of the ventricular aditus by inflammation, scarring or tumour. As the sealed cavity contains mucous glands, an expanding mucus-filled cyst is formed. This laryngocele may expand into the paraglottic space and extend superiorly to expand the aryepiglottic fold and reach the vallecula (internal laryngocele). Acute respiratory obstruction may result especially if the contents of the cyst become infected. The cyst may also expand through the thyrohyoid membrane at the point of entry of the internal laryngeal neurovascular bundle to appear as a lump in the neck overlying the thyrohyoid membrane (external laryngocele).

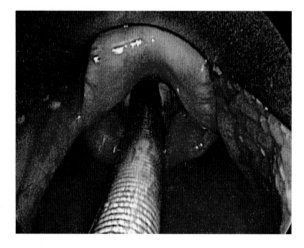

Fig. 6.1.2 Endoscopic view with a 0° rigid telescope of the laryngeal inlet, or aditus, under general anaesthesia

6.1.1.4   Glottis

The glottis includes the paired true vocal cords, the anterior and the posterior commissure, and the rima glottidis between them. The rima glottidis is the fissure between the vocal cords anteriorly and the arytenoid cartilages posteriorly. Its shape is roughly triangular during quiet breathing, widens to a pentagon with deep inspiration, and narrows to a slit during phonation and a Valsalva manoeuvre. It is bounded behind by the mucosa passing between the arytenoid cartilages at the level of the vocal cords. The rima glottidis is customarily divided into two regions: an anterior intermembranous part, which makes up about three fifths of its anteroposterior length and is formed by the underlying vocal ligament, and a posterior intercartilaginous part, which is formed by the vocal processes of the arytenoid cartilages. The average sagittal diameter of the glottis in the newborn is 0.7 cm, in the adult male is 23 mm and in the adult female is 17 mm. It is the narrowest part of the larynx and of the whole upper airway. Its width and shape vary with the movements of the vocal cords and arytenoid cartilages during respiration and phonation. During adduction (or closure) of the vocal cords, like in phonation or during a Valsalva manoeuvre, the rima glottidis becomes virtual, owing to the contact of the two vocal cords on the midline. During maximal abduction (or opening), like in deep breathing or sniffing, the rima glottidis reaches its maximum width (Fig. 6.1.3).

The free thickened upper edge of the cricovocal membrane forms the vocal ligaments. It stretches back on either side from the mid level of the thyroid angle to the vocal processes of the arytenoid cartilages. When it is covered by mucosa, it is termed the 'vocal cord'. The vocal cords form the anterolateral edges of the rima glottidis and are concerned with sound production. The complex microanatomy of the true vocal fold allows the loose and pliable superficial mucosal layers to vibrate freely over the stiffer structural underlayers. The mucosa overlying the vocal ligament is thin and lies directly on the vocal ligament, and so the vocal cord appears pearly white in vivo. It is loosely attached to the ligaments: oedema fluid readily collects in this potential space in disease. Known as Reinke's space, it extends along the length of the free margin of the vocal ligament and a little way onto the superior surface of the cord. The site where the vocal cords meet anteriorly is known as the anterior commissure (Fig. 6.1.4). Fibres of the vocal ligament pass here through the thyroid cartilage to blend with the overlying perichondrium, forming Broyles's ligament. Each vocal ligament is composed of a band of yellow elastic tissue related laterally to vocalis muscle.

The mucous membrane is loosely attached throughout the larynx and can accommodate considerable swelling, which may compromise the airway in acute infections. At the edge of the true vocal cords the mucosal covering is tightly bound to the underlying ligament, so oedema fluid does not pass between the upper and lower compartments of the vocal cord mucosa. Any tissue swelling above the vocal cord exaggerates the potential space deep to the mucosa (Reinke's space), causing accumulation of extracellular fluid and flabby swelling of the vocal cords (Reinke's oedema). Smoking and vocal abuse may initiate such changes.

Aberrant muscle balance during phonation may cause initial contact during vocal cord apposition to occur at a point at the junction of the anterior third and the posterior two thirds of the vocal ligament. Excessive trauma at this point, for example when singing with poor technique or forcing the voice, may produce subepithelial haemorrhage or bruising, and subsequent pathologic changes such as subepithelial scarring ('singer's nodes').

6.1.1.5   Subglottis

The subglottis extends from 1 cm below the free edge of the vocal cords to the lower border of the cricoid cartilage. Its walls are lined by respiratory mucosa, and are supported by the cricothyroid ligament above and the cricoid cartilage below. Prolonged intubation, trauma or inadequate endoscopic manoeuvres can ulcerate the mucosa and submucosa of this area, exposing the underlying cricoid cartilage to the risk of chondritis, chondronecrosis and subsequent circumferential scarring. This process is the base for the formation of subglottic and/or tracheal stenoses.

6.1.1.6   Skeletal Framework

The skeletal framework of the larynx is formed by a series of cartilages interconnected by ligaments and fibrous membranes (Figs. 6.1.5, 6.1.6), and moved by a number of muscles. The cartilaginous structures which form its framework are the epiglottis, thyroid cartilage, cricoid cartilage and arytenoid cartilages. The thyroid cartilage, cricoid cartilage and epiglottis are single cartilages, whereas the arytenoid cartilages are paired.

The larynx is slung from the U-shaped hyoid bone by the *thyrohyoid membrane* (*and ligaments*) and *thyrohyoid muscles*. The hyoid bone itself (the only bone of our body not connected to other bones through articular joints) is a U-shaped bone, open backwards and attached to the mandible and tongue by the suprahyoid muscles, namely the hyoglossus, mylohyoid, geniohyoid and digastric muscles, to the styloid process by the stylohyoid ligament and muscle, and to the pharynx by the middle constrictor. Three of the four strap muscles of the neck, the omohyoid, the sternohyoid and the thyrohyoid, find attachment to it, only the sternothyroid fails to gain it.

The *epiglottis* is a feather-shaped fibroelastic cartilage lying behind the root of the tongue. It is attached ante-

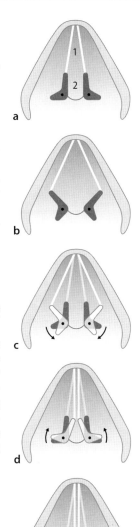

Fig. 6.1.3a–e Relation between the vocal cords and the arytenoid cartilages. **a** The position of the rima glottidis in quiet respiration. The intermembranous part of the rima glottidis seems triangular and the intercartilaginous part rectangular. **b** Forced inspiration. Both parts of the rima glottidis seem triangular. **c** Abduction of the vocal cords. The *arrows* show the movement of the abducted, retracted and laterally rotated arytenoid cartilages. Both parts of the rima glottidis seem triangular. **d** Adduction of the vocal cords. The *arrows* show the movement of the medially rotated arytenoid cartilages induced by the cricoarytenoid muscles. **e** Closure of the rima glottidis. The *arrows* show the movement induced by the transverse arytenoid muscles, without rotation of the arytenoid cartilages

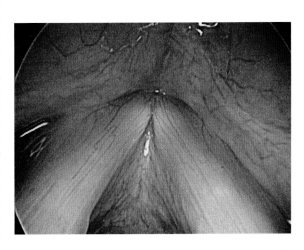

Fig. 6.1.4 Endoscopic view with a 70° rigid telescope of the anterior commissure under general anaesthesia

riorly to the body of the hyoid by the hyoepiglottic ligament and below to the back of the thyroid cartilage by the thyroepiglottic ligament, immediately above the vocal cords. Its sides are attached to the arytenoid cartilage by the aryepiglottic folds (containing the aryepiglottic muscle) which run backwards to form the margins of the vestibule, or *aditus*, of the larynx. Its free upper anterior surface projects above the hyoid bone (suprahyoid epiglottis) and is covered by mucosa (the epithelium is nonkeratinized, stratified, squamous), which is reflected onto the base of the tongue and the lateral pharyngeal walls as a median glossoepiglottic and two lateral glossoepiglottic folds. The depression on either side between these folds is the *glossoepiglottic vallecula*. The inferior half of the epiglottis (infrahyoid epiglottis) is the posterior boundary of the pre-epiglottic space, a fat-filled visceral space of the larynx, comprising the hyoepiglottic ligament above, the thyrohyoid ligament and upper half of the thyroid cartilage anteriorly, and the epiglottis itself with its thyroepiglottic ligament posteroinferiorly. In the sagittal plane the pre-epiglottic space is triangular in shape, whereas in the axial plane it has a U shape open backwards. Posterolaterally, the pre-epiglottic space communicates with the lateral paraglottic space, a fat-filled laryngeal visceral space that, on each side, comprises the thyroid ala and the vocal muscle at the glottic plane, and the quadrangular membrane at the level of the false vocal fold. Even though some subtle connective membranes have been microscopically observed at the junction between the pre-epiglottic and the lateral paraglottic spaces, some authors consider these as a unique anatomical entity. The major function of the epiglottis is to help prevent aspiration during swallowing. The epiglottis is displaced posteriorly by the tongue base retropulsion and laryngeal elevation. This causes the su-

perior free edge of the epiglottis to fall over the laryngeal inlet, which, in conjunction with sphincteric closure of the larynx at the supraglottic and glottic levels, closes off the laryngeal vestibule. The epiglottis is not essential for swallowing, which occurs with minimal aspiration even if this cartilage is destroyed by disease or removed by a surgical procedure as for supraglottic cancer excision, nor it is essential for respiration or phonation.

The *thyroid cartilage* is the largest of the laryngeal cartilages. It consists of two quadrilateral laminae whose anterior borders fuse along their inferior two thirds at a median angle (of approximately 90° in adult males, and 120° in women and children), forming the subcutaneous laryngeal prominence (Adam's apple). This projection is most distinct at its upper end, and is well marked in postpubertal men but is scarcely visible in children and women. Attached to each lamina posteriorly are the superior and inferior cornua. The superior cornua are attached to the greater horns of the hyoid bone by the thyrohyoid ligaments, found in the context of the thyrohyoid membrane. The inferior cornua form a synovial joint with the cricoid cartilage (the cricothyroid joint). At the junction of each superior cornu with its respective thyroid ala is a cartilaginous prominence, the superior tubercle. The superior tubercle is of significance because it marks the point 1 cm below which the superior laryngeal artery and nerve cross over the lamina to pierce the lateral aspect of the thyrohyoid membrane. The relationship of the internal laryngeal structures to the surface anatomy of the thyroid cartilage is important in surgical planning, for example when planning the placement of the window for thyroplasty or before cutting the thyroid cartilage transversally during open-neck horizontal supraglottic laryngectomy. The level of the vocal fold lies a

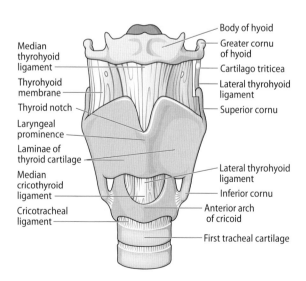

Fig. 6.1.5 Anterolateral view of the laryngeal cartilages and ligaments

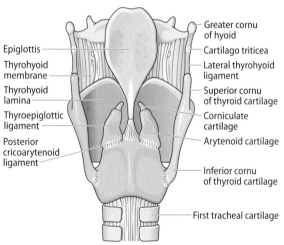

Fig. 6.1.6 Posterior view of the laryngeal cartilages and ligaments

little bit closer to the lower border of the thyroid cartilage lamina than to the upper border, more than at its exact midpoint.

The *cricoid cartilage* is attached inferiorly by the *cricotracheal membrane* to the trachea, and articulates with the thyroid cartilage and the two arytenoid cartilages by synovial joints. It is the only complete ring of cartilage throughout the respiratory tract. It is signet-ring-shaped, deepest behind. Its posterior part, also called 'cricoid plate', is covered by the posterior cricoarytenoid muscles and by the hypopharyngeal mucosa of the postcricoid area. The upper oesophageal sphincter is located at this level. The anterior portion of the cricoid cartilage, also called 'cricoid arch', is covered by the cricothyroid muscles. It represents the most important surgical landmark when emergency cricothyroidotomy is performed. The cricothyroid membrane represents the most superficial portion of the airway and the easiest point in it to gain access to it during an airway emergency, even without adequate surgical instrumentation and assistance. Owing to the anatomy of the airway, a congenital malformation of the cricoid cartilage may result in severe narrowing of the subglottic airway and respiratory obstruction.

The paired pyramidal *arytenoid cartilages* sit one on each side of the posterior 'signet' (or plate) of the cricoid cartilage. They have an upper projection covered by the corniculate cartilage, an anterior one called 'vocal process', made of elastic cartilage on which the vocal ligament and thyroarytenoid muscle are attached, and a posterolateral muscular process which allows insertion of the posterior and lateral cricoarytenoid muscles. Movements of the arytenoid cartilages on the underlying cricoid plate (made possible by the intrinsic laryngeal muscles and the cricoarytenoid joint) are reflected as movements of the vocal cords (essentially, adduction or closure and abduction or opening).

In addition to the above-mentioned major laryngeal cartilages, there are two paired cartilaginous nodules at the inlet of the larynx: the *corniculate cartilage*, lying at the apex of the arytenoid cartilage, and the *cuneiform cartilage*, a flake of cartilage within the margin of the aryepiglottic fold. These likely serve to provide additional structural support to the aryepiglottic folds.

The thyroid cartilage, cricoid cartilage and most of the arytenoid cartilages consist of hyaline cartilage and may therefore become calcified. This is a postpubertal process which initially involves the lower and posterior part of the thyroid cartilage, and subsequently spreads to involve the remaining cartilages. Calcification of the arytenoid cartilage starts at the base. The degree and frequency of calcification of the thyroid and cricoid cartilages appear to be less in females, in which the ossification process usually starts later in life. There is some evidence to suggest that a predilection for tumour invasion may be enhanced by calcification of the laryngeal cartilages. By contrast, the vocal processes of the arytenoid cartilage and the epiglottis are made of fibroelastic cartilage and never ossify during life.

6.1.1.7 Laryngeal Joints

The most important joints of the larynx are the cricoarytenoid and the cricothyroid. They are both diarthrodial joints with a capsule, a synovial lining and extracapsular ligaments. The cricoarytenoid joint is the primary moving structure of the intrinsic larynx. The arytenoid cartilages articulate with the cricoid cartilage, forming multiaxial joints (making possible at least three distinct arytenoid movements: sliding from posterior to anterior, rocking from lateral to medial, and twisting or rotation along a vertical axis perpendicular to the articular facet). The action of movement at the cricoarytenoid joints changes the distance between the vocal processes of the two arytenoid cartilages and between each vocal process and the anterior commissure. The combined action of the intrinsic laryngeal muscles on the arytenoid cartilages alters the position and shape of the vocal folds. Each cricoarytenoid joint sits at a 45° angle with the horizontal plane on the cricoid cartilage. Subluxation or frank luxation of this joint after laryngotracheal trauma or postintubation damage can cause ipsilateral vocal fold fixation, to be taken into account in the differential diagnosis of recurrent nerve palsy.

The cricothyroid joint is formed from the articulation of the inferior cornua of the thyroid cartilage with facets on the cricoid lamina. The two major actions at this joint are anteroposterior sliding and rotation of the inferior thyroid cornu upon the cricoid cartilage. Cricothyroid muscle contraction pulls the thyroid alae anteriorly with respect to the cricoid cartilage and closes the anterior visor angle between the thyroid and the cricoid arch. This motion increases the distance between the anterior commissure and the vocal processes of the arytenoid cartilages and serves to lengthen and tense the vocal folds. This joint can be manipulated to assist in pitch control in cases of paralytic dysphonia and to provide vocal fold tightening like in changing the voice in case of male to female transsexuals.

6.1.1.8 Soft Tissues

The skeletal framework of the larynx is interconnected by ligaments and fibrous membranes, of which the thyrohyoid, cricothyroid, cricotracheal, quadrangular and cricovocal (or conus elasticus) membranes are the most significant. The thyrohyoid, cricothyroid and cricotracheal membranes are external to the larynx, whereas the paired quadrangular and cricovocal membranes are internal. Inside the larynx are also found two ligaments: the hyoepiglottic and thyroepiglottic.

The cricovocal membrane connects the thyroid, cricoid and arytenoid cartilages. Its upper edge is attached anteriorly to the posterior surface of the thyroid cartilage and behind to the vocal process of the arytenoid cartilage. Between these two structures, the upper edge of the membrane is thickened slightly to form the *vocal ligament*. Anteriorly, the membrane thickens, as the *cricothyroid membrane*, easily felt subcutaneously at palpation.

The muscles of the larynx may be divided into intrinsic and extrinsic muscles. The intrinsic muscles are responsible for altering the length, tension, shape and spatial position of the vocal folds by changing the orientation of the muscular and vocal processes of the arytenoid cartilages with the fixed anterior commissure. As a result of these movements, the glottis is opened during inspiration, closed during phonation and closed with supraglottic reinforcement during deglutition. The intrinsic muscles are the cricothyroid, posterior and lateral cricoarytenoid, transverse and oblique interarytenoid, aryepiglottic, thyroarytenoid and its subsidiary part, vocalis, and thyroepiglottic muscles. The intrinsic laryngeal muscles may be placed in three groups according to their main actions: three major vocal fold adductors (thyroarytenoid, lateral cricoarytenoid, and interarytenoid muscles), one abductor (posterior cricoarytenoid muscles), and one tensor (cricothyroid muscle). The posterior and lateral cricoarytenoid muscles and oblique and transverse interarytenoid muscles vary the dimensions of the rima glottidis. The cricothyroid, posterior cricoarytenoid, thyroarytenoid and vocalis muscles regulate the tension of the vocal ligaments. The oblique interarytenoid, aryepiglottic and thyroepiglottic muscles modify the laryngeal inlet. Bilateral pairs of muscles usually act in concert with each other. The posterior cricoarytenoid muscle anatomy serves as a key landmark for arytenoid adduction surgery aimed at the closure of the posterior glottal chink after standard medialization thyroplasty.

The cricothyroid muscle is the only intrinsic laryngeal muscle of the larynx supplied by the external branch of the superior laryngeal nerve. The recurrent laryngeal nerve innervates all the other intrinsic muscles. All these muscles (both adductors and tensor) have a sphincter action; the only exception is represented by the abductor muscle, the posterior cricoarytenoid muscle, which, by rotating the arytenoid cartilages outwards, separates the vocal cords (Fig. 6.1.7).

The extrinsic muscles connect the larynx to neighbouring structures and are responsible for moving it vertically during phonation and swallowing. They include the infrahyoid strap muscles, i.e. thyrohyoid, sternothyroid, sternohyoid and omohyoid muscles, and the inferior constrictor muscle of the pharynx. The role of the extrinsic muscles during respiration appears variable. The larynx has been seen to rise, descend or barely move during inspiration. The extrinsic muscles can affect the tone and pitch of the voice by raising or lowering the larynx, and the geniohyoid muscle (together with the suprahyoid muscles, generally considered as part of the floor of the mouth) elevates and anteriorly displaces the larynx, particularly during deglutition.

6.1.1.9   Vascular Supply

The blood supply of the larynx is derived mainly from the superior and inferior laryngeal arteries arising, respectively, from the superior thyroid artery (branch of the external carotid artery) and the inferior thyroid artery (branch of the thyrocervical trunk, from the subclavian artery). The venous drainage passes superiorly via the superior thyroid vein to the internal jugular vein and inferiorly via the inferior thyroid vein to the brachiocephalic vein.

6.1.1.10   Lymphatic Drainage

The supraglottis has a rich, partly multilayered capillary lymphatic network, converging on the anterior insertion of the aryepiglottic fold and leaving the larynx in a small collections of vessels along the superior neurovascular pedicle of the larynx. Submucous and pre-epiglottic horizontal anastomoses have been found in the midline of the larynx and are responsible for bilateral and/or contralateral lymph node metastases, frequently observed in supraglottic carcinoma. The supraglottis drains to the upper deep cervical lymph nodes (levels IIA–III) and then to

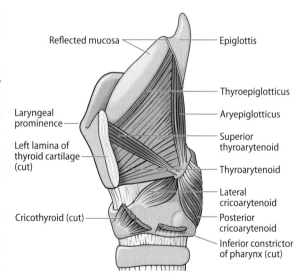

Fig. 6.1.7 Left lateral aspect of the muscles of the larynx

the mediastinal lymph nodes (level VI), some lymphatics passing via small nodes lying on the thyrohyoid membrane. Below the cords, drainage is to the lower deep cervical nodes (levels III–IV), partially via nodes on the front of the larynx and trachea (level VI), one of them rather constant and called the Delphian node, located in front of the cricothyroid or cricotracheal membranes. The vocal cords themselves act as a complete barrier separating the two lymphatic areas, even though posteriorly there is free communication between them. A laryngeal carcinoma may thus seed throughout the whole lymphatic drainage area of the larynx. The upper deep cervical lymph nodes act as pathways for spread of malignant tumours of the supraglottic larynx: up to 40% of these tumours will have undergone such spread at the time of clinical presentation. The glottis is very poorly endowed with lymphatic vessels, which means that 95% of malignant tumours confined to the glottis will cause a change in voice or airway obstruction but will not show clinical signs of spread to adjacent lymph nodes at presentation. The subglottic capillary network is not as dense as the supraglottic one, but its density is more than that observed at the level of the glottic plane. Tumours of the subglottic larynx will often spread to the chain of paratracheal and recurrent lymph nodes (level VI) prior to clinical presentation. Even in this laryngeal subsite, bilateral and contralateral metastatic spread are frequently encountered in the case of malignant tumours.

6.1.1.11 Nerve Supply

The nerve supply of the larynx is of great practical importance and comprises the superior and recurrent laryngeal nerves, branches of the vagus nerve (cranial nerve X).

The *superior laryngeal nerve* exits the vagus just below the nodose ganglion, and passes deep to the internal and external carotid arteries, where it divides. Its internal (sensory) branch pierces the thyrohyoid membrane together with the superior laryngeal vessels to supply the mucosa of the larynx down to the vocal cords. The external (motor) branch passes deep to the superior thyroid artery to supply the cricothyroid muscle. During thyroidectomy, ligation of the superior pedicle of the thyroid gland may pose at risk for the anatomical integrity of the external branch of the superior laryngeal nerve, thus causing some weakness of phonation owing to the loss of the tightening effect of the cricothyroid muscle on the cord. Selective ligation of every branch of the superior thyroid vessels when they enter the upper pole of the thyroid lobe allows avoidance of undue lesion to this nerve.

The *recurrent laryngeal nerves* have a different course on each side. The right nerve arises from the vagus as this crosses the front of the subclavian artery, passes deep to and behind this vessel then ascends behind the common carotid to lie in the tracheo-oesophageal groove accompanied by the inferior laryngeal vessels. The nerve then passes deep to the inferior constrictor muscle of the pharynx to enter the larynx behind the cricothyroid articulation. The left nerve arises on the arch of the aorta, winds below it, deep to the ligamentum arteriosum, and ascends to the trachea. It then lies in the tracheo-oesophageal groove and is distributed as on the right side. The recurrent laryngeal nerves supply all the ipsilateral intrinsic laryngeal muscles, apart from the cricothyroid muscle (supplied by the external branch of the superior laryngeal nerve), and the mucosa below the vocal cords (Fig. 6.1.8). The recurrent laryngeal nerves, at the level of the tracheo-oesophageal groove, are usually behind the terminal branches of the inferior thyroid artery. Occasionally, however, the nerve lies in front of these vessels or passes between them. Careful dissection (possibly with the aid of magnification by surgical loops) of the distal branches of the inferior thyroid artery, with attention paid to the preservation of the superior and inferior parathyroid vascularization (entirely depending on the inferior thyroid artery), allows identification of the recurrent laryngeal nerve. Proximal ligation of the inferior thyroid artery (as it emerges behind the common carotid artery) is technically easier, usually preserves the recurrent laryngeal nerve, but can cause permanent iatrogenic hypoparathyroidism. The left recurrent laryngeal nerve, in its thoracic course, may become involved in a bronchial or oesophageal carcinoma, or in a mass of enlarged mediastinal nodes, or may become stretched over

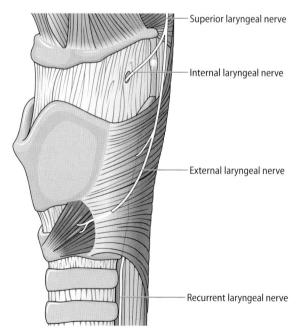

Superior laryngeal nerve

Internal laryngeal nerve

External laryngeal nerve

Recurrent laryngeal nerve

Fig. 6.1.8 Nerve supply to the larynx

an aneurysm of the aortic arch. The enlarged left atrium in advanced mitral stenosis may produce a recurrent laryngeal palsy by pushing up the left pulmonary artery, which compresses the nerve against the aortic arch. Either nerve, in the neck, may be damaged by an advanced thyroid carcinoma or malignant lymph nodes. For these reasons, loss of voice due to unilateral recurrent palsy must be always regarded as an ominous symptom requiring careful investigation of the entire course of the vagus and recurrent laryngeal nerves.

Unilateral complete palsy of the recurrent laryngeal nerve (more commonly on the left side owing to its increased length) leads to paralysis of all the laryngeal muscles on the affected side with the exception of the cricothyroid. The patient may be asymptomatic or have a hoarse, breathy voice. The hoarseness may be permanent or may become less severe with time as the opposite cord develops the ability to hyperadduct and appose the paralysed cord and thus close the glottis during phonation and coughing. Clinically, the position of the vocal cord in the acute phase after section of the recurrent laryngeal nerve is very variable. Stridor is more common after bilateral lesions but by no means does it represent the rule; indeed the cords may be sufficiently abducted for there to be little problem with airway obstruction. With great surprise for beginners, bilateral vocal cord palsy is usually associated with a better quality of voice than unilateral vocal cord dysfunction, owing to the tendency of the vocal cords to assume an adducted position which allows a relatively good (but static) glottic closure. Even food inhalation and liquid inhalation are exceptional after bilateral vocal cord palsy, but are sometimes observed in unilateral paralysis (particularly in the presence of a vagal lesion with simultaneous impairment of the superior and inferior laryngeal nerves).

6.1.1.12   Histology

The laryngeal epithelium is mainly a ciliated, pseudostratified respiratory epithelium where it covers the inner aspects of the larynx, including the posterior surface of the epiglottis, and it provides a ciliary clearance mechanism shared with most of the respiratory tract. However, the vocal cords are covered by non-keratinized, stratified squamous epithelium, an important variation which protects the tissue from the effects of the considerable mechanical stresses acting on the surfaces of the vocal cords during phonation, deglutition and coughing. The highly specialized functions of the vocal cords explain their peculiar anatomical microstructure. Deep to the epithelium, a stratified arrangement of connective tissue allows the mucosa to vibrate upon the underlying vocal ligament and muscle. Below the epithelial basal membrane, the superficial layer of the lamina propria (the so-called Reinke

space) is loosely arranged with collagen and elastic fibres that allows a uniform and optimal sharing of the forces produced during epithelium vibration, thus reducing to a minimum the impedance to vibration. The intermediate and deep layers of the lamina propria are denser and more compact, formed by highly concentrated and thicker collagen bundles. The intermediate and deep layers of the lamina propria together constitute the vocal ligament. The vocal ligament and the underlying vocal muscle form the body of the vocal cord, whereas the epithelium represents the cover (body-cover theory). The cover vibrates on the underlying body thanks to the presence of Reinke's space. Moreover, an elastic gradient is provided to the vocal cords even in the anterior–posterior direction. In fact, lamina propria is thickened at the two ends of the membranous vocal cord, forming the anterior and posterior maculae flavae. These structures are mainly formed by elastic fibres. They cushion the vocal folds and provide extra strength at regions of maximal stress, those of connection of the vocal ligament to the anterior commissure of the thyroid cartilage anteriorly and to the vocal process of the arytenoid cartilage posteriorly. Moreover, maculae flavae generate connective tissue such as collagen and elastin in the lamina propria.

The exterior surfaces of the larynx which merge with the hypopharynx and oropharynx (including the anterior surface of the epiglottis) are also subject to the abrasive effects of swallowed food, and are therefore covered by non-keratinized stratified squamous epithelium. The laryngeal mucosa has numerous mucous glands, especially over the epiglottis, where they pit the cartilage, and along the margins of the aryepiglottic folds anterior to the arytenoid cartilages, where they are known as the arytenoid glands. Many large glands in the saccules of the larynx secrete periodically over the vocal cords during phonation. The free edges of these folds are devoid of glands and their stratified epithelium is vulnerable to drying, thus requiring the secretions of neighbouring glands. Hoarseness due to excessive speaking is due to partial temporary failure of this secretion. Taste buds, like those in the tongue, occur on the posterior epiglottic surface, aryepiglottic folds and less often in other laryngeal regions.

6.1.2   Anatomy of the Hypopharynx

6.1.2.1   Generalities

The hypopharynx (or laryngopharynx) is the lowermost portion of the pharynx and, in the craniocaudal direction, it follows the rhinopharynx and the oropharynx. It is part of the digestive tract, but it has strict anatomical, functional and pathologic relationships with the larynx. The hypopharynx is a 5-cm-long cone-shaped tube, wide superiorly (about 4 cm) and rapidly narrowing in the post-cricoid and cervical oesophagus area (1.5 cm). It extends from the tip of the epiglottis superiorly to the inferior edge of the cricoid cartilage. Anteriorly it communicates with the larynx which, in fact, is posterolaterally surrounded by the two funnel-shaped piriform sinuses and by the postcricoid area. The hypopharynx is anteriorly limited by the marginal structures of the laryngeal inlet and the posterior surface of the larynx; superiorly it is continuous with the oropharynx. Laterally it is separated from the common carotid artery, the internal jugular vein and the vagus nerve by the inferior constrictor muscles and the piriform sinus (bounded medially by the aryepiglottic fold and laterally by the internal surface of the thyroid ala and the thyrohyoid membrane), a pair of spaces with the shape of upside-down pears, with the apex (or stem of the pear) located inferiorly, at the level of the inferior limit of the cricoid cartilage, and the superior border corresponding to the pharyngoepiglottic fold (Fig. 6.1.9). Posteriorly the constrictor muscles separate the hypopharynx from the prevertebral fascia and the bodies of the third to the sixth cervical vertebra. Inferiorly the hypopharynx opens into the oesophagus at the level of the upper oesophageal sphincter. The piriform sinuses on each side, the posterior pharyngeal wall and the postcricoid region form the three designated anatomical sites within the hypopharynx. Their boundaries, however, overlap and their demarcation is somewhat arbitrary.

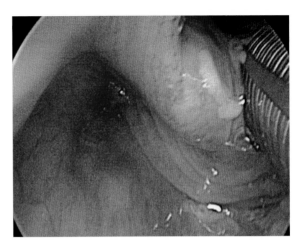

Fig. 6.1.9 Endoscopic view with a 70° rigid telescope of the left piriform sinus under general anaesthesia

6.1.2.2 Soft Tissues

The hypopharynx is essentially a muscular tube (whose epithelial lining consists of non-keratinized stratified squamous epithelium, whereas the lamina propria of mucosa contains scattered lymphoid aggregates and mucoserous glands) with strict relationships with some of the components of the cartilaginous laryngeal framework previously described, particularly the thyroid and cricoid cartilages. The funnel-shaped muscular segments forming the entire pharyngeal tube are overlapped at their lower end by the segment below, even though all segments are inserted posteriorly into a tendinous median raphe. The inferior constrictor muscle is divided into a superior thyropharyngeal part (inserting on the thyroid lamina at the level of the oblique line) and an inferior cricopharyngeal one (inserted at the junction between the cricoid arch and plate). The cricopharyngeus muscle encircles the hypopharynx more or less in an axial plane, in contradistinction to the angulated course of the fibres of the other constrictors. It does not have a posterior midline raphe, therefore being continuous from its left to right sides. The cricopharyngeus muscle is the major component of the upper oesophageal constrictor and, with its tonic contraction, maintains a constant level of closing pressure,

approximating the pharynx to the cricoid plate. During swallowing, the cricopharyngeus muscle relaxes, thus permitting passage of the bolus from the hypopharynx to the cervical oesophagus. On the posterior midline of the inferior end of the hypopharynx, a triangular dehiscence (known as Killian's triangle) comprises the superior oblique muscle fibres of the thyropharyngeus muscle and the inferior horizontal ones of the cricopharyngeus muscle. A pharyngoesophageal pouch (or Zenker's diverticulum) may develop at this weak point owing to abnormal pressure during swallowing for altered function of the upper oesophageal sphincter.

The craniocaudal movements of the hypopharynx are made possible by the presence of three paired muscles (stylopharyngeus, salpingopharyngeus and palatopharyngeus) radiating into the pharyngeal wall from outside at the level of the oropharynx. Even the stylohyoid and styloglossus muscles are responsible for pharyngeal elevation during swallowing. On the other hand, a true intrinsic longitudinal muscle in the hypopharynx does not exist and only begins at the level of the upper oesophageal sphincter. Surrounding the hypopharynx, the parapharyngeal and retropharyngeal spaces, filled with loose areolar connective tissue, allows this organ to freely move with respect to the fascia overlying the prevertebral muscles, vertebral column and adjacent tissues.

6.1.2.3 Vascular Supply

The hypopharynx receives arterial branches from the ascending pharyngeal artery (branch of the external carotid artery) and the superior and inferior thyroid arteries. The venous drainage is accomplished by a number of small venous vessels forming a submucosal plexus and draining into the mid and distal portion of the internal jugular vein.

6.1.2.4 Lymphatic Drainage

The hypopharynx has a quite rich mucosal and submucosal lymphatic capillary network, explaining the high propensity of tumours of this organ to precociously metastatize to adjacent lymph nodes. This is either via an inconstant retropharyngeal lymph node (Rouvier's node) and then to the deep middle and lower jugular lymph nodes (levels III–IV) or directly to the latter group. The piriform sinuses and postcricoid area also drain to the recurrent or paratracheal lymph nodes (level VI), thus gaining a connection to the lymphatic system of the thoracic cavity.

6.1.2.5 Nerve Supply

A number of branches leave the vagus nerve in the midportion of the neck, cranially to the emergence of the superior laryngeal nerve, to innervate the pharyngeal musculature. These branches arborize and intercommunicate with branches of the glossopaharyngeal nerve to form a plexus enveloping the constrictor musculature of the pharynx. This plexus, along with additional contributions from the vagus nerve, continues along the oesophagus and into the remainder of the alimentary tract. Disruption of this plexus or its contribution from the vagus nerve has a deleterious effect on the constrictor activity and sensation of the pharyngeal musculature and mucosa, with ensuing deterioration of the swallowing function.

6.1.3 Physiology of the Larynx and Hypopharynx

During respiration at rest, the laryngeal valve is open (abducted position of the vocal cords) and the air comes in and out through its lumen without an active participation of the larynx in the process itself. During high-volume respiration, the glottis is actively abducted and tensed thanks to the contraction of the posterior cricoarytenoid and cricothyroid muscles. In this way, the cross-sectional area of the glottic plane is considerably widened and the resistance to the airflow reduced.

The human larynx, when acting as a sphincter or closed valve, does a lot more than protect the airway. It comprises several important reflexes for protection of the airway against external stimuli and foreign bodies (glottic closure reflex). These reflex mechanisms are relayed by the mucosal (sensory afferent), myotatic and articular receptors of the larynx via both the superior and the recurrent laryngeal nerves. The strongest of the laryngeal reflexes is that of laryngospasm (a response to mechanical stimulation). Other reflexes include those producing cough, apnoea, bradycardia and hypotension. The glottic closure reflex is one of the most crucial events during swallowing. It is reinforced by supraglottic closure of the epiglottis (thanks to retropulsion of the base of the tongue and laryngohypopharyngeal elevation), and adduction of the false vocal folds and aryepiglottic folds. Simultaneous mediolateral and craniocaudal squeezing of the hypopharyngeal muscular tube allows a bolus to enter the postcricoid area. The relaxation of the cricopharyngeus muscle transmits the bolus to the cervical oesophagus. After its passage, the cricopharyngeus muscle comes back to its tonic closure, thus avoiding retrograde regurgitation of the bolus. At this time, the vocal cords are abducted again. An effective glottic closure is also needed to produce an adequate Valsalva manoeuvre, essential in a number of different physiologic functions such as defecation, urination, parturition, coughing, weight lifting and jumping.

Sound production requires that several mechanical properties be met. There must be adequate breath support to produce sufficient subglottic pressure. There must also be adequate control of the laryngeal musculature to produce not only glottic closure, but also the proper length and tension of the vocal folds. Finally, there must be favourable pliability and vibratory capacity of the tissues of the vocal folds. Once these conditions are met, sound is generated from vocal fold vibration. The detailed contribution, timing and recruitment of each of the above-described laryngeal muscles in the production of sound have been studied. The intrinsic laryngeal muscles are not only highly specialized for their particular vector of action, but they are also controlled for the timing of the onset of contraction, and the degree of recruitment and fade during phonation. Actual phonation is a complex and specialized process that involves not only brainstem reflexes and the muscular actions described above, but high-level cortical control as well. Accessory effects such as lung capacity, chest wall compliance, pharyngeal, nasal, and oral anatomy and subsequent mental status also play a role. The process begins with inhalation and subsequent glottal closure. An increase in subglottic pressure follows until the pressure overcomes the glottal closure force and air is allowed to escape between the vocal folds. Once air passes between the vocal folds, the body-cover concept of phonation takes effect. The body-cover theory describes the wavelike motion of the loose mucosa of the vocal folds over the stiffer, more densely organized vocal ligament and vocalis muscle. This motion is known as the mucosal wave. The wave begins infraglottically and is propagated upward to the free edge of the vocal fold and then laterally over the superior surface. Eventually, the inferior edges become reapproximated owing to both a drop in pressure at the open glottis and the elastic recoil of the tissues themselves. The closure phase is also propagated rostrally. With the vocal folds fully approximated, subglottic pressure may again build and the cycle is repeated.

Suggested Reading

1. Armstrong WB, Netterville JL (1995) Anatomy of the larynx, trachea, and bronchi. Otolaryngol Clin N Am 28:685–99

2. Berkovitz BKB, Moxham BJ, Hickey S (2000) The anatomy of the larynx. In: Ferlito A (ed) Diseases of the larynx. Chapman and Hall. London, pp 25–44

3. Dorland NW (2003) Dorland's illustrated medical dictionary, 30th edn. Saunders Philadelphia

4. International Anatomical Nomenclature Committee (1989) Nomina anatomica, 6th edn. Churchill Livingstone, New York

5. Shah J (2003) Head and neck surgery and oncology, 3rd edn. Mosby, Edinburgh

6. Standring S, Ellis H, Berkovitz BKB (2005) Larynx. In: Standring S, Ellis H, Berkovitz BKB (eds) Gray's anatomy: the anatomical basis of clinical practice, 39th edn. Elsevier, Philadelphia, pp 633–646

6.2 Office Examination

CHRISTIAN SITTEL

6.2.1 Office Examination and Laryngoscopy

6.2.1.1 Definition

Office examination and laryngoscopy are tools for the initial evaluation of a patient with a complaint referable to the larynx on an outpatient basis using a minimal amount of equipment. They can be used by any otolaryngologist or motivated physician having acquired these skills. With use of indirect techniques, the following structures can usually be visualized: base of tongue, lingual and laryngeal surface of the epiglottis, aryepiglottic folds, arytenoid prominences, true and false vocal cords. The postcricoid part of the hypopharynx and the piriform sinuses are not subject to examination using indirect techniques.

6.2.1.2 Examination

Any patient with a laryngeal complaint warrants a complete examination of the head and neck including otoscopy, rhinoscopy, inspection of the oral cavity, oropharynx and nasopharynx and palpation of the neck. The larynx is palpated by moving it lateral over the anterior vertebral bodies, producing normal laryngeal crepitus. Palpation during swallowing allows an appreciation of the laryngeal excursion in deglutition. The thyroid lobes can be assessed by palpating them along either side of the trachea just below the larynx.

6.2.1.3 Laryngoscopy

Mirror Examination

Since its presentation by Manuel Garcia in 1855, this procedure has changed little. The equipment required is minimal and consists of a headlight (alternatively a head mirror and an external light source) and a laryngeal mirror. The patient sits facing the examiner with a straight back, leaning slightly forward at the waist. The laryngeal mirror is warmed and tested for temperature on the back of the hand. The patient's tongue is grasped using a gauze, and the back of the mirror is used to elevate the uvula. With the light focused on the mirror, the supraglottic and glottic structures can be visualized. The patient is then asked to vocalize a sustained *e*, thus tilting the epiglottis forward and bringing the vocal folds into apposition.

Endoscopic Examination

Indirect laryngoscopy using rigid or flexible endoscopes provides superior visualization of endolaryngeal structures, requires less compliance and facilitates documentation; therefore, endoscopic examination is the routine standard of larynx examination in Europe today.

Rigid telescopes are available with a 90° or 70° angled lens at the tip. For optimal optical quality a diameter of 9 mm should be chosen; for children smaller instruments down to 2.6-mm diameter should be at hand. The technique of the procedure is identical to that of the indirect mirror examination. Though it is performed more easily, it still requires patient cooperation. When applicable, indirect laryngoscopy using rigid endoscopes offers image quality superior to that of any other modality, making it the best option for documentation purposes.

Flexible fibre-optic laryngoscopy offers the advantage of being feasible in non-compliant populations such as small children and seriously ill, demented or psychiatric patients. In patients who are not able to tolerate the aforementioned techniques owing to gagging, flexible endoscopy is usually possible. There is a wide variety of instruments available. In general, a fibre-optic endoscope for diagnostic purposes should not be longer than 30 cm. There should be no additional channel for suctioning to facilitate disinfection. A separate high-intensity light source is necessary. After the patient's nose has been decongested and anaesthetized, the tip of the instrument is passed along the floor of the nose under permanent visualization into the nasopharynx. The patient is asked to breathe through the nose and the endoscope is angled downwards, until the base of the tongue and the supraglottic and glottic structures are visualized. Passing the glottis to investigate the subglottic region may elicit laryngospasm and must be performed only in a setting where medically trained assistance personnel and intubation equipment are readily available.

6.2.2.1   Definition

Laryngeal electromyography (LEMG) comprises a set of electrophysiological procedures for diagnosis, prognosis and treatment of laryngeal movement disorders, including laryngeal dystonias, vocal fold paralysis and other neurolaryngological disorders. It is performed by otolaryngologists, often in collaboration with a neurologist. LEMG requires special skills and equipment as well as considerable experience, although no formal training exists for the laryngeal electromyographer. LEMG may provide useful information that cannot be obtained by other techniques, but still is not available as a routine examination in every ENT department in Europe.

6.2.2.2   Technique

Electromyography evaluates the integrity of the motor system by recording action potentials generated in the muscle fibres. Principally, all five major laryngeal muscles (thyroarytenoid muscle, lateral cricoarytenoid muscle, posterior cricoarytenoid muscle, interarytenoid muscle, cricothyroid muscle) lend themselves to electrophysiological examination, with the thyroarytenoid muscle being investigated most frequently. This muscle may be approached in the awake patient either transcutaneously or transorally. For the transcutaneous approach, bipolar concentric needle electrodes are passed through the cricothyroid membrane, then the tip of the needle is angled to the affected side laterally and superiorly 30–45°. If the patient coughs, which indicates penetration of the airway space, the needle is withdrawn and repositioned. Increase of LEMG activity while the patient is phonating validates correct electrode position. If no muscle activity is detectable, electrode displacement cannot be discriminated from complete vocal fold paralysis using the transcutaneous technique.

For transoral LEMG, bipolar hooked-wire electrodes are available. The hooks at the end of these thin flexible wires act as barbs, keeping the electrode in place once it has been positioned in the muscle. Electrodes are positioned using a special device for application, which is inserted into the endolarynx under endoscopic guidance with the needle tip being secured in the applicator. Surface anaesthesia of the oropharynx and endolarynx prior to the procedure is mandatory. When the applicator is positioned correctly above the mediodorsal aspect of the vocal fold, the tip of the needle is pushed into the thyroarytenoid muscle. Owing to the hooks at the distal end of the wire, the electrode remains in position when the applicator is withdrawn. Although this technique allows better control over electrode position, it is more time-consuming, significantly more expensive and technically more difficult.

LEMG recordings are made visible on a monitor and are made audible through a loudspeaker. The findings are characterized as normal silent resting potential, voluntary motor unit potential, spontaneous fibrillation potential and polyphasic reinnervation potential. The absence of any electrical activity either on electrode insertion or on attempted voluntary motion is called 'electrical silence'. Normal voluntary action potentials are diphasic or triphasic and are extremely variable in amplitude. Spontaneous fibrillation activity is defined as involuntary potential generated by a single muscle fibre, indicating axonal degeneration; however, this symptom of degeneration does not appear earlier than 10–14 days after injury. Polyphasic motor units have four or more phases and herald nerve regeneration.

6.2.2.3   Clinical Applications

LEMG has been shown to be useful for localizing the thyroarytenoid muscle for transcutaneous injection of botulinum toxin A in the treatment of spasmodic dysphonia. Electrophysiological examinations of the larynx offer the only option to differentiate vocal fold paresis and paralysis from mechanical fixation. With limitations, LEMG is useful for the assessment of prognosis of vocal fold paresis and paralysis. Furthermore, LEMG may be helpful in diagnosis and evaluation of diseases affecting the neuromuscular junction or systemic neuropathic and myopathic disorders involving the larynx.

Suggested Reading

1.   Sataloff RT, Mandel S, Mann EA, Ludlow CL (2004) Practice parameter: laryngeal electromyography (an evidence-based review). J Voice 18: 261–274
2.   Munin MC, Murry T, Rosen CA (2000) Laryngeal electromyography. Otolaryngol Clin North Am 33: 759–770

6.3 Inflammatory Diseases and Lasers

MARC REMACLE

6.3.1 Inflammatory Diseases

6.3.1.1 Definition

The term "laryngitis" does not refer to a specific disease but rather to an inflammation of the larynx arising from any given cause.

6.3.1.2 Aetiology

The most frequent causes are:
* Infection
* Voice misuse or overuse
* Gastro-oesophageal reflux

Laryngitis is often multifactorial and more than one of these causes can be identified.

Among other potential causes, we find:
* Allergies
* Acute or chronic rhinosinus infections
* Vomiting
* Aspiration
* Irritation due to inhalation

Infection

In adults infection may be:
1. Viral: Adult infection of the larynx is most often of viral origin, accompanied by general malaise and/or fever. The symptoms are dysphonia, coughing and the sensation of globus. Herpetic laryngitis, which occurs most often in immune-depressed subjects, is characterized by vesicles or painful ulceration of the larynx.
2. Bacterial: Bacterial laryngitis is the usual complication of a viral laryngitis. The most common germs are streptococcus, staphylococcus, pneumococcus and type B *Haemophilus influenzae*. The laryngitis may be pseudomembranous and, if associated with tracheitis, mimics diphtheria.
   Epiglottitis affects one adult in 100,000 per annum. It affects the entire supraglottic area. It develops less rapidly than in children. The cherry-red swollen epiglottis, like a "thumb sign", leads to dysphagia, pain and

increased temperature. The voice has that "hot potato" quality. This dyspnoea is not systematic, but represents a serious factor. Diagnosis is based on nasopharyngeal fibroscopy. In fact it corresponds to a septicaemia of type B *Haemophilus influenzae*, whose origin is to be found in the subglottic region.
3. Mycotic
   - Candidosis: Laryngitis candidosis is caused by:
     * Steroids
     * Wide-spectrum antibiotics
     * Diabetes
     * Alcohol
     * Prolonged intubation
     * Caustic or infectious irritation of the larynx
     * Immunodepression
   Inhaled steroids cause superficial candidosis, which can be recognized by an erythematic larynx and a pale, friable exudate. On the other hand, in cases of immunosuppression or acquired immunodeficiency (AIDS), we observe invasive forms involving neighbouring organs, septicaemia, bleeding and obstruction of the larynx.
   - Aspergillosis: The severity of the attack depends on immunocompetence. It may mimic a laryngeal carcinoma.
   - Other very rare mycoses: Blastomycosis, histoplasmosis, coccidioidomycosis and sporotrichosis.
3. Tuberculosis: This has been on the increase for the last 20 years and is provoked by the tuberculosis mycobacterium (Koch's bacillus). It generally occurs as a condition secondary to a pulmonary infection. Infected secretions from the lung contaminate the larynx, or the bacterium may pass through the blood system. The pulmonary infection may pass unnoticed. Clinical appearance is highly varied. We may observe simple hyperhaemia, monocorditis, exudative oedema of the vocal cords or an ulceration of different parts of the larynx. Tuberculosis may mimic laryngeal cancer, for which it forms part of the differential diagnosis.
4. Syphilis: Laryngeal localizations of syphilis are both rare and highly polymorphic. It is caused by *Treponema pallidum*.
5. AIDS: This opens the door to specific infections of the larynx, incurring, among other things, the return of both tuberculosis and syphilis.

In children infection may be:

1. Viral
   - Acute oedematous subglottic laryngitis: This is the most frequent type of acute dyspnoeic laryngitis. It occurs in children from 1 to 3 years of age. The viruses that cause it are myxovirus, parainfluenza viruses 1 and 3, rhinovirus, adenovirus and echovirus. One may also find the respiratory syncytial virus in babies. Bacterial origin is rare.

     Above all, viral infection is observed in autumn and winter, although it may occur at any time of the year with the emergence of a local epidemic. The context of febrile rhinopharyngitis may be missing. The diagnosis is clinical. Dyspnoea will often occur at night. Inspiratory bradypnoea and dyspnoea are accompanied by crowing. Coughing will be raucous and barking. The voice is normal or somewhat deeper. Swallowing is normal. General health is maintained. Temperature is moderate, around 38°C. Treatment should be started as soon as possible. It is based, for example, on oral corticotherapy with betamethasone, at a dose of 0.3 mg/kg. It should be carried out over several days and may be repeated after 30 min if symptoms persist. Urgent hospitalization is recommended if there is no rapid improvement, as emergency intubation or tracheotomy may be necessary. Relapse is frequent, though of diminishing gravity. Factors such as gastro-oesophageal reflux, allergies and adenoiditis should be avoided.
   - Stridulous or spasmodic laryngitis: This is the least serious type. Its function is still poorly known. The causes are probably various: reflux, allergy, inflammation and psychological influences. It occurs in short crises of dyspnoeic laryngitis, mostly nocturnal. It may be accompanied by a suffocating cough with cyanosis. Spontaneously resolving within a few minutes, such a bout never exceeds 1 h. Relapse is frequent. Oral corticotherapy may be used (betamethasone, 0.125 mg/kg per day) for a few days accompanied by a humidifier in the bedroom. It may accompany enanthemata, measles or chicken pox. It should therefore be considered a serious sign.

2. Bacterial
   - Epiglottitis or subglottic laryngitis: As in adults, this is largely provoked by type B *Haemophilus influenzae* and results in an inflammation, not only of the glottis, but also of the entire subglottic larynx. Treatment has been markedly improved since the commercialization of the vaccine in 1992. One should, however, not ignore it, since a delay in diagnosis can have serious consequences.

     It primarily affects children between 3 and 6 years of age and follows a bout of rhinopharyngitis. Dyspnoea and a sensation of stretching are quickly very noticeable. The child spontaneously takes up a seated position with the head forward. The mouth falls open to allow the saliva that is too difficult to swallow to dribble out. The voice has a muffled quality. The child is often ill at ease and anxious, with a general disposition very different from the normal. This is an indication for urgent hospitalization. Only an ENT specialist in a hospital environment can carry out transnasal fibroscopy. Intubation is indicated. This is a difficult procedure, which can also only be carried out by an anaesthetist familiar with paediatric endoscopy. Steroids are of little effect on their own. Intravenous antibiotherapy effective against *Haemophilus influenzae* is administered, such as cefotaxime (Claforan), 200 mg/kg per day.
   - Bacterial laryngotracheobronchitis, called "pseudomembranous", is rare but serious. It is provoked by staphylococcus, *Haemophilus influenzae*, streptococcus and *Branhamella catarrhalis*. When complicating an otherwise banal subglottic laryngitis, it adds a septic table and dyspnoea by obstructing the larynx and trachea with pseudomembranes. Diagnosis can be pronounced after endoscopy. It is sometimes necessary to remove the pseudomembranes, but this is not an act without implications, since it may be accompanied by bleeding or even toxic shock as germs are mobilized. At any rate, the reappearance of these is a general rule.

     Intubation and antibiotherapy based on oral smears taken together with the endoscopy are indispensable until healing is complete.
   - Specific infectious laryngitis: Diphtheric laryngitis is extremely rare nowadays, though one should keep it in mind in the case of children of migrant communities. It is caused by the diphtheria corynebacterium. It is characterized by
     - Weakness
     - Generally altered state
     - Tachycardia
     - Rough cough
     - Smothered voice
   - Pseudomembranous laryngitis: Measles affects young children from the age of 1 year and occurs as dyspnoea, which is induced by an ulceronecrotic and pseudomembranous laryngitis.

Allergy

The dilation of vessels and increase in capillary permeability through the effect of histamine causes an inflammation of the laryngeal mucosa. Exposure to inhaled allergens may trigger laryngeal oedema. This is generally of a minor nature, with light hoarseness and a sensation of scratchiness in the throat.

Nasal obstruction due to allergic rhinitis also provokes buccal breathing with resultant dryness of the vocal cords and the pharyngeal mucosa. The severity of the inflammation may even lead to an obstruction of the larynx. Among the factors, the following are also found:

- Foodstuffs
- Medications: conversion enzyme inhibitors, anti-inflammatory non-steroids, aspirin and penicillin
- Insect bites and stings

Angioneurotic oedema, or Quincke's oedema, corresponds to a sudden swelling of the face and neck, which represents a danger to the larynx area.

A hereditary variant exists which is transmitted by an autosomic dominant mode. The resultant deficit in C1 esterase is responsible for its liberation in vasodilating polypeptides. Treatment is based on oxygenation, epinephrine, steroids and antihistamines. Androgenic derivatives, such as danazol, increase the level of C1 esterase to constitute a prophylactic treatment.

Toxic Inhalation

The inhalation of toxic vapours may irritate the larynx and chronic exposure may lead to metaplasia. It is suspected that chronic exposure may induce cancers. However, there are few studies in the literature explaining acute reactions to specific toxins and how to deal with the problem. From the clinical point of view, diagnosis is considered evident if the laryngitis can be linked to a specific exposure. Any patient presenting with a laryngitis of obscure cause should be questioned on their professional or environmental exposure to inhaled toxins.

Reflux

Laryngopharyngeal reflux is a common cause of non-infectious laryngitis. Symptomatology and mechanisms are different from those for oesophagitis and gastro-oesophageal reflux. Since the oesophageal mucosa is most often intact, the patient with a secondary laryngitis with reflux will not complain of pyrosis, belching or regurgitation. The reflux often occurs when standing up. Symptomatology consists of a cough, dysphonia, throat clearing and, occasionally, dysphagia. In cases of nocturnal reflux, patients tell of awaking with a bad taste in the mouth and a sensation of having an obstruction in the throat. This symptom is induced by too heavy meals, taken too late in the evening and accompanied by alcohol consumption. Dysphonia is exacerbated by microtraumatism caused by the voice effort.

The clinical signs are to be found, above all, at the posterior part of the larynx with oedema of the arytenoids and posterior commissure with secretions. Significant acid reflux can lead to an ulceration of the mucosa and granuloma.

pH-metry with a double probe remains the examination method of choice. It may, however, give negative findings, owing to the intermittent nature of the reflux, or laryngeal lesions may be induced by reflux with a pH value higher than that responsible for an oesophagitis.

In borderline cases, a test treatment with a proton pump inhibitor can be proposed, possibly associated with a prokinetic drug.

Voice Misuse

Misuse or overuse of the voice (muscle tension dysphonia) may cause laryngitis. Shouting and loud singing involving high intraglottic pressure may result in a traumatic laryngitis. Above all, such pressure bears upon the posterior part of the glottis where the mucosa rests directly on the arytenoid cartilage. Oedema at this point inhibits correct closure of the vocal cords, with a resulting breathiness. The patient will generally try to compensate for this by increasing the pressure, which further exacerbates the oedema. The swelling at the posterior part of the larynx is felt as an obstruction, leading to frequent attempts to "clear" the throat. In short, a vicious circle of vocal overuse develops.

Systemic Diseases

The larynx may be affected by certain systemic, idiopathic, inflammatory diseases:

- Rheumatoid arthritis affects the larynx in 30% of cases, causing, in its acute phase, laryngeal congestion and oedema. Chronic arthritis results in a loss of mobility caused by fibrosis, with occasional rheumatoid nodules. Treatment is medical. The nodules are operated on if they cause dysphonia. Ankylosis of the vocal cords may require tracheotomy or endoscopic enlargement at the level of the posterior part of the glottis.
- Erythematosus lupus is an autoimmune disease in which circulating immune complexes alter the vessels, the connective tissue and the mucosa. Principal signs of the disease are arthritis, skin rash and nephritis.
- Relapsing polychondritis is a painful chronic inflammation, which first affects the external ears, the nose and, subsequently, the larynx. It involves a progressive destruction of the cartilages coupled with a progressive stenosis of the larynx. It is treated with dapsone and steroids.
- Pemphigus and pemphigoid are two distinct autoimmune diseases which occur in the form of blisters with ulceration of the epithelia and/or mucosa. Pemphigus attacks the epithelium, while pemphigoid attacks the subepithelial tissue. Chronic pemphigoid may provoke severe laryngeal stenosis and ocular complications. Treatment is based on steroids, methotrexate and cyclophosphamide. Plasmapheresis is recommended for severe cases of pemphigus.
- Sarcoidosis is a granulomatous idiopathic disease. Dysphonia comes with the development of nodules in

the submucosa. Local injection of steroids may be useful in cases where systemic treatment fails.

- Wegener's granulomatosis is a necrotic granulomatosis that affects the airway, inducing glomerulonephritis; 8.5% of cases are observed in the trachea and subglottis.
- Amyloidosis is provoked by extracellular deposits of fibrillar proteins in the tissues. It may be primary and idiopathic, or secondary to a systemic disease such as rheumatoid arthritis or tuberculosis. Usually it is asymptomatic, although the deposits may induce dysphonia or even a dyspnoea requiring surgical ablation. Complete ablation is difficult and local recurrence is frequent.

Chronic Laryngitis

Classically speaking, distinction is made between "red" types of laryngitis, where inflammatory phenomena predominate, and the "white" types, otherwise known as keratoses.

- Pseudomyxomatous laryngitis, or Reinke's oedema, occurs mostly in smokers, and is associated with an overuse of the voice. The lesion can be found on the upper face of the vocal cords, from the anterior commissure to the vocal processes. The inferior face and the ventricle are respected. The cords show a whitish, translucent aspect. The lesions are generally bilateral. A ventricular eversion may develop. The presence of associated dysplasia is quite rare.
- White laryngitis occurs principally in three types: leucoplakia, white pachydermia and horny papilloma in adults. The white colour is due to the keratinization of the surface (Fig. 6.3.1).

The leucoplakic lesion is flat, like a candle-wax stain, of pearlescent or grey colour and with slightly vague contours. It may be single or multiple, localized or diffuse. The adjacent mucosa is usually inflamed.

In white pachydermia, the lesion has a tumourlike aspect. It is of a chalky greyness with clearly defined limits. Its surface is irregular. It feels hard when palpated and the suppleness of the vocal cords may be altered.

Malignant transformation can be suspected with the following aspects:
- Irregularity of surface
- Induration of the cord
- Ulceration
- Haemorrhages
- Significant inflammation of the surrounding area
- Microcapillary anomalies

The distinction between horny papilloma and pachydermia is most often histological. Papilloma occurs in the form of a mass that is either greyish or of a granulated

rose colour, highly exophytic, with a characteristic spicular surface. Its base is large and well defined. It can be most easily found on the anterior part of the vocal cord or on the anterior commissure. The free edge of the vocal cord may be affected, showing a sawtoothed aspect.

Characteristically, the tumour is of a hard consistency. It is most often single and does not show a tendency to spread.

The term "precancerous state", when applied to lesions of the vocal cords, refers to those lesions of the epithelium that precede an invasive carcinoma. Clinically speaking, they look like a chronic laryngitis, and correspond histologically to changes ranging from simple hyperplasia to carcinoma in situ. They are usually termed "dysplasia". However, the principal problem, both diagnostic and therapeutic, lies in their relationship to invasive cancer:

1. Aetiological factors
   - Tobacco: This is an important causal factor in the development of precancerous lesions and, more specifically, in the keratinization of the mucosa. The risk of developing dysplasia of the vocal cords is 7 times more significant in a smoker than in a non-smoker.
   - Asbestos: Work undertaken on the role played by asbestos has produced contradictory findings; however, the influence of asbestos seems to conjugate with that of tobacco.
   - Other incriminatory factors: Nickel, wood dust, chrome, arsenic and sulphuric acid.
   - Alcohol: This seems to play a role in laryngeal carcinogenesis. Its potentialization and its active synergy with tobacco are often mentioned. Alcohol can act like a solvent, facilitating the penetration of the epithelium by tobacco carcinogens. In cases of massive and prolonged absorption, alcohol favours nutritional deficiencies, in particular that of vitamin A, which plays a protective role in maintaining the mucosa.

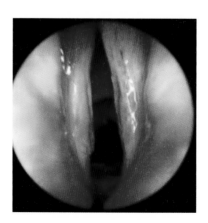

Fig. 6.3.1 Chronic laryngitis

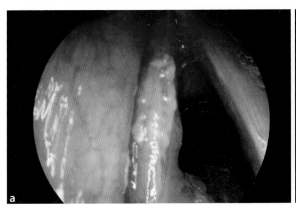 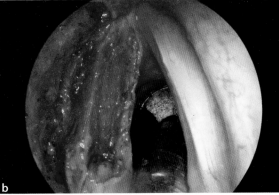

Fig. 6.3.2a,b Chronic keratosis: **a** at laryngoscopy; **b** following laser excision

– Papilloma viruses: In contrast to precancerous lesions of the uterine cervix, numerous questions remain as to the possible role of papilloma viruses in the development of laryngeal dysplasia. Detection of human papilloma virus in cancer of the larynx occurs, according to the series records, in 5–54.1% of cases.

2. Reflux: The role of gastro-oesophageal reflux has been mentioned for quite a while. Several studies have concluded its causality in the appearance of cancerous lesions, but these findings are controversial. Gastro-oesophageal reflux causes inflammatory reactions, which may induce cellular modifications (metaplasia, keratinization), but the development of dysplasia is rarely noted in the absence of other known risk factors.

3. Dysplasia corresponds to an alteration of cellular maturation. It can be observed on hyperplastic mucosa, whether keratinized or not. It expresses itself in more or less pronounced anomalies of cell morphology, as well as by an alteration of the stratification and structure of the malpighian epithelium.

Various classifications for gradation of dysplasia have been published allowing a step-by-step gradation of these changes, and taking into account the intensity of the changes observed. They are all based on modifications to the tissue architecture and cell morphology. Classification in three stages or grades is the most rec-

ognized. It is based on histological criteria, clinical criteria having little value (Fig. 6.3.2). This classification assimilates severe dysplasia and carcinoma in situ:
– Grade 1: hyperplasia and/or keratosis with or without mild dysplasia
– Grade 2: moderate dysplasia
– Grade 3: severe dysplasia or carcinoma in situ

Carcinoma in situ may be defined as a histological entity having the morphological character of a cancer, but whose spread is limited to the place of its appearance.

The distinction between carcinoma in situ and micro-invasive carcinoma is a difficult one. Crossing of the basal membrane is the most recognized criterion.

Several studies have shown that keratoses without atypical phenomena rarely develop into carcinoma (from 2 to 5% of cases), and this only after a long period of latency. The percentage of invasive cancer development increases with the presence of cellular atypia. The degree of atypia is the principal prognostic factor in the evolution of such lesions. The risk of evolution towards invasive carcinoma increases with the degree of dysplasia. A rate of degeneration of, respectively, 2, 12 and 23% for stages I, II and III has been advanced. In the absence of treatment, it has been shown that 63–90% of carcinoma in situ develop into an invasive carcinoma within an average of 5 years.

Diffuse forms of dysplasia are more serious and evolve more frequently towards an invasive carcinoma. The more clearly differentiated forms of severe dysplasia tend more significantly towards recurrence or evolution to invasive carcinoma than the less differentiated forms.

The relationship simple hyperplasia, dysplasia, carcinoma in situ and invasive carcinoma does not seem to be mandatory. Kleinsasser's chart, from 1963, takes into account the possible evolutionary modalities (Fig. 6.3.3).

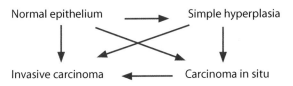

Fig. 6.3.3 Kleinsasser's chart

Of course, a lesion cannot be recognized as precancerous unless it has been entirely removed, thus formally eliminating any associated carcinoma. The correlation between dysplastic lesions and cancer is a statistical one; no single element available today permits us to prejudge the evolution of a particular case.

6.3.2 Specific Lesions

6.3.2.1 Reinke's Oedema

This is a lesion principally situated in the superficial chorion of the vocal cord, which is invaded by a generally quite fluid oedema. The vocal cord has a ballooned aspect. In dysplasia cases, the epithelium will, of course, require resection for histological analysis, but most often it can be conserved. The surgical principle is that of suctioning the oedema through an incision of the superior side of the vocal cord (Gould–Hirano technique). Resection of the excess epithelium after suction should be so parsimonious as to allow the bared chorion of the vocal cord to be recovered after redraping.

It is recommended before the incision to coagulate the microvessels of the vocal cord with the laser, thus diminishing bleeding, which would often otherwise be troublesome.

Next, an incision of the epithelium in the superior side of the vocal cord, at its junction with the ventricular floor, is realized. After this the free edge of the epithelium is drawn towards the medial line with heart-shaped forceps and the oedema is suctioned. Finally the epithelium is redraped onto the chorion and any excess epithelium is resected. Some surgeons prefer, at this point, to fix the microflaps with a few drops of fibrin glue. Except in special cases, both vocal cords are operated on in one session, but one must take care not to harm the anterior commissure, so as to avoid the development of synechia.

A far clearer and higher voice is often obtained. Attaining such results can sometimes be more difficult, especially in cases of bilateral intervention. It is advisable to warn the patient in serious cases of Reinke's oedema that the vocal recovery may be long (4–6 weeks in a majority of cases). The extent of this healing period must be known to the patient and must be taken into account for the surgical decision.

6.3.2.2 Hypertrophic Laryngitis

This is an indication for subepithelial cordectomy (type 1) or decortication, according to the classification of the European Laryngological Society. Subepithelial cordectomy consists in the resection of the epithelium and the superficial lamina propria. The surgical procedure spares the deeper tissue, and therefore the vocal ligament.

Since, depending on the degree of severity, the entire epithelium is affected, it is necessary to perform a complete resection; thus, the risk of leaving a dysplastic or even cancerous zone in place is avoided. In rarer cases, in which epithelial changes only affect part of the vocal cord, the clinically normal epithelium is left in place.

Inasmuch as subepithelial cordectomy ensures a histological examination of the entire epithelium, its role is, above all, diagnostic. It may be therapeutic if the histological results confirm the presence of either hyperplasia or dysplasia. Such lesions are, by definition, limited to the epithelium. This technique is not sufficient for dealing with invasive carcinomas; however, for carcinoma in situ, in cases where there is no doubt of a possible microinvasion, this type of cordectomy may suffice, though under reserve of close clinical monitoring and, if necessary, an endoscopy.

Subepithelial cordectomy may be carried out as a phonosurgical intervention: 0.1-s single pulse, "superpulse", at 2–3 W, with a focal distance of 400 mm. If Acublade can be used, subepithelial cordectomy may be undertaken with a superpulse or ultrapulse beam, of 1–2-mm length, incision depth of 0.2 mm, in single pulse mode, which corresponds to a power of 10 W over a period of 0.16 s.

6.3.3 Which Laser Should Be Used?

Even if trials have been carried out using other types of laser, notably the potassium triphosphate laser, the CO_2 laser remains the workhorse in laryngology. Laser action takes place in a gaseous mixture. The transmitted wavelength is 10,600 nm (which places it in the infrared band, with an invisible beam). This wavelength is responsible for the fact that the CO_2 laser beam is absorbed by water and glass. Living tissue, which contains 70% water, is therefore highly absorbent, and the coagulation and vaporization effects of the CO_2 laser are both very superficial and visible.

At a temperature of around 100°C, cells explode owing to the evaporation of the intracellular and pericellular water. This destructive effect acts like a cut if the beam is sufficiently sharp. In first-generation CO_2 lasers, the beam diameter was sometimes in excess of 1 mm, whereas the latest models offer a spot dimension of 250 µm for use in laryngology. The size of the cut, that is to say the amount of tissue destroyed, is thus 3 times less.

Progress has been made in the production of CO_2 lasers by way of optimizing the sectioning effect. These CO_2 laser wavelengths have been called "superpulse" or "ultrapulse". The principle is to produce peaks of high power, between 400 and 500 W, over a very short time

(1 ms). After each peak there is an off period, known as the thermal relaxation time, to allow the tissue to cool. The off periods are calculated in such a way as to ensure the average power delivery required over a desired time, for example 3 W in 1 s.

Use of the scanner enables the laser beam to be delivered in a far more regular and rapid way than the human hand could manage. The scanner consists of a unit which is connected between the arms of the laser and the micromanipulator. This component contains a set of mirrors off which the laser is bounced as it traverses the scanner. These mirrors are mobile on their own axis and are guided by software included in the laser unit.

Thanks to the scanner, the beam can rapidly sweep a surface. Each passage permits it to vaporize an average of 100 µm. This function is very useful, for example, in the treatment of papillomatosis. The software guiding the scanner can also guide the beam on an incision line, which can be programmed for length, depth of cut as well as form (straight line or curve). If the length is a "real" dimension, the depth is, however, based on the average water content of human tissues; thus, the higher the water content, the deeper the incision. The energy is thereby distributed evenly and rapidly throughout the length of the incision. The section line is far more regular and it has been measurably demonstrated that the induced thermal effects at the edge of the lesion are now half those of earlier equipment. It was also found necessary to redesign the micromanipulator, so as to enable the beam to be guided left and right via a "joystick". The whole system goes under the name of Acublade.

Use of Acublade involves a change to the parameter procedure for the laser: one now has to think in terms of length and depth of incision as well as in operational time. The software then calculates the necessary power. This is higher (around 10 W) than with the micropoint, because the energy is distributed far more rapidly along the length of the incision line. It is, of course, possible to increase or reduce the power suggested should one wish to do so.

Suggested Reading

1. Dworkinn JP (2008) Laryngitis: types, causes, and treatments. Otolaryngol Clin North Am 41(2):419–436
2. Joniau S, Bradshaw A, Esterman Z, Carney AS (2007) Reflux and laryngitis: a systematic review. Otolaryngol Head Neck Surg 136(5):686–692
3. Remacle M, Lawson G, Watelet JB (1999) Carbon dioxide laser microsurgery of benign vocal fold lesions: Indications, techniques, and results in 251 patients. Ann Otol Rhinol Laryngol 108(2):156–164
4. Remacle M, Lawson G, Nollevaux MC, Delos M (2008) Current state of scanning micromanuiplator applications with the carbon dioxide laser. Ann Otol Rhinol Laryngol 117(4):239–244
5. Sliva L, Damrose E, Bairao F, Nina ML, Junior JC, Costa HO (2008) Infectious granulomatous laryngitis: a retrospective study of 24 cases. Eur Arch Otorhinolaryngol 265(6):675–680

6.4 Mucosal Disease of the Glottis

JESÚS HERRANZ, JAVIER GAVILÁN BOUZAS,
CARLOS VÁZQUEZ BARRO, AND LOURDES MARTÍN MÉNDEZ

6.4.1 Glottic Symptoms

Dysphonia is the most frequent clinical symptom of laryngeal disorders. Vocal abuse and vocal misuse predispose one to acute or chronic dysphonia. Vocal abuse includes excessive talking, throat clearing, coughing, inhaling of irritants, smoking, screaming, and yelling. Vocal misuse is improper voice usage such as speaking too loudly, or at an abnormally high or low pitch. Frequent vocal abuse and misuse can damage the vocal folds and cause temporary or permanent changes in vocal function and voice quality.

To produce a clear and clean tone, the vocal cords must come together with minimum tension, vibrating with a soft respiratory flow. Incorrect voice production implies that the vocal cords must vibrate under excessive tension. If high-tension adduction is present, much larger respiratory pressure is needed to make the vocal cords vibrate. This condition induces inflammation and permanent changes in the vocal cords, leading to dysphonia. Permanent changes may result in the identification of certain lesions, namely nodules, polyps or Reinke's oedema and cysts. Treatment is directed to teach the patient how to avoid vocal abuse and misuse. Although lesions are sometimes reversible after rehabilitation, surgery may be necessary to remove irreversible structural changes.

6.4.2 Vocal Cord Structure

The vocal cord structure is a complex system of epithelial, connective and muscular elements designed to control the aerodynamic forces involved in a highly specific function such as voice production. Minor alterations in the structure of the vocal cord are responsible for dramatic changes in voice production leading to dysphonia.

Detailed studies on vocal cord structure, along with stroboscopic analysis, have shown the importance of the multilayered structure of the true vocal cord for its mechanical properties as a vibrator element. According to Hirano, the vocal cord has five different layers, each one with specific and different functions:

1. The most external layer is the epithelium, squamous cell type, whose purpose is to maintain the vocal cord shape.
2. Underneath the epithelium is the lamina propria, with three different layers. The superficial layer of the lamina propria corresponds to Reinke's space and consists mainly of loose fibres and matrix which can be regarded as a mass of soft gelatin.
3. The intermediate layer of the lamina propria consists mainly of elastic fibres that run parallel to the edge of the vocal cord. It can be regarded as a bundle of soft rubber bands.
4. The deep layer of the lamina propria consists mainly of collagenous fibres that run parallel to the vocal cord edge. From the mechanical point of view, it can be regarded as a bundle of cotton threads.
5. Finally, the vocalis muscle constitutes the main part of the vocal cord. From the mechanical standpoint, it can be regarded as a bundle of stiff rubber bands, with the stiffness changing according to the degree of muscle contraction.

These five different structures have their own biomechanical properties according to their stiffness. They can be grouped into three different sections: the cover (epithelium and superficial layer of the lamina propria), the transition (intermediate and deep layers of the lamina propria) and the body (fibres of vocalis muscle). From the vocal edge to the muscle the stiffness increases owing to the tissue composition. The outer layer is more fluid-like, whereas the inner layers are more elastic.

Mucus, produced in the epithelium superior and inferior to the vocal cord edge, is a critical element for the mucosa of the vocal cord to vibrate.

6.4.3 Vocal Nodules

Vocal nodules are bilateral, chronic thickenings of the vocal cord epithelium, usually located at the junction of the anterior third with the middle third (Fig. 6.4.1). They develop more frequently in women and male children, and in people with occupations with highly demanding vocal

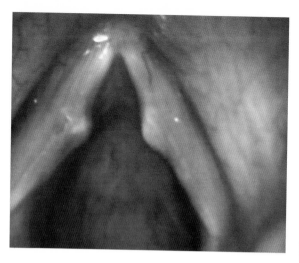

Fig. 6.4.1 Vocal nodules

activity (teachers, singers, salesman, etc.). They are also more frequent in children with a cleft palate.

Around 10–20% of patients with nodules have other vocal cord pathologic conditions such as anterior commissure microwebs that, if undetected, can be the reason for treatment failure.

A forceful vibration causes trauma at the membranous portion of the vocal cord, leading to oedema of the submucosa. Persistent trauma during phonation may lead to thickening of the epithelium and fibrosis at the level of Reinke's space.

Nodules are closely related to voice misuse. It is well known that the anterior two thirds of the vocal cords take part in the vibration. If vibration is forced owing to an excessive subglottic pressure, or long-lasting use, an acute inflammation will occur in the area where vibration is more intense, i.e. at the junction of the anterior third and middle third of the vocal cord. Initially the nodule is a light soft thickening at the membranous portion of the vocal cord. If trauma persists, acute inflammation becomes chronic, with thickening affecting the epithelium and submucosal hyalinization. These changes are not reversible.

Permanent or intermittent dysphonia is the usual symptom, sometimes associated with unspecific pharyngeal symptoms. Singers show difficulty in achieving high tones. Other voice symptoms are breathy voice, need for frequent throat clearing, and coughing and tightness tension while singing.

On examination, the vocal nodules are usually bilateral, shiny white, with a wide base, and located at the junction of the anterior third and middle third of the vocal cord, with voice distortion not always related to nodule size. Acute nodules are usually oedematous and translucent, whereas chronic nodules are white and fibrotic. Under stroboscopic examinations, acute nodules disap-

pear with vocal cord tension, whereas chronic nodes stop mucosal wave progression.

Although there is no agreement on which is the best treatment for vocal nodules, it is important to remember that nodules are usually a consequence of vocal misuse and for this reason speech therapy is essential for treatment.

If dysphonia is not important for the patient, rehabilitation and vocal hygiene (lubrication of the vocal folds, hydration, respiratory coordination) is the initial part of treatment. Surgery is indicated in cases where dysphonia is not acceptable for the patient, or when the nodules do not disappear after speech therapy.

6.4.4 Vocal Polyps

Polyps are benign lesions usually located at the vocal edge of the vocal cord, impeding vocal cords meeting while adducting (Fig. 6.4.2). Polyps are usually larger than nodules, with a wide or narrow pedicle, and may have a contact lesion in the contralateral vocal cord.

They appear mainly in adult males, and vocal abuse and a noisy environment at work are risk factors. Other factors related to polyps are aspirin intake, anxiety and extroverted behaviour.

Polyps are the consequence of a violent and short voice strength that leads to the rupture of capillaries in the submucosa, with subsequent haemorrhage. If after this haemorrhage voice misuse continues, the initial lesion can evolve to a haemorrhagic polyp or, after some time, to a fibrotic polyp. Excessive sphincteric function of the larynx (weight lifting, glassblowing, etc.) can also induce polyp formation.

Dysphonia is usually abrupt, coincident with the vocal abuse. Later on, dysphonia can be intermittent or continuous, depending on the polyp structure and localization. Vocal range is reduced and conversational voice appears muffled, with difficulty to achieve high-pitched tones. Polyps can become large, producing even glottis obstruction.

They are usually unilateral, located in the membranous portion of the vocal cord, with a contact ulcer in the contralateral vocal cord. Polyps are usually larger than nodules, and at the beginning they may have a haemorrhagic aspect (Fig. 6.4.3). Large polyps move up and down in the glottis along with the respiratory movements.

Laryngeal polyp treatment is usually surgical upon patient request. Microsurgical technique is directed to polyp removal by cutting its pedicle and avoiding disrupting the vocal ligament. Endoscopic laser removal has also been proposed .

Medical treatment is not important in polyp treatment, other than changing or removing the possible harmful

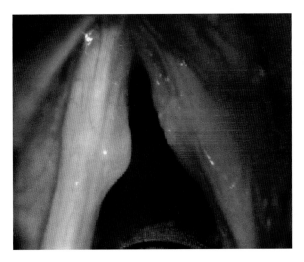

Fig. 6.4.2 Left vocal cord polyp and contralateral contact lesson

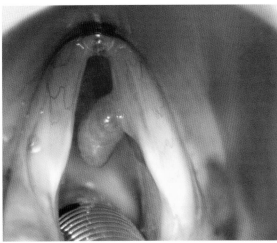

Fig. 6.4.3 Right vocal cord polyp

medications taken by the patient (aspirin, warfarin). If gastropharyngeal reflux is present, adequate antireflux measures should be applied.

Although speech therapy is not essential, postsurgical rehabilitation is recommended to teach the patient good vocal hygiene habits.

6.4.5 Reinke's Oedema

Reinke's oedema is a unilateral or bilateral swelling of the vocal cord characterized by the accumulation of gelatin-like material in Reinke's space (Fig. 6.4.4). Vocal cord mobility is preserved, but patients have a low-pitched voice.

Its cause is related to chronic irritation of the larynx leading to oedema, vascular congestion and capillary stasis in the submucosa. Other causes such as chronic sinusitis, hypothyroidism and exposure to industrial or environmental irritants have also been considered. Patients with Reinke's oedema are usually heavy smokers, vocal misusers, and have a long history of dysphonia.

Reinke's oedema is thought to appear owing to accumulation of fluid, a consequence of poor lymphatic drainage, vascular congestion and venous stasis. A mechanical cause has also been considered.

Microscopically, the basal membrane is thickened, with oedematous areas containing variable amounts of polysaccharides, thickening of the vascular walls and fibrin deposits.

The voice characteristics of a patient with Reinke's oedema are similar to those of heavy smokers and vocal misusers, having long-lasting dysphonia. Vocal pitch is low, with females having a male tone. Speech parameters include a narrow vocal range as well as a reduction in the fundamental frequency. Occasionally, the oedema may be big enough to reduce the glottic space, causing dyspnoea.

Laryngoscopy typically shows fusiform oedema in both vocal cords. Sometimes a yellow fluid content can be seen through the vocal cord mucosa.

Stroboscopic examination shows a complete glottic closure, with asymmetric movement of the vocal cords, and an overexpressed mucosal wave, whose stiffness is severely reduced.

Initial measures are directed to avoid irritants and follow speech therapy. Voice improvement takes time, and should be monitored periodically by indirect laryngoscopy. In advanced cases, or when conservative measures do not improve the voice, surgery is indicated.

Separate procedures for each vocal cord, to avoid web formation at the anterior commissure, are no longer con-

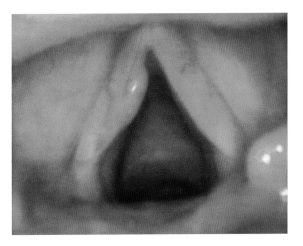

Fig. 6.4.4 Left vocal cord Reinke's oedema

sidered if the mucosal removal is from no further than the anterior macula flava.

Stripping should be avoided owing to the multiple microadherences between the mucosa. Surgery should include a cordotomy in the superior aspect of the vocal cord, and aspiration of the fluid present in Reinke's space. Redundant mucosa is removed with microscissors.

6.4.6 Vocal Cord Cysts

Cysts in the vocal folds are typically white, subepithelial, spherical, unilateral lesions located in the middle third of the vocal cord (Fig. 6.4.5). They appear in approximately 5% of adults with voice disorders. The cyst content can be serous, mutinous or keratin. In the lattermost case, the cyst is called an epidermoid cyst and it is usually more adherent to the deep structures of the submucosa. Vocal cord surgery can induce the development of an epidermoid cyst by placing epithelium under the mucosa during the procedure.

Vocal cord cysts can be congenital or acquired. Congenital cysts develop from epithelial rests buried underneath the mucosa that grow over the years. Acquired cysts appear as a consequence of mucosal gland obstruction. Spontaneous rupture of the cyst is thought to be the origin of sulcus vocalis.

The symptoms are similar to those produced by nodules. Vocal misuse is a frequent clinical characteristic, with dysphonia as the most constant clinical symptom. Spontaneous opening of the cyst produces a sudden improvement of voice quality.

Patients usually have a long-lasting history of dysphonia and vocal abuse. Laryngoscopy shows a white, soft, smooth, fusiform elevation of the middle third of the vocal cord, sometimes with a contralateral vocal cord contact lesion. Small vessels on the vocal cord surface running towards the cyst can be found.

Epidermoid cysts are larger, ovoid, yellow and sometimes bilateral, with greater effect on voice quality than retention cysts, which tend to be smaller, white and unilateral.

Stroboscopic examination shows an increase of the fundamental frequency with the characteristic stop of the mucosal wave in the cyst area, maintaining a normal wave progression in the mucosa anterior and posterior to the cyst. Sometimes, vocal cord cysts can only be found during surgical exploration of the vocal cord.

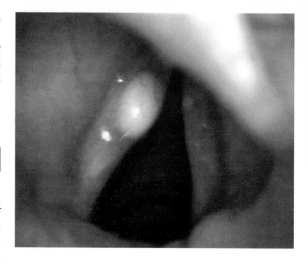

Fig. 6.4.5 Left vocal cord cyst

Surgery is the treatment of choice. Speech therapy is indicated to improve voice habits in the postoperative period. Surgery includes a superior cordotomy and cyst detachment from the underlying mucosa. Corticoid injections in the vocalis muscle have also been recommended to avoid postoperative inflammation and adherence between the epithelium and the vocal ligament.

Suggested Reading

Bouchayer M, Cornut G, Witzig E, Loire R, Roch JB, Bastian RW (1985) Epidermoid cysts, sulci, and mucosal bridges of the true vocal cord: a report of 157 cases. Laryngoscope 95:1087–1094

Dikkers FG, Schutte HK (1991) Benign lesions of the vocal folds: uniformity in assessment of clinical diagnosis. Clin Otolaryngol 16:8–11

Hirano M, Bless DM (1993) Videostroboscopic examination of the larynx. Singular, San Diego

Roch JB, Cornut G, Bouchayer M (1989) Modes of appearance of vocal cord polyps. Rev Laryngol Otol Rhinol (Bord) 110:389–390

Shapshay SM, Rebeiz EE, Bohigian RK, Hybels RL (1990) Benign lesions of the larynx. Should the laser be used? Laryngoscope 100:953–957

Tillmann B, Rudert H, Schunke M, Werner JA (1995) Morphological studies on the pathogenesis of Reinke's edema. Eur Arch Otorhinol 252:469–474

6.5 Benign Neoplasms and Other Tumours of the Larynx

PATRICK J. BRADLEY

6.5.1 Introduction

The presence of a mass lesion within the larynx can provoke numerous acute, chronic, progressive or even life-threatening symptoms. These symptoms may be minimal or dramatic and are a reflection of the tumour site and size. In assessing the patient with a potential laryngeal tumour, a thorough history should be taken with particular emphasis on the age of the patient, the temporal course of the symptom complex, the presence of infection, any previous surgery or trauma, and the presence or absence of respiratory, vocal or swallowing symptoms, all of which will give clues as to the nature and extent of any tumour. Certain tumours have a site-specific predilection, but in principle the supraglottis is the site most frequently involved (85%), followed by the glottis and the subglottis. Although the experienced laryngologist may be able to make an accurate clinical diagnosis by outpatient nasendoscopy, evidence suggests that the accuracy of diagnosis based on visual examination alone can be subject to some variation.

The initial decision to operate depends upon detailed visual inspection of the lesion, histological diagnosis and a need to establish that the tumour is not malignant. Also, a contemporary meticulous endoscopic examination of the entire upper aerodigestive tract is required to assess the size, position, consistency and extent of any tumour, in addition to excluding any concurrent aerodigestive tract disease. All swelling located within the larynx, although some may appear to be benign in appearance, must always be confirmed histologically prior to any further planning of treatment. Modern radiological imaging may demonstrate the anatomic extent of the mass lesion and/or its vascularity; biopsy findings when typical of a particular benign disease are reassuring to the patient and the treating clinician. The differentiation of benign from malignant tumours is vital. Paragangliomas, neurofibromas, chondromas, etc. have malignant variants, with certain granular cell tumours, haemangiopericytomas and others having histological features that mimic those of malignant disease. Reliance on expert histopathologists is crucial for accurate and appropriate patient treatment selection and ultimate outcome.

Furthermore, information relating to endoscopic and surgical access and potential for resection should be carefully considered in planning future definitive surgical management. Indications for surgery beyond this first therapeutic step include failure of conservative measures, symptomatic relief, maintenance of organ function and concern about any potential for malignant transformation. A number of benign tumours have a predilection to recur if they have been incompletely removed either in months or even in years after removal—papillomas, oncocytic tumours, pleomorphic adenoma, lymphangiomas, neurofibromas, fibromatosis, paragangliomas and rhabdomyomas—and patients should be informed of the results of surgery, so if symptoms return they can be re-referred and examination may be performed. Ultimately the method by which resection is undertaken is dependent upon both tumour and patient factors and the experience of the operating surgeon and facilities available.

6.5.2 Classification

The definition of non-cancerous, or benign, tumours of the larynx requires some elaboration. The early laryngologists proposed that, as true proliferative neoplasms were often clinically indistinguishable from non-proliferative inflammatory or hyperplastic growths, the term "benign tumour" should be used to encompass all abnormal growths of tissue within the larynx that lacked malignant or metastatic properties. In the 1950s, this concept was revised, identifying that vocal fold nodules, laryngeal polyps, cysts and non-specific granulomas to be mucosal reactive inflammatory disorders and therefore non-neoplastic in nature.

Notwithstanding these various viewpoints, the principals of management remain analogous. A nomenclature based on the authoritative surgical head and neck pathological tomes is shown in Table 6.5.1. True benign neoplastic tumours of the larynx are rare (Table 6.5.2). Four large series have reported patients diagnosed and treated over differing periods of time, but the majority of benign neoplasms (80–92%) were squamous papillomas, thus supporting the observation that the other benign lesions

Table 6.5.1 Pathological classification of benign laryngeal tumours

Origin
Epithelial
Squamous epithelium
Recurrent respiratory papillomatosis
Keratinised papilloma
Glandular
Pleomorphic adenoma
Oncocytic tumour
Non-epithelial
Vascular
Haemangioma
Lymphangioma
Cartilage and bone
Chondroma
Osteoma
Giant cell tumour
Muscle
Leiomyoma
Rhabdomyoma
Angiomyoma
Epithelioid leiomyoma
Adipose
Lipoma
Neural
Neurilemmoma
Neurofibroma
Schwannoma
Paraganglioma
Granular cell
Pseudotumours
Fibroma
Inflammatory fibroblastic
Amyloid
Laryngeal cysts

Table 6.5.2 Benign laryngeal tumours (reported large series [1–5])

Series duration (years)	Median 23.5 years, range 12–45 years
Total true proliferative tumours	1,211
Total squamous papilloma	1,061 (87.6%)
Non-squamous papilloma	
Adenoma	4
Chondroma/osteochondroma	19
Fibroma	6
Fibromatosis	1
Fibrous histiocytoma	6
Granular cell	16
Haemangioma	27[a]
Lipoma	9
Lymphangioma	4
Myxoma	0[a]
Neurilemmoma	4
Neurofibroma	6
Nodular fasciitis	1
Oncocytoma	35
Others	5
Paraganglioma	5
Rhabdomyoma	2
Total	150 (12.3%)

[a]Some series included child and adult papillomas, some haemangiomas and myxomas were excluded because they were considered inflammatory rather than neoplastic and one series consisted of an accumulation of two time periods.

6.5.3.1 General Considerations

Squamous papillomas are the most common benign tumours of the larynx. Barnes [1] classifies papillomas into two histological types, keratinised and non-keratinised. Keratinised papillomas (papillary keratosis) occur mainly in adults and are mostly solitary lesions that arise from the true vocal cord. The majority of keratinised papillomas are not related to viral infection but are associated with smoking and can be associated with malignant transformation. Keratinised papillomas variably recur following simple excision.

or neoplasms are rarely encountered. This chapter concentrates on those lesions considered to be "true" benign proliferative neoplastic tumours, and reserves the management of reactive mucosal and inflammatory lesions for another discussion.

Recurrent respiratory papillomatosis (RRP), or non-keratinised papilloma, is the most frequently occurring benign laryngeal neoplasm. The estimated incidence is around four per 100,000 population in children and one to two per 100,000 population in adults. A disease of viral origin, RRP is both a neoplastic and an infectious phenomenon caused by the human papilloma viruses (HPV). More than 90 subtypes of HPV are recognised, with HPV-6 and HPV-11 most commonly found in laryngeal papilloma. RRP occurs in response to mucosal infection with HPV and can develop on any mucosal surface of the upper aerodigestive tract.

RRP has a tendency to form at anatomic sites of junctions between squamous and ciliated epithelium: papillomas occur most often at the nasal valve, the nasopharyngeal surface of the soft palate, the laryngeal surface of the epiglottis, the upper and lower margins of the ventricle, the under surface of the vocal folds, the carina and bronchial spurs. The most frequently affected site at diagnosis in both the paediatric and adult population is the larynx.

The incidence of RRP is bimodal, giving rise to two distinct forms: juvenile onset and adult onset. Juvenile-onset RRP is more aggressive than the adult form Most investigators consider RRP to be of adult onset if the patient is older than 16–20 years of age at diagnosis. Adult-onset RRP is diagnosed most frequently between the ages of 20 and 40 years and shows a slight male preponderance.

The incidence of carcinoma developing in patients with RRP is reported at between 1 and 7%. Laryngeal cancer complicating RRP has an increased association with HPV-11, HPV-16 and HPV-18 infection, previous exposure to radiation and in patients with the juvenile-onset RRP variant. As patients with RRP can also be heavy smokers and drinkers, larger studies are required to clarify any causal or synergistic relationship that may exist between HPV, and or its subtypes, RRP and carcinogenesis.

6.5.3.2   Indications

The main indications for surgery in RRP are the need for histological diagnosis, the maintenance of an adequate airway and the preservation of laryngeal and vocal function. As RRP represents an as yet undefined alteration of mucosal immunosurveillance rather than a simple mechanical change, surgery for the disease is rarely curative even after en bloc resection of the papillomatous epithelium. The philosophy of surgery for RRP must be altered accordingly. In this situation the tenet of "less is more" applies. Removal of disease most commonly occurs under general anaesthesia. Some patients with mild disease may require only a few treatments. Patients with more aggressive variants can require monthly or bimonthly

surgery to promote disease regression. This is one reason why newer office-based procedures are gaining popularity (see later).

6.5.3.3   Specific Assessment

The most common presenting symptom of RRP in adults is some degree of hoarseness or dysphonia and sometimes shortness of breath. These voice changes may be subtle and can persist for many years.

Occasionally adult-onset RRP may behave like the more aggressive juvenile variant. Here the patient may develop progressive dyspnoea, stridor and even acute life-threatening airway compromise. Preoperatively it is useful to evaluate the location and morphology of the papilloma using a flexible nasendoscope.

Macroscopically, papillomas are pink or white, sessile or exophytic, pedunculated or broad-based (Fig. 6.5.1a). Occasionally the papilloma develops across a wide field, appearing like a carpet or velvety sheet of disease, requiring high levels of magnification to localise it accurately. As the disease can affect different anatomic sites within the larynx, it is important for the surgeon to be comfortable with several different surgical methods and instruments.

6.5.3.4   Surgical Techniques

In treating RRP, the menu for surgical options includes microsurgical cold steel, carbon dioxide (CO_2) laser, microdebridement and office-based angiolytic laser treatment. As new techniques have developed, some investigators have preferred one method over another. The approaches for surgical removal of RRP remain controversial. It should be remembered that no surgical method has been shown to eradicate RRP and therefore it remains a chronic disease where surgical techniques and instrumentation should be selected to enable the surgeon to achieve the goals of surgery.

CO_2 Laser

CO_2 laser operative techniques are described in detail elsewhere. Precise operation of the laser will depend on the location and the morphology of the lesion or lesions. Generally speaking, for bulky lesions a defocused spot in continuous mode is utilised. Narrow-focus spot size and pulsed mode reserved for areas where minimal damage to laryngeal structures is desired. In this method the laser is set to the lowest power setting (2–3 W) that will allow adequate vaporisation of tissue. The time exposure is set to 1 s and the spot size diameter is set to 0.3 mm. The laser is then applied in brush strokes in an anterior to posterior direction to the broad surface of the papillomas. This

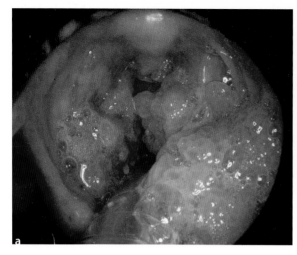

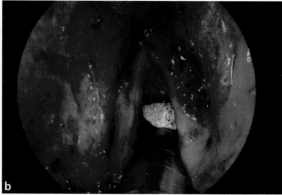

Fig 6.5.1 a Squamous papillomas involving glottis and supraglottis. **b** After CO_2 laser excision

causes superficial vaporisation and carbonisation of the surface of the lesion. The char is removed with a saline-soaked neurosurgical patty ("the brush") and microsuction, and at high magnification the depth of removal can easily be assessed and the laser is used in repeated brush strokes until the uninvolved submucosal layer is identified (Fig. 6.5.1b).

Angiolytic Laser Treatment

The philosophy of angiolytic laser treatment for RRP appears a sound one. In theory, laser energy between wavelengths of 500 and 600 nm is selectively absorbed by intravascular oxyhaemoglobin, resulting in coagulation of target tissue vasculature. Early results showed that compared with the CO_2 laser, the pulsed dye laser was capable of comparable levels of disease regression and a reduced risk of normal tissue damage. A further advantage of the pulsed dye laser is that it can be deployed in the office setting under conditions of local anaesthesia.

It may be that utilising cold steel, microdebridement or the CO_2 laser as an initial treatment strategy with angiolytic laser therapy reserved for maintenance or follow-up surgery will evolve. Some predict that outpatient-based angiolytic laser therapy will supplant CO_2 laser ablation as the primary mode of follow-up surgical management for RRP.

Microdebrider

The microdebrider as a surgical instrument is composed of suction, angled oscillating blades and irrigation. Adaptation of the powered microdebrider system for laryngeal use in RRP was first reported in 1999 and it has been deployed in the larynx under suspension laryngoscopy or in conjunction with a handheld Hopkins rod. Refinements and a proliferation in instrument design have led to a

growth in popularity and supporters claim several safety advantages over the CO_2 laser.

6.5.3.5 Adjuvant Therapy

General Considerations

Some progress is being made toward developing effective medical treatments for RRP and it is hoped that surgical treatments will one day be outdated. Current antiviral adjuvant treatments in limited use for RRP include cidofovir, α-interferon and indole-3-carbinol. Novel agents undergoing phase III trials include fusion proteins (heat shock protein E7) and cyclooxygenase-2 inhibitors (celecoxib). Furthermore, prophylactic immunisation against HPV infection, as licensed for cervical HPV infection in young women, is now quite possible, although large populations would need to be treated to prevent one case. There are currently no formal guidelines, and no substantial randomised controlled trials of adjuvant therapy in RRP. The decision to offer adjuvant therapy therefore must be individualised and based upon the frequency of surgical interventions, the morbidity of frequent surgeries and the recurrence pattern of the papillomas, balanced against the possible risks and side effects of these agents (e.g. possible mutagenic effects of cidofivir).

Cidofovir

The use of the intralesional antiviral agent cidofovir (1-[(S)-3-hydroxy-2-(phosphonomethoxy)propyl]cytosine dihydrate) in RRP was first described in 1995. Since then numerous studies have reported favourable results in terms of disease regression and remission following direct intralesional injection in adults. Interpretation of these and other data is complicated by wide variation in the total dose given (2–57 mg), frequency (2–8 weeks) and duration of treatments (months to years) and the concurrent use of surgical and other adjuvant treatments. In addition, the heterogeneity in case series between adult and juvenile populations further confounds interpretation of outcomes.

The precise dose, frequency of administration and duration of treatment of cidofovir in adults with RRP is unclear. Furthermore, informed consent detailing the potential side effects, including nephrotoxicity and carcinogenesis risks, should be obtained. Concerns over long-term efficacy and potential side effects of malignant transformation mandate adequately powered randomised, controlled trials.

α-Interferon

The interferons are a group of naturally occurring proteins produced by the body in response to infection.

Interferons may be classified as alpha, beta or gamma and are named after their ability to interfere with viral replication. These substances have been synthesised for clinical use using recombinant DNA techniques. In therapeutic doses, interferon can produce considerable side effects, including flulike symptoms such as fatigue, headache and aches and, less regularly, hypothyroidism, arthritis, thrombocytopenia and psychiatric disturbances. Since 1981 various studies have demonstrated the usefulness of α-interferon in severe RRP requiring frequent surgical interventions.

6.5.3.6   Specific Recommendations

It is important to remember that RRP is not typically cured by surgical removal of disease and the infectious nature of RRP will eventually manifest itself by recurrence. An aggressive surgical strategy therefore will not lead to reduced recurrence or a chance of cure. It should also be understood that RRP is limited to the surface epithelium. The principles of surgery, irrespective of the technique chosen, should be tailored to precise and careful removal of disease with consideration of preservation of underlying structures and vocal function. This is particularly important in relation to the glottis and subglottis, where overaggressive ablation can result in severe scarring and dysfunction. Preservation of even small areas of mucosa with intact superficial lamina propria may make a huge difference to voice outcomes. Extreme care should be taken in the areas of the anterior and posterior commissure. Papillomas should not be removed from both sides of the anterior or posterior commissure simultaneously as this can lead to web formation. An anterior commissure spatula or retractor should be used to protect one side of the anterior commissure while laser ablation or laser excision is performed on the other side.

6.5.4   Haemangioma

Laryngeal haemangiomas are rare but important as they may present with significant airway obstructive symptoms. Haemangiomas occur in two groups: paediatric (10%) and adult (90%) types. The paediatric type is typically subglottic. The pathogenesis of haemangiomas remains controversial as to whether they represent a true neoplasm or a congenital abnormality. Their behaviour at times may be aggressive and they may be considered to be a malignant neoplastic lesion. When such lesions occur in the adult, they usually arise on or above the vocal cords, and patients present with vague and often extended histories of hoarseness and occasional dysphagia. These tumours are more frequent in men (60–70%), and the majority are of the cavernous type of haemangioma, the other being capillary type. The tumours are mostly rounded, projecting or pedunculated, purplish growths arising on or above the vocal cords. Occasionally they are larger sessile tumours that extend submucosally into the laryngopharynx. As a rule the only symptom is hoarseness, and they rarely progress to the point of causing respiratory narrowing or obstruction. Although most angiomas are benign growths, some are multicentric and the term "haemangiomatosis" is applied, and may be part of a variety of clinical syndromes such as Rendu–Weber–Osler and the Sturge–Weber dyscrasia.

Surgery is the treatment of choice, but potential severe haemorrhage during biopsy or excision is well documented. Since the introduction of laser therapy for vascular lesions, the management of laryngeal haemangiomas has proven very useful. The use of photocoagulation with the Nd:YAG laser has offered the clinician an effective alternative therapy that is minimally invasive and has few complications. Success also has been reported with the use of CO_2 laser excision, and occasionally the use of the laser may require staging and time spacing of the surgical procedure to allow a complete resolution of the postoperative laryngeal tissue inflammation and oedema, and some patients may require a temporary tracheostomy during the course of these laser procedures.

6.5.5   Haemangiopericytoma

These are rare, but highlighted as they can present diagnostic as well as histological dilemmas. These lesions present as a supraglottic cyst-like mass, which is usually identified with a vascular-type appearance. The mass is firm, solid, pedunculated or nodular, usually well circumscribed, in a submucosal location, measuring up to 4 cm in greatest diameter. The surface is covered by intact epithelium with dilated vessels. Histologically the tumour has few mitoses. Occasional increased cellularity, pleomorphism and mitotic activity are associated with recurrences or metastases in other anatomic locations. The differential diagnosis includes haemangioma, angiosarcoma, glomus tumour, fibrous histiocytoma, leiomyoma, synovial sarcoma, malignant melanoma, leiomyosarcoma, spindle cell squamous cell carcinoma and mesenchymal chondrosarcoma.

Surgical treatment is to be recommended and may necessitate a total laryngectomy, but lesser surgical procedures have been described. Sadly, long-term follow-up of such cases is lacking to support a laryngeal conservation surgical approach in the light of difficulties with histopathological diagnosis.

6.5.6 Leiomyoma

This extremely rare neoplasm usually occurs in the supraglottic larynx, with the ventricle and false cord most often involved, although leiomyomas of the subglottis and trachea have been described. These tumours arise from smooth muscle, and are peculiar in that there is little smooth muscle in the larynx, compared with other parts of the head and neck. The tumours are usually sessile, bulging or polypoidal red-brown masses, measuring up to 5 cm in maximum diameter. These masses are usually covered by an intact smooth surface epithelium, with a conspicuous vascular arborising pattern, although ulceration is noted in larger lesions.

Microscopically, leiomyomas are distinctly encapsulated masses located in the submucosa, composed of spindle cells arranged in fascicles, whorls and intersecting bundles. Three different types of leiomyomas are recognised: these are the "common" leiomyoma, the vascular leiomyoma (angiomyoma) and the epitheloid leiomyoma (leiomyoblastoma). All three have been identified in the larynx.

The differential diagnosis rests with benign peripheral nerve sheath tumours, neurilemmomas and neurofibromas, nodular fasciitis, fibromas and leiomyosarcoma. However, any of the spindle cell tumours (inflammatory myofibroblastic tumour, contact ulcer, fibrosarcoma, spindle cell squamous cell carcinoma, synovial sarcoma) should also be considered.

6.5.7 Rhabdomyoma

These tumours in the larynx arise from striated muscle and are divided into two subtypes based on histological features, and not upon the patient's age at presentation: the adult type and the fetal cellular type. The current definition of rhabdomyoma is a benign neoplasm of striated muscle tissue, consisting usually of polygonal, frequently vacuolated (glycogen-containing) cells with a fine granular, deeply acidophilic cytoplasm resembling myofibrils cut in cross-section.

Adult rhabdomyomas occur more frequently in men than in women (4:1), with reported ages affected having a range from 16 to 76 (mean age 52). The adult type presents as a single lobulated, polypoidal or pedunculated, non-encapsulated lesion and is tan-yellow to deep grey-red-brown. Occasionally these lesions may be multifocal—there may have a lesion in more than two locations in the head and neck, including the larynx. They may measure up to 7.5 cm in greatest dimension, but most usually in the 1–3-cm range. The lesions have been most frequently located to the supraglottis or vocal cord. There is also a fetal cellular type of rhabdomyoma with similar presentations that may affect the head and neck region in elderly men, but is usually found in preadolescent patients; there is also a fetal myxoid type that is found in the head and neck region in children, especially in the postauricular region, but it has also been reported in the adult larynx.

The benign differential diagnosis in the adult type of tumour includes granular cell tumour, oncocytoma, paraganglioma, hibernoma and alveolar soft-part sarcoma. They are characterised by the presence of sarcolemma sheath, rod-like cytoplasmic bodies and cross striations.

6.5.8 Lipoma

Benign lipomas are commonly encountered in a wide variety of locations throughout the body. It is estimated that 13% of lipomas occur in the head and neck. Laryngeal lipomas are very rare, mostly occurring in adult-aged male patients, with fewer than 100 cases reported, and when present are most frequently located to the aryepiglottic fold.

In general, these lesions present like cystic lesions, encapsulated, smooth, and usually pedunculated. Symptoms are few and uncharacteristic, making accurate diagnosis difficult. Clinically they can be confused with other benign lesions, such as retention cysts or laryngocoeles. There has been no report of malignant transformation of solitary lipoma, whereas malignant change in multiple lipomas of the larynx and the pharynx has been described.

6.5.9 Neurofibromas and Neurilemmomas or Benign Schwannomas

Benign nerve tissue tumours are uncommonly found in the larynx. There are two classes of benign neurogenic tumours of the larynx: schwannoma and neurofibroma, with schwannomas being more frequent. Since the first reported case of laryngeal schwannoma in 1925, more than 130 cases of laryngeal tumours of neural origin had been reported up to the mid-1990s, but it is difficult to distinguish the exact number of neurilemmomas and neurofibromas.

The majority of schwannomas present in the parapharyngeal space, with schwannomas in the head and neck accounting for 25–45% of those identified clinically. The larynx remains a rare site. These tumours in the larynx may present at any age, with a slight female preponderance. Almost all benign neurogenic tumours of the larynx arise in the supraglottis, the true vocal cord may be involved, with fewer than ten cases reported.

They are more likely to affect sensory nerves than motor nerves and differ from neurofibromas in that the latter are unencapsulated, do not cause symptoms and may be associated with neurofibromatosis type II.

Neurilemmomas affect both sexes equally, and they occur most often during the fifth to sixth decades of life. Neurilemmomas typically affect nerve sheaths but not usually the nerve fibres. Neurofibromas may be single or multiple; multiple lesions characterise neurofibromatosis type I.

It is important to distinguish between neurofibromas and schwannomas. The recurrence rate is greater for neurofibromas, and malignant transformation from neurofibroma to malignant neurosarcoma occurs in approximately 10% of cases, whereas malignant degeneration of schwannomas is extremely rare. CT and MRI are useful to aid with diagnosis, revealing not only the extent, but the degree of lipomatous element as well. Compared with CT, MRI offers superior soft tissue definition and better visualisation of the laryngeal musculature.

The characteristic finding is a round submucosal bulge arising from the false cord and/or aryepiglottic fold, obstructing the view of the ipsilateral true vocal cord. Symptoms are dependent on the site of origin. Most neurogenic tumours of the larynx originate in either the aryepiglottic fold or the false cord. In these locations, the nerve of origin is likely to be the recurrent laryngeal nerve or the internal branch of the superior laryngeal nerve. The tumour as it expands will distort the lateral larynx and will eventually close the airway and cause dysphonia. There are no characteristic features suggestive of neurilemmoma on simple inspection, although CT and MRI will delineate between benign and malignant tissue in the larger tumours. Pathological diagnosis is dependent on three criteria: the presence of a capsule, identification of Antoni A and B areas and a positive reaction of the tumour for S-100 protein.

Ideally, a neurilemmoma should be totally excised, but anatomic constraints sometimes make this difficult. The preferred method is microlaryngeal endoscopic excision with either conventional microlaryngeal endoscopic instrumentation or the use of the CO_2 laser. The open approach may be necessary for larger lesions. The treatment should be individualised with alternatives for an open approach via a transhyoid, laryngofissure or a lateral pharyngotomy approach.

6.5.10 Salivary Gland Tumours

Benign pleomorphic salivary adenoma of the larynx has been reported more than 40 times; another series of 11 cases have been reviewed in the Japanese literature. Males predominate slightly, with an age range from 15 to 82 years, most patients presenting in the fifth to seventh decades. The type and severity of symptoms depends on the size and location of the tumour mass—with dysphonia and dyspnoea symptoms being most common, some cases have been diagnosed en passant. The supraglottis is by far the most common site, followed by the subglottis and the glottis. Within the supraglottis, the epiglottis is the most common site, located to the laryngeal surface most commonly. Only one case has involved the whole of one side of the larynx from the valleculae to the ventricle. The tumour presented as a mass with mucosal deformity without ulceration. The tumour may be pedunculated.

The differential diagnosis must include angioma, fibromas, cylindroma, lymphoma, schwannoma, aberrant thyroid, vestigial cyst and internal laryngocoele. Two cases have been reported of carcinoma arising in a pleomorphic adenoma within the larynx.

Surgical removal is curative and will depend on the location and size of the tumour. The majority have been approached by a conservation surgical approach with cure—which have included endoscopic surgery including the laser, external approach via a laryngofissure or later pharyngotomy. However, if the tissue analysed is misinterpreted, or an is error made, then a more extensive surgical approach may result and several such occurrences have been reported. Importantly, the use of radiotherapy alone in a few cases did not shrink the tumour.

6.5.11 Oncocytoma

Solitary oncocytoma masses are extremely rare and few have been reported in the literature. Oncocytic hyperplasia by contrast is frequently diagnosed in elderly patients, and is most commonly reported in the supraglottis. Oncocytic lesions range from a solid proliferation to a thin-walled cyst, lined by multiple layers of cuboidal epithelium. Oncocytic lesions of the larynx manifest themselves as a morphological spectrum of changes, including surface metaplasia of the respiratory or squamous epithelium, solitary oncocystic "adenomas" (neoplasms), multifocal "hyperplastic" masses and cysts lined by oncocytes. Each of these entities is within the benign spectrum of oncocytic lesions, without any treatment implications. However, oncocytic change/metaplasia can be diagnosed if present diffusely or multifocal throughout the larynx. If there is a solid proliferation of oncocytes, the designation of adenoma can be used. Many cysts of the larynx are lined by oncocytes, and a clear distinction between saccular or ductal cyst and oncocystic papillary cystadenoma may not always be possible.

6.5.12 Necrotising Sialometaplasia

Two cases of necrotising sialometaplasia of the larynx have been reported. One case occurred in the subglottis and the other in the false cord. It is suggested that this process is associated with other diseases or processes, a secondary process, occurring in the larynx at the same time and another cause in proximity should be sought, such as cancer. It is thought that the likely pathogenesis is the result of vascular compromise to the affected area.

6.5.13 Paraganglioma

Neuroendocrine neoplasms of the larynx can be divided into two main groups: those of epithelial origin (carcinoid and neuroendocine carcinoma) and those of neural type (paraganglioma). Paragangliomas are uncommon, slow-growing, generally benign tumours. They arise from the paraganglion cells derived from the neural crest as part of a diffuse neuroendocrine system. To date 76 cases have been agreed as fulfilling the specific criteria laid down to make an accurate diagnosis.

In the larynx there are two paired paraganglia: the superior and the inferior. The superior paraganglia are 0.1–0.3 mm in diameter and are situated in the false cord fold along the course of the superior laryngeal artery and nerve. The inferior paraganglia are 0.3–0.4 mm in diameter and are found near the lateral margin of the cricoid cartilage in the cricotracheal membrane along the course of the recurrent laryngeal nerve.

Typically, these tumours arise from the superior paraganglia (82%) and have a right-sided and female predilection (3:1). Only 11 cases of subglottic paraganglia have been reported, again with a female preponderance. An uncommon case demonstrating a transventricular location occurring with a fixed vocal cord presented a diagnostic challenge. The majority of laryngeal paragangliomas present during the fourth to sixth decades, with an age range of 5–90+ years.

Examination reveals a red or blue swelling, lobulated, submucosal, smooth mass in the false cord. Rarely are they associated with a neck mass, unless they are large enough to herniate through the thyrohyoid membrane. The lesion bleeds excessively if it is biopsied. Diagnosis can be made by radiological imaging and angiography.

Histologically, paragangliomas are characterised by chief and sustentacular cells. Electron microscopy shows neural secretory granules. Chief cells stain positive for chromagranin and synaptophysin. The presence of mitotic activity does not correlate with the clinical behaviour.

The goal of treatment is eradication with preservation of maximal laryngeal function. Cryosurgery has been attempted, but laryngofissure or radiation has been required following this procedure; no long-term follow-up of such cases has been documented. Endoscopic removal has been employed by several surgeons, but has been associated with frequent recurrences. The successful use of the CO_2 laser has been reported in a 4 cm × 4 cm × 3 cm mass in the supraglottis, with a 2-day postintubation period and a protracted hospital stay, with a 5-year tumour-free follow-up. Open surgery has in the past achieved excellent tumour control with preservation of laryngeal functions, even when the tumour is located in the subglottis. Radiation has not been reported as successful to date.

6.5.14 Granular Cell Tumours

Granular cell tumours are uncommon benign lesions that can be determined anywhere in the body. They have a predilection for the upper aerodigestive tract. Fifty percent of all cases occur in the head and neck region. The incidence of granular cell tumours in the larynx is 3–10% of cases in adults, and it is extremely rare in children.

In the head and neck, the anterior tongue and the larynx are the most common and second most common sites of these tumours. In the larynx, granular cell tumours are located on the posterior third of the vocal cord. Symptoms depend on the location and size of the tumour, with the most common symptom being dysphonia, and frequently they may be diagnosed in asymptomatic persons. The histopathological origin and cause of this tumour are unknown. A recent report suggests a neurogenic origin.

Macroscopically, these tumours are described as greyish-yellow, smooth but firm, well circumscribed, polypoidal or sessile. Fifty to 65% of laryngeal granular cell tumours have pseudoepitheliomatous hyperplasia, which can lead to misinterpretation owing to the similarity of these lesions to squamous cell carcinoma. Granular cell tumours are not malignant and a malignant transformation has so far never been reported, but laryngeal malignant granular cell tumours have been recorded. They metastasise early and the prognosis is not good. In a 34-year-old man, a histologically benign granular cell tumour has been reported that recurred with rapid growth.

The original tumour was characterised by atypia and pagetoid extensions into the epithelium. It is suggested that such cases be followed up very closely. Tumours are described that behave in a benign manner, and others behave more aggressively, with local tissue destruction, and have the potential to metastasise.

Treatment is local excision by endoscopic, transoral or laryngofissure methods appropriate to the site of the lesion. The recurrence rate after resection with free margins has been reported to be 8%; however, this increases to 21–50% with positive margins. The use of frozen sections has been used to aid endoscopic excision using the CO_2 laser and should be considered where there is pathological support for such a technique.

6.5.15 Giant Cell Tumours

This lesion is a true neoplasm and is presumed to be part of a series of tumours more frequently reported in long bones: the fibrohistiocytic series. In the larynx, giant cell tumours arise in the osteocartilaginous supporting structures of the larynx proper; they do not seem to be discrete soft tissue masses. A recent review suggests that 18 true cases have been reported. The lesion involves adult males, in their third to sixth decades, with female patients not having been reported to date. Presenting problems include the presence of a slowly growing mass and dysphonia.

On examination, a mass is usually palpable, most commonly originating in the thyroid cartilage. Endoscopically, the lesions have proven to be deeply seated with an overlying intact mucosa. CT scanning reveals a mass with a density intermediate between that of muscle and fat, which may or may not show come central cystic change. The multinucleated giant cell type is more likely to show malignant features than the smaller mononuclear cell type. In all laryngeal giant cell tumours reported, however, tumours with both cell types have been cytologically benign.

Older reports suggest radiotherapy may be used to control these tumours; modern therapy would suggest either a laryngectomy or a hemilaryngectomy both to achieve local control and to obtain sufficient tissue to confirm the pathological diagnosis.

6.5.16 Chondroma

Laryngeal chondromas are uncommon and are seen most often in the sixth to seventh decades of life. The most frequent site is the cricoid cartilage, then the thyroid cartilage and uncommonly the epiglottis. The exact number reported is unknown because it is difficult or impossible to separate the benign chondroma from low-grade chondrosarcoma; it is suggested that both patterns may overlap, and a single tumour can contain both patterns. This occurred because of the smallness of the biopsy specimen, and may not be representative of the whole or entire tumour. It is therefore recommended that if the cartilage tumour is suspected, then the whole of the tumour is excised and subjected to histopathology. The treatment and prognosis of chrondroma and those of low-grade chondrosarcoma are similar. Should an excised chondroma recur, there serious be doubt of the accuracy of the initial diagnosis—it had probably been a low-grade chondrosarcoma all along.

Surgery has always been the treatment of choice for laryngeal cartilage tumours. Most authors claim conservative surgery is the appropriate treatment for low-grade tumours as well as chondromas. Even in cricoid lesions, conservative treatment through a laryngofissure is possible, when the tumour involves less than half the cartilage. Radiotherapy for laryngeal cartilage tumours is controversial, and the experience is limited to 12 cases, with only two cases of documented long-term follow-up. Recent reports have described CO_2 laser therapy as a procedure to deal with recurrences, or even with primary lesions.

6.5.17 Non-neoplastic Laryngeal Tumours

6.5.17.1 Hamartomas

According to the WHO classification (1991), a hamartoma is a "developmental anomaly characterised by the formation of a tumour-like mass composed of mature tissue elements that are normally present in the location where it is found but occurring in abnormal proportions or arrangements" [6]. Hamartomas of the head and neck are uncommon, but have been described in the sinonasal tract, nasopharynx, oral cavity, oropharynx, larynx, hypopharynx, cervical oesophagus, ear, parotid gland, trachea, parathyroid gland and eye. They may be unifocal or multifocal. The term "pleiotropic hamartoma" is used to indicate the presence of multiple hamartomas in different sites in a given patient. Hamartomas of the larynx are very rare. Presently it is suggested that there are only 11 cases of well-documented hamartoma of the larynx. Males are more involved than females, with age peaks in early childhood and middle age (39–56 years). Of the 11 cases accepted as hamartomas of the larynx, six involved patients aged 16 years or more. The main symptoms of laryngeal involvement are similar to those of other benign mass lesions—dysphonia, dyspnoea and dysphagia.

Microscopically, the tissues show a disorganised architectural pattern with mesenchymal derivatives alone, or with superadded epithelial elements. Hamartomas of the larynx are mainly composed of cartilage and fibromuscular tissue. Fatty tissue and nerve elements are often seen. No features of malignancy are present. The dominant tissue defines the lesion, for example as cartilage hamartoma or myxochondromatous hamartoma. Such lesions need to be differentiated from choristoma, teratoma and rhabdomyoma, among others.

6.5.17.2 Pseudotumours or Pseudoneoplastic Lesions

From a practical point, pseudoneoplastic lesions of the larynx may be divided broadly into two groups: (1) growths that present clinically as mass lesions, but by histological examination are readily diagnosed and are appropriately classified as benign non-neoplastic lesions, and (2) benign lesions that may show histopathological features suggestive of neoplasia. The latter group may be further divided into lesions that are *clinically* suspicious and those that present a *microscopic* dilemma. Some are discussed next.

Inflammatory Fibroblastic Tumours

Inflammatory myofibroblastic tumours can be polypoid, pedunculated, spherical, lobular or nodular, with a smooth external appearance. They may be confined to the immediate submucosal region, and are not truly invading. They are firm in consistency, fleshy, and gritty on a cut surface, grey-yellow or tan-white, and may measure up to 3 cm in the greatest dimension. To date only ten cases of inflammatory myofibroblastic tumours have been reported in the larynx.

The most common site is the vocal cord. These lesions are usually located on the true vocal cord, although the subglottis and upper trachea can be involved. The lesions may demonstrate a myxomatous appearance, but do not exhibit necrosis or haemorrhage. Histopathologically, special stains confirm the diagnosis. The differential diagnosis centres around spindle cell squamous cell carcinoma, but inflammatory fibrosarcoma, nerve sheath tumours, nodular fasciitis and non-specific inflammation must also be excluded.

Fibroma

Fibromas generally present as a polyps or nodules, either sessile or pedunculated in attachment, soft or firm, and their size is dependent on the duration and intensity of exposure to the irritating factors. Most lesions are covered by an intact epithelium, often exhibiting keratosis, and can measure up to 4 cm. Many fibromas involve Reinke's space (superficial lamina propria), and arise from the anterior two thirds of the vocal cord.

Fibromas, probably represent a reactive change and are not true neoplasms. With removal of the putative underlying insult, healing may occur after surgical excision. All lesions removed from the larynx require histopathological examination and a diagnosis is essential for patient management and prognosis.

Amyloidosis

Isolated amyloidosis (without plasmacytoma) frequently occurs along the false vocal cord, although any portion of the larynx can be affected. The term "amyloidosis" is used to indicate an extracellular accumulation of homogenous protein-derived fibrillary and eosinophilic material, with well-defined histochemical characteristics. When amyloidosis involves the supraglottic or glottic region, the lesion demonstrates an elevated, smooth or bosselated, polypoidal, mucosa-covered, firm mass. Subglottic amyloidosis presents as a more generalised, diffuse swelling. Multifocal deposits occur quite frequently.

Surface ulceration has been reported in more extensive and larger lesions. The mass is firm, with a waxy, translucent cut surface ranging in colour from tan-yellow to red-grey. It is reported that up to 15% of patients who demonstrate laryngeal amyloidosis may have amyloid deposits in other head and neck sites.

It is important when they are diagnosed that patients are screened for the possibility that they may have tumour-forming amyloid, primary systemic amyloidosis (diagnosed by serum or urine immunoelectrophoresis or rectal biopsy), secondary amyloidosis (associated with some other predisposing disease) and plasmacytoma, whether it be solitary or part of multiple myeloma. The most common amyloid lesions seen in the larynx are amyloid deposition alone, localised amyloid deposit or amyloid tumour (without associated lymphoproliferative disorder).

Most authors agree that surgery should be the treatment of choice of laryngeal amyloidosis. Surgical procedures include external partial laryngectomy or microlaryngeal excision. An alternative surgical technique is the use of CO_2 laser excision.

Laryngeal Cysts

The gross appearances of cysts in the larynx are often determined by the point of origin in the larynx and the type of cyst (saccular, retention/inclusive, ductal, vascular or traumatic). The cyst can be considered external or internal to the larynx based upon the degree of compression of the larynx by the cyst and the extent of the disease within the larynx. Cysts generally do not communicate with the interior of the larynx. A laryngocoele (an air-filled herniation or dilatation of the saccule) can be either internal or external to the larynx, communicating with the lumen. Saccular cysts (anterior or lateral) are submucosal and do not communicate with the lumen, but instead are filled with mucus or acute inflammatory elements.

Cysts occur in all regions of the larynx, with retention cysts most often located in the epiglottis, saccular cysts in the false cord and traumatic cysts in the arytenoid region. The size of the cysts depends on the location; small cysts are usually found on the vocal cords, whereas larger cysts are found attached to the epiglottis, pushing the larynx to one side, or projecting into the hypopharynx.

Cyst walls of fibrous connective tissue vary in thickness. The lining helps to differentiate the cysts into a variety of subtypes. Most cysts are lined by squamous or respiratory epithelium (retention and saccular), and a few cysts are lined by fibrous connective tissue. Those with an admixture of both mesodermal and endodermal layers qualify as congenital or embryonal cysts. A proposal has been suggested that all laryngeal cysts can be classified into congenital, retention and inclusion cysts.

All cyst lesions should be considered for a confirmatory histopathological diagnosis, a biopsy can confirm the clinical suspicion of a benign diagnosis, before patient reassurance can be given with confidence.

6.5.18 Summary

Benign tumours present uncommonly in the larynx, but should be considered and excluded by a thorough history of the symptoms, local physical signs within the larynx, appropriate endoscopic examination with appropriate biopsy and confirmation of the histopathological diagnosis before embarking on patient management. The management of benign tumours should aim at function preservation, with ensuing complete excision of the tumour most often performed by endoscopic excision, using the laser as a tool. Patients should be warned and advised that after surgery in certain diseases there is a risk of tumour recurrence, and should seek appropriate laryngeal evaluation should their symptoms return or their anxieties require alleviation.

References

1. Barnes L (2001) Diseases of the larynx, hypopharynx, and oesophagus. In: Barnes L (ed) Surgical pathology of the head and neck, 2nd edn. Dekker, New York, pp 151–154
2. Glanz H, Schulz A, Kleinsasser O, Schulze W, Dreyer T, Arens C (1997) Benign lesions of the larynx: basic clinical and histopathological data. In: Kelinsasser O, Glanz H, Olofsson J (eds) Advances of laryngology in Europe. Elsevier, Amsterdam, pp 3–14
3. Holinger PH, Johnston KC (1951) Benign tumors of the larynx. Ann Otol Rhinol Laryngol 60(2):496–509
4. Narozny W, Mikaszewski B et al. (1995) Benign neoplasms of the larynx. Auris Nasus Larynx 22(1):38–42
5. New GB, Erich JB (1938) Benign tumors of the larynx: a study of 722 cases. Arch Otolaryngol Head Neck Surg 28:841
6. Rinaldo A, Mannara GM, Fisher C, Ferlito A (1998) Hamartoma of the larynx: a critical review of the literature. Ann Otol Rhinol Laryngol 107:264–267

Suggested Reading

1. Andrus JG, Shapshay SM (2006) Contemporary management of laryngeal papilloma in adults and children. Otolaryngol Clin North Am 39(1):135–158
2. Arens C, Glanz H et al. (1997) Clinical and morphological aspects of laryngeal cysts. Eur Arch Otorhinolaryngol 254(9–10):430–436
3. Dikkers FG (2006) Treatment of recurrent respiratory papillomatosis with microsurgery in combination with intralesional cidofovir—a prospective study. Euro Arch Otorhinolaryngol 263(5):440–443
4. Guilemany JM, Alos L, Alobid I, Bernal-Sprekelsen M, Cardesa A (2005) Inflammatory myofibroblastic tumour in the larynx: clinicopathological features and histogenesis. Acta Otolaryngol 125(2):215–219
5. Martines F, Martines E, Caamitjana CF, Perello Scherdel E (2007) Inflammatory myofibroblastic tumour of the larynx: case report. Ann Otorhinolaringol Ibero 34(2):210–208
6. Wenig BM, Devaney K, Bisceglia M (1995) Inflammatory myofibroblastic tumour of the larynx. Cancer 76(11):2217–2229
7. Wenig BM, Devaney K, Wenig BL (1995) Pseudoneoplastic lesions of the oropharynx and larynx simulating cancer. Pathol Annu 30(1):143–187

6.6 Laryngeal Cancer

DOMINIQUE CHEVALIER AND JEAN-LOUIS LEFEBVRE

6.6.1 Definition

Malignant tumours of the larynx: The majority of malignancies 95% are squamous cell carcinomas; other primary malignant tumours include salivary gland tumours, neurological tumours and chondromas. Other malignant tumours may metastasize to the larynx (secondary)—malignant melanoma, hypernephroma—and general or systemic malignancies may manifest themselves in the larynx—non-Hodgkin's lymphoma.

6.6.2 Aetiology/Epidemiology

Laryngeal cancer is frequent and currently represents 3% of male cancers in Europe. The incidence of laryngeal cancer is higher in men than in women (6:1), although the incidence in women is rising owing to the increased prevalence of smoking tobacco and alcohol indulgence. These cancers usually manifest themselves during the second half of life, with a peak incidence in the fifth and sixth decades (on average, 55 years for men and 60 years for women) [6].

Other causes cited include dietary deficiencies, and environmental exposure may also contribute to carcinogenesis, but their exact roles are not well understood. The possibility of a genetic predisposition continues to be investigated. Genotypic and phenotypic deficiencies in the metabolism of tobacco-related and other carcinogens as well as abnormalities in DNA repair mechanisms may also play an aetiological role.

6.6.3 Symptoms

Patients with cancer of the larynx commonly present with a history of a sore throat, dysphonia, dysphagia, referred otalgia and/or a neck mass or a combination of these. Dysphonia is a common symptom of glottic carcinoma. Patients with a supraglottic and/or glottic cancer often complain of a foreign-body feeling in the throat. Progressive dysphagia, initially for solid foods and later for liquids, is frequently seen in patients with supraglottic cancer. When patients present with symptoms of severe dysphagia and dyspnoea, most usually have an advanced-stage cancer most commonly with laryngeal cartilage invasion. Weight loss may result from invasion of the pharynx in advanced-stage tumours.

Palpable cervical lymphadenopathy is frequent at the time of diagnosis, more so with supraglottic than with glottic cancers, and these palpable or involved nodes are most often located in the subdigastric (level IIa) and mid-jugular (level III) nodal levels.

Thorough examination must be performed in every patient presenting with palpable lymph nodes who has a persistent sore throat, dysphonia, dysphagia or otalgia, particularly when known risk factors (alcohol abuse and/or tobacco use) are documented or suspected from the patient's history.

6.6.4 Diagnosis

6.6.4.1 Physical Examination

The oral cavity and the oropharynx must be examined to detect a possible second primary cancer, and dental status must also be assessed. Indirect laryngoscopy remains the basic diagnostic procedure and, when necessary, is complemented by an examination with a rigid endoscope or a flexible fibre-optic scope. The fibre-optic laryngoscope is particularly useful in patients with an uncontrollable gag reflex. The patients must be examined during both respiration and phonation. This examination provides global information on the site and size of the tumour, as well as the mobility of the vocal cords. While tumours of the vocal cord and the ventricular fold are usually easily visualized by indirect mirror examination, tumours located in the ventricle, the subglottis, the trachea and the epiglottis may escape detection. Attention must be paid to indirect signs such as mucosal oedema or erythema, which may suggest an underlying or deeper abnormality and must initiate further investigation, most commonly direct visualization at direct laryngosopy and the performing of a biopsy.

Palpation of the neck is necessary to detect adenopathy. The size, site and mobility of all nodes should be documented. Examination of the neck may also reveal signs of direct extension of the cancer into the tissues of the neck. Pain generated by the movement of the thyroid cartilage is highly suggestive of an extension into the neck.

Most patients currently with such symptoms and signs are investigated by radiological imaging, including a computed tomography (CT) scan or a magnetic resonance imaging (MRI) scan.

6.6.4.2 Direct Pharyngolaryngoscopy

Direct endoscopic examination of the pharynx, larynx and oesophagus is performed under general anaesthesia. It is conducted with rigid endoscopes and with rigid telescopes to improve the quality of the mucosal assessment particularly in the case of a small cancer [2]. It is an indispensable diagnostic tool and has several goals:

- It allows for multiple mucosal biopsies for histological examination.
- It provides an accurate evaluation of the superficial tumour spread.
- The systematic examination of the entire upper aerodigestive tract and the oesophagus allows for detection of synchronous cancers.

6.6.4.3 Diagnostic Imaging

Imaging techniques are becoming more precise and are now used routinely in conjunction to complement the clinical and the endoscopic assessment of patients with laryngeal carcinomas.

CT is currently the most useful imaging modality, particularly the helical CT technique, which is simple, fast and allows multiplanar reconstruction [7]. The goal of CT is to accurately assess the location and size of the primary cancer and to evaluate extension to the neck either directly or through lymphatic metastasis. CT examination must be performed from the nasopharynx to the upper mediastinum first without and thereafter with intravenous contrast enhancement. In the case of small laryngeal tumour, CT is preferably performed before the endoscopy and the biopsies, to avoid inflammation, which may result in an overestimation of the cancer infiltration. CT also allows for the use of dynamic manoeuvres such as the Valsalva manoeuvre and phonation.

A cancer of the vocal cord or the ventricle may extend into the paraglottic space, and supraglottic cancer can extend to invade the pre-epiglottic space. Pre-epiglottic extension is easily detected after image reconstruction in the sagittal plane. Laterally, laryngeal cancer may extend to the thyroid cartilage, which acts as a temporary barrier against extension in the neck. Although CT usually demonstrates cartilage destruction when it is massive, it often fails to detect limited invasion of cartilage but this may be suggested by the presence of cartilage sclerosis. The helical CT scan technique allows exploration in the same session of the upper aerodigestive tract and the lung.

Metastatic lymph nodes are frequently encountered with carcinoma of the supraglottis. The probability of metastatic involvement of a lymph node is associated with the following criteria seen on imaging:

- Size greater than 10 mm (12 mm in the subdigastric area)
- Central necrosis with heterogeneity and peripheral enhancement
- Circular shape

In the evaluation of carcinoma of the subglottis, a CT scan yields important information regarding superior mediastinal and retropharyngeal lymph nodes where clinical examination is not feasible.

MRI is performed with the use of an anterior neck coil and application or use of a protocol, which consists of axial T2, weighted fast spin echo and T1-weighted spin echo images. Then, following intravenous administration of gadolinium, axial, sagittal and coronal T1-weighted spin echo images are obtained. MRI is more sensitive in detecting minimal neoplastic invasion to the cartilage than CT [1], but CT is more specific. MRI has superior resolution for demonstrating soft tissue details. Nevertheless, owing to its susceptibility to motion-induced artefacts, MRI is not routinely performed in staging of cancer of the larynx.

Ultrasonography is helpful for assessment of the cervical lymph nodes. It is a simple, non-invasive, rapid and high-sensitivity technique for the detection of subclinical lymph node metastasis, but its reliability is operator-dependent. It is a useful method for the follow-up and can be combined with fine-needle aspiration to confirm histological invasion.

6.6.5 Therapy

6.6.5.1 Surgery

Surgery in early-stage glottic and supraglottic cancers may be performed endoscopically using either traditional surgery or the CO_2 laser to perform partial laryngeal surgery [3]. In more advanced stage disease the decision to perform surgery, either endoscopic or external, is based upon the expertise available, the practice of the local department, or in some centres patients are treated by radiotherapy with or without chemotherapy.

The following partial procedures have been described and are indicated for the surgical treatment of glottic cancer:

- Cordectomy, when feasible, can frequently be performed by an endoscopic approach. It is indicated for vocal cord cancer without deep infiltration.
- Frontolateral laryngectomy is performed less frequently and currently is indicated when the tumour is located to the anterior commissure.
- Anterior frontal laryngectomy with epiglottoplasty is indicated for the treatment of a bilateral vocal cord tumour without deep infiltration.
- Supracricoid partial surgery is indicated for the treatment of T2 and selected T3 glottic carcinomas particularly when deep infiltration is suspected.
- Hemiglossectomy is indicated for T2 glottic cancer and is an alternative to supracricoid partial surgery.

The following partial procedures are indicated for the treatment of supraglottic cancer:

- Horizontal supraglottic laryngectomy is indicated for the treatment of a tumour limited to the epiglottis without deep extension to the pre-epiglottic space or involving the ventricle. In selected cases this procedure can be extended to include larger tumours that involve the base of the tongue or the upper part of the piriform sinus.
- Supracricoid partial laryngectomy with cricohyoidopexy is indicated for a tumour extended to the inferior part of the pre-epiglottic space or involving the ventricle or the glottis with normal mobility of both arytenoid cartilages.

Total laryngectomy is indicated for tumours demonstrating massive invasion of the larynx.

As a rule, partial surgical techniques are always combined with radical or modified ipsilateral neck dissection. Contralateral neck dissection is necessary when the primary tumour involves the supraglottis.

6.6.5.2 Radiotherapeutic Treatment

Definitive Irradiation
Definitive irradiation techniques vary according to the primary site and tumour extension within or outside the larynx, as well as the likely involvement of the neck.

Radiotherapy sources are either cobalt-60 or 4–6-MV electron beams. Patients are treated in a supine position after 3D dosimetry.

Tumours strictly limited to the glottic area are treated by small 5 cm × 5 cm lateral opposite and parallel fields [5].

Two lateral opposite and parallel fields including the larynx and both necks treat tumours invading or originating from the supraglottic area. More extensive tumours require modification of the treatment fields depending on their local anatomic involvement.

Tumours invading or originating in the subglottis are treated by two lateral opposite and parallel fields including the larynx and both necks and the upper mediastinum.

The conventional treatment consists of one fraction of 2 Gy per day, 5 days per week for a total of 65–70 Gy. Radiotherapy may also be delivered with a hyperfractionated schedule (two fractions per day) for a total of 70–80 Gy.

Postoperative Irradiation
Postoperative irradiation is indicated when there is proven extension of the tumour outside the larynx or when there is the presence of cervical nodal involvement. A 60-Gy dose is delivered to the surgical bed and up to 70 Gy is delivered to the areas of positive margins or of positive lymph nodes using a technique of two lateral opposite and parallel fields.

6.6.5.3 Medical Treatment

The most frequently used drugs are cisplatin (or carboplatin as a substitute), 5-fluorouracil or, in a palliative setting, methotrexate. There are three treatment options: induction, adjuvant or concomitant chemotherapy.

Most clinicians have nearly abandoned the use of adjuvant protocols. Induction chemotherapy in the past failed to improve the survival and disease control, but recently discussion of its use in larynx preservation has reopened (see below). Concurrent chemotherapy has significantly resulted in improved patient survival but generates moderate to severe mucositis [4].

With the appearance of taxanes and targeted therapies (in particular cetuximab), the concept of expanding medical treatments continues to be advocated by some physicians.

6.6.5.4 Larynx Preservation

There are three possibilities to avoid performing a total laryngectomy:

1. Induction CT followed in good responders by irradiation. The randomized trials carried out on this basis have shown that survival was not jeopardized and that around 60% of the larynx could be preserved.
2. Concurrent chemoirradiation. One randomized American trial (RTOG) has shown that this strategy

provided a higher larynx preservation rate but also a higher mucosal toxicity, while survival remained unchanged.

3. Induction chemotherapy followed by concurrent chemoirradiation in good responders. This promising strategy is under evaluation.

6.6.6 Prognosis

1. T1–T2
   - Local control over 85%
   - Five-year survival for supraglottis around 70% and for glottis around 80%
2. T3
   - Local control over 80%
   - Five-year survival for supraglottis around 60% and for glottis around 70%
3. T4 resectable
   - Local control over 66%
   - Five-year survival for supraglottis around 40% and for glottis around 50%
4. T4 non-resectable: local control and 5-year survival below 30%

References

1. Castelijns JA et al. (1998) Invasion of laryngeal cartilage by cancer: comparison of CT and MRI imaging. Radiology 167:199–206
2. Chevalier D et al. (1997) Endoscopic evaluation of glottic cancer. Ann Otolaryngol Chir Cervicofac (Paris) 114:197–198
3. Eckel HM et al. (1998) Potential role of transoral laser surgery for larynx carcinoma. Lasers Surg Med 23:79–86
4. Forastiere AA et al. (2003) Concurrent chemotherapy and radiotherapy for organ preservation in advanced laryngeal cancer. N Engl J Med 349:2091–2098
5. Franchin G et al. (2003) Radiotherapy for patients with early-staged glottic carcinoma: univariate and multivariate analyses in a group of consecutive, unselected patients. Cancer 98 (4):765–772
6. Mollen Jensen O et al. (1990) Cancer in the European Community and its member states. Eur J Cancer 26:1167–1256
7. Robert Y et al. (1996) Helical CT of the larynx a comparative study with conventional CT scan. Clin Radiol 51:882–885

6.7 Trauma to the Laryngeal and Tracheal

NORBERT KLEINSASSER

6.7.1 Definition

Traumata of the larynx and trachea are heterogeneous sequelae of blunt, perforating or endoluminal forces affecting the head, neck or mediastinum.

6.7.2 Aetiology/Epidemiology

Laryngeal or tracheal trauma may result from internal, endoluminal or external forces, the lattermost being rarer.

Endolaryngeal and endotracheal injuries caused by intubation mechanisms may lead to:
- Haematoma of the soft tissue
- Lacerations, perforations and ruptures of, e. g., the vocal cords (Fig. 6.7.1)
- Dislocation of arytenoid cartilage

Endoluminal trauma caused by endotracheal anaesthesia or respirator treatment may lead to:
- Intubation granulomas
- Postintubation cysts
- Pigment inoculation into the mucosa
- Synechias between vocal cords or between false cords
- Scar stenosis on the posterior wall of the larynx
- Subglottic membranous stenosis
- Funnel-shaped laryngotracheal or tracheal stenosis
- Partial or total obliteration of the larynx and/or trachea

Further reasons for endoluminal traumata include the ingestion of xenobiotics (e.g. caustic lyes, acids, gases), endolaryngeal surgery and a variety of other surgical and diagnostic procedures.

External traumata are heterogeneous in terms of their mechanisms and consequences. External trauma due to the impact of blunt objects or tearing may lead to:
- Endoluminal soft tissue lesions (Fig. 6.7.2)
- Fractures of the thyroid/cricoid/tracheal cartilage
- Ruptures of the laryngeal, laryngotracheal and tracheal ligaments
- Combined fractures and ruptures with soft tissue lesions

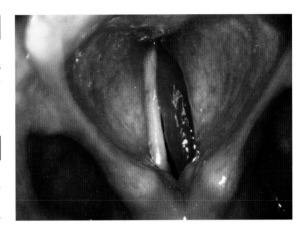

Fig. 6.7.1 Laryngeal contusion with hematoma of the right vocal fold after blunt laryngeal trauma at endoscopy

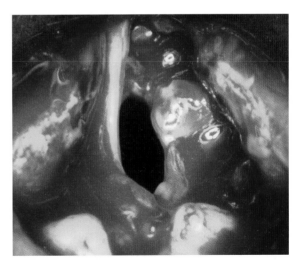

Fig. 6.7.2 Laryngeal rupture (type 2) seperation of right arytenoid from right vocal cord

External trauma due to perforating forces may lead to:
- Lacerations of the larynx, trachea and neck tissue as well as the laryngeal nerves (Fig. 6.7.3)
- Dyspnoea

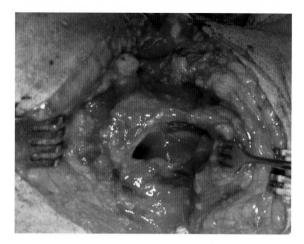

Fig. 6.7.3 Supraglottic separation after attempted Suicide with knife

- Aspiration, air embolism and pneumothorax
- Bleeding of major vessels
- Tracheoarterial and tracheo-oesophageal fistulas

Additional reasons for external trauma to the larynx and trachea are coniotomy, tracheostomy, dilational tracheotomy, partial resections as well as other surgical and diagnostic procedures. Furthermore, trauma to the functional precursors of the larynx, e. g., to the inferior or to the superior laryngeal nerve, is also of major importance.

6.7.3 Symptoms

Symptoms of laryngeal and tracheal traumata vary widely according to the diversity of the origin and severity. In addition to the individual history, common indicators for laryngeal and/or tracheal trauma in many cases may be:
- Hoarseness
- Dyspnoea, cyanosis
- Stridor
- Crepitation
- Haemoptysis and coughing attacks
- Soft tissue emphysema
- Haematoma
- Strangulation marks
- Pain, fear, shock
- Open ruptures and fractures, dislocations
- Bleeding, aspiration, desoxygenation
- Cardiopulmonal arrest

Clearly, the onset of symptoms in regard to the history of trauma is also of critical importance, especially in endoluminal trauma.

6.7.4 Complications

Besides the respiratory and circulatory complications mentioned already in acute laryngeal and tracheal trauma, long-term sequelae have to be monitored and combated. These include:
- Formation of scars and stenosis
- Impairment of voice, deglutition and ease of breathing

6.7.5 Diagnosis

6.7.5.1 Recommended European Standard Diagnostic Steps

- Detailed history taking (e. g. onset of symptoms, type of force, previous surgery)
- Inspection
- Palpation
- Indirect endoscopy with rigid and/or flexible scopes
- Microlaryngoscopy and tracheobronchoscopy

6.7.5.2 Additional/Useful Diagnostic Procedures

- Auscultation and percussion of the thorax
- X-ray of the thorax and neck
- CT scan of the thorax and neck
- High-resolution CT scan of the larynx
- Blood oxygen saturation monitoring
- Pulmonary functional test
- MRI in children
- Fluorescence MRI for functional evaluations

6.7.6 Therapy

6.7.6.1 Conservative Treatment

Recommended European Standard Therapeutic Steps
- Preservation of respiratory and circulatory functions
- Antiphlogistics (steroids and non-steroids)
- Analgesics

Additional/Useful Therapeutic Strategies
- Cooling
- Inhalation
- Voice and deglutition therapy

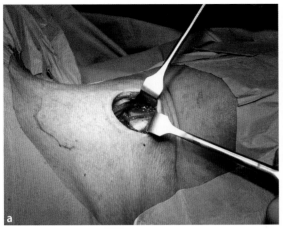 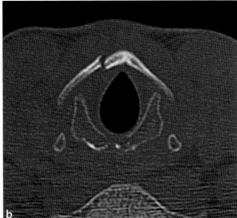

Fig. 6.7.4 a Fracture of thyroid cartilage on CT imaging. **b** Fractured thyroid cartilage at open reduction prior to fixation (same patient 4a)

6.7.6.2 Surgical Treatment

Recommended European Standard Surgical Procedures

In addition to the preservation of the respiratory and circulatory functions, as well as the care for soft tissue lesions, sequelae of trauma to the larynx and trachea have to be minimized, remedied or repaired by surgical means. These sequelae include endoluminal soft tissue lacerations and ruptures, dislocations of laryngeal or tracheal elements, scars, stenosis and obliterations. Surgical procedures include:

- Endolaryngeal microsurgery (e. g. readaptation of soft tissue lesions, resolution of scars)
- Endoscopic surgery of the trachea
- Endo-extraluminal repositioning and fixation of fragments

Additional/Useful Surgical Strategies

- Glottic enlargement procedures
- Subglottic enlargement procedures
- Tracheal and tracheolaryngeal segment resections
- Temporary tracheostomy
- Tracheal and/or tracheolaryngeal stents

6.7.7 Differential Diagnosis

Whereas in acute external laryngeal and tracheal trauma the history of the patient provides the best indication for the source of complaints, after endoluminal trauma diagnosis may be harder to achieve. Here the following symptoms that are often associated with trauma, e. g., hoarseness and dyspnoea, may be evaluated:

- Functional lesions of the laryngeal nerves
- Neoplastic or infectious and allergic diseases
- Systemic, cardiopulmonary or central and psychogenic affections

6.7.8 Prognosis

In severe laryngeal and/or tracheal trauma, major vessels of the neck and/or intrathoracic organs may also be compromised, threatening respiration, circulation and, therefore, life. Thus, in a situation of progressive symptoms, securing vital functions is mandatory. Still, some patients succumb to external laryngeal trauma before they can be treated. For those surviving the immediate trauma, exact diagnosis and implementation of therapy require a thorough understanding of the trauma. By these means, the strategic end points of prognosis, such as ease of breathing, décanulement, and voice quality may be very much influenced by the quality of initial and long-term treatment.

Additional Reading

Butler AP, Wood BP, O'Rourke AK, Porubsky ES (2005) Acute external laryngeal trauma: experience with 112 patients. Ann Otol Rhinol Laryngol 114 (5): 361–368

Graonka MA, Kleinsasser O (1996) Intubation damage to the larynx. Manifestations, comments on pathogenesis, treatment and prevention. Laryngorhinootologie 75(2): 70–76

Kleinsasser NH, Priemer FG, Schulze W, Kleinsasser OF (2000) External trauma to the larynx: classification, diagnosis, therapy. Eur Arch Otorhinolaryngol 257 (8): 439–444

Lee WT, Eliachar R, Eliachar I (2006) Acute external laryngotracheal trauma: diagnosis and management. Ear, Nose Throat J. 85(3): 79–84

Mussi A, Ambrogi MC, Ribechini A, Lucchi M, Menoni F, Angeletti CA (2001) Acute major airway injuries; clinical features and management. Eur J Cardiothorac Surg 20(1): 46–51

Verschuerment DS, Bell RB, Bagheri SC, Dierks EK, Potter BE (2006) Management of laryngo-tracheal injuries associated with craniomaxillofacial trauma. J Oral Maxillofac Surg 64(2): 203–214

6.8 Laryngeal and Tracheal Stenosis in Children and Adults

GYÖRGY LICHTENBERGER

6.8.1 Supraglottic Laryngeal Stenosis

6.8.1.1 Definition

The mildest form of a supraglottic laryngeal stenosis is the supraglottic web between the false vocal cords. The laryngeal entrance, the epiglottis and the false vocal cords and both arytenoidal regions are seldom destroyed so seriously that it would result in severe stenosis. However, this rear change may be a consequence of chemical damage; the resultant scar narrows the lumen or there is obvious no lumen.

6.8.1.2 Aetiology

1. Trauma (accident) from the outside (for example a car accident, the wheel crashing against the hyoid bone and the ossified thyroid cartilage)
2. Chemical damage to the laryngeal entrance (lyes, acids, insecticides)
3. Infections
   - Tuberculosis
   - Scleroma
   - Diphtheria
   - Syphilis
   - Typhus
   - Fungi
   - Scarlatina
4. Boeck sarcoidosis
5. Pemphygoid
6. Wegener's granulomatosis
7. Amyloid

6.8.1.3 Symptoms

At the beginning or in mild cases symptoms are dysphonia and dyspnoea, or with increasing narrowing of the lumen loss of voice (aphonia) or severe breathing difficulties at rest.

6.8.1.4 Diagnosis

1. History (development of the stenosis, type of force, previous surgery).
2. Inspection of the neck, breathing rate and difficulty, evidence of cyanosis.
3. Palpation of the laryngeal anatomy.
4. Auscultation and percussion of the thorax.
5. Indirect laryngoscopy, magnifying indirect laryngoscopy, nasolaryngotracheoscopy.
6. Imaging
   - Plain X-ray
   - CT scan
   - MRI
   - Virtual endoscopy in selected cases
7. Direct microlaryngoscopy, with or without the use of telescopes and/or magnification. The employment of anaesthetic may use intubations or jet ventilation or a preliminary tracheostomy.

6.8.1.5 Additional Diagnostic Procedures

- Blood oxygen saturation monitoring
- Pulmonary functional test
- Examination for gastro-oesophageal reflux disease (GORD)

6.8.1.6 Therapy

Conservative Treatment
This is only possible in patients with early acute cases presenting within hours! If this situation occurs, by examining the supraglottic part of the larynx, one can see that there is a swelling and oedema on the epiglottis and aryepiglottic fold and on the false cords. It is very important to try to check the mobility of the vocal cords. Influencing this situation with medication is possible only for fresh cases in the acute stage. It can be used if there is only subfusion of the mucosa and oedema and the patient suffers only from mild dyspnoea.

The respiratory and circulatory functions can be preserved by:

- Oxygen supply
- Humidification
- Steroids
- Inhalation
- Analgesics

Surgical Treatment

1. External trauma
   - Acute: Resulting in damage to the cartilage and laceration of the supraglottic mucosa. Depending on the severity, tracheotomy and thyrotomy should be performed in fresh cases along with debridement. Adaptation and suturing of mucosal edges should be performed, preserving as much of the structures as possible and reconstruction with miniplates or stenting should be performed to keep the reconstructed lumen.
   - Chronic: In cases after developed scarring destroyed the entrance of the larynx, supraglottic laryngectomy or step-by-step reconstruction of the larynx is indicated, but only after scar formation has definitely finished.
2. Internal trauma: Topical damage leading to severe oedema with exudation

6.8.1.7   Complications

1. Resulting from untreated cases
   - Loss of airway, dyspnoea requiring a tracheotomy.
   - Loss of voice, roughness, hoarseness or aphonia.
   - Swallowing difficulties seldom occur unless there is additional injury associated with the pharynx or upper oesophagus.
2. Resulting from treated cases
   - General: Pneumothorax may develop if the air route for exhaling is not sufficient by using jet anaesthesia.
   - Local: Delayed wound healing, wound splitting, restenosis, rescarring.

6.8.1.8   Prognosis

This depends on the need for tracheostomy, whether the patient could have been decannulated after the treatment or not. The voice after the management is mostly good if the supraglottic larynx is reconstructed. In cases where only the entrance of the larynx has been destroyed, the patient has good chances after supraglottic laryngectomy has been performed.

6.8.2   Glottic Laryngeal Stenosis

6.8.2.1   Anterior Commissure Web

Definition

Congenital: The anterior commissure web is one of the mildest forms of congenital laryngeal malformation. This is mostly thin membrane, but the anterior part may run deep in the subglottic region. The necessary intervention depends on the enlargement of the membrane. Urgent intervention is mostly not needed. However, in enlarged cases where the vocal cords can no longer be identified, immediate intervention is necessary owing to severe asphyxia.

Acquired: These webs may be different, in some cases very large and very thick. A mucous or fibrous anterior commissura web may develop. It may be small or large, thin or thick. Generally the solution of the mucosal web is easier.

Aetiology

The congenital webs result from the lack of the resorption of the proliferating epithelium in the intrauterine period of 7–8 months.

The acquired webs result from infections such as:

- Tuberculosis
- Syphilis
- Scleroma
- Diphtheria
- Typhus
- Scarlatina
- Fungi and from:
- Pemphygoid
- Boeck sarcoidosis
- Amyloidosis

They also result from:

- Different types of external trauma of the thyroid cartilage
- Surgical intervention (partial laryngectomy): endolaryngeal microsurgery, damaging the mucous membrane of the anterior commissure, for instance mucosal damage after removal of papilloma from this region
- Prolonged intubation

Symptoms

The symptoms depend on the size of the web and on concomitant changes in the larynx. (A concomitant change may be, for example, insufficient glottic closure developed after laser cordectomy enlarged in the anterior commissure. In such cases to achieve a good result it is not enough just to eliminate the web; it is also necessary to manage the glottic gap with medialization or augmentation.) Thin and small webs mostly cause nothing or only mild dysphonia. If the web is big and thick, both dysphonia and dyspnoea may be present.

Diagnosis
See Sect. 6.8.1.4.

Therapy

Conservative Treatment
In acute acquired cases right after the damage has been revealed, there is the chance to cover the rough deepithelized surface with fibrin glue to try to prevent adhesions or one can use mitomycin C.

Surgical Treatment
Only very thin anterior commissure membranes may be cured by simple dissection of the membrane, using a laser or microscalpel. In other cases it is necessary after dissection, and division of the web, to fix a silicon sheet or keel with endo-extralaryngeal sutures in the anterior commissure for 2–3 weeks without tracheostomy. An open procedure with preliminary tracheotomy is mostly not necessary even in cases of enlarged and bigger scarred webs. Tracheotomy is necessary only in rare cases, if the patient is suffering from severe dyspnoea, but the solution of these webs even in these cases may be performed endoscopically.

Complications
1. Resulting from untreated cases: Without the management of a big web, there may be narrowing the laryngeal lumen. Cardiopulmonary consequences should be taken in consideration
2. Resulting from treated cases
   - General: Pneumothorax may develop, if the air route for exhaling is not sufficient by using jet anaesthesia.
   - Local
     - Infection: When endoscopic procedures using endo-extralaryngeal suture fixation of the keel or sheet are performed, the stitching canal around the thread, below and above the anterior commissure, may be infected if the patient is not covered with antibiotics and the keel or sheet is not removed within 3–4 weeks after the implantation.
     - Rescarring may occur if the position of the keel was not adequate.

Prognosis
The prognosis is mostly very good if the web was not running deep below the anterior commissure. With a thick and an especially thick web below the anterior commissure, it should be taken into account that repeated procedures may be necessary to achieve optimal results because the web may only partially have been eliminated.

6.8.2.2 Posterior Commissure Stenosis

Definition
The posterior commissure stenosis is a finding resulting from a process fixing the vocal cords in paramedian position.

Aetiology
- Congenital: Rarely occurs.
- Acquired: Posterior commissure stenosis develops most usually as a consequence of prolonged intubation or previous laryngeal surgery.

Symptoms
The symptoms are not dependent on the enlargement of the scar in the posterior commissure, because a small scar results the same paramedian position of the vocal cords as would a bigger scar. Dyspnoea is a consequence of the narrow glottic chink due to the paramedian position of the vocal cords, and is independent of the enlargement of the scar. (However the solution and the methods introduced for the management of the stenosis depend on the enlargement of the scar.)

Diagnosis
See as before and in addition:
- EMG to reveal whether there is only fixation of the vocal cords by scars or if there is a combined disease with fixation and paralysis of the vocal cords
- Palpation of the arytenoid cartilages by direct microlaryngoscopy to reveal cricoarytenoid joint fixation

Therapy
If the patient has not been tracheotomized yet and the scar is less than 5 mm, it is possible after dissection of the scars by using the laser or microscalpel to temporarily lateralize both vocal cords until reepithelization of the mucosa of the posterior larynx for 3–4 weeks (Fig. 6.8.1). If the patient has already been tracheotomized and the scar in the posterior commissure is bigger than 5 mm but less than 10 mm, after preliminary tracheostomy the scar

fixing the vocal cords in paramedian position should be dissected, and an individually shaped soft silicon stent should be placed and fixed in the larynx for 3–4 weeks to prevent readhesion.

If there is a unilateral cricoarytenoid ankylosis or subluxation of the joint, the consequence is only dysphonia. If there is a bilateral cricoarytenoid ankylosis, posterior cricoid split and autologous costal cartilage homograft interposition is to fix into the posterior part of the larynx.

Complications

- General: When performing endoscopic procedures using suture fixation for temporary lateralization without tracheotomy in jet anaesthesia, pneumothorax may develop in very rare cases.
- Local: The stitching canal around the thread may be infected if an antibiotic is not administered or the

threads or the stent fixed by the threads is not removed 4 weeks after putting in the sutures.

Prognosis

The results are very good without any kind of tracheotomy with temporary bilateral endo-extralaryngeal lateralization of the vocal cords after endoscopic dissection of the scar, if the scar in the posterior commissure is not bigger than 5 mm and there is normal activity in the vocal cords as checked by EMG.

The prognosis is still good if the scar in the posterior commissure is bigger than 5 mm but less than 10 mm. In such cases, however, a temporary tracheotomy is necessary, because the lumen of the larynx has to be filled up with a silicon stent for 3–4 weeks and fixed by endo-extralaryngeal sutures. In these cases both the breathing and the phonation may be fully restored. If the scar is bigger than 10 mm and involved or destroyed one or both

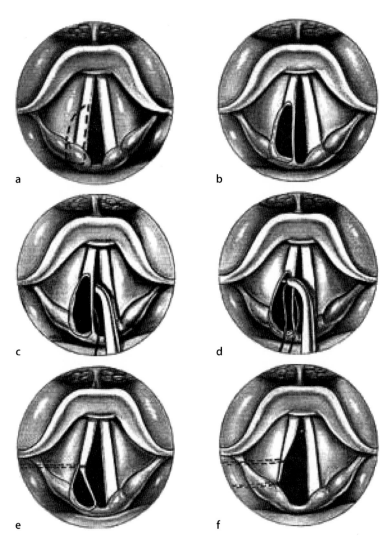

a

b

c

d

e

f

Fig. 6.8.1a–f Reversible endo-extralaryngeal lateralization, bilateral

arytenoid cartilages, the breathing results may be good after introducing open procedures; however, there are poorer phonation results.

6.8.2.3   Interarytenoid Scar Bridge

Definition
The interarytenoid scar bridge is a finding fixing the vocal cords in paramedian position.

Aetiology
- Congenital: Occurs rarely.
- Acquired: The interarytenoid scar bridge in nearly all cases is a consequence of prolonged intubation or previous surgery in the posterior larynx.

Symptoms
Dyspnoea.

Diagnosis
- History (development of the stenosis, type of force, previous surgery).
- Indirect laryngoscopy, magnifying indirect laryngoscopy, nasolaryngotracheoscopy.
- Direct microlaryngoscopy, with or without the use of telescopes and/or magnification. The employment of anaesthetic may use intubations with jet ventilation or a preliminary tracheostomy.

Additional Diagnostic Procedures
- Blood oxygen saturation monitoring
- Pulmonary functional test
- Examination for GORD

Differential Diagnosis
It is very important to differentiate the interarytenoid scar bridge from the bilateral vocal cord paralysis and from the posterior commissure stenosis. These scars are mostly not seen by indirect laryngoscopy. Therefore, direct laryngoscopy is mostly necessary to see not only the paramedian position of the vocal cords, but also to reveal the scars. If there is only a scar bridge, it is always a sulcus between the scar bridge and the posterior wall of the larynx. This sulcus may be detected by using a probe. If there is a real posterior commissure stenosis, there is no sulcus; the posterior part of the larynx is totally filled up by scar.

Therapy
If the patient has not been tracheotomized yet, it is possible just to dissect the scar bridge by using the laser or microscalpel. In contrast to posterior laryngeal stenosis, an additional surgical procedure is not necessary.

Complications
- General: When performing endoscopic procedures without tracheostomy, pneumothorax may develop in very rare cases.
- Local: Never happens.

Prognosis
The prognosis is mostly very good, with complete recovery.

6.8.2.4   Bilateral Cricoarytenoid Ankylosis

Definition
Ankylosis of the cricoarytenoid joints is a finding fixing the vocal cords usually in paramedian position.

Aetiology
Ankylosis of the cricoarytenoid joints may be consequence of prolonged intubation or chronic synovial joint diseases.

Symptoms
- Dyspnoea if both joints are involved
- Dysphonia if only one side joint is involved or there is only dislocation

Diagnosis
As before.

Therapy
1. Conservative: Depends on the cause of the ankylosis. In synovial joint diseases with administration of steroids the condition may be improved.
2. Surgical
   - If the patient has not been tracheotomized yet, it is possible to perform laser arytenoidectomy endoscopically and partial removal of the median and lateral thyroarytenoid muscles submucosally and lateralization of the preserved median mucous membrane by using endo-extralaryngeal sutures.
   - Cordotomy is not the method of choice, because this procedure for the management of bilateral an-

kylosis is not sufficient, as the position of the fixed arytenoids will not change. The other problem with this procedure is that there is granuloma formation after the operation and the defect created is filled up again with scars, resulting in an inadequate lumen.

Complications

As before.

Prognosis

The prognosis is mostly very good, with complete recovery of the breathing but with more or less impaired voice.

6.8.2.5   Bilateral Vocal Cord Paralysis

Definition

Bilateral vocal cord paralysis is a finding where the vocal cords are in paramedian position. There is no electric activity in the vocal cords. The paresis or paralysis may be the consequence of mostly direct damage of the recurrent laryngeal nerve.

There are acute (temporary) and chronic (definitive) cases.

Aetiology

- Congenital
- Surgery (neck, thoracic, cardiac, spinal, brainstem, etc.)
- Infections, mostly virus infection
- Degenerative processes
- Tumours (brainstem, mediastinal, chest, lung, oesophagus)

Symptoms

Symptoms are dependent on the white of the glottic chink. The paralysed vocal cords are mostly in paramedian position; however, the white of the glottic chink is different.

Diagnosis

As before.

Therapy

1. Conservative: There is mostly no chance for conservative treatment. However, in some cases there is a slight possibility to widen the lumen by local administration of Botox in the cricothyroid muscles to reduce the tension of the vocal cords, resulting in a little enlargement of the glottic chink.
2. Surgical
   - In acute cases: Within 2 weeks after the onset if the EMG samples are still not reliable, it is possible to perform the reversible vocal cord lateralization without tracheostomy in jet anaesthesia or in controlled apnoea using two endo-extralaryngeal sutures. With this technique one vocal cord is lateralized, as long as the function does not return (Fig. 6.8.2).
   - In chronic cases: Two weeks after the onset when the definitive paralysis has been proven by EMG–electroneuronography or if the immobility of bilateral vocal cord is older than 1 year, there are possibilities for irreversible glottis dilating operations such as
     - Arytenoidectomy
     - Submucosal cordectomy
     - Removal of a triangle of the vocal cord/s by using the laser
     - Preparation and submucosal removal of the anterior two third of the arytenoid cartilage and partial submucosal resection of the median and lateral thyroarytenoid muscles. After this procedure has finished, the medially preserved mucous membrane is turned laterally and fixed gently with two endo-extralaryngeal sutures. The threads should be removed 21 days after lateralization. To this time the laterally adapted mucosa will keep this position laterally, ensuring sufficient glottic chink (Fig. 6.8.3).

   These reversible and irreversible techniques could be performed without tracheostomy with jet anaesthesia.

Complications

- General: When performing endoscopic procedures without tracheostomy in jet anaesthesia, pneumothorax may develop in very rare cases.
- Local: Mild haemorrhage and oedema may develop, but very rarely. The stitching canal around the thread may be infected if an antibiotic is not administered or if the threads are not removed 3 weeks following the laterofixation.

Prognosis

The prognosis is mostly good, with adequate airway and differently reduced voice quality; however, the voice is adequate but seldom normal!

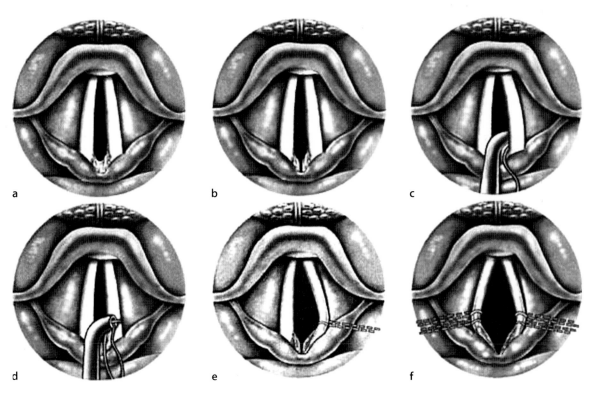

Fig. 6.8.2a–f Reversible endo-extralaryngeal lateralization, right side

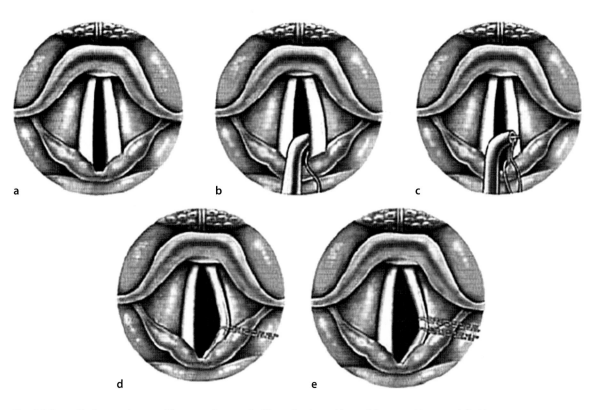

Fig. 6.8.3a–e Endo-extralaryngeal laryngomicrosurgical lateralization with partial arytenoidectomy, left side

6.8.3 Subglottic Laryngeal Stenosis (Cricotracheal Stenosis)

6.8.3.1 Definition

Subglottic laryngeal stenosis (cricotracheal stenosis) is a finding causing mild or severe dyspnoea as a consequence of a narrow airway in the subglottic region of the larynx or in the cricotracheal region.

6.8.3.2 Aetiology

As before (see Sect. 6.8.1.2):
- Congenital: The congenital subglottic stenosis is caused mostly by malformation of the cricoid cartilages. It may be concentric, elliptic and oval in craniocaudal direction. This stenosis may be membranous and cartilaginous. The most serious version of this malformation is congenital atresia.
- Acquired: As before. The stenosis is caused in adults mostly by prolonged intubation.

6.8.3.3 Symptoms

- In the most serious congenital cases, immediate intervention is necessary to save the life of the newborn.
- Moderate dyspnoea at the beginning or in mild cases, and life-threatening dyspnoea in serious cases.

6.8.3.4 Diagnosis

- Congenital: In severe congenital cases, rigid tracheobronchoscopy is mandatory.
- Acquired: As before (see Sect. 6.8.1.4).
- In addition: MR, virtual endoscopy in selected cases.

6.8.3.5 Classification of the Stenosis

The grading of the stenosis is recommended according to the classification of Myer, Connor and Cotton.

6.8.3.6 Therapy

1. Conservative: Mostly there is no chance for conservative treatment. However, in some cases there is a slight possibility to widen the lumen by local administration of mitomycin C.

2. Surgical
   - In congenital cases: With dilatation and laser surgery, a definitive good result cannot be achieved.
   - In acquired cases: There is the chance in selected cases to perform laser surgery to widen the lumen; however, in most of the cases, operation with an open procedure is necessary.

There are a large range of surgical procedures:
- Posterior cricoid split
- Posterior cricoid split with augmentation using costal cartilage autograft
- Anterior cricoid split and augmentation with costal cartilage autograft
- Anterior cricoid split and augmentation of the anterior cricotracheal region with septal cartilage autograft
- Anterior cricoid split and augmentation of the anterior cricotracheal region with the transposed part of the hyoid bone supplied with the sternohyoid muscle stem.
- Castellated incision and reconstruction
- Cricotracheal resection and thyreotracheal anastomosis

6.8.3.7 Complications

- General: When performing resection with elimination of the stoma and immediate anastomosis using jet anaesthesia, pneumothorax may develop if the air route for exhaling is not sufficient by using jet anaesthesia.
- Local: When performing augmentation techniques using autografts, wound infection, rejection of the graft and rescarring may occur. When performing resection and anastomosis, wound splitting, restenosis and rescarring may occur.

6.8.3.8 Prognosis

The prognosis depends on the severity, length and multiplicity of the stenosis.

6.8.4 Tracheal Stenosis

6.8.4.1 Definition

Tracheal stenosis is a finding causing moderate or severe dyspnoea as a consequence of a narrow airway in the trachea.

6.8.4.2 Aetiology

1. Congenital
   - Atresia or agenesis of the trachea (very rare disease, no chance of survival)
   - Concentric or eccentric mucosal-membranous stenosis not involving the cartilage
     - Fibrous stenosis involving partly the cartilage as well
     - Tracheomalacia
     - Malformation of the trachea (hypoplasy from cricoid to carina, tunnel-shaped stenosis, segmental stenosis)
2. Acquired
   - Incorrect creation of the tracheotomy opening
   - Inappropriate cuff-induced necrosis resulting in stenosis: prolonged intubation

6.8.4.3 Symptoms

The symptoms depend on the degree of the stenosis and may be mild or severe dyspnoea or asphyxia.

6.8.4.4 Diagnosis

1. Congenital: Rigid tracheobronchoscopy
2. Acquired: Flexible and rigid tracheoscopy
   - Plain X-ray
   - CT scan
   - MR
   - Virtual endoscopy in selected cases (Fig. 6.8.4)

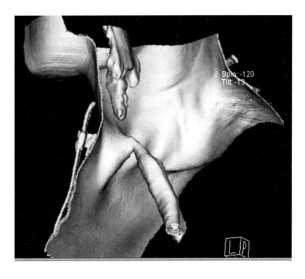

Fig. 6.8.4 3D picture of suprastomal tracheal stenosis

6.8.4.5 Therapy

- Tracheostomy
- Balloon dilatation technique in selected cases
- Laser resection by mucous-membranous stenosis
- Resection and end-to-end anastomosis (Figs. 6.8.5–6.8.6)
- Anterior tracheal split and augmentation with septal cartilage homograft
- Anterior tracheal split and augmentation with costal cartilage homograft

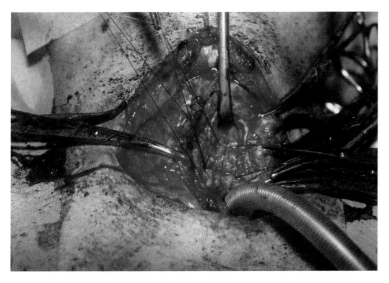

Fig. 6.8.5 Suturing of the back wall of the trachea after resection of the stenotic segment

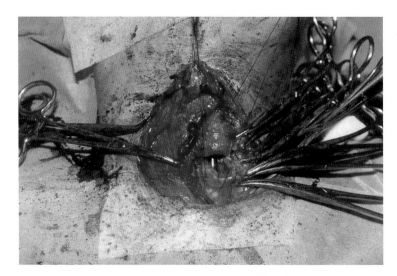

Fig. 6.8.6 Suturing of the anterior wall of the trachea

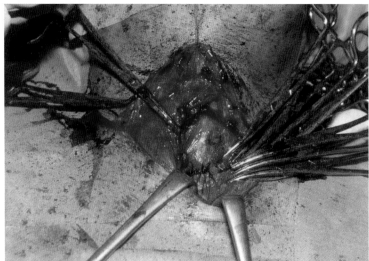

Fig. 6.8.7 Suturing after completing the anastomosis

- Castellated incision and reconstruction
- Pericardial tracheoplasty
- Slide tracheoplasty in strictly selected cases
- Rotary door flap technique
- Implantation of Montgomery T-tube

6.8.4.6   Complications

- General: Pneumothorax may develop if the air route for exhaling is not sufficient by using jet anaesthesia.
- Local: Rejection of the grafts by augmentation technique, wound infection, wound splitting and rescarring by resection and end-to-end anastomosis.

6.8.4.7   Prognosis

- No chance of survival with atresia and agenesia
- Very pure prognosis with malformation of the trachea
- Good prognosis for patients with circumferential mucous-membranous stenosis
- Good prognosis in cases where the stenosis is no longer than five rings

Suggested Reading

1. George M, KLang F, Pasche P, Monnier P (2005) Surgical management of laryngotracheal stenosis in adults. Eur Arch Otorhinolaryngol 262(8):609–615

2. Lichtenberger G (2003) Comparison of endoscopic glottis-dilating operations. Eur Arch Otorhinolaryngol 260(2):57–61

3. Lichtenberger G, Sittel C, Merati AL, Remenyi A (2007) Endoscopic technique to mark the site of tracheal stenosis for resection. J Laryngol Otol 121(8):790–793

4. Mandour M, Remacle M, Van de Heyning P, Elwany S, Tantawy A, Gaafar A (2003) Chronic subglottic and tracheal stenosis: endoscopic management vs. surgical reconstruction. Eur Arch Otorhinolaryngol 260(7):374–380

5. Monnier P, George M, Monod ML, Lang F (2005) The role of CO_2 laser in the management of laryngotracheal stenosis: a survey of 100 cases. Eur Arch Otorhinolaryngol 262(2):602–608

6. Sapundzhiev N, Lichtenberger G, Eckel HE, Friedrich G, Zenev I, Toohill RJ, Werner JA (2008) Surgery of adult bilateral vocal fold paralysis in adduction: history and trends. Eur Arch Otorhinolaryngol 265(12):1501–1514

6.9 Laryngeal Nerve Disorders

HANS EDMUND ECKEL

6.9.1 Definition

The larynx has two major functions. It acts as a sphincter to close the lower airway during deglutition, preventing aspiration of food and saliva, and serves secondarily as the organ of voice. Airway protection is phylogenetically the oldest and most essential function of the larynx. A failure to permanently protect the lower airway is a potentially life-threatening condition, since it results in chronic aspiration and subsequent pneumonia. Phonation is defined as sound production by means of vocal fold vibrations resulting from the tracheal air stream during expiration. Besides, the larynx also stabilizes the thorax by preventing exhalation, and helps to compress the abdomen during coughing.

To adequately comply with these physiological needs, laryngeal function relies on afferent (sensory) and efferent (motor) innervation. Nerve supply to the larynx (and pharynx) is provided by branches of **cranial nerve X (vagus nerve)**. The vagus nerve exits the skull through the jugular foramen and then bilaterally branches off the pharyngeal nerve, the superior laryngeal nerve and the recurrent laryngeal nerve. The pharyngeal nerve enters the pharynx and divides into the pharyngeal plexus to supply all of the striated muscles of the soft palate and the pharynx except for the m. tensor veli palatini and the m. stylopharyngeus (which are innervated by cranial nerves V and IX, respectively). The superior laryngeal nerve innervates the cricothyroid and the inferior constrictor muscles. The recurrent laryngeal nerves supply all of the intrinsic muscles of the larynx except the m. cricothyroideus. On the right, the recurrent laryngeal nerve loops around the subclavian artery and then turns upward again to the larynx, while the left recurrent laryngeal nerve passes under the aortic arch and then returns upward to the larynx. Parasympathetic fibres of cranial nerve X also innervate smooth muscles of the airway and gut, providing signals to open the airway during breathing, to produce bronchoconstriction, and also to coordinate peristalsis of the oesophagus.

Sensation from the vocal cords and the larynx below this level is carried by sensory fibres of the recurrent laryngeal nerve. Sensation above the vocal folds is transmitted by the superior laryngeal nerve.

Disorders of laryngeal nerve supply lead to a variety of **phonatory**, **respiratory** and **deglutition disorders**, resulting from impaired sensitivity of the larynx, from movement disorders of the vocal cords, and from impairment of pharyngo-oesophageal bolus transport during deglutition.

"Paralysis" is the term used to describe the complete loss of voluntary motor function (movement) due to neural or muscular disorders, whereas **paresis** is a reduced, but incomplete abolition of voluntary movement. "Palsy" is an older term that has been used interchangeably with either "paralysis" or "paresis"; its use is now restricted to historical diagnoses that have been retained in conventional use such as Bell's palsy.

In clinical laryngology, nerve disorders are by far more frequently found than muscle disorders, the latter usually not being limited to laryngeal muscles. Nerve injuries are categorized according to morphological alterations, nerve functionality, and the ability for spontaneous recovery. The classification of nerve injury is usually based on electromyographic findings.

The mildest condition is **neurapraxia**. Neurapraxia is defined as dysfunction and/or paralysis without loss of nerve sheath continuity and peripheral Wallerian degeneration. Neurapraxia will usually result in a more or less complete recovery of voluntary muscular action.

Axonotmesis is determined by damage to the axons with preservation of the neural connective tissue sheath (endoneurium, epineurium), with consecutive distal Wallerian degeneration. Axonotmesis in the recurrent laryngeal nerve almost invariably results in so-called misdirected reinnervation. This means that axons will eventually regenerate and finally reach laryngeal muscles, but not their physiological targets. Instead, reinnervation follows an accidental pattern. Some axons will finally gain access to their initial target muscle, while others will be directed towards others, sometimes antagonistically acting muscles. Axonotmesis usually results in paralysis without muscular atrophy.

Neurotmesis is the most severe class of nerve injury. It occurs when the axon and surrounding connective tissue components are hurt and disrupted. Recovery through axonal regeneration cannot occur. Neurotmesis will therefore result in paralysis with muscular atrophy.

Combined types of nerve injuries (e.g. neurapraxia with coexisting axonotmesis in some axons) are common. These combined types of nerve lesions hamper reliable prognostic information solely from electromyography.

6.9.2 Aetiology/Epidemiology

Vocal cord paralysis may result from lesions at the central nervous system (nucleus ambiguous and its supranuclear tracts), or the main trunk of the vagus nerve and its two laryngeal branches (inferior or "recurrent" laryngeal nerve and superior laryngeal nerve). Intracranial tumours or haemorrhages and demyelinating diseases cause central paralysis. Neoplasms at the base of the skull and trauma of the neck cause vagus paralysis. Isolated paralysis of the inferior or superior laryngeal nerve is caused by cervical or thoracic lesions.

Paralysis of the vagus nerve or, more commonly, of the inferior laryngeal nerve most frequently occurs after **surgical procedures in the neck** (especially involving the thyroid gland) and upper mediastinum. It may also be caused by **malignant tumours** invading the larynx, hypopharynx, oesophagus, thyroid, or tracheobronchial tree and other malignant neoplasms in the lower neck or upper mediastinum. Neurogenic laryngeal stenosis may also develop during the course of viral inflammations or as a result of central nervous system processes (cerebral or skull-base tumours, injuries, surgical procedures in the lateral skull base). The preoperative recognition of concomitant superior laryngeal nerve paralysis on one side is important because it is a contraindication for surgical measures (especially arytenoidectomy) that could result in increased aspiration.

Previous surgery, mostly thyroid surgery, is the most common cause of laryngeal nerve paralysis. Revision thyroidectomy bears a particularly high risk for inferior and also superior laryngeal nerve trauma. The rate of immediate postoperative unilateral recurrent laryngeal nerve paresis following primary thyroid surgery for benign disease is approximately 2–7%; the rate of permanent paralysis has been reported to range from 0.5 to 4%. In revision surgery, and in operations for malignant conditions of the thyroid gland, unilateral recurrent laryngeal nerve paresis occurs in some 10–20% of all interventions. Bilateral vocal fold paralysis is obviously seen far less frequently. Surgery of the cervical spine via an anterior approach, surgery of the larynx, pharynx, cervical oesophagus and the upper mediastinum, and carotid artery surgery can typically result in laryngeal nerve or even vagus nerve injury. Other conditions causing laryngeal nerve palsies include:

- Lesions of the brainstem
- Neurovascular disorders (stroke) and other central nervous disorders
- Demyelinating disorders of the peripheral nervous system (Guillain–Barré syndrome)
- Lateral skull-base lesions (trauma, tumour)
- Sequelae of skull-base surgery
- Cervical spine injury or surgery
- Degenerative motor unit disorders (e.g. amyotrophic lateral sclerosis)
- Infectious diseases of the affected nerves
- Neurotoxins (e.g. lead)
- Primary neurogenic tumours (e.g. schwannoma)
- Malignant tumours of the thyroid, larynx, pharynx, trachea, oesophagus, bronchus, thymus, and other malignant tumours of the neck and mediastinum
- Traumatic lesions of the neck
- Aortic aneurysm

If, in spite of complete diagnostic workup, no aetiologic factor can be found, the paralysis is labelled as **idiopathic**.

Viral neuronitis probably accounts for most cases of idiopathic vocal cord paralysis. However, a complete diagnostic workup is needed if the cause of laryngeal nerve impairment cannot readily be derived from the patient's history or obvious medical findings.

Difficulty in swallowing (dysphagia) is a relatively common presenting complaint in the practice of otolaryngology. It is reasonable to expect that, with the growing percentage of older individuals in the overall population, the numbers will increase in the future. Swallowing of food may be **obstructed** by mass lesions in the oral cavity, oropharynx, hypopharynx or oesophagus or by disturbances of neuromuscular regulation, especially absent or delayed opening of the upper oesophageal sphincter (cricopharyngeus muscle) during swallowing. Delayed relaxation of the cricopharyngeus muscle results in the formation of hypopharyngeal diverticula (so-called Zenker's diverticula) with typical regurgitation of food hours after eating.

Aspiration may result from loss of substance, especially in the larynx, e.g. after a supraglottic partial laryngectomy, or it may have a neurogenic cause, e.g. lesions of the superior laryngeal nerve or vagus nerve, sequelae from a stroke (infarct or haemorrhage), closed head injuries, anoxic encephalopathy and depression of the central nervous system resulting from intoxication. Neurogenic aspiration usually results from the loss of laryngeal sensitivity, and of cough and swallow reflexes.

6.9.3 Symptoms

Vagus nerve paralysis or dysfunction of its laryngeal and pharyngeal branches results in loss of vocal cord abduction or adduction, and in uncoordinated bolus transport during deglutition. It may affect phonation and respiration, and food, fluids and saliva may be aspirated into the trachea.

Unilateral paresis of the vagus or recurrent laryngeal nerve is usually associated with impaired abduction of the vocal cord or immobility in a paramedian position. It results in immediate hoarseness and breathiness of voice, since incomplete vocal fold adduction causes a constant glottal gap during phonation precluding adequate contact of the paralysed vocal fold with the normally mobile fold. Inadequate glottic closure produces a breathy and rough voice with a weak cough resulting from failure of the mobile vocal fold to approximate the paralysed fold during adduction. Synchronous aspiration, frequently associated with the vocal fold fixed in an intermediate position (somewhat more lateral than the paramedian position), is always suggestive of combined inferior and superior laryngeal nerve paresis. If patients complain about airway problems, these are usually related to phonation ("phonatory leakage"). Inspiratory stridor, otherwise typical for central airway stenosis, is not encountered.

In contrast, simultaneous **bilateral recurrent nerve paralysis** frequently leads to functional glottic stenosis with the vocal folds in a fixed paramedian position. The predominant symptom is airway compromise. This can range from unnoticeable to mild dyspnoea, inspiratory stridor and respiratory distress, even without exertion. Acute airway obstruction resulting from bilateral vocal fold immobility (e.g. following thyroidectomy) sometimes requires reintubation or tracheotomy. Bilateral vocal fold paralysis is a potentially life-threatening condition that frequently requires some kind of surgical intervention to prevent acute asphyxiation or pulmonary consequences of chronic central airway obstruction. In contrast to unilateral vocal cord paralysis, voice quality is not the primary concern in these patients. Voice quality is usually only mildly affected (if just the recurrent laryngeal nerves are involved).

Dysphagia may occur with any one of three main symptoms:
1. Obstruction (impairment of bolus transport)
2. Aspiration (inhalation of food particles or saliva)
3. Globus sensation (vague feeling of fullness in the throat, often perceived subjectively as "difficult swallowing" although solid foods and fluids are still swallowed normally)

6.9.4 Diagnosis

In most patients presenting with laryngeal palsies, the underlying condition is obvious from the patient's history (e.g. recurrent laryngeal nerve paresis following thyroidectomy). In patients with unclear cause of the underlying condition, a complete diagnostic workup is compulsory. The diagnostic protocol for these patients includes indirect mirror laryngoscopy, zoom laryngoscopy and/or transnasal flexible laryngoscopy, lung function tests (expiratory peak flow, resistance), voice analysis, laryngeal electromyography, tracheobronchoscopy and suspension laryngoscopy with tactile assessment of arytenoid cartilage mobility.

If the cause of the condition remains unclear, a comprehensive diagnostic workup of the thyroid gland including [^{99m}Tc]pertechnetate scintiscanning, ultrasound of the neck, and related laboratory tests (TSH) is indicated. If thyroid assessment remains inconclusive, chest CT scans and a barium swallow with fluoroscopy should be obtained. If additional signs of neurogenic disorders are present, MRI studies of the brain and additional laboratory tests (including complete blood count and CSF examination) should be considered. In patients with suspected inflammatory nerve disorders or joint disease, additional laboratory tests, including a blood cell and a differential blood cell count, determination of an acute phase indicator (usually C-reactive protein), tests for Lyme disease antibodies, rheumatoid factor, antinuclear antibodies and antineutrophil cytoplasmatic antibodies and renal, liver and electrolyte studies, are sometimes helpful.

The use of laryngeal electromyography has been advocated to classify the severity of neural damage, to establish a prognosis for nerve recovery and to differentiate neurogenic palsy from vocal fold immobility caused by arytenoid fixation. While it has been helpful in many cases, it is not considered a routine diagnostic tool by many laryngologists. Its prognostic accuracy is limited to patients with neurotmesis.

Delayed relaxation of the cricopharyngeus muscle during swallowing can occasionally lead to dysphagia, which is often accompanied by secondary aspiration. A diverticulum is not (yet) demonstrable in all cases. The disorder is more common in older individuals. Video cinematography is generally necessary to make a diagnosis.

6.9.4.1 Recommended European Standard Diagnostic Steps

- Detailed history taking (previous surgery?)
- Inspection
- Palpation

- Indirect endoscopy with rigid and/or flexible scopes
- Thyroid gland workup
- Ultrasound of the neck

6.9.4.2 Additional/Useful Diagnostic Procedures

- Stroboscopy
- Microlaryngoscopy, pharyngo-oesophagoscopy, and tracheobronchoscopy
- CT scans of thorax and lateral skull base
- Pulmonary function test
- Voice analysis
- Laryngeal electromyography
- Barium swallow with fluoroscopy
- MRI studies of the brain
- Laboratory tests

6.9.5 Therapy

6.9.5.1 Conservative Treatment

Isolated **unilateral vocal cord paralysis** results in a hoarse and breathy voice. Initially, voice rest is indicated for some days. If the onset of the paresis has been acute, medical treatment is indicated. It includes oral steroids and non-steroidal antiphlogistics, and antiviral or antibiotic agents if an infection is suspected. All patients should be offered logopaedic counselling shortly after the onset of the paresis to avoid functional maladjustment. If vocal cord immobility persists, logopaedic treatment is indicated. It usually restores vocal function within 2–3 months.

Once the acute respiratory compromise caused by **bilateral recurrent nerve paralysis** of recent onset has been overcome, most patients can breathe well at rest and during mild physical exertion. High-dose intravenous steroids are used in the early phase of this disorder. Once the patient has adjusted to the glottic narrowing, mild physical training should be encouraged to enable the thoracic muscles to overcome increased inspiratory airway resistance. Upper airway stenosis involving surface areas of no more than 50 mm^2 can be overcome using adequate respiratory compensation, but any additional narrowing below this limit will result in hypoventilation, inappropriate oxygen uptake and retention of carbon dioxide.

For the treatment of deglutition disorders, rehabilitation therapy is the basis of **dysphagia management**. Following the placement of a nasogastric feeding tube or a percutaneous enteral feeding tube, logopaedic rehabilitation uses compensatory strategies to reduce the risk of aspiration:

- Oral feeding with consistency modifications (thickened liquids increase oropharyngeal control and decrease difficulties with mastication).
- Modifying volume and tempo of food presentation.
- Head rotation (the ipsilateral pharynx is closed, forcing the food bolus to the contralateral pharynx, while cricopharyngeal pressure is decreased).
- Holding the chin down during deglutition to narrow the airway entrance.
- Supraglottic swallow: This technique uses simultaneous swallowing and breath-holding, closing the vocal cords and protecting the airway. The patient thereafter can cough to expel any residue in the laryngeal vestibule.
- Thermal stimulations can be performed in which icing of the anterior faucial arches may help to decrease the delay of pharyngeal swallow.
- Mendelsohn manoeuvre: This manoeuvre is a form of supraglottic swallow in which the patient mimics the upward movement of the larynx by voluntarily holding the larynx at its maximum height to increase the duration of the cricopharyngeal opening.

Additional exercises are used to increase muscle tone and to improve coordination and strengthening of muscles of the jaw, lips, cheek, tongue, soft palate and vocal cords.

The following are recommended European standard therapeutic steps:

1. For voice improvement in unilateral vocal cord paralysis
   - Initial voice rest
   - Oral steroids and non-steroidal antiphlogistics
   - Antiviral or antibiotic agents if an infection is suspected
   - Logopaedic voice rehabilitation
2. For airway improvement in bilateral vocal cord paralysis
   - Nasotracheal intubation for acute airway distress
   - High-dose intravenous steroids and non-steroidal antiphlogistics
   - Antiviral or antibiotic agents if an infection is suspected
   - Mild physical training once the patient has adjusted to the glottic narrowing
3. For deglutition disorders
   - Feeding via a nasogastric tube or PEG
   - Modifications in food consistency and viscosity
   - Postural manoeuvres to modify the flow of the bolus
   - Modifications in volume and tempo of food presentation
   - Supraglottic swallow
   - Exercises to increase muscle tone and to improve coordination

6.9.5.2 Surgical Treatment

Isolated **unilateral vocal cord paralysis** only very rarely requires surgery to improve the patient's voice. A persistent glottic gap despite logopaedic treatment may result from misdiagnosed combined paralysis of the inferior and superior laryngeal nerve, or in elderly patients with additional functional voice disorders.

Most patients with **bilateral vocal cord paralysis** can breathe well at rest and during mild physical exertion. Once the acute respiratory compromise caused by bilateral recurrent nerve paralysis of recent onset has been overcome by adaptation of the respiratory muscles, the indication for glottis-expanding surgery in these cases is based on:

- A lack of exercise tolerance
- The potential risk to the patient from sporadic respiratory inflammations (flulike infections) that may cause swelling of the already-tight glottis

With few exceptions, glottis-expanding surgery is indicated for bilateral recurrent nerve paralysis to restore at least partially the patient's exercise tolerance and reduce the risk of asphyxiation due to respiratory infections. As long as the degree of respiratory compromise is acceptable to the patient at rest and during mild exercise, it is reasonable to wait for approximately 9 months after the onset of paralysis to watch for spontaneous recovery of nerve function.

Although extralaryngeal surgical procedures (lateral fixation with its numerous variants) were once the standard treatment for bilateral vocal cord paralysis, endoscopic techniques have advanced considerably since the advent of endolaryngeal laser surgery. Today, endoscopic procedures have largely replaced open laryngeal surgery in the treatment of this disorder.

Arytenoidectomy is very effective for expanding the airway if the surgeon can completely remove the arytenoid cartilage and completely divide the conus elasticus as far as the cricoid cartilage. Even a partial arytenoidectomy is believed to provide satisfactory airway enlargement. The drawbacks of this technique include frequent transient aspiration and the risk of cricoid chondritis in patients who have had previous radiation to the neck.

Cordectomy is as effective as arytenoidectomy for airway restoration. There is no risk of aspiration with this procedure, but there may be a greater adverse effect on voice quality than after arytenoidectomy.

Posterior cordectomy, in which the vocal cord is divided in the area of the vocal process of the arytenoid cartilage combined with division of the conus elasticus, is considered by many laryngologists to be the best compromise between expanding the airway and preserving voice quality.

Temporary lateral fixation of the vocal cord as described by Lichtenberger is a potentially reversible procedure for airway expansion. Once nerve function has recovered, the endoscopically performed lateral fixation of the vocal cord can be reversed.

As a rule, modern endoscopic laser operations to expand the glottis are considered to be reliable techniques for airway restoration. Generally they can be performed without a temporary tracheotomy, making them easier for patients to tolerate. However, any surgical widening of the glottis trades voice for airway. Therefore, a compromise must be found between retaining voice quality and restoring an adequate airway.

The **treatment of Zenker's diverticula** has become an established domain of minimally invasive surgery during recent years. These diverticula develop as a result of deficient or delayed relaxation of the cricopharyngeus muscle during swallowing. Until a few years ago, open cricopharyngeus myotomy combined with diverticulectomy through a left transcervical approach was the standard surgical treatment for Zenker's diverticula. Although endoscopic myotomy (division of the posterior part of the annular cricopharyngeus muscle) was described as early as 1917, the endoscopic approach was abandoned later owing to excessive complications. Today, the complications and results of endoscopic myotomies appear to be comparable to or better than those achieved with open surgery. In addition, endoscopic myotomy obviates the need for an external neck incision and practically eliminates the risk of recurrent nerve paralysis. Patients are fed through a temporary nasogastric tube or by temporary parenteral nutrition for 2–7 days after surgery. In all cases, oral contrast examination with a water-soluble medium (Gastrografin) should be done before the resumption of oral intake to exclude paravasation into the upper mediastinum.

Recommended European Standard Surgical Procedures

1. For voice improvement in unilateral vocal cord paralysis
   - Vocal fold augmentation using fat, collagen or disperse silicone
   - Medialization thyroplasty using autologous cartilage or laryngeal implants (e.g. Friedrich's titanium implant)
2. For airway improvement in bilateral vocal cord paralysis
   - Temporary tracheotomy
   - Posterior cordectomy
   - Temporary or permanent laterofixation of one vocal cord
   - Endoscopic arytenoidectomy

3. For deglutition disorders
   – Laryngeal elevation (thyrohyomandibulopexy)
   – Medialization thyroplasty (to reduce the glottic gap)
   – Myotomy of the cricopharyngeal muscle

Additional/Useful Surgical Strategies

A number of alternatives to laser surgery are available for the treatment of Zenker's diverticula and cricopharyngeal dysfunction. Endoscopic myotomy with a stapler has been recommended. The device is an automatic stapler of the type commonly used in open abdominal surgery. A special stapler has been developed for the treatment of Zenker's diverticula and can be introduced and operated through a diverticuloscope. It divides the common wall between the diverticular sac and oesophagus, simultaneously closing the wound surfaces on both sides with staples. This technique is supposed to prevent leakage into the mediastinum. Because of the way the stapler is designed, a part of the wound always remains open at the lowest point of the incision. Open myotomy is always available as an alternative to endoscopic myotomy in cases where it is important to avoid opening the pharynx. The surgery is done through a left transcervical approach, like the classic operation for treating a Zenker's diverticulum. Following meticulous division of the cricopharyngeus muscle, the pharyngeal mucosa is left intact and the walls of the diverticulum are left in place.

An elegant, minimally invasive treatment option is to temporarily paralyse the cricopharyngeus muscle by the localized injection of botulinum toxin. The advantage of this method is that it is practically free of complications when carried out correctly. The disadvantage is that its effect lasts only a few months, after which time the treatment may have to be repeated (generally necessitating brief general anaesthesia). Thus, botulinum toxin injection is not a permanent treatment option. It does, however, provide an ideal test method in equivocal cases to determine whether the proposed surgical division of the cricopharyngeus muscle will improve the patient's symptoms. If the symptoms improve following transient paralysis of the muscle with botulinum toxin and then worsen again after the effect has subsided, the patient can be scheduled for a definitive cricopharyngeal myotomy.

For severe aspiration (e.g. following mass lesions of the brainstem or paralysis of the lower cranial nerves), surgery is needed to separate the airway from the alimentary tract. Surgical procedures that may be used in this context include:
- Tracheotomy
- Medialization thyroplasty (to reduce the glottic gap)
- Myotomy of the cricopharyngeal muscle
- Closure of the larynx

- Laryngotracheal separation
- Total laryngectomy

6.9.6 Differential Diagnosis

Impaired movement of the cricoarytenoid cartilage with immobility of the vocal cord and airway obstruction may occur as a consequence of disorders of the cricoarytenoid articulation, of interarytenoid fibrous adhesion, or of both. Immobility of the cricoarytenoid joint may arise from arytenoid cartilage dislocation during laryngotracheal intubation and consequent ankylosis, from arthritis or from tumorous infiltration in laryngeal and hypopharyngeal carcinoma. Interarytenoid fibrous adhesion most commonly results from prolonged or traumatic tracheal intubation. The tube causes a decubitus with chondritis and consequent scar tissue formation involving the arytenoid cartilages and the interarytenoid area resulting in severe impairment of both cricoarytenoid joints' motility and laryngeal stenosis. Electromyography may provide additional information, but is probably not mandatory in long-standing vocal cord immobility, or if clear signs of arytenoid cartilage fixation have been seen during endoscopy.

6.9.7 Prognosis

There are two aspects to the prognosis of vocal fold palsy: vocal cord mobility and phonatory/respiratory/deglutitive function. Imperfect function of the intrinsic laryngeal muscles may be compensated for, with only minimal impact on vocal ability. It is well known that phonation can be unaffected in patients who have vocal folds that move apart or come together only weakly. For idiopathic palsies, a rate of less than 50% for partial and complete recovery can be expected, but phonatory function will largely recur to normal in a significantly higher percentage of cases. In patients with vocal fold palsy, the detection of well-defined signs of neural degeneration on electromyography allows for the prediction of poor functional outcome with high reliability in an early phase of the disease process. In the presence of electromyographic signs of neural degeneration, the decision for definitive surgical interventions such as thyroplasty or vocal fold augmentation in unilateral or partial cordectomy in bilateral vocal fold paralysis can be made safely at an earlier stage of the disease process. However, the absence of degenerative alterations on electromyography does not necessarily indicate recovery to a normal or near-normal functional level.

Suggested Reading

1. Blitzer A (1992) Neurological disorders of the larynx. Thieme, Stuttgart

2. Fried MP, Ferlito AA (2007) The larynx, 3rd edn. Plural, San Diego

3. Remacle M, Eckel HE (2009) Surgery of the larynx and trachea. Springer, Berlin

4. Sen P, Kumar G, Bhattacharyya AK (2006) Pharyngeal pouch: associations and complications. Eur Arch Otolaryngol 263(5):463–468

5. Shama H, Connor NP, Ciucci MR, McCullack TM (2008) Surgical treatment of dysphagia. Phys Med Rehabil Clin N Am 19(4):817–835

6.10 Basic Surgical Procedures on the Respiratory Tract: Laryngoscopy, Tracheoscopy and Including Tracheostomy

PATRICK J. BRADLEY

6.10.1 Direct Laryngoscopy

6.10.1.1 Definition

Direct laryngoscopy aims at the examination of the larynx by direct techniques to evaluate the patient's complaint or altered laryngeal function, to make a clinical diagnosis, either by inspection or by biopsy of the physical abnormality, and if possible to correct that complaint or altered function by performing a therapeutic procedure.

6.10.1.2 Preoperative Preparation

Most adults undergoing direct laryngoscopy will have the procedure performed under a general anaesthetic. However, in certain circumstances the procedure may be performed under local anaesthetic with intravenous sedation.

6.10.1.3 Procedure

The procedure is generally undertaken after the patient has been evaluated by indirect laryngoscopy and the evaluation also may have included some form of diagnostic imaging such as CT or MRI scanning. On occasions if an obstructing laryngeal lesion is likely to be identified or found, the patient should be warned that a tracheostomy may be necessary, or if the examination procedure becomes more difficult! Complications (see Sect. 6.10.1.12) should be explained to each patient preoperatively.

6.10.1.4 Indications

- Precise location and diagnosis of lesions of the larynx
- Biopsy of laryngeal lesions—keratoses, leucoplakia, neoplasms
- Removal of "mass lesions"—by surgical dissection or by the use of a laser
- As an adjunct to some other therapeutic procedure

6.10.1.5 Goals

The primary goal of laryngoscopy is to provide an unobstructed view of the larynx for diagnosis and/or treatment or as part of a procedure to align the upper-airway tract for bronchoscopy. The selection of the scope is based on the type of the lesion, its anatomical considerations, such as size and location, and the type of procedure likely to be performed.

6.10.1.6 Anaesthesia

Endoscopy of the larynx can be performed under local or general anaesthesia. The selection of anaesthesia is based on the preference of the patient and the surgeon and the patient's health. Certain considerations will dictate the type of technique used: supraglottic tumours will contraindicate local anaesthetic; uncooperative patients cannot be examined under local anaesthetic. Rigid endoscopy of the larynx, trachea or bronchus is best performed under general anaesthesia. Continuous monitoring of the patient's pulse, blood pressure and other vital signs is "a must" when undertaking such an examination as it is very stressful on the patient's cardio/respiratory system.

The Technique of Local Anaesthesia Application
The additional use of intravenous sedation is considered by some to be very important in the technique of local anaesthetic use for the procedure of direct laryngoscopy. Equipment for emergency intubation and/or tracheostomy must be to hand for immediate use for the duration of the procedure. The use of atropine may help to minimise or prevent vagal stimulation and also helps to dry the oral and oropharyngeal mucosa, which maximises the effect of topical anaesthesia.

After informed instructions to the patient have been given, the oral and oropharyngeal mucosa is sprayed with topical anaesthetic. If one is using the technique of patient-assisted indirect laryngoscopy, the supraglottic area and vocal cords are sprayed directly with local anaesthetic. Several applications may be required to achieve adequate anaesthesia with suppression of the gag reflex; the use of inhalation techniques may help to anaesthetise the subglottis and trachea.

Should adequate topical anaesthesia not have been achieved, the superior laryngeal nerves can be anaesthetised through the mucosa of the piriform sinus by the application of cotton wool pledgets soaked with local anaesthetic or by direct external injection of the nerves which are located below the greater cornu of the hyoid bone.

Techniques of General Anaesthesia

- In adults the usual technique is to intubate the larynx, with a small-bore tube, and the surgeon works around the endotracheal tube by displacing it anteriorly or posteriorly with the rigid endoscope. The use of a cuffed endotracheal tube prevents the airway from becoming contaminated with blood or other fluids during the procedure.
- The insufflation technique allows patients to remain in a deep level of anaesthesia by insufflating anaesthetic agents into the hypopharynx while the patient spontaneously breathes. This has the advantage that the larynx is unobstructed, but the surgeon and the assistants are exposed to inhalation agents throughout the procedure. This technique is used mainly in children.
- Forced inhalation (jet anaesthesia) of anaesthetic gases and oxygen can also be used. Inhalation can be administered at a normal inspirational rate or at a more rapid rate (high-frequency jet ventilation). Usually the patient is paralysed to allow easier ventilation, and this allows for smaller volumes of anaesthetic gases to be used and reduces the exposure of the theatre staff to anaesthetic gases.
- If tracheoscopy or bronchoscopy is to be performed, the patient can be ventilated through the bronchoscope to maintain a controlled airway.

6.10.1.7 Instrumentation

Three basic types of laryngoscopes are available. They include scopes with an open or a side slit, narrow-tipped scopes to view the anterior commissure and opening of the laryngeal ventricle, and a variety of laryngoscopes which are used for the technique of suspension laryngoscopy. In general, the procedure to be performed and the location and size of the lesion will dictate the technique and type of laryngoscope used.

The *side laryngoscopes* are best placed in the valleculae to hold the base of the tongue, allowing the larynx to be exposed for bronchoscopy.

The *anterior commissure laryngoscope* is designed to visualise the anterior glottis, the subglottis and the laryngeal ventricle. It is narrowest at the mandible and therefore allows a better view anteriorly.

Microscopic laryngoscopes are designed for binocular vision, magnification through a microscope and manual manipulation of the larynx. Other scopes used are larger and provide as much exposure as possible, such as the distensible laryngoscope.

The technique of suspension laryngoscopy aims to stabilise the laryngoscope separate from the use of a second surgeon or assistant to hold the scope during the procedure. The laryngoscope can be suspended from a stand separate from the table, from a stand attached to the table or from the patient's body.

Once the larynx has been visualised, the surgeon can opt for better lighting and visualisation by using telescopes or a microscope. The best view is to be had using the microscope, and with both hands available for instrumentation. A focal length of 400 mm should be used for laryngeal work.

6.10.1.8 Positioning the Patient

Positioning the patient is of primary concern for good or optimum laryngoscopy. The patient may be put in the "sniffing position" described by Jackson. The neck is flexed forward on the chest and the head is extended on the neck. The occiput is positioned in a plane somewhat higher than the table. The use of a shoulder roll or pillow under the patient is frequently all that is required and gives optimum positioning.

6.10.1.9 Technique of Lanyngoscopy

Protection of the teeth or upper alveolus from local trauma is important. This can be accomplished by the use of a tooth guard or a gauze pad that will evenly distribute the pressure from the scope. The upper teeth should not be used as a fulcrum for leverage of the scope, as it is being passed distally. It is better to elevate the whole head rather than use leverage on the teeth to avoid dental trauma.

The technique is as follows:
- The scope is grasped in the left hand (right-handed surgeons!) and the mouth is opened with the right hand by placing the thumb on the lower incisors and the index finger on the upper incisors.
- The scope is passed down the right gutter of the oropharynx, displacing the tongue to the left. Care must be taken not to crush the tongue between the lower incisors and the scope.

- The thumb of the right hand is also used to guide and advance the scope. Depending on the size and type of the laryngoscope, it can usually be placed in the valleculae or under the epiglottis.
- Advancing the scope must be performed under direct vision and with appropriate use of suction to clear away any mucus or other fluids that may occlude the view at the working distal end of the scope!

A variety of micro and macro laryngeal instruments have been described for laryngeal surgery. Supplementary armrests can be used to make the position of the surgeon's arms more comfortable and the hands steadier. The use of anterior laryngeal pressure, or pressure on the thyroid cartilage, by using a swab placed on the thyroid cartilage to protect the skin and by applying sticky tape over this swab and with traction downwards towards the operating table, and anchoring the sticky tape to the table, will aid with better visualisation of the anterior commissure. If a good view is still not possible, an alternative scope should be used. Palpation of the internal laryngeal structures is important to rule out arytenoid fixation and to evaluate the nature and length of laryngeal stenoses. It is also best to size the subglottis with instruments calibrated to perform such functions, as visualised estimations of the subglottis are notoriously inaccurate.

6.10.1.10 Biopsy

Frequently, local mucosal abnormalities are detected in the larynx which explain the patient's symptoms and support the indication for having performed a laryngoscopy. However, the pathological nature of these lesions requires histopathological examination and as a result they need to be excised. The excision of such lesions may be performed using cupped "grabbing" biopsy forceps and angled microscissors or currently more frequently using forceps and microdissection using a CO_2 laser. The location of the lesion, if it is on the vocal cord, and its excision may have a significant effect on laryngeal function, especially voice, and a minimal but adequate amount of tissue must be removed to minimise local trauma and healing, but the amount must be adequate for diagnostic and therapeutic measures to eradicate the local abnormality. The technique of hydrodissection may aid in achieving these goals: the injection of a small quantity of saline into the "normal" surrounding mucosa, thereby lifting the mucosal lesion off the vocal ligament, will minimise the local thermal and surgical trauma inflicted by the use of surgery or a CO_2 laser.

It should be remembered that leucoplakia, or white lesion, occurs most frequently on the vocal cords, and as such "all" such lesions must be biopsied to confirm their true nature. If the lesion is considered small enough, it should be excised totally, pinned out on a card, orientated in direction and marked, and subjected to serial sectioning by the pathologist. It is recognised that a "pinch" biopsy may not be fully representative of the whole lesion. Should the lesion be diffuse and not suitable for single-stage excision, multiple biopsies or sequential excisions should be recommended, and should be processed as described above. The use of digital photography of such lesions, prior to biopsy, has not only aided greatly communication between surgeons and patients, but also may be used as a "road map" for surgeons and pathologists.

6.10.1.11 Postoperative Care

It is of the utmost importance that the surgeon and the patient are comfortable with the postoperative plan. If there are worries about airway compromise or imminent obstruction, the patient must be admitted, the nursing staff warned of these concerns, the patient placed under nursing observation and connected to a pulsed oxymeter and the patient must be observed for several hours before a state of high concern can be lowered. Sometimes the use of antibiotics and steroids may be considered. Humidification of the inhaled air and voice rest may help prevent crust formation at the site of surgery.

6.10.1.12 Complications

The rate of complications of laryngoscopy following direct or suspension laryngoscopy is difficult to estimate as only major complications have been recorded and the recordings are usually retrospective. It has been reported that the incidence of minor complications such as dental injuries or minor bleeding ranges from 9 to 31%. It has been recorded that dental injuries expected to be to the upper teeth may also be recorded in the lower jaw as well. Major complications defined as complications requiring hospitalisation—reintubation, tracheostomy, pneumothorax, etc.—have reported incidences of up to 20%. The likelihood of complications is dependent on the indication for and urgency of laryngoscopy, whether any associated surgical manoeuvres were performed and the experience of the anaesthetist and the operating surgeon. Associated with suspension laryngoscopy is the risk of temporary nerve lesions—injury to the lingual and hypoglossal nerves—considered to be due to local pressure applied for a considerable length of time; occasionally these nerve palsies can be permanent. Temporary palsies may take a median of 8 weeks to recovery—it is therefore recommended that patients should be informed about these risks before the operation.

6.10.2 Tracheobronchoscopy

6.10.2.1 Indications

The history is crucial in evaluation of a patient and the indications for tracheobronchoscopy. The indications are best thought of as diagnostic and therapeutic.

Indications are airway obstruction (severity, progression, cyanotic episodes, periods of sleep apnoea), problems with eating (coughing, choking, etc.) and abnormalities seen on X-rays. The indications may be different in children and in adults.

Children and Adults

- Airway difficulty or obstruction, dyspnoea or stridor
- Recurrent or atypical croup
- Recurrent pneumonia or bronchitis
- Weak or absent cry
- Apnoeic or cyanotic attacks
- Abnormalities seen on X-rays—distortion or pressure on the trachea or bronchi
- Bleeding—haemoptysis

Therapeutic Indications

- Establish an airway
- Removal of a foreign body—mucus, organic or inorganic
- Bronchial toilet
- Removal of "tumours"

6.10.2.2 Goals

The goals of tracheobronchoscopy are to secure the airway and provide as good visualisation of the airway as possible for diagnostic and therapeutic measures. The instrumentation must provide a mechanism for adequate ventilation of the patient during the procedure.

6.10.2.3 Instrumentation

Two types of instruments are available for the examination of the lower airway—the trachea and bronchi:

1. Flexible scopes are available that can be small enough to examine both children and adults and that allow for the use of suction, the use of a steerable tip and also for biopsies to be performed at the same time. The flexible scope is best considered as a diagnostic instrument and has limited therapeutic utility.

2. Rigid bronchoscopes with or without the use of telescopes have improved the visualisation and expanded the range of indications for therapeutic interventions.

Flexible and rigid endoscopic instruments may be used complementarily, or one instrument may be preferred for a particular situation. The relative advantages and disadvantages of flexible and rigid bronchoscopes are compared in Table 6.10.1.

6.10.2.4 Technique

Flexible Bronchoscopy

Flexible bronchoscopy can be performed with the patient in a sitting or recumbent position. The supine position is more comfortable for the patient and examiner, and also the patient is less likely to suffer a vasovagal attack. This procedure can be undertaken in almost all patients; however, the very young may be distressed and this procedure should probably be done using a general anaesthetic.

The scope can be passed through the nose, either anaesthetised or not. The nose is preferable to the mouth, as it is easier for the patient to cough, the patient may continue to vocalise and the scope is less likely to be damaged. The larynx and hypopharynx may need to be anaesthetised to suppress local sensitivities and suppress cough.

When using the flexible scope, three manoeuvres allow the scope to be "driven" in the desired direction:

1. First, the shaft of the bronchoscope is rolled between the thumb and the finger. Placing a C loop in the bronchoscope will allow easy rotation.
2. Second, the scope is advanced by walking the scope with the fingers and the thumb.
3. The third manoeuvre is to control the tip of the scope with flexion and extension. The head of the scope is held between the third and fifth fingers and the thenar eminence of the right hand. The control is operated with the tip of the thumb and the first finger is used to control the suction portal.

The bronchoscope, as the nasendoscope, should be passed through the nose between the middle and inferior turbinates. The area under the middle turbinate is the most sensitive portion of the nasal airway. Difficulties of "turning the corner" in the pharynx may be helped by extending the neck, pulling the tongue forward and insufflating air into the pharynx. The larynx can be easily passed through, if and when it is anaesthetised, and using the inspiratory cycle when the cords are abducted. As the scope is passed down the trachea, it must remain centred in the lumen. The bronchi are examined in an orderly manner commencing on one side, usually the right,

Table 6.10.1 Relative advantages and disadvantages of flexible and rigid bronchoscopes

Area of comparison	Flexible scope	Rigid scope
Preparation of patient	Topical anaesthesia	General anaesthesia
Approach	Transnasal	Transoral
Ventilation	Around the scope	Through the scope
Physical abnormalities	Easier examinations	Difficult examinations
Intubated patient	Possible through nasal examination	Not possible, no nasal examination
Examination of Upper Respiratory Tract	Trans-nasal examination Less distortion	No nasal manipulation Requires exposure of supraglottis and glottis
	Good view of supraglottis and glottis	Good view of posterior commissure
Examination of Lower Respiratory Tract	Can view distally Difficulty with Ventilation	Cannot view small airways Ventilation through scope
Airway trauma	Less potential	Greater potential
Airway surgery	Contraindicated	Wide application
Biopsy	Small samples only	Big biopsies/all patients
Bronchoalveolar lavage	Widely performed	With small scope only
Bedside examination	Common	Uncommon
Foreign body removal	Contraindicated	Superior
Diagnosis of supraglottitis	Contraindicated	Indicated
Massive haemoptysis	Contraindicated	Superior control
Risks	Low	Higher
Size of scope	Dependent on outer diameter	Dependent on inner diameter
Costs	No OR/anaesthetic costs	OR/anaesthetic costs
Durability	Relatively fragile	Durable/telescopes fragile

OR operating room

and then the other side is examined. The anatomy must be clearly understood before commencing such examinations, because when using the flexible scope the orientation is dependent on knowing where you have been.

Rigid Bronchoscopy

The basic instrument for rigid examination of the airway is a tracheoscope (bronchoscope without the ventilation ports) or a ventilation bronchoscope of the appropriate size for the patient and the anticipated condition. The larynx should be exposed with a side laryngoscope placed in the valleculae. The larynx needs to be entered atraumatically, whatever method or instruments are being used.

Once it is in the trachea, the bronchoscope is held in the left hand, between the thumb and first finger, and the long finger rests on the plane behind the central incisors. This allows stabilisation of the head and fixes the bronchoscope to the mouth.

The orientation of the leading edge of the bronchoscope is crucial to prevent laryngeal trauma. The scope may be inserted through the laryngoscope to the level of the larynx, rotated to 90° to the left or right and the leading edge of the scope is centred in the larynx by looking directly at the true vocal cord. The bronchoscope is advanced through the larynx and rotated back when the subglottis is entered. The examination must be performed under apnoea or spontaneous ventilation with the insufflation technique as there is no way to ventilate the patient. Careful technique and haemostasis are essential to prevent oedema and spasm of the airway during recovery from anaesthetic.

As the bronchoscope is advanced, the trachea is examined. Careful attention is directed to the width and shape of the subglottis. The tracheal rings are carefully examined for consistency in their shape and whether there is evidence of a complete tracheal ring. The trachea is examined for any evidence of collapse, tracheomalacia or compression from external structures such as vascular rings or the thyroid gland. The overlying mucosa should be pink with small vessels present that clearly delineate the underlying cartilage. The carina when seen is usually sharp and clearly delineated. A widened carina may be secondary to a mass; lymph node mass at the bifurcation. Once at the carina, the bronchi can be seen. The head is rotated to the left to access the right main bronchus and to the right for the left mainstem bronchus. The examination of the right and left main bronchus will reveal the segmental bronchi. It may be necessary to rotate the scope to visualise each of the segmental bronchi openings. It is at this stage that the complementary use of the flexible bronchoscope may be used to examine in more detail the small bronchi.

6.10.2.5 Biopsy

Biopsy of the trachea or bronchial lesions can be performed through a rigid bronchoscope, blindly or under direct vision with biopsy forceps. If there is significant bleeding, the rigid scope is the ideal instrument to have in place as it allows for the use of suction and ventilation, and occasionally the application of cautery.

6.10.2.6 Postoperative Care

- The recovery room must be well equipped and communication with all of the staff is paramount to a stressful recovery.
- Humidification is usually delivered.
- Steroids may be given when airway distress is anticipated, and should be given preoperatively to be effective when required!
- Elevation of the head or the prone position may help improve the airway.
- The oral or nasal airway may help until the patient is fully alert.

6.10.3 Tracheostomy

The term "tracheotomy" is used to refer to the creation of a surgical opening into the trachea for the purposes of maintaining a patent airway or to assist with ventilation. "Tracheostomy" is used to describe the opening itself, the stoma. The tube that is placed through the tracheal opening is referred to as the "tracheostomy tube".

6.10.3.1 Procedures

Minitracheostomy

This technique may be useful in ambulatory patients in need of continuous oxygen therapy. A 5-Fr plastic catheter is inserted through the first to second tracheal rings and oxygen is administered.

Cricothyroidotomy (Minitracheostomy)

Needle cricothyroidotomy is a technique that requires less dissection and therefore results in decreased haemorrhage in the emergency situation. The trachea is entered by creating a channel through the cricothyroid membrane and the lumen is maintained by the insertion of a small tracheostomy tube.

Percutaneous Tracheostomy

The term "percutaneous tracheostomy" is used to refer to the fashioning of a tracheostomy, using a trochar and/ or guide wire to identify the tracheal lumen and a series of progressively enlarging bougies or a specially designed instrument to allow introduction of a tracheostomy tube. All of these percutaneous tracheostomy procedures lack a surgical dissection of skin flaps, division of strap muscles and formal identification of the thyroid isthmus.

Surgical Tracheostomy

The placement of a tracheostomy tube into the trachea in a formal manner by a skilled surgeon has many advantages over the rather simple and quicker procedures described above. The placement of a tracheostomy tube is positioned by good surgical exposure and good control of the process and its consequences. In a meta-analysis, percutaneous tracheostomy was associated with a higher prevalence of perioperative complications and especially perioperative deaths and cardiorespiratory arrests. Postoperative complication rates were higher with surgical tracheostomy.

6.10.3.2 Indications

- Acute upper respiratory obstruction
- Elective when a potential upper respiratory obstruction may occur postoperatively
- For airway control following surgery or trauma
- Part management of lower respiratory ventilation and toilet
- Conversion from prolonged tracheal intubation
- Chronic upper respiratory obstruction—sleep apnoea
- Ventilation of patients with respiratory distress syndrome

- Management of airway in patients with laryngeal tumours or stenoses
- Aid to the removal of impacted tracheal foreign body

6.10.3.3 Preoperative Preparation

In the case of acute obstruction, an emergency airway can be achieved by a cricothyroidotomy or tracheal puncture with a large-bore needle or cannula. Once the airway has been secured, a formal surgical tracheostomy in the operating room can be preformed, once the patient has been stabilised medically.

If there is need to perform a surgical tracheostomy in an acute emergency—life and death situation—a midline skin incision over the trachea with the patient in a supine position and the neck extended will allow for a rapid, wide exposure approach to the trachea; the thyroid isthmus can be divided under direct vision on the way through! There is profuse bleeding, but with appropriate assistance and adequate suction the trachea can entered in seconds and the haemorrhage can be controlled electively once the airway has been stabilised!

In the chronic upper airway obstruction scenario, the optimum place for the creation of a surgical tracheostomy is in the operating room. It should be avoided in the emergency room, intensive care unit or more so on the ward, unless exceptional circumstances prevail.

All patients must be positioned in a supine position with a bolster between the shoulder blades with the head extended. The addition of intravenous sedation may be of great help, and it is imperative that the patient's vital signs, pulse and blood pressure be continuously monitored during and after the procedure.

6.10.3.4 Anaesthesia

General anaesthesia with an endotracheal tube is preferred.

Local anaesthetic may be the only technique possible as patients have presented with significant airway compromise and may be considered too ill for a general anaesthetic. The injection of local anaesthetic must be local to the skin and the deeper structure in the midline. Injections deviating from the midline or excessive use of local anaesthetic may result in overspill into the neighbouring tissues and cause paralysis of the recurrent laryngeal nerve and increase the respiratory distress further—making a semiurgent surgical procedure into a catastrophe!

6.10.3.5 Technique

- A horizontal incision is made midway between the cricoid cartilage and the suprasternal notch, laterally to the anterior border of the sternomastoid muscles.
- The strap muscles are identified and the investing fascia is divided in the midline, allowing the muscles to be retracted laterally.
- The thyroid isthmus is identified overlying the second to the fourth tracheal rings. It is recommended that *all* thyroid isthmi be divided to aid with cannulation and decannulation of the tracheostomy tube.
- The pretracheal fascia is incised and the anterior tracheal wall and the cricoid cartilage and the upper three tracheal rings are exposed.
- Should the procedure be performed under local anaesthetic, it is important that all haemorrhage be controlled at this stage *before* the trachea is opened. Before opening into the trachea, one should warn the patient that local anaesthetic is going to be injected into the trachea and coughing may be precipitated. This may precipitate additional respiratory distress, and it may be necessary to open the trachea and place the tracheostomy tube quickly to relieve the situation.
- In patients whose tracheostomy is being performed under general anaesthetic, the injection of local anaesthetic aids with suppression of coughing in the postoperative recovery period. The patient must also be preoxygenated prior to opening into the trachea.
- The use of a tracheal hook may aid with exposure of the trachea, by elevation of the first tracheal ring caudally. A small window of cartilage, approximately 1-cm diameter, is excised from the anterior wall midline of the trachea, usually the third tracheal ring, and a midline tracheotomy is created. Trousseau tracheal dilators can then be inserted to hold the tracheostomy open, while the tube is being passed. In children, the minimum amount of surgical trauma is recommended to the thin and growing trachea to prevent possible subsequent stenosis.
- The tracheostomy tube, whose cuff integrity has been previously tested, is inserted into the stoma. The obturator is removed and the presence of the tube in the lumen is ensured by the anaesthetist or by passing a suction catheter into the trachea. Once the tube is established within the tracheal lumen, the tube can be secured by the placement of tapes around the patient's neck or by placement of sutures at each end of the tracheostomy tube flange.

There are advocates for the use of the Bjork tracheal flap, which is inferiorly based, brought out onto the skin and sutured to the neck skin edge using non-absorbable sutures. This is said to aid with changing the tracheostomy tube and with the ability to find the tracheal lumen in the early postoperative period should the tube become displaced. Others advocate the placement of lateral traction sutures, for reasons similar to those given above.

Paediatric tracheostomies create some unique problems. When the child is hyperextended, the pleura may be moved from its intrathoracic position into the lower neck, as can also the brachioinnominate artery. The placement of the incision should therefore be higher in the necks of children.

6.10.3.6 Postoperative Care

Frequent suctioning is necessary in the early stages of tracheostomy to keep the airway clear. Sterile technique is mandatory and care is taken not to traumatise the tracheal mucosa. It is not necessary to place dressing about or below the tracheostomy site, as this will encourage surgical emphysema in the early phase, and aid with wound maceration in the later stage.

Humidification is essential to prevent drying of secretions in the trachea. Meticulous care of the tracheostomy wound is essential to avoid infection.

Change of the tracheostomy tube should be performed by the surgeon who performed the surgery, or by an experienced nurse in about 3–5 days after placement. The tracheostomy wound should be matured enough for a clear tract to have been created from the skin to the trachea. A tracheostomy hook, Trousseau dilator, a good source of light or a head light, and appropriate suction must be available at the time of this change. In addition, a tube one size smaller should be available in case trouble ensues and reintubation with a tube of the original size is too tight.

6.10.3.7 Complications

Complications are common; most are usually self-limiting and easily managed by appropriate nursing care. However, there are some complications that are fatal, and early signs of imminent problems should be ignored at the clinician's peril! Complications are best considered to be immediate (within the first 24 h), intermediate (while the patient is still in hospital and within the first 4 weeks) and late (after discharge) (Table 6.10.2).

6.10.3.8 Closure of the Tracheostoma Scar/Fistula

Tracheostomies are indicated and created to treat a specific need of a patient. The creation of a tracheostomy may therefore be either temporary or permanent. If a tracheostomy which has been performed in a standard way has been maintained for months or years, it may result in serious damage to the laryngotracheal complex. The difference between a temporary and a permanent tracheostomy is essentially one in which the stoma is designed for long- or short-term patency. Measures must be taken to prevent contracture or collapse of the stoma edge, and to minimise or avoid rough surfaces, cartilage, granulations, infection or pain. In a mature tracheostoma, the gap between the surface of the anterior cervical skin and the trachea should be circumferentially lined by either skin or mucus membrane. This gap should be short and stable, obviating the need for a permanent placed tube to maintain patency.

However, the majority of tracheostomies are temporary and when the indication for placement is no longer

Table 6.10.2 Complications of tracheostomy

Immediate (Within 24 hrs)	Intermediate (Within first 4 weeks)	Late (After Hospital Discharge)
Haemorrhage (usually venous)	Dislodgement/Displacement of the Tracheostomy Tube	Tracheal stenosis
Air Embolism	Surgical Emphysema	Difficulty with decannulation
Apnoea	Pneumothorax	Tracheo-cutaneous Fistula
Cardiac Arrest	Pneumomediastinum	
Local damage:	Scabs and crusts	
Thyroid Cartilage	Infection	
Cricoid Cartilage	Tracheal Necrosis	
Recurrent Laryngeal N.	Tracheo-arterial fistula	
	Tracheo-oesophageal fistula	
	Dysphagia	

present or has been corrected, the tracheostomy tract, or more specifically a fistula, should heal once the tracheostomy tube is removed. Most fistulae heal spontaneously, if they have been present for 12 weeks or less. If the tract heals by secondary intention, the skin is thin, irregular, unsightly and frequently becomes attached to the trachea by fibrous tissue, resulting in the scar moving up and down when the patient swallows. Not infrequently a patent fistula persists and tracheal secretions will continue to be expelled onto the neck skin surface, causing continuing frequent infections of the local skin and trachea and resulting in the patient being conscious of a poor neck scar and cosmesis.

In such cases surgery is indicated and closure must aim to be single-staged, aiming to separate the anterior tracheal wall from the neck skin. The fistula tract needs to be excised completely, to include the old scarred skin edge, the fistula or tract and the edge of opening into the trachea. The strap muscles can be mobilised and medialised, sutured together, thus separating the trachea from the neck skin. The neck skin should be freshened and, if necessary, rotated or plastied by local releasing incisions, to allow non-tension closure of "new skin" over the old tracheostomy site. It must be remembered that this wound is now a potential space under which air can flow from the open trachea and cause massive surgical emphysema or even haematoma. This wound can be approximated by untied sutures, around a corrugated drain, or even a tracheostomy tube, and the sutures can be closed electively once the patient's breathing and cooperation has been stabilised. The skin sutures can be placed and closed using local anaesthetic, and the wound/process must be "covered" by the use of broad-spectrum antibiotics.

Suggested Reading

1. Bradley PJ (2009) Bleeding around a tracheostomy wound: What does it all mean? J Laryngol Otol 123:952–956
2. Caruso DM (2009) Percutaneous dilational tracheostomy. J Burn Care Res 30(1):194–195
3. Kern EB (2003) The preoperative discussion as a prelude to managing a complication. Arch Otolaryngol Head Neck Surg 129:1163–1165
4. Klussmann JP, Knoedgen R, Wittekindt C et al. (2002) Complications of suspension microlaryngoscopy. Ann Otol Rhinol Laryngol 111:972–977

6.11 Laryngeal, Hypopharyngeal and Tracheal Imaging

MARKUS JUNGEHÜLSING AND JOHANNES HIERHOLZER

6.11.1 Clinical Symptom Investigation

The primary diagnosis of disease of the hypopharynx and larynx is based on clinical examination, 90° rigid endoscopy as well as flexible (fibre-optic) endoscopy of the region, followed by endoscopic procedures such as microlaryngoscopy. Assessment of the condition of the mucous membrane can certainly be achieved with these methods, and also by taking tissue samples for subsequent histological tests. Valuable evidence regarding the manoeuvrability of the vocal cords can be obtained from phonetic investigations and measurements such as stroboscopy and electromyography.

Ultrasound for bedside investigation is easy and reliable, and gives information on neck soft tissue conditions such as lymph node swelling or metastasis or primary tumour extension, whereas laryngeal cartridge and air often inhibit depiction of lesions within the laryngeal and hypopharyngeal space.

Conventional swallows with barium or water-soluble contrast media, supplemented by video cinematography or high-frequency cinematography, are employed for assessment of the swallowing process (Fig. 6.11.1).

The main application of cross-sectional imaging techniques—computed tomography (CT), magnetic resonance imaging (MRI) and ^{18}F-fluorodeoxyglucose (FDG) positron emission tomography (PET)—is for the assessment of deep-seated lesions and tumours, which in most cases are primarily detected through endoscopy. This can also give a simultaneous evaluation of the status of the cervical lymph nodes, particularly whether they are involved or not in malignant metastatic disease. Further applications of the above-mentioned imaging techniques are for the diagnosis of traumatic and inflammatory lesions.

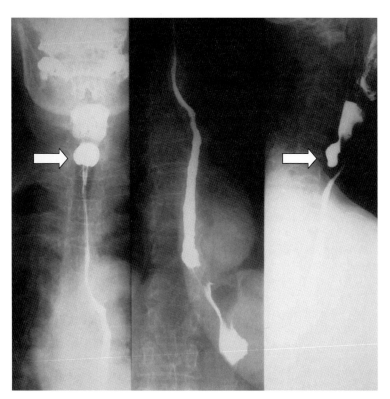

Fig. 6.11.1 Barium swallow in a patient suffering from Zenker's diverticulum. Typical prevertebral contrast agent accumulation

6.11.2 Imaging

6.11.2.1 Ultrasound

Modern ultrasound allows for detailed imaging of many anatomical structures and pathological processes of the head and neck. Unfortunately, lesions of the larynx, pharynx and trachea are located to a large extent in the sonographic acoustic shadow, behind the sometimes calcified cartilages, are surrounded by air and therefore cannot be visualised. Whereas ultrasound is widely regarded as the imaging method of choice for the evaluation of diseases of the thyroid, salivary glands (parotid gland, submandibular gland and sublingual gland), lymph nodes, muscles and soft tissues of the head and neck, it is of restricted use in the evaluation of laryngeal and pharyngeal lesions. Nevertheless, real-time ultrasound examination allows for dynamic assessment of congenital and tumorous lesions, inflammation and abscesses processes, abnormal lymph nodes, cysts, muscle hypertrophy and post-traumatic conditions outside the cartilage.

6.11.2.2 Conventional Radiography and Digital Subtraction Angiography

In conventional radiography, the laryngeal skeleton is only adequately recognisable when ossification of the primary cartilaginous structures has already commenced. However, since this process of ossification has already commenced in adolescents, the thyroid and cricoid cartilages can be satisfactorily demonstrated as a rule. Despite this, taking conventional radiographic imaging of the larynx and hypopharynx remains restricted when evaluating cases of suspected trauma. Obtaining images in two planes is to be recommended as is, if necessary, performing imaging in a lateral view so as to observe changes in the lumen of the respiratory tract associated with inspiration and expiration. Particular attention should be paid to the prelaryngeal, paralaryngeal and retrolaryngeal soft tissue and the cervical vertebral bodies and a separation of more than 5 mm between cervical vertebrae (Fig. 6.11.2) and the laryngeal tract should be investigated further with CT images.

An interesting application of digital subtraction angiography is when there are suspicions of trauma or tumour with unstoppable bleeding and subsequent embolism using platinum coils or coated stents.

6.11.2.3 Computed Tomography

CT comes into play for tumours, traumatic lesions and postoperative complications. In contrast to MRI, CT is valued because it is better at distinguishing between bone or cartilaginous erosion and destruction by a tumorous infiltration. Apart from this, a CT examination can be carried out considerably faster and therefore is less of a strain on patients who are frequently uncooperative and restless.

Distinguishing between vessels and tumours and the surrounding soft tissue is made easier with the use of injection of a contrast medium containing iodine. As a rule, it is not necessary to carry out a simple examination without contrast medium. The image display can be adjusted according to the purpose of the investigation by selecting a suitable "window" (e.g. bone or soft tissue windows). Before any contrast agent injection, TSH and creatinine clearance have to test normal to prevent thyroid problems as well as renal failure.

There are limitations in the lower-jaw region because artefacts from metal limit the clarity of the image after dental work particularly in this region. Positioning the patient with forced dorsal extension of the head with the corresponding gantry angle helps in such cases. Alternatively, artefacts can be minimised using slices parallel to the jawline.

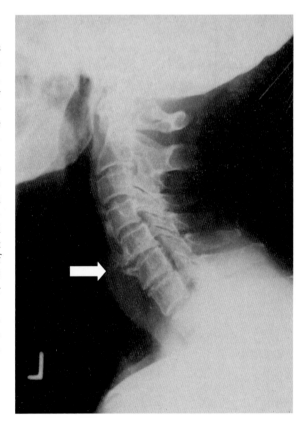

Fig. 6.11.2 Native planar X-ray detects an osteophyte (*arrow*) causing swallowing disorders and globus nervosus

High-resolution thin-slice CT with 1- or 2-mm slice thickness can be of use for specific queries related to the laryngeal skeleton. It is possible to assess the manoeuvrability of the vocal cords by examining E-phonation or the Valsalva technique.

To confirm a tumorous infiltration, a constant, demonstrable asymmetry or a unilateral restriction of movement must be observed. In this way, valuable additional information can be obtained, particularly after radiation therapy or laser treatment of small tumours.

Spiral CT recording is the basis for so-called virtual endoscopy, whereby endoscopy of the respiratory tract is simulated using a three-dimensional reconstruction algorithm. However, initial studies showed that small glottal tumours cannot be adequately revealed, particularly in the presence of artefacts caused by swallowing. A potential use is imaging the distal regions in cases of stenosis where endoscopy is not possible.

6.11.2.4 Magnetic Resonance Imaging

In general, superconductive tomograms between 0.5 and 1.5 T are used routinely, the advantage of higher field strength being a better signal-to-noise ratio and the possibility of faster sequencing. It is obligatory to use a receiving magnet for the throat. The investigation matrix should not exceed 256 × 256 pixels and the thickness of the axial slices is between 2 and 5 mm. Simple T1-weighted sequencing is very useful for differentiating between tumours and fatty tissue in the subglottal region. The slice thickness should not exceed 2 mm (Figs. 6.11.3, 6.11.4).

After contrast medium injection (gadolinium diethylenetriamine pentaacetic acid, Gd-DTPA), all malignant tumours show a significant increase in signal in comparison with the various surrounding structures because of the increased vascularisation (Fig. 6.11.5). Because Gd-

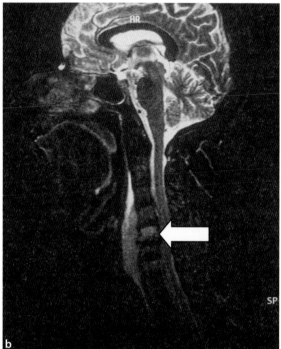

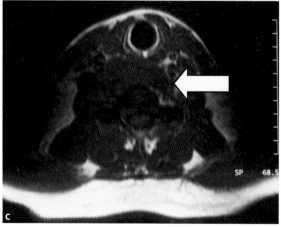

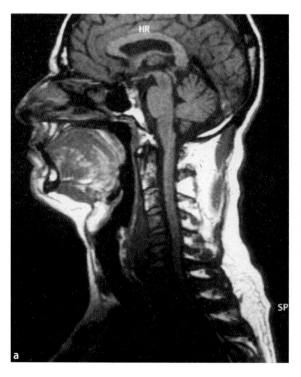

Fig. 6.11.3a–c Sometimes even very rare tumours may cause swallowing disorders, as in this patient suffering from multiple myeloma with vertebral column spongiosal infiltration (**b**, *arrow*) and spread to the retropharyngeal soft tissue (**c**, *arrow*). **a** T1-weighted sagittal sequence, **b** T2-weighted slice, **c** transverse section

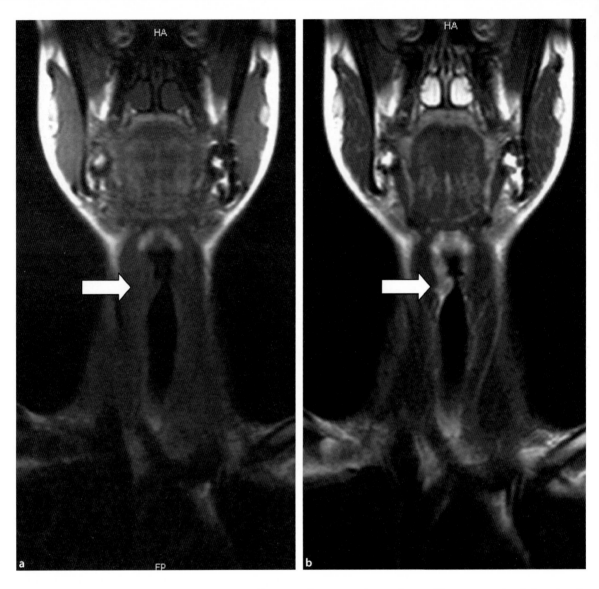

Fig. 6.11.4 a T1-weighted coronal slice of an 18-year old woman suffering from T2 laryngeal carcinoma of the sinus Morgagni. **b** Coronal inversion recovery sequences as "search sequences" for as yet unknown lesions. Hyperintense signal alteration allows further confirmation with use of axial slices with a thin-slice system (3 mm)

DTPA injection is known to cause renal failure in rare cases as well, creatinine clearance should be checked before any administration. However, the increased enrichment of normal mucosa or inflamed mucosa at a breadth of several millimetres makes it difficult to detect small submucosal tumours.

With respect to this, sequencing with spectral fat saturation has been proven to be useful. In this way it is possible to combine the fat saturation with T1- and T2-weighted sequencing, thereby improving T2 contrast with simple sequencing, giving better contrast between contrast-medium-enriched tissue and surrounding fat with gadolinium. Nevertheless, MRI can lead to overestimation of tumour size in isolated cases when there is inflammatory granulation tissue bordering the tumour.

Lymphatic tissue and glandular tissue also give an impressively high increase in intensity with T2-weighted sequences. Moreover, they demonstrate advantages in the evaluation of an invasion of cartilaginous tissue. On the whole, MRI appears to give better sensitivity for the

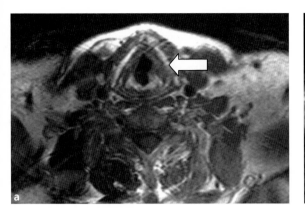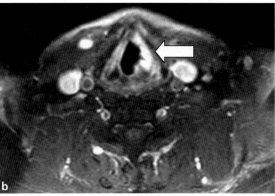

Fig. 6.11.5 a T2 laryngeal squamous cell carcinoma, T1-weighted axial 3-mm slices showing irregular borders of the right vocal fold. **b** After contrast medium injection (0.2 mmol gadolinium diethylenetriamine pentaacetic acid/kg body weight), the tumour shows a significant increase in signal in comparison with the various surrounding structures because of the increased vascularisation

diagnosis of cartilage invasion than CT, but with lower specificity.

T2-weighted turbo-spin-echo sequences have such a short test time that they are part of every routine protocol. A disadvantage is the higher susceptibility to artefacts in addition to the lower signal-to-noise ratio.

MRI has advantages over CT in that it produces better differentiation between soft tissue structures and it is possible to view anatomical and pathological structures in all desired planes without repositioning the patient. A further advantage is the absence of any radiation dose, so progress can be monitored frequently without any problems.

6.11.2.5 ^{18}F-Fluorodeoxyglucose Positron Emission Tomography

To the morphological details depicted by CT, FDG-PET adds metabolic information. The PET–CT image fusion technique combines morphological images with metabolic tracer uptake images. The so-called trapping of FDG in tissues using glucose as an anaerobic power supply renders visible tissues using high amounts of glucose for metabolism, such as malignant tumours. Applied to patients suffering from malignant tumours of the upper aerodigestive tract, FDG-PET allows depiction of even small malignant lesions (Fig. 6.11.6). FDG-PET is useful in patients suffering from carcinoma of unknown origin and in patients with iatrogenic changes after surgery and radiation therapy, such as scarring and fibrosis, and suspected tumour recurrence. Nevertheless, the investigation is expensive and should be reserved for patients with the above-mentioned problems.

6.11.3 Pathology of the Larynx and Pharynx

Clinical frequency in particular must be taken into consideration in the context of differential diagnosis. Squamous cell carcinoma is seen most often, and among malignant tumours is significantly in the foreground (Figs. 6.11.4, 6.11.5). One should also consider inflammatory processes, which can be viral, bacterial or fungal. In addition, laryngoceles (Fig. 6.11.7) and Zenker's diverticulum (Fig. 6.11.1) are among the most frequently seen lesions. Previous trauma or incorporated foreign bodies should be ruled out through anamnesis. Other lesions are seen significantly less frequently.

Congenital malformations such as atresia, hypoplasia, stricture, stenosis or laryngeal malaise are also to be considered. Benign tumours such as haemangioma or papilloma are also seen rarely in this region. Amyloidosis or other tumours such as angiofibroma, chondroma, rhabdomyoma or fibroma are considered rarities, as are sarcoma or a metastatic invasion of the hypopharynx or larynx. Finally, disease secondary to tuberculosis, Boeck sarcoidosis or Wegener granulomatosis should be mentioned.

6.11.3.1 Cysts and Inflammatory Lesions

The differential diagnosis includes cysts, celes, swelling and necrotic tumours. There is a characteristic topographic position of laryngoceles in relation to the laryngeal ventricle (Figs. 6.11.7, 6.11.8), where cysts or abscesses can develop ubiquitously. Whereas the wall of an

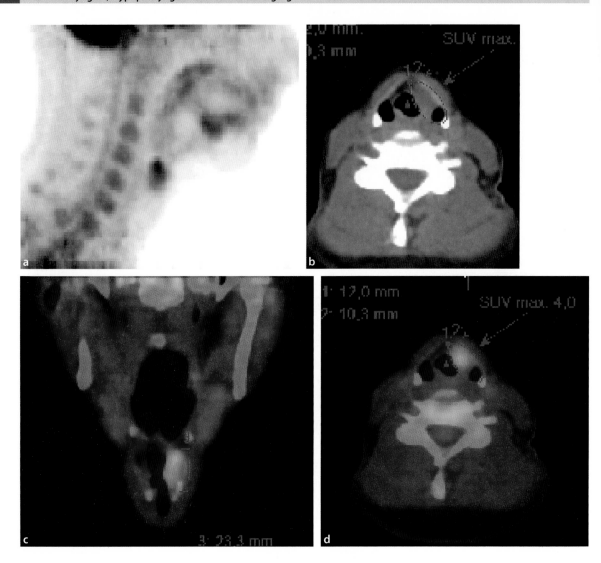

Fig. 6.11.6a–d 18-FDG-PET and PET-CT fusion images in a patient suffering from small cell carcinoma of the larynx. **a** 2 hours after injection of 370 MBq 18-Fluoro-deoxy-glucose, positron emission tomography is performed. Note the high tracer accumulation of the larynx in sagittal images. **b** coronar CT scan in the same patient. *Red circle*: swelling of the left vocal fold. **c** coronar and **d** transversal PET – CT fusion images. The high tracer uptake is now clearly projected on the left vocal fold swelling.

abscess or decaying necrotic tumour seems thicker, the wall of a cyst appears thin and homogenous (Fig. 6.11.9). In addition, tumours often have solid components and an irregular basic form.

Further, the density and observed signal are indicative of the inner structure. Serous liquid, as seen in cysts or celes, has a tomographic density of less than 30 Hounsfield units (HU), whereas an abscess with protein-rich exudation has a density of more than 30 HU. MRI gives corresponding indicators through an increased signal in T2-weighted sequences (Fig. 6.11.10). With lesions containing gas, one should at first suspect a laryngocele. Gas-containing blisters are seen with collapsing abscesses and decaying necrotic tumours. Cervical soft tissue emphysema as a consequence of pneumothorax or laryngeal trauma is an important consideration (Fig. 6.11.11). With both CT and MRI it should be possible to provide a diagnosis through characteristically low density values (less than 100 HU) and with loss of signal in all sequences without any problem.

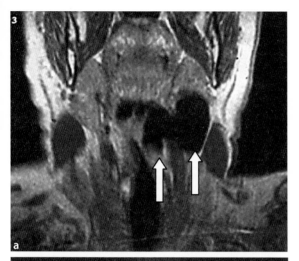

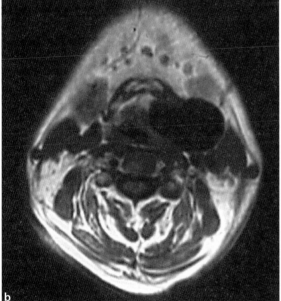

Fig. 6.11.7 a T1-weighted coronal slice in a patient suffering from a combined inner and outer laryngocele. The cele is filled with air and therefore shows no signal. **b** The T1-weighted transverse section shows the typical orientation of the cele between laryngeal and cricoid cartilage, following the upper laryngeal nerve through the thyrohyoid membrane

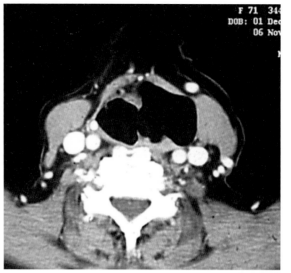

Fig. 6.11.8 CT scan of a combined inner and outer laryngocele. Filled with either gas or liquid, they demonstrate sharp edges on CT and different density depending on what they contain

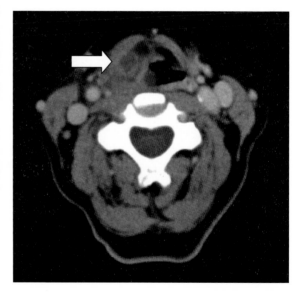

Fig. 6.11.9 Coronal slice of a patient suffering from vallecular abscess after iodine contrast agent administration. Note the increased density of the cystic wall in comparison with the low-density serous liquid

Laryngocele

A laryngocele results from dilation of the laryngeal ventricle, which can be either present at birth or acquired during adulthood (often by glass-blowers or players of wind instruments). Paralaryngeal inner laryngoceles can be distinguished from outer laryngoceles by the egg-tim-er configuration or perforation of the thyroid membrane (Fig. 6.11.7). Correspondingly, excavations cranially can appear as laryngoceles. Filled with either gas or liquid, they demonstrate sharp edges on CT and different density depending on what they contain (Fig. 6.11.8). Equally, the

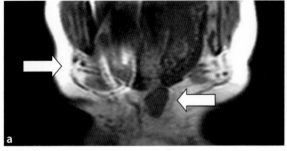 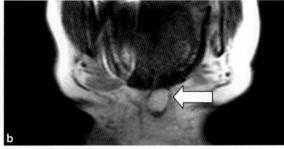

Fig. 6.11.10a,b T1- and T2-weighted coronal slices of a small medial cervical cyst, filled with fluid, *in loco typico*. *Left arrow* a typical metal artefact caused by teeth filling, *right arrow* cyst and hyoid bone

combined application of T1- and T2-weighted sequences in MRI allows the differentiation between liquids with different protein content and gas. Of clinical importance is the bilateral presence in up to 20% of cases and also the frequent association with malignant tumours or tuberculosis.

Paralaryngeal and Parapharyngeal Abscess

A paralaryngeal abscess can occur as a complication of laryngitis, but is mostly seen with weakened immunity or poor general health and in particular after trauma or injury through ingestion of foreign bodies (Fig. 6.11.9). In advanced cases it is associated with a secondary extralaryngeal inflammatory reaction affecting the lymph nodes in the region, in addition to compression of the airway with stridor on inspiration.

Epiglottitis

A balloonlike swelling of the epiglottis with thickened mucosa and narrowing of the respiratory tract are indications of acute epiglottitis. These changes are often recognisable on conventional X-ray with lateral projection. Primarily, such observations are not an indication to perform imaging, since in the acute stage an immediate clinical intervention is required. In complicated cases, however, performing CT or MRI is justified to plan the intervention.

Laryngitis

With laryngitis, as with epiglottitis, thickened mucosa and narrowing of the respiratory tract are to be seen. Morphologically, an oedema of the laryngeal mucosa reveals itself as thickening on imaging, which can be either

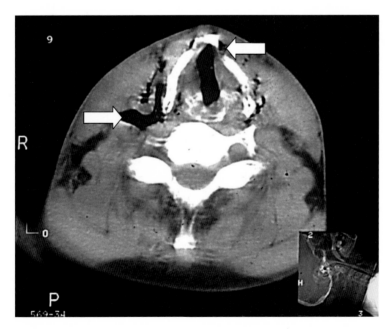

Fig. 6.11.11 Cervical soft tissue emphysema as a consequence of laryngeal trauma. CT shows characteristically low density values (less than 100 HU). Note the emphysema (*left arrow*) and the laryngeal cartilage fracture (*right arrow*)

locally restricted to the vocal folds (Reinke oedema) or diffusely affecting the entire larynx (Quincke oedema).

The latter is often observed in the context of an allergic reaction, primarily after intravenous administration of contrast medium. Acute virus-induced subglottal stenosing laryngitis in children (pseudo-Krupp) is a special case worthy of note.

6.11.3.2 Chronic Inflammatory Changes

Laryngeal Tuberculosis

Laryngeal tuberculosis may involve the larynx, demonstrating inflammation and thickening of the epiglottis by granuloma formation. CT and MRI evaluation of such cases demonstrated an infiltrative growth without cartilage destruction.

Arthritis/Perichondritis

The arytenoid cartilage and the interarytenoid region are the areas with a predisposition to perichondritis and arthritis. A thickening of the mucous membrane with diffuse oedema and contrast medium uptake in CT and MRI can be observed. An association with rheumatoid arthritis is seen as a rarity, but in these cases a contrast medium enrichment of the fatty tissue surrounding the cartilaginous structures can be seen. Of particular clinical importance is the accurate differentiation between radiogenic perichondritis and a residual tumour, which can be established using MRI.

6.11.3.3 Tumours

To determine whether there is any tumour invasion of the larynx, coronal slices are particularly useful in MRI, and clearly show asymmetry or infiltration of the laryngeal ventricle (Fig. 6.11.4). This phenomenon can already be seen with small glottal tumours, and with a more advanced stage of tumour the tendency is more towards a central necrosis.

Becker et al. [1] stated that sclerosis of the cartilage which can be proven tomographically is the most important observation for tumours. Further important proofs of malignancy are extralaryngeal tumour growth, tumour close to non-ossified cartilage, erosion or cell destruction, irregular edges and obliteration of bone marrow.

Characteristically, there is primarily high signal intensity in haemangioma with T2-weighted sequences, in addition to the clear enhancement with intravenously administered contrast medium. Tumours with a chondrogenic matrix show only a relatively low enhancement, but are generally diagnosed from their typical growth

from the thyroid or cricoid cartilage (Fig. 6.11.11). These are to be differentiated from iatrogenic or postoperative changes such as from fat injection, which are well demonstrated with MRI, particularly with T1-weighted sequences.

Cartilage Destruction

A main criterion for establishing the stage of malignant tumours is whether there is infiltration of the laryngeal skeleton. The differential diagnosis in cartilage destruction of the larynx is between tumour infiltration by squamous cell carcinoma or primary chondroma/chondrosarcoma and inflammatory processes such as Wegener granulomatosis, perichondritis, osteosclerosis and arthritis of the cricoarytenoid joint, and also thyroid cartilage fracture and physiological ossification. When unilateral sclerosis is seen on CT, a tumorous infiltration is to be suspected; osteoradionecrosis can also be clearly demonstrated by raised density on CT. Early-stage infiltration with incomplete ossification is shown better with MRI, where above all T2-weighted sequences show subtle dishomogeneity.

Squamous Cell Carcinoma

Asymmetrical and infiltrative growth with unclear edges and an inhomogeneous inner structure is the sign of malignant tumours seen on imaging. This can include infiltrative as well as exophytic growth formations. Various subgroups are also differentiated histologically, including verrucous carcinoma, spinalioma and basal cell carcinoma. Different criteria for these tumours were compiled in a review, but these cannot be seen as pathognomonic on their own in atypical growths. The relatively early tendency towards central necrosis is indicative of squamous cell carcinoma. Bone and cartilage destruction is evident on CT. A significant contrast medium uptake by the tumour and possible narrowing of the respiratory tract can also be seen on CT and MRI (Figs. 6.11.4, 6.11.5).

The sensitivity and specificity of the accurate assessment of the tumour stage is significantly improved using CT and MRI in comparison with the sole use of endoscopy.

Zbaren et al. [2] in a study on classification of laryngeal tumours achieved an accuracy of 80–87% in contrast to 55% (laryngeal tumour) and 36% (hypopharyngeal tumour) by clinical methods. On the whole, CT and MRI were seen as of equal value, MRI having better sensitivity, but CT having better specificity. Other studies support these findings on the whole and confirm the value of both procedures for the diagnosis of tumorous infiltration of the pre-epiglottal space.

The diagnosis of hypopharyngeal carcinoma and supra- and subglottal laryngeal carcinoma is often only made after the initial detection of cervical lymph node metastases. Hoarseness is the first main symptom of glottal laryngeal carcinoma, whereas an irritation of the lymph nodes in the region is only seen as a later development.

The prognosis of laryngeal and hypopharyngeal tumours after radiotherapy is more dependent on tumour volume than on its stage. In this study, 85% of patients with smaller tumours were free of residual cancer over a 2-year observation period.

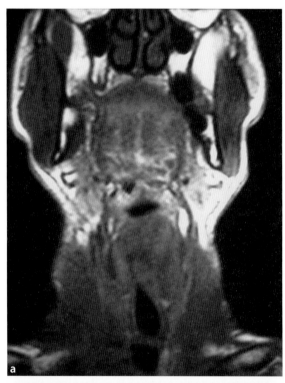

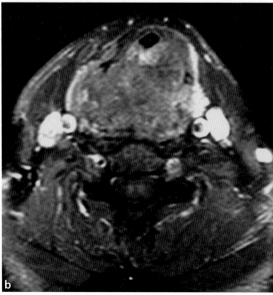

Rare Malignant Tumours

Rare tumours of the larynx are rhabdomyosarcoma, fibrosarcoma and adenoid cystic carcinoma. Important indicators can be uncharacteristic location of the direction of growth of the lesions, which either stem from muscle or tendons or grow along them. An important differential diagnosis to be made, however, is chondrosarcoma (Fig. 6.11.12), which is discernible through its typical growth from the thyroid or cricoid cartilage, and through its high degree of differentiation it has in most cases a better prognosis.

Not to be forgotten are the very rare laryngeal metastases which may include malignant melanoma, breast cancer as well as kidney cancers. Kaposi's sarcoma has also spread to involve the larynx and reportedly grows two-dimensionally with no ossicular destruction and through its good vascularisation shows a high contrast medium uptake on CT and MRI, without evidence of involvement of local lymph nodes or secondary metastases. The sharp edges and fast growth in addition to the association with HIV are further diagnostic features.

Rare Benign Lesions

Other rarely seen lesions are fibroma, angiofibroma, rhabdomyoma and lipoma, only the lattermost of which can be confidently diagnosed through its typical density/signal on CT or MRI (Fig. 6.11.13). Haemangioma and lymphangioma can be identified with CT through their calcified pepper-and-salt matrix caused by focal thrombosis. With an adenoma, a smooth edge with a homogenous in-

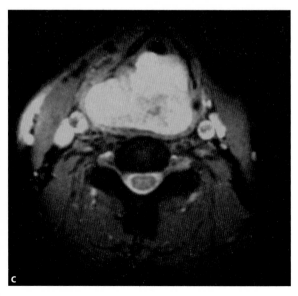

Fig. 6.11.12a–c Chondrosarcoma of the larynx shows only a relatively low enhancement with gadolinium diethylenetriamine pentaacetic acid (**b**), but a strong signal intensity in T2-weighted images (**c**)

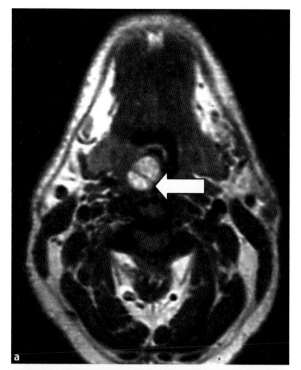

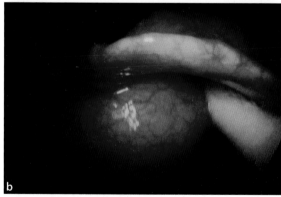

Fig. 6.11.13 a T1-weighted transverse image of a pedunculated fibrolipoma of the arytenoid fold. High signal intensity of lipomatous tissue, typical septal intersection (*arrow*). **b** Findings during laser surgery

ner structure is seen. On imaging it shows a slow and suppressing growth with average contrast medium uptake. Amyloidal infestation of the laryngeal mucous membrane is a further rarity, and shows an absence of contrast medium uptake with swelling surrounding the mucosa.

Papilloma/Polyp

Virus-induced papilloma is frequently seen in children. These tumours have a smooth edge and morphology similar to a cauliflower, and are located anteriorly to the plicae vestibularis or vocalis, reaching to the subglottal space. Diffuse papilloma growth in the larynx is known as juvenile papillomatosis. A differentiation between this and a mucous membrane polyp is not possible through imaging, because these also tend to grow in the anterior region of the plicae vocales.

Chondroma

A chondroma, normally stemming from the cricoid cartilage, shows a characteristic amorphological calcification matrix, and is best confirmed through CT. Further diagnostic features are the smooth edges with narrowing of the respiratory tract and low contrast medium uptake.

6.11.3.4 Recurrent Nerve Paresis

After a clinical assessment, the following overview of possible causes should be excluded or confirmed by CT or MRI:

- Iatrogenic after thyroid surgery
- Malignant processes of the thyroid, oesophageal or lung cancer
- Aortic arch aneurysm
- Metastatic disease
- Trauma
- Neurotropic recurrent nerve infection

Owing to the number of possible causes of paresis of the recurrent nerve, the area necessary to be examined is large, including cervical structures as well as the entire mediastinum. Similarly, with no positive findings seen with endoscopy, a CT examination is the first method of choice to check for tumours.

6.11.3.5 Malformations

Congenital malformations cause typical clinical symptoms and are usually diagnosed by endoscopy. Diaphragma laryngis, a sail-like connection between the vocal cords, laryngeal fissure in cartilage lamella fusion dysfunction and laryngeal malaise may also be found on imaging.

6.11.3.6 Trauma and Foreign Bodies

Clinically, with changes induced by trauma, one differentiates between injury from the outside, such as gun, knife or strangulation wounds (Fig. 6.11.14), and injury from the inside through scalding, foreign bodies or iatrogenous injury.

In the larynx and hypopharynx, fracture of the thyroid cartilage is the most common traumatic injury. A broadening of the laryngeal and paratracheal soft tissue

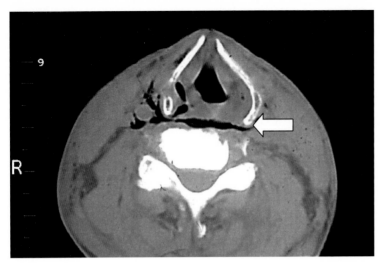

Fig. 6.11.14 Strangulation wound in a patient seen in a coronal CT scan. Note the prevertebral emphysema of the neck soft tissue

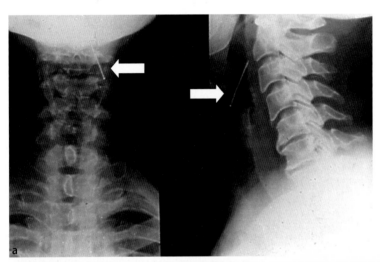

Fig. 6.11.15 **a** Conventional X-ray on two planes in a patient who swallowed a needle by mistake. The needle is located in the upper hypopharynx (*arrows*). **b** This 1-year-old boy swallowed a one Deutschmark coin. The coin was stopped in the upper oesophageal narrowing. Endoscopic findings on the *right*

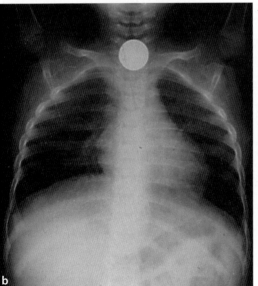

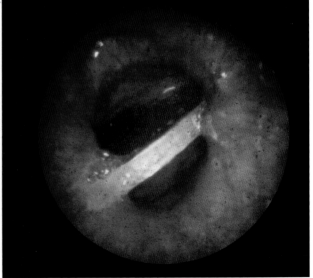

on conventional X-ray is a primary observation to be made. In general, a fracture line as well as a surrounding haematoma or dislocation of the arytenoid cartilage from its normal position or a non-physiological rotation is endoscopically ruled out, but may be also demonstrable by CT (Fig. 6.11.11). The possible direct observations with a dislocation of the arytenoid cartilage are, among others, swelling of the aryepiglottic folds and fixation of the vocal folds during E-phonation or Valsalva technique.

Conventional X-ray in two planes in acute situations provides the location of X-ray-dense foreign bodies or associated changes in soft tissue (Fig. 6.11.15). It is not possible, however, to exclude the presence of materials which do not give a shadow (glass, wood, plastic, etc.) and that are therefore not detectable by conventional X-ray. In these cases a CT scan is recommended, through which additional perifocal-associated reactions or haemorrhage can be seen.

6.11.3.7 Changes Caused by Surgery

An important consideration for differential diagnosis in the head and neck region is problems resulting from therapeutic intervention. Of great importance are reconstructive plastic surgery procedures such as skin grafts, fat removal or implantation of muscle or metal, as well as sclerotic and fibrous changes caused by irradiation and radiochemotherapeutic protocols.

The most important aid for differential diagnosis is accurate documentation of results, in particular comparison with preinterventional findings and interdisciplinary consultations.

Total extirpation of the larynx is a radical surgical intervention, where breathing is maintained by tracheotomy (Fig. 6.11.16). Still more radical is laryngopharyngectomy and reconstruction of the pharynx using stomach pull-up surgery or microanastomosed tubular jejunal interpositions, leaving a completely changed cervical anatomy (Figs. 6.11.17, 6.11.18).

Typical signs seen during or immediately after radiation therapy are diffuse inflammatory or oedemous changes in the region being targeted. Indicators of chondroradionecrosis are regularly seen on the thyroid and cricoid cartilage, and interfere with the diagnosis of residual tumour growth with secondary invasion of cartilage. Scarred retractions and osteosclerosis of the cartilage can be chronic changes seen months to years after radiation therapy. Above all, MRI, through its high soft tissue definition, is particularly suitable for imaging surgical reconstruction and differentiation of scarring, postradiation therapy changes and residual tumour growth. FDG-PET–CT is restricted to patients in whom it is not possible to differentiate between scarring, fibrosis and recurrent tumour growth.

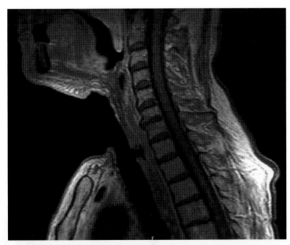

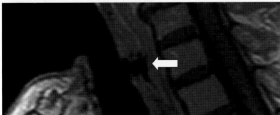

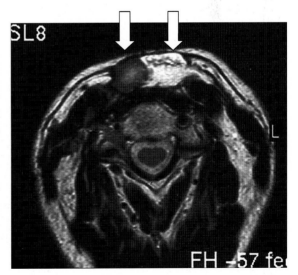

Fig. 6.11.16 T1-weighted sagittal section demonstrating the anatomical changes after laryngectomy. Note the silicon voice fistula (Provox 2) within the dorsal, membranaceous part of the trachea (*arrow*), connecting tracheal and oesophageal lumen

Fig. 6.11.17 T1-weighted section in a patient with laryngopharyngectomy and microanastomosed tubular jejunal interposition. *Left arrow* jejunum, *right arrow* peritoneal and vascular pedicle

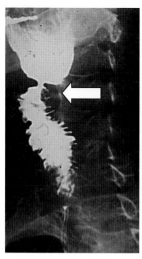
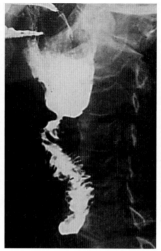
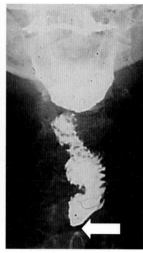

Fig. 6.11.18 Same patient as in Fig. 6.11.16. Barium swallow, video cinematography. Note the jejunal mucosal relief. Slight proximal and distal stenosis (*arrows*)

6.11.4 Trachea

The most frequent clinical signs of tracheal disease are stridor, cough and haemoptysis. These different disease manifestations are usually caused by stenosis. Stenosis itself is caused by stricture, scarring tumour growth or trauma. Possible differential diagnosis of stridor includes tracheitis and (pseudo) Krupp, particularly with subglottal location and concentric narrowing. In addition, an infiltration/constriction with thyroid gland tumour, goitre and stricture through scarring after intubation are to be considered in this region. An intraluminal stenosis is an indication of primary tracheal infection or scarred granulation tissue following injury through intubation or surgical tracheotomy. Tracheal malaise expresses itself with a characteristic slot-shaped stenosis of the trachea caused by a deficiency in the stability of the cartilaginous skeleton. The tracheal bifurcation, particularly the right main bronchus, is noted as the typical location of incorporated foreign bodies. Mediastinal lymph nodes or other tumorous infections can lead to a supracarinal extrinsic compression.

Tumorous lesions of the trachea include benign tumours such as fibroma, chondroma, papilloma, hypertrophy through scarring, mucous membrane polyp or an amyloid tumour and malignant tumours, including squamous cell carcinoma, adenocarcinoma and adenoid cystic carcinoma. Metastasis from another primary tumour can also be seen in the trachea in rare cases. All tumours can arise ubiquitously, with no characteristic topography. Normally, growth of a chondroma stemming from the tracheal cartilage is obvious and also shows an increased density with irregular calcification on CT.

In general, CT provides adequate imaging of a tracheal stenosis. Fluctuation of the lumen on inspiration and expiration (seen in tracheal malaise) is well demonstrated by X-ray.

Calcification of the tracheal cartilaginous cords is regularly seen in patients of advanced age, and normally is of no significance for differential diagnosis. In such cases, the entire length of the trachea, including the tracheobronchial bifurcation, can be affected. Calcification of the tracheal cartilage is therefore often only mentioned as an observation on X-ray of the thorax.

6.11.4.1 Trauma-Induced Changes

Conventional imaging of the cervical spine in two planes is best suited for the primary diagnosis of a neck fracture.

For assessment of the posterior edge and inward bleeding of the spine, CT (2-mm slice thickness) is often necessary. Equally, with conventional imaging, a haematoma in the prevertebral space can be diagnosed through thickening of the soft tissue shadow, but the exact extent of this is provided by CT, and with MRI direct damage to the myelin can be seen.

Direct injury with perforation of the oesophagus can be revealed with iodine contrast agent swallow following trauma, as in a traffic injury. Penetrating injuries with exposure of the trachea can lead to dislocation of the tracheal cartilaginous skeleton with soft tissue haematoma and perifocal oedema and also cervical soft tissue emphysema.

More and more frequent are lesions caused by inadequate dilational tracheotomy procedures (Fig 6.11.19), causing scarring and stricture of the trachea with subsequent events of dyspneoa.

6.11.4.2 Tracheitis

An initial viral infection with catarrh problems can lead to acute tracheobronchitis. Of decreasing importance is bacterial diphtheria (Krupp) with characteristic whitish

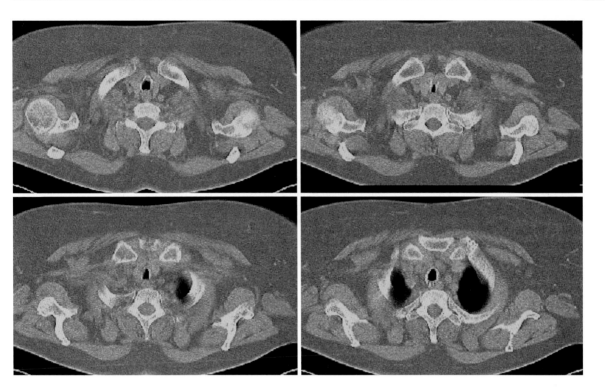

Fig. 6.11.19 CT (3-mm adjacent coronal slices) of the upper trachea in a patient 2 months after temporary percutaneous dilatational tracheotomy. Inadequate tracheotomy has caused severe narrowing of the tracheal diameter

deposits in the gum region. Thickened mucous membrane in the affected region is demonstrable on CT and MRI. Subglottal stenosing viral laryngotracheitis, also known as "pseudo-Krupp", manifests itself above all in early childhood and the children suffer from a dry, often described as "barking" cough with stridor on inspiration, leading to cyanosis and acute fear of asphyxiation in advanced cases. Environmental toxins and allergies have also been discussed as possible causes of this disease. With conventional imaging, stenosis in the region of the subglottal larynx and the length of the trachea is generally adequately represented for diagnosis. In addition, MRI is also useful for diagnosis in children because of the lack of radiation. A chronic cough can lead to a tracheitis sicca through exogenous damage of the mucous membrane, and in general a diagnosis can be made clinically with no need for initial imaging.

6.11.4.3 Tracheal Tumours

Stenosis of the trachea with alteration of the surrounding soft tissue indicates primarily an intratracheal tumour. One differentiates between benign tumours (fibroma, chondroma and papilloma) and hypertrophy with scarring and constriction following a previous trauma or radiotherapy. Alternatively, malignant tumours (squamous cell carcinoma, adenocarcinoma and adenoid cystic carcinoma) are indicated by destruction of the tracheal cartilage and unsharp edges. Furthermore, relapsing polychondritis may cause thickening of the tracheal cartilage. These primary tracheal tumours are to be differentiated from external infiltration, e.g. from a thyroid gland carcinoma. Through a diffuse or nodal goitre, the trachea can be displaced or misshapen, and then it is known as a sabre-shaped trachea.

An endotracheal goitre can arise from dystrophy of the thyroid gland tissue, normally located in the cranial portion of the trachea. If a smooth-edged constriction of the tracheal lumen is seen without infiltrative growth, a further diagnostic tool available is thyroid gland scintigraphy after indication from CT (without iodine contrast agent) or MRI. Further, so-called pseudotumours such as mucous membrane polyp or amyloid tumour can be observed.

6.11.5 Summary

Clinical examination and endoscopy alone can provide basic assessment for differential diagnosis of laryngeal, hypopharyngeal or tracheal lesions. Further imaging, including of the mediastinum, is indicated particularly for recent onset of recurrent nerve paresis. While conventional radiological imaging is adequate for trauma to start with, CT and MRI assist with therapy planning and assessment of the stage of development of solid lesions. Of particular importance is the differentiation between inflammatory and tumorous processes. The most frequently seen tumorous process in this region is squamous cell carcinoma, and the role of imaging lies here in the assessment of deep infiltration and lymph node involvement. Both pieces of information are used for the correct grading of tumour stage, which is necessary for further therapy planning, the main two branches of which are primarily radiation therapy and surgical intervention. Several studies have reported CT and MRI to be procedures of equal rank, with sensitive assessment of cartilage invasion provided by MRI and higher specificity in CT. For patients unable to cooperate, CT should be chosen because of the lower number of movement artefacts and shorter test time.

Generally, differentiation between rare tumour manifestations, such as chondroma/chondrosarcoma, Kaposi's sarcoma and polyp/papilloma and other rare lesions, are effectuated by histological examinations during endoscopy, but modern tomography techniques may add necessary information. Imaging and endoscopy are thus to be seen as complementary techniques and are not in competition with one another. FDG-PET and FDG-PET–CT should be reserved for patients with carcinoma of unknown primary site and patients with extended post-therapeutic anatomical changes and suspected malignant tumour recurrence.

References

1. Becker M, Burkhardt K, Dulguerov P, Allal A (2008) Imaging of the larynx and hypopharynx. Eur J Radiol 66(3):460–479
2. Zbaren P, Becker M, Lang H (1997) Staging of laryngeal cancer: endoscopy, computed tomography and magnetic resonance versus histopathology. Eur Arch Otorhinolaryngol 254(Suppl 1):S117–S122

Suggested Reading

1. Jungehulsing M, Scheidhauer K, Pietrzyk U, Eckel H, Schicha H (1999) Detection of unknown primary cancer with fluor-deoxy-glucose positron emission tomography. Ann Otol Rhinol Laryngol 108(6):623–626
2. Lell M, Baum U, Greess H, Nomayr A, Cavallaro A, Koester M, Bautz W (2001) Multi-slice spiral CT of the head and neck region. Rontgenpraxis 53(4):157–163
3. Schmidt M, Schmalenbach M, Jungehulsing M, Theissen P, Dietlein M, Schroder U, Eschner W, Stennert E, Schicha H (2004) 18F-FDG PET for detecting recurrent head and neck cancer, local lymph node involvement and distant metastases. Comparison of qualitative visual and semiquantitative analysis. Nuklearmedizin 43(3):91–101
4. Sittel C, Gossmann A, Jungehulsing M, Zahringer M (2001) Superselective embolization as palliative treatment of recurrent hemorrhage in advanced carcinoma of the head and neck. Ann Otol Rhinol Laryngol 110(12):1126–1128

Voice Disorders

Edited by Patrick J. Bradley

7.1 Voice Disorders: Classification

PATRICK J. BRADLEY

There is huge variation in what is accepted as a 'normal voice'. Defining its essential characteristics is problematic as there is a continuum between a normal and a disordered voice. A normal voice is essentially unremarkable in quality and permits adequate communication without undue effort or discomfort.

'**Hoarseness**' is a term that describes an abnormal quality of the voice which may be rough, harsh, breathy, weak or strained.

A **voice problem**, or **dysphonia**, can be defined as any impairment, limitation in activity or restriction in participation (World Health Organisation) as a result of a structural or functional abnormality of the voice mechanism.

The prevalence of dysphonia in the UK has been reported as 2.5%, although other studies have estimated this to range between 0.8 and 15%. There is a higher prevalence of voice disorders (18–32%) in certain occupational groups such as teachers, call-centre workers and performers, where there is a requirement to use the voice for prolonged periods, especially at raised intensity levels. In children, voice problems tend to affect more males than females, but in adults the reverse is true, with the highest number of patients being in the 20–40-year-old age group. The commonest voice complaints are outlined in Table 7.1.1.

7.1.1 Aetiology of Voice Problems

Voice problems can be broadly classified into four main categories: structural/neoplastic, inflammatory, neuromuscular and muscle tension imbalance (Fig. 7.1.1). Many patients will have evidence of more than one of these conditions contributing to their voice condition and this may change at different phases in the chronology of the condition. For example a vocal fold polyp (structural/neoplastic cause) may arise as a result of primary muscle tension imbalance as a result of voice abuse, e.g. shouting when suffering from a viral upper respiratory tract infection (inflammation). The presence of a polyp can in turn cause secondary physical trauma to the vocal folds (inflammation) and a muscle tension imbalance to compensate for the alteration in the biomechanical prop-

erties of vocal folds. An important part of the assessment of a patient is the determination of which of these four conditions are present, which are primary and which are secondary and which are actually contributing to the patient's voice complaint.

7.1.2 Guidelines and Referral Pathway into Secondary Care

Examination of the larynx is rarely possible in the GP surgery without special endoscopic equipment. As laryngeal visualisation is the key examination to the diagnosis of voice disorders for which most patients will need to be referred. Patients with persistent hoarseness or a change in their voice for 3 weeks, who are smokers, aged 50 years or older, and heavy drinkers should have an urgent chest X-ray to exclude a recurrent laryngeal nerve palsy sec-

Table 7.1.1 Commonest voice complaints

Change in voice quality (hoarseness, roughness and breathiness)
A deeper or higher-pitched voice that is not appropriate for the age and sex
Problems controlling the voice described as pitch breaks, squeaky voice or the voice cutting out
Difficulty making oneself heard in a noisy environment or in raising the voice
Effort in producing voice
Reduced stamina of the voice or one that tires with use
Difficulties or restrictions in the use of voice at different times of the day or related to specific daily, social or occupationally related tasks
A reduced ability to communicate effectively
Difficulty in singing
Throat-related symptoms (soreness, discomfort, aching, dryness, mucus) particularly related to voice use
The consequent emotional, psychological effects caused by the above

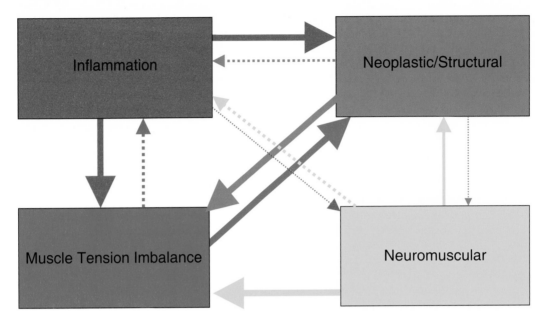

Fig. 7.1.1 Aetiological categories of voice disorders and their interactions

ondary to lung cancer. Those with positive findings on X-ray should be referred urgently to a lung cancer specialist team. Those with negative findings or with other upper aerodigestive tract symptoms should be referred to a head and neck cancer specialist team. Other patients should be seen in a specialist benign voice disorders clinic. These may be run by a laryngologist, voice therapist or as a joint multiprofessional voice clinic.

7.1.3   Methods of Assessment

A comprehensive assessment of a patient with a voice problem will include the items listed in Table 7.1.2 for an accurate diagnosis to be made and an appropriate management plan to be constructed.

The first aim of the consultation is to identify the presence of the four main aetiological factors (Fig. 7.1.1). Important points to consider in the history are outlined in Table 7.1.3. During the consultation clues as to the psychological well-being of the patient may also become apparent. During the recount of the history, it is essential to listen to the voice quality, whether it is rough, breathy, weak or strained, to assess the appropriateness of the pitch for the age and sex of the patient, whether the voice is too loud or too soft and whether the characteristics of the voice are constant or intermittent. This auditory perceptual analysis can be done more formally using validated assessment schemes, e.g. GRBAS, voice profile analysis.

Table 7.1.2 Assessment of a patient with a voice problem

Essential assessment of a voice patient
Detailed clinical history
Auditory perceptual evaluation of the voice quality
Flexible nasoendoscopic examination of vocal tract
Structure
Function
Videolaryngostroboscopic assessment of vocal fold vibration
Neck inspection and palpation
Lymphadenopathy and other masses
Increased muscle tension and imbalance
Larynx position in neck and relationship of the thyroid and cricoid cartilages
Neck, back and overall body posture
Breathing patterns during speech
Neurological assessment—psychological assessment
Further investigations and assessment
Diagnostic microlaryngoscopy
Quality of life measures using validated questionnaires
Objective measurements of vocal function, e.g. acoustic, electolaryngographic and aerodynamic measures, electromyography
24-h dual-site pH monitoring with impedance
Oesophagogastroduodenoscopy

A flexible endoscope allows inspection of the vocal tract from the nasal cavity to the larynx and also assessment of speech, singing and non-phonatory tasks such as coughing. It is the preferred technique in neuromuscular and muscle tension imbalance disorders. A rigid endoscope placed on the tongue provides better quality, more magnified images and is better for examining the structure and function of the vocal folds. In addition, the use of stroboscopic light improves the accuracy of the diagnosis of structural/neoplastic, inflammatory and some neuromuscular cases by about 30%. Recording the images digitally means that they can be stored, easily retrieved and played back in slow motion. The neck should be examined for neck masses, abnormalities of the shape and movement of the laryngeal cartilages and tenderness of the extralaryngeal muscles as this may indicate the presence of increased muscle tension.

Objective measures of the voice or laryngeal function can provide supportive diagnostic information and be used as outcome measures. Electromyography is helpful in detecting paresis and in the differential diagnosis of cricoarytenoid joint fixation from vocal cord palsy. A diagnostic microlaryngoscopy is occasionally helpful in cases of persistent chronic laryngitis or when outpatient laryngoscopy is not possible. Investigations of laryngopharyngeal reflux include 24-h pH with proximal and distal probes coupled with oesophageal impedance measurements and occasionally oesophagogastroduodenoscopy.

7.1.4 Treatment Options

The treatment options (Table 7.1.4) for a patient with a voice problem will depend on the diagnosis, the reasons for seeking referral, the vocal requirements and the risk/benefit of any intervention. More conservative measures are usually tried first as many patients either respond or do not want further treatment once they have had an explanation of their voice condition. If the diagnosis is not clear at the initial consultation, a trial of simple vocal hygiene measures, medical treatment or voice therapy may be tried. Primary surgery is usually only performed for suspected neoplastic lesions, leucoplakia (white mucosal lesions) and many cases of papillomas, polyps and vocal cord palsy. Other structural lesions may require surgery if more conservative measures fail. Postoperative voice therapy is frequently required for optimal results.

7.1.5 Structural/Neoplastic Conditions

Structural or neoplastic conditions are where there is a structural abnormality or mass lesion involving part of the larynx (Table 7.1.5). This type of condition may involve any layer from the inner mucosal surface to the outer cartilage of the larynx. The effect on the voice will depend on the effects of the lesion on vocal fold vibra-

Table 7.1.3 Important points in history

Voice problem, e.g. abnormal quality, pitch, loudness, loss of voice function	Past and current medical history, including conditions affecting the respiratory, gastro-oesophageal, neurological, musculoskeletal and endocrine systems
Onset and duration	Psychological and psychiatric conditions
Constant/intermittent	Effects of drugs[a]
Relieving and exacerbating factors	Reduced laryngeal secretions and mucosal drying, e.g. anticholinergics, diuretics
Voice requirement in terms of	Irritant, e.g. bronchial inhalers
Fine precision and control	Androgenic, e.g. danazol
Voice projection	Predisposition to infection, e.g. *Candidosis* from steroid inhalers
Continuous periods of use	Predisposition to gastro-oesophageal reflux
Social history, hobbies and lifestyle factors	Central nervous system, e.g. Parkinsonism secondary to antipsychotics
Smoking and alcohol consumption	
Dietary habits	
Caffeine and fluid intake	

[a]For frequently prescribed medications and effects on voice and speech, see http://www.ncvs.org/ncvs/info/vocol/rx.html.

Table 7.1.4 Treatment options for patients with voice problems

Reassurance/education	Medical treatment
Vocal hygiene, lifestyle and dietary advice	Antibiotics are rarely effective
Stop smoking	Antifungal medication if *Candidosis* is suspected
Cut out excessive alcohol	Antireflux medication
Limit caffeine intake	Proton pump inhibitor
Drink 1.5–2 l of water/day	0.5 h before breakfast and evening meal
Reduce intake of fatty foods	For a minimum of 2 months
Avoid eating within 3 h of going to bed	Alginates after meals and at night
Avoid irritants, e.g. dust, chemicals	Botulinum toxin injection for spasmodic dysphonia
Ensure the atmosphere is moist	Surgery
Use steam inhalations	Phonosurgery/microlaryngoscopy
Avoid throat clearing	Diagnostic
Avoid damaging voice use	Biopsy
Screaming/yelling	Glottoplasty
Talking above background noise for prolonged periods	Medialisation surgery
Voice therapy	Laryngeal framework surgery
Patient education	Thyroplasty
Relaxation techniques to reduce muscle tension	Injection techniques
Improve efficiency of vocal function	Transoral laser resection
Change vocal behaviour	
Counselling	
Laryngeal manual therapy	
Advice on coping strategies	
Advice on amplification aids	
Specialist therapy	
Singing lessons	
Voice craft	

tion and glottic closure. If the vocal fold vibration is disorganised, this will tend to cause a rough voice, whereas if glottic closure is incomplete, the voice may have a more breathy quality. Superficial mucosal lesions are thought to be congenital (sulcus vergeture), secondary to inflammation (cysts, sulcus vocalis, mucosal bridges, granulomas), surgical trauma (intubation granulomas, scarring), or physical trauma, e.g. voice abuse with inflammation (nodules, ectasia, polyps, pseudocysts, Reinke's oedema). Androgens can cause the female larynx to irreversibly enlarge and severe hypothyroidism can cause the vocal folds to become thickened. The anatomical structure of the vocal fold and false cords can become distorted by benign and malignant neoplasms or from deformities of the laryngeal skeleton from external trauma.

The diagnosis is usually made with videolaryngostroboscopy or occasionally on diagnostic microlaryngosco-py. In some cases adequate improvement in vocal function may be achieved with vocal hygiene and lifestyle advice, voice therapy and treatment of inflammation. However, surgical resection is often required and a microlaryngoscopy and biopsy should always be performed where malignancy is a possibility.

7.1.6   Inflammatory Conditions

Inflammation of the larynx can be broadly classified into infective and non-infective causes (Table 7.1.6). In acute infective cases, the laryngitis may be part of an upper respiratory tract infection or occasionally secondary to rhinosinusitis or a lower respiratory tract infection. Fungal infections from *Candida albicans* can result from

Table 7.1.5 Structural or neoplastic conditions

Benign	Inflammatory mass
Mucosal deposits/thickenings	Papillomatosis
Nodules	Granuloma
Polypoid nodules	Arytenoid
Reinke's oedema	Pyogenic
Pseudocyst	Rheumatoid deposits
Deficits/tethering	Amyloid
Cysts	Laryngeal framework trauma
Epidermoid	Neoplasms
Mucus retention	Laryngoceles
Sulcus vocalis	Mixed/reactive
Sulcus vergeture	Malignant/premalignant
Mucosal bridge	Epithelial
Scarring	Hyperkeratosis
Microvascular lesions	Dysplasia
Ectasia	Squamous cell carcinoma
Haemorrhagic polyp	Minor salivary gland
Endocrinological	
Hypothyroidism	
Androgenic	

the incorrect use of steroid inhalers or in cases of immunosuppression. Other causes of hoarseness in asthmatics have been attributed to drying or irritant effects of some inhalers, muscle tension imbalance and laryngopharyngeal reflux.

Laryngitis can also be due to a variety of other non-infective causes, of which laryngopharyngeal reflux is thought to be one of the commonest causes. Laryngopharyngeal reflux is more likely if the hoarseness is worse in the morning and when it is associated with other symptoms, such as chronic cough, phlegm in the throat, throat clearing, globus sensation and difficulty swallowing liquids and tablets. The diagnosis of laryngopharyngeal reflux is usually made on the basis of the history, laryngeal findings, exclusion of other causes and response to a therapeutic trial of antireflux medication (Table 7.1.6). The absence of heartburn does not exclude laryngopharyngeal reflux as a cause.

Simple physical trauma due to increased friction between poorly lubricated vocal folds from prolonged shouting, inadequate fluid intake, dehydrating agents or exposure to irritants such as smoke and chemicals can also cause laryngitis. Laryngitis may also cause huskiness, reduced pitch, loss of part of the range of the voice, pitch instability, an increased effort to speak, vocal fatigue and pain or discomfort on speaking.

'Laryngitis' is term used to describe anything from a few prominent vessels on the vocal folds to gross oedema, erythema, ulceration or leucoplakia of the whole laryngopharyngeal mucosa. Stroboscopy is useful in determining the presence and degree of stiffness of the mucosa of the vocal fold on vibration. Localised stiffness may indicate a structural abnormality such as an intracordal cyst or sulcus. A generalised absence of a mucosal wave is highly suspicious of an infiltrative process including carcinoma and tuberculosis.

Infective cases may settle spontaneously or require appropriate antibacterial (e.g. broad-spectrum antibiotics) or antifungal treatment (e.g. 14-day treatment with amphotericin lozenges 100 mg every day, nystatin suspension 1 ml every day or fluconazole 50 mg once daily). Many cases of non-infective laryngitis can be treated with appropriate advice about voice use or voice rest, lifestyle and diet (Table 7.1.4). In non-responsive cases or where there is impairment of the mucosal wave, a diagnostic microlaryngoscopy including biopsy or incision and exploration of Reinke's space (cordotomy) may be required.

7.1.7 Neuromuscular Conditions

Neuromuscular conditions (Table 7.1.7) arise when any part of the neural pathway or function of the vocal muscles is impaired.

True hypofunctional conditions occur when there is global reduction in vocal muscular activity. The voice is generally weak, the pitch range reduced and the voice tires with use. Examples include Parkinson's disease, myasthenia gravis and bulbar palsy. Hyperfunction of vocal muscles associated with speech tasks is seen in spasmodic dysphonia, which is a focal dystonia and gives a staccato quality to the voice. Hyperfunction is also seen in pseudobulbar palsies, chorea and spastic dysphonia secondary to cerebrovascular accidents.

Voice problems may be the first signs of a more generalised neuromuscular disorder such as Parkinson's disease, motor neurone disease, multiple sclerosis and myasthenia gravis. Neuromuscular disorders should always be considered in cases where the vocal folds look normal but the pattern does not fit with a muscle tension dysphonia, fails to respond to voice therapy or there is progressive worsening of the dysphonia.

The voice in more general neurological conditions, e.g. Parkinson's disease and myasthenia gravis, may be improved with systemic treatment for those conditions. Spasmodic and spastic dysphonia can often be relieved by intralaryngeal injections of botulinum toxin for up to 3 months. Unilateral palsies and paresis may respond to voice therapy, although they often require a surgical procedure to medialise the vocal cord. This can be achieved either by injecting a material such as autologous fat or a polymethylsiloxane elastomer into the vocal cord or by placing a shim through a window in the thyroid cartilage (thyroplasty).

The commonest neuromuscular conditions, however, are unilateral vocal cord palsies or paresis affecting the recurrent laryngeal, superior laryngeal or vagus nerves. It is important to investigate the cause of the palsy and in particular exclude bronchial, oesophageal and thyroid carcinomas, which account for nearly a third of cases. Surgical

Table 7.1.6 Inflammatory causes

Infective	Non-infective
Primary—laryngeal	Laryngopharyngeal reflux
Viral	Allergy
Bacterial (including tuberculosis)	Trauma/irritation
Fungal, e.g. *Candida albicans*	Physical, e.g. phonotrauma
Secondary	Fumes/chemical
Pulmonary infections	Smoke
Rhinosinusitis	Laryngeal dehydration
	Drugs
	Direct irritant, e.g. asthma inhalers
	Indirect dry, e.g. antimuscarinics
	Autoimmune, e.g. Sjogren's syndrome
	Non-specific

Table 7.1.7 Neuromuscular conditions

Hypofunctional	Mixed or variable hypo/hyperfunctional
Parkinson's disease	Vocal cord palsy/paresis
Myasthenia gravis	Motor neurone disease
Bulbar palsy	Multiple sclerosis
Hyperfunctional	Control/coordination
Spasmodic dysphonia	Tremor
Pseudobulbar/spastic dysphonia	Myoclonus
Chorea	Cerebellar lesions

trauma following thyroidectomy, oesophageal, thoracic and cervical spine procedures accounts for almost another third. A viral neuropathy is thought to account for many 'idiopathic cases' where no specific cause is identified. Patients with a palsy or paresis will often complain of weak voice, effortful phonation, throat discomfort or vocal fatigue as the vocal folds fail to meet and vibrate effectively. The voice may sound breathy, unstable or high pitched, and the patient may complain of choking episodes (particularly with liquids) as a consequence of glottic incompetence. Laryngeal examination will reveal that the vocal cord is immobile on the affected side with compensatory overactivity on the functioning side. In cases of paresis, there may only be a subtle asymmetry of abduction and adduction. This asymmetry may only be apparent after repetitive vocalisation and by observing that the affected side 'lags behind' the normal side. Stroboscopy may reveal an asymmetry of the phase and amplitude of the mucosal wave and apparent bowing on the affected side.

7.1.8 Muscle Tension Imbalance Conditions

Primary muscle tension imbalance is when there is inefficient use of the vocal apparatus causing either episodic dysphonia or aphonia (Table 7.1.8). This may manifest itself as an imbalance either between specific synergists and antagonists or between one side of the larynx and the other or as a global increase in tension of the intrinsic and extrinsic laryngeal muscles. Primary muscle tension imbalance may result from increased demands on the voice or producing the voice with a poor technique. Ineffective vocal fold vibration can result from poor posture and breathing patterns, too much inappropriate muscular effort or failure of relaxation of the laryngeal muscles.

Muscle tension imbalance is also not infrequently due to psychological conditions such as anxiety, stress and depression or true conversion disorders. Symptoms can include inappropriate voice pitch for age and sex, bizarre, whispery or strained voice qualities, limitations of pitch range, effortful phonation, voice fatigue and vocal tract discomfort. Primary muscle tension imbalance can also lead to structural abnormalities such as vocal fold nodules. Conversely, in secondary muscle tension imbalance more muscular effort is required to overcome a structural, inflammatory or neuromuscular disorder and reducing this effort often makes the dysphonia worse.

The diagnosis of muscle tension imbalance is usually based on the history, by listening to the way in which the history is recounted, the laryngeal appearance and the response to vocal therapy exercises. Often the voice quality is variable and out of proportion to the laryngeal findings. The larynx may look relatively normal but there may be evidence of dynamic glottic and supraglottic constriction or splinting of the vocal folds apart with no airflow.

Treatment of primary muscle tension imbalance (Table 7.1.4) is with reassurance, vocal hygiene advice, voice therapy, specialist therapy, osteopathy and occasionally counselling.

7.1.9 Conclusion

Voice problems are multifactorial in origin. Although a detailed history may point to the diagnosis, in many cases it is impossible to exclude malignancy and other physical abnormalities without a laryngeal examination. In primary care, the risk of malignancy needs to be carefully assessed and an urgent referral made if it is a possibility. In other cases, with an obvious primary cause, simple lifestyle, vocal hygiene and dietary advice or a therapeutic medical trial is worth considering (Table 7.1.4). All other cases need referral for laryngeal examination. In terms of treatment, some patients may just require reassurance and simple advice. Those who are more symptomatic and want help require a more comprehensive assessment with laryngostroboscopy. Close multiprofessional team working is essential for effective and efficient patient management. Regional access to more specialised investigations and treatment should also be available.

Table 7.1.8 Muscle tension imbalance

Primary	Secondary
Vocal demands/strain	Inflammation (including postinfection problems)
Occupational	Structural/neoplastic (including end-stage hyperfunction)
Inadequate vocal skills	Neuromuscular
Psychogenic	Breathing disorders
Anxiety/'stress'	Postural abnormalities
Conversion dysphonia/aphonia	Congenital laryngeal anatomical abnormalities
Puberphonia/mutational voice disorder	Presbylaryngis

Suggested Reading

1. Carding P (2003) Voice pathology in the United Kingdom. Br Med J 327:514–515
2. Jecker P, Orloff LA, Mann WJ (2005) Extraoesophageal reflux and upper respiratory tract diseases. ORL J Otorhinolaryngol Relat Spec 67:185–191
3. MacKenzie K, Millar A, Wilson JA, Sellars C, Deary IJ (2001) Is voice therapy an effective treatment for dysphonia? A randomised controlled trial. Br Med J 323:658–661
4. National Centre for Voice and Speech (1999) Frequently prescribed medications and effects on voice and speech. http://www.ncvs.org/ncvs/info/vovol/rx.html
5. Vaghela HM, Fergie N, Slade S, McGlashan JA (2005) Speech therapist led voice clinic: Which patients may be suitable? Logopedics Phoniatrics Vocology 30(2):85–89
6. World Health Organisation (1998) Towards a common language for functioning and disablement. Report ICIDH-2. World Health Organisation, Geneva

7.2 Voice Evaluation and Respiratory Function Assessment

PHILIPPE H. DEJONCKERE

7.2.1 Introduction

The voice laboratory can be considered an essential tool for the assessment and treatment evaluation of voice patients and for clinical research on voice disorders. Whereas the medical examination focuses on the primary aetiologic diagnosis (cancer, infection, neurologic disease, reflux, and so forth), the voice laboratory provides a functional diagnosis and offers multidimensional information concerning the characteristics, limitations, and possibilities for change of disturbed voice production.

Several specific questions may be answered from the information obtained in the voice laboratory:

- Is a given voice or voice function measurement to be considered as normal (within normal limits) or pathologic?
- If the voice or voice function is to be considered pathologic, how severe is the alteration?
- Which aspects or mechanisms of voice production are concerned with the voice disorder? How does the primary (medical) cause or lesion explain the components of voice production which are perceived or analysed as deviant (e.g. by limiting vocal fold closure or by eliciting irregular vibrations related to vocal fold asymmetry), and how does it account for the patient's complaints (e.g. voice fatigue or compensation mechanisms)?
- What is the result of a comparison of voice production at two or more times (e.g. before and after therapy), or in two or several situations or voicing conditions (spontaneously vs. louder, or when doing an Isshiki manoeuvre, or when applying a defined therapeutic technique)? Have the changes returned the voice to normal function as indicated by voice measurement?

These questions are relevant in daily clinical practice, because they make the dialogue between clinician and patient less abstract and more reality-based. They are also essential for research purposes (comparing outcomes of treatments) and, when necessary, to support medical decisions in legal proceedings. The clinician's and the patient's expectation is that the voice laboratory provides objective documentation of the condition of the voice. This concept of objective documentation is of major importance, although limitations remain with regard to standardization of procedures and normative values among laboratories.

Attempts to reach more uniformity and standardization in basic methods for functional assessment of pathologic voices continue to be a major issue among voice scientists. The purpose of laboratory standardization is to allow relevant comparisons when communicating the results of voice treatment (e.g. a phonosurgical technique) or when presenting a new or improved instrument or procedure for investigating the pathologic voice (e.g. a new algorithm for noise computation or for periodicity perturbation). The need for standardization has been illustrated in a study comparing vocal fold augmentation with medialization laryngoplasty to treat unilateral vocal fold paralysis. Although an abundant literature is available on this topic, an adequate meta-analysis is limited by the great diversity in assessing functional outcomes.

7.2.2 A Prerequisite: Recording a Voice Sample

Audio recording is the most important basic requisite for voice quality assessment. Once a high-quality recording has been performed, it can be stored and remains available—as a document—for performing at a later time additional investigations, such as blind perceptual evaluation by a panel or sophisticated acoustic analyses. It is essential that all recordings of voice patients are filed as an archive, where it is easy to retrieve an earlier voice sample. A digital recording system should be used to store signals, unless analogue-to-digital conversion and storage is directly performed by the computer. All commercially available computer systems for acoustic voice analysis record directly and store the voice samples. A sampling frequency of at least 20,000 Hz is recommended. The recordings should be made ideally in a sound-treated room, but a quiet room, with ambient noise permanently less 50 dB, is acceptable. The mouth-to-microphone distance needs to be held constant at 10 cm. A (miniature) head-mounted microphone offers a clear advantage, but a harmonica holder is also effective. Off-axis positioning (45–90° from the mouth axis) reduces aerodynamic noise from the mouth in speech.

An example of a protocol for standard recording is:

- /a:/ at (spontaneous) comfortable pitch/loudness, recorded three times to evaluate variability of quality.
- /a:/ slightly louder, to evaluate the possible change in quality (plasticity) and the slope of the regression line of frequency against sound pressure level.
- A single sentence or a short standard passage.

Phonetic selection can be useful, e.g., a short sentence with:

- Constant voicing (no voiceless sounds and to be spoken without interruption)
- No fricatives

A sentence such as "We mow our lawn all year" can be analysed by the computer program for sustained vowels, and as it contains no articulation noise, there is no biasing of harmonics-to-noise computations. Computation of percentage voiceless (normal in this case is 100%) is useful for neurologic voices or spasmodic dysphonia. Further, it allows easy determination of the mean habitual fundamental speaking frequency.

Another example of a criterion for phonetic selection could be a multiplication of voice onsets, as they are critical in disturbed voices. Such criteria are not language-linked.

A standard reading passage should also be recorded, whenever possible. Two classic and often used reading passages for English-speaking persons are "The Rainbow Passage" (a phonetically selected passage including all the speech sounds of English) and "Marvin Williams" (an all-voiced passage).

7.2.3 Perception

Existing research does not support the substitution of instrumental measures for auditory-perceptual assessment. To be valuable, however, perceptual assessment should follow a standard procedure, as does the voice recording. A currently used scale for making perceptual judgements is the GRBAS scale, which rates grade, roughness, breathiness, asthenicity, and strain on a 0–3 scale. The rating is made on current conversational speech or a reading passage. The severity of hoarseness is quantified under the parameter G (grade relates to the overall voice quality, integrating all deviant components). Two main components of hoarseness may be identified, as shown by principal component analysis:

1. Breathiness (B): an auditive impression of turbulent air leakage through an insufficient glottic closure, including short aphonic moments (unvoiced segments).
2. Roughness or harshness (R): an impression of irregular glottic pulses, of abnormal fluctuations in fundamental frequency, of separately perceived acoustic impulses (as in vocal fry), including diplophonia and register breaks. When present, diplophonia can also be noted as "d."

These parameters have shown sufficient reliability (inter- and intrarater reproducibility). A reliability analysis by Webb et al. provided further evidence to support the GRBAS scale as a simple reliable measure for clinical use. The behavioural parameters asthenicity (A) and strain (S) appear to be less reliable. The remaining simplified scale, GRB, then becomes similar to the RBH scale (*Rauhigkeit* for "roughness", *Behauchtheit* for "breathiness", and *Heiserkeit* for "hoarseness"), used in German-speaking countries.

For reporting purposes, a four-point grading scale is convenient (0 for normal or absence of deviance; 1 for slight deviance; 2 for moderate deviance; 3 for severe deviance), but it is also possible to score on a visual analogue scale of 10 cm, possibly with anchoring points.

It is proposed to use the term "dysphonia" for any kind of perceived voice disorder: the deviation may concern pitch or loudness, as well as timbre or rhythmic and prosodic features. "Hoarseness" is limited to deviant voice "quality" (or timbre), and excludes pitch, loudness, and rhythm factors. A limited number of voice disorder categories, such as those related to mutation or transsexuality, are specifically concerned with pitch and register. Rhinophonia is a specific abnormality of resonance and needs to be reported separately, if present. Tremor is a characteristic temporal feature, and must also be reported separately, whenever it is present. A special protocol is required for substitution voices: it includes the criteria "intelligibility", "voicing" and "fluency", which are usually less relevant for common dysphonias.

Perceptual evaluation—if averaged among several blinded raters—is very well suited to demonstrate treatment efficacy in voice pathology.

7.2.4 Vocal Fold Imaging

7.2.4.1 Videolaryngostroboscopy

Videolaryngostroboscopy is the main clinical tool for diagnosing the cause of voice disorders, but it can also be used to assess the quality of vocal fold vibration and thus evaluate the effectiveness of a treatment. Figure 7.2.1 shows nine steps of a schematic vibration pattern, as observed in a male modal register. The laryngoscopic view (Fig. 7.2.1, *right*) is correlated with a frontal section at the midpart of the glottis (Fig. 7.2.1, *left*). Stroboscopy involves a video-perceptual series of judgements and ratings (e.g. glottic closure, regularity, symmetry, mucosal wave).

The pertinence of stroboscopic parameters is based on a combination of reliability (inter- and intraobserver reproducibility), nonredundancy (from the factor analysis), and clinical sense (relation to physiologic concepts).

The basic parameters are:

1. Glottal closure: Quantitative rating using a four-point grading scale, or a visual analogue scale of 10 cm (see earlier). It is recommended the type of insufficient closure also be recorded and categorized.
   - Longitudinal: Over the whole length of the glottis and without sufficient adduction.
   - Dorsal (posterior triangular chink): It is however important to consider that a slight dorsal insufficiency—even reaching into the membranous portion of the glottis—occurs in about 60% of middle-aged healthy women during normal voice effort. Fifty percent of the women close the glottis completely during loud voice.
   - Ventral.
   - Irregular.
   - Oval: Over the whole length of the glottis, but with a dorsal closure.
   - Hourglass-shaped.

   Rating of glottal closure has been found very reliable. Objective quantitative measurements are also possible.

2. Regularity: Quantitative rating of the degree of irregular slow motion, as perceived with stroboscopy.

3. Mucosal wave: Quantitative rating of the quality of the wavelike movement of the vocal fold cover (epithelium and superficial lamina propria) over the vocal fold body (ligament and muscle), accounting for the physiologic function of the layered structure of the vocal folds.

4. Symmetry: Quantitative rating of the "mirror" motion of both vocal folds. Usually asymmetry is caused by the limited vibratory quality of a lesion (e.g. diffuse scar, or localized cyst or leucoplakia).

For each stroboscopic parameter, a four-point grading scale (0 is no deviance; 3 is severe deviance), or a visual analogue scale can be used.

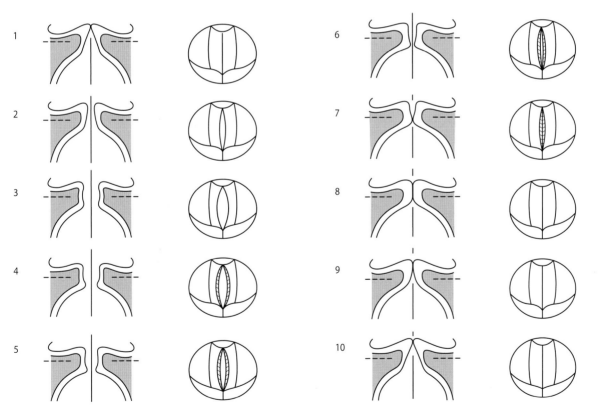

Fig. 7.2.1 Nine steps of a schematic vibration pattern, as observed in a male modal register. The laryngoscopic view (*right*) is correlated with a frontal section at the midpart of the glottis (*left*). Steps 5–7 demonstrate the aspect of the mucosal wave

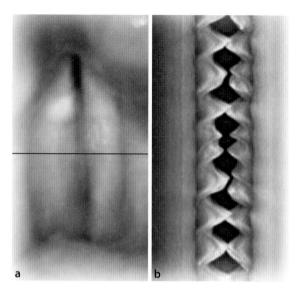

Fig. 7.2.2a,b Videokymography (single line camera scan). **a** The traditional laryngoscopic image during phonation: with normal (not stroboscopic) light, the glottis appears unsharp, owing to vibration of the vocal fold edges. With a kymograph camera, a single horizontal line can be selected and monitored at high speed (approximately 8,000 per second). The displayed image (**b**) is composed by putting the successive high-speed line images below each other, demonstrating the vibration of the selected level of the vocal folds over time

Videostroboscopy can be documented on a hard copy, and can thus be archived. Rating "a posteriori" is possible.

It is classically recommended to observe and record videostroboscopic pictures in different voicing conditions. For example, the degree of glottal closure usually increases with raised loudness. However, this basic rating concerns the comfortable pitch and loudness.

For comparisons (pretreatment/posttreatment), it is recommended to use the same kind of endoscope (rigid or flexible; if rigid with the same angle). Laryngostroboscopic ratings and measurements have been found to be relevant for documenting therapeutic effects.

7.2.4.2 Digital High-Speed Pictures

With modern technology, it has become possible to capture and store digital vocal fold images at a rate of 2,000 (and more) per second with sufficient definition (several hundred pixels) and to display the image sequence at a rate of, e. g., 20 per second, immediately after capture. This procedure does not seem to be appropriate for routine use in the diagnosis of voice problems, as a long review time is needed for a short sequence, further without simultaneous sound. A specific indication for digital high-speed

photography is the analysing and understanding of the vibratory characteristics in aperiodic voices, during voice onsets, accidents (breaks), or in the case of diplophonia or triplophonia.

7.2.4.3 High-Speed Single-Line Scanning

High-speed single-line scanning (videokymography) is an imaging technique for investigating vocal fold vibration, especially when the vibration is irregular and when the focus is on accidents or short events in this vibration so that conventional stroboscopy is unsuitable. A modified video camera selects a single horizontal line from the whole image and monitors it at high speed (8,000 per second). The displayed image is composed by putting the successive high-speed line images below each other, demonstrating the vibration of the selected ventrodorsal level of the vocal folds over time. This type of (multiline) display provides relevant information for comparing the vibration amplitude/mucosal wave of both folds and for understanding diplophonia, as well as for analysing vibratory irregulations (http://www.kymography.com/) (Fig. 7.2.2).

7.2.5 Aerodynamics

Aerodynamic analysis of voice production includes measurement of airflow, air pressure, and their relationships during phonation. Using appropriate instrumentation, a number of derived measurements can provide information regarding vocal efficiency. For certain measurements, only a stopwatch is needed.

7.2.5.1 Phonation Airflow

The simplest aerodynamic parameter of voicing is the maximum phonation time (MPT) in seconds. It consists of the prolongation of a /a:/, for as long as possible after maximal inspiration, and at spontaneous, comfortable pitch and loudness. It is one of the most widely used clinical measures in voice assessment worldwide. A prior demonstration is necessary, and three trials are required, the longest being selected for comparison to the norm. As it concerns an "extreme" performance, it has been shown to be very sensitive to learning and fatigue effects. Further, in good voices, the duration of "apnoea" can become the limiting factor, rather than the available air. Children show significant lower values of MPT, as their lung volume is smaller. A reduction of possible bias, e. g. supportive respiratory capabilities compensating for poor membranous vocal fold closure, is possible by computing the equation

Averaged phonation airflow or PQ = vital capacity (ml)/MPT (s), where PQ is the phonation quotient.

Vital capacity (VC) is defined as the volume change at the mouth between the position of full inspiration and complete expiration. It can be measured in a reliable way by using a hand-held spirometer. VC depends, in normal subjects, on anthropometric factors, and is, e.g., quite strongly correlated with height. It is also sensitive to lung disease, especially for patients with carcinoma. As VC is not directly related to voice quality, it is meaningful to take it into account, certainly if children are investigated.

The mean airflow rate can also be measured by using a pneumotachograph. This device provides a direct measurement of the mean airflow rate (ml/s) for sustained phonation over a comfortable duration, usually 2–3 s, at the habitual pitch and intensity level, and following habitual inspiration. A pneumotachograph consists of a hand-held mouth tube (possibly connected to a mask) within which is placed a fine mesh wire screen to create a (small) resistance to airflow. This resistance results in a pressure difference across the screen that can be measured with a differential pressure transducer: the pressure difference increases with the flow.

Pathophysiologic backgrounds and normative values have been reported by Hirano, Verdolini, Colton and Casper and Woo et al.

The variation of averaged phonation air flow considerably varies among normal subjects, and there is a large overlapping range of values in normal and dysphonic subjects. This limits the value for diagnostic purposes. Nevertheless, when comparing glottal function before and after surgical intervention or nonsurgical voice training techniques, airflow measurement may be useful in monitoring therapeutic effects, e.g. in the case of paralytic dysphonia, or when microlaryngeal phonosurgery is performed. The method is especially useful for demonstrating changes in a single test subject over time.

For comparisons (pretreatment/posttreatment), it is recommended to use the same kind of technique (PQ or mean airflow rate measured by pneumotachography).

Flow glottography consists of an inverse filtering of the oral airflow waveform. The basic tool is a high-frequency pressure transducer incorporated within an airtight Rothenberg mask. The inverse filtering procedure removes the resonant effects of the vocal tract and produces an estimate of the waveform produced at the vocal folds. The special advantage of this technique is that it differentiates and, after calibration, quantifies the leakage airflow (the DC component of the airflow) and the pulsated (AC) airflow. Leakage airflow is an important concept: it assumes that there is an opening somewhere along the total length of the vocal folds through which air escapes. Calibration is critical for reliable measurements. Flow glottography can also be used to analyse the voice onset.

7.2.5.2 Subglottal Air Pressure

Measurements of subglottal air pressure made using oesophageal balloons or pressure transducers, transglottal catheters, or tracheal puncture are semiinvasive or invasive and limited to research situations. An accurate estimation of subglottal pressure can be obtained by measuring the intraoral air pressure produced during the repeated pronunciation of /pVp/ syllables (that is, a vowel between two plosive consonants). A thin catheter is introduced in the mouth through the labial commissure, sealed by the lips, and not occluded by the tongue. If there is no closure of the vocal folds, the intraoral air pressure should be similar to the pressure elsewhere in the respiratory tract. During the production of a voiceless consonant, the vocal folds are abducted and should not impose any significant obstruction to the airflow from the lungs. Thus, the pressure behind the lips is the same everywhere and reflects the pressure available to drive the vocal folds if they were to vibrate. This technique also allows measurement of the phonation threshold pressure, the minimum pressure required to initiate phonation. Pressure is usually reported in pascals: 1 Pa is equal to $1 N/m^2$; 1 kPa is equivalent to 10 cm of H_2O.

7.2.5.3 Efficiency of Phonation

Together with airflow and vocal intensity, subglottal air pressure can be used to estimate the efficiency of phonation. Obviously, reduced efficiency is expected to induce voice fatigue. Vocal efficiency is defined as the ratio of the acoustic power to the aerodynamic power and can be estimated by dividing the acoustic intensity of the utterance by the product of the air pressure and the airflow used to produce the utterance.

7.2.5.4 Flow–Volume Loops

The spirometer is important for investigating cases in which voice problems are associated with laryngeal obstruction, as in bilateral abduction paralysis, stenosis caused by extensive webs and scars, cancer, or even severe Reinke's oedema. The flow–volume loop is generated when measurements of a maximum forced expiration and a maximum forced inspiration are plotted on a graph with flow rates on the ordinate and lung volume on the abscissa (Fig. 7.2.3). Lack of effort is easy to detect, because there is reduced flow at the beginning of the expiratory curve and the inspiratory curve is abnormal (Fig. 7.2.3b). Obstructing lesions of the larynx are easily detected and quantified because the morphology of the flow–volume loop is altered: variable extrathoracic obstruction (as in bilateral vocal fold paralysis) manifests itself as a decrease in inspiratory flow only (Fig. 7.2.3c), while a fixed obstruction of the upper airway, as in the case of extensive laryngeal cancer, is objectivated and quantified by a symmetric reduction of inspiratory and expiratory flow (Fig. 7.2.3d).

7.2.6 Acoustics

Acoustic measures provide in an objective and noninvasive way a lot of information about vocal function. Increasingly, these measures have become available at affordable cost, and appear to have succeeded very well in monitoring changes in voice quality over time, e.g. before and after treatment. Acoustic measures reflect the status of vocal function and do not relate specifically to various voice disorders, because basic biomechanical changes resulting in acoustic features can be induced by various types of lesions or dysfunctions.

7.2.6.1 Visible Speech

Acoustic analysis can firstly be used to make the voice and speech visible, e.g. in spectrograms (Fig. 7.2.4). This visual representation may be a considerable aid to the perception and description of the voice characteristics. Spectrograms are also useful for comparing normal phonation with phonation characterized by excessive noise. Commercially available software packages provide synchronized displays of the microphone signal and the spectrogram, showing the frequency distribution of acoustic energy over time. A choice can be made between narrowband filtering (frequency resolution, mainly demonstrating fundamental frequency, harmonics, interharmonic and high-frequency noise, subharmonics) and broadband filtering (temporal resolution, mainly demonstrating periodicity, but also formant location). The addition of visible speech to the perceptual evaluation of pathologic voices is an interesting clinical asset to significantly

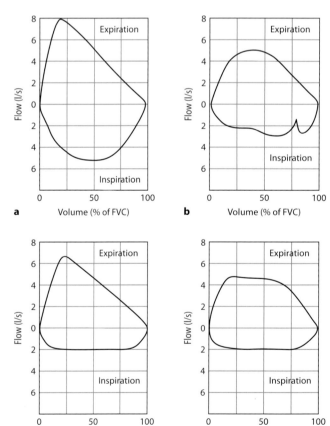

Fig. 7.2.3a–d Flow–volume curves: measurements of a maximum forced expiration and a maximum forced inspiration are plotted with flow rates on the ordinate and lung volume on the abscissa. In normal respiration (**a**), the expiratory flow curve decays linearly. When effort is poor, the initial slope of part of the expiratory curve decreases (**b**); the inspiratory curve is also abnormal. A variable extrathoracic obstruction (**c**) decreases only the inspiratory flow rate. In the case of fixed obstruction of the upper airway (**d**), inspiratory and expiratory flow rates are both reduced

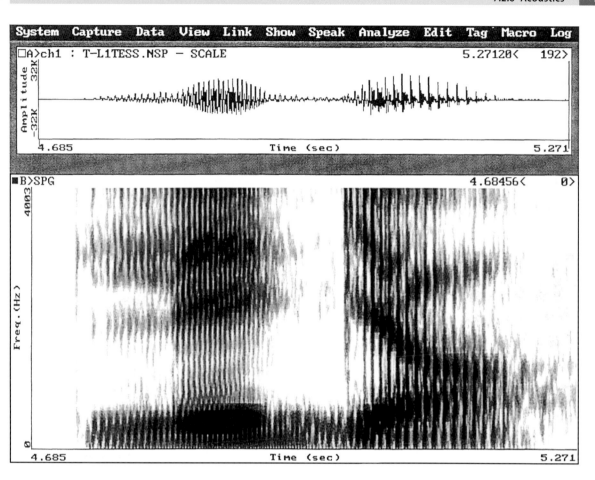

Fig. 7.2.4 Visible speech or sonography, as displayed by the Computerized Speech Lab (Kay Elemetrics, Lincoln Park, NJ, USA). Microphone signal (*top*). Frequency display (0–4,000 Hz) over time (about 0.6 s) (broadband filtering with time resolu-tion). This kind of display provides qualitative information about noise components, regularity of glottal pulses, fundamen-tal frequency shifts, subharmonics, voice onsets, formant loca-tion and formant shifts

enhance reliability. Affordable computer software is cur-rently available that provides the spectogram in quasi real time while the physician is conversing with the patient. Voice characteristics such as sound pressure level, funda-mental frequency, and formant central frequency can also be displayed over time for analysis of singing voice. Fast Fourier transform graphics can also be visualized in quasi real time, as long-time average spectra.

7.2.6.2 Acoustic Parameters

Acoustic analysis can also provide precise numerical values for many voice parameters, from averaged funda-mental frequency to sophisticated calculations for noise components or tremor features.

Factor analysis allows the large number of acoustic pa-rameters to be reduced to a limited number of clusters:

1. Short-term fundamental frequency perturbation
2. Short- or medium-term amplitude perturbation and voiceless segments
3. Harmonics-to-noise ratio
4. Long-term frequency and amplitude modulation
5. Very long term amplitude variation
6. Subharmonics
7. Tremor

Perturbation measures (in period and amplitude) as well as the harmonics-to-noise computations on a sustained vowel (/a:/) at comfortable frequency and intensity ap-pear as the most robust measures, and seem to determine the basic perceptual elements of voice quality: grade,

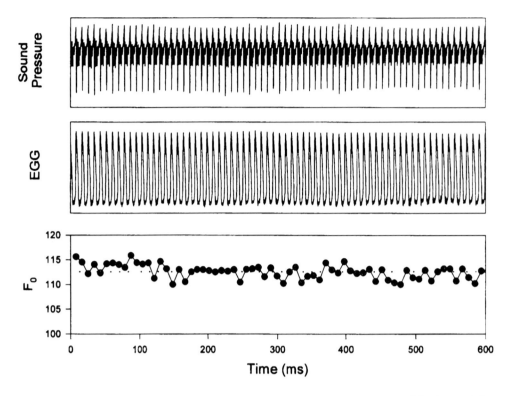

Fig. 7.2.5 Normal male voice, sustained /a:/: microphone signal, electroglottogram, and fundamental frequency plot with time. Normal voice is characterized by slight (less than 1%) random variation of the fundamental frequency. In most cases of disorder, this aperiodicity (jitter) increases

roughness, and breathiness. Nevertheless, correlations with perceptual data remain usually moderate. Jitter is computed as the mean difference between the periods of adjacent cycles divided by the mean period; it is thus a fundamental frequency related measurement (Fig. 7.2.5). For shimmer, a similar computation is made on peak-to-peak amplitudes. Voice breaks must always be excluded. For pathologic voices, the coefficients of variation of jitter and shimmer for a sustained /a/ are on the order of 20–30% for successive single trials as well as trials on different days. A general limitation is the systems employed for acoustic analysis cannot (or not in a reliable way) analyse strongly aperiodical acoustic signals. Perturbation measures of less than about 5% have been found to be reliable. Only "quasi-periodic" voices are suited for perturbation analysis. Therefore, visual control of the period definition on the microphone signal is always necessary: even in regular voices, a strong harmonic or subharmonic may account for erratic values. Alternatives from the field of nonlinear dynamics, such as the Lyapunov coefficient, have been proposed for analysing "chaotic" or "bifurcated" signals. Also for substitution voices, special acoustic approaches of frequency perturbation have been proposed.

Acoustic measurements on a sustained /a/ mainly provide information about the mechanics of the voice instrument (its quality as an oscillator: that what phonosurgery can improve), while perception mainly provides information about vocal behaviour (including, e. g., coordination between breath support and laryngeal mechanics, as in onsets and offsets): that what voice therapy can improve. Periodicity analysis of running speech is expected to be more closely related to perception and behaviour: very promising results have been presented by Fourcin and Abberton, who used the electroglottography (EGG) signal (see Sect. 7.2.8) for period detection.

Another approach for quantifying the regularity of vocal vibrations is cepstrum analysis: the cepstrum is the inverse spectrum of the fast Fourier transform. The magnitude of the cepstrum peak reflects the stability of the fundamental frequency (Fo).

For signal-to-noise ratio computations (normalized noise energy, harmonics-to-noise ratio, cepstrum peak, etc.) there is currently insufficient standardization of the optimal algorithm(s), as well as insufficient knowledge of normative values, for widespread clinical use. The harmonics-to-noise ratio was also found to be a less suitable parameter for demonstrating the effects of therapy.

Rhinophonia is a particular resonance characteristic of the voice. It may be present without concomitant articulation disorder. Acoustic nasometry provides objective measurements by (schematically) computing the ratio between nasal and whole (nasal + oral) voice sound pressure levels.

7.2.6.3 Phonetography/Voice Range Profile

The phonetogram plots the dynamic range (dBA) as a function of fundamental frequency range (Hz), documenting the extreme possibilities of voice. These extremes are of importance for professional voice users, especially singers, but they must be interpreted with care because the acoustic energy is related to the spectral distribution. Normative values for children and teachers have been defined by Heylen et al..

Computerized systems make possible real-time measurement and display of fundamental frequency versus sound pressure level and also of quality parameters such as jitter. Jitter results in various colour gradations within the voice area, showing specific altered zones, or register boundaries (Fig. 7.2.6). Such computerized systems can also provide range profiles of current speech, possibly coupled with provocation tests, such as the task of reading at a controlled, louder intensity. These profiles are expected to be relevant for occupational voice users.

The highest and lowest frequencies and the softest intensity (A-weighted measurements at 30 cm) seem most sensitive for changes in voice quality, the latter being related to phonation threshold pressure. The measurement of the lowest frequency allows one to compute the fundamental frequency range. Such a "three-point range profile" can be obtained without completing a (time-consuming) whole voice range profile. However, as these three points represent "extreme" performances, they are, as well as MPT and VC, very sensitive to learning and fatigue effects.

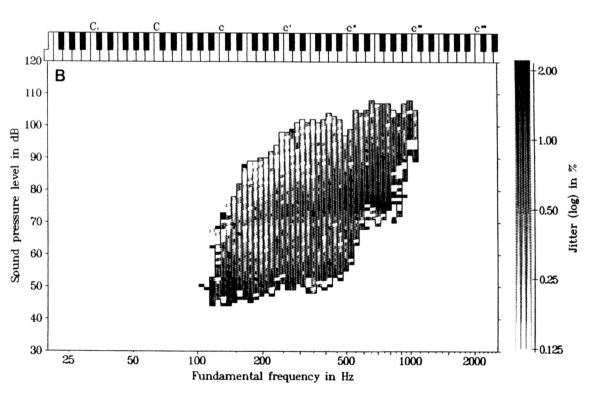

Fig. 7.2.6 Computerized phonetogram (voice range profile), with a grey scale indicating the amount of jitter (normal female voice). The more jitter, the darker the area. The horizontal axis represents the fundamental frequency in hertz (or musical tones on a keyboard) and the vertical axis represents the sound pressure level, measured at 30 cm (dBA). This plot combines information about extreme possibilities of voice as well as on an aspect of voice quality

7.2.7 Subjective Evaluation by the Patient

Although subjective by definition, self-evaluation is of great importance in clinical practice. Careful quantification is needed for self-evaluation to be compared and correlated with the objective assessment provided by the voice laboratory. The purpose of subjective self-evaluation is to determine the deviance of voice quality and the severity of disability or handicap in daily professional and social life and the possible emotional repercussions of the dysphonia.

The basic aim is to differentiate the deviance of voice quality *stricto sensu*, and the severity of disability/handicap in daily social or, if relevant, professional life. A voice handicap index can be computed on the basis of patient's responses to a carefully selected list of questions; it also investigates the possible emotional repercussion of the dysphonia. For patients with substitution voices, a slightly corrected version has been used. However, for the basic protocol, a minimal subjective evaluation can be provided by the patient himself or herself on a double visual analogue scale of 100 mm: the impression about voice quality *stricto sensu*, and the impression about the repercussion of the voice problem on everyday social and, if relevant, professional life and activities. "0" (maximal left) means normal voice on the first scale and no handicap (related to voice) in daily life on the second scale. "100" (maximal right) means extreme voice deviance on the first scale and extreme disability or handicap in daily social (and, when relevant, professional) activities, as rated by the patient himself/herself. A comparative study does not suggest that the exhaustive questionnaire is more reliable than the simple scales. Some criticism is required when comparing different kinds of disorder. The US Voice Handicap Index and the translations into different European languages appear to be equivalent, which means that the results from studies from the various countries included can be compared.

7.2.8 Adjuvant Techniques

7.2.8.1 Electroglottography

Electroglottography (or electrolaryngography) (EGG) is a method for monitoring vocal fold contact, rate of vibration, and perturbation of regularity during voice production (Fig. 7.2.7). The major advantage of EGG is that it does not interfere with the physiologic processes of speaking or singing. The signal originates from two electrodes lightly placed on the speaker's neck at the level of the thyroid cartilage. Pitch extraction from the EGG waveform is particularly reliable—as far as there is at least partial vocal fold contact during the vibration cycle—because

the waveform is unaffected by vocal tract resonances and environment noise.

The main applications of EGG are:

- Fundamental frequency computations (range, regularity, distribution, display across time, cross plots, etc.), as long as there is a vocal fold contact
- Voice onset time
- Pre- and postphonatory laryngeal gestures
- Closed phase information (hyperkinetic vs. hypokinetic adduction)
- Voice range profile of spontaneous speech (falsetto excluded)
- Triggering of a stroboscopic light source

In the case of vocal fold paresis, laryngeal electromyography is a predictor of laryngeal electromyography.

7.2.8.2 Electromyography

Electromyography is an electrophysiologic investigation of neuromuscular function. The main indications are mobility disorders (especially reduced mobility). Neuromuscular pathologic conditions in laryngeal muscles do not basically differ from neuromuscular pathologic conditions in other muscles, so it is recommended that these investigations be performed in cooperation with a general myographist. In a supine patient with the neck extended, the thyroid muscle is approached by insertion of a concentric needle electrode through the cricothyroid ligament The needle electrode is then angled cranially 45° and laterally 20° to an approximate depth of 1.5–2 cm. The cricothyroid muscle is reached by inserting the electrode off the midline close to the inferior border of the thyroid cartilage. Electromyography is also to be used for monitoring botulinum injections in vocal muscles. An evidence-based review has been provided by Sataloff et al.

7.2.9 The Basic Protocol for Functional Assessment of Voice Disorders

The protocol described was recommended by the European Laryngological Society, especially for investigating efficacy of (phonosurgical) treatments and evaluating new assessment techniques.

This proposal is an attempt to reach better agreement and uniformity concerning the basic methods for functional assessment of pathologic voices. The purpose is to allow relevant comparisons with the literature when presenting/publishing the results of any kind of voice treatment, e. g. a phonosurgical technique or a new/improved instrument or procedure for investigating the pathologic voice.

A few basic principles served as guidelines:

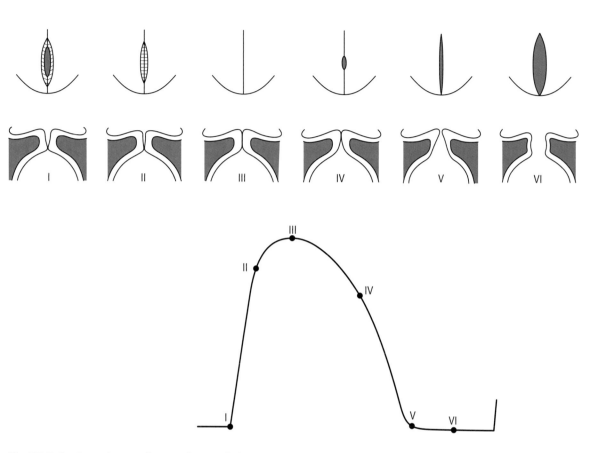

Fig. 7.2.7 An electroglottographic waveform, with the corresponding laryngoscopic view and the frontal section through the mid-portion of the glottis. Point III corresponds to the minimal impedance that is maximal closure of the glottis

1. Voice function is multidimensional.
2. A (minimal) set of basic requirements for presenting (publishing) results of voice treatments is necessary, in order to make comparisons and meta-analyses possible.
3. New and more sophisticated measurement or evaluation techniques and procedures are to be encouraged, but the basic set needs to be performed in all cases, for comparison.
4. The recommendations must be suited for all "common" dysphonias, but a few specific categories of voice disorders need a specific protocol for increasing sensitivity: e.g. substitution voices and spasmodic dysphonia.
5. In the basic set or *truncus communis* for the assessment of common dysphonias, the following components need to be considered. All of them provide quantitative data.
   - Perception
   - Videostroboscopy
   - Acoustics
   - Aerodynamics/efficiency
   - Subjective rating by patient

When substitution voices and spasmodic dysphonias are investigated, elements such as intelligibility and fluency should be added. Further, scales and algorithms should be adjusted for the dimensions "perception", "videostroboscopy" and "acoustics".

6. Each of the above items has its own specific relevance when reporting results or statistics, as it provides a particular insight (multidimensionality). Combined scores or indexes,[1] integrating these or other data into one single value, may be useful, but optimal evaluation and understanding of the treatment effect also requires the intrinsic comparison of the scores for the different components. The first implementation studies pointed

---

1 The Dysphonia Severity Index (DSI), was constructed by logistic regression (Fisher discriminant analysis) and combines the highest fundamental frequency (Fo) (Hz), softest intensity, MPT, and jitter (%), according to the formula DSI = 0.13 × MPT + 0.0053 × highest Fo – 0.26 × lowest intensity – 1.18 × jitter (%) + 12.4. For normal voices the DSI is +5, for severely dysphonic voices it is –5.

out that, for some patients, treatment effects can considerably vary from one dimension to another.

7. In the assessment of treatment outcomes, a maximal objectivity must be constant care. However, even objective data, such as audio recordings or videolaryngostroboscopic pictures, may be subjectively rated and interpreted. Nevertheless, for research purposes, it remains possible to considerably improve the validity by (1) averaging the ratings of a panel and (2) rating blindly, that means without knowing what is, e.g., before and after treatment.

8. Although the present guideline only concerns basic, nonsophisticated approaches, it is not to be considered as the ultimate way to basically assess the voice function. Further implementation studies as well as further research work are necessary, and are warmly encouraged by the Committee on Phoniatrics of the European Laryngological Society.

9. Instrumentation is kept to a minimum, but is considered essential for professionals performing phonosurgery. The ENT surgeon can be assisted in performing this basic set of measurements by a qualified and trained speech therapist.

10. In summary, two of the dimensions are to be considered as objective (as far as the subject is normally cooperating)—aerodynamics and acoustics; two dimensions are objective but rated subjectively by the examiner (however, ratings can be made blindly by a panel!)—recording of a voice sample and videostroboscopy; and one dimension remains totally subjective (self-rating by the patient).

Implementation of this protocol demonstrates the clinical relevance of each item, and the low redundancy. When investigating treatment effects, the correlations between the before and after changes for the different parameters are weak. Multidimensional information about changes induced by therapy help clinicians to achieve a better understanding of the actual way in which a treatment works.

The following is an example of a report for the proposed basic protocol:

- Women, 26, diagnosed with vocal fold nodules, before treatment
- Perception: G34; B52; R18d
- Stroboscopy: Clo 40hs; Reg10; MW25; Sym0
- Aerodynamics: PQ 285 ml/s (MPT 13 s).
- Acoustics: Ji 1.2%; Shi 6.1%; Fo range c–g1; softest intensity 53 dBA 30 cm
- Subjective evaluation: Vo30; Dis50

The explanation is as follows:

- *Perception* is rated on three visual analogue scales of 100 mm: grade, roughness and breathiness. Grade is scored 34/100, etc. 0 always means normality (no de-

viance) and 100 means extremely deviant. Diplophonia is present (d).

- *Stroboscopy* is rated on four visual analogue scales of 100 mm: closure, regularity, quality of mucosal wave, and symmetry. For closure, if abnormal, a categorical choice is also recommended: in this case an hourglass-shaped pattern. Symmetry is normal in this case.
- *Aerodynamics*: PQ (ml/s) and MPT (s). VC here was 3,705 ml.
- Acoustics: Jitter (%) and Shimmer (%) on a sustained /a:/, at comfortable pitch and loudness. c corresponds to 131 Hz and g1 to 392 Hz. As for phonetography, the distance to the microphone needs to be 30 cm.
- *Subjective evaluation* is provided by the patient herself on a double visual analogue scale of 100 mm. The first scale concerns the impression of voice quality *stricto sensu* (e.g. 30/100, slight to moderate), while the second one concerns the impression of the repercussion of the voice problem on everyday social and, if relevant, professional life and activities (e.g. 50/100, moderate to severe).

Suggested Reading

1. Dejonckere PH (2000) Perceptual and laboratory assessment of dysphonia. Otolaryngol Clin North Am 33:731–750
2. Dejonckere PH, Bradley P, Clemente P, Cornut, G, Crevier-Buchmann L, Friedrich G, Van De Heyning P, Remacle M, Woisard V (2001) A basic protocol for functional assessment of voice pathology. Eur Arch Otorhinolaryngol 258:77–82
3. Dejonckere PH, Crevier-Buchman L, Marie JP, Moerman M, Remacle M, Woisard V (2003)
4. Implementation of the European Laryngological Society (ELS) basic protocol for assessing voice treatment effect. Rev Laryngol Otol Rhinol 124:279–283
5. Fourcin A, Abberton E (2008) Hearing and phonetic criteria in voice measurements. Clinical applications. Logoped Phoniatr Vocol 33(1):35–48
6. Sataloff RT, Mandel S, Mann EA, Ludlow CL (2004) Practice parameter: laryngeal electromyography (an evidence-based review). J Voice 18:261–274
7. Speyer R, Wieneke GH, Dejonckere PH (2004) The use of acoustic parameters for the evaluation of voice therapy for dysphonic patients. Acta Acust United Acust 90:520–527
8. Webb AL, Carding PN, Deary IJ, MacKenzie K, Steen N, Wilson JA (2004) The reliability of three perceptual evaluation scales for dysphonia. Eur Arch Otorhinolaryngol 261:429–434
9. Wuyts F, De Bodt M, Molenberghs G, Remacle M, Heylen L, Millet B, Van Lierde K, Raes J, Van de Heyning PH (2000) The Dysphonia Severity Index: an objective measure of quality based on a multiparameter approach. J Speech Lang Hear Res 43:796–809

7.3 Phonosurgery

GERHARD FRIEDRICH

7.3.1 Definition

The term "phonosurgery" refers to any surgery designed primarily for the improvement or restoration of voice. Phonosurgery is therefore not defined by the surgical method but by the intended operative goal. In addition to this narrow definition, the term "phonosurgery" is often also used in a wider sense (Table 7.3.1). Primary phonosurgery means improvement or restoration of voice as the only indication, whereas in secondary phonosurgery the surgical procedures for improvement or restoration of voice are additional, while the indication for surgery is different (e.g. histology, oncologic principles). Owing to the source–filter theory, voice is a result not only of laryngeal sound production but also of resonatory effects of the vocal tract. Hence, phonosurgery could be expanded to surgery of the vocal tract as "phonetic surgery" or "phonetosurgery". The classification and following statements are restricted to primary phonosurgery (Table 7.3.2).

7.3.2 Indication

Phonosurgery differs clearly in its intentions form traditional laryngeal surgery, which is performed because of vital indications. It is therefore necessary to define basic principles for the indication for phonosurgery. One precondition is a sufficient diagnosis and documentation of the disordered voice, which unfortunately is not always done (see Sect. 7.2). As the aetiopathogenesis of voice disorders is multidimensional, phonosurgery is only one part of the complex treatment of voice disorders and must be combined with various non-surgical methods together in a complex/global rehabilitation programme. Indication for phonosurgery must be based on functional points of view, not on morphology. The phonosurgeon must have knowledge of functional orientated investigation of the voice/vocal organ and additional/alternative treatment regimes or must work in close cooperation with someone having this knowledge. Phonosurgical interventions should never simply focus on the appearance of the vocal folds but should aim at improvement of voice adapted to the individual requests and needs of the patient. As phonosurgery is not vitally indicated, counselling and informed consent must rather be orientated to functional surgery than to surgery in, e.g., laryngeal cancer.

7.3.3 Vocal Fold Surgery

7.3.3.1 Definition

Surgical procedures performed directly on the vocal folds with the aim of improving the vibratory movement/restoration of the normal mucosal wave or correction of vocal fold position and/or tension.

7.3.3.2 Approach

Phonosurgery on the vocal folds usually requires magnification. Phonosurgery via the direct endoscopic approach under general anaesthesia can be performed using an operating microscope (phonomicrosurgery) or a telescope connected to a video camera. Phonosurgery via the indirect endoscopic or percutaneous approach under local anaesthesia can be performed either with a flexible

Table 7.3.1 Different types and definitions of phonosurgery

	Primary	Secondary
Phonosurgery (surgery of the larynx)	Phonosurgery (in the restricted sense)	For example excision of leucoplakia, glottic widening in bilateral RNP
"Phonetosurgery/phonetic surgery" (surgery of the vocal tract)	For example velopharyngoplasty	For example adenoidectomy/tonsillectomy in cleft palate

Table 7.3.2 Classification of (primary) phonosurgery

Vocal fold surgery

Laryngeal framework surgery

Neuromuscular surgery

Reconstructive surgery

– Partial defect of the larynx

– Total loss of the larynx

Table 7.3.3 Vocal fold surgery—approaches

Endolaryngeal
   Indirect
   Direct

External
   Open neck
   Percutaneous

transnasal fibrescope or with a transoral telescope, possibly combined with stroboscopy. The endoscopic approach under general anaesthesia is currently preferred by most phonosurgeons for the vast majority of procedures (Tables 7.3.3, 7.3.7, 7.3.8).

7.3.3.3   Procedures

Different methods are used to address the different lesions properly (Table 7.3.4). The basic principle of phonosurgery is to maintain or even improve the functional structure of the vocal fold by respecting its layered structure. This is achieved by means of minimal tissue excision, minimal disruption of the superficial layer of the lamina propria and preserving the epithelium intact, especially at the vibratory margin. This has led the concept of the mi-

Table 7.3.4 Vocal fold surgery—procedures

Incision

Excision

Dissection (microflap)

Augmentation

Injection/implantation

Vaporization

Coagulation

Injection of pharmaceutical agents

Suction

Stenting

Mobilization

croflap technique, which itself sometimes is divided into subgroups such as mini-microflap, subepithelial microflap, medial and lateral microflap. These techniques have completely replaced the former technique of resecting the epithelium—so called stripping or decortication or now better subepithelial cordectomy—and have thus contributed substantially to the nowadays good and predictable outcome of phonosurgery. The instrumental choice is a matter for the surgeon. Most surgeons currently favour cold instruments but new developments such as the Acuspot micromanipulator and Acublade software allow similar postoperative progress and functional outcome using a CO_2 laser compared with cold instrument surgery.

7.3.3.4   Aetiopathogenesis

Two major aetiopathogentic groups are addressed by vocal fold surgery: vocal fold lesions with redundant pathological tissue impairing the vibratory movement (Table 7.3.5) and vocal fold movement disorders with inappropriate position and/or tension of the vocal fold (Table 7.3.6). As a result of the complex pathogenesis of the voice, there is naturally also an overlapping of the two groups.

In epithelial lesions the primary aim of surgery is complete epithelial resection for histological purposes (Table 7.3.5). This surgical procedure therefore is secondary phonosurgery as it has been defined (Table 7.3.1). Benign vocal fold lesions with the same histological components (fibrosis, vascular ectasia and oedema) are grouped under the heading "exudative lesion of Reinke's space". In terms of vocal fold movement disorders (Table 7.3.6), this work is restricted to lesions amenable to vocal fold surgery.

7.3.3.5   Types

The different types of vocal fold surgery in terms of disorder, therapeutic aim, procedure and approach are listed in Tables 7.3.7 and 7.3.8. Surgical instruments (e.g. cold instruments, CO_2 laser, microdebrider) or injectable materials (e.g. fat, collagen) are not taken into account, because they are essentially operator-dependent and usage may vary with time. Certain instruments, substances, drugs or implants are still at an experimental stage.

7.3.4   Laryngeal Framework Surgery

7.3.4.1   Nomenclature

Laryngeal framework surgery is the general term for this whole group of phonosurgical procedures which describe surgical modification of the structure of the larynx and recognizes the importance of the functional implications

Table 7.3.5 Vocal fold lesions impairing the vibratory movement

Epithelium
Papillomatosis
Chronic hypertrophic laryngitis
– Hyperplasia
– Dysplasia
– Carcinoma in situ
Carcinoma

Lamina propria
Exudative lesions affecting Reinke's space
– Nodule
– Polyp
– Pseudocyst
– Reinke's oedema
Cyst
– Epidermoid
– Mucous retention
Sulcus ("open cyst")
Mucosal bridge
Atrophy/scar
– Congenital ("sulcus, vergeture")
– Acquired
– Presbyphonia
Vascular
– Ectasia
– Varicosity
– Hematoma

Arytenoid
Granuloma

Anterior commissure
Glottal web, microweb

Table 7.3.6 Movement disorders of the vocal folds

Vocal fold immobility
– Paralysis/paresis
– Cricoarytenoid joint disorders
Neurologic
– Tremor/spasmodic dysphonia
Dysfunctional
– Hyperfunctional/hypofunctional
– Dysphonia plicae ventricularis

of these procedures. Laryngoplasty has also been introduced as a generic term for laryngeal framework surgery which refers to the functional aspect of the procedure. In this sense laryngoplasty is more or less synonymous with laryngeal framework surgery but is more suited for use in daily practice for reasons of simplicity. A certain confusion is sometimes created because the term "injection laryngoplasty" is also used for injection augmentation techniques. Thyroplasty is a subgroup and refers to laryngeal framework surgery which involves alteration or modification of the thyroid cartilage exclusively.

7.3.4.2 Definition

Surgical procedures performed on the laryngeal skeleton and/or inserting muscles for correction of position and/or tension of the vocal folds, aiming at an improvement of vibratory movements of the vocal folds or reduction of unmodulated/turbulent phonatory airflow or alteration/modification of vocal pitch. This can be achieved by correction of glottic insufficiency, reduction of vocal fold imbalance, increase or decrease of glottic aperture and change of vocal fold tension.

7.3.4.3 Approach

An external approach is used.

7.3.4.4 Types

The types are listed in Tables 7.3.9 and 7.3.10 and are described as follows:

- Approximation laryngoplasty: As insufficient glottic closure is one of the most common causes of dysphonia, glottal narrowing procedures are the most widely performed types of laryngeal framework surgery. Glottic insufficiency with dysphonia but also aspiration are the primary indications.
- Expansion laryngoplasty: The indication for this procedure is for glottal widening in cases where the glottis is functionally overclosed such as in adductor spasmodic dysphonia. The aim of the procedure is to improve the voice, not to improve the respiratory status like in glottic stenosis or bilateral vocal fold paralysis.
- Relaxation laryngoplasty: The indications for this type of procedure are pathologic tightened or stiffed vocal folds such as adductor spasmodic dysphonia or sulcus/vergeture, or an inappropriately high-pitched voice such as those seen in mutational voice disorders. The indications for this procedure are rare as voice pitch disorders usually react well to voice therapy; it is therefore mostly part of a combination laryngoplasty (Table 7.3.10). The common principle is to shorten the distance between the vocal fold attachments and thereby reduce the tension of the vocal folds.
- Tensioning laryngoplasty: This is the antagonistic procedure to relaxation and is indicated in abnormal lax

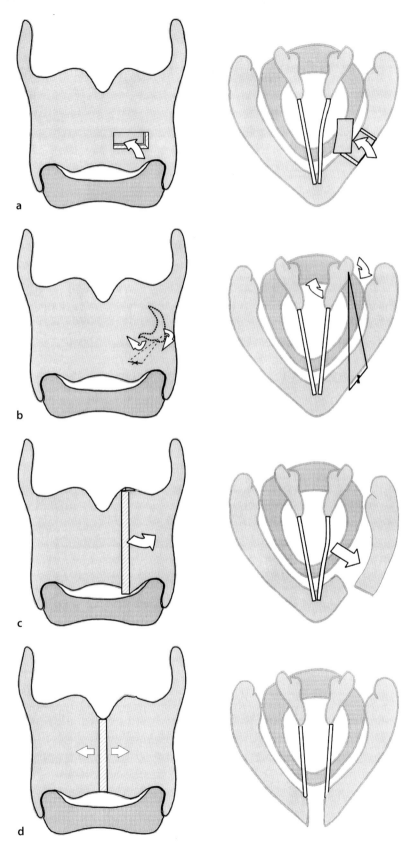

Fig. 7.3.1 Different types of Laryngeal Framework Surgery. **a** Medialization Thyroplasty. **b** Arytenoid Adduction (rotation technique). **c** Lateralization Thyroplasty (lateral approach). **d** Lateralization Thyroplasty (medial approach)

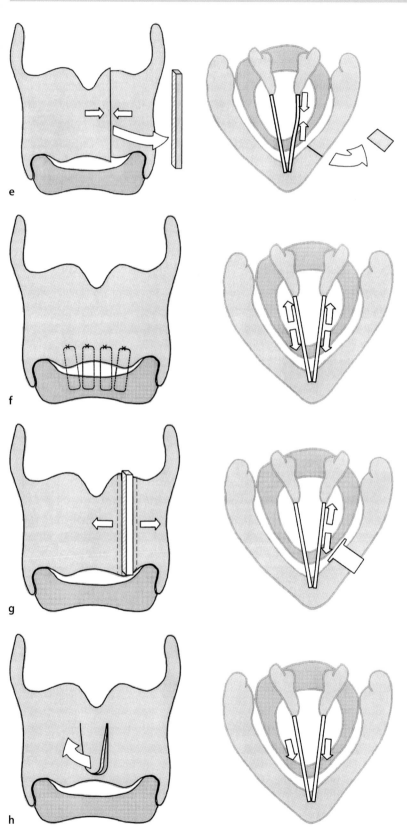

Fig. 7.3.1 (*continued*) Different types of Laryngeal Framework Surgery. **e** Shortening Thyroplasty (lateral approach). **f** Cricothyroid Approximation. **g** Elongation Thyroplasty (lateral approach). **h** Elongation Thyroplasty (medial approach). (Figure from Friedrich G., De Jong F.I.C.R.S., Mahieu H.F., Benninger M.S., Isshiki N. (2001) Laryngeal framework surgery: a proposal for classifikation and nomenclature by the Phonosurgery Committee of the European Laryngological Society Eur Arch Otorhinolaryngol, 375:1–8)

Table 7.3.7 Vocal fold lesions impairing vibratory movements. Phonosurgical procedures aiming at improvement of vibratory movements/restoration of the normal mucosal wave. Procedures less often performed or less recognized are shown in *italics*

Disorder	Procedure	Approach	
Exudative lesions of Reinke's space			
Nodule	Dissection and excision	Endolaryngeal	Direct
Polyp			*Indirect*
Pseudocyst			
Reinke's oedema	Dissection and suction (and excision)	Endolaryngeal	Direct
Cyst			
Epidermoid	Dissection an excision	Endolaryngeal	Direct
Mucous retention			
Sulcus ("open cyst")	Dissection, excision (and augmentation)	Endolaryngeal	Direct
Mucosal bridge	Excision	Endolaryngeal	Direct
	Dissection and gluing		
Atrophy/scar			
Congenital ("sulcus vergeture")	Dissection, excision (and) augmentation	Endolaryngeal	Direct
Acquired	*Implantation*		
Presbyphonia	Augmentation	Endolaryngeal	Direct
	Implantation		
Vascular			
Ectasia	Coagulation and/or excision	Endolaryngeal	Direct
Varicosity	Vaporization	Endolaryngeal	Direct
Hematoma	Incision and suction	Endolaryngeal	Direct
Arytenoid granuloma	Excision	Endolaryngeal	Direct
	Tension reduction		
	(botulinum toxin injection)		
Glottal web, microweb	Incision (and stenting)	Endolaryngeal	Direct

Table 7.3.8 Movement disorders of the vocal folds. Phonosurgical procedures aiming at correction of the position and/or tension of the vocal folds. Procedures less often performed or less recognized are shown in *italics*

Disorder	Procedure	Approach	
Vocal fold immobility			
Paralysis/paresis	Augmentation	Endolaryngeal	Direct
			Indirect
		External	*Percutaneous*
	Implantation	*Endolaryngeal*	*Direct*
		External	*Open neck*
Cricoarytenoid joint disorders	Augmentation	Endolaryngeal	Direct
			Indirect
		External	*Percutaneous*
	Implantation	*Endolaryngeal*	*Direct*
		External	*Open neck*
	Mobilization	Endolaryngeal	Direct
			Indirect
		External	*Open neck*

Table 7.3.8 (*continued*) Movement disorders of the vocal folds. Phonosurgical procedures aiming at correction of the position and/or tension of the vocal folds. Procedures less often performed or less recognized are shown in *italics*

Disorder	Procedure	Approach	
Neurologic			
Tremor/spasmodic dysphonia	Injection (botulinum toxin)	Transcutaneous	Percutaneous
		Endolaryngeal	Direct
			Indirect
	Thyroarytenoid muscle excision/coagulation	*Endolaryngeal*	*Direct*
Dysfunctional			
Hyperfunction	*Injection (botulinum toxin)*	*Endolaryngeal*	*Direct*
			Indirect
Hypofunction	*Augmentation*	*Endolaryngeal*	*Direct*
Dysphonia plicae ventricularis	*Excision*	*Endolaryngeal*	*Direct*
	Injection (botulinum toxin)	*Endolaryngeal*	*Direct*
			Indirect

or bowed vocal folds such as in presbyphonia or as is seen in inappropriately low pitched voices including paralysis of the cricothyroid muscle, androphonia in women and male to female transsexualism. The basic principle here is to increase the distance between the vocal fold attachments.

- Combination laryngoplasty: The different types of laryngoplasty can be favourably combined to achieve an optimal functional result (Table 7.3.10).

7.3.5 Neuromuscular Surgery

7.3.5.1 Definition

Surgical procedures performed on the laryngeal neuromuscular structures to restore motility and/or tension of the vocal folds.

7.3.5.2 Approach

External, endolaryngeal and percutaneous approaches are used.

7.3.5.3 Methods

Surgical and pharmaceutical (botulinum toxin) are used.

Table 7.3.9 Laryngeal framework surgery—classification and nomenclature

Approximation laryngoplasty
Medialization thyroplasty (thyroplasty type I)
Arytenoid adduction
– Rotation (pull) techniques
– Fixation techniques (adduction arytenopexy)

Expansion laryngoplasty
Lateralization thyroplasty
– Lateral approach (thyroplasty type IIa)
– Medial approach (thyroplasty type IIb, expansion of the anterior commissure, midline lateralization thyroplasty)
Vocal fold abduction
– Suture technique
– Resection technique (thyroarytenoid myectomy)

Relaxation laryngoplasty
Shortening thyroplasty
– Lateral approach (thyroplasty type III)
– Medial approach (anterior commissure retrusion)

Tensioning laryngoplasty
Cricothyroid approximation (thyroplasty type IVa, cricothyroid subluxation)
Elongation thyroplasty
– Lateral approach (thyroplasty type IVb)
– Medial approach (springboard advancement, anterior commissure advancement, anterior commissure laryngoplasty)

Table 7.3.10 Combination laryngoplasty (examples)

Combination	Purpose	Indications
Medialization TPL + arytenoid adduction (rotation)	Medialization of the entire vocal cord (anterior and posterior)	Open posterior glottis – High vagal paralysis – RLN paralysis with lateralized arytenoid – Non-rotating arytenoid
Bilateral medialization TPL	Medialization of both membranous vocal cords	Open anterior glottis – Bilateral vocal cord weakness (presbyphonia, etc.) – Bilateral loss of muscle mass – Tremor-induced AbSD
Medialization TPL + tensioning LPL	Stretching of vocal cord with medialization of affected side	Unilateral SLN weakness
Medialization TPL + arytenoid adduction (fixation)	Medial vocal cord fixation	Anterior dislocation of arytenoid cartilage Arytenoid fracture Failed arytenoid adduction (rotation) (cricoarytenoid joint ankylosis)
Bilateral relaxation LPL	Relaxation of both vocal cords	Too-high-pitched male voice Stable AdSD in males
Medialization TPL + relaxation LPL	Relaxation and Increased mass of one vocal cord	High-pitched, presbyphonic male voice

TPL thyroplasty, *LPL* laryngoplasty, *RLN* recurrent laryngeal nerve, *AbSD* abductor-type spasmodic dysphonia, *SLN* superior laryngeal nerve, *AdSD* adductor-type spasmodic dysphonia

7.3.5.4 Types

The different procedures of neuromuscular surgery are listed in Table 7.3.11. Except for chemodenervation, all types of neuromuscular surgery are currently being investigated in animal experiments and/or controlled clinical studies but are not applicable in clinical routine. But—in contrast to the methods of vocal fold surgery or laryngeal framework surgery—this group of phonosurgery comprises the only methods that enable a complete *restitio ad integrum* of a denervated or neuromuscular malfunctioning larynx.

7.3.6 Reconstructive Surgery

Reconstructive surgery (Table 7.3.12) consists of surgical procedures for restoring the voice after loss of functional structures or the entire larynx. In contrast to the other procedures of phonosurgery, the functional goal is primarily aimed at the restitution of oral communication rather than voice improvement.

7.3.7 Closing Remarks

This statement is the result of a consensus of the European Laryngological Society aiming at recommending the adoption of a common language for phonosurgery. In this respect the author would like to particularly acknowledge the contributions of Marc Remacle on classification of vocal fold surgery, Jean-Paul Marie on neuromuscular surgery and Christof Ahrens on reconstructive surgery and of course of numerous other colleagues who have participated in discussions within the European Laryngological Society. All methods and techniques mentioned are in many cases only one option for addressing the problem. There may be alternative and even preferable surgical procedures or combinations of various techniques, whether simultaneously or consecutively, to reach the best outcome (Tables 7.3.10, 7.3.13). This review covers all reported techniques to enable comparison and discussion. No recommendations or estimations of the different methods are given in here. It also does not imply that the author of this section endorses all the techniques reviewed.

Table 7.3.11 Types of neuromuscular surgery. Procedures less often performed (in humans) are shown in *italics*

Suppressive procedures

Nerve resection (unilateral)
- RLN trunk resection
- Selective intralaryngeal branch resection (in spasmodic dysphonia)

Chemodenervation (botulinium toxin)
- Global
- Unilateral or bilateral
- Selective

Laryngeal reinnervation

Muscle reinnervation

Non-selective reinnervation (not functional)
- *Nerve trunk anastomosis (ansa hypoglossi, or other strap muscle nerve, RLN, X, XI; XII)*
- *Mixed (with passive procedure (augmentation; medialization LPL) or with selective denervation)*

Selective reinnervation (functional)
- *Adductor muscles (ansa hypoglossi, XII, RLN, external branch of the SLN, nerve muscle pedicle)*
- *Abductor muscles (ansa hypoglossi, RLN, X, phrenic nerve, nerve muscle pedicle)*
- *Mixed (selective contemporary denervation; passive procedure associated: LFS)*
- *Both adductors and abductors; unilateral or bilateral*

Muscle transposition
- *Cricothyroid muscle transposition*
- *Strap muscle to the arytenoid*

Sensory reinnervation

Nerve transfer
- *SLN*
- *Superficial cervical plexus*
- *V, IX, X*

Innervated mucous flap transfer

Electrical stimulation

Nerve stimulation
- *RLN*
- *Vagus nerve*
- *Ansa hypoglossi*

Muscle stimulation
- *Posterior cricoarytenoid*
- *Adductors*

Restoration of a reflex bow
- *Sensory receptor*
- *Type of motor stimulation*

Table 7.3.12 Types of reconstructive surgery

Scar formation and webs at the glottic level

Anterior
  Laryngeal keel
  Alternating mucosal flaps
  Buccal mucosal flap
  Mitomycin C

Posterior
  Laminotomy of the cricoid
  Laryngeal keel
  Postcricoid flap
  Mitomycin C, temporary laterofixation

Partial defects

Primary glottic reconstruction
  Augmentation by injection
  Simple ventricular fold flap unilateral / bilateral
  Augmented ventricular fold flap (thyroid cartilage)
  Combined ventricular fold – partial epiglottic flap
  Sliding epiglottic flap

Secondary glottic reconstruction
  Augmentation by injection or implantation
  Medialisation thyroplasty (mod.: superior approach, enlarged thyroplasty)
  Sliding flap with/ without implantation
  Cervical skin flap
  Prelaryngeal muscle flap

Total defect

Tracheopharyngeal shunts
  Tracheopharyngeal Anastomosis
  Microvascular grafts (Radial forearm flap, Jejunum graft)
  Voice prosthesis

Larynxtransplantation

Table 7.3.13 Phonosurgical procedures due to diagnosis and indication

Diagnosis/indication	Goal	Methods
Lesions on the vocal fold impairing the vibratory movements	Improvement of vibratory movements by excision or dissection	VFS

Pathologic position, shape and/or tension of the vocal folds
  Glottic Insufficiency
  Loss of tension and/or vocal pitch too low
  Pathologic tension and/or vocal pitch too high
	Improvement of vibratory movements by correction of position shape and/or tension	LFS
		VFS
		NMS

Loss of functional structures	Restoration of oral communication	RCS NMS VFS

VFS vocal fold surgery, *LFS* laryngeal framework surgery, *NMS* neuromuscular surgery, *RCS* reconstructive surgery

Additional Reading

1. Dailey S., Diagnostic and therapeutic pitfalls in phonosurgery. Otolaryngol Clin Nth Am 2006; 39 (1): 11–22.
2. Friedrich G., Basic principles for indications in phonosurgery. Laryngorhinootologie 1995; 74(11): 663–5.
3. Friedrich G, Remacle M, Birchall M, Marie JP, Arens C., Defining phonosuregry; a proposal for classification and nomenclature by the Phonosurgery Committee of the European Laryngological Society (ELS). Eur Arch Otorhinolaryngol 2007; 264 (10): 1191–1200.
4. Isshiki N, Mechanical and dynamic aspects of voice production as related to voice therapy and phonosurgery, Otolaryngol Head Neck Surg 2000; 122 (6): 782–93.
5. Zeitels SM, Healy GB., Laryngology and phonosurgery. N Engl J Med 2003; 349 (9): 882–92.

Diseases of the Thyroid Gland: Diagnostics and Treatment

Edited by Matti Anniko

8.1 Hashimoto's Thyroiditis

ANDRÉS COCA AND CARLOS SUÁREZ

8.1.1 Definition

Hashimoto's thyroiditis is commonly characterized clinically as painless, diffuse enlargement of the thyroid gland occurring predominantly in middle-aged women. Patients are often euthyroid, but hypothyroidism may occur.

8.1.2 Incidence

The clinical disease is more frequent than Graves's disease when mild cases are included. The incidence is three to six cases per 10,000 population per year, and the prevalence among women is at least 2%.

8.1.3 Aetiology

The thyroid parenchyma is diffusely replaced by a lymphocytic infiltrate and fibrotic reaction. An autoimmune phenomenon may be seen in most patients. These patients have serum antibodies reacting with thyroglobulin and thyroid peroxidase, and against an unidentified protein present in colloid. Many patients have cell-mediated immunity directed against thyroid antigens.

All theories also emphasize a basic abnormality in the immune surveillance system, which in some way allows autoimmunity to develop against thyroid antigens, and as well against other tissues, including stomach, adrenal, and ovaries, in many patients with thyroiditis.

It is suggested that Hashimoto's thyroiditis, primary myxoedema, and Graves's disease are different expressions of a basically similar autoimmune process. This response may include cytotoxic antibodies, stimulatory antibodies, blocking antibodies, or cell-mediated immunity. Thyrotoxicosis is viewed as an expression of the effect of circulating thyroid stimulatory antibodies. Hashimoto's thyroiditis is predominantly the clinical expression of cell-mediated immunity leading to destruction of thyroid cells, which in its severest form produces thyroid failure and idiopathic myxoedema.

The gland involved in thyroiditis tends to lose its ability to store iodine, produces and secretes iodoproteins that circulate in plasma, and is inefficient in making hormone. Thus, the thyroid gland is under increased TSH stimulation, fails to respond to exogenous TSH, and has a rapid turnover of thyroidal iodine.

8.1.4 Diagnosis

Diagnosis include the finding of a diffuse, smooth, firm goitre in a young woman, with strongly positive titres of thyroglobulin antibody and/or thyroid peroxidase antibody and a euthyroid or hypothyroid metabolic status.

8.1.5 Therapy

A patient with a small goitre and euthyroidism does not require therapy unless the TSH level is elevated. The presence of a large gland, progressive growth of the goitre, or hypothyroidism indicates the need for replacement thyroid hormone. Surgery is rarely indicated. Development of lymphoma, though very unusual, must be considered if there is growth or pain in the gland involved.

8.2 Graves's Disease

ANDRÉS COCA AND CARLOS SUÁREZ

8.2.1 Definition

Graves's disease includes thyrotoxicosis, goitre, exophthalmos, and pretibial myxoedema, but can occur with one or more of these features. Thyrotoxicosis may also be produced by toxic multinodular goitre, toxic adenomas, excessive thyroid hormone ingestion, or several other rare syndromes.

8.2.2 Incidence

The incidence of Graves's disease is reported to be one to two cases per 1,000 population per year, with higher frequency in women.

8.2.3 Aetiology

The cause of Graves's disease is still unknown. Graves's disease is a disease of "autoimmunity", but the final cause of autoimmunity remains unclear. A strong hereditary tendency is present. Inheritance of human leucocyte antigens B8, DR3, DQ 2, and DQA1*0501 predisposes an individual to Graves's disease. Psychic trauma, sympathetic nervous system activation, strenuous weight reduction, and iodide administration have been associated with the onset of Graves's disease, but without a proven aetiologic role. The abnormal immune response is characterized by the presence of antibodies directed against thyroid tissue antigens, including antibodies that react with the thyrotrophin receptor by binding to the receptor. Antibodies can act as an agonist and stimulate the thyroid. The best known of the antibodies is the serum factor LATS, now known as TSAb. Hypersecretion of TSH is not a cause of Graves's disease, and serum TSH is typically suppressed to or near zero.

It has been shown in active Graves's disease that T lymphocyte suppressor cell function is diminished and suppressor cell number is reduced. Specific T suppressor cells controlling thyroid autoantibody production may also be diminished. The goitre, lymphocyte infiltrate, and antithyroid antibodies, with the exception of thyroid-stimulating antibodies, overlap with features of Hashimoto's thyroiditis.

The thyroid gland is hyperfunctioning in Graves's disease, and its action is not suppressed by administration of exogenous triiodothyronine. The pituitary response to TRH is also suppressed. The gland is unusually responsive to small doses of iodide, which both block further hormone synthesis and inhibit release of hormone from the gland.

Thyrotoxicosis itself is associated with pathologic changes including damage to muscles and mild damage to the liver. Graves's disease is associated with hyperplasia and lymphoid infiltrates in the thyroid, generalized lymphoid hyperplasia, and the specific changes of infiltrative ophthalmopathy and pretibial myxoedema.

8.2.4 Symptoms

The classic features of thyrotoxicosis are nervousness, diminished sleep, tremulousness, tachycardia, increased appetite, weight loss, and increased perspiration. In Graves's disease these symptoms and signs are associated with goitre, occasionally with exophthalmos, and rarely with pretibial myxoedema.

8.2.5 Diagnostic Procedures

Physical findings include fine skin and hair, tremulousness, a hyperactive heart, Plummer's nails, muscle weakness, accelerated reflex relaxation, occasional splenomegaly, and often peripheral oedema. Autoimmune vitiligo or hives may coexist.

The disease typically begins gradually in adult women and is progressive unless treated. Muscle weakness is frequent, myasthenia may coexist, and hypokalaemic periodic paralysis may be induced by thyrotoxicosis. Hypercalciuria is frequent, but severe osteitis fibrosa or osteomalacia and fractures are rare. Kidney stones rarely occur. Thyrotoxicosis can cause congestive heart failure. Mitral valve prolapse occurs with increased frequency in toxic patients. Atrial tachycardia and fibrillation are commonly caused by thyrotoxicosis. Normocytic anaemia is found. Diarrhoea occurs, but malabsorption is unusual. Minimal liver damage and hyperbilirubinaemia may be induced. Amenorrhoea or anovulatory cycling is common in women, and fertility is reduced. Oxygen consumption is greatly increased, lipid production and turnover are accelerated, and plasma total lipid and cholesterol levels tend to be low.

8.2.6 Complications

Thyrotoxicosis in untreated cases leads to cardiovascular damage, bone loss and fractures, or inanition, and can be fatal. The long-term history also includes spontaneous remission in some cases and eventual spontaneous development of hypothyroidism if autoimmune thyroiditis coexists and destroys the thyroid gland. Diagnosis of the classic form is easy and depends on the recognition of the cardinal features of the disease and confirmation by such tests as those for TSH and free thyroxin index.

8.2.7 Therapy

The available forms of treatment include surgery, drugs, and ^{131}I therapy. Antithyroid drugs are widely used. About one third of the patients undergoing long-term antithyroid therapy achieve permanent euthyroidism. Drugs are the preferred initial therapy in children and young adults.

Total or subtotal thyroidectomy is a satisfactory form of therapy but is used infrequently. The combined use of antithyroid drugs and iodine makes it possible to prepare patients adequately before surgery. Many young adults, especially males, are treated by surgery if antithyroid drug treatment fails.

Radioactive iodine is considered to be the best treatment. Evidence to date indicates the risk of late carcinogenesis must be near zero. Dosage is calculated on the basis of ^{131}I uptake and gland size. Most patients are cured by one treatment. The principal side effect is hypothyroidism.

Thyrotoxicosis in children is best handled initially by antithyroid drug therapy. If this therapy does not result in a cure, surgery may be performed. Treatment with ^{131}I is accepted as an alternative form of treatment. Neonatal thyrotoxicosis is a rarity. Antithyroid drugs, propranolol, and iodide may be required for several weeks until maternally derived antibodies have been metabolized.

8.3 Other Causes of Thyrotoxicosis

ANDRÉS COCA AND CARLOS SUÁREZ

8.3.1 Toxic Adenoma

Toxic adenomas are characterized by a single hyperactive nodule in the thyroid leading to clinical and biochemical thyrotoxicosis.

Autonomous or toxic adenomas are considered to originate from somatic mutations in the gene of G_s alpha protein or the gene of the thyrotropin receptor. In toxic adenoma only a hot nodule is visible on the thyroid scan. The frequency of toxic adenoma in patients with hyperthyroidism ranges between 1.5 and 44.5%. The possibility of developing thyrotoxicosis in a patient with a hot nodule with a diameter of 3 cm or larger is 20% in 6 years. This risk is substantially less for smaller nodules. Also, older patients with a hot nodule are more likely to become toxic as compared with younger patients. Definitive treatment consists of surgical removal of the nodule, administration of ^{131}I, or percutaneous administration of ethanol into the nodule. The likelihood of malignancy in a toxic nodule is very low.

8.3.2 Painless Thyroiditis

Thyrotoxicosis due to painless thyroiditis is an autoimmune thyroiditis due to lymphocytic infiltration of the thyroid and is identical to postpartum thyroiditis. About half of the patients pass through four classic phases consisting of thyrotoxicosis, euthyroidism, hypothyroidism, and back to euthyroidism. The other half of the patients do not become hypothyroid or, for a small minority, remain hypothyroid. Biochemically, characteristics include uptake of radioactive iodine being absent in the thyrotoxic phase and high serum thyroglobulin levels. Clinical thyrotoxicosis is mild and treatment with beta blocker agents is often sufficient. Sometimes addition of prednisone is necessary. Relapses may be seen. Although complete recovery is the rule, these patients are at high risk of developing hypothyroidism in later years. Permanent follow-up is therefore necessary.

8.3.3 Thyrotoxicosis Factitia

Thyrotoxicosis factitia (thyrotoxicosis due to surreptitious ingestion of thyroid hormone) is primarily a psychiatric disorder. Diagnosis must be suspected. Patients usually deny thyroid hormone tablet ingestion. Characteristically, thyroid uptake of radioactive iodine is low or absent and thyroglobulin is not detectable in the serum. The thyroid is usually small or absent on palpation. Treatment of the psychiatric disorder is difficult. Another form of excessive thyroid hormone intake is the "hamburger thyrotoxicosis". Subjects became thyrotoxic and showed characteristic serum abnormalities due to inclusion of thyroid in ground beef.

8.3.4 Induced Thyrotoxicosis

Thyrotoxicosis may be seen in association with elevated serum human chorionic gonadotrophin (hCG) activity in 1–2% of normal pregnant women. hCG has low intrinsic thyroid stimulating activity, and hCG acts on the human thyroid cell through the TSH receptor. Desialylation of hCG renders it more biologically active. In hydatidiform mole disease however, high levels are found in patients' serum. When values are above 300,000 U/l, thyrotoxicosis is likely. Surgical removal of the mole renders the patient euthyroid.

8.3.5 Induced Thyrotoxicosis

Administration of moderate or high doses of iodine may induce thyrotoxicosis in patients with or without apparent pre-existing thyroid disease. Iodine may be derived from iodine solutions, radiographic contrast agents, and medications. A notorious iodine containing agent is the anti-arrhythmic drug amiodarone. Owing to its structure, it may block pathways of thyroid hormone metabolism and action, leading to hypothyroidism, but it can also cause hyperthyroidism owing to its iodine content.

Amiodarone may also cause disruption of thyroid follicles, resulting in thyrotoxicosis owing to release of stored iodothyronines.

sists of surgery with postoperative external irradiation. Administration of dopamine antagonists or somatostatin analogues has been shown to be successful as well.

8.3.6 Aberrations in TSH Secretion

Inappropriate TSH secretion by a TSH-secreting pituitary tumour may cause hyperthyroidism. Treatment of the pituitary tumour will lead to euthyroidism. The prognosis is better in patients with microadenoma. Treatment con-

8.3.7 Metastasis

Rarely, metastases of follicular carcinoma may result in thyrotoxicosis with suppressed activity of the thyroid gland. Treatment of the metastases with radioactive iodine will ameliorate thyrotoxicosis.

8.4 Multinodular Goitre

ANDRÉS COCA AND CARLOS SUÁREZ

8.4.1 Incidence

Perhaps the most common of all the disorders of the thyroid gland is multinodular goitre. Even in non-oedemic regions it is clinically detected in about 4% of all adults beyond the age of 30. The disease is much more common in women.

8.4.2 Aetiology

Multinodular goitre is thought to be the result of primarily two factors. The first factor is genetic heterogeneity of follicular cells with regard to function (i.e. thyroid hormone synthesis) and growth. The second factor is the acquisition of new qualities that were not present in mother cells and become inheritable during further replication. Mutations may occur in follicular cells leading to constitutively activated adenomas and to thyrotoxicosis. These factors may lead to loss of anatomical and functional integrity of the follicles and of the gland as a whole. These processes ultimately lead to goitre formation and are accelerated by stimulatory factors. These stimulatory factors may be TSH, brought about by events such as iodine deficiency, inborn errors of thyroid hormone synthesis, goitrogens or local tissue growth-regulating factors. These basic and secondary factors may cause the thyroid to grow and gradually evolve into an organ containing hyperplastic islands of normal glandular elements, together with nodules and cysts of varied histologic pattern.

8.4.3 Symptoms

Nodular goitre is most often detected simply as a mass in the neck, but at times an enlarging gland produces pressure symptoms on the trachea or oesophagus. Occasionally tenderness and a sudden increase in size herald haemorrhage into a cyst. Thyrotoxicosis develops in a large proportion of these goitres after a few decades. A rare complication is the paralysis of the recurrent laryngeal nerve.

8.4.4 Diagnosis

The diagnosis is based on the physical examination. Thyroid function test results are normal or reveal subclinical or overt hyperthyroidism. Thyroid autoantibodies are usually absent or present at low levels, excluding Hashimoto's thyroiditis. Imaging procedures may reveal distortion of the trachea, calcified cysts, or impingement of the goitre on the oesophagus. From 4 to 17% of multinodular thyroids removed at operation contain foci that on microscopic examination fulfil the criterion of malignant change.

8.4.5 Treatment

If a clinically and biochemically euthyroid multinodular goitre is small and produces no symptoms, treatment is not necessary. If the clinically euthyroid goitre is unsightly, shows subclinical hyperthyroidism, or is causing pressure symptoms, treatment with ^{131}I is successful in virtually all cases but causes hypothyroidism to varying degree. Surgery is an acceptable alternative. The efficacy of thyroxine treatment after surgery, to prevent regrowth, is uncertain.

Overt toxic nodular goitre is usually treated with radioactive iodine. A gratifying reduction in the size of the goitre and control of the thyrotoxicosis may be expected. Hypothyroidism often ensues. Surgery is an alternative.

8.4.6 Colloid Goitre

The term "colloid goitre" is applied to glands composed of uniformly distended follicles appearing as a diffuse enlargement of the thyroid gland. The condition is found almost exclusively in young women. With time it may gradually develop into a multinodular goitre which becomes increasingly prominent as the decades pass. Appropriate therapy, if required, is the timely administration of thyroid hormone, which may be continued for several years.

8.4.7 Intrathoracic Goitre

An intrathoracic goitre is usually an acquired rather than a developmental abnormality. It may come about in embryonic life by a carrying downward into the thorax of the developing thyroid anlagen, or in adult life by protrusion of an enlarging thyroid through the superior thoracic inlet into the yielding mediastinal spaces. These lesions may produce pressure symptoms and may also be associated with hyperthyroidism. If the goitre is too large for treatment with ^{131}I, the appropriate therapy is resection of the goitre through the neck, if possible. Attachment of the intrathoracic goitre to the gland in the neck ordinarily proves the site of origin and provides a method for its easy surgical removal.

8.4.8 Infectious Thyroiditis

The thyroid may be the seat of an acute or chronic suppurative or nonsuppurative inflammation. Infectious thyroiditis is a rare condition. Its signs are heat, pain, redness, and swelling, and special ones conditioned by local relationships, such as dysphagia and a desire to keep the head flexed on the chest to relax the peritracheal muscles. The treatment is that for any febrile disease, including specific antibiotic. Surgical drainage may be necessary and a search for a pyriform sinus fistula because of a third branchial cleft malformation should be made, particularly in children with thyroiditis involving the left lobe.

8.4.9 Subacute Thyroiditis

Subacute (granulomatous) thyroiditis is a more common and protracted disease that usually involves the thyroid symmetrically. The gland is swollen and tender, and the systemic reaction may be severe, with fever and an elevated erythrocyte sedimentation rate. During the acute phase of the disorder, tests of thyroid function reveal a diminished thyroidal radioactive iodine uptake and increased serum concentrations of thyroxine, triiodothyronine, and thyroglobulin. The cause of this disease has been established in only a few instances in which a viral infection has been the initiating factor. There may be repeated recurrences of diminishing severity. Usually the function of the thyroid is normal after the disease has subsided. Subacute thyroiditis may be treated with rest, non-steroidal anti-inflammatory drugs or aspirin, and thyroid hormone. If the disease is severe and protracted, it is usually necessary to resort to administration of glucocorticoids, but recurrence may follow their withdrawal.

8.4.10 Riedel's Thyroiditis

Riedel's thyroiditis is a chronic sclerosing replacement of the gland that is exceedingly rare. The process involves the immediately adjacent structures, making any surgical attack very difficult. The cause is unknown, and no treatment is available beyond resecting the isthmus of the thyroid gland to relieve the symptoms of tracheal or oesophageal compression. Sarcoid may involve the thyroid, and amyloid may be deposited in the gland in quantities sufficient to cause goitre. In all of these diseases, it may be necessary to give the patient levothyroxine replacement therapy if the function of the gland has been impaired.

8.5 Thyroid Regulation and Dysfunction in the Pregnant Patient

ANDRÉS COCA AND CARLOS SUÁREZ

8.5.1 Incidence

Pregnancy has profound effects on the regulation of thyroid function in healthy women and patients with thyroid disorders. Overt thyroid dysfunction occurs in 2–3% of pregnancies, but subclinical thyroid dysfunction (both hyperthyroidism and hypothyroidism) is probably more prevalent and frequently remains undiagnosed. Maternal alterations of thyroid function due to iodine deficiency, hypothyroidism, and hyperthyroidism have important implications for fetal/neonatal outcome.

8.5.2 Aetiology

Pregnancy increases the metabolic rate, blood flow, heart rate, and cardiac output, and various subjective sensations such as fatigue and heat intolerance that may suggest the possibility of coexistent thyrotoxicosis. Other metabolic changes which also impact the hypothalamic pituitary thyroid system are the potential direct stimulation of the maternal thyroid by hCG, as well as the accelerated metabolism of thyroxine, presumably due to increased placental deiodination enzymes.

8.5.3 Therapy

In patients with hypothyroidism, it is important to recognize that the therapeutic requirements for exogenous thyroxine are increased by 50% on average during pregnancy. This should be taken into account in the management of such patients.

The main causes of thyrotoxicosis in pregnancy include Graves's disease and gestational non-autoimmune transient. The natural history of Graves's disease is altered during pregnancy, with a tendency for exacerbation in the first trimester, amelioration during the second and third trimesters, and typically a rebound during the postpartum period. These changes are the consequences of partial immune suppression during gestation with a rebound during the postpartum period.

Fetal and neonatal hyperthyroidism is due to the transplacental transfer of maternal stimulating TSH-receptor antibodies (TRAb). The diagnosis of fetal (and neonatal) hyperthyroidism is usually made on the basis of fetal tachycardia, accelerated bone age, and intrauterine growth retardation. It may occur in infants born to women with active Graves's disease, but also in women who have had prior definitive cure of their disease by surgery or radioactive iodine treatment, but who maintain high titres of TRAb.

8.6 Thyroid Carcinoma

ANDRÉS COCA AND CARLOS SUÁREZ

8.6.1 Incidence

Thyroid carcinoma is unusual among human malignancies (less than 1%) but is the most frequent endocrine cancer, accounting for about 5% of thyroid nodules. Thyroid nodules are very frequent in the general population and, according to the method of detection and the age of the patients, their prevalence may approach 20–50% of the general population. Thyroid cancer is one of the human cancers with quickly increasing incidence. A history of previous radiation therapy to the head and neck region, or accidental exposure to ionizing radiation (e.g. Chernobyl nuclear accident) is known to increase dramatically the risk for a well-differentiated carcinoma of the thyroid.

8.6.2 Papillary Carcinoma

The most common type of thyroid cancer is papillary carcinoma, which represents 70–80% of all thyroid cancers and, together with follicular carcinomas, arises from follicular cells of the thyroid. Women are more commonly affected than men, and the average age at diagnosis is around 40 years. Multicentric carcinomas are often present secondary to intraglandular lymphatic spread. Lymphatic metastasis to the neck nodes are also very common. Usually, papillary carcinomas show a slow growing pattern. Papillary carcinoma has the best prognosis of the thyroid malignancies, with a cancer specific mortality at 10 years from 5 to 10%. Despite this excellent prognosis, there is a group of patients who will die from progressive disease. High-risk patients include those older than 45 years, with a carcinoma size larger than 4 cm, extrathyroidal involvement, and distant metastasis.

8.6.3 Follicular Carcinoma

Follicular carcinomas represents 10–20% of all thyroid cancers, and spread more commonly by haematogenous dissemination, but few of them show multicentric disease or neck node metastasis. Follicular carcinomas have a higher propensity for local aggressiveness and a faster rate of growth. The worse prognosis for patients with follicular carcinoma is due to the more common association with advanced age and advanced disease.

8.6.4 Medullary Carcinoma

Medullary carcinoma arises from the C cells that secrete calcitonin. At presentation, the thyroid swelling may be associated with neck node clinical or microscopic metastasis in up to 70% of patients. In addition to the spread to regional lymph nodes, this type of carcinoma has the ability to metastasize to bone, liver, and lungs. Rarely, patients may present with symptoms due to secretion of neuroendocrine substances. Medullary thyroid cancer represents around 5% of all thyroid cancers, and often is a component of multiple endocrine neoplasia syndromes types 2A and 2B due to mutation of RET proto-oncogene. The overall survival for patients with medullary carcinomas is from 50 to 60% at 10 years. Prognosis is most accurately predicted by TNM tumour classification, and the presence of lymph node metastases has a dominant influence on survival.

8.6.5 Anaplastic Carcinoma

Anaplastic carcinoma is nowadays uncommon and represents less of 5% of all thyroid cancers. Anaplastic carcinoma is a very aggressive tumour that shows an extensive local invasion and neck and distant metastasis, with a mean survival of 6 months.

8.6.6 Therapy

It is known that the primary therapy for thyroid carcinoma is surgery. The optimal initial operation is controversial and surgeons have to decide how much thyroid tissue must be removed. However, the last reviews suggest that most patients are best served by total thyroidectomy followed by the administration of radioiodine to destroy any remaining thyroid tissue and microscopic foci of tumour.

Patients with a thyroid nodule have to undergo a complete history and physical examination of the thyroid and the neck, laboratory evaluation, fine needle aspiration cytology, neck ultrasonography, and thyroid gammagraphy. A CT scan image is only obtained when there is great suspicion of malignancy owing to physical findings such as vocal cord palsy.

8.7 Surgical Options for Thyroid Malignancy

ANDRÉS COCA AND CARLOS SUÁREZ

8.7.1 Solitary Thyroid Nodule

Patients with a solitary thyroid nodule with suspicion of malignancy must undergo a hemithyroidectomy with intraoperative pathologic diagnosis. If pathologic analysis confirms carcinoma, a total thyroidectomy must be performed. Subtotal thyroidectomy, in which several grams of thyroid tissue is preserved along the posterior capsule is an inadequate procedure for patients with thyroid carcinoma.

Microscopic regional lymph node metastases of papillary carcinoma occur in up to 80% of patients. However, only 35% have cervical or mediastinal node metastases that are detected at the time of initial surgery. Because microscopic modal disease is rarely of clinical importance or subsequent radioiodine administration ablates these occult foci, prophylactic neck dissection does not improve long-term outcome.

Neck dissection must be performed when there is a diagnosis of papillary carcinoma with visibly involved nodes. Preoperative cervical ultrasound can detect clinically non-palpable, metastatic nodes in up to 20% of patients with papillary carcinoma, including those with primary tumours less than 1 cm in diameter. Lateral compartment nodes containing metastases detectable by ultrasound are associated with a shortened relapse-free survival, whereas those only found by histologic examination do not predict altered outcomes. Owing to these facts, we recommend lateral node dissection in papillary carcinomas of the thyroid based upon intraoperative gross involvement or preoperative ultrasound detection.

Cervical nodal metastases are rare in patients with follicular carcinoma, patients with the Hürthle cell variant may have nodal disease (which predicts a worse outcome) and should have a neck dissection. There is controversy about how to manage the central compartment of the neck in papillary and Hürthle cell cancer. The American Thyroid Association recommends routine central neck dissection and the National Comprehensive Cancer Network recommends central neck dissection only in the presence of grossly positive metastases.

During the operation, the lymph nodes should be inspected, and any suspected of containing carcinoma should be biopsied. If nodes in the central compartment are found to contain carcinoma, dissection of lymphatics and tissue in that compartment should be performed, and if nodes in the lateral compartment are found, dissection of these areas should be performed.

8.7.2 Medullary Thyroid Carcinoma

Management of medullary thyroid carcinoma varies from treatment of differentiated thyroid carcinomas. Because this tumour is multifocal and bilateral in virtually all patients with hereditary disease and in at least 20% of patients with sporadic disease, total thyroidectomy has been the logical treatment of choice. As medullary thyroid carcinoma occurs in 0.6% of thyroid nodules, it has been suggested that all patients undergoing assessment for nodular thyroid disease should have at least basal calcitonin measurement to avoid the undesirable surprise of the incidentally discovered medullary thyroid carcinoma. It must be emphasized that it is mandatory that all patients undergoing surgery for medullary thyroid carcinoma should have preoperative measurement of urinary catecholamines to exclude a phaeochromocytoma, even when there is no specific evidence to suggest the thyroid tumour is of the hereditary variety.

The central neck compartments should be dissected in all pT1 tumours. If central disease is sufficiently gross to be apparent either on ultrasound or intraoperatively, both lateral nodal compartments should also be dissected. The lateral nodal dissection should be performed with preservation of the spinal accessory nerve, sternomastoid muscle, and internal jugular vein unless any of these structures are actually invaded by tumour.

All pT2–4 tumours should be treated by complete central and bilateral lateral compartmental excision. Although a strategy of resecting only significant and clinically involved nodes may, at times, be reasonable in the treatment of differentiated thyroid carcinoma where there are backup treatment modalities including radioactive iodine, such a conservative policy has no place in the management of medullary thyroid carcinoma, a tumour which does not take up radioiodine.

8.7.3 Anaplastic Thyroid Cancer

Anaplastic thyroid cancer makes up about 2% of all thyroid cancers. It begins in the follicular cells of the thyroid. The cancer cells tend to grow and spread very quickly. Anaplastic thyroid cancer is very hard to control, often requires a very aggressive treatment plan with surgery, radiation, and sometimes even chemotherapy. It often requires the patient to have a tracheostomy to maintain the airway.

8.7.4 Surgery for Invasive Disease

The primary tumour or local and regional metastases may invade the muscles, trachea, recurrent laryngeal nerves, larynx, oesophagus, thoracic duct, or carotid artery. It is essential that a careful preoperative and intraoperative evaluation is performed, including symptom-guided imaging studies.

We can perform conservative procedures such as vertical hemilaryngectomy for unilateral laryngeal cartilage invasion, or circumferential tracheal resection for subglottic invasion may allow maintenance of function. Extensive intraluminal invasion may necessitate total laryngectomy.

Suggested Reading

1. Abalovich M, Amino N, Barbour LA, Cobin RH, De Groot L, Glinoer D, Mandel SJ, Stagnaro-Green A (2007) Management of thyroid dysfunction during pregnancy and postpartum: an Endocrine Society clinical practice guideline. J Clin Endocrinol Metab 92:S1–S47

2. Ballantyne AJ (1994) Resections of the upper aerodigestive tract for locally invasive thyroid cancer. Am J Surg 168:636–639

3. Cooper DS, Doherty GM, Haugen BR, Kloos RT, Lee SL, Mandel SJ, Mazzaferri EL, McIver B, Sherman SI, Tuttle RM (2006) The American Thyroid Association Guidelines Taskforce. Management guidelines for patients with thyroid nodules and differentiated thyroid cancer. Thyroid 16:109–142

4. Derwahl M, Studer H (2001) Nodular goiter and goiter nodules: where iodine deficiency falls short of explaining the facts. Exp Clin Endocrinol Diabetes 109:250–260

5. Hodgson NC, Button J, Solorzano CC (2004) Thyroid cancer: is the incidence still increasing? Ann Surg Oncol 11:1093–1097

6. Kasagi K, Kousaka T, Higuchi K, Iida Y, Misaki T, Alam MS, Miyamoto S, Yamabe H, Konishi J (1996) Clinical significance of measurements of antithyroid antibodies in the diagnosis of Hashimoto's thyroiditis: Comparison with histological findings. Thyroid 6:445–450

7. Krohn K, Führer D, Bayer Y, Eszlinger M, Brauer V, Neumann S, Paschke R (2005) Molecular pathogenesis of euthyroid and toxic multinodular goiter. Endocr Rev 26:504–524

8. Miller FR, Otto RA (eds) (2003) Disorders of the thyroid. Otolaryngol Clin N Am 36:1–233

9. Zingrillo M, Torlantano M, Ghiggi MR, Frusciante A, Varraso A, Liuzzi A, Trischitta V (2000) Radioiodine and percutaneous ethanol injection in the treatment of large toxic thyroid nodule: a long-term study. Thyroid 10:985–990

8.8 Surgery of the Thyroid Gland

JOHAN WENNERBERG AND HANS GERTZÉN

8.8.1 Anatomy

The thyroid gland consists of two lobes positioned antero-laterally to the larynx and trachea (Fig. 8.8.1). During embryogenesis the thyroid rudiment descends from the base of the tongue, and the remnant can be seen as the thyroglossal duct. An isthmus just below the cricoid cartilage unites the lobes. It normally weighs 15–30 g. The average size of a lobe is 2 × 2.5 × 4 cm (width × thickness × height). Anteriorly the gland is covered by the sternothyroid and sternohyoid muscles (the strap muscles). Laterally are the internal jugular vein and the common carotid artery.

The major blood supply to the thyroid is cranially from the superior thyroid artery, the first branch from the carotid artery, and caudally from the inferior thyroid artery, a branch from the thyrocervical trunk. It is important to note that the superior thyroid artery runs down to the superior pole in close proximity to the superior laryngeal nerve (SLN). It supplies sensory innervations to the supraglottic larynx (internal branch), and motor innervation to the cricothyroid muscle (external branch). The venous drainage of the thyroid gland is by the veins parallel to the arterial pedicles, and with a separate middle thyroid vein draining directly into the internal jugular vein. The lymphatic drainage is predominantly into the para- and pretracheal lymph nodes and secondarily into the jugular nodes (levels III, IV and V).

The recurrent laryngeal nerve (RLN) innervates the intrinsic laryngeal muscles and provides sensory inner-

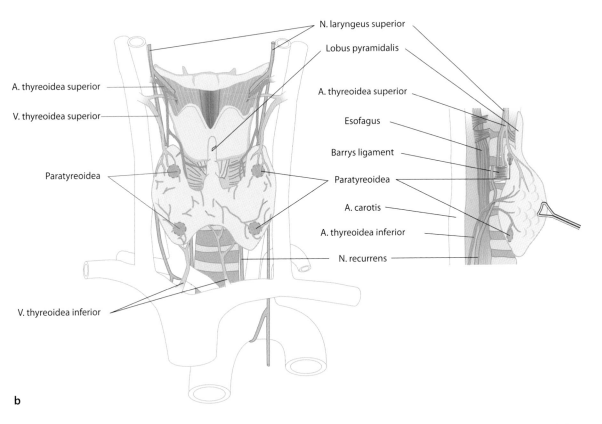

b

Fig. 8.8.1 Anatomy of the thyroid gland (Adapted with permission from Anniko M [2006] Otolaryngology. Liber AB, Stockholm. ©AB Typoform)

vation to the glottic larynx. It has great variability in its course and relationship to adjacent anatomical structures. It commonly runs in the tracheal–oesophageal groove, and usually passes deep to the inferior thyroid artery. It can however also be in front of the artery, and even pass between branches of the artery. In approximately 1% of cases, on the right side, the nerve is nonrecurrent. The RLN can divide into two or more branches of 1–2 cm, before entering the larynx.

The location of the parathyroid glands is variable. The superior pair is less variable and usually in or near the capsule posterior to the upper third of the thyroid gland. The inferior pair is more variable, about 40% being located in the tissue immediately adjacent, anterior or posterior, to the lower pole of the thyroid gland. Regarding superior and inferior parathyroids 2–5% will be located subcapsular of the thyroid.

8.8.2 Physiology

The regulation of thyroid hormone production is a complex of pathways and feedback mechanisms involving the hypothalamic–pituitary–thyroid axis. The functional unit is the thyroid follicle, composed of cubic thyroid epithelial cells surrounding a colloid-containing lumen.

Thyrotropin-releasing hormone (TRH) from the hypothalamus stimulates the anterior pituitary to release thyroid-stimulating hormone (TSH). This in turn stimulates the thyroid to synthesise the thyroid hormone-binding thyroglobulin, and the synthesis and release of thyroid hormones, primarily T_4 (thyroxine) but also T_3 (triiodothyronine). In the peripheral blood, T_4 and T_3 are bound to carrier proteins; less than 0.5% is free. In peripheral tissues, T_4 is metabolised (de-iodinated) to T_3, which is the major effector of biological effects. Both T_4 and T_3 inhibit in a negative feedback loop TSH release.

If hormone synthesis is suppressed, then the normal gland has a supply of hormone sufficient for 3–4 weeks. The peripheral supply of T_4 bound to carrier protein lasts for a shorter period and after, e.g. a total thyroidectomy, clinical signs of hypothyroidism can be seen after approximately 3 weeks.

In between the thyroid follicles are the parafollicular C cells. They are embryologically derived from the ultimobranchial bodies and produce the peptide hormone calcitonin, which is responsible for maintenance of osseous structure by control of bone resorption. Calcitonin lowers serum Ca^{2+}.

8.8.3 Epidemiology

8.8.3.1 Goitre

Simple or colloid goitre, a diffuse enlargement of the gland later evolving into multinodular goitre due to asymmetrical focal hyperplasia, involution, haemorrhage and scarring reflects the effects of increased levels of TSH secondary to decreased output of thyroid hormone. The most common cause is iodine deficiency. The prevalence of goitre worldwide is highly variable. High incidence of goitre is seen in, e.g. the mountainous regions around the world where alimentary intake of iodine is low. In all EU countries, table salt is iodinated.

8.8.3.2 Thyroid Nodule

Isolated thyroid nodules are very common. Clinical examination suggests a prevalence of 1–7%. In the prospective Framingham study in Massachusetts, the estimated lifetime risk of developing a thyroid nodule was estimated to be between 5 and 10%. In an autopsy series from Malmoe, Sweden, comprising 821 thyroid glands, the reported nodule prevalence was 49.5%. Regardless of the "true" incidence of thyroid nodules, the critical question is whether a detected nodule is malignant. Other prevalence studies of goitre in women over 50 years of age have reported approximately 2% visible nodules, 14% are palpable, 40% are found with US, and ca. 50% discovered at autopsy.

8.8.3.3 Thyroid Carcinoma

As for goitre there are wide variations in incidence between countries. Thyroid cancer is two to four times more frequent in females than in males. The annual incidence of thyroid cancer ranges from 1.2 to 2.6 per 100,000 men and 2.0 to 3.8 per 100,000 women.

In countries where the dietary iodine intake is adequate, differentiated carcinoma (papillary and follicular) accounts for more than 85% (68% papillary and 17% follicular). In regions with lower iodine intake, papillary carcinoma account for about 40%, with follicular carcinoma being more frequent. In regions where iodine repletion has been introduced, there has been an increase in papillary carcinoma compared with follicular carcinoma.

Genetic factors play a role in the development of thyroid cancer. Some oncogens (MYC and FOS) are seen in all carcinomas, whereas others are primarily found in papillary thyroid cancers (RET/PTC, MET, TRK). The oncogene p53 predisposes one to the anaplastic type of thyroid cancer.

8.8.3.3.1 Risk Factors

Epidemiological studies indicate several different risk factors for thyroid carcinoma:

- Obesity (women, but not men)
- Low alimentary iodine intake
- Certain familial syndromes (e.g. familial polyposis coli, Gardner's syndrome)
- Hormonal and reproductive status (increased risk associated with late menarche and high parity)
- Ionising radiation (especially in childhood)

Experiences from Hiroshima and Nagasaki, from nuclear fall-out after atmospheric testing as well as from external radiation towards the neck has clearly demonstrated an increased risk for thyroid carcinoma, the latency period being 15–20 years. Findings after the Chernobyl accident, however, indicate that the latency period for children (<10 years of age) is considerably shorter, less than 5 years. Children tend to get papillary cancer, and the younger the patient the more aggressive the tumour.

8.8.4 Clinical Evaluation

All thyroid enlargements should be evaluated, independently of how long the history of goitre or an isolated nodule is.

The inquiry into the patient's medical history should include information of previous neck irradiation, how rapid the growth has been, and symptoms of compression or of invasion in adjacent structures, such as hoarseness (recurrent nerve), dysphagia (oesophagus) or haemoptysis (trachea). A laryngeal examination is a mandatory part of the clinical examination, and vocal cord mobility should carefully be evaluated.

Laboratory assessment is an important part of the workup. Determination of thyrotropin (S-TSH), and serum-free T_4 (S-fT_4) allows judgement as to whether the patient is euthyroid. Most patients with thyroid nodules are euthyroid. If a malignant enlargement is suspected S-thyroglobulin and sometimes calcitonin should be indicated. It is important to know that immediately after an FNA serum thyroglobulin (S-Tg) will be false positive for at least a month. The blood sample thus has to be collected before FNA.

8.8.5 Imaging

The thyroid and the surrounding neck spaces can be visualised using different techniques: radionuclide scanning, US, CT and MRI.

8.8.5.1 Radionuclide Scanning

Using radioisotopes, commonly [99m]technetium or [123]iodine, was once a cornerstone in the workup but has gradually fallen out of favour. Approximately 80% of nodules are cold on scintigraphy, 5% are hot, and the remaining "intermediate". Scintigraphy cannot differ between malignant and nonmalignant cold nodules. About 10–20% of cold nodules are malignant. If the nodule however is hot, then the risk for malignancy is less than 1%. A radionuclide scan is also of value in guiding the FNA.

8.8.5.2 Ultrasound

The US technique has successively been refined the recent 10–15 years. It is a simple and cheap investigation. Using colour-coded Doppler technique vessels can be imaged, and in combination with FNA, it allows high precision in sampling. Due to high resolution, 3-mm nodules can be visualised. Therefore, there is a considerable risk of over-diagnosis.

Nodules can be solid or cystic on US. Purely cystic nodules are reported to carry a lower risk of malignancy (<3%) than predominantly solid nodules do (~10%). Using US-guided FNA, semisolid cysts can be evacuated and aspiration directed toward the solid component.

8.8.5.3 Computed Tomography

An important generalisation in thyroid imaging is that neither CT nor MRI can differentiate benign thyroid adenoma from thyroid malignancy based on primary imaging findings. Colloid cysts cannot, e.g. be differentiated from goitre or carcinoma that has undergone cystic degeneration. Ancillary findings, however, such as nodal metastasis, cartilaginous or bony destruction, allow the identification of malignancy.

MRI is the preferred imaging tool when thyroid imaging is required presurgically when suspicion of malignancy exists. CT is not recommended in this setting. CT without iodine-enhanced examination gives poor morphological information, and iodine-contrast-enhanced CT makes [131]iodine therapy impossible up to 3 months. MRI can also be of value in the follow-up after surgery of thyroid carcinoma. However, if availability of MRI is low, then it can be an unnecessary delay for the patient.

8.8.5.4 Positron Emission Tomography

Integrated CT-PET scan with [18]FDG tracer is lately the method of choice for thyroidectomised patients with no clinical signs of recurrent local or metastatic tumour, but elevated values of thyroglobulin, where CT or an iodine scan has not been able to show any recurrence. The same can be said of medullary carcinomas with pathologic values of calcitonin.

In some centres CT-PET scan is used in the basic investigation of medullary carcinoma as soon as the cytology is proved.

In summary, the better the uptake is on iodine scanning, the less the possibility of uptake on CT-PET scan. In the future we will see better CT-PET scans with amino acid or iodine tracers.

8.8.5.5 Fine-Needle Aspiration Cytology

All euthyroid patients presenting with a thyroid tumour should have an FNA as a mandatory part of the diagnostic procedure. If possible, the puncture should be guided by US or radionuclide scanning. The needle should be 0.4–0.7 mm, and puncture can be done with or without an aspiration handle.

It is important to be aware of the strength and weakness (the sensitivity and specificity on one's own hospital) of FNA. Overall (benign and malignant tumours together):

$$\text{sensitivity} = \frac{\text{true positives}}{\text{true positives} + \text{false negatives}} = 0.5 \text{ to } 0.6$$

and

$$\text{specificity} = \frac{\text{true negatives}}{\text{true negatives} + \text{false positives}} > 0.95.$$

The sensitivity is higher for medullary and undifferentiated carcinoma than it is for papillary and follicular carcinoma. The major weakness of thyroid FNA lies in the diagnosis of papillary and follicular carcinomas. The specificity of FNA of thyroid tumours however, is high enough to permit surgical intervention after cytodiagnosis of malignancy.

The cytological diagnosis follicular neoplasia is an absolute indication for surgery, because 20% of these will show up as follicular carcinomas in histology. This is due to the definition of a follicular carcinoma, which is histologic: infiltration of the capsule and/or vascular invasion, which cannot be seen in the cytology specimen. Caution should be with patients treated with antithyrotoxic agents, because these agents make the reading of the cytology very difficult (false-positive carcinomas).

Table 8.8.1 Malignant lesions of the thyroid

Histopathology	Frequency (%)	Age of presentation
Papillary carcinoma	60–70	30–60 years
Follicular carcinoma	10–20	45–70 years
Medullary carcinoma	5–10	
Familiar form	10	From 10 years of age
Sporadic	90	>50 years
Anaplastic carcinoma	5–10	>55 years

8.8.5.6 Malignant Thyroid Tumours

Thyroid carcinoma exhibits a wide variation in biological aggressiveness and prognosis (Table 8.8.1), ranging from anaplastic carcinoma with close to 100% mortality within a year after diagnosis, to the much more common papillary carcinoma found in young female patients with a very favourable 20-year prognosis, which means normal life expectancy in located (T1–T3) tumours after radical surgery.

8.8.5.6.1 Papillary Carcinoma

This is the most common of thyroid carcinomas, accounting two thirds of incident cases. The age-related incidence curve is bimodal, exhibiting two peaks (Fig. 8.8.2). It is two to three times more common in females compared with males. Ionising radiation is a known risk factor; after the nuclear power plant accident in Chernobyl, there was a high rise in childhood papillary carcinoma.

The presenting symptom is usually an asymptomatic neck mass, typically located in the thyroid, but it can present in the neck. Up to half of patients have a neck metastasis at the time of diagnosis, and an enlarged lymph node can be the first sign of the disease. The second most common metastatic location is the lungs. Metastasis to the skeleton is uncommon.

Papillary carcinoma arises from the follicular cells of the gland. Histopathologically it is characterised by a papillary proliferation of thyroid epithelium. The tumour cells exhibit characteristic nuclear features, with an empty appearance of the nuclei described as optically clear, pale, ground glass, resembling "Orphan Annie eyes" These features can be diagnosed by FNA. There are variants of papillary carcinoma as, e.g. the follicular variant with a predominantly follicular growth pattern but associated with the nuclear changes seen in papillary carcinoma.

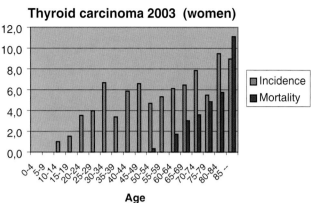

Fig. 8.8.2 Age-standardised incidence and mortality of thyroid carcinoma in Sweden 2003 for different age groups (data from Cancer Incidence in Sweden, Centre for Epidemiology, The National Board of Health and Welfare)

Papillary carcinoma is often multifocal. Papillary microcarcinoma is a termed applied to an incidentally identified intrathyroidal papillary carcinoma smaller than 10 mm in diameter. It is found during thyroid surgery for other, benign diseases or at autopsy. The malignant potential is considered very low, and usually it does not require measures other than follow-up more vigilant and thyroid hormone substitution.

Prognostic Factors
Young age, female gender, absence of metastatic (M⁺) DNA diploidy and radical surgery as well as small tumours are all favourable prognostic factors. Nodal (N⁺) spread does interestingly not change the outcome in younger (<45 years) patients. "Tall" cell type and aneuploidy worsens the prognosis markedly.

Treatment
An overview is given in Table 8.8.2 of treatment options in relation to tumour stage.

8.8.5.6.2 Follicular Carcinoma
Follicular carcinoma is the second most common of the differentiated thyroid carcinomas. It accounts for 10–20% of incident cases. There is an increased incidence in areas with endemic goitre. In contrast to papillary carcinoma, lymphoglandular spread is uncommon; the predominant pattern of spread is hematogenous to the lungs and bone. However, when nodal spread is present it has an unfavourable, negative impact on prognosis.

As for papillary carcinoma, the presenting symptom is usually a slow-growing, asymptomatic neck mass, located

Table 8.8.2 Treatment overview of papillary carcinoma

Tumour status	Re-operate, if possible	¹³¹I treatment	External radiotherapy	Hormone suppression
Occult carcinoma (tumour is <10 mm)	–	–	–	+ (Only substitution is necessary)
"Low risk" (completely removed intrathyroidal carcinoma without low-diff ca)	–	–	–	+
"High risk" (close margins, pT4, pN3, low-differentiated cancer)	+	+	–	+
Macroscopically remaining carcinoma	+	+	+	+
Nonresectable carcinoma		+	+	+
Inoperable, distant metastases	Individualised treatment			

Table 8.8.3 Overview of follicular carcinoma

Tumour status	Re-operate, if possible	^{131}I treatment	External radiotherapy	Hormone suppression
Occult carcinoma (pT1 N0)	–	–	–	+
Macroscopically radical thyroidectomy without signs of remnant thyroid on scintigraphy	–	+	–	+
Macroscopically radical thyroidectomy but with signs of remnant thyroid on scintigraphy	+	+	–	+
Macroscopically remaining carcinoma	+	+	+	+
Nonresectable carcinoma		+	+	+
Inoperable, distant metastases	Individualised treatment			

in the thyroid gland. While FNA is of value in the diagnosis of papillary carcinoma, it is of little help in distinguishing follicular adenoma from follicular carcinoma, and the cytologic result is follicular neoplasia. The presence of capsular and/or vascular invasion in histology makes it a follicular carcinoma. The size of the tumour is not of the same importance as for papillary carcinoma, since even small follicular carcinomas can result in distant metastasis.

Hürtle cell carcinoma is a variant of follicular carcinoma. It is also referred to an oncocytic carcinoma. The cells are derived from follicular epithelium. The cells are large, containing abundant cytoplasm with small hyperchromatic nuclei. The cytoplasm turns pink on hematoxylin and eosin (H&E) staining and contains numerous mitochondria. Hürtle cells are believed to represent a common metaplastic change in damaged follicular epithelium. They are characteristically found in Hashimoto's disease, and, more importantly, may form neoplastic and non-neoplastic nodules.

Hürtle cell carcinoma in general has the same prognosis as has follicular carcinoma. Metastasis however usually does not take up iodine; thus metastatic Hürtle cell carcinoma has a worse prognosis than metastatic follicular carcinoma does.

Treatment

An overview of treatment options in relation to tumour stage is given in Table 8.8.3.

8.8.5.6.3 Medullary Thyroid Cancer

This cancer is derived from the parafollicular C cells and accounts for about 5–10% of all cancers of the thyroid gland. One interesting detail of this cancer is that it exists as a hereditary autosomal dominant trait, which that has been linked to a defect in chromosome 10. Family members are usually screened using the Ret/MTC oncogen. Screening was previously carried out using calcitonin after stimulation with pentagastrin.

Before any surgery pheochromocytomas must be excluded during workup because of high risk of hypertensive crisis with arrhythmias and perioperative death. Lymph node engagement (manifest and subclinical) is common (50%) bilaterally and in the mediastinum.

8.8.5.6.4 Anaplastic Thyroid Cancer

Anaplastic thyroid cancer is the most aggressive of all thyroid cancers. Although only 5% of all thyroid cancers are anaplastic, this cancer can hardly ever be cured; only very few survive longer than 1 year after diagnosis. Most patients with this cancer are elderly. The treatment is a combination of chemoradiotherapy and palliative surgery, mainly to keep the airway open.

8.8.5.7 Classification of Thyroid Carcinoma

Thyroid cancer can be staged in several different ways. The most common system is the TNM classification. T represents the tumour, N is regional lymph nodes and M is distant metastasis. Please note that this classification can only be used for carcinomas.

In Europe the UICC classification is the most common. The sixth edition (2002) has some changes for thyroid cancer:

T1	Tumour is ≤2 cm.
T2	Tumour is 2–4 cm.
T3	Tumour is >4 cm, or any tumour with minimal extrathyroid extension (sternothyroid muscle or perithyroid soft tissues)
T4a	Tumour extends beyond the thyroid capsule and invades any of the following: subcutaneous soft tissues, larynx, trachea, oesophagus, recurrent laryngeal nerve.

T4b	Tumour invades prevertebral fascia, mediastinal vessels, or encases the carotid artery.
T4a*	(Anaplastic carcinoma only) Tumour is limited to thyroid, surgically respectable.
T4b*	(Anaplastic carcinoma only) Tumour extends beyond the thyroid capsule, unresectable.

The changes regarding regional lymph nodes are:

NX	Regional lymph nodes cannot be assessed.
N0	No regional lymph nodes
N1	Regional lymph node metastasis
N1a	Metastasis in level VI
N1b	Metastasis in other levels
M0	No distant metastasis
M1	Distant metastasis

The combination of T and N gives stages I–IV.

Several systems can be used to evaluate the prognosis for a patient with cancer of the thyroid gland. In some cases the prognosis is good and in others poor. Remember that these systems refer to large groups of patients, and an individual with high stage or with poor scores may live a normal life and have a normal life span. A bad prognosis does not mean that the situation is hopeless.

One of the most commonly used systems has been proposed by EORTC (European Organisation for Research and Treatment of Cancer). This system has been criticised for making age a too-important criterion.

Other prognostic systems are the MACIS score (distant *m*etastasis, patient *a*ge, *c*ompleteness of resection, local *i*nvasion, and tumour *s*ize, only applicable for papillary cancer; Dr. Ian Hay, Mayo Clinic, Rochester, Minn.); and the Shaha score (follicular cancer only) that Ashok Shaha at The Memorial Sloan Kettering Hospital in New York, N.Y., has proposed.

These prognostic systems take into account the extent of primary tumour, M[+], histopathology and degree of differentiation, age and radical surgery. Differences in opinion between pathologists thus affect the results of the scoring systems. Sending specimens to specialised pathologists for second-opinion readings can help reduce this problem.

8.8.5.8 Treatment of Thyroid Carcinoma

If cytology is positive for cancer or there is suspicion of cancer (including follicular neoplasia) in the cytological specimens, then surgery should be carried out (Fig. 8.8.3).

Surgery is also recommended for cysts larger than 4 cm due to a higher-than-normal frequency of malignancy. Goitres compressing the windpipe or oesophagus are also candidates for surgery.

Surgery is usually the first-line treatment for malignancies of the thyroid gland. The most common operation is a total thyroidectomy (the entire thyroid is removed). The exception is small papillary tumours, where hemithyroidectomy is probably the best surgical treatment for females under 45 years of age. Postoperative radioiodine therapy is given to all patients with a follicular cancer and to patients with large papillary cancers.

External beam radiation is only given to nonradically operated patients or T4 tumours.

8.8.5.8.1 Surgical Technique

Surgical treatment requires meticulous dissection using bipolar cautery, surgical loupes with headlight, or microscope. The recurrent laryngeal nerves must be identified and saved if not invaded by cancer. When dissecting the cranial pole and the superior thyroid artery, it is imperative not to injure the superior laryngeal nerve. The parathyroid glands, responsible for the regulation of calcium, must be identified and saved with intact blood supply or autotransplanted, diced into 1-mm slices or cubes to suture to marked pockets in the sternocleidomastoid muscle. Frozen sections should be obtained from the parathyroid glands to confirm that the tissue is indeed from the parathyroid gland and without any signs of cancer infiltration.

A suspicious node is also sent for frozen section and if positive, a modified selective neck dissection is performed. The external jugular vein should be followed in the neck, and all enlarged nodes should be removed. This should be carried out bilaterally. If the cancer is small, then a lobectomy and isthmusectomy might be sufficient in papillary cancer. If the tumour is a medullary cancer, then the upper part of the mediastinum should be examined because metastasis to the mediastinum will be found in approximately 50% of the cases.

In benign retrosternal goitre, the blood supply from the superior and inferior thyroid arteries is usually accessible in the neck. If the upper pole, the strap muscles and the isthmus are all divided, then there will be better space for gentle finger dissection and traction of the retrosternal part of the gland. If there is suspicion of malignancy, then the surgeon should be prepared to perform a sternal split for better access.

Anaplastic thyroid cancer is treated with chemotherapy (usually Adriamycin), external radiation therapy and palliative surgery with tumour debulking to reduce breathing difficulties and problems with swallowing. Most patients will succumb within a year, due to distant metastasis.

Algorithm for solitary, palpable thyroid nodule in an euthyroid patient. (normal TSH)   **Fig. 8.8.3** Diagnostic strategy

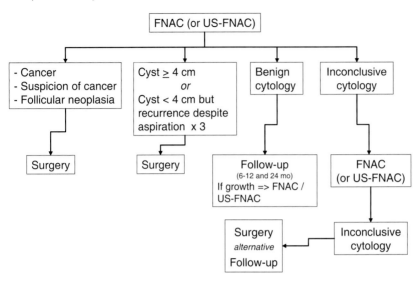

Algorithm for multinodular goitre

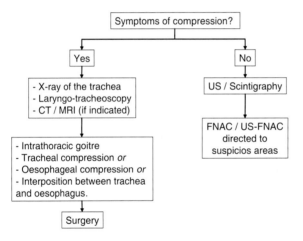

8.8.5.8.2 Complications

Paralysis of a vocal cord should not occur in more than 1–3% of all surgical cases with the exception of cases where the nerve or parathyroid glands are embedded in the tumour. Bilateral paralysis of the vocal cords causes acute respiratory stridor, and the situation might call for reintubation and a temporary laterofixation.

A speech pathologist should evaluate patients with paralysis of a vocal cord. Voice exercises may significantly improve voice quality. If both vocal cords are paralytic, then the patient might require a tracheotomy. Paralysis may be temporary if the nerve (or nerves) has not been severed intentionally in order to remove the tumour. Permanent surgery (e.g. vocal cord laterofixation) may be

considered after about 1 year. Good breathing will improve voice quality.

The SLN may be damaged during surgery and will cause voice quality problems (reduced tone and pitch, a disaster for a singer). The findings at laryngoscopy after damage to the external branch of the SLN are not as obvious as after RLN palsy. Such damage produces changes, manifested by lower voice pitch, range and fatigability.

The most serious complication is postoperative airway obstruction due to laryngeal oedema. It can rapidly be life threatening and is usually caused by postoperative bleeding with wound haematoma. It requires immediate action, with reintubation (if possible) and opening of the wound with evacuation of the haematoma. If intubation is not possible, then access to the trachea can be gained by the opened wound.

Postoperative hypocalcemia is not uncommon, and reported in between 7 and 25% of cases. Most cases are usually asymptomatic. Patients operated on for total or subtotal thyroidectomy should be monitored every 6–8 h in the immediate postoperative period, either with albumin and serum calcium or with ionised calcium levels. Nadir should be seen within 72 h. Mild hypocalcemia can be treated with oral calcium supplementation, for depletion more severe, with calcium glubionate intravenous. Permanent hypoparathyroidism is uncommon, and it requires treatment with vitamin D and a consultation of an endocrinologist.

8.8.5.8.3 Follow-Up

The rational for follow-up after treatment of differentiated thyroid carcinoma is threefold. Thyroid-hormone-suppression therapy with T_4 needs to be monitored, and in cases with postoperative hypoparathyroidism, Ca^{2+} metabolism and its medical treatment need to be followed. Thyroid carcinoma requires lifelong follow-up.

Signs of recurrence should be sought and identified with clinical examination, US of the neck and serum S-thyroglobulin level measurement if a total thyroidectomy has been performed. If the S-thyroglobulin level is rising, then a ^{131}I whole-body scan is indicated and can be done directly after Thyrogen injection without cessation of T_4 by the patient. Thirdly the patient treated for a malignant disease mostly needs psychological support. It is well known that patients successfully treated for malignant disease might develop anxiety and/or depression postoperatively.

Patients treated for papillary or follicular carcinoma should be followed lifelong; when a 20-year-old patient becomes 60 years old, the risk of recurrence is multifold, which has been seen in long–follow-up series. The first year, the patient should be seen three to four times, two times the second and third year, and then yearly. A chest X-ray is recommended yearly the first 3 years, then year 5 for papillary carcinomas and every second to third year for follicular carcinoma. Thyroglobulin (in patients operated with a total thyroidectomy) and TSH should be monitored yearly up to 10 years, and then with increasing intervals lifelong.

Patients operated with a hemithyroidectomy for benign disease should have their TSH and T_4/T_3 checked after 3 months and again after 6 months. However if there is histopathological signs of chronic Hashimoto's thyroiditis, consideration of T_4 substitution should be given more weight.

If there is a rise in TSH, then the patient should have T_4 substitution. If TSH/T_4 is normal, then the patient should be informed about signs of hypothyroidism and recommended to contact his or her general practitioner if hypofunction is suspected.

Head and Neck Tumors

Edited by Matti Anniko

9.1 Cysts and Benign Tumours of the Neck

MATTI ANNIKO

9.1.1 Congenital Disorders

The most common congenital lesions are medial (thyroglossal) and lateral (branchial) cysts and fistulae. In addition, haemangiomas, lymphangiomas and dermoid cysts can occur. Congenital malformations of the neck are comparatively rare and present as neck masses that typically present in the two first decades of life.

Fistulae and cysts of thyroglossal origin are also known as thyroglossal duct/tract remnants, and median neck cysts/fistulae. Those of branchial origin are referred to as branchial cleft cysts/sinuses/fistulae.

9.1.1.1 Definition/Aetiology/Histology

Branchial cleft cysts and fistulae are classified as first, second, third and fourth branchial cleft abnormalities, although the second branchial cleft cyst/fistula is the most common.

The first branchial cleft cyst/fistula is located either in the preauricular region usually anterior to the pinna, or posterior to or inferior to the angle of the mandible.

The second branchial cleft cyst or its opening is found along the anterior border of the sternocleidomastoid muscle.

A third branchial cleft cyst is very rare, but also appears along the anterior border of the sternocleidomastoid muscle. The tract passes laterally to the common carotid artery, posteriorly to the internal carotid artery and deviates medially, and finally opens (reaches) at the pyriform sinus.

A fourth branchial cleft cyst/fistula is extremely rare and has very complex anatomy. It begins at the apex of the pyriform sinus and exits the pharynx caudally to the superior laryngeal nerve, the cricothyroid muscle and the thyroid cartilage. These fistulae open to the skin anteriorly to the lower portion of the sternocleidomastoid muscle. Usually these fistulae can never be excised totally. The opening from the pyriform sinus is designed to seal further connections outside the pharynx.

Cysts may occur in any location along the path of sinuses and fistulae associated with all four branchial cleft anomalies:

- Median neck cysts/fistulae are infrahyoidal remnants of the thyroglossal duct apparatus, which normally obliterates by the end of the eighth embryonic week and become completely reabsorbed. Its site of origin persists as the foramen caecum at the base of the tongue. Although they can be situated anywhere along the midline from the foramen caecum to the suprasternal region, the majority occur in the proximity of the hyoid bone. The most common presentation of the thyroglossal duct cyst is an upper midline (fluctuating) cervical mass that occurs during the first decade of life. Roughly 75% of cases present during the first 5 years of life, with equal distribution between sexes. Fistulae – if occurring – manifest early in infancy as draining dimples, which will retract during swallowing.
  Histopathologically, the majority of specimens demonstrate squamous or respiratory columnar epithelium. Up to 20% of the lesions have been reported to contain thyroid tissue.
- Lateral neck cysts/fistulae arise from remnants of the second, third and fourth branchial arches. They can be connected with the ipsilateral tonsil. Clinically, branchial cysts/fistulae are usually located at the superior–anterior margin of the sternocleidomastoid muscle (upper neck triangle). Most branchial cysts are found in older children and adults as a fluctuating neck mass. There is no gender or laterality predominance. Bilateral presentation is rare.
- Histopathologically, branchial cysts characteristically appear as stratified squamous and/or a mixture of squamous and respiratory epithelium with lymphoid follicles.

9.1.1.2 Symptoms

- Median neck cysts/fistulae
  - Recurrent supralaryngeal cystic swelling, 1 to 3 cm in size, painless and non-tender. Depending on the size, protrusion of the tongue is possible.
  - Approximately 10–15% demonstrate infection (reddening, pain) (Fig. 9.1.1).
  - Fistula formation (pus drainage) is only present after infection of the cyst and maceration of the lin-

ing skin, since there is no normal communication of the thyroglossal duct tract to the skin during development.

- Lateral neck cysts/fistulae
  - Bothersome, well-visible tumour, often of changing size and feelings of pressure (Fig. 9.1.2).
  - Bacterial infection (from the tonsil) is common, causing pain, abscess or phlegmon formation. After diagnostic puncture, a persistent fistula may occur.

9.1.1.3   Complications

- Median neck cysts/fistulae
  - Abscess formation, large cysts at the base of the tongue may cause dyspnoea, dysphagia or even sore throat symptoms.
- Lateral neck cysts/fistulae
  - Abscess, infiltrating phlegmons involving jugular vein
- In patients older than 40 years, malignant transformation of branchial cleft cysts is possible (the so-called branchiogenic carcinoma; see Sect. 9.7).

9.1.1.4   Diagnosis: Recommended European Standard

- Inspection
  - Colour
  - Size
  - Is skin maceration present?
- Palpation
  - Bimanual palpation of the floor of the mouth and tongue (in cases of median cysts/fistulae)
  - Bimanual palpation of the lateral neck cyst together with the ipsilateral tonsil: is there a common mobility?
  - Is it hard? Inflexible? Mobile? Fluctuating?
- If a fistula, explore the fistula by using a silver probe.
- Hypopharyngo-laryngoscopy is used to identify the foramen caecum.
- Ultrasound
  - Is the tumour solid or fluid filled?
- Fine-needle aspiration cytology

9.1.1.5   Additional/Useful Diagnostic Procedures

- Fine-needle aspiration cytology
- X-ray after filling of the fistula with contrast (in thyroglossal fistulae)
- Contrast MRI (in branchial cleft cysts)
- Scintigraphy if an ectopic thyroid is suspected

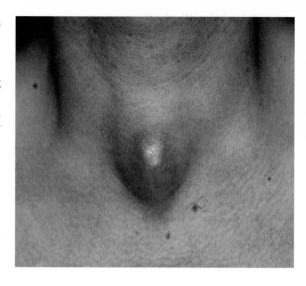

Fig. 9.1.1 Infected thyroglossal cyst located in the midline. Overlying skin is macerated, and there is a risk for spontaneous rupture of the abscess. (Photo courtesy of Prof. W. Arnold, Technical University of Munich, Germany)

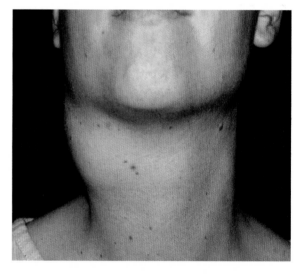

Fig. 9.1.2 Branchial cyst from the second cleft. Swelling is obvious in the upper half of the right side of the neck, with the major mass along the anterior margin of the sternocleidomastoid muscle. (Photo courtesy of Prof. W. Arnold, Technical University of Munich, Germany)

9.1.1.6   Differential Diagnosis

The physician must first consider the patient's age group. Within each group, the incidence of congenital, inflammatory and neoplastic disease must be considered. Paediatric patients generally exhibit inflammatory disease and congenital neck masses more often than they do neoplastic masses. In contrast, in older adults neoplastic disease should be the first consideration, with less emphasis on inflammatory or congenital masses. Young adults fall somewhere between these two groups.

- Median neck cyst/fistulae
  - Lymph node
  - Dermoid cyst
  - Thyroid tissue
- Lateral neck cysts/fistulae
- Unspecific or specific lymphadenopathy
- Metastatic carcinoma in cervical lymph nodes
- Malignant lymphoma
- Paraganglioma
- Haemangioma
- Lymphangioma
- Dermoid cyst
- Laryngocele

9.1.1.7 Treatment: Recommended European Standard

The definitive therapy for branchial anomalies is complete surgical excision. Injection of sclerosing solutions should not be performed except for fourth branchial cleft fistulae.

- Median cyst or fistula
  - Surgical removal
    - It is important to follow the epithelial trunk up to the hyoid bone. At least the central part of the hyoid bone must be removed. If the epithelial trunk continues cranially, it must be followed up to the tongue base.
- Lateral neck cyst or fistula
  - Should be removed at initial diagnosis, since repeated infections make later surgery more difficult
    - The epithelial tract passes superiorly and laterally to the common carotid artery, whereafter the tract turns medially between the internal and external branches. The tract ends close to the middle constrictor muscle, or can have an internal opening in the tonsillar fossa. The cyst and the entire fistula must be resected up to the tonsillar region to avoid recurrences. If the patient is over 40 years of age, tonsillectomy is recommended because of the high risk for tonsillar carcinoma with metastatic spread.

9.1.1.8 Prognosis

- Median neck cyst and fistula
  - If completely removed, the patient is considered cured. If the middle portion of the hyoid bone in not resected, recurrence will usually happen. All

cysts and tracts must be examined histopathologically for rare instances of concomitant neoplastic disease, especially if the patient has received prior neck irradiation.

- Lateral neck cyst or fistula
  - Surgical removal usually cures the patient. However, if surgery is not radical with complete removal of the cyst or fistula, there is a high incidence of recurrence.
- With increasing age, one has to consider malignancy (cystic metastases) as an increasingly important differential diagnosis of a lump in the neck; this makes the surgical excision even more relevant. In some international reports, up to 25% or all "branchial cysts" have been reported to be histopathologically malignant in individuals older than 40 years of age. A malignant transformation of a lateral branchial cyst itself is extremely unusual, and only a few cases have been reported in the international literature.

9.1.2 Vascular Anomalies

9.1.2.1 Haemangiomas

A haemangioma is the most common vascular tumour in children. Histopathologically, haemangiomas are benign but show proliferation of endothelial cells and mitoses. Around 85% of all infantile haemangiomas manifest themselves in the first few weeks of life. The life cycle for such a lesion has three phases: proliferative (rapid growth from 2 weeks to 1 year), involuting (slow regression from 1 to 7 years) and involuted (complete regression after 8 years of age). Approximately 50% of infantile haemangiomas are completely resolved by 5 years of age, and 70% by 7 years of age.

A haemangioma presents as a skin lesion or cystic mass. A change in size is noticeable when the child strains or cries. The lesion is compressible, and causes surrounding skin to appear bluish.

This tumour is diagnosed with MRA. A CT is not always characteristic. Fine-needle cytology confirms the diagnosis.

Treatment is indicated if there occurs pressure of the haemangioma on adjacent structures, for instance, nose, around the eyes or in the subglottic area. In addition, cosmetic considerations are important. Interventional radiology with sclerosing agents can be helpful preoperatively. Systemic steroid therapy has been tried, with varying rates of success.

9.1.2.2   Lymphangiomas (Cystic Hygromas)

Lymphangiomas, or cystic hygromas, are congenital malformation of lymphatic channels. The majority of these lesions occur in the neck. They are regarded as developmental anomalies of the jugular lymphatic sac. Lymphangiomas are classified into three types: lymphangioma simplex (capillary-sized, thin-walled lymphatics), cavernous lymphangioma (dilated lymphatic spaces) and cystic hygroma (lymphatic cysts ranging from a few millimetres to several centimetres in diameter).

Lymphangiomas manifest themselves in the same way as haemangiomas do, but can become very extensive and infiltrate the soft tissues of the neck and oral cavity (Fig. 9.1.3). Lymphatic malformations are usually present in infancy, with 90% being detected before 2 years of age.

Diagnosis is by way of clinical examination, ultrasound, CT scan and/or MRI. Fine-needle cytology is utilised to confirm the diagnosis.

Throughout the decades, therapy has included surgical resection, sclerotherapy, incision and drainage, aspiration and radiation therapy. When complete surgical excision is possible, it is a legitimate option, although recurrences can occur. If possible, surgery should be postponed until the child is 3–4 years old. However, if symptoms of compression appear or the child suffers recurrent infections, surgery may be indicated at an earlier age.

9.1.2.3   Vascular Malformations

These benign vascular tumours have normal histopathological endothelium but an altered vascular morphogenesis. The malformation can be capillary, arterial, venous, lymphatic or a mixture of these manifestations.

A multidisciplinary approach is needed for optimal treatment (otorhinolaryngology–head and neck surgery, dermatology, radiology, paediatrics). During recent years, an interventional radiology approach with embolisation and sclerosing has been more successful than were many earlier techniques.

9.1.3   Infections

9.1.3.1   Lymphadenopathy

9.1.3.1.1   Acute Infections

Infections with bacteria and/or viruses initially cause a reaction in Waldeyer's ring of the oropharynx and as the next step, an involvement of the upper jugular lymph nodes. If the infection is initially restricted to the teeth or oral cavity, submental and submandibular lymph nodes become involved. Severe infections can induce abscesses

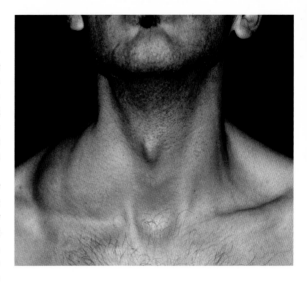

Fig. 9.1.3 Lymphangioma in the right side of the neck (supraclavicular area). (Photo courtesy of Prof. W. Arnold, Technical University of Munich, Germany)

in lymph nodes. Treatment of bacterial infections is with antibiotics.

One has to consider the risk for development of phlegmon of the mouth floor, with possible further complications such as trismus and breathing difficulties because of swelling of the pharynx.

9.1.3.1.2   Chronic Lymph Node Disease

Chronic lymph node disease is caused by both bacteria and viruses. One has to consider toxoplasmosis, tularaemia, brucellosis and sarcoidosis. The most common causes for chronic lymph node disease are nowadays due to atypical mycobacteria, *Mycobacterium tuberculosis* and HIV.

Fine-needle aspiration can aid in diagnosis. If this is not conclusive, the entire lymph node should be removed.

Atypical Mycobacteria

Atypical mycobacteria are found in children who have not received vaccination against tuberculosis. Atypical mycobacteria are resistant to antibiotics and chemotherapeutics. The clinical entity is very characteristic, presenting as an enlarged lymph node and eventually fixation of it to the overlying skin, which can become inflamed. Sometimes, spontaneous fistulation takes place. The treatment is to excise the lymph node (at times including some overlying skin) or to perform curettage to remove the infected tissue.

Tuberculosis

M. tuberculosis infection of the head and neck is relatively rare. Neck involvement often occurs simultaneously with pulmonary disease. These affected lymph nodes can be found anywhere along the jugular lymph node chain, but usually are along its caudal region and the posterior fossa. The tonsils can be the primary route of entry. Generally, diagnosis is confirmed by fine-needle aspiration, although an open lymph node extirpation might be necessary. A pulmonary X-ray is essential. Further handling is outside the scope of otorhinolaryngology–head and neck surgery.

Submandibular Abscess

A submandibular abscess is also known as Ludwig's angina. The infection is anatomically located between the floor of mouth and hyoid bone, where the superficial neck fascia is fastened inferiorly. Patients experience considerable swelling of the submandibular region, high fever, dysphagia and at time, trismus. The abscess must be drained by incision, and further antibiotic treatment is necessary. The origin of the abscess is often dental, which must be treated by a dentist. Further details are given in Sect. 5.1.

Parapharyngeal Abscess

A parapharyngeal abscess originates from the tonsils, peritonsilar region or near the molars in the mandible. The infection spreads downwards between the deep and middle fascia of the neck, towards the pyriform sinus. Thus, it is not a peritonsilar abscess. Patients have trouble with swallowing, and the abscess can mimic an upper-airway obstruction including trismus. Treatment is by surgical incision, drainage and antibiotics. Further details are given in Sect. 5.1.

Retropharyngeal Abscess

A retropharyngeal abscess generally originates in the parapharyngeal region, but instead of continuing into the parapharyngeal space, it spreads into its neighbouring area – the retropharyngeal space – and then proceeds downwards into the mediastinum. Treatment is surgical drainage and antibiotics. Further details are given in Sect. 5.1.

Cervical Necrotising Fasciitis

Cervical necrotising fasciitis is a very serious infection, with its origin in the oral–pharynx region. The infection tends to spread to all fasciae and muscle tissues in the neck. The morbidity and mortality of this disease can be quite high. The treatment needs a rapid intervention – within hours if possible – with antibiotics and surgical excision of infected tissues and opening of all fasciae for decompression. Hyperbaric oxygen treatment is a valuable complementary tool, if available.

Diagnostic procedures for these infections include:
- Clinical examination
- Peripheral blood smear including sedimentation rate
- Bacterial culture from infected area (nasopharynx or tonsils may be the entry route)
- Specific serologic tests (depending on type of infection suspected)
- Ultrasound investigation
- Fine-needle aspiration for cytology
- Excisional biopsy of lymph node (if other procedures failed to give diagnosis)
- Blood culture (if symptoms of sepsis)

9.1.4 Primary Tumours of the Neck

9.1.4.1 Peripheral Nerve Neoplasms

Peripheral nerve neoplasms are known as neurofibromas, fibrogliomas, neuromas, neurilemomas, schwannomas and von Recklinghausen's disease.

These tumours originate from neural crest cells, which differentiate either into Schwann cells or into sympathicoblasts. The former gives rise to neurofibromas and schwannomas, whereas sympathicoblasts can develop into paragangliomas (chemodectomas). Traumatic neuromas represent an abnormal attempt by an injured nerve to regenerate, and histologically show proliferation of entangled endoneural and peripheral tissue, Schwann cells and regenerating axons.

Neurofibromas frequently occur in multiple locations; they are not limited to the neck region. The most recognized condition is von Recklinghausen's disease, with multiple manifestations in the body, including the skull base and spinal cord.

Schwannomas are usually benign, although malignant transformation has been known to occur. The lesion is situated along a peripheral nerve. Such tumours can be painful, and the best treatment is excision. Most schwannomas of the neck originate from the vagal nerve.

Von Recklinghausen's disease (neurofibromatosis) is a variant of neurofibromas with café au lait spots and multiple neurofibromas. This disease is an autosomal dominant one, with variable penetrance. It may be associated with other neurologic abnormalities or developmental anomalies such as glioma and spina bifida.

These tumours most commonly appear as a mass in the lateral neck. Pain and neurologic dysfunctions are rare. Fine-needle aspiration is of help, but the diagnosis is mainly established histologically when the neck mass is removed. MRI or CT scan imaging delineates the lesion.

If possible, the tumour – diagnosis is primarily by fine-needle aspiration – should be surgically removed, but with an attempt to preserve the integrity of the nerve

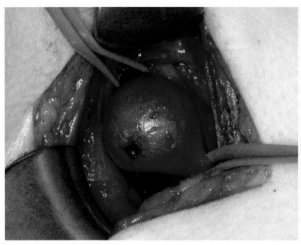 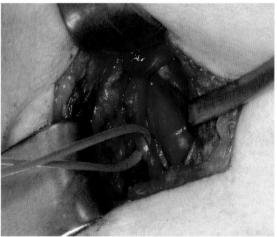

Fig. 9.1.4 Vagal neurinoma of the left side. The solid tumour is removed without damaging the vagal nerve, which is embraced by the vessel loop. (Photo courtesy of Prof. W. Arnold, Technical University of Munich, Germany)

origin (Fig. 9.1.4). Since approximately 10% of all cases become malignant (developing into sarcomas), debulking is also of value. As most Schwannomas originate from the vagal nerve, surgical excision may cause palsy of the vocal cord of the same side.

9.1.4.2 Paragangliomas

Paragangliomas are composed of cells (chemoreceptors) sensitive to pH changes in the blood, as well as to oxygen and carbon dioxide concentrations. Such cells are distributed in many areas of the head and neck region: carotid bifurcation, along the vagal nerve, in the larynx and the temporal bone, amongst others. According to international literature, multiple localizations occur in the neck in 15–20% of cases. Approximately 3% of all paragangliomas originate from the vagal nerve. Carotid paragangliomas arise from the carotid body located near the bifurcation of the common carotid artery. In older literature, many of these tumours were reported hormonally active, producing cathecholamines, whilst literature more recent does not support this assumption to the same degree.

Peripheral nerve tumours are benign and non-painful neck masses. However, malignancies have been reported in 5–8% of cases, and these tumours can give rise to metastases spread haematologically.

Under most circumstances, the otolaryngologist–head and neck surgeon can make an appropriate differential diagnosis quickly, based on patient history and clinical examination.

The paraganglioma tissue is very well vascularized. Diagnosis can be clinically suspected by its classical localization in the carotid bifurcation and is later confirmed by MRA (Fig. 9.1.5). Fine-needle aspiration can be difficult to interpret but can support the clinical findings.

Treatment is by surgery in most cases. A preoperative embolisation significantly reduces surgical blood loss. In elderly patients (older than 70 years of age), in lieu of primary surgery, yearly follow-ups are the accepted treatment.

9.1.4.3 Lipomas

A lipoma is benign, encapsulated, subcutaneous collection of adipose tissue. It is unclear if this lesion represents a true benign neoplasm, malformation or hyperplasia of adipose tissue. In general, lipomas are non-infiltrating and rarely recur even after enucleation. However, it can be difficult, even histopathologically, to separate a very unusual low-grade malignant liposarcoma from a benign lipoma.

A lipoma occurs as an asymptomatic slowly growing mass movable against the overlying skin, soft and often lobulated. It is unusual in the neck region. Palpation gives the clinical diagnosis. Sometimes ultrasound can be used but is not necessary.

The clinical diagnosis can be confirmed by fine-needle aspiration for cytology and – if extensive – by MRI of the neck.

A special variant of lipoma is Madelung's disease, characterized by excessive accumulation of fat in the neck (Fig. 9.1.6). Excess fat is seen predominantly in the posterior part of the neck, under the trapezius and sternocleidomastoid muscles, in the supraclavicular fossa and/or the anterior part of the neck (supra- or infrahyoid regions). Even the superior mediastinum and the prevertebral space can be involved in such an accumulation.

Treatment consists of surgical removal if the lipoma interferes with aesthetics or function.

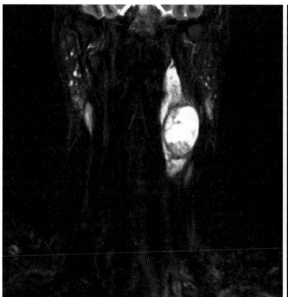
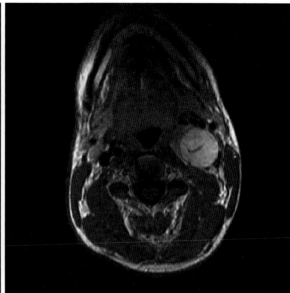

Fig. 9.1.5 MRA of the neck showing a paraganglioma located at the carotid bifurcation

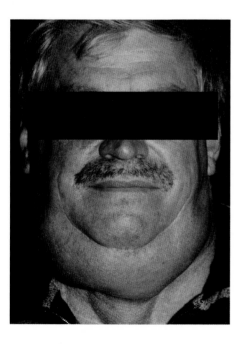

Fig. 9.1.6 Massive infiltration of the neck by fat (Madelung's disease). (Photo courtesy of Prof. W. Arnold, Technical University of Munich, Germany)

Suggested Reading

Acierno SP, Waldhausen JH (2007) Congenital cervical cysts, sinuses and fistulae. Otolaryngol Clin North Am 40:161–176

Ahuja AT, King AD, Chan ES, Kew J, Lam WW, Sun PM, King W et al (1998) Madelung disease: distribution of cervical fat and preoperative findings at sonography, MR, and CT. AJNR Am J Neuroradiol 19:707–710

Bauland CG, Smit JM, Ketelaars R, Rieu PN, Spauwen PH (2008) Management of hemangiomas of infancy: a retrospective analysis and treatment protocol. Scand J Plast Reconstr Surg 42:86–91

Boedeker CC, Ridder GJ, Schipper J (2005) Paragangliomas of the head and neck: diagnosis and treatment. Fam Cancer 4:55–59

Caccamese JF, Coletti DP (2008) Deep neck infections: clinical considerations in aggressive disease. Oral Maxillofac Surg Clin North Am 20:367–380

Choi SS, Zalzal GH (1995) Branchial anomalies: a review of 52 cases. Laryngoscope 105:909–913

Erickson D, Kudva YC, Ebersold MJ, Thompson GB, Grant CS, van Heerden JA, Young WF Jr (2001) Benign paragangliomas: clinical presentation and treatment outcomes in 236 patients. J Clin Endocriol Metab 86:5210–5216

Fihman V, Raskine L, Petitpas F, Mateo J et al (2008) Cervical necrotizing fasciitis: 8-year's experience of microbiology. Eur J Clin Microbiol Infect Dis 27:691–695

Kang GC, Song C (2008) Forty-one cervicofacial vascular anomalies and their surgical treatment: retrospection and review. Ann Acad Med Singapore 37:165–179

Kohut MP, Hansen M, Pribaz JJ, Mulliken JB (1998) Arteriovenous malformations of the head and neck: natural history and management. Plast Reconstr Surg 102:643–654

Lin ST, Tseng FY, Hsu CJ, Yeh TH, Chen YS (2008) Thyroglossal duct cyst: a comparison between children and adults. Am J Otolaryngol 29:83–87

Luna-Ortiz K, Rascon-Ortiz M, Villavicencio-Valencia V, Granados-Garcia M, Herrera-Gomez A (2005) Carotid body tumours: review of a 20-year experience. Oral Oncol 41:56–61

MacArthur CJ (2006) Head and neck hemangiomas of infancy. Curr Opin Otolaryngol Head Neck Surg 14:397–405

Metry D (2004) Update on hemangiomas of infancy. Curr Opin Pediatr 16:373–377

Mondin V, Ferlito A, Muzzi E, Silver CE, Fagan JJ, Devaney KO, Rinaldo A (2008) Thyroglossal duct cyst: Personal experience and literature review. Auris Nasus Larynx 35:11–25

Myssiorek D, Ferlito A, Silver CE, Rodrigo JP, Baysal BE, Fagan JJ, Súarez C et al (2008) Screening for familial paragangliomas. Oral Oncol 44:532–537

Ozcan C, Görür K, Talas D, Aydin O (2005) Intramuscular benign lipoma of the sternocleidomastoid muscle: a rare cause of neck mass. Eur Arch Otorhinolaryngol 262:148–150

Schroeder JW Jr, Mohyuddin N, Maddalozzo J (2007) Branchial anomalies in the pediatric population. Otolaryngol Head Neck Surg 137:289–295

Young WF Jr (2006) Paragangliomas: clinical overview. Ann NY Acad Sci 1073:21–29

9.2 Malignant Tumours of the Neck

MATTI ANNIKO

9.2.1 Definition

Most neck masses in adults – except for thyroid cancer – are metastatic squamous cell carcinomas located in lymph nodes, with their primary origin the regional aerodigestive tract. In contrast, most cervical masses in the paediatric population are nonmalignant.

- Malignant tumours of the neck
  - Primary neck lesions
    - Lymphoma
    - Sarcoma
    - Salivary gland carcinoma
      - Adenocarcinoma
    - Thyroid carcinoma
      - Papillary adenocarcinoma
      - Follicular carcinoma
      - Hürthle cell tumour
      - Medullary carcinoma
      - Anaplastic carcinoma
    - Parathyroid carcinoma
    - Branchial cleft cyst carcinoma
      - Squamous cell carcinoma
    - Thyroglossal duct cyst carcinoma
      - Squamous cell carcinoma
    - Cutaneous malignancies
      - Squamous cell carcinoma
      - Basal cell carcinoma
      - Malignant melanoma
    - Metastatic disease
    - From head and neck area
    - Of infraclavicular origin
      - Lung
      - Kidney
      - Prostate
      - Stomach
      - Breast
      - Gonad

9.2.2 Diagnosis

The critical distinction is between metastatic squamous cell carcinoma and other masses.

Fine-needle aspiration cytology is generally a valuable diagnostic tool. Fine-needle aspiration cytology is, however, inadequate for definitive diagnosis and subcategorisation of lymphomas, which must be diagnosed via excisional nodal biopsy.

Thick-needle biopsy (to obtain material for histopathology) can be helpful for classification of a malignancy; it is usually not needed for cervical lesions, but rather for the base of the tongue, larynx and the pyriform sinus.

Further investigation of the neck is done with MRI, PET-CT or CT. These imaging techniques often also reveal involvement of nodes that are not readily palpable, e.g. the retropharyngeal nodes (see Chap. 9, Sect. 9.3).

- Diagnostic procedures
  - Recommended European standard
    - Clinical examination (can be repeated – most important)
    - Endoscopy and biopsy (often used for CUP syndrome and for search of second primary occult tumours (see Chap. 9, Sect. 9.7)
    - Ultrasound examination (differentiates solid from cystic masses – very useful in congenital and developmental lesions)
    - CT, MRI, MRA (if involvement of the CCA or ICA is suspected) or PET-CT
    - Chest radiograph
    - Sentinel node imaging (its value regarding head and neck cancer is still under evaluation)
    - Fine-needle aspiration cytology (initial diagnostic procedure; experienced cytopathologist needed)
    - Thick-needle biopsy for histopathology (limited indications)
    - Open biopsy (performed only after workup is completed and if a diagnosis is not evident; a "guided" biopsy may be needed in the nasopharynx, base of the tongue, pyriform sinus or tonsils [tonsillectomy])

- Excision biopsy (needed for lymphomas; otherwise, often combined with frozen sections and continued with some type of neck dissection)

9.2.3 Primary Site

The spread of head and neck carcinoma is similar to that of inflammatory disease, generally following an orderly, lymphatic pattern. The probability of lymphatic spread of squamous cell carcinoma in the head and neck area is related to the abundance of capillary lymphatics in the given primary site. The densest capillary networks of lymphatics are found in the nasopharynx, tongue and hypopharynx. Thus, the rate of metastases from these sites is high. In contrast, the larynx and paranasal sinuses have a sparse lymphatic network and therefore, a lower rate of metastases.

Patients with metastases in multiple cervical lymph nodes (more than four) located at different levels in the neck, particularly in the lower neck, and with extracapsular spread are the most likely to develop systemic disease.

Current investigations suggest a strong correlation between tumour thickness and regional node involvement. So far, this has been evaluated only for oral cavity tumours. Lesions less than 1.5-mm thick developed cervical metastases in less than 2% of cases, whereas the incidence increased to 33% for lesions 1.5- to 3.5-mm thick, and further increased to around 60% for lesions more than 3.5 mm in thickness. Thus, an oral carcinoma classified as T2 but with a thickness of 2 mm should be of less concern than should a T1 carcinoma with a thickness of 10 mm. The issue of tumour thickness and depth of invasion demonstrates a significant weakness of our current staging system for primary tumours.

9.2.4 Bilateral Spread of Squamous Cell Carcinoma

Lesions in the midline area (base of the tongue, posterior pharyngeal wall, supraglottic larynx) tend to metastasise, with a higher incidence of bilateral spread than do lesions in well-lateralised primary sites (e.g. lateral tongue), with mainly an ipsilateral spread. However, surgery and radiation can alter lymphatic flow.

9.2.5 Treatment

See Chap. 9, Sects. 9.5, 9.6 and 9.7.

9.3 Malignant Lymphomas in the Ear, Nose and Throat Area

ANNA LAURELL

9.3.1 Definition

Malignant lymphomas arise from the lymphatic system, which is widespread, mobile tissue with complex maturation. The precursor cells are located in the bone marrow, and the lymphoid stem cells differentiate into two distinct lymphatic lineages of T- and B-cell types, respectively. Lymphomas arise from both lineages, but not at all in proportion to their respective masses, and with large differences in incidence in children and adults, and in the Western countries in contrast to Asia and Latin America.

9.3.2 Incidence

The incidence of lymphoma varies in different parts of the world, but is approximately in seventh place in order of malignancies in the Western world. Large differences in lymphoma subtype occur in different parts of the world, and in also in children as compared with adults. In adults, 85% of the lymphomas are of B-cell derivation and 15% of T-cell origin worldwide, but in the Western countries, the proportion of mature T-cell lymphomas is only 5% [3]. In Asia and Latin America, conversely, certain subtypes of T-cell lymphomas account for a relatively higher proportion than do T-cell lymphomas. The absolute majority of T-cell lymphomas in adults are of a mature, peripheral type and portend a generally much worse prognosis than do the B-cell lymphomas [4].

In children, the situation is markedly different than it is in adults. Children have high prevalence of immature precursor T- and B-cell lymphomas/leukemias and Burkitt's lymphoma, whereas anaplastic large-cell lymphoma and Hodgkin's lymphoma are the major lymphomas for mature groups. Indolent B-cell lymphomas and peripheral T-cell lymphomas are rare in children [5].

9.3.3 Aetiology

The different B-cell lymphomas are thought to correspond to different stages in B-cell differentiation. The naïve B cells migrate from the bone marrow and home to nodal and extranodal areas, directed by homing receptors in the tissue. Maturation takes place in the germinal centres of the lymph nodes and the extralymphatic areas after antigenic encounter, and then recirculation occurs, which results in widespread disease in many lymphomas. Less is known of the intricate T-cell differentiation and trafficking, and since these diseases are comparatively rarer, knowledge regarding them is sparse. The WHO's 2008 classification of malignant lymphomas comprises a large number of subgroups, all defined by morphological, immunological and genetic markers, and the classification is used worldwide [6].

9.3.4 Diagnostic Biopsy

The ear, nose and throat (ENT) area is a common site of presentation in malignant lymphomas, accounting for about a third to half of all diagnostic biopsies. The area has dense and well-developed lymphatic tissue, and the presence of a tumour is easily detected in the head and neck region. The extranodal lymphatic areas of the upper aerodigestive tract are frequently involved with lymphoma, and next to the gastrointestinal region, they are the second most common site of localised extranodal presentation.

A lymphoma should be suspected in the case of a non-tender, enlarged lymph node without signs of infection. Mononucleosis in young adults can give rise to menacing lymphoid hyperplasia, and this should always be borne in mind and excluded by EBV serology. Reactive nodes can easily be identified with fine-needle biopsy supported with flow cytometry to show B polyclonality. However, Hodgkin's lymphoma is common in adolescence and notoriously difficult to diagnose with a fine-needle aspirate. The gold standard diagnostic procedure for all lymphomas is a knife biopsy. This method should ensure enough collection of material for the extensive pathological workup with morphology, immunohistochemistry, flow cytometry and ancillary techniques (cytogenetics, molecular genetics, gene-expression arrays) needed to meet the meticulous WHO classification requirements [7].

The biopsy technique is of utmost importance, since lymphoma tissue is much frailer than are nodes involved with cancer. Diagnosis is based on morphology and immunology, and the biopsy must be handled with an atraumatic technique as to not to disturb the pattern of lymphoma involvement in the tissue. Fresh material is optimal for extended molecular analyses, but routine immunohistopathology is adequately accomplished with formalin-fixed tissue. Radical excision is not favoured, and (possibly disfiguring) surgery should be avoided, since chemotherapy with or without radiotherapy is the gold standard of treatment.

9.3.5 Lymphoma Classification, World Health Organisation 2008

The entire group is now designated "malignant lymphomas" – formerly non-Hodgkin's lymphoma – and the present WHO classification has evolved during the past decades from a plethora of different systems. This vastly complex classification separates the malignant lymphomas into immature and mature lymphoid neoplasms [6]. Immature, precursor lymphoid neoplasms of T- and B-cell type (pre-**a**cute B-/T-cell **l**ymphoblastic **l**eukaemia [ALL] or lymphoma) – especially the B-cell type – frequently manifest with nodal involvement in children, but the clinical picture is dominated by the leukaemia, and thus not further commented on here.

Mature lymphomas are categorised into B-cell and T-/NK-cell neoplasms, and further subdivided into 30 and 18 subtypes, respectively. The two most frequent B-cell lymphomas in the Western countries are diffuse large B-cell lymphoma (DLBCL) and follicular lymphoma (FL), accounting for roughly a third each, which are followed by mucosa-associated lymphoma (MALT), making up 10% of cases [8]. Hodgkin's lymphoma is a distinct entity with B-cell origin, and the very rare histiocytic and dendritic neoplasms are grouped separately. T-cell lymphomas are dominated by peripheral T-cell lymphoma (PTCL), angioimmunoblastic lymphoma (AILT) and anaplastic large-cell lymphoma (ALCL), together constituting 75% of the T-cell types [4]. Finally, immunodeficiency-associated lymphoproliferative disorders covering a broad spectrum from nonmalignant to overt lymphoma are classified separately.

9.3.6 Staging of Lymphoma

Patients with newly diagnosed lymphoma should undergo staging with a CT scan, MRI or PET scan of the neck, thorax and abdomen; bone marrow biopsy and aspiration; haematology; and blood chemistry [9]. The presence (B) or absence (A) of general symptoms (drenching night sweats, fever and 10% weight loss within 3 months)

should be noted. Stage of disease is defined according to the Ann Arbor (Michigan, USA) staging system, and for localised extranodal disease (primarily extranodal [Pe]) according to Musshoff's staging system. Localised tumours should also be described according to the tumour–node–metastasis (TNM) system, which more accurately relates to tumour bulk and extent.

Staging can be rather narrow if patient performance or comorbidity precludes curative treatment, or if the procedures do not influence choice of therapy. On the other hand, staging more extensive is used to define localised disease when radiotherapy is planned. Probably due to homing mechanisms, there is a propensity for lymphoma spread from Waldeyer's ring to the gastrointestinal tract. In the case of isolated tonsillar involvement, gastroscopy with biopsy is recommended.

9.3.7 Treatment of Lymphoma

Surgery has its place only as a diagnostic procedure, and chemotherapy is the treatment of choice. In all B-cell lymphoma subtypes, addition of antibodies against B cells (anti-CD20, rituximab) to chemotherapy regimens has increased cure rates (10–15% over chemotherapy alone) and substantially prolonged remissions.

Many B-cell lymphomas are curable diseases, like DLBCL and Burkitt's lymphoma, but others are incurable; however, they often have good prognoses due to the lethargic progressive behaviour of the particular lymphoma, such as FL, chronic lymphatic leukaemia (CLL) and MALT. In such indolent lymphomas with asymptomatic disease, treatment can even be deferred until symptoms occur.

Localised aggressive DLBCL with extranodal (primary extranodal, or stage Pe I) or nodal (stage I) is preferentially treated with a shorter course of rituximab and **c**yclophosphamide (Cytoxan), Doxorubicin (Adriamycin, **H**ydroxydaunomycin), vincristine (**O**ncovin), and **p**rednisolone [CHOP]) chemotherapy for three to four cycles, and additional involved field radiotherapy, 2–30 Gy per fraction, or alternatively, full immunochemotherapy [10]. Extended field radiotherapy alone should be avoided in a curative setting. If radiotherapy alone is chosen, the dose is increased to 2–40 Gy per fraction. In localised indolent lymphoma (FL, MALT, CLL), the involved region with a few-centimetre margin is irradiated at 2–30 Gy per fraction.

In Hodgkin's lymphoma stage I–II, radiotherapy is still mandatory as consolidation after chemotherapy with A(B)VD (**A**driamycin [doxorubicin], **b**leomycin, **v**inblastine, **d**acarbazine) or BEACOPP (**b**leomycin, **e**toposide, **A**driamycin, **O**ncovin, **p**rocarbazine, **p**rednisolone) [11].

Generalized indolent B-cell lymphomas such as FL and marginal zone lymphoma of the MALT type are initially treated with less intense, single-agent alkylating drugs, e.g. chlorambucil with or without rituximab, since the approach is palliative. In younger patients, rituximab with CHOP-like regimens are preferred. Lymphocytic lymphoma is identical to CLL in the bone marrow, and treated with fludarabine and cyclophosphamide to obtain remission, or chlorambucil in the palliative setting [12].

Disseminated aggressive B-cell lymphoma dominated by DLBCL is approached with curative intent, and treated accordingly with combination chemotherapy with standard regimen rituximab–CHOP (R-CHOP) for 6 cycles every 3 weeks. Intensification with shortening of the interval to 2 weeks is performed in poor-risk patients, and made possible with the support of granulocyte colony-stimulating factor (G-CSF) [10].

Mantle-cell lymphoma is an aggressive lymphoma for which longstanding remission is obtainable only in younger patients who can endure aggressive, multiagent chemotherapy including rituximab and CHOP-like regimens in combination with the antimetabolites cytarabine and Methotrexate (hyper-CVAD), and consolidation with high-dose chemotherapy and autologous stem cell support. In the elderly, rituximab in addition to CHOP or DHAP (cisplatin, cytarabine, dexamethasone) or FC (fludarabine, cyclophosphamide) are less toxic alternatives [13].

Burkitt's lymphoma in Western countries is also called *sporadic BL* and distinct from the African *endemic BL* in pathogenetic, molecular and clinical aspects, but it is morphologically indistinguishable. It is by far the fastest proliferating of all lymphomas, and it is treated with extensive regimens including high doses of alkylating agents and antimetabolites, and intensive dosing according to the Berlin–Frankfurt–Münster (BFM) Group, hyper-CVAD or ALL protocols [14]. It is of utmost importance to start therapy immediately at diagnosis, since this is the most curable of all lymphomas (in the young) if treatment can be completed according to schedule. The cure rate is well above 80% in the younger-age population. Hyper-CVAD is also feasible in patients older than 40 years; with the addition of optimal supportive care and growth factors, and with the introduction of rituximab, the prognosis is almost equivalent to that of younger people [15]. Due to high tumour cell decay, pretreatment with steroids and protection with rasburicase to prevent tumour lysis syndrome is mandatory.

T-cell lymphomas in the ENT region (though rare) are of several subgroups. ALCL occurs in two types, with or without the translocation t(2;5) involving the *ALK* gene. The translocation portends a good prognosis despite often-widespread nodal and extranodal involvement in ENT bone, soft tissue and skin. ALCL ALK⁺ occurs predominantly in children and adolescents. ALCL ALK⁻, on the other hand, is dominantly a widespread nodal disease and has a much poorer prognosis. AITL is primarily a generalised nodal disease in the middle-aged, with extranodal involvement of almost any site with B symptoms and signs of cytokine release. T-cell lymphomas not otherwise specified account for approximately 30% of the PTCL in Western countries, and occur almost exclusively in adulthood, with widespread nodal and extranodal disease. In generalised T-cell lymphoma (noncutaneous, non-ALK⁺), the prognosis is much worse than in B-cell lymphoma, and standard CHOP results in only a 10–20% rate of long-term survival. Addition of etoposide, consolidation with high-dose chemotherapy, anti-CD52 antibody (alemtuzumab) and new drugs are still under study [4].

In conclusion, the site of disease has little importance for choice of treatment; the decisive factors are

- Histological type of lymphoma
- Stage of disease

In addition, different prognostic scores and cytogenetic markers are used to modulate treatment intensity, such as the international prognostic index (IPI) for DLBCL, follicular IPI (FLIPI) for FL and several factors for Hodgkin's disease. In CLL, del(17p) and del(11q) mutations harbinger a bad prognosis, and in ALC lymphoma, the existence of the t(2;5) translocation is a marker of good prognosis. However, the lymphoma presentation (below) is done from a clinical viewpoint from the perspective of site of presentation, starting with lymph nodes and proceeding to the extranodal areas, in order of frequency of involvement.

9.3.8 Lymph Nodes

Cervical, supraclavicular, preauricular and occipital lymph node involvement can occur as part of generalised lymphadenopathy or isolated in almost any lymphoma subtype. If no other lymphoma spread is evident at staging, and curative radiotherapy is planned, efforts should be done to exclude involvement of the presumed site draining to the affected lymph node. Extended investigation of Waldeyer's ring with biopsy or tonsillectomy if grossly affected, and inspection/biopsy of the nasopharynx should be performed in cases of affected cervical nodes.

The three most common subtypes of adult nodal lymphomas are all of B-cell type:

1. DLBCL
2. FL
3. Lymphocytic lymphoma/CLL

Together, these constitute three quarter of all cases [16]. In young adults, Hodgkin's lymphoma is the most frequent, presenting as indolent, hard, multiple nodes. A large, fast-growing lymph node in an adolescent should give rise to suspicion of Burkitt's lymphoma. Mononucleosis should be a differential diagnosis, and this EBV-driven lymphadenopathy could give rise to dangerous nodes, often with gross tonsillar enlargement and airway obstruction. Biopsy from lymph nodes in patients with mononucleosis should be avoided, since the pathology is alarming and could give rise to a preliminary misdiagnosis of lymphoma.

FL in cervical lymph nodes is usually part of a generalised lymphadenopathy, and treated with rituximab with or without chemotherapy at progression. The 10-year survival rate is excellent, but the disease is not eradicated with current therapy.

DLBCL is an aggressive but curable (65%) lymphoma if treated with rituximab and short-term polychemotherapy (CHOP). If truly localised, the prognosis is excellent, with an 80% cure rate. The risk of occult involvement of additional nodes is however much greater in nodal than in extranodal disease. Increased staging efforts could be performed with PET in cases with nodal stage I [9].

9.3.9 Waldeyer's Ring

Lymphoma involvement of the tonsils is either unilateral or bilateral. Symptoms of thickness, harshness, slurred speech and airway obstruction can rapidly progress in aggressive lymphoma. A differential diagnosis of EBV infection should always be the first choice for adolescents, but not for the elderly, for whom it is very unlikely. A diagnostic tonsillectomy should be performed if no obvious lymph node is accessible for biopsy. B-cell types dominate, as in all other sites. The most frequent type is the DLBCL, which can be confined to this site or the draining lymph node, i.e. stage Pe I–II. In children or adolescents, Burkitt's lymphoma rarely occurs; however, it is important to implement special precautions, and there is urgency in starting treatment within a few days of diagnosis. Indolent lymphomas such as lymphocytic lymphoma/CL and FL, and mantle-cell lymphoma could involve the tonsillar region, often then bilaterally and usually as part of disseminated disease [17].

Extramedullary plasmocytoma occurs in the upper aerodigestive tract of the nasopharynx, oropharynx, sinus and larynx. In contrast to osseous plasmocytoma, the disease seldom progresses to myeloma, and radiotherapy, 2–40 Gy per fraction, provides excellent local control. Spread to the contiguous cervical lymph nodes occurs in 15% of cases, and an abnormal monoclonal immunoglobulin (M component) in plasma – usually IgA – occurs in 20% of cases [18].

9.3.10 Salivary Glands

Salivary gland lymphomas account for 5–10% of all salivary gland tumours. The parotid and (less commonly) the submandibular glands are primarily involved, but rarely affected as a part of generalised lymphoma. Usually, unilateral swelling occurs, and fine-needle biopsy should be performed to minimise the subsequent surgery to a diagnostic biopsy. MALT lymphoma is one of the most common types, and contralateral spread occurs due to specific homing. As in thyroid lymphoma, there is a correlation with autoimmune disease and Sjögren's syndrome, and the occurrence of MALT lymphoma in the salivary gland. MALT lymphoma of the salivary gland is an extremely indolent disease; therapy should be minimised, and radiotherapy even withheld if an excision biopsy is performed, to avoid aggravating preexisting sicca. As common as MALT is the aggressive DLBCL, mainly in the parotid; if localised to the gland (Pe I), it can be treated with radiotherapy alone. Chemotherapy with rituximab and CHOP might be a more attractive alternative, to avoid dryness of the mouth. FL and mantle-cell lymphoma might occur in the salivary glands and then as part of an intraglandular lymph node and predominantly as part of widespread nodal disease, and should be treated accordingly.

9.3.11 Oral Cavity

Involvement of the gingiva buccal mucosa, palate or underlying bone is common with DLBCL. Symptoms of swelling, chewing discomfort, ill-fitting dental prosthesis disorder, ulceration, pain and peripheral nerve dysfunction are analogue to those of cancer in the oral cavity. Potentially disfiguring surgery should be avoided, and local staging is best performed with MRI. Primary origin in the underlying bone structures should intensify staging concerning widespread bone involvement and/or bone marrow infiltration. As in the case of sinonasal involvement, Burkitt's lymphoma, plasmablastic lymphoma and T-cell lymphomas of the AILT subtype are differential diagnoses. Mantle-cell lymphoma and indolent lymphomas of MALT type and FL occur infrequently.

9.3.12 Thyroid Gland

The thyroid gland is a relatively infrequent extranodal site of lymphoma, occurring mainly in the elderly. Two subtypes of B-cell lymphoma dominate. The first and most frequent thyroid lymphoma is DLBCL. The disease usually presents as a rapidly growing goitre in elderly women, with symptoms similar to those of large-cell anaplastic cancer of the thyroid. In contrast, if truly localised, it is highly curable with rituximab and CHOP, or radiotherapy despite local aggressiveness. It is important to diagnosis DLBCL rapidly, which is simplest by fine-needle aspiration that is followed by biopsy – not via a thyroidectomy. Disseminated disease must be treated with rituximab and CHOP.

The second most frequent thyroid lymphoma is marginal zone lymphoma arising from MALT lymphoma. The lymphoma is by lymphoepithelial lesions (LEL). These occur in the setting of chronic inflammation and autoimmune disease. Patients with Hashimoto's thyroiditis have a threefold increase of lymphoma and a 70-fold increase of thyroid lymphoma. The disease is mainly localised and spreads primarily to draining cervical nodes, and present as indolent swelling. Plasmacytic differentiation of MALT lymphoma can result in a small M component in the plasma. Local radiotherapy, 2–30 Gy per fraction, is the treatment of choice in localised disease (Pe I–II). Transformation from MALT to DLBCL is sometimes histologically evident, and treatment should be directed according to the most aggressive component [19].

9.3.13 Paranasal Sinus

Painful swelling and destruction of the surrounding bone with involvement of the orbit or nasal cavity or the maxilla are the symptoms of aggressive lymphoma in the sinus, much the same as in cancer. By far, the most common type is DLBCL, and it is often localised; however, extensive spread of the disease is indication for primary radiotherapy. Due to the sinus's proximity to the CNS, intrathecal prophylaxis is optional in addition to R-CHOP. Remission can be difficult to define, and additional radiotherapy is often administered when there is bone involvement [20]. Other, rarer histologies at this site are T-cell lymphoma and Burkitt's lymphoma. In HIV-positive patients, aggressive EBV-positive plasmablastic lymphoma occurs in the sinonasal and oral cavity, often with multifocal bone involvement [21]. T-/NK-cell lymphomas – identical with the nasal type, with local destructive growth – are rare in Western countries, but frequent in Asian populations.

9.3.14 Nasal Cavity

The aggressive lymphoma variants in the nasal cavity present with symptoms of pain, epistaxis, local destructive growth and facial swelling, and the more indolent ones present with chronic nasal obstruction, with nasal speech and snoring. In the Western countries, B-cell lymphomas dominate. Most common in the nasal cavity is not only the aggressive DLBCL, but also mantle-cell lymphoma, indolent-lymphoma-like FL, lymphocytic lymphoma/CLL and extramedullary plasmocytoma.

The unique lymphoma entity for this site is nasal-type T-/NK-cell lymphoma, formerly called *lethal midline granuloma*. This is the dominant lymphoma in Asian and South American populations, but it is infrequent in the native European and Western populations. The tumour is closely related to EBV, and can occur posttransplantation and in immunosuppressive states. Lymphoma growth is angiocentric, destroying the vascular bed with prominent necrosis and destruction, invading bone and the adjacent sinuses. Aggressive chemotherapy combined with high-dose radiotherapy is often curative in localised disease, but the prognosis in extended disease is dismal [4].

9.3.15 Larynx

The larynx is a rare site of lymphoma involvement. In the case of indolent MALT histology, gastroscopy should be performed to exclude mutifocality. Peripheral T-cell lymphoma and DLBCL (or any) histology is possible [22].

9.3.16 Special Situations

9.3.16.1 Posttransplantation Lymphoproliferative Disorders

Immunodeficiency states – inherited, acquired or iatrogenic – greatly increase the risk of lymphoma. The most common clinical situation is post-allogeneic transplantation. In almost all cases, EBV-driven lymphoproliferation due to defective T-cell surveillance is the pathogenetic mechanism. The risk of developing PTLD is greatest in patients who are EBV-negative before transplant. The risk is also related to the type and intensity of immunosuppressive regimen. The morphological picture is that early lesions polymorph into plasmacytic hyperplasia– or mononucleosis-like cells, and then increasingly monomorph, following the pattern of DLBCL, Burkitt's lymphoma or plasma cell lymphoma types. In addition, T-cell lymphomas and Hodgkin's lymphoma occur posttransplant [23]. Tonsillar and cervical node involvement is frequent in early-onset PTLD, and manifests with disturbingly fast-growing lymphomas and airway obstruction. First, immunosuppression should be reduced, and then PTLD treated with rituximab alone. Chemotherapy should be withheld from those who fail to regress [24].

References

3. Han X, Kilfoy B, Zengh T et al. (2008) Lymphoma patterns by WHO subtype in the United States, 1973–2003. Cancer Cause Control 19:841–858

4. Armitage J et al. (2008) International peripheral T-cell and natural killer/T-cell lymphoma study: pathology and clinical outcomes. J Clin Oncol 26:4124–4130

5. Hochberg J, Waxman IM, Kelly KM, Morris E, Cairo MS (2009) Adolescent non-Hodgkin lymphoma and Hodgkin lymphoma: state of the science. Br J Haematol 144:22–40

6. Swerdlow SH, Campo E, Harris N, Jaffe ES et al. (eds) (2008) WHO classification of tumours of haematopoietic and lymphoid tissues. IARC Press, Lyon, France:

7. Ellis DW, Eaton M, Fox RM, Junejas S, Leong AS, Miliauskas J, Norris DL, Spagnolo D, Turner J (2005) Diagnostic pathology of lymphoproliferative disorders. Pathology 37:434–456

8. A clinical evaluation of the International Lymphoma Study Group classification of non-Hodgkin's lymphoma. The Non-Hodgkin's Lymphoma Classification Project. (1997) Blood 89:3909–3918

9. Cheson BD (2008) Staging and evaluation of the patient with lymphoma. Hematol Oncol Clin North Am 22:825–837, vii–viii

10. Armitage J (2007) How I treat patients with diffuse large B-cell lymphoma. Blood 110:29–36

11. Eich HT, Müller RP, Engenhart-Cabillic R, Lukas P, Schmidberger H, Staars S, Willich N, German Hodgkin Study Group (2008) Involved-node radiotherapy in early-stage Hodgkin's lymphoma. Definition and guidelines of the German Hodgkin Study Group (GHSG). Strahlenther Onkol 184:406–410

12. Kay NE, Rai KR, O'Brien S (2006) Chronic lymphatic leukaemia: current and emerging treatment approaches. Clin Adv Hematol Oncol 4(Suppl):S1–S10; quiz, S11–S12

13. Gill S, Richter D (2008) Therapeutic options in mantle-cell lymphoma. Leuk Lymphoma. 49:398–409

14. Blum KA, Lozanski G, Byrd JC (2008) Adult Burkitt leukemia and lymphoma. Blood 104:3009–3020

15. Thomas DA, Faderi S, O'Brien S et al. (2006) Chemoimmunotherapy with hyper-CVAD plus rituximab for the treatment of adult Burkitt and Burkitt-type lymphoma or leukemia. Cancer 106:1569–1580

16. Anonymous (1997) A clinical evaluation of the International Lymphoma Study Group classification of non-Hodgkin's lymphoma. The Non-Hodgkin's Lymphoma Classification Project. Blood 89:3909–3918

17. Laskar S, Mohindra P, Gupta S, Shet T, Muckaden MA (2008) Review. Non-Hodgkin lymphoma of the Waldeyer's ring: clinicopathologic and therapeutic issues. Leukemia Lymphoma 49:2263–2271

18. Soutar R, Lucraft H, Jackson G, Reece A, Bird J, Low E, Samson D (2004) Guidelines on the diagnosis and management of solitary plasmacytoma of the bone and solitary extramedullary plasmacytoma. Br J Haematol 124:717–726

19. Mack LA, Pasieka JL (2007) An evidence-based approach to the treatment of thyroid lymphoma. World J Surg 31:978–986

20. Laskin JL, Savage KJ, Voss N, Gascoyne RD (2005) Connors JM. Primary paranasal sinus lymphoma: natural history and improved outcome with central nervous system chemoprophylaxis. Leukemia Lymphoma 46:1721–1727

21. Colomo L, Loong F, Rives S, Pittaluga S, Martinez A, Lopez-Guillermo A, Ojanguren G, Romagosa V, Jaffe ES, Campo E (2004) Diffuse large B-cell lymphoma with plasmablastic differentiation represent a heterogeneous group of disease entities. Am J Surg Pathol 28:736–747

22. Veelken AS, Schmitt-Gräff A, Maier W, Richter B (2007) Multifocal extranodal mucosa-associated lymphoid tissue lymphoma affecting the larynx. Ann Otol Rhino Laryngol 116:257–261

23. Harris NL, Ferry JA, Swerdlow SH (1997) Posttransplant lymphoproliferative disorders: summary of Society for Hematopathology Workshop. Semin Diagn Pathol 14:8–14

24. Elstrom RL, Andreadis C, Aqui NA, Ahya VN, Bloom RD, Brozena SC, Olthoff KM, Schuster SJ, Nasta SD, Stadtmauer EA, Tsai DE (2006) Treatment of PTLD with rituximab or chemotherapy: The University of Pennsylvania Experience. Am J Transplant 6:569–576

9.4 Clinical Examination and Diagnostic Techniques in Head and Neck Oncology

JOCHEN A. WERNER

9.4.1 Introduction

Careful clinical examination in the case of suspected malignoma plays a central role in the planning of specific therapies. It is well known that patients with carcinoma of the upper aerodigestive tract develop metachronous secondary carcinoma in up to 40% of cases. This circumstance influences decisively the diagnosis and treatment concept of mucosal head and neck cancer. However, it must be mentioned clearly that the prognosis of patients suffering from head and neck cancer does not mainly depend on the primary tumour, but on the presence or absence of lymphogenic metastasis. Thus the identification of lymphogenic metastasis, the description of the location of lymph node metastases and—which is especially important for the further course of the disease—the detection of distant metastases plays an important role in addition to the detection of the primary tumour. Only the entire assessment of these findings allows a therapeutic regime adapted to the stage of the tumour disease according to international standards.

It is clear that the overview of clinical examination methods described in the following passages cannot encompass the numerous other techniques important for addressing oncologic questions in exceptional cases. However, the goal of this chapter is to focus on the most important clinical examination methods, and to give even residents of otorhinolaryngology tools of how to become valid examiners in the field of head and neck oncology.

In cases of carcinomas of the upper aerodigestive tract, in particular one aspect must be considered carefully, which is the occurrence of secondary cancers. They are defined according to the criteria of Warren and Gates, and must be confirmed histologically. Secondary carcinomas are divided into two different types. The first type is synchronic secondary carcinomas, occurring simultaneously with the primary tumour disease. The second type describes metachronic secondary carcinomas, occurring in the further course of malignant disease of the upper aerodigestive tract. The incidence of synchronic secondary carcinomas is estimated at 7–10%. It must be excluded that the secondary carcinoma is a metastasis of the primary tumour. The frequency of developing metachronic secondary carcinomas is reported in the literature for patients with malignant tumours of the head and neck at 10–40%. The incidence per year amounts to 3–7%. The risk in developing secondary carcinomas increases with each year after primary treatment. A clear tendency to manifest secondary carcinomas of the aerodigestive tract can be observed when the primary tumour is located in the area of the oral cavity, the oropharynx or hypopharynx. In 16–18% of these cases, patients manifest secondary carcinomas. In comparison, the probability of developing secondary carcinomas in cases of epipharyngeal cancer amounts to about 8%. Due to the high risk of developing secondary carcinomas in cases of tumours located in the mentioned areas (oral cavity, oropharynx, hypopharynx and even larynx) a long-term follow-up of these tumour patients should be planned.

The location of the secondary carcinoma is decisive for the prognosis. Secondary carcinomas located in the lung or the oesophagus have nearly always very poor or even infaust prognoses, whereas secondary carcinomas of the oral cavity or the larynx can often be treated with curative purpose if they are diagnosed at an early stage.

9.4.1.1 Introduction to TNM Classification

In order to achieve an international standard of tumour classification, each anatomic region is described according to the following scheme:

- Classification according to the procedure for determination of the T, N and M stages. Additional methods for more precise determination prior to therapy can be applied
- Anatomic regions and subregions, if necessary
- Definition of the regional lymph nodes
- TNM: clinical classification
- G: histopathological grading
- Staging
- Brief summary

9.4.1.1.1 Regional Lymph Nodes

The definition of the N stage is the same for all head and neck regions, except the nasopharynx and thyroid gland. Lymph nodes located in the midline are taken as ipsilateral, except when concerning the thyroid gland.

9.4.1.1.2 Distant Metastases

The definition of the M stage is the same for all head and neck regions. The categories M1 and pM1 can be specified as follows:

Pulmonary	PUL
Osseous	OSS
Hepatic	HEP
Brain	BRA
Lymph nodes	LYM
Bone marrow	MAR
Pleura	PLE
Peritoneum	PER
Adrenals	ADR
Skin	SKI
Other	OTH

9.4.1.1.3 Histopathological Grading: G Grading

The definitions of G categories are the same for all head and neck locations, except the thyroid gland:

GX	Grade cannot be assessed
G1	Well differentiated
G2	Moderately differentiated
G3	Poorly differentiated
G4	Undifferentiated

9.4.1.1.4 R Classification

The presence or absence of residual tumours after therapy is described by R classification. The following definitions are the same for all head and neck locations:

RX	Presence of residual tumour cannot be assessed
R0	No residual tumour
R1	Microscopic residual tumour
R2	Macroscopic residual tumour

9.4.1.1.5 L: Lymphatic Vessel Invasion

LX:	Lymph vessel invasion cannot be assessed
L0:	No lymphatic vessel invasion
L1:	Lymphatic vessel invasion

9.4.1.1.6 V: Venous Invasion

VX:	Venous invasion cannot be assessed
V0:	No venous invasion
V1:	Microscopic venous invasion
V2:	Macroscopic venous invasion

9.4.2 Ear

In addition to clinical examination, a detailed anamnesis is important for reconstruction of prior events. Questions must be asked about:

- Unclear sensation of pressure
- Pain
- Outflow of liquid or secretions from the auditory canal (otorrhea)
- Hearing loss
- Vertigo
- Ringing in the ears

Prior to every examination the outer appearance of the auricle must be observed with regard to its structure and if necessary, palpation must be performed. The difference must be made between congenital and acquired structural changes.

9.4.2.1 Inspection and Palpation

9.4.2.1.1 Inspection

The auricle, the mastoid and the entrance of the auditory canal are examined with regard to:

- Redness
- Swellings
- Ulceration
- Fistulae
- Malformations
- Tumorous neoplasms
- Scars
- Crusts
- Fluids

9.4.2.1.2 Palpation

Examination by palpation of the outer auricle as well as the surrounding structures also includes palpation of the mastoid process, generally performed bimanually and bilaterally. Attention must be paid to unilateral swellings as well as pain on pressure or percussion of the planum mastoideum or the mastoid tip. Further, the auricle should be examined with regard to pain on pressure of the tragus or pain on tension of the auricle. Bimanual palpation of the pre- and retroauricular lymph nodes as well as lymph nodes in the area of the maxillary angle completes the palpatory examination of the outer ear.

9.4.2.2 Otoscopy

Otoscopy allows the examination of the deeper parts of the acoustic meatus, the tympanic membrane as well as defects of the tympanum and part of the eardrum.

The acoustic meatus is about 3 to 3.5 cm long and consists of an outer cartilaginous as well as an inner bony part. Bending and narrowness of the meatus characterise the transition of cartilaginous to bony part. In order to examine completely the tympanum by otoscopy, the auricle must be drawn in a posterior–superior direction to bring the cartilaginous part of the meatus in line with the bony meatus. Otoscopy can be performed generally by means of otoscopes with integrated source of light, a head lamp with otoscope or a microscope, which gives the clearest examination results.

The directing of the otoscope is performed with the left hand when examining the right as well as the left ear in order to have the right hand for handling instruments, the microscope and for positioning the head. Examining the right as well as the left ear, the otoscope is taken between thumb and index finger. When the right ear of the patient is examined, the middle finger is placed in the cymba, and the ring finger is positioned on the posterior surface of the auricle, lifting the auricle by tension in the posterior direction. Otoscopy of the left ear is performed by positioning the middle finger in the cymba and pressing it against the anthelix.

9.4.2.3 Functional Tests

9.4.2.3.1 Cochlear Diagnosis

The tuning fork tests according to Rinne and Weber are performed in order to distinguish between transmission hearing loss and sensorineural hearing loss. Rinne's test allows a comparison between air conduction and osteotympanic conduction of the same ear. A tuning fork (435 Hz) is put into vibration and placed on the mastoid process. When the patient no longer hears the sound of the tuning fork, it is immediately held in front of the same ear, without being put into vibration again. Healthy persons hear the sound again because air conduction is better than osteotympanic conduction (positive Rinne's test).

By means of Weber's test the osteotympanic conduction can be checked. For this purpose the vibrating tuning fork is placed on top of the skull and the patient is asked on which side the sound is heard. Healthy individuals hear the sound on both ears or in the middle of the head. However, this is also the case in a symmetric inner ear hearing loss.

In order to detect a fixation of the ossicular chain, as, for example, to diagnose otosclerosis, the so-called Gellé's test is performed. In this context, the vibrating tuning fork is placed laterally at the cranial vault, and then the acoustic meatus is closed in an airtight fashion with a Politzer's bag. Compressing the bag leads to an air column on the tympanum; this stiffens the ossicular chain and impairs its motility. Healthy individuals with a flexible ossicular chain will notice a change in the loudness of the sound of the tuning fork. However, if the ossicular chain is initially fixed, then the compression will not have an influence on the loudness of the tuning fork sound (negative Gellé's test).

Audiometry allows verifying the quantitative extent of the hearing loss. Herewith the so-called tone hearing is checked. Pure sounds in octave or quint intervals are offered, and the auditory threshold and the discomfort threshold are verified by volume regulation. In the context of further differential diagnosis of sensorineural hearing loss verified by audiography, so-called suprathreshold hearing tests may be indicated. Those are the recruitment measurement described by Vogler, the noise audiometry described by Langenbeck, the short increment sensitivity index (SISI) test described by Jerger, and auditory field scaling (Metz recruitment) as well as otoacoustic emissions (OEA). Finally so-called auditory fatigue tests can detect neural hearing loss. These tests as well as speech audiometry and objective hearing tests are not focussed in this context because they are less important for the field of oncologic diagnosis. Of course, such knowledge is essential even for head and neck oncologists, considering the fact that some chemotherapeutics are possibly ototoxic. In this context, stapedius reflex diagnosis may also be important, as the functioning of the facial nerve must sometimes be examined from an oncologic point of view.

9.4.2.3.2 Vestibular Diagnosis

Three classic vestibular tests verifying the function of the vestibular system without experimental stimulation are spontaneous nystagmus, provocation nystagmus and positional nystagmus. Spontaneous nystagmus and provocation nystagmus are checked through the so-called Frenzel's glasses, which inhibits fixation by glasses of 15 dioptres. The spontaneous nystagmus is hereby verified in the five main lines of vision: straight ahead, to the left, to the right, upward and downward. The triggering of a provocation nystagmus is also performed by means of Frenzel's glasses, by placing the patient in the position, in which vertigo occurs by shaking the head, quickly lying down and then sitting up, as well as the positional test. The positional test reveals nystagmus occurring in supine position, and in the right or left lateral position, to detect

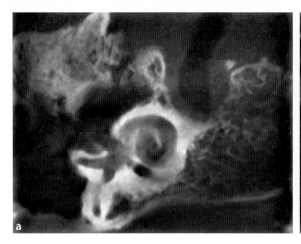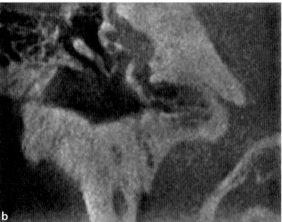

Fig. 9.4.1 a Digital volume tomography clearly visualizes cochlea and oval window. **b** Digital volume tomography clearly visualizes normal moulded right body of the incus

positional nystagmus in the context of a benign paroxysmal positional vertigo.

The experimental vestibular tests include the thermal test, the rotatory test and the test of a fistula symptom. The thermal vestibular test allows the testing of each vestibular organ. Cold and warm rinsing checks the peripheral irritability. The rotatory test verifies the function of both vestibular organs at the same time, and the functional balance or dysfunction is assessed. In the case of a marginal tympanic lesion occurring after chronic otitis media epitympanica, or of course also in the case of cancer of the temporal bone, the test of the pressory fistula symptom should be performed in order to verify a circumscribed destruction of the labyrinthine capsule. In the case of a positive fistula symptom, the indication for emergency intervention is made to avoid diffuse labyrinthitis and possible endocranial complications.

A Politzer's bag is placed (airtightly) into the auditory canal, and at the same time the eye movement is observed through Frenzel's glasses. In the case of a fistula of semicircular duct, a nystagmus movement to the bad side is provoked on the side where Politzer's bag is placed and compressed. When the bag is released, aspiration leads to nystagmus to the other side.

9.4.2.4 Imaging Techniques

The modern techniques of computed tomography (CT) and magnetic resonance imaging (MRI) have mostly substituted the formerly performed conventional radiological imaging of the skull. CT scans permits the delineation of bony structures of the middle ear and the labyrinth. Its indication is made further in cases of suspected skull fractures in order to detect intracranial bleeding and in cases of dural disruption. CT scan is also indicated to re-

veal otogenous cerebral abscesses or glomus tumours and bone destruction in cases of middle ear tumours or erosion of the sinus shell.

MRI is the method of choice for detail of acoustic neurinomas. MRI is performed after application of the contrast agent gadolinum-diethylene triamine penta-acetic acid (Gd-DTPA). MRI is also indicated for detection of vascular volvuli, the exact course of the vestibular and facial nerves, the description of liquid-filled spaces of the inner ear as well as inflammatory endocranial complications and the extent of glomus tumours.

Current developments in the field of digital volume tomography (DVT) will possibly further optimise the description of the otobasis in the next years. Compared with conventional CT with a high radiation exposure, devices available up to now allow a three-dimensional description of the otobasis, with an excellent resolution and only 3–5% of the conventional radiation exposure. This procedure can preoperatively reveal necrotic changes in the area of the ossicular chain, its joints, or erosions in the area of the semicircular ducts, the cochlea, and the canal of the facial nerve (Fig. 9.4.1a,b).

9.4.2.5 Cancer of the Auricle

Tumours of the auricle can be observed frequently; they can be well detected and treated, whereas tumours of the acoustic meatus occur rarely and remain often undetected. Early diagnosis and differentiation between benign tumour and precancerous neoplasms and malignomas of the auricle are important for the prognosis. Due to its location the auricle is exposed to the sun, and so epithelial actinic tumours of the skin occur frequently. The difference must be made between squamous cell carcinomas of the auricle and those of the acoustic meatus; those of the auricle occur 10 to 30 times more frequently. Regarding malignant masses of the ear, squamous cell carcinomas occur most frequently and about twice as frequently as basal cell carcinomas. Although squamous cell carcinomas of the auricle may develop in the area of the whole auricle, generally mainly the helix and the border of the anthelix are concerned.

Clinical manifestation of auricular cancer shows a destructing, exophytically and endophytically growing tumour that is solid with partly hyperkeratotic and exulcerating parts. This tumour, which is solid on palpation, destroys bones and cartilages. Carcinomas of the auricle have a comparably high metastatic frequency, with up to more than 15% infiltrating the parotid and craniojugular draining lymph nodes. Hematogenous metastatic spread is observed in the further course of the disease.

The frequency of malignant melanomas of the head and neck amounts to about 10% in male and female patients. With regard to the total amount of malignant melanoma, its presence in the area of the auricle amounts to 12–18% and with retroauricular location, to 27%. The concha, tragus, and antitragus are mostly involved while the nodular malignant melanoma occurs most frequently at approximately 50%, followed by superficially growing melanoma with 30% and the lentigo malignant melanoma with 20%.

Genetic disposition, exposition to ultraviolet light as well as chronic irritations plays a decisive role in the development of malignant melanomas. The differentiation to similarly pigmented skin neoplasms is performed according to the ABCDE rule:

A	Asymmetry
B	Border irregularity
C	Colour variation
D	Diameter larger than 5 mm
E	Elevation

The clinical occurrence of melanoma is often maculous asymmetric and irregular neoplasms measuring more than 5 mm in diameter, with diffuse margins and regular pigmentation of light brown to deep-black colour. In addition, suspect must be itchiness, signs of regression, inflammatory margins, vertical growth, ulceration and bleeding. The lymphogenic frequency of malignant melanomas of the skin amounts to 19–32% in cases of higher tumour thickness (>4 mm). The incidence of lymph node metastases of malignant melanomas of intermediary tumour size (1.5–3.9 mm) amounts to about 7%.

Based on extensive investigations of the sentinel node concept, meanwhile-funded knowledge on the main metastatic directions of melanomas located in the area of the skin has been established. Melanomas located in the area of an imaginary coronary preauricular line from the vertex to the anterior cervical soft parts metastasise mainly into the parotid gland and levels I–III, while melanomas located between an imaginary pre- and postauricular coronary line may metastasise into the parotid gland as well as levels I–V. Melanomas located behind the imaginary postauricular coronary line metastasise most frequently into levels II–V as well as in occipital lymph nodes.

Regarding malignant melanomas, additional differentiation must be made. Local metastases are recurrences in the surgical scar and/or satellite metastases in close proximity of the primary tumour (<2 cm). Transit metastases are located at a distance of more than 2 cm between the primary and regional lymph node station. Distant metastasis generally occurs in the lung, the brain and the liver. Regarding the prognoses of patients, the difference is made according to the number and type of metastatically affected organs between limited disease (less than organs affected) and extensive disease (more than organs affected).

9.4.2.6 Cancer of the Acoustic Meatus and Temporal Bone

Isolated tumours of the acoustic meatus occur rarely. However, contemporary involvement of the acoustic meatus in cases of initial auricular cancer is frequently observed. Such a contemporary involvement of the acoustic meatus generally has an influence on the therapeutic concept, primarily because simple excision is no longer possible. In contrast to tumours of the auricle, isolated tumours of the acoustic meatus often remain undetected, and they are treated as otitis externa for an extended time.

Squamous cell carcinomas of the skin of the acoustic meatus are the most frequently occurring malignant tumours of the acoustic meatus. In contrast, adenoidcystic carcinomas, adenocarcinomas and basal cell carcinomas occur more rarely. Clinically carcinomas of the acoustic meatus manifest as exulcerating, painful, nonhealing neoplasms of the skin of the acoustic meatus. Very frequently, bleeding and secondary infections with chronic purulent otorrhea occur. With this in mind each nonhealing, exulcerating or granulating neoplasm of the acoustic meatus must be biopsied with the operating microscope. In addition to incisional biopsy, sonography of the lymphatic drainage region, CT or MRI of the skull as well as neurologic examination should be performed for preoperative diagnosis of squamous cell carcinomas of the external acoustic meatus. Frequently, significant extension into the depth can be diagnosed and compared to the findings verified initially in the area of the external acoustic meatus. Meatal bones, mandibular joint, mastoid, middle ear, facial nerve and the skull base might already be affected. The metastatic rate of squamous cell carcinomas located in the area of the external acoustic meatus is very high if extended tumour growth has occurred and amounts to about 40%. In cases of temporal bone invasion, deafness and labyrinth deficiency as well as peripheral paresis of the facial nerve may occur. Further otogenous sinus thrombosis as well as otogenous sepsis are possible. Even extradural abscesses, subdural empyema, otogenous meningitis or otogenous cerebral abscesses, or finally ostitis and osteomyelitis with pyramidal pyesis with thrombosis of the cavernous sinus and impaired cerebral nerves III–VI may occur. Finally invasion of the auditory tube and the pharynx as well as thrombosis of the cavernous sinus, the carotid sinus and the petrosal sinus is possible.

9.4.2.7   Tumour Classification

T staging as suggested by Pascher and Stell:

T1	Tumour limited to the original location, no paresis of the facial nerve, no bone destruction
T2	Tumour growth beyond the primary location, clinically manifest by paresis of the facial nerve or radiologically detected bone destruction, no tumour growth beyond the limits of the primary organ
T3	Clinical or radiological indication of tumour growth into surrounding structures (dura, skull base, parotid gland, maxillary joint, etc.)
T4	Patient showing findings that are insufficient for classification, including those patients who were examined and treated in other places

9.4.3   Nose and Nasopharynx

The major group of carcinomas of the outer nose are the epithelial carcinomas, as it is the case also for other facial tumours. Actinic exposition by ultraviolet radiation most probably contributes to the genesis of the diseases. Squamous cell carcinomas of the outer nose ranks second in the frequency of malignant tumours of the outer nose, and occur in advanced age. The mostly nodular, ulcerating skin neoplasms show rapid growth with exulcerating growth destroying cartilage and bone. Lymphogenic metastasis occurs in the submandibular and parotid lymph nodes.

In contrast to that, basal cell carcinomas (Fig. 9.4.2), which are the most frequently occurring malignancies of the outer nose, do not show metastatic behaviour. Basal cell carcinomas of the outer nose occur mainly between the sixth and seventh decade. Due to locally infiltrative growth, basal cell carcinomas belong to a group of malig-

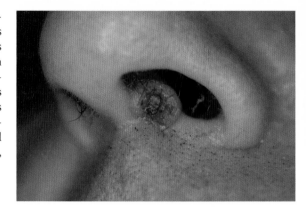

Fig. 9.4.2 Basal cell carcinoma of the left side of the nose

nant neoplasms that might cause significant destruction despite missing metastatic patterns. It is typical for the disease that nodules develop at the beginning with subsequent pearly margins and areal ulceration. Frequently small telangiectasia occurs; however, the exact extent is often underestimated due to subcutaneous growth.

Tumours of the nasal cavity and the paranasal sinuses often manifest by nasal obstruction, recurrent epistaxis, headache, a closed rhinophonia or even by a tubal ventilation disorder associated with serotympanon and conductive hearing loss. In advanced stages, swellings of the cheek and the medial ocular angle may occur, a displacement of the bulbus with diplopia, exophthalmos as well as severe headache in cases of penetration of the skull base with infiltration of the dura.

In addition to the diagnostic procedures described in the following passages, the suspicion of lymphoepithelial carcinoma of the nasopharynx may lead to Epstein–Barr virus (EBV) serology. Nasopharyngeal carcinomas are frequently associated with EBV, an infection that may be diagnosed by an immunoglobulin (Ig)A increase (in contrast to an IgM/IgG increase in cases of infectious mononucleosis). In addition to clinical examination and the imaging diagnosis, an incisional biopsy should be performed under local anaesthesia in order to introduce an appropriate therapy.

9.4.3.1   Inspection and Palpation

The assessment of the inner and outer nose as well as the nasopharynx starts with the careful inspection and palpation of the nose as well as surrounding structures such as cheek, lip and eye. First obvious changes of the form of the nose such as scoliotic nose, hump nose, saddle nose, leptorrhine or broad nose must be described as well as changes in the area of the nasal bridge. In cases of basal cell carcinoma or squamous cell carcinoma of the skin located in the area of the nose, attention must be paid to the extension to the lower eyelid and/or in the direction of the nasal ala, because such findings are important for further operative procedures. Along with a description of the size of the malignant lesion, the clinically assessable extent of a possible ulceration, sometimes even with complete penetration in endonasal direction, should be made. Of course it must also be documented if the carcinoma located exteriorly has invaded the endonasal space.

Findings located endonasally must be considered with regard to pain above the paranasal sinuses in addition to major morphological changes. Concerning the maxillary sinus, pain on pressure above the facial maxillary wall in the area of the exit of the infraorbital nerve, or pain on percussion above the premolars must be verified. Regarding the frontal sinus, pain or lack thereof on pressure in the area of the medial ocular angle, in the area of the anterior skull base or the anterior wall of the frontal sinus must be examined. The diagnostic point for pain for the ethmoid sinus is located in the area of the medial ocular angle. Pain due to processes in the area of the sphenoid sinus generally manifests itself by a pressure sensation as well as pain in the area of the middle of the skull, on the head, and at times in the back of the head. Percussion on the vertex can increase these pains. If thrombophlebitis of the angular vein has occurred, then high sensitivity to pressure can be observed in the course of the angular vein at the nasal clivus. This is a warning signal because of the risk of cavernous thrombosis. As well inspection of the nose, the motility of the eye and/or exophthalmos should be checked in order to exclude orbital involvement. An associated swelling of the cheek may indicate a lymph oedema and/or the penetration of a sinonasal carcinoma.

Of course in cases of all deeply penetrating carcinomas of the facial skin, particular attention must be paid to sensibility, especially in the area of the area innervated by the infraorbital nerve.

Finally a careful inspection and palpation of the hard and soft palates should be performed to clinically verify an oral penetration in cases of advanced malignancies of the nasal cavity and the maxillary sinus.

It must also be mentioned that in cases of possible tumour extent into the sphenoid sinus, careful examination of the function of cerebral nerves must be performed.

Anterior Rhinoscopy

Anterior rhinoscopy is used for assessment of the nasal vestibule and the nasal cavity. Care must be taken that the speculum is not spread too widely because otherwise, anterior rhinoscopy with the speculum might be very painful for the patient. In any case, contact to the turbinates and the nasal mucosa must be avoided.

Generally, the speculum is handled with the left hand (by right-handers). The speculum is inserted with tilted and closed branches into the nasal cavity and spread in front of the piriform aperture. Then the right hand of the examiner bends the head into different examination positions. After local anaesthesia, incisional biopsy can be performed in cases of masses that reach into the nasal cavity and can be seen via anterior rhinoscopy. For this purpose, special punches are usually used.

Posterior Rhinoscopy

Posterior rhinoscopy is used for assessment of the posterior nasal parts including the choanae, the posterior turbinate ends as well as the posterior edge of the vomer. Finally posterior rhinoscopy or postrhinoscopy allows the assessment of the nasopharynx.

Formerly, posterior rhinoscopy was generally performed by means of a mirror placed above the mouth. Today this procedure has mostly substituted by the application of rigid 70 or 90° optics or with the flexible endoscopes available.

Endoscopy

Significant clinical inspection or examination of the posterior nasal parts including the choanae, the posterior turbinate ends as well as the posterior edge of the vomer and the nasopharynx performed in a conscious patient is only possible by means of endoscopy. Routinely, the nose and the nasopharynx are examined with rigid 0 and 30° optics and if necessary, with flexible endoscopes.

Prior to rhinoscopy, the nasal mucosa should be decongested and additionally superficial anaesthesia must be performed. A mixture of, for example, 1% Pantocain® as well as decongesting nose drops (e.g. Otriven®) is recommended. After 5–10 min, the endoscope can be inserted carefully and progressed via the inferior, perhaps also middle meatus, to examine the posterior nasal parts. In addition to a detailed inspection of the nasopharynx and the nasopharyngeal folds, flexible endoscopy even allows examination of the transition to the oropharynx as well as the posterior surface of the soft palate.

The endoscopic examination of the nasal cavity and the nasopharynx is often imperatively included in the panendoscopy. Herewith the transnasal examination of the nasal cavity is performed not only with the 0°, but also with the 30° optic. The nasopharynx is examined transnasally by means of flexible endoscopy or the above-mentioned optics and transorally with the 70 or 90° optic. Each suspect mucosal neoplasia must be assessed by biopsy. In cases of suspected, possibly submucosally located tumour in the area of the nasopharynx, sometimes the palpatory examination of the nasopharynx under velotraction is obligatory for diagnosis.

9.4.3.2 Examination of the Paranasal Sinuses

Sufficient decongestion of the middle nasal meatus frequently permits an inspection of the ethmoid infundibulum as well as the natural maxillary ostium and the anterior ethmoid sinus. Further examinations of the paranasal sinuses, however, must be performed by ultrasound or radiological diagnostic procedures. The last-mentioned radiological procedures are particularly significant. In this context CT and—in cases of certain indications— MRI must be mentioned. CT scans are appropriate for verification of bony lesions, whereas MRI is indicated for determination of the extent of soft tissue processes.

9.4.3.3 Functional Tests

Obstructing processes of the nasal cavity lead to an objectively quantifiable reduction of the passage of the nasal airways, which can be verified by rhinomanometry. Additionally, malignant lesions in the area of the rhinobase are often associated with a reduction of the smelling capacity. In this context a subjective smelling test is not only reasonable, but essential. This qualitative orienting check that is normally done in clinical practices is performed by offering different substances prior and subsequent to decongestion of the nasal mucosa. Those substances are put separately in front of each nostril.

The difference must be made between odorous substances that exclusively activate the olfactory nerve as, for example, coffee, vanilla, wax, cinnamon and lavender. Other smelling substances activate the trigeminal nerve. Those are among others: menthol, acetic acid, and formalin. Finally there are odorous substances with additional sense of taste as, for example, chloroform and pyridine.

In cases of complete loss of the smelling sensation, the pure smelling substances are not realised at all; odorous substances from the other groups can at least be sensed and/or tasted.

9.4.3.4 Imaging Techniques

Due to the availability and for correct determination of the extent by means of CT, the conventional radiological diagnosis has nearly lost its importance nowadays. For assessment of bony lesions as well as relations between bony and soft parts, CT today is the method of choice. In order to better differentiate soft tissue and the exact delimitation between tumour and surrounding soft tissue, MRI is superior to CT scan in cases of tumours of the paranasal sinuses and the nasopharynx.

9.4.3.5 TNM Classification

9.4.3.5.1 T Staging (Nasopharynx)

T1	Nasopharynx
T2	Soft parts of oropharynx and/or nasal cavity

T2a	Without parapharyngeal extension
T2b	With parapharyngeal extension
T3	Infiltration of bony structures and/or paranasal sinuses
T4	Intracranial extension and/or cranial nerve, infratemporal fossa, hypopharynx, orbit, masticator space

9.4.3.5.2 T Staging (Maxillary Sinus)

T1	Tumour limited to maxillary sinus mucosa with no erosion or destruction of bone
T2	Tumour causing bone erosion or destruction including extension into the hard palate and/or middle nasal meatus, except extension to posterior wall of maxillary sinus and pterygoid plates

9.4.3.5.3 T Staging (Nasal Cavity and Ethmoid Sinus)

T1	Tumour restricted to any one subsite, with or without bony invasion
T2	Tumour invades two subsites in a single region or extending to involve an adjacent region within the nasoethmoidal complex, with or without bony invasion
T3	Tumour invades the medial wall or floor of the orbit, maxillary sinus, palate or cribriform plate
T4a	Tumour invades any of the following: anterior orbital contents, skin of nose or cheek, minimal extension to anterior fossa, pterygoid plates, sphenoid or frontal sinuses
T4b	Tumour invades any of the following: orbital apex, dura, brain, middle cranial fossa, cerebral nerves other than (V_2), nasopharynx or clivus

9.4.3.5.4 Staging (Nasopharynx)

Stage 0	Tis	N0	M0
Stage I	T1	N0	M0
Stage IIA	T2a	N0	M0

Stage IIB	T1	N1	M0
	T2a	N1	M0
	T2b	N0, N1	M0
Stage III	T1	N2	M0
	T2a, T2b	N2	M0
	T3	N0, N1, N2	M0
Stage IVA	T4	N0, N1, N2	M0
Stage IVB	Each T stage	N3	M0
Stage IVC	Each T stage	Each N stage	M1

9.4.3.5.5 Staging (Nasal Cavity and Paranasal Sinuses)

Stage 0	Tis	N0	M0
Stage I	T1	N0	M0
Stage II	T2	N0	M0
Stage III	T3	N0	M0
	T1	N1	M0
	T2	N1	M0
	T3	N1	M0
Stage IVA	T4a	N0	M0
	T4a	N1	M0
	T1	N2	M0
	T2	N2	M0
	T3	N2	M0
	T4a	N2	M0
Stage IVB	T4b	Any N	M0
	Any T	N3	M0
Stage IVC	Any T	Any N	M1

9.4.4 Oral Cavity and Oropharynx

In the majority of cases, malignant tumours of the lip are located on/in the lower lip. In more than 90% of the cases those tumours are squamous cell carcinomas. Tumours of the upper lip are most often basal cell carcinomas. More than 90% of cancer of the oral cavity and the oropharynx are squamous cell carcinomas that frequently develop on the floor of precanceroses and especially leukoplakia and erythroplakia. A main characteristic of squamous cell carcinomas of the oral cavity, the tongue, and the oropharynx—and this is also true for all other squamous cell carcinomas located in the area of the upper aerodigestive tract—is their early and highly frequent lymphogenic metastatic spread into regional lymph nodes. This knowledge not only influences the therapeutic strategy, but also the differentiated staging of cervicofacial lymph nodes that accompanies each tumour suspicion. Therefore the

examiner must take into consideration that not only the stage of the primary tumour has prognostic relevance for the 5-year survival and the overall survival, but also the stage of the affected cervicofacial lymph nodes.

9.4.4.1 Inspection and Palpation

In the context of inspection of the lips, the oral cavity and the oropharynx, care must always be taken that dental protheses are removed. By means of a front lamp, a frontal reflector or optimally under microscopic view, the buccal mucosa is examined. The lip and the cheeks are carefully lifted with the spatula in order to assess the parotid secretory ducts that have their openings opposite to the second upper molar. For better examination of the floor of the mouth as well as the secretory ducts of the submandibular glands, the patient is asked to lift the tongue (Fig. 9.4.3). Additionally the tongue is pushed to the side by means of the spatula to inspect the lateral floor of the mouth. The motility check of the tongue includes extending the tongue. Herewith the tongue deviates to the paralysed side in cases of paresis of the hypoglossal nerve (Fig. 9.4.4). By putting the spatula on the body of tongue and carefully, however effectually, pressing it down, the oropharynx with palatine arches, tonsils and posterior wall of the pharynx can be examined. Along with the description of the mucosal surface, the assessment can answer the question whether present tonsils are symmetric and/or luxable and/or coated and/or ulcerated. According findings must be verified regarding possible lesions of the mucosa of the posterior pharyngeal wall as well as the soft palate. The

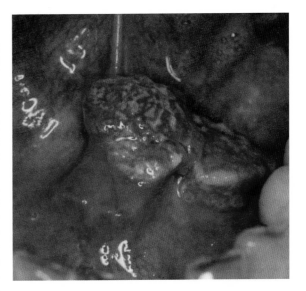

Fig. 9.4.3 Small squamous cell carcinoma of the floor of the mouth

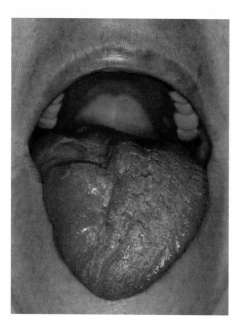

Fig. 9.4.4 Paralysis of the hypoglossal nerve with resulting atrophy of the right part of the tongue and diverging of the tongue to the affected side

9.4.4.2 Endoscopy

The endoscopic examination of the oral cavity and the oropharynx is an essential part of the panendoscopy. By means of the microscope, the oral cavity and the tongue are carefully examined with regard to mucosal lesions. Biopsies are performed from suspicious areas. In the context of direct microlaryngoscopy, the base of tongue and the epiglottic vallecula are also examined. As described previously, palpation is included in the diagnostic procedure in cases of suspected malignomas.

9.4.4.3 Functional Tests

Extending the tongue allows verification of the motility of the tongue. In cases of paresis of the hypoglossal nerve (Fig. 9.4.4), the tongue deviates to the paralysed side. In order to check the motility of the soft palate, phonation of the letter A is required. In cases of paresis of the glossopharyngeal nerve, the soft uvula and the soft palate deviate to the healthy side. A gustatory test is performed by adequate stimulation of the tongue. Aqueous solutions of glucose, saline, citric acid and quinine are dripped on the tongue. This is not performed at random but in certain area of the tongue and the oral cavity: the so-called taste zones. Glucose (sweet) is dripped on the lateral tip of the tongue. Aqueous saline solution is applied to the dorsum of tongue. Citric acid as well as quinine is applied to the area of the vallate papillae representing the border between the body of tongue and the root of tongue. With the chemical gustatory test the identification of certain taste modalities is examined. After eating, smoking or teeth brushing, at least 1 hour must pass before a test.

Further gustatory tests can be performed by electrogustometry. Constant anodic power can evoke a sour metallic sensation at the taste receptors of the tongue. Electrogustometry offers methodical advantages versus chemical tests because lateral differences can be better quantified and precisely situated stimulation is possible. The duration of stimulation is about 0.5–1.5 s. Ten seconds must separate two stimulations. The amperage amounts to 3–300 µA, while the normal stimulation on the tip of the tongue is about 8 µA. Objective gustatory tests are possible, however very complex, and are only offered in large centres to clarify difficult questions posed by experts.

9.4.4.4 Imaging Techniques

CT scan with a bone window is necessary for detection of bony erosions. MRI is mainly indicated for carcinomas located in the area of the tongue and the base of tongue in order to verify the extent of infiltration of the

motility of the soft palate can be checked by phonation of the letter A, which can be repeated several times if necessary. In contrast to hypoglossal paresis, soft uvula and the palatine arches deviate to the healthy side in cases of paresis of the glossopharyngeal nerve. For examination of the base of tongue as well as the posterior surface of the soft palate, the laryngeal speculum or the laryngoscopic examination in the area of the floor of the tongue with the 90° optic, or flexible endoscopy via the nose is recommended. At the same time, flexible transnasal endoscopy can be very helpful.

Palpation is essential in the diagnosis because carcinomas of the oral cavity and the oropharynx might grow in the submucosa. Often this tumour location shows submucosal growth reaching largely beyond the clinically visible limits, which must be verified diagnostically. Those carcinomas are frequently associated with more or less extended pain due to an accompanying bacterial infection in this area. Thus a real palpatory examination is often only possible under general anaesthesia. In the last-mentioned cases, the suspicious areas should be palpated with the index finger; in the area of the floor of the mouth, bimanual examination is recommended to verify differences in the consistency. Palpation allows drawing conclusions concerning the extent, motility, consistency and pain, if palpation is performed on the conscious patient.

base of tongue. MRI can also be very helpful for assessment of possible periosteal infiltration of neighbouring bony structure. Ultrasonographic control of the cervicofacial lymph nodes is essential, completed by fine-needle aspiration (FNA) cytology, if needed, in order to verify the lymph node status preoperatively.

9.4.4.5 TNM Classification

9.4.4.5.1 T Staging (Lip, Oral Cavity)

T1	≤2 cm
T2	>2–4 cm
T3	>4 cm
T4a	Tumour invades adjacent structures (e.g. through cortical bone, into deep (extrinsic) muscle of the tongue [genioglossus, hyoglossus, palatoglossus and styloglossus], maxillary sinus, skin of face)
T4b	Tumour invades masticator space, pterygoid plates, or skull base and/or encases internal carotid artery

9.4.4.5.2 T Staging (Oropharynx)

T1	≤2 cm
T2	>2–4 cm
T3	>4 cm
T4a	Tumour invades the larynx, deep/extrinsic muscle of tongue, medial pterygoid hard palate or mandible
T4b	Tumour invades the lateral pterygoid muscle, pterygoid plates, lateral nasopharynx, or skull base or encases carotid artery

9.4.4.5.3 Staging (Lip, Oral Cavity)

Stage 0	Tis	N0	M0
Stage I	T1	N0	M0
Stage II	T2	N0	M0
Stage III	T3	N0	M0
	T1	N1	M0
	T2	N1	M0
	T3	N1	M0

Stage IVA	T4a	N0	M0
	T4a	N1	M0
	T1	N2	M0
	T2	N2	M0
	T3	N2	M0
	T4a	N2	M0
Stage IVB	T4b	Any N	M0
	Any T	N3	M0
Stage IVC	Any T	Any N	M1

9.4.4.5.4 Staging (Oropharynx, Hypopharynx)

Stage 0	Tis	N0	M0
Stage I	T1	N0	M0
Stage II	T2	N0	M0
Stage III	T3	N0	M0
	T1	N1	M0
	T2	N1	M0
	T3	N1	M0
Stage IVA	T4a	N0	M0
	T4a	N1	M0
	T1	N2	M0
	T2	N2	M0
	T3	N2	M0
	T4a	N2	M0
Stage IVB	T4b	Any N	M0
	Any T	N3	M0
Stage IVC	Any T	Any N	M1

9.4.5 Larynx, Hypopharynx and Upper Oesophagus

According to the location of the tumour, malignomas of the larynx show different symptoms. Hoarseness is one of the early symptoms of glottic cancer, whereas it only manifests in supraglottic and subglottic cancer when the glottis is infiltrated. Unspecific symptoms such as dysphagia, cough, haematorrhea, globus sensation and pain may also indicate laryngeal malignoma. Dyspnoea, however, only occurs at a more advanced tumour stage. At this point, it must be mentioned that supraglottic cancer can show uni- or bilateral cervical lymph nodes metastases as a first symptom. Only in the context of tumour search the primary carcinoma can be verified in the area of the supraglottis. With this background, as for all other carcinomas of the upper aerodigestive tract, the assessment of the preoperative cervical lymph node stage belongs to the established diagnostic concept in order to introduce an appropriate therapy.

The clinical examination of the conscious patient is traditionally performed with a laryngeal speculum. Herewith, the patient is required to extend the tongue. The tongue is taken with the left hand and slightly drawn out while the right hand of the examiner introduces a warmed-up mirror in direction of the uvula. Under slight lifting of the uvula and the invitation to the patient to phonate the sound /hee/, the glottic level can be examined. A more detailed overview can be achieved by laryngoscopical examination with an angled 90° optic or flexible endoscopy of the larynx via the nose. In order to differentiate superficial or infiltrating carcinoma, stroboscopy is recommended as a procedure of differential diagnosis.

Stroboscopy of the larynx allows a differentiated assessment of the vocal fold vibration during phonation. The principle of stroboscopy is based on visual illusion. According to Talbot's rule the human eye is not able to differentiate impressions of less than 0.2 s. Each light impression leaves maximally one positive after-image with duration of 0.2 s; e.g. two different impressions cannot be assessed separately if the interval is shorter than 0.5 s. Thus vocal fold vibrations occurring with very high frequency cannot be assessed by indirect laryngoscopy or microlaryngoscopy. With the aid of a stroboscope, they can be observed and assessed. When a rapidly and regularly vibrating vocal fold is illuminated during phonation with short flashes of the same frequency as the vocal fold vibration, this will happen in the same phase of vibration. Regarding the image, the vocal folds seem to be standing in the phonation level. This is the reason why the vocal folds seem to be stagnant in the illuminated vibration phase. In contrast, the image of the vocal folds seems to be moving in cases of phase shift. For general orientation, first stroboscopy is performed in the moving image by means of a laryngeal microphone. The flash period is longer than the vibration period of the vocal folds. In slow motion the different pitches and intensities of the vocal fold vibrations become evident. In cases of congruence of the flash and the vibration periods, a stagnant image results, as previously explained. The findings achieved by video stroboscopy of a normal vocal fold vibration are based on three different movements. First there are horizontal oscillations in the medial-to-lateral direction, then a hinted vertical vibration going from caudal to cranial in direction, and finally a wave-like motion of the median vocal folds with opening of the glottis from caudal-to-cranial direction, which is called lateral displacement. The normal physiologic vibration of the vocal folds is characterised by regular equal motion of middle amplitude, a complete closing phase and clear mucosal displacement.

In deep frequencies, the vocal folds expand to their total length and breadth and show clear lateral displacements. In comparison to that, the lateral displacement and the amplitude decrease with higher pitches. Increasing loudness, however, leads to wider amplitude, and the lateral displacement becomes more significant. The vocal folds are tense when phonation is performed in the volume of voice performed. The assessment criteria for the stroboscopic findings are glottal closing, symmetry of vibrating vocal folds, amplitude, lateral displacement, periodicity as well as phonatory standstill when amplitude and lateral displacement can no longer be detected. This phonatory standstill must not be confused with impaired or suspended motility of the vocal folds between phonation and respiration. If the phonatory standstill lasts for more than 2 or 3 weeks, then vocal fold carcinoma must be suspected. Differential diagnosis must exclude laryngitis as well as postoperative dysphonia with scarring. In cases of inflammatory disease, however, the phonatory standstill must have subsided after 3 weeks.

Direct microlaryngoscopy with incisional biopsy for histologic diagnosis is indicated for every clinically suspect lesion. The necessity for histologic examination is also true for suspected carcinomas of the hypopharynx and the upper oesophagus. In those cases dysphagia, regurgitation, pressure, or retrosternal pain, and even pain radiating into the ipsilateral ear may occur as first symptoms of hypopharyngeal cancer.

9.4.5.1 Microlaryngoscopy

Today, microlaryngoscopy is a standard method applied worldwide for detection of malignant processes and their pre-stages (Fig. 9.4.5). At the same time it is used for diagnosis and therapy of numerous benign laryngeal processes.

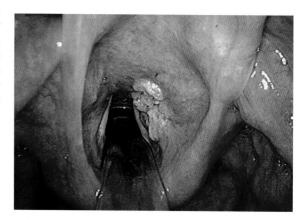

Fig. 9.4.5 T2 carcinoma of the larynx

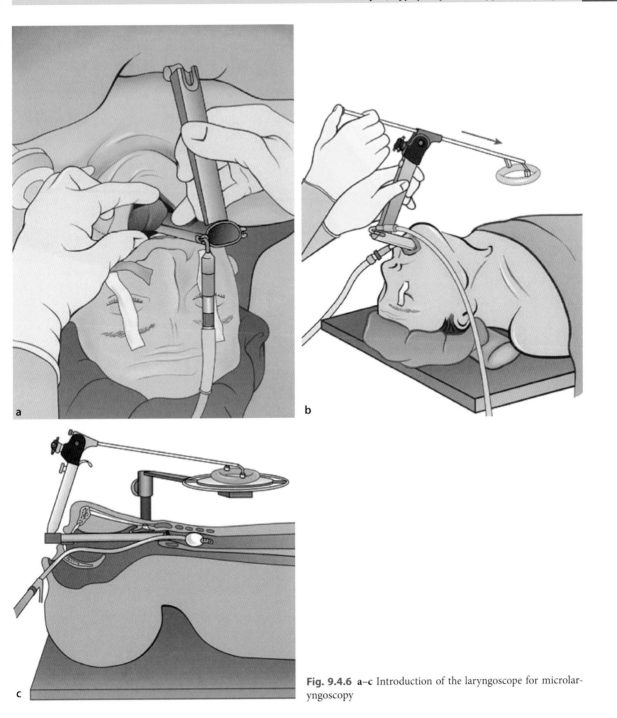

Fig. 9.4.6 a–c Introduction of the laryngoscope for microlaryngoscopy

The patient should lie flat on the table. After intubation and insertion of the maxillary tooth guard, the head of the completely relaxed patient must be flexed dorsally as far as possible. It is recommended for the right-handed surgeon to introduce the laryngoscope from the right, with the endotracheal tube placed on the left (Fig. 9.4.6a).

The position of the tube can be controlled digitally in the patient's pharynx. Care is taken to prevent the tongue from being caught between teeth and laryngoscope. The laryngoscope is guided with the tip to the glottis, following the intubation catheter (Fig. 9.4.6b,c). If the laryngoscope is optimally set, then the vocal cords are in full view from the anterior commissure to the tips of the vocal processes. Sometimes the anterior commissure cannot be overlooked completely due to anatomical conditions that do not allow adequate adjustment of the larynx. In such a case the field to be overlooked can be adjusted either with a laryngoscope with slightly elevated tip or examined by means of an angular optic. In many cases, however, it is sufficient to impose slight pressure on the larynx in order to adjust the anterior commissure. Even the examination of the ventricles can be optimised by laterally imposing pressure, by pressing the tip of the laryngoscope against the ventricular fold in the lateral direction. Also in this context the angular optic can give additional information, as it proved of value for the inspection of the laryngeal epiglottic surface and the subglottic space. The posterior wall of the larynx can be well examined by pushing the endotracheal catheter into the anterior commissure. This positioning also allows an examination of the postcricoid region.

A short and stiff neck, a very prominent base of tongue being firm on palpation, long protrusive teeth of the upper jaw as well as dislocations of the larynx can make microlaryngoscopy rather difficult or even impossible. Those exceptional cases commonly influence the decision of the therapy that the originally planned tumour resection must be performed from the exterior.

Before commencing the operation, photographic and/or video demonstration is made with the aid of the operating microscope or a photoendoscope. Generally, the documentation can be recorded directly via the operating microscope or via a rigid photo optic. The video demonstration enables the anaesthesiologist and operating room staff as well as surgeons in training or visitors to follow the operation on the screen. It provides for faster and more effective cooperation with the scrub nurse. In the case of a haemorrhage for example, an experienced nurse will be able to act swiftly and appropriately. A further advantage is the objective documentation of preoperative, intraoperative and postoperative findings or the continuous recording of the operation for teaching purposes.

9.4.5.2 Oesophagoscopy

The technique of oesophagoscopy can be performed with a rigid tube or a flexible oesophagoscope. The indications for both methods overlap. Finally the choice of the endoscope is also influenced by the experience of the examiner. Generally, it can be stated that the rigid oesophagoscope can be applied diagnostically as well as therapeutically; it is the instrument of choice for foreign-body extraction. From a diagnostic point of view, fibre endoscopy under local anaesthesia must be considered superior. This technique is often combined to gastroduodenoscopy.

9.4.5.2.1 Rigid Oesophagoscopy

Rigid oesophagoscopy is performed with the patient's head slightly lifted and reclined. After insertion of the laryngoscopy spatula, the oesophagoscope is introduced from the right corner of the mouth and directed behind the arytenoid protuberances, which in this position can be slightly shifted with the tip of the instrument. The rigid oesophagoscope is carefully advanced until the oesophageal mouth is seen as an oval fissure. With introduction of the tube behind the arytenoid cartilage, the examination has to be performed through the endoscope; the laryngeal spatula is then removed. After penetration of the upper oesophageal sphincter, the tube is advanced carefully with two fingers, without any effort into the oesophagus; the patient should be completely relaxed. The inspection of the mucosa and incisional biopsy is performed while drawing back the oesophagoscope under view with the double spoon or a punch. Possible bleeding is controlled by application of a vasoconstrictor.

9.4.5.2.2 Flexible Oesophagoscopy

For flexible oesophagoscopy, the patients should be fasting, and the patient's current blood clotting status known. Intravenous sedation with, e. g. 5–10 mg midazolam (Dormicum®), facilitates not only ease of the examination for the patient, but also for the examiner. After repositioning the patient in left lateral position, extended mucosal anaesthesia of the pharynx is performed with lidocaine (Xylocain®) spray. Further metal dental protection should be inserted into the upper jaw. It is also recommended to apply anaesthetising gel to the oesophagoscope, e. g. lidocaine (Xylocain® gel), and then to introduce it through the mouth and the pharynx into the oesophagus. The flexible oesophagoscope is inserted from the side with the right hand of the examiner. The patient is asked to breathe deeply and to swallow at the same time. After passing through the oesophageal mouth the oesophagoscope is advanced visually. The visual field must be cleaned by *suction and air insufflation*. With further advancing, the distal end of the oesophagoscope is always directed to the centre of the oesophagus, with the handhold. As in the context of rigid endoscopy, the oesophagus is inspected carefully when drawing the instrument back. If necessary, the oesophagus is displayed by air insufflation. For incisional biopsy, special forceps are advanced through the instrumentation canal and applied visually. After incisional biopsy, forceps are carefully drawn back.

9.4.5.3 Imaging Techniques

The diagnostic methods of examination of the hypopharynx and larynx correspond generally to the ones of the oesophagus, while CT scan and MRI give the best overview when applied with contrast agents, in the context of assessment of the tumour extent. In the area of the hypopharynx, MRI can be superior to CT scan because it allows a better differentiation of the soft parts and thus facilitates the discernment of the tumour versus surrounding healthy tissue. This procedure, however, can be impaired within the entire region by swallowing artefacts. In the oesophagus, generally CT is sufficient due to the neighbouring pulmonary tissue. In cases of special questions in the area of the larynx, e.g. infiltration of the preepiglottic space regarding a process located in the area of the anterior commissure, thin-section tomography of the larynx is essential.

9.4.5.4 TNM Classification

9.4.5.4.1 T Staging (Hypopharynx)

T1	≤2 cm, limited to a subregion
T2	>2–4 cm or more than one subregion
T3	>4 cm or with hemilaryngeal fixation
T4a	Thyroid/cricoid cartilage, hyoid bone, thyroid gland, oesophagus, central cervical soft parts
T4b	Prevertebral fascia, internal carotid artery, mediastinal structures

9.4.5.4.2 T Staging (Supraglottis)

T1	One subregion, normally mobile vocal folds
T2	Mucosa of more than one subregion of supraglottis/glottis or mucosa or one area outside the supraglottis, no laryngeal fixation
T3	Limited to the larynx with fixation of the vocal folds and/or invasion of the post-cricoid region, preepiglottic tissue, paraglottic space, low-grade thyroid cartilage erosion
T4a	Tumour invades the thyroid cartilage and/or invades tissues beyond the larynx (e.g. trachea, soft tissue of neck including deep extrinsic muscle of the tongue, strap muscles, thyroid or oesophagus)
T4b	Tumour invades prevertebral space, encases carotid artery or invades mediastinal structures

9.4.5.4.3 T Staging (Glottis)

T1	Limited to the vocal fold(s), normally mobile vocal folds
T1a	One vocal fold
T1b	Both vocal folds
T2	Growth into supraglottis or subglottis, limited mobility of the vocal folds
T3	Fixation of the vocal folds, extent to the preepiglottic space, low-grade erosion of the thyroid cartilage
T4a	Tumour invades the thyroid cartilage and/or invades tissues beyond the larynx (e.g. trachea, soft tissues of neck including deep extrinsic muscle of the tongue, strap muscles, thyroid or oesophagus)
T4b	Tumour invades prevertebral space, encases carotid artery or invades mediastinal structures

9.4.5.4.4 T Staging (Subglottis)

T1	Limited to subglottis
T2	Normal or limited mobility
T3	Vocal fold fixation
T4a	Tumour invades cricoid or thyroid cartilage and/or invades tissues beyond the larynx (e.g. trachea, soft tissues of the neck including deep extrinsic muscle of the tongue, strap muscles, thyroid or oesophagus)
T4b	Tumour invades prevertebral space, encases carotid artery or invades mediastinal structures

9.4.5.4.5 Staging (Larynx)

Stage 0	Tis	N0	M0
Stage I	T1	N0	M0
Stage II	T2	N0	M0
Stage III	T3	N0	M0
	T1	N1	M0
	T2	N1	M0
	T3	N1	M0

Stage IVA	T4a	N0	M0
	T4a	N1	M0
	T1	N2	M0
	T2	N2	M0
	T3	N2	M0
	T4a	N2	M0
Stage IVB	T4b	Any N	M0
	Any T	N3	M0
Stage IVC	Any T	Any N	M1

9.4.5.4.6 Staging (Oropharynx, Hypopharynx)

Stage 0	Tis	N0	M0
Stage I	T1	N0	M0
Stage II	T2	N0	M0
Stage III	T3	N0	M0
	T1	N1	M0
	T2	N1	M0
	T3	N1	M0
Stage IVA	T4a	N0	M0
	T4a	N1	M0
	T1	N2	M0
	T2	N2	M0
	T3	N2	M0
	T4a	N2	M0
Stage IVB	T4b	Any N	M0
	Any T	N3	M0
Stage IVC	Any T	Any N	M1

9.4.6 Tracheobronchial System

9.4.6.1 Tracheobronchoscopy

Compared to oesophagoscopy, tracheobronchoscopy can also be performed under general anaesthesia or under local anaesthesia. In this context, flexible tracheobronchoscopy in local anaesthesia serves for prognostic purposes, e. g. in cases of stenosis; however it is not appropriated for foreign-body extractions.

9.4.6.2 Rigid Tracheobronchoscopy

Rigid tracheobronchoscopy is performed under intubation anaesthesia. The patient is in supine position with reclined head and relaxation. The patient is not intubated via an intubation tube, but the rigid tube is inserted through the glottis into the trachea after initial mask ventilation, and at the same time oxygen inhalation anaesthetic is applied. Differently angled optics can be inserted through this endoscope, permitting high imaging quality as well as the transtracheal or transbronchial extraction of foreign bodies. This is the method of choice for the purpose of foreign-body extraction and for transtracheal or transbronchial puncture of mediastinal lymph nodes or tumours. The diameter of the bronchoscope should correspond to the diameter of the ungual phalanx of the little finger of the patient. The rigid bronchoscope is shifted through the glottis and advanced into the trachea, up to the bifurcation. Then inspection first of the right and then of the left main bronchus is performed as well as further inspection of the bronchial arborizations with differently angled optics.

9.4.6.3 Flexible Tracheobronchoscopy

Flexible tracheobronchoscopy is generally performed with a thin fibre endoscope after premedication and preparations as for oesophagoscopy. Herewith the fibre endoscope is also inserted through the glottis and the trachea. A thin (about 6 mm in diameter) fibre endoscope allows biopsy sites located more peripherally in the subsegmental bronchi. Foreign-body extraction, however, is not always possible, as already explained. In comparison to rigid tracheobronchoscopy with optics, the imaging is clearly of reduced quality. Flexible endoscopes are mainly applied in the context of intensive care in cases of long-term intubation for control of the tracheal mucosa.

9.4.7 Major Salivary Glands

The diagnosis of diseases of the salivary glands includes first a detailed anamnesis verifying duration and course of a possibly occurring swelling of the gland in the sense of continuous growth or a swelling on ingestion. Further, pain and redness of the skin, intermittent pain due to ingestion, xerostomia or additionally occurring paresis of the facial nerve must be assessed pathognomically, especially for malignant tumours of the parotid gland. Additional concomitant symptoms such as gnathospasm or associated eye diseases and articular complaints must be assessed as well as condition after irradiation of the head and neck. Internal diseases such as hypertonia, hyperthyreosis or diabetes mellitus as well as regularly taken medications, as for example, antihistamines, beta-blockers, anticholinergics or antidepressants, must be questioned. Inspection and palpation includes the description of glandular swellings in the sense of diffuse, painful and possibly short-term or even localised and long-term masses. The palpatory comparison between the right and the left side reveals uni- or bilateral glandular growth. Further, the orifice of the excretory duct of the parotid gland, which is located opposite to the second molar of the upper jaw, must be inspected, and after pressure on the parotid gland the secretion must be examined microscopically. The caruncula with the orifice of the submandibular/sublingual gland is located in the anterior floor of mouth paramedian to the insertion of the frenulum. Even there the secretion expressed by pressing on the submandibular gland should be examined microscopically. Care must be taken in cases of protrusion of the lateral wall of the pharynx of the soft palate, or the tonsillar region in the case of a so-called iceberg tumour, a deeply located tumour of the retromandibular area and the pharyngeal process of the parotid gland.

Imaging examination includes first B-mode sonography as a screening examination in order to differentiate cystic and solid processes and the detection of calculi. Ultrasonography can be completed by FNA biopsy. In this context, care must be taken that in about 10–20% of the cases false-positive or false-negative results are achieved, which can be explained by the frequently complex cellular image of the single-tumour entities. An additional imaging technique is the plain radiography of the floor of the mouth. This procedure is performed tangentially and laterally in cases of suspected calculi of the submandibular gland or the parotid gland. The detection of calculi, however, is only successful when the concretions contain sufficient calcium. Further sialography is possible in cases of negative findings of plain radiography. Herewith the contrast agent application is performed via a plastic catheter (diameter of 1 mm) that is inserted into the excretory duct of the salivary gland. Previous local anaesthesia for example with Gingicain® spray is recommended. Sialography shows the calculi generally as round, negative contrasts. In the case of chronic recurrent sialadenitis, the image shows a "leafy tree" with calibre differences. Malignant neoplasms can be accompanied with ductal evulsion and the outflow of contrast agent into the glandular parenchyma, while benign tumours can be detected due to displacement of the ducts filled with contrast agent. In the case of Sjögren's syndrome the image of a leafless tree appears in the final stage of the diseases due to rarification of the ductal system.

Sjögren's syndrome is caused by an immune reaction against the excretory duct epithelia of the salivary and the lacrimal glands. Sometimes concomitant symptoms such as pharyngitis, laryngotracheitis, rheumatic arthropathia, allergic vascular purpura, or periarteritis nodosa make the diagnosis difficult. If only xerostomia or xerophthalmia occur, primary Sjögren's syndrome is diagnosed. Secondary Sjögren's syndrome is present when additional diseases of rheumatoid character occur. Patients suffering from Sjögren's syndrome have a significantly higher risk

(in about 5% of the cases) do develop MALT (mucosa-associated lymphoid tissue) lymphoma or another non-Hodgkin's lymphoma resulting from lymphatic infiltrations of the lympho-epitheliomatous lesions. This makes life-long follow-up of these patients essential.

The assessment of the salivary quantity (sialometry) and an analysis of the secretion (sialosemeiology) permits drawing conclusions about the disease, as, for example, in the case of Sjögren's syndrome. After previous sufficient local anaesthesia with Gingicain® and probe of the excretory duct, a plastic catheter measuring 1 mm in diameter is introduced into the glandular excretory duct. Then the saliva is collected for 10 min prior and subsequent to stimulation, respectively, with ascorbic acid. For this purpose, the free end of the plastic catheter is inserted into a plastic tube outside the mouth. The quantity of the collected fluid allows drawing conclusions regarding the quantitative secretion of the gland. The qualitative analysis of the secretion (e.g. electrolyte composition) can be performed chemically.

In the case of a suspected tumour, MRI of the salivary glands and/or CT are/is the method(s) of choice in order to objectify the exact extent of the mass into adjacent structures (skull base, parapharyngeal space).

9.4.8 Neck

For squamous cell carcinomas of the upper aerodigestive tract, the presence of lymph node metastases is the most important prognostic factor. Often only palpation is used in order to determine cervical lymph node swellings. Because of the low sensitivity of physical examination, a neck showing no metastases on palpation (clinical N0 neck) bears the risk of hiding so-called occult metastases. Furthermore, some malignancies of the head and neck develop contralateral metastases, especially when the primary tumour is situated near the midline, or it has even surpassed it. With this background, the procedures that are used in the diagnosis of cervical lymph node enlargement are described and their significance discussed critically in the context of determining cervical lymph node metastases.

9.4.8.1   Inspection and Palpation

The first condition for the evaluation of lymph node swelling in the head and neck is a very carefully obtained patient history and physical exam with information on duration of the swelling, change in size, presence or absence of pain, possibility of displacement, possible origins of the disease and any pretreatments. Inspection and palpation are the base of each medical examination and should be performed prior to every technical examination. For examination of the neck the patient should undress the upper part of the body and remove jewellery. The patient should sit straight up because this position allows optimum examination conditions. Special attention must be paid to scars that are sometimes very difficult to identify.

The palpation of the neck is performed simultaneously on both sides, e. g. bimanually to compare the two sides. Usually the patient sits and the examiner stands in front of or behind the patient. The palpation of single lymph node regions is performed with one hand while the other hand guides the head of the patient or exposes deeply situated tissue by counter-pressure. For palpation of the supraclavicular lymph nodes, the patient should cough or strain because these manoeuvres will reveal palpable changes in the lymph nodes. The pre- and postauricular lymph nodes are mainly situated superficially and can be palpated with the fingertips.

9.4.8.2 B-Mode Sonography

During the last two decades, ultrasonography has developed into an indispensable method in the diagnosis of diseases of the head and neck region. Technical advances in sonographic equipment as well as colour Doppler and duplex sonography make sonography undoubtedly the imaging procedure of choice for the morphologic examination of cervical soft tissues in Europe. B-mode sonography has high sensitivity in the detection of enlarged lymph nodes. Including ultrasound-guided FNA cytology, the sensitivity amounts to 93–95% and the specificity to 87–93%. Investigators have reported it to be superior to palpation (60%), CT (83%) and MRI (83%). Its application is useful in differential diagnosis, surgical planning and the postoperative care of the neck. For examination of the cervical region, high-resolution probes (5–7.5 MHz) with a width of about 1 cm and a length of 4–5 cm should be used. By means of the small contact, surface challenging areas like the paramandibular region can be depicted without significant artefacts.

Sonographic examination of the lymph nodes is evaluated in terms of localisation, size in transverse and longitudinal diameters, shape, echo characteristics, grouping and perfusion pattern, and pulsatility as seen in the colour Doppler. In B-mode sonography, lymph nodes appear from echoless to mainly homogenous structures. They are oval or round, mostly clearly limited and of different sizes. In the context of the entire clinical situation (symptoms, palpation and inspection), a certain percentage of sonographically and/or clinically detected lymph nodes can be described. However, at this time, there are no safe sonomorphological criteria, especially for lymph nodes smaller than 8 mm, that allow pathognomonic diagnosis or guarantee a precise differential diagnosis of malignancy. In order to ascertain the diagnosis and to ex-

clude malignant diseases, in almost every case a cytologic examination is necessary.

9.4.8.2.1 Sonographic Criteria

The sonographic assessment of lymph nodes considers localisation, size, contour, delineation, density and the internal structure. Benign lymph nodes are generally strictly delimited and are bean-shaped as well as homogenous and moderately echogenic. Further benign criteria are the sharp limitation of the hilar vessel (Fig. 9.4.7) and an only indicated or even missing distal sound reinforcement.

Cervical lymph node metastases are generally low echogenic, round or bean-shaped. Although metastatically affected lymph nodes often have a diameter of more than 10 mm (Fig. 9.4.8), this fact alone is no criterion for malignancy. In this context the short/long axis ratio is important. If it is ≥2, then this is an indication for malignancy. Another criterion of malignancy is a missing hilar vessel image. Nearly always, a distal sound reinforcement can be detected. Considering all criteria of distinction, the detection of hilar vessel image is highly significant; the ratio of short/long axis is significant.

In the context of staging examinations, all enlarged lymph nodes must be suspected malignant. This is very important because in 40% of cases, lymph nodes with a diameter of less than 10 mm were found involved by cancer, with some showing extracapsular spread.

9.4.8.2.2 Sonographically Controlled FNA Cytology

In the last years, sonography has been performed more and more in combination with aspiration cytology to im-

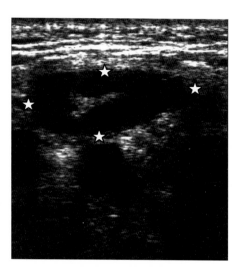

Fig. 9.4.7 Typical appearance of a benign lymph node with central hilar vessel and exact limitation

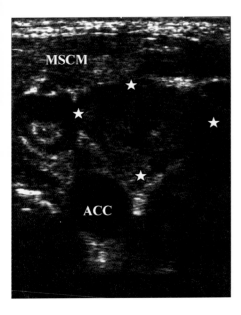

Fig. 9.4.8 Typical appearance of a round, centrally necrotic lymph node metastasis. *MSCM* sternocleidomastoid muscle, *ACC* carotid artery

For core biopsy, special aspiration cannulas (Tru-Cut system: 11.4 cm long, 14-G diameter) are used. Aspiration must generally be performed under sterile conditions. Local anaesthesia is required, in contrast to FNA. Prior to the introduction of the aspiration cannula an incision should be made with a scalpel to avoid adding small skin parts to the specimen. The biopsy specimen is fixed with formalin, and after embedding in paraffin it is examined histologically.

An error sometimes made is choosing the wrong lymph node to be aspirated. Lymph node size and morphology help predict the metastatic behaviour of the primary tumour. Similar to core needle biopsy, cytology represents only the part of the tumour where the cell aspiration has been performed. Aspiration of lymph node areas not harbouring tumour cells, the aspiration of liquid parts, or a very low number of tumour cells in the aspiration lead to false-negative results. Theses difficulties occur especially in smaller (<5 mm) or necrotic lymph nodes.

The complication rate of FNA cytology and core biopsy is very low. The risk of seeding tumour cells of malignant tumours in the needle tract is considered very low as well.

9.4.8.2.3 Future Technical Development of Sonography

The significance of the *colour-coded duplex sonography* for differential diagnosis of lymph node diseases, the differentiation of reactive lymphadenitis from cervical lymph node metastases, has not been completely clarified. The initial hope to increase significantly the sensitivity by evaluating lymph node perfusion and establishing characteristic perfusion parameters is not yet fully rea-

prove the assessment of cervical tumours. FNA is a diagnostic method that is very easy to perform. It is rapidly available, cost-effective, can be performed on an outpatient basis, is minimally morbid for the patient and can easily be repeated if necessary. The advantage of ultrasound-directed FNA in comparison to palpatory aspiration is that tumour tissue is aspirated visually. This is particularly important if the tumour is small and localised in the deeper cervical levels and cannot be assessed by palpation. Lymph nodes of a size of 3–4 mm diameter or lymphomas situated very close to vessels can be aspirated specifically. Furthermore, the differentiation can be made if the cellular aspiration is gained from a solid or cystic part of the lymph node, which can be of significant diagnostic importance for necrotic lymph node metastases.

The differentiation is made between FNA and core biopsy. The core biopsy is performed by aspirating a tissue cylinder that is sufficient for histologic examination, whereas FNA takes cells from the tissue aggregate that can then be diagnosed cytologically (Fig. 9.4.9).

For FNA, a 20-ml syringe is used that is fixed to a syringe holder so that high suction is possible, using one hand for aspiration. Needles 22 or 23 G with an external diameter of 0.7 or 0.8 mm are attached to the syringe. Cells or cell groups are aspirated from the tissue aggregate by suction and moving up and down of the needle. After discontinuation of the aspiration the vacuum is broken with the cannula still in the tumour. Thus the theoretically possible seeding of tumour cells in the needle tract can be avoided.

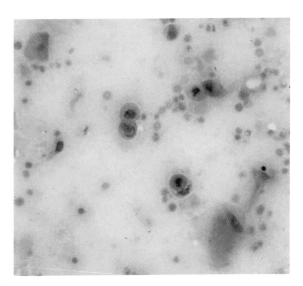

Fig. 9.4.9 FNA cytology of a metastasis

lised. Possibly the introduction of contrast enhancers can achieve a higher degree of accuracy.

To what extent the *application of signal* amplifiers leads to an increased specificity of the colour-coded duplex sonography in the diagnosis of enlarged cervical lymph nodes is not evident, and must be proven by prospective studies with greater numbers of cases.

Clinical experience with *three-dimensional sonography* of the head and neck has been limited. Identical sensitivity and specificity concerning the preoperative diagnosis of cervical lymph node metastases can be shown in comparison to B-mode sonography. This procedure, when used to detect questionable vascular infiltration of the carotid artery, is very useful. Three-dimensional sonography could also contribute to an improved sensitivity in ultrasound-guided FNA cytology.

Tissue harmonic imaging makes use of the nonlinearity of sound created in tissue and allows correction of the defocusing, phase-shifting effects. This new technology (Ultrasound system Elegra®, Siemens, Erlangen, Germany) allows an improved spatial resolution with contrasting of deeply situated tissue. The conventional B-mode sonography can thus be optimised, especially in obese patients and in cases of lymphoedema or anatomic changes after surgical interventions. The basis for this technique is the sending of subsequent, inverted ultrasound impulses so that the regressive signals of the pulses and the linear echo cancel out each other. The resulting images appear clearer and sharper. *Contrast harmonic imaging* allows the description of the smallest vessels in colour-coded duplex sonography without motion artefacts or over-radiation by adjacent bigger vessels. Initial experience with this technique is very encouraging.

In *sono-CT real-time compound imaging,* pulses in addition to the vertical sending of the probe are sent and received. Via digital processing of the received signals with very high computer capacity, an image is composed in real-time that is created from the single images of different sound angles and summed up (compound technique). The resolution and quality of the image is improved with this technique in comparison to the traditional B-mode imaging. Clinical experience with this technique in patients suffering from cancer of the head and neck is virtually nil.

9.4.8.3   Imaging Techniques

9.4.8.3.1   CT and MRI

Since their clinical introduction into the diagnostic routine, CT and MRI have both been applied for evaluation of enlarged cervical lymph nodes and tumorous masses. CT is generally preferred over MRI. It is available at any time, free from motion artefacts, and is easier to interpret

by the head and neck surgeon. Furthermore, CT is indicated in all patients who suffer from claustrophobia and have other contraindications (e.g. cardiac pacemaker, metallic implantations) for MRI.

In the CT scan, normal lymph nodes are seen as well-defined, generally long and oval masses. They reveal a homogeneous density comparable to vessels, with hypodense values equivalent to muscle. They can be distinguished from round vascular structures only after administration of intravenous contrast agents. The description of lymph nodes sized ≥5 mm is possible with newer CT equipment; however, it depends significantly on the determined slice thickness. The diameter of benign lymph nodes is generally less than 10 mm, while the lymph nodes in region II may be larger due to persistent tonsillar tissue.

After intravenous contrast enhancement, the density is higher in inflammatory diseases and malignant lymphomas than in metastases. Malignant lymphomas are most often well circumscribed, have a homogeneous density and do not reveal rim enhancement after contrast application. In lymph node metastases, central necrosis occurs early and presents as a hypodense area in the CT scan. Central necrosis and rim enhancement are only nonspecific criteria because they also occur in inflammatory lymph node diseases with necrosis or abscess formation.

In comparison to CT scanning, MRI better defines soft tissue due to its high tissue contrast. For assessment of smaller cervical lymph nodes, a slice thickness of 3 mm is recommended, especially in the clinically most interesting regions, generally the levels II and III. The scans should always be performed in two levels from the skull base to the clavicle. The contrast application of Gd-DTPA is helpful in assessing tumour necrosis within lymph nodes and also for better delineation of the primary tumour.

9.4.8.3.2   Dynamic Scintigraphy of Lymphatic Drainage

In the head and neck, lymphoscintigraphy has been used for the preoperative description of the lymphatic drainage of carcinomas. In this area, however, the detection of lymph node metastases by this method is less important, because B-mode sonography is a more reliable and less costly technique for routine staging. The aim of lymphoscintigraphy of squamous cell carcinomas of the head and neck is more the description of lymphatic drainage direction in order to obtain further information regarding the extent of neck dissection.

Lymphatic drainage in the neck occurs depending on the localisation of the primary tumour. By means of lymphoscintigraphy it can thus be verified if the metastatic spread is limited to the predominant lymphatic direction or if other lymph node regions and/or the contralateral side must be included into the treatment concept. This is important for the N0 neck because selective neck dissection would only be performed in neck lymph node areas where the chance of metastatic spread is high. Furthermore, in the case of advanced ipsilateral metastatic spread, and therefore potentially exhausted transport capacity of the lymphatic fluid, contralateral lymphatic spread can also be detected.

The results of lymphoscintigraphy have shown in up to 70% of cases a good description of ipsilateral and/or contralateral lymphatic drainage with anatomic allocation to defined cervical lymph node regions. In about 30% of the examined patients no lymphatic drainage could be detected. The authors explain this fact by reduced lymphatic drainage due to intraoperative tissue compression by the endoscopy instruments. Other reasons might include suspended lymphatic drainage because of tumour infiltration in lymph nodes as well as posttherapeutically transformed or missing lymph vessels. At this point it must be stressed that the radionuclide is taken up in reduced quantity or not at all by the lymph nodes that are affected by a metastases and possibly have capsular rupture. Another disadvantage of dynamic lymphoscintigraphy is that only tumour localisations in the region of the oral cavity and the oropharynx allow the application of the radionuclide without additional anaesthesia.

Summing up the experiences collected up to date, it may be stated that lymphoscintigraphy in the double-tracer technique allows the exact allocation of a described lymphatic drainage to the anatomic structures of the head and neck, and can thus be helpfully applied in the preoperative diagnosis paradigm to augment other imaging procedures. For primary detection of cervical lymph nodes, however, it is not appropriate.

9.4.8.3.3 Sentinel Node Concept

The purpose of the sentinel node concept is to identify the lymph nodes draining the lymph fluid of the tumour region in patients showing no clinical evidence of lymphogenic metastasis. This purpose is justified in patients who might have occult metastasis in the first lymph node station due to tumour size and location. Regarding the terminology, a difference must be made between classic *sentinel node biopsy* and *lymphatic mapping*. Sentinel node biopsy implies the identification and extirpation of an isolated tracer accumulating lymph node. Lymphatic mapping means the detection and resection of more radiotracer accumulating lymph nodes.

The description of the regional lymphatic drainage of a malignant tumour of the head and neck by means of scintigraphic procedures is not new. Fisch performed the first detailed studies on these procedures. The effort associated initially with lymphoscintigraphy of the head and neck to detect metastatically affected lymph nodes of malignant tumours was abandoned because it became obvious that in particular, metastatically affected lymph nodes cannot or only insufficiently be described by scintigraphy.

In the context of sentinel node biopsy, scintigraphy is performed in patients in whom there is no clinical indication of lymphogenic metastatic spread for identification of the lymph node draining the lymph fluid of the tumour region. This procedure is justified in patients who are suspected of having an occult metastatic spread into the first lymph node station, due to the size and location of the tumour. Thus scintigraphy of the lymph draining pathways of a primary tumour of the upper aerodigestive tract serves to identify this so-called sentinel lymph node, which is maintains physiological integrity. Only the subsequent histological examination reveals possible metastatic involvement in the sense of micrometastasis or limited macrometastasis.

As the value of this new diagnostic and therapeutic procedure depends on the assured detection of the true sentinel node, detecting the sentinel node in the head and neck along with the disperse radiation of the neighbouring primary tumour presents an enormous challenge. While the tracer can be injected in local anaesthesia in cases of easily accessible oral carcinomas, pharyngeal and laryngeal carcinomas can only be exposed completely under general anaesthesia. It has been shown that because of better exposure of the primary lesion and reduced movement of the relaxed patient (e. g. pharyngeal reflex, motility of the tongue), the precise injections can be realized as well for carcinomas of the oral cavity. This more clearly marked drainage region contributes to the value of this method. Due to the density and direction of the initial lymph vessels in the primary tumour region, a preferred drainage in one or more of those lymph node stations exists for each location of a primary tumour of the upper aerodigestive tract, so that one primary tumour may have more first-draining lymph nodes. Thus the authors think that one to three hot nodes should be excised and examined histologically in order to minimise the number of false-negative results.

The topographic analysis of the intraoperatively identified sentinel node confirms the classic description of the regional lymphatic drainage of carcinomas of the upper aerodigestive tract. So pharyngeal and laryngeal carcinomas metastasise mainly into level II and less frequently into level III. Carcinomas of the anterior oral cavity mainly drain into level I and less frequently into level II. According to these findings it can be expected that dissection of the according cervical lymph node levels can include the majority of clinically occult metastases.

Regarding the significance of the sentinel lymphadenectomy for carcinomas of the head and neck, critical and careful verification is essential if the method described for other tumour entities can be transferred to head and neck carcinomas. A first step regarding the comparability of the examination results is to standardise the procedures. Otherwise, the techniques performed by different groups can vary significantly with important consequences for the oncologic treatment concepts for the patients. For example, for the isolated lymph node extirpation performed in few centres, no valid data exists. Regarding the significant prognostic importance of an overlooked lymphogenic metastatic spread with cloudy reduction of the 5-year survival rate, such a standardised procedure should be elaborated, in the form of controlled prospective studies, as the sentinel node concept is still in an experimental stage for this tumour entity.

9.4.8.3.4 Positron Emission Tomography

Positron emission tomography (PET) is a noninvasive procedure for measuring biochemical processes in tissue. In contrast to morphologic imaging (CT, MRI), PET results detail function in organs and tissues. In PET scanning the radiopharmaceuticals are labelled with a so-called positron-emitting radionuclide. Those are extraordinarily transient elements occurring in organic material. The most common are ^{15}O ($t_½$: 2 min); ^{13}N ($t_½$: 10 min); ^{11}C ($t_½$: 20 min) and as a substitute for hydrogen, ^{18}F ($t_½$: 110 min). Numerous detectors arranged in a circular array and calibrated according to complex reconstruction algorithms in section images can measure the radiation resulting from decay of the PET nuclides.

Studies concerning the significance of PET for lymph node diagnoses are very few. However, in studies thus far, PET revealed an accuracy in the detection of cervical lymph node metastases to similar to CT or MRI. The sensitivity amounted to 71–90% while the specificity varied between 77 and 100%. In contrast to pretherapeutic diagnosis, PET seems to have some advantages in the posttherapeutic assessment of cervical lymph node status. The sensitivity of revealing recurrent or residual lymph node metastases is estimated to be more than 90%. Because some of the patients with a locoregional recurrence suffer from distant metastases, those can be identified reliably by means of whole-body PET. This procedure is of significant importance in planning further diagnosis and therapy.

9.4.8.4 Lymph Node TNM Classification

N staging (regional lymph nodes) is categorized as follows:

NX	Regional lymph nodes cannot be assessed
N0	No regional lymph node metastases
N1	Metastases in solitary ipsilateral lymph nodes, ≤3 cm

N2	Metastases in solitary ipsilateral lymph nodes, >3 cm, ≤6 cm, or in multiple ipsilateral lymph nodes, none >6 cm, or in bilateral or contralateral lymph nodes, none >6 cm of maximal size
N2a	Metastases in solitary ipsilateral lymph nodes, >3 cm but ≤6 cm
N2b	Metastases in multiple ipsilateral lymph nodes, none >6 cm of maximal size
N2c	Metastases in bilateral or contralateral lymph nodes, none >6 cm of maximal size
N3	Metastases in lymph nodes, >6 cm of maximal size

9.4.9 Special Diagnostic Procedures

Considering their microscopic and endoscopic aspects, tumorous neoplasms, especially leukoplakia, chronic laryngitis with its different grades of dysplasia and even some highly differentiated carcinomas and papillomatous diseases, cannot be reliably graded and classified with regard to their gravity. Even intraoperative examination frequently leaves uncertainty, so that finally only histological examination of specimens leads to a reliable diagnosis. The improved early detection of preneoplastic mucosal lesions (ideally even in the sense of screening) would allow therapeutic approaches at a significantly lower tumour stage. In this context possible new diagnostic procedures could be autofluorescence endoscopy and fluorescence endoscopy with the use of photosensitisers such as 5-aminolaevulinic acid (ALA).

9.4.9.1 Autofluorescence Diagnostics

During the last decades, several efforts were made to verify different endogenic fluorophores of malignant and benign tissue. However, due to the complexity of the emitted light, no real success was achieved. Given this, autofluorescence diagnosis is performed using a monochromatic or very narrow spectral exciting light to focus on one or more strong fluorophoric agents. The so-called LIFE system (light-imaging fluorescence endoscope) was the procedure that was applied first in 1990 for bronchoscopy. It was a monochromatic helium cadmium laser with an exciting wavelength of 442 nm, focussing on the fluorophore protoporphyrin IX. The in vivo tissue excitement via a xenon lamp (D-light no. 20-133201, Storz, Tuttlingen, Germany) used a wavelength of 375–440 nm. In addition to fluorescence exciting light, this source of light delivers white light so that both lights can be used by manually switching or by foot switch. Healthy mucosal areas present in the autofluorescence mode of the D-light system typically as green-bluish light. In comparison, benign as well as malignant mucosal lesions are revealed differently. Malignomas appear mainly as greyish, brownish green; the main characteristic is the toning down or even lack of the typical green-bluish colour of the mentioned mucosal area. Also, precancerous mucosal lesions appear similar, so that autofluorescence endoscopy allows early detection of preneoplastic lesions in comparison to white light endoscopy. The additional spectral analysis of the different fluorescences allows better quantification of fluorescence examination results and thus objectifies them. Recently, success has been achieved in the differentiation of carcinomas and healthy mucosa. With the aid of different photosensitisers, even the fluorescence of malignant tissue can be reinforced. In this context, ALA-induced fluorescence diagnosis must be mentioned.

Comparing autofluorescence endoscopy and 5-ALA endoscopy, the above-mentioned procedure seems to have several advantages regarding the sensitivity.

9.4.9.2 Fluorescence Diagnosis of Neoplasms

With its background, 5-ALA–induced fluorescence diagnosis has gained in importance during the last years. The special violet light, which is used for activation of the tissue specific green autofluorescence and the red protoporphyrin IX fluorescence, originates from xenon light (D-light/AF-system, Storz). This source of light can also be used as a white light source. The changing application of both lights can be controlled by a foot switch or by hand. The fluorescence detection requires the use of certain, specially conceived endoscopes (Storz, Tuttlingen, Germany) and an electric modified colour CCD camera (Telekam SL-PDT, Storz, Tuttlingen, Germany). For activation of the fluorescence, a filter combination can be used with the D-light/AF-system, which limits the emission of the lamp to a spectrum between 375 and 440 nm. For fluorescence an appropriate filter in the ocular of the endoscope can completely or partly eliminate detection of the reflected activation light. Biopsies are excised during fluorescence diagnosis from the tumour (the tumour margins as well as surrounding healthy tissue). In order to detect a correlation between histopathological diagnosis, biopsy, and macroscopic red fluorescence of the excised biopsy the subjectively assessed intensity of the fluorescence should be graduated into high, moderate, and low.

Although 5-ALA–induced fluorescence diagnosis allows a more exact description of the tumour edges than by white light endoscopy, the examiner must bear in mind different sources of irritation that do not always make possible reliable reproducibility. Independently from the tumour location and 5-ALA application, significant differences of the fluorescence contrast can the detected macroscopically. Bigger tumour surfaces regularly lead to lower fluorescence intensity than smaller surfaces. Bleaching of the fluorescence can be observed in more advanced oropharyngeal and hypopharyngeal carcinomas during examination. Rather disturbing are unspecific fluorescence uptakes due to bacterial infections or fungi, especially in the area of the oral cavity. Smaller bleeding, occurring for example, after minimal contact by the endoscopic instruments in cases of ulcerating tumours of the mucosa, leads to a nearly complete obliteration of the fluorescence. With this in minds, all results obtained by application of 5-ALA fluorescence diagnosis must be evaluated with special care.

9.4.10 Follow-up in Head and Neck Squamous Cell Carcinoma Patients

The extent and type of follow-up of head and neck cancer patients varies in each department. Careful anamnesis, local inspection as well as palpation of the neck are essential for every follow-up examination. Each examination should include the assessment of the (ear, nose and throat) ENT-specific stage, endoscopy or microlaryngoscopy, as well as sonography of neck in patients with low risk of recurrence. Patients with a high risk in developing tumour recurrences may additionally undergo control CT or MRI, with description of the tumour region including the local lymphatic drainage pathways. Sonography of the lymphatic drainage region is indicated in short intervals in the case of treatment option(s). A second control CT scan can be planned in the second year of tumour follow-up. The same is true for control panendoscopy; however, even in this context the procedures of the single institutions vary enormously.

Sonography of the cervical soft parts, possibly completed by colour-coded duplex sonography and in cases of suspected lymph node metastasis, ultrasound-guided FNA cytology, should be performed in the context of each follow-up examination as long as treatment option exists. Chest X-rays are ignored increasingly by some institutions because of its limited significance and the extraordinarily poor prognosis in cases of present pulmonary metastases. In cases of indication for imaging, a thorax CT scan should be performed. Performance of bone scintigraphy and sonography of the upper abdomen is indicated dependent on the respective disease; however, it no longer belongs to the standard.

Tumour follow-up is an important part of the daily routine in ENT departments that are active in the field of oncology. Due to the relatively high risk in developing secondary carcinomas and the often very good therapeutic options (depending on the location and the tumour stage), follow-up should be planned long term, perhaps even life long. Particular attention must be paid to the question of whether the possibility of neck dissection exists in cases of second intervention. Those patients who might probably have curative therapy options should be summoned in 4- to 6-week intervals during the first year after surgery, in the second year every 2–3 months, in the third to fifth year every 3–6 months and afterwards every year. Patients who have undergone primary neck dissection and who must expect missing curative therapeutic options in cases of tumour recurrence should be seen every 3 months during the first and second year, in the third year every 6 months, and afterwards in yearly intervals. Independently from the size of the primary tumour and the detection of lymphogenic metastasis at the time of diagnosis, sonography of the neck should be performed during the first 2 years. In the case of a suspected tumour, extended diagnosis is indicated. The application of invasive or noninvasive methods should be decided individually.

In the context of prognosis and treatment strategies, serologic parameters for detection of distant metastases of squamous cell carcinomas of the upper aerodigestive tract may be helpful.

Our own studies showed that serologic follow-up of individual patients revealed in cases of recurrences, and in particular in cases of distant metastasis the cytokeratin fraction 21-1 (CYFRA 21-1), value of the serum increases significantly. Herewith the individual increase of the CYFRA values must be compared to the individual postoperative level. In contrast to pulmonary carcinomas, squamous cell carcinomas of the upper aerodigestive tract seem to have no comparable cutoff value. Based on these results, CYFRA 21-1 in the context of tumour follow-up is appropriate as a parameter in the course of the disease for early detection of distant metastases. The serologic control of CYFRA 21-1, which is currently not yet integrated in the clinical routine, could be performed at the time of first diagnosis, 8 weeks, and 6 months after therapy as well as once per year afterwards.

9.5 Interpretation of Relevant Imaging

ÅKE BODESTEDT

9.5.1 General Section

9.5.1.1 Introduction

Imaging plays an important role in the evaluation of cancer of the head and neck. It is required for tumour staging, therapy monitoring and in detecting tumour recurrence. Imaging results in the upgrading of tumour stages in a significant number of cases, and directly affects the surgical approach and planning of radiotherapy (RT). Optimal tumour staging and assessment of tumours in the head and neck is a multidisciplinary task. For the radiologist, close collaboration with the surgeon and oncologist is important; to, they benefit from a sound understanding of the possibilities and limitations of contemporary imaging techniques.

A basic understanding of some technical concepts and terms in radiology is helpful in this respect.

Imaging modalities can be grossly characterised as morphological or functional. The most commonly used methods are described in this chapter.

Cross-sectional imaging with CT and MRI are the basic morphological imaging modalities. Ultrasound (US) can also be used to evaluate tumours. Conventional radiography (X-ray) is of limited use for cancer assessment. However, a barium swallow is routinely given when assessing the hypopharynx and oesophagus. Panoramic radiographs are used to evaluate the jaws, but they are gradually being replaced by CT. Highly vascularised tumours may require angiography and embolisation prior to surgery.

The limitations of morphological imaging in cancer assessment are well known. Benign lesions cannot reliably be distinguished from malignant tumours. As these methods depend on size criteria to determine the presence of a mass, small tumours and micrometastases often escape detection. Detection of recurrent disease is difficult because of scarring due to surgery and radiation therapy.

In recent years, much interest has been focused on metabolic and functional imaging methods having the potential to overcome the limitations of conventional imaging. These modalities will probably play an increasing role in cancer evaluation.

Today, MRI is more than simply a morphological imaging method; pathology at cellular and molecular levels can be assessed as well. Changes in molecular diffusion, e.g. in malignant tumours, can be studied with appropriate sequences (diffusion-weighted MRI). One can also use MRI to acquire quantitative spectra of various metabolites in a volume of tissue (MR spectroscopy [MRS]). Recent studies indicate that these methods may become useful both for staging and for therapy monitoring of malignant tumours.

In nuclear medicine, a radioisotope-labelled substance, when injected, accumulates in different soft tissues depending on the specific carrier used. Various methods exist. Bone scintigraphy utilising technetium (Tc99m-labelled phosphate) is well established and is highly sensitive in detecting metastatic bone deposits. PET using ^{18}F-labelled deoxyglucose ([18]FDG) is currently the dominant method. PET detects tissue having increased metabolism. With PET-CT, metabolic and anatomical information is displayed in separate image sets but can also be "fused" in a third set of images to display both metabolic and anatomical information.

9.5.1.2 Imaging Modalities

9.5.1.2.1 CT

Development of the CT technique has been very rapid during the last few years, and helical (or spiral) CT scanners are now in general use. These are usually equipped with multiple detector rows (*multi*detector CT [MDCT]) to allow acquisition of several parallel image sections (*multi*slice CT [MSCT], *multi*channel CT [MCCT]). The most recent generation of these rapid scanners can simultaneously generate images up to 0.64 mm thick each half-second of rotation of the X-ray tube, producing 128 images per second. The thorax and abdomen can thus be scanned during one breath-hold. The entire neck can be scanned in a few second, and the technique is therefore less sensitive to image artefacts caused by patient motion, swallowing or phonation.

During CT scanning the patient is normally lying supine on the examination table, which is then moved at a constant speed through the tunnel-shaped CT gantry. The gantry holds the X-ray tube and, on the opposite side, the X-ray detectors. During the table motion the tube rotates, thereby forming a spiral relative to the patient. The detectors register what remains of the X-rays after they have passed through the patient's body. The CT scanner computes the difference between the radiation that left the X-ray tube and the radiation that reached the detectors and thus what was absorbed, or attenuated, while passing through the patient. This attenuation, which is proportional to the electron density of the various tissues, provides the basis for the image contrast and can also be quantified in the CT image.

As air does not absorb X-rays, the attenuation is virtually nonexistent, and air thus appears black on the image; dense bone with high attenuation will thus appear white. Soft tissues, with medium attenuation, appear on the image as different shades of grey. Fluid appears dark while fat, with even lower attenuation, is almost black. Soft tissue contrast in MDCT is, however, inferior to that of MRI, by which, on the other hand, cortical bone is less clearly depicted.

During the spiral movement of the X-ray tube and detectors (relative to the patient), attenuation data are collected from a large number of angles (projections) per tube rotation. This results in data acquisition of a volume. Cross-sectional images are then computed (reconstructed) from this volume, using mathematical algorithms to calculate the electron density at each point in the image plane, e.g. image slice. Image quality is dependent on tube current and voltage, slice thickness, table speed and the reconstruction process.

In this image reconstruction, different software programs may be chosen, depending on the desired properties in the final image. Bone and soft tissue reconstruction algorithms allow optimal visualisation of high-density skeletal structures and soft tissues, respectively. The three-dimensional (3D) data thus collected can be reconstructed into images of varying slice thickness and overlap. High-quality multiplanar reconstructions (MPR) and 3D display views with only marginal loss of spatial resolution can be produced. MPR are usually reformatted in the coronal plane to allow reading of the images from front to back and in the sagittal plane from right to left. The coronal reformatted images are particularly valuable for interpretation of CT of the head and neck.

Intravenously injected contrast medium containing iodine is routinely used. The high-electron-density contrast agent absorbs X-rays and therefore appears white on images. In the neck, contrast enhancement of vessels and vascular lesions facilitates image interpretation and delineation of pathology (Fig. 9.5.1). The contrast medium is normally excreted in the urine, but in patients with impaired kidney function the nephrotoxic effect of the medium must be considered.

Modern MSCT has thus significantly improved image quality and shortened examination time, therefore increasing patient throughput. The entire neck can be scanned in a matter of seconds. Total patient examination time is a few minutes.

Other clinical applications of MDCT are vascular examinations generating 3D angiographic images, virtual endoscopy, and angioscopy. In dental CT, images of dentition are reconstructed utilising special software programs.

One drawback is the use of ionising radiation; although most patients who are considered for MDCT are elderly, and the potentially harmful effect of the radiation dose seldom constitutes a problem. For some applications, e.g. MDCT of the nasal sinuses, a low-dose examination procedure may be considered, especially for younger patients.

Artefacts from dental restoration can make evaluation of the oral cavity and floor of the mouth suboptimal (Fig. 9.5.2) but may be effected by repeated scanning, varying the angulation of the CT gantry.

9.5.1.2.2 MRI

MRI is a complex imaging modality but has inherent high flexibility. It offers better soft tissue resolution than does CT, but examination time is considerably longer.

Although a detailed technical description is beyond the scope of this chapter, an attempt is made to explain certain basic physical terms and concepts. Some background knowledge will be helpful in understanding MR image interpretation.

MRI is based on the magnetic properties of protons in atomic nuclei. In medical MRI, the hydrogen nucleus is used, as hydrogen constitutes two thirds of all atoms in the human body. When a patient is placed in a strong external magnetic field, the hydrogen nuclei align themselves in the direction of that field. The strength of the external magnetic field is measured in units of Tesla. A radiofrequency pulse (RF pulse) is then applied, which disturbs the alignment of these nuclei. When the RF pulse is switched off, the nuclei reorient themselves to equilibrium and a lower energy state. In this process of nuclear relaxation, a radiofrequency wave is released. This constitutes the fundamental resonance phenomenon on which all MRI is based.

The emitted signal (or echo) can be recorded and displayed. An object emitting a strong signal appears bright, while objects giving a weak signal or none appear dark. Spatial localisation of such a signal is accomplished by applying a complex system of magnetic coils (gradient fields).

In MRI, a number of parameters influence image contrast and signal intensity, e.g. proton density, T_1 and T_2 effects, magnetic susceptibility and flow. Their relative contribution to image contrast and signal intensity can be manipulated by varying the emitted RF pulse and gradient fields, using different pulse sequences.

Two important tissue parameters determining image contrast are T_1 and T_2 relaxation. Relaxation time varies

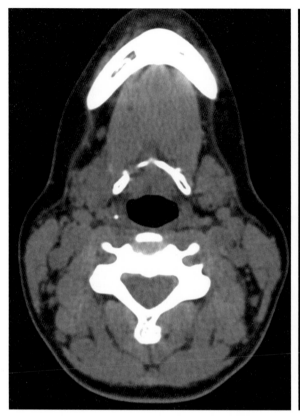 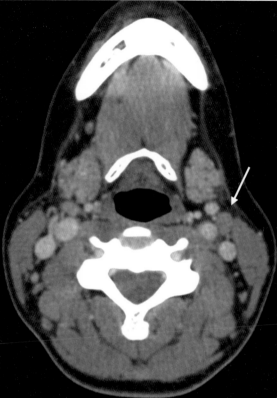

Fig. 9.5.1 Noncontrast CT (*left*) versus contrast-enhanced CT (*right*): axial slice at the level of the submandibular glands and the hyoid bone. Vessel enhancement aids image interpretation. A non-enlarged lymph node on the left side (*arrow*) at the an-terior border of the sternocleidomastoid muscle is more easily identified. Note that low-density fat can be easily differentiated from other soft tissues of intermediate density

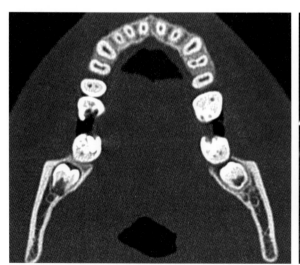 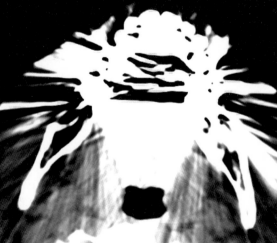

Fig. 9.5.2 *On the left*, axial CT slice of the mandible and teeth. *On the right*, the same level in another patient. Artefacts from dental restorations causes severe image degradation

in different tissues according to their chemical properties. T_1 relaxation is a function of how quickly the stimulated nuclei revert to their basic energy level after the RF pulse is switched off. T_2 relaxation is dependent on the loss of phase coherence of the nuclei when the RF pulse is switched off. Selection of an appropriate pulse sequence can generate an image that is predominantly T_1-weighted or T_2-weighted. The images so produced will have differing soft tissue contrast properties.

T_1-weighted images delineate anatomy very clearly: fluid is dark; soft tissue generally emits an intermediate signal, while fat generates a strong signal that thus appears very bright. Inherent sharp contrast between soft tissues and fat enables us to discern lymph nodes and even peripheral nerves in the neck. The T_2-weighted image is recognised by the very strong signal emitted by most fluids, e.g. cerebral spinal fluid (CSF) and oedema, which will appear white on the images. This makes it an excellent tool for the evaluation of the central nervous system (CNS) and detection of pathological changes (Fig. 9.5.3).

As cortical bone and air have low proton densities, e.g. few mobile protons, they emit no signal, and therefore appear black. Although "invisible", cortical bone structure (if not too thin) can often be delineated, as it is surrounded by soft tissues and bone marrow, which do generate a

signal. Soft tissue signal in cortical bone may therefore indicate tumour invasion and bone destruction.

Another commonly used technique is fat suppression, whereby the signal from fatty tissue can be suppressed. Fat will then appear dark, and lesions surrounded by fat can thus be rendered more conspicuous (Fig. 9.5.4).

The influence of flow on image contrast is rather complex. Fast-flowing blood generates no signal and hence appears black on imaging. Slow-flowing blood emits a stronger signal and therefore causes vessel enhancement. This latter phenomenon is utilised to produce images of magnetic resonance angiography (MRA).

MRI produces two-dimensional (2D) image slices in any chosen plane. True volume (3D) is also possible, allowing the production of ultrathin (submillimeter) slices. External magnets more powerful generate a stronger recordable signal. Additional local coils (surface coils) placed over a region of interest on the patient's body further intensify the signal. Consequently, thin slices and images with high spatial resolution can be produced. Intravenous administration of a paramagnetic contrast agent (gadolinium) is helpful in many cases, enhancing the signal from tissues of interest (Fig. 9.5.5). Gadolinium is not dependent on kidney function.

An interesting and new intravenous contrast agent in MRI imaging is ultrasmall superparamagnetic iron oxide

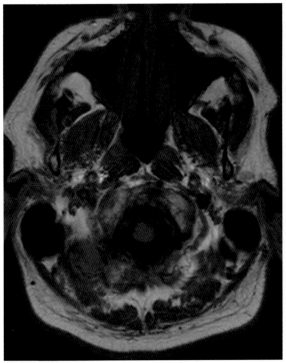 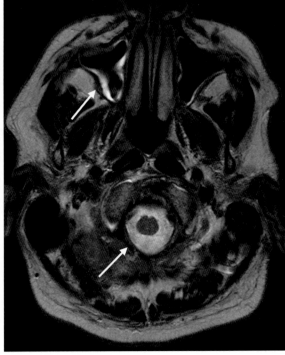

Fig. 9.5.3 The different contrast properties between T_1- (*left*) and T_2-weighted (*right*) images in MRI. Note the high signal from CSF and the slightly swollen mucosa of the right maxillary sinus on the T_2-weighted image (*arrows*). Fat is relatively bright on both images. Muscles are of intermediate density, but appear somewhat darker on the T_2-weighted images

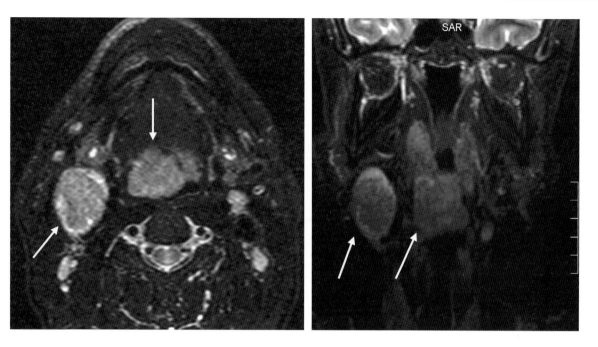

Fig. 9.5.4 Axial (*left*) and coronal (*right*) T_2-weighted MRI images with fat suppression. Cancer of the base of the tongue and a metastatic gland on the right side of the neck (*arrows*). Suppression of the surrounding high-fat signal makes these lesions more conspicuous

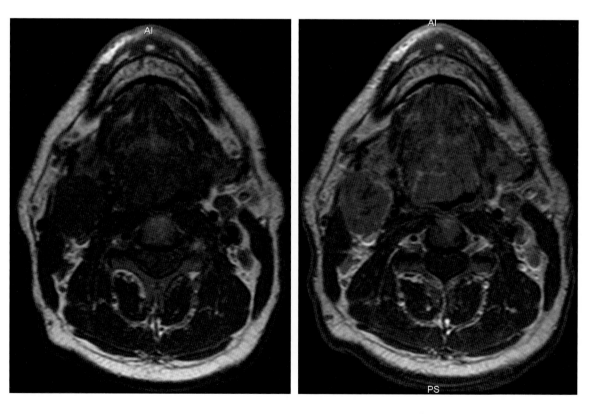

Fig. 9.5.5 The same case presented in Fig. 9.5.4. Native T_1-weighted image before (*left*) and after (*right*) administration of intravenous contrast. Enhancing lesions surrounded by fat may occasionally be more difficult to delineate, as they acquire similar signal intensity as does fat

(USPIO). These iron particles are taken up and phagocytosed by normally functioning lymph nodes. The particles cause local magnetic field effects, reducing T_2-weighted signal intensity. The patient must be examined before and after administration of the contrast agent. On the postcontrast exam, a normal lymph node loses its signal and appears dark on images, whereas metastatic nodes have lost their macrophages and will show no signal loss. In this way, metastatic disease in nonenlarged lymph nodes can be detected. This is not possible with conventional imaging with CT and MRI, which rely mainly on size criteria.

9.5.1.2.3   Ultrasound

The main application of US in malignancies of the head and neck is for the evaluation of lymph nodes (Fig. 9.5.6). US can also be used as a complement to CT or MRI in the case of a suspect node. US-guided FNA biopsy is the most accurate method for diagnosis of lymph node metastases. If required, biopsy of the primary tumour can be made as well.

US can be used for tumour evaluation, but there are certain limitations when defining deep tumour extent. In addition, US waves cannot penetrate bone, and certain tumours are therefore not completely accessible for evaluation. However, US is extensively used for the evaluation of thyroid–parathyroid disease and of the salivary glands. Advanced tumours growing outside the gland's capsule and deep tumour extent are best assessed with CT or MRI.

9.5.1.2.4   Conventional X-Ray Imaging

Plain film is of limited use for the evaluation of head and neck cancer. Various soft tissues have similar electron densities, and they cannot be differentiated on the image. However, plain film is still used in the evaluation of sinusitis, where intermediate-density soft tissue in the sinus is distinctly contrasted against air and bone. Occasionally a tumour might be discovered this way.

For skeletal and dental evaluation, panoramic radiography of the jaws is still routinely used. Bone destruction and dental status are assessed (Fig. 9.5.7). Dental restoration is important before planned surgery or radiation therapy.

Standard chest radiography may be performed when pulmonary metastases are suspected.

Fluoroscopy, with barium or iodinated contrast medium, is often the initial radiographic exam in the evaluation of a patient with dysphagia. A barium swallow will yield both anatomic and dynamic information. The high-density contrast agent will outline the mucosa of hypopharynx and oesophagus. Superficial mucosal lesions that might escape detection by CT or MRI can be visualised. Dynamic analysis includes evaluation of motion, distensibility and pliability of the mucosal wall (Fig. 9.5.8).

9.5.1.2.5   Angiography and Interventional Procedures

In conventional angiography, contrast medium is injected into the arteries, delineating blood supply in highly vas-

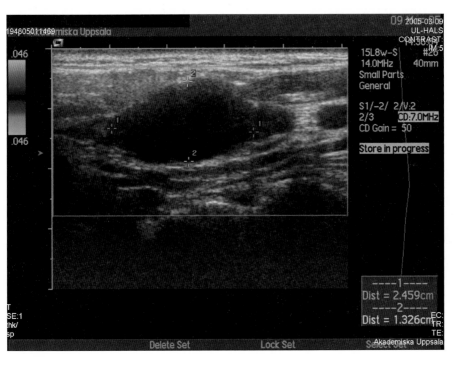

Fig. 9.5.6 Ultrasound image demonstrating a mass of low echogenicity in the neck. This represents an enlarged gland, which can be easily identified because it is surrounded by fat of high echogenicity

cularised tumours prior to surgery. Preoperative embolisation can also be performed, reducing blood supply and tumour volume and thereby simplifying surgery and reducing the risk of bleeding complications (Fig. 9.5.9).

9.5.1.2.6 PET and PET-CT

PET is a functional nuclear imaging technique that generates images based on the different functional characteristics of various tissues, e.g. metabolism.

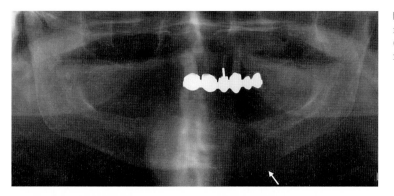

Fig. 9.5.7 Panoramic radiograph of the mandible demonstrating bone destruction (*arrow*) secondary to a carcinoma of the floor of the mouth

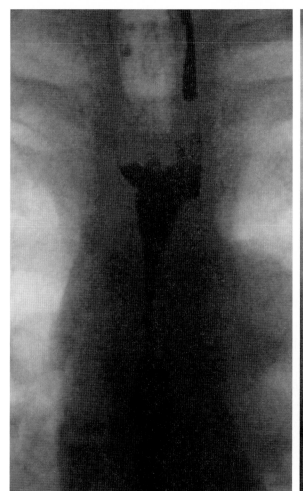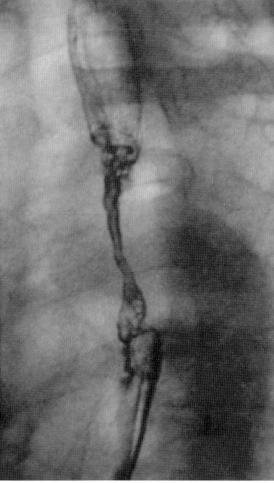

Fig. 9.5.8 Barium swallow showing a stricture of the middle part of the oesophagus. Mucosal irregularity and destruction indicate a malignant tumour

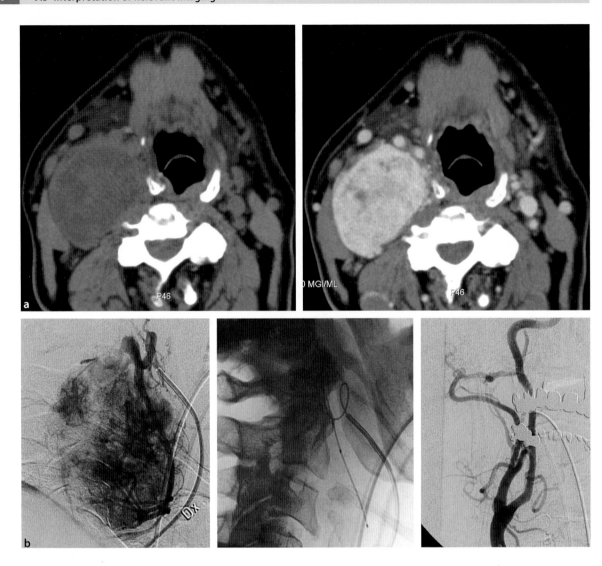

Fig. 9.5.9 a Axial CT image before (*left*) and after administration of intravenous contrast (*right*). A large, well-circumscribed tumour in the right carotid space displaces the ECA and ICA ventrally. Intense contrast enhancement indicates a highly vascularised lesion. Imaging suggests a paraganglioma, possibly originating from the vagal nerve. **b** The same case as on previous images. *On the left*, intense tumour blush after administration of intravenous contrast consistent with paraganglioma (glomus). *In the middle*, microcatheter placed in feeding arteries from the ECA prior to embolisation. *On the right*, postparticulate embolisation image with the catheter in the CCA. The tumour is fully devascularised

Most malignant tumours show increased glycolytic activity. The PET substance, or PET tracer, which is used mainly for oncological PET imaging, is therefore ^{18}FDG, which accumulates more in malignant tumours than in most normal tissues. ^{18}FDG is injected intravenously, and the PET camera examination is performed about an hour later. During this resting period the patient must refrain from physical activity and talking, since false-positive results in the form of ^{18}FDG accumulation in muscle tissue and larynx may otherwise occur. PET radionuclides are usually produced in a cyclotron and are short-lived (half-life of 110 min for ^{18}F and 20 min for ^{11}C). The use of ^{11}C tracers for PET therefore requires in-house production.

Important factors for tumour detection are the ^{18}FDG uptake in the lesion, compared with that of the surrounding tissues, and also tumour size. The physical resolution of the PET camera is about 0.5 cm.

False-negative results may therefore be expected for tumours that are small and/or show low ^{18}FDG uptake, e. g. micrometastases. The radioactivity concentration in the images can be correlated to the injected ^{18}FDG dose and the patient's distribution volume (mostly body weight) in order to create images of standardised uptake value (SUV). When comparing SUV from various PET examinations it is important to consider on which time postinjection the SUV recalculation is based. With most standard ^{18}FDG PET protocols, a tumour SUV exceeding 3 usually indicates malignancy. SUV carries prognostic information in squamous cell carcinoma.

In the head and neck area, variable ^{18}FDG uptake is frequently seen in nasal turbinates, pterygoid and extraocular muscles, salivary glands and lymphoid tissue, which must be taken into consideration during image interpretation. Other potential pitfalls are, as previously mentioned, not only physiological muscle uptake, but also inflammatory lesions. This renders diagnosis of residual and recurrent disease unreliable for at least 3 months after ending external radiation therapy.

Because of the variable ^{18}FDG accumulation in normal tissues, the localisation of an abnormal uptake can sometimes be difficult due to lack of anatomical reference structures. In this respect the new generation of PET-CT scanners is an improvement, producing three sets of images, viz. PET, CT and a fusion image series of PET and CT, providing both functional and detailed anatomical information in the same set of images.

^{18}FDG-PET has proved useful for the primary staging of head and neck tumours, but also has the potential to distinguish recurrent malignant neoplasms from postoperative changes and radiation fibrosis. Surgery and radiation treatment result in distortion of normal anatomy and in soft tissue changes, making image interpretation difficult when using conventional radiological methods. Serial imaging with CT and MRI is therefore often required to detect tumour recurrence, e. g. enlargement over time. By contrast, ^{18}FDG-PET can detect recurrence when CT or MRI is inconclusive.

In head and neck cancer, ^{18}FDG-PET is most frequently utilised to detect recurrent and residual disease. However, PET is not recommended for evaluation of salivary gland tumours that generally have low FDG uptake, thereby resulting in poor sensitivity.

Another important PET application currently being investigated is therapy monitoring (tumour response evaluation). Not only can the tumour SUV before treatment indicate the therapy outcome, but also it can indicate a decrease in the tumour accumulation of ^{18}FDG during treatment, and compared with pretherapy ^{18}FDG-PET, can indicate therapeutic response. This metabolic response usually precedes by far any reduction in tumour volume measured by conventional radiological methods. By contrast, lack of SUV reduction suggests a change of therapy.

PET can also be used to search for unknown primary tumours, in lymph node staging and for detection of distant metastases (Fig. 9.5.10). PET-CT can facilitate directed biopsies and guide surgical or radiation treatment planning.

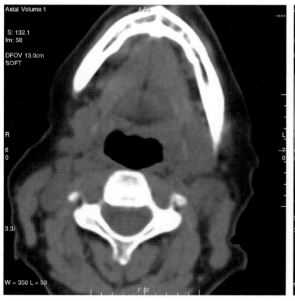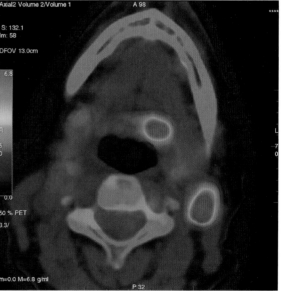

Fig. 9.5.10 PET-CT in search of a primary occult tumour. *On the left*, a native CT image reveals an enlarged gland on the left. *On the right*, a "fused" PET-CT image. Increased 18FDG uptake is seen not only in the metastatic gland, but also in the base of the tongue on the left side. Biopsy revealed a primary squamous cell carcinoma. Conventional diagnostic CT prior to the PET-CT examination detected only the enlarged gland. The primary tumour was not identified, probably because of its small size (1 cm)

9.5.1.3   Role of Imaging in Cancer Assessment

9.5.1.3.1   Pretreatment Imaging

The primary role of the radiologist is to assess local tumour extent and size, identify cervical metastases and, when relevant, signs of distant spread. Diagnosis is only a secondary consideration. In clinical practice the existence of a tumour is usually known prior to imaging. CT and MRI should not be used to exclude early cancer. In general, a biopsy will be necessary in the final staging process.

The importance of radiological analysis is dependent on the site of the lesion. Superficial and mucosal malignancies are investigated primarily by visual inspection, palpation and endoscopy. Imaging in these cases is complementary and focused on deep submucosal and nodal spread (Fig. 9.5.11). On the other hand, a deep-seated central skull base tumour or a retropharyngeal lymph node can be visualised and evaluated only by means of imaging. Tumour extension in certain critical areas cannot be visualised by endoscopy or palpated, yet will have a direct impact on staging and treatment. Imaging serves as a valuable complement in these clinical "blind spots", e.g. subglottic spread in glottic carcinoma or cartilage destruction (Fig. 9.5.12). In patients presenting with hoarseness but negative findings on endoscopy, a CT scan of the chest may be indicated to rule out a tumour engaging the recurrent laryngeal nerve (Fig. 9.5.13).

Clinical findings at inspection, palpation and endoscopy should be conveyed to the radiologist. In preoperative imaging when the resectability of a tumour is to be evaluated, the surgeon should specify in his/her request the clinical problem and key anatomic areas to be investigated. This is especially true of MRI in which the exam is tailored to solve a specific clinical problem. Knowledge of the clinical findings is also necessary for optimal image interpretation.

The radiologist must be familiar with the TNM system and the principles of nodal staging and classification. This knowledge will ensure effective communication with the clinicians. For example, in nodal classification, suspected metastatic nodes should be identified and related to specified anatomic structures. This will provide the clinician with information necessary when deciding the appropriate type of neck dissection. Nodal surveillance in nonsurgical treatment is also simplified. Imaging-based tumour and nodal classification systems have been developed and are now being partly incorporated in clinical classification systems. Consequently, even closer cooperation between clinicians and radiologists will be required in the future.

In the diagnostic workup, evaluation of the chest is usually performed using plain films or CT to rule out lung metastases. CT is more sensitive than is conventional radiography. The examination will also serve as a useful baseline study for future chest scanning. Distant metastatic spread to liver and bone can also occur.

Imaging should be performed prior to biopsy. Biopsy-induced changes may cause difficulties in image interpretation.

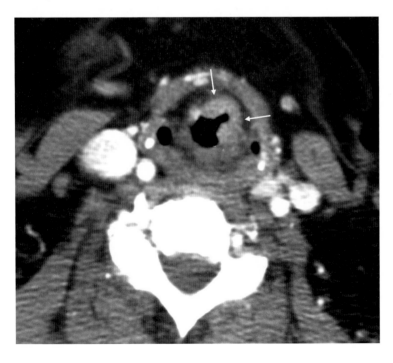

Fig. 9.5.11 Axial CT slice demonstrates a supraglottic cancer diagnosed with endoscopy (*arrows*). There is thickening and enhancement of the mucosa but no signs of deep spreading. The adjacent laryngeal fat is preserved

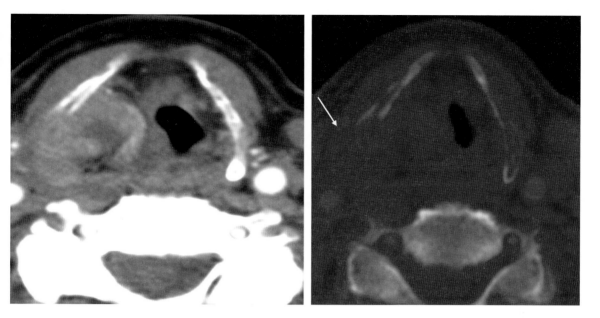

Fig. 9.5.12 *On the left,* contrast-enhanced CT shows an enhancing mass on the right side of the hypopharynx. *On the right,* a CT bone window displays obvious destruction of the adjacent thyroid cartilage (*arrow*)

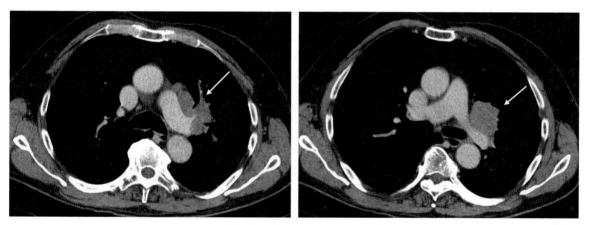

Fig. 9.5.13 Patient with paresis of the left vocal cord. CT of the chest shows a primary carcinoma in the left lung (*arrows*), adjacent to the aortic arch and left pulmonary artery, affecting the left recurrent laryngeal nerve

9.5.1.3.2 Posttreatment Imaging

Detection of recurrent disease is a challenge for both clinician and radiologist. Appropriate image interpretation requires knowledge of the various treatment options and their appearances on the radiographs. Surgery and RT induce soft tissue changes that must be identified by the radiologist and need to be distinguished from recurring or persistent disease.

The radiologist must be familiar with the various surgical procedures currently available, including radical, modified and selective neck dissections. These procedures can often be readily recognised on the images, but in some instances cannot be correctly identified, e.g. in selective neck dissection. Scar tissue in the incision area may be misinterpreted as recurring disease.

In reconstructive surgery, pedicled flaps or free flaps can be used. Muscle and subcutaneous fatty tissue can be identified on the radiographs, but evaluation of tumour recurrence after extensive surgery can be challenging. As a rule, the clinician should tell the radiologist which type of surgery has been performed to avoid misinterpretation.

Early detection of tumour recurrence is important, as it will improve the patient survival rate and palliation. As posttreatment changes and reconstructive flaps make palpation difficult, a baseline surveillance CT or MRI exam is recommended prior to clinical examination. It should be performed 4–6 weeks after surgery or RT, when the immediate soft tissue changes have subsided. Further surveillance may include a scan 6 months after treatment and then once a year. The vast majority of recurrences develop within the first 3 years. However, the relatively high incidence of metachronous and synchronous tumours may necessitate lifelong annual checkups.

In cases of suspected recurrence, US- or CT-guided biopsy should be performed.

As PET scanners are becoming increasingly available, they are used more often when conventional imaging fails to confirm a mass as being either a recurrence or scar tissue. Although PET is highly sensitive it has limited specificity, which can result in false-positive results. An interval of at least 4–6 months after treatment is recommended before performing a PET scan. Inflammatory changes in a previously treated tumour site will show increased [18]FDG uptake. The same is true of reactive or inflamed lymph nodes.

False negatives derive from the inability of PET to detect small tumourous deposits and micrometastases. After radiation therapy, an interval of 4 months is recommended before PET scanning is performed, as false negatives may otherwise result.

9.5.1.4 Tumour Evaluation with CT and MRI

9.5.1.4.1 CT and MRI in Cancer Assessment
Both CT and MRI can be used in the primary diagnostic workup process. The methods are competitive, but also complementary; both have advantages and disadvantages.

MDCT has proved its value in tumour evaluation, and it adequately defines the extent of disease in most instances. Cortical bone destruction is visualised excellently. Examination times are considerably shorter than with MRI, so patient movement is therefore a minor problem.

MRI clearly has advantages in certain situations, such as when intracranial or perineural tumour spread is to be assessed (Fig. 9.5.14). MRI can sometimes detect marrow involvement before any cortical bone destruction is evident on CT. MRI can also identify cortical bone destruction; the normal signal void (black) of cortical bone is then replaced by tumour with intermediate signal.

MRI examination takes considerably longer than CT does. Patient movement is liable to cause artefacts, which is a problem, particularly in cases of obstructive tumours of the head and neck, when swallowing and dyspnea can impair image quality. The confined examination tunnel renders 10% of the patients claustrophobic.

CT and MRI can be complementary methods in tumour evaluation. An initial CT exam may reveal a nasopharyngeal tumour, showing signs of bone destruction of the skull base. MRI should then be performed to delineate intracranial spread. On the other hand, if MRI was used primarily and revealed signs of intracranial tumour spread, CT may be used to evaluate the extent of bone destruction (Fig. 9.5.15).

The preferred method is also influenced by the patient's ability to cooperate, as mentioned above, and by

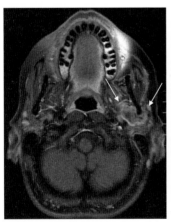 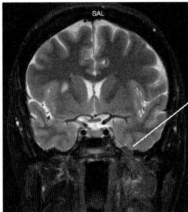 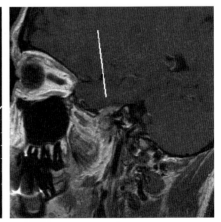

Fig. 9.5.14 *On the left*, an enhancing primary adenoidcystic cancer of the parotid gland (*arrows*), demonstrated on, T_1-weighted MRI images. *In the middle*, T_2-weighted images demonstrate perineural tumour extension along nervus maxillaris through the oval foramen. *On the right*, a contrast-enhanced T_1-weighted scan shows intracranial extension

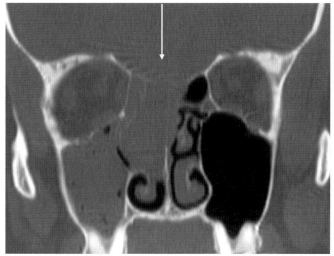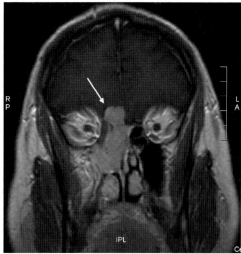

Fig. 9.5.15 *On the left*, an adenocarcinoma of the ethmoid sinuses. CT (bone window) shows an expansile lesion with bone destruction of the anterior skull base and possible intracranial tumour extension (*arrow*). The opacification of the right maxillary sinus is secondary to obstruction and stagnant secretions. *On the right*, a T_1-weighted MRI image shows an enhancing mass with obvious intracranial tumour extension (*arrow*)

local availability and experience. A good approach for the clinician to employ when considering which method to use is to consult the radiologist responsible for the exam.

9.5.1.4.2 Pretreatment Image Interpretation

The delineation of a tumour is dependent on the contrast between tumour and surrounding soft tissues. In the head and neck, fat provides excellent contrast, as it has very low density (dark) on CT and emits a strong signal (bright) on MRI. Obliteration or displacement of these fat planes indicates the presence of a tumour.

On CT images without intravenous contrast, tumours usually cannot be distinguished from muscle, as they have similar intermediate attenuation. Lymph nodes of normal size as well as enlarged metastatic nodes are of intermediate density. Squamous cell carcinomas show similar density whether well or poorly differentiated.

As MRI has better soft tissue resolution, interfaces between tumour and soft tissue can sometimes be more clearly identified. MRI is particularly useful for delineating tumour from surrounding mucosa and retained secretions in the sinonasal cavities (Fig. 9.5.16).

The signal patterns of malignant masses are, however, unspecific and variable. Signals from squamous cell carcinomas and nonmucosal soft tissue tumours are usually of intermediate intensity. Tumour necrosis is revealed by a signal pattern similar to that of fluid, e.g. dark on T_1-weighted images and bright on T_2-weighted images.

Intravenous contrast agents are used routinely in CT. Contrast enhancement is different in different tissue. Vessels in the neck are easily identified, as they enhance more than surrounding structures and thus appear bright on the images. Most importantly, the vessels can be delineated from adjacent lymph nodes. Squamous cell carcinomas are vascular, and contrast enhancement of the primary tumour can make them more conspicuous, delineating them from surrounding muscle. Tumour and lymph node necrosis can be identified, as these avascular areas will not enhance (Fig. 9.5.17).

With MRI, an intravenous contrast agent (gadolinium) is often used for tumour evaluation. However, tumour enhancement does not always elicit additional information concerning tumour extent. The contrast agent will intensify the T_1 signal, and vascularised tissue appears brighter on the image. Intravenous administration of contrast can occasionally render a lesion less conspicuous, as it may emit the same bright signal as surrounding fat emits. Fat suppression may be advantageous in such cases.

Once a tumour has been detected, the radiologist should try to identify the lesion's site of origin. How nearby structures and spaces are displaced will help the radiologist to make his decision. Knowledge of the anatomical contents of the cervical space in question will narrow the list of possible differential diagnoses. In larger trans-spatial masses the site of origin may be difficult to identify.

It must be understood that differentiation between a malignant and a benign lesion cannot be based solely on radiographic findings. There is considerable overlap in the morphological appearance of tumours (Fig. 9.5.18). An obviously infiltrating lesion and findings of necrotic lymph nodes will of course make the diagnosis of a ma-

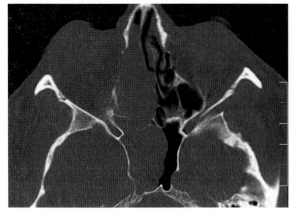
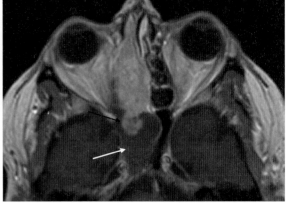

Fig. 9.5.16 *On the left*, an axial CT slice. Opacification of the ethmoid and sphenoid sinuses on the right side. On the right side, corresponding T_1-weighted, contrast-enhanced MR image. Enhancing tumour (*black arrow*) in the ethmoid sinuses can be easily delineated from retained, non-enhancing secretions of low signal in the dorsal aspect of the sphenoid sinus (*white arrow*)

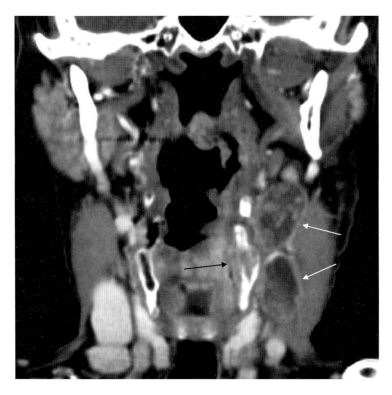

Fig. 9.5.17 Coronal CT slice. Two enlarged glands on the left side of the neck with peripheral contrast enhancement and central necrosis (*white arrows*). These represent metastases from a primary carcinoma of the sinus piriformis. There are also signs of thyroid cartilage destruction (*black arrow*)

lignant tumour more, or even quite, certain. On the other hand, a finding of a clearly delineated mass without enlarged lymph nodes does not rule out malignancy.

Imaging Keypoints in Tumour Evaluation
- Are there signs of expansion, with displacement of adjacent structures?
- What is the spatial localisation of the lesion?
- Is the lesion clearly or poorly delineated, with signs of infiltration into adjacent spaces?

- Are there signs of expansion, infiltrative spread and necrosis, indicating malignancy?
- Is there a single lesion or mutifocality?
- Are there secondarily enlarged nodes in expected locations?
- Are there signs of bone destruction, bone remodelling or sclerosis?
- Is the lesion involving primarily soft tissue or bone?
- Is there intense contrast enhancement, indicating a highly vascularised tumour?

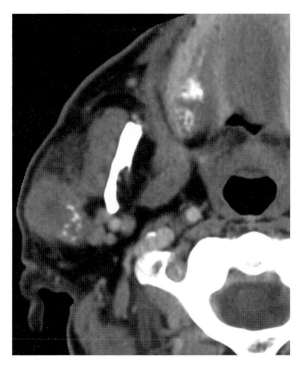

Fig. 9.5.18 Axial CT slice after administration of intravenous contrast. An enhancing, well-circumscribed mass with calcifications is seen in the dorsal aspect of the parotid gland. This case represents a low-grade mucoepidermoid cancer. However, a benign pleomorphic adenoma may have an identical appearance

9.5.1.4.3 Posttreatment Image Interpretation

In the early postoperative period, inflammatory soft tissue reactions and haemorrhage may occur. Surgical procedures alter the anatomy and cause scar tissue formation. Immediate postoperative changes usually subside after 4–6 weeks, but in some patients can persist for months or even years. Vascularised scar tissue can cause contrast enhancement resembling that of a recurrent tumour.

RT generally causes soft tissue oedema, revealing a reticular pattern in subcutaneous fat. Postirradiation chronic sialadenitis is common, and the glands on the irradiated side diminish and become more cellular and fibrotic. Radiation-induced change is of course dependent on the dose administered, but there is considerable variation among patients in the degree of RT reaction. Such changes are usually delayed, becoming most pronounced 4–6 weeks after treatment. In most cases, these changes will resolve during subsequent months. In some patients soft tissue changes can persist for years or indefinitely.

When evaluating the response to RT it is important to compare pretreatment versus posttreatment scans. The primary tumour response may differ from nodal response.

On CT and MR imaging the reticular pattern of subcutaneous fat and mucosal swelling is well visualised.

Furthermore, increased attenuation of the subcutaneous fat is often seen on CT.

Irradiated salivary glands appear small and highly attenuated on CT. With MRI the signal will be weaker than normal.

Recurrences usually occur along margins of the operative site, in the surgical bed or within reconstructed flaps. As stated above, persistent soft tissue changes make detection of recurrent or persistent disease more difficult. The only reliable morphological criterion in CT and MRI is the increased soft tissue mass in consecutive scans. Soft tissue fullness due to oedema can be distinguished on imaging, but solid tumour on CT has attenuation similar to muscle. In MRI signal patterns vary and are unspecific. Soft tissue fullness that is unchanged or decreases in size does not indicate cancer. These changes should be interpreted as posttreatment healing. An important exception is stable tumour size during chemotherapy. When therapy ceases, the tumour may start to grow again.

9.5.1.4.4 Limitations and Pitfalls with CT and MRI

MRI is more sensitive than CT is for detecting tumour infiltration, but is less specific. MRI tends to overestimate tumour size due to concomitant peritumoral oedema, whereas CT tends to underestimate it.

Cancer in a nonenlarged lymph node can go undetected unless necrosis is identified. On the other hand, fat-containing lymph nodes can be mistaken for necrosis. Lymphoid hypertrophy may be mistaken for a tumour. Reactively enlarged lymph nodes cannot be distinguished from metastatic involvement.

In the jaws, coexisting periodontal inflammatory disease must be ruled out. Radiation-induced changes in bone marrow and cartilage cause similar interpretation difficulties.

9.5.2 Specific Section

9.5.2.1 Paranasal Sinuses

- Sinonasal malignancies have usually reached an advanced stage at presentation, with bone destruction and extension beyond the confines of the sinus.
- Concomitant infection is not unusual. It can overshadow both clinical presentation and findings at imaging.
- Small tumours without bone destruction may be misdiagnosed by the radiologist as inflammatory polypoid disease.
- Squamous cell carcinoma typically causes bone destruction, but it can be found in other malignancies. Bone destruction is not uncommon in infections more aggressive tumours.

- Imaging should focus on deep tumour spread. Signs of extension outside the sinus walls and involvement of the skull base should be assessed.
- Metastatic nodes must be identified, especially those so deeply seated that they cannot be clinically assessed.

9.5.2.1.1 Imaging

- CT and MR are complementary methods. Axial, coronal and sagittal imaging planes are useful.
- Both CT and MR can detect bone erosion; CT detects primarily cortical erosion, while MRI reveals marrow infiltration. Involvement of the thin bony walls surrounding the sinuses is best demonstrated by CT.
- MRI is preferred to CT for demonstrating dural, intracranial and perineural tumour spread.
- MRI is useful when distinguishing tumour from surrounding mucosa and retained secretions in the sinuses, as these entities show similar density on CT.

Imaging Key Points

- Is there destruction of the posterior wall of the maxillary sinus?
- Is there tumour extension into the fossa pterygopalatina (the most important landmark)?
- Is there involvement of the maxillary nerve and perineural spread to foramen rotundum, ovale and middle fossa?
- Is there extension into the fossa infratemporalis or nasal cavity?
- Is there orbital tumour extension via inferior orbital fissure?
- Is there engagement of the floor of the anterior cranial fossa and orbit?
- Evaluation of key lymph nodal groups: sinonasal malignancies usually metastasise to retropharyngeal, submental, submandibular and upper jugular lymph nodes.

9.5.2.2 Nasopharynx

- In nasopharyngeal cancer the symptoms are insidious. Early cervical lymph node metastases are common.
- Lymphadenopathy to upper jugular nodes or posterior triangle nodes is the most common clinical presentation.
- Tumour obstruction of the Eustachian tube can lead to middle ear effusion or otomastoiditis I.
- Tumours can escape detection by the endoscopist, due to minimal mucosal engagement.
- Detection of tumour extension to skull base, perineural spread and metastatic nodes is crucial.
- Persistent adenoid tissue can be a differential problem at imaging, though it is rarely seen beyond the age of 30 years.

9.5.2.2.1 Imaging

- Imaging should complement endoscopy.
- CT and MRI are complementary methods, and multiplanar image displays are useful.
- CT and MRI are used to detect skull base involvement and bone erosion.
- Dural, intracranial and perineural tumour spread is best evaluated with MRI.

Imaging Key Points

- In the early stages, the only findings on imaging might be soft tissue asymmetry, obliterating the normal outline of torus tubarius, fossa of Rosenmüller and the Eustachian tube.
- In advanced tumours signs of skull base invasion should be assessed.
- Is there bone destruction in the nasopharyngeal roof and intracranial involvement?
- Does the tumour spread into sphenoid sinuses and further to clivus?
- Is there tumour extension into sinus cavernosus?
- Is there tumour spread to fossa pterygopalatina?
- Is there involvement of V_3?
- Are there signs of inferior submucosal spread along lateral pharyngeal walls?
- Is nodal engagement evident? Usually higher jugular nodal chains are involved and, in advanced cases, posterior cervical nodes.
- Are there enlarged retropharyngeal nodes?

9.5.2.3 Larynx and Hypopharynx

- Patients with laryngeal and hypopharyngeal cancers usually present with symptoms of hoarseness or swallowing difficulties.
- These tumours are usually revealed and diagnosed by endoscopy.
- In patients with swallowing problems, a barium swallow may be the initial procedure.
- Various surgical procedures have been developed, aiming to preserve the voice and ability to swallow. Adequate image interpretation requires that the radiologist has a sound knowledge of existing treatment options.
- Imaging is performed to determine deep tumour spread in relation to specific anatomic landmarks and to detect cartilage destruction. These landmarks are similar for both laryngeal and hypopharyngeal cancers.

9.5.2.3.1 Imaging

- Imaging is complementary to endoscopy.
- CT or MRI is recommended, and images in axial and coronal planes are most useful.

- Image distortion secondary to patient movement and swallowing can be a problem, especially with MRI.
- Superficial mucosal lesions are best detected by endoscopy. However, if a barium swallow had been performed initially, then it might have revealed mucosal irregularities or lack of pliability of the pharyngeal wall, indicating tumour infiltration. In such cases, endoscopy should be performed.

Imaging Key Points

- In supraglottic lesions, imaging should focus on contraindications against supraglottic laryngectomy in order to preserve the voice.
- Is there caudal transglottic extension across laryngeal ventricle?
- Are there signs of cartilage invasion, extralaryngeal spread, sinus pyriformis involvement and significant tongue extension? Is there evidence of pre-epiglottic invasion?
- In glottic carcinomas, imaging is directed chiefly at selecting candidates for voice-sparing surgery by vertical hemilaryngectomy and cordectomy.
- Imaging findings of a tumour invading the anterior commissure, the posterior commissure or paraglottic fat will rule out cordectomy.
- Contraindications to vertical hemilaryngectomy are transglottic spread, cartilage invasion, subglottic extension to upper margin of cricoid cartilage, involvement of the commissures or cricoarytenoid joint and paraglottic fat invasion.
- In the less common subglottic tumours, imaging should assess cartilage invasion and inferior extension into the trachea.
- Key nodal groups to be evaluated are jugular and paratracheal nodal chains.

9.5.2.4 Oral Cavity and Oropharynx

- In oropharyngeal carcinomas, the tongue base and the tonsils are the most common locations.
- In most instances, mucosal extension can be assessed clinically.
- Imaging in these cases is performed to assess submucosal spread and nodal involvement.
- In the oral cavity the exact location of the primary tumour is important in image evaluation, as patterns of spread as well as treatment options differ.
- Mandibular invasion requires careful evaluation. Marrow changes observed at imaging may be secondary to dental disease and may not indicate malignancy.
- Mandibular assessment after radiation therapy can be challenging. Marrow changes can result from radiation fibrosis, osteoradionecrosis, osteomyelitis or periodontal disease.

- Evaluation of dental status should be performed to provide a basis for posttreatment dental restoration.
- Gingival cancers may occasionally be detected primarily by the dentist at intraoral X-ray imaging.

9.5.2.4.1 Imaging

- CT or MRI can be used in primary tumour assessment. Axial and coronal scans are most useful. Sagittal images are valuable in tongue base tumours.
- Dental amalgam can cause distortion of CT images of the oropharyngeal area; in these instances MRI is recommended.
- Image distortion caused by patient movement or swallowing is not uncommon and can be problematic, especially with MRI.
- Mandibular assessment can be performed with either CT or MRI.
- For pretreatment dental status assessment, dental CT, intraoral images and panoramic radiographs are used.

Imaging Key Points

- *Tongue*: Is there a relationship with the neurovascular bundles? Is there tumour extension across the midline or into the floor of the mouth?
- *Tongue base*: Is there engagement of ipsilateral neurovascular bundle, floor of the mouth and tumour extension across the midline? Are there signs of pre-epiglottic fat invasion?
- *Floor of the mouth carcinoma*: Tumours can obstruct Wharton's duct. Is there evidence of mandibular invasion? Is there deep invasion along mylohyoid and hyoglossus muscles, and engagement of ipsilateral or contralateral neurovascular bundle? Is there tongue base invasion and possible extension into the soft tissues of the neck?
- *Tonsillar, soft palate and posterior wall carcinoma*: Is there evidence of submucosal extension into parapharyngeal space and nasopharynx? Is there tongue base extension, bone erosion or pre-vertebral muscle invasion, or skull base extension in advanced tumours?
- *Carcinomas of gingival and hard palate, buccal and retromolar trigone tumours*: Are there signs of bone erosion, or perineural spread?

9.5.2.5 Salivary Glands

- Salivary gland tumours are relatively uncommon.
- The salivary glands have a complex embryogenesis, and the histological appearance of tumours is quite variable.
- Malignancies are carcinomas, malignant nonepithelial tumours, malignant lymphomas and secondary tumours.

- Wide varieties of benign and tumour-like conditions exist. In clinically indeterminate lesions, imaging cannot reliably distinguish benign from malignant tumours.
- Imaging is indicated in advanced and deep-seated lesions to assess deep tumour extent and metastatic nodes.
- Imaging might not be necessary in superficial smaller lesions of the parotid gland, as primary surgical resection is the preferred treatment.

9.5.2.5.1 Imaging
- CT, MRI and US can be used.
- MRI is probably the best method for assessment of deep tumour extension, and it will detect perineural spread better than CT will.
- US is of limited value for evaluating advanced tumours with deep extracapsular spread.

Imaging Key Points
- The most common low-grade salivary gland malignancies develop pseudocapsules. These lesions are well circumscribed on imaging, and therefore they appear benign. An infiltrating mass is, however, more probably a high-grade malignancy.
- Tumour location and extent in relation to critical areas should be evaluated, e. g. neurovascular structures, signs of skull base invasion or perineural spread or intracranial extension.

9.5.2.6   Cervical Lymph Nodes

- The detection of metastatic lymph nodes is of crucial importance for both pre- and posttreatment tumour evaluation.
- Imaging is a complement to clinical examination.
- Imaging detects adenopathy in a significant number of patients, and nodes outside typical treatment areas can be identified.
- Imaging is necessary in the staging procedure, which predicts survival and has an influence on treatment planning (TNM staging).
- The location of nodes allows of the appropriate selection of proper type of neck dissection (nodal classification).
- Identification of metastatic nodes is based on size criteria derived from findings on imaging with CT and MRI. Lymph node enlargement is an unspecific finding, however.

- Unilateral lymph node involvement can be found in metastatic carcinoma, lymphoma, granulomatous disease and local infections. Diffuse nodal involvement suggests systemic infectious processes or possibly lymphoma.
- Nodal necrosis is highly suggestive of metastatic disease but can be seen in lymphomas or infectious processes.
- Functional imaging with PET and CT-PET may become a useful tool for detecting metastatic spread in nonenlarged nodes.

9.5.2.6.1 Imaging
- In morphological imaging, CT, MRI and US can be used.
- With US, suspect nodes can be biopsied.
- Routine neck examination with CT and MRI should include the skull base and extend down to the manubrium. Axial and coronal images should be evaluated.
- Imaging should be performed prior to biopsy of suspect nodes.
- Bleeding and inflammatory changes can cause difficulties in interpreting images of the primary lesion.

Imaging Key Points
- Is there presence of pathologically enlarged lymph nodes >1 cm? (Exceptions are jugulodigastric nodes, where a size of 1.5 cm is allowed.)
- Are there signs of nodal necrosis or extracapsular spread?

References

1. Som PM, Curtin HD (2003) Head and neck imaging, 4th edn, Mosby, St. Louis, MO
2. Harnsberger HR, Wiggins RH, Hudgins PA, Michel M, Swartz J, Davidson HC, Macdonald A et al. (2004) Diagnostic imaging: head and neck, 1st edn. Amirsys, Salt Lake City, Utah
3. Myers EN, Suen JY, Myers JN, Ehab Y, Hanna N (2003) Cancer of the head and neck, 4th edn. Saunders, Philadelphia, PA
4. Oehr P, Biersack H-J, Coleman RE (2004) PET and PET-CT in oncology. Springer, Berlin Heidelberg New York
5. Yousen DM (1998) Head and neck imaging. Mosby, St. Louis, MO

9.6 Head and Neck Tumours

ERIK BLOMQUIST

9.6.1 Introduction

There does note seem to be any standard or universally accepted treatment approaches to patients with head neck cancer. Therapy recommendations vary between geographic regions as well as between institutions and physicians [6]. It has been said, "Clinical oncology is based largely on empirical data rather than on inviolable scientific truths".

This lack of consensus seems, however, to have diminished during recent years, especially when patients presented initially with an advanced disease, e.g. stage III or IV [26]. Neoadjuvant chemotherapy and concomitant chemoradiotherapy have won wider acceptance in those cases in which primary surgery is not the choice because of the difficulties of performing a radical tumour resection. For earlier stages at which the patient is operable, the common strategy in most centres is radical resection, which is followed by in many patients postoperative radiotherapy. Many exceptions to that general rule exist; earlier stages of laryngeal cancer are best treated with curative intended radiotherapy, and small tongue cancers may be successfully treated with brachytherapy alone—mostly iridium-192 implants—if the technique is readily available.

Yet in spite of the increasing amount of information gathered in many clinical studies on the effect of chemotherapy in patients with head and neck squamous cell carcinoma (HNSCC), currently surgery and radiotherapy are the only treatment modalities achieving local control and (often) cure in many head and neck cancer patients. Ongoing studies should further elucidate the expected, improving effect of combinations with chemotherapy and radiotherapy [12].

Relatively new tools in the field are monoclonal antibodies and drugs interfering with various receptors involved in stimulating cell proliferation; among them, the epidermal growth factor receptor (EGFR) is stirring much interest [4,13]. As well as the specific influence on the disease of each new modality, which so far seems moderate, an overall improvement in local control and survival may be attained with new combinations of different drugs.

9.6.2 Histopathology

The majority of tumours in the head and neck region are squamous epithelial carcinomas, and most prospective treatment studies in the field concern patients with these tumours [3, 25].

Tumours of the salivary gland show a panorama of different histological types—mostly adenocarcinomas—in which the subgroups of mucoepidermoid cancers and adenoidcystic cancers are the most common. "Pure" adenocarcinomas are more infrequent. Different types of sarcomas may appear in low frequencies as well as different types of lymphomas, thyroid cancers and mucosal malignant melanomas. (Those tumours are discussed elsewhere in this volume.)

9.6.3 Aetiology

Smoking habits and overconsumption of alcohol have strong correlations with the incidence of HNSCC [7]. For oral carcinomas, human papilloma virus (HPV) may play a role in the development of cancer [19]. EBV has (for some time) been detected in nasopharyngeal carcinomas; it is likely involved with the carcinogenesis.

9.6.4 Incidence

Patients with tumour in the head and neck region account for about 2.5–3% of the total cancer incidence in Europe and the United States. The median age for head and neck tumour debut is around 65–66 years, compared with the overall cancer incidence with a median age of 57–58 years.

(See Sect. 9.6.8 for common tumour locations of the head and neck.)

This implies that comorbid diseases are comparatively more common in patients with head and neck cancer than in younger cancer patients. This might affect treatment strategies for cure for the older patient group, e.g., the presence of heart, lung and kidneys diseases, aging diabetes, atherosclerosis and generally poor health may be responsible for lowered compliance with perceived difficult and physically more demanding treatment.

9.6.5   Examination

The importance of adequate patient examinations cannot be stressed enough. The patient's medical history is the number one priority on the list of investigations. Older patients with memory difficulties may need the assistance of (accompanying) relatives or friends to understand better the evolvement of the tumour. The speed of tumour development is an important factor when the treatment decision is made. The occurrence of comorbid diseases and current medication will naturally also interfere with the patient's expected tolerance for a physically demanding treatment. Signs and symptoms should guide further examination. The goal should be to have the tumour classified according to the Union Internationale Contre le Cancer (International Union against Cancer) (UICC) TNM classification [30] with at least a cytological specimen for proper diagnosis. More convincing is usually a biopsy with enough tumour tissue for a complete histopathological examination.

An examination is not complete if the physical aspect of it is not done properly [10]. This involves inspection and palpation of available sites, and endoscopy of the mouth, nose, pharynx, nasopharynx, larynx and hypopharynx if necessary. A palpation of the neck bilaterally is also compulsory in order to find lymph nodes with tumour involvement. Some tumours may grow exophytically into the lumen, and they are not always fully represented in CT or MRI images. This fact makes endoscopic findings especially important if the patient is recommended radiotherapy as the primary treatment.

Examinations with CT and/or MRI for the entire head and neck region are important for categorising the extension of the disease at the site and for the detection of lymph node metastasis. If PET is available, then the infiltration of the tumour in the surrounding tissue and the location of certain lymph node metastases may be better clarified.

After a full examination the TNM status of the tumour should be assessed as a basis for treatment decision, prognosis and as tool for future comparing of results. The full extension of the disease defines the basis for the decision whether radical surgery is possible, and also for the treatment volume in radiotherapy. If distant metastases are diagnosed, then curative treatment is no longer possible. However, local radiotherapy of the primary tumour may still be given for palliative reasons. The total volume of the tumour disease, including both the primary and eventual metastases, also has prognostic value.

Older patients may have increased difficulty with complying, due to lowered resistance to the physical and emotional stress of treatment. It is as important as in younger patients to explain carefully the intention and side effects of the treatment. A well-informed patient who declines treatment must be respected as well in cases where a strong pressure to treat stems from family members. In cases of dementia it is up to the judgement of the responsible physician to find the appropriate level of palliation.

9.6.6   Oncological Treatment

9.6.6.1   Curative Versus Palliative Intention

Before treatment decision, all patients must be carefully examined, with cytological and/or histopathological analysis regarding type of tumour, and classification of localisation, size and possible metastasis of the tumour according to the UICC TNM system [30]. The patient's general condition and the presence of other diseases are of course also important for the treatment decision. Elderly age may also hamper successful outcome of treatment, but it is not a definite contraindication to curative intent. The combination of surgery and radiotherapy must be considered in the entire evaluation of treatment modalities. Curative versus palliative intention must be decided before start of treatment. A common round with ENT surgeons, radiotherapists, dentists and pathologists is a recommended for such a discussion.

9.6.6.2   Reflections on Surgery

The aim of surgery is a total removal of the tumour and, if present, locoregional metastases, to attain local control. The possibilities for larger resections, e. g. operation in patients with large cancers, have expanded tremendously during the last decades by the application of microneurovasculature-free transfer techniques [9].

The surgical alternatives may be listed as follows:
- Primary closure
  - No reconstruction is made. Avoidance of undue tension to avoid broadening of surgical scars is important.
- Skin grafts
  - Primary application in small defects of the oral cavity and ear, maxillectomy cheek flap, temporalis fascia flap or coverage of muscle.
- Local skin flaps
  - Local skin flaps are primary applied in the reconstruction of external facial defects and are characterised by superior colour, contour and texture.

- Regional flaps
  - Mainly three types of flaps may be categorised: the pectoralis major, latissimus dorsi and trapezius. The pectoralis major myocutaneous flap remains the major myocutaneous pedicled tissue transfer in head and neck reconstructions. This flap is based on the pectoral branch of the thoracoacromial artery of the second portion of the axillary artery.
- Microneurovasculature-free flaps
  - The free flap is a composite block of tissue perfused by a defined anatomic vascular pedicle and it subsequent myocutaneous or fasciocutaneous perforating vessels.

9.6.6.3 Oncological Modalities

In an oncology department, different treatment modalities may be used. Radiotherapy is the standard modality for cure, with or without combination with surgery. Different approaches may be utilised:

1. Radiotherapy
   a. Preoperative irradiation
      i. The standard schedule is 2 Gy day^{-1}, 10 Gy week^{-1}, for a total dose of 50 Gy.
      ii. Arguments for: sterilises the tumour bed, shrinks tumour adherent to bone, simplifying curatively intended surgery and less hypoxic regions, which can reduce the effect of irradiation
      iii. Arguments against: delays surgery, impairs and prolongs healing
   b. Postoperative irradiation
      i. Depends on type of tumour and the presence of free margin at the resection
      ii. Generally 2 Gy day^{-1}, 10 Gy week^{-1}, for a total dose to 50–66 Gy, is given.
      iii. Most common regime for patients with advanced tumours
   c. Curative per se
      i. Used in cases in which surgery is not possible because of the size and growth pattern of the tumour or general medical condition that prohibits anaesthesia, and/or an expected life-threatening postoperative condition
      ii. The standard schedule is to give 2 Gy day^{-1}, 10 Gy week^{-1}, for a total dose of 66–70 Gy.
   For alternative regimes, see Sect. 9.6.7.
2. Chemotherapy
   Only a few cytostatics have a pronounced effect on tumours in the head and neck region. These include cisplatinum, carboplatin, 5-fluorouracil (5-FU), methotrexate, leucovorin, mitomycin and some taxanes. The cytotoxic drugs interfere with certain steps in cellular growth and replication cycles. The most common drug is cisplatin, alone or in combination with 5-FU, in patients with squamous epithelial carcinoma [12,27]. With induction or neoadjuvant chemotherapy, the following conclusions have been drawn:
   a. A high response rate may be achieved (up to 90%); although most studies show no certain improvement of local control and survival.
   b. Distant metastases may be less frequent.
   c. Induction chemotherapy may allow for organ preservation in some patients.
   d. The role of chemotherapy outside clinical trials needs to be defined.

Chemotherapy may be administered temporally in different ways:
- Adjuvant: after other treatment modalities
  - Results: questionable effect on survival and local control; mostly used in a palliative setting.
- Neoadjuvant: before other treatment modalities
  - Results: in some series, an effect has been observed on survival and local control.
- Concomitant: during radiotherapy, mostly given intermittently
  - Results: slight effect on tumour control in advanced cases thus far. Local control may increase 4–8% compared with radiotherapy [22, 29].
3. "Immunological" treatment
   In patients with advanced cancers there is still a strong need for further improvement of therapy. EGFR, a member of the ErbB family of receptor tyrosine kinases, is abnormally activated in epithelial cancer, including head and neck cancer. Radiation increases the expression in cancer cells, and blocking of EGFR signalling sensitises cells to radiation [13].
   A paper on the introduction of monoclonal antibodies targeting EGFR (cetuximab) given concomitant with radiotherapy [4] has recently been published. In patients with advanced cancer, an improvement in local control was found, without increased toxic effects.
   It seems highly probable that a development of substances directed against other cellular or vascular targets will be developed. The integration of these new treatment tools in the clinical routines necessitates clinical trials, in which primary objectives should be frequency of local control, improved survival and toxic effects.

9.6.7 Radiobiology

Cell death is the major effect of ionising radiation relevant to radiation therapy. It occurs in two distinct modes [18]:

1. Reproductive cell death
2. Interphase death by apoptosis

The target for the radiation injury is the DNA molecule. It is generally agreed that the induced double-stranded breaks (DSB) and the chromosome aberrations that occur because of the DSB lead to cell death. Irradiated cells may appear morphologically intact and metabolically functional, and undergo lysis only when attempting mitotic division. This may happen at the first division or after several divisions. These are seen via clonogenic studies in cell cultures.

Less frequent is radiation damage not linked to mitosis. This interphase death by apoptosis occurs within hours after exposure of irradiation. The dying cells separate into clusters of membrane-bound apoptotic bodies, which are phagocytosed by adjacent cells or macrophages. Experimental evidence suggests that apoptosis plays an important role in tumour and normal tissue response to various forms of cancer treatment, including radiotherapy. The serous cells of the salivary and lacrimal glands are highly susceptible to apoptotic death, which explains the xerostomia and xerophtalmia that develop after relatively low doses of radiation in the head and neck region.

Most mammalian cells are not altered by radiotherapy by the doses used clinically. However, tissues with a normal rapid turnover may express radiation injury rather soon after exposure. This is the case with most epithelia and the bone marrow.

When cells are exposed to radiation in experimental systems with analysis of the clonogenic survival, the plotted curve in most cases expresses an initial slope, the "shoulder", which is followed by a straight line if the measuring points are given in semi-logarithmic form. The shoulder corresponds to the dose range of conventional dose fractionation. When the radiation dose is fractionated the shoulder on the survival curve reconstitutes itself. Cells surviving the first dose of radiation respond to subsequent radiation as if they had never been irradiated. The total dose given with repeated fractionation will then totally eradicate the tumour, provided there are not too many clonogenic cells. The result also implies a sparing effect on the normal tissue, whose tolerance is generally the limit to radiotherapy treatment.

To account for the shoulder of the survival curve, different mathematical models have been developed. The trend has been towards the linear–quadratic survival curve equation:

$$S = e^{-\left(\alpha D + \beta D^2\right)}$$

where S is the surviving fraction of cells, D is the dose and α and β are constants representing cell killing by single hit (irreparable damage) and double hit (reparable damage). The α and β values may be found in tables showing data for acute and late effects for different tumours and tissues. A parameter $\frac{\alpha}{\beta}$ is the dose (in Grays) at which the α and β components of logarithmic cell kill are equal. Typical values for $\frac{\alpha}{\beta}$ are 1–4 Gy for so-called late-responding normal tissues and 5–20 Gy for tumours and so-called early responding tissues.

In order to compare the effect of fractionation schedules with different overall treatment times and size of fractions, the cumulative radiation effect (CRE) formula may be used.

$$\mathrm{CRE} = \frac{1}{D \times N^{-0.24} \times T^{-0.11}},$$

where D is the dose, N is the number of fractions, and T is the overall treatment time.

9.6.7.1 Fractionation in Radiotherapy

The rationale for fractionation in radiotherapy is based on the five R's of radiobiology: repair, reoxygenation, redistribution, regeneration and radiosensitivity [28]:

1. *Repair.* E.g. sublethal lesions are repaired if enough time is allowed between fractions. Treatment fractions may need to be well separated, to not compromise repair in normal tissue.
2. *Reoxygenation.* The presence of hypoxic cells may reduce the effect of irradiation and change with shrinkage of the tumour, so that more cells are oxygenated and are thus more sensible to radiotherapy. Administration of the total dose in many fractions increases that possibility of additional cell killing.
3. *Redistribution.* Actively dividing cells, e.g. cancer cells, may have different sensitivities to radiation during the cell cycle. Repeated small fractions increase the chances to hit every cell. Adequate time between fractions may, however, be necessary for allowing cells to redistribute into sensitive phases of the cell cycle.
4. *Regeneration.* Both normal tissue and tumours respond to radiation with repopulation. The capability to regenerate is dependent on the number of stem cells available for recruitment. Regeneration is the major determinant in deciding the optimal length of a radiotherapy course. Protraction of the total duration of irradiation may spare the patient an acute side effect, but it may also allow the tumour to proliferate out of control.
5. *Radiosensitivity.* Intrinsic radiosensitivity differs between tumour cells and normal tissue types, and strongly determines the final surviving frction of tumour cells. It can account for the variable responses of tumours.

9.6.7.2 Modes of Radiation Delivery

1. External irradiation
   Conventional dose fractionation has evolved empirically over the years. It is generally implicated to mean 1.8–2.0 Gy day^{-1}, five times a week, for a total dose between 60 and 70 Gy for 6–8 weeks. Attempts have been made to improve the therapeutic ratio by giving more than one fraction per day. Two distinct approaches are made:

   a. *Accelerated fractionation.* The overall treatment time is reduced, but the total dose is kept close to the conventional total dose. The basic concept is to prevent tumour cell regeneration during treatment.

   b. *Hyperfractionation.* The overall time is conventional, but the total dose increased by two or more daily fractions. The basic concept is to increase the tolerance to normal tissue, thus improving the therapeutic ratio.

   The two strategies may be combined.

2. Brachytherapy
   Low-dose-rate *continuous irradiation* by implantation of a radioactive nuclide—preferably iridium-192—combines the benefits of hyperfractionation and accelerated fractionation.

   Low-dose-rate continuous irradiation is equivalent to a large number of very small fractions, reducing the duration of treatment much more than can be achieved with the external beam technique. The volume of the high dose can also be kept small, sparing the normal surrounding tissue, provided the technical skill is available for implantation [1, 20].

9.6.7.3 Radiotherapy in Practice

Modern radiotherapy centres generally have at least two additional therapy units. Most common are linear electron accelerators, which can deliver beams of electrons and photons of different energies. With a combination of modified beams, in theory any target in the body should be available for irradiation. The selection of treatment technique, the combination of electron and photons of various energies, and the ratio of the given dose of each beam depend on the maximum depth of the lesion to be treated. A variation of combined treatment is that of an additional, or "boost", therapy, which uses reduced portals to raise the total dose in a limited volume to reduce the risk of late tissue side effects [2].

1. Imaging for radiotherapy
   Dose planning requires a CT scan (preferably one with contrast) of the head and neck. In most cases the CT scan is done with the patient in supine position and the head in a fixation device made of a thermoplastic material. The CT images are exported to a dose planning system in which the target is outlined by the responsible physician. The results from the full examination of the patient must be available during the planning procedure, e.g. MRI, PET, US and endoscopies.

2. Target definition
   It is essential to know the extension of the primary tumour and metastasis, independently of the aim of the treatment (e.g. curative per se, pre- or postoperative, or palliative) to be able to define the target of irradiation.

   a. Treatment volumes
      The treated tumour volumes should be addressed according to international standard as clarified in the International Commission of Radiation Units and Measurements (ICRU) Report 50 [14]:

      i. *Gross target volume* (GTV) is the solid tumour as found in clinical examination and on CT, MRI or PET images.

      ii. *Clinical target volume* (CTV) equals GTV plus the infiltrating margin as judged by the responsible physician.

      iii. *Planning target volume* (PTV) equals GTV plus a few-millimeter margin for body movements and the penumbra on the radiation fields.

      It may also be practical when treating patients with head and neck cancer to distinguish between a primary volume regarding the primary tumour or the PTV after surgery and a secondary volume consisting of the involved neck nodes with a margin or a suspected volume for possible microscopic disease. For microscopic disease a total dose in general of 50 Gy in 1.8- to 2-Gy fractions is considered satisfactory to achieve local control.

3. Beams for radiotherapy
   Radiotherapy is given with high-energy beams of ionising radiation [2]. The most widely used types of radiation are:

   a. *Photons*, or electromagnetic radiation, are a deeply penetrating radiation used for most targets in the head and neck region. The characteristic dose build-up near the surface is important for dose sparing of the skin. Photon beams for radiotherapy can either be X-rays generated by bremsstrahlung from high-energy electron beams or gamma rays from radioactive sources. The high-energy electron beams are produced by accelerators (linear accelerators are dominating the field).

   b. *Electrons* are charged particles with short to moderate depth penetration. This type of radiation is mainly used for superficial targets, mostly in or beneath the skin. The accelerators producing photon beams can also deliver clinical electron beams.

c. *Protons*, or hydrogen ions, are heavier charged particles, available only at a few radiotherapy centres in the world. Protons have physical properties with a well-defined range that enables dose delivery, which is more conformal to the target volume than can be achieved with photons and electrons. The energy and range of the protons can be varied to cover both superficial and deep target locations. The accelerators for protons are mainly cyclotrons and synchrotrons, which are much larger than the clinical electron accelerators.

4. Delivery techniques

Irradiation to a tumour may technically be done in different ways. External radiation delivered from an accelerator is the most common technique. Brachytherapy makes use of radioactive sources in which the radiation emanates from an internally, exactly located source in the tumour or adjacent to the tumour. The most common generator of electrons and photons utilised in almost all radiotherapy units are linear accelerators. A minimum dose of 4 MV is generally required, with a choice of higher energies to at least 15 MV.

5. External beam therapy

The most common modes utilised are:

a. Conformal techniques (3D CRT)

The principle is to match more closely the shape of the high-dose region to that of the target volume, thus minimising the dose to surrounding normal tissue and, in particular, the dose to organs at risk, e. g. the brain stem, the spinal cord, the eye lens, retina and the optical nerves. Even a lateralised two-field technique utilised in patients with small tongues or tonsillar cancers can be delivered in conformed fashion.

b. Intensity modulated radiotherapy (IMRT)

IMRT may be looked upon as a more technically advanced form of conformation. In principle it is a multifield, multisegmented technique that enables a steeper fall-off of high dose around the target, compared with more traditional conformal approaches. The advantages are the possibility to stick to the same treatment technique during the entire course of radiotherapy and significantly reduce the dose to salivary glands, thus partially avoiding dry mouth (xerostomia). A drawback may be the resulting dose bath of low-radiation doses of larger volumes of the surrounding tissue. Utilising IMRT does probably display the best advantage in patients in advanced stages when both sides of the neck have to been treated.

6. Brachytherapy

Three distinct types of brachytherapy exist:

a. *Intraluminal or intracavitary* location of radioactive sources, for example, in treatment of nasopharynx cancer. This enables that high doses with a steep fall of dose can be administered as a compliment (boost) to external radiotherapy, in order to increase the probability of local control in, e. g. cases of nasopharyngeal cancer.

b. *Interstitial* therapy implies surgical introduction of radioactive sources. The source used must have a small diameter to allow penetration in the tissue. Typical targets are cancer in the tongue; there, small tumours may be treated solely with interstitial therapy or utilised as a boost to external therapy, for example, in patients with cancer of the base of the tongue.

Traditionally, radioactive sources have been manoeuvred by hand by surgeons and radiotherapists. This naturally exposed the staff to high radiation doses. Most centres now use different forms of afterloading techniques, with flexible wires or compressed air carrying the radioactive source from a containing machine to an exact location in the tumour or close to the target. This necessitates the presence of preformed channels through the tumour, with the insertion of plastic tubes through which the radioactive source can travel. A surgical intervention has thus to be made after dose planning and before treatment to secure the optimal position and movement of sources.

The radiation may be delivered as a low-dose rate (LDR,) typically 7–20 Gy/day, or a high-dose rate (HDR) of 30–40 Gy/day. The most popular nuclide for implantation in the head and neck seems to be the iridium-192 HDR source, with a half-life of 74 days and principal gamma-ray energy of 370 keV. Iridium-192 is made in small cylinders to fit in the afterloading system.

c. *Surface applicators* may be used for small circumscript tumours of the skin, e. g. cancer of the eyelids.

7. Immobilisation and positioning

During radiotherapy the marks and settings made during the simulation secure reproducibility in every fraction. Certain quality assurance measures are also made regarding the performance of each accelerator. The method of repeated taking of portal films is gradually changing to the use of electronic portal imaging devices (EPID). This technique permits visualisation of any deviation in the setup of the patient. Other methods with fiducial markers for stereotactic setup are also utilised.

A typical time for positioning is between 5 and 10 min. A treatment field may be given in less than a minute. For irradiation with an IMRT approach, the total time for the patient on the treatment couch may be about 20 min.

Before dose planning starts the patients head has to be immobilised in a fixation device. These are generally individually made of certain thermoplastic materials that can be made malleable by, e.g. immersion a water bath (60°C), and then applied to the patient's head, where the material stiffens as it cools in the chosen position. This position will be the same through the entire process of preparing and realisation of the radiotherapy.

8. Treatment planning

The designation of portals and their combination is generally made by a hospital physicist or dosimetrist. The choice of energy and consequential dose distributions are naturally dependent on available accelerators and location of the target [23].

The patient is taken to CT, where the fixation device is applied again, and images are made for dose planning. These are exported to the computers, which handle the mathematical algorithms for dose calculations and actual data on the available accelerators energies and dose distributions. The aims of the treatment planning are the following [23]:

a. Localisation of the tumour volume and definition of target (GTV, CTV, PTV)
b. Measurement of the patient's outline
c. Determination of the optimal treatment configuration with particular clinical constraints
d. Calculation of the dose distribution
e. Preparation of an unambiguous set of treatment instructions for the radiographers

After the approval of the responsible physician, the dose plan is exported to the simulator, where the patient again has the fixation device applied while in the supine position. The proposed treatment is simulated in each beam direction, and beam entry marks are made preferably on the fixation device but if necessary, also on the skin. The simulation is verified with X-ray images from each portal. Thus it should be easy to repeat the treatment at every fraction in standardised fashion. The radiotherapy may start immediately after that the simulation is done.

9.6.7.4 Clinical Requirements for Radiotherapy

A radiotherapy schedule, in order to be curative, must fulfil the requirements below in order to achieve a reasonable number of patients with local control:

1. *Total dose*. The doses below are the those usually given:
   a. Preoperative radiotherapy: 2 Gy/day, 10 Gy/week, for a total dose of 50 Gy.
   b. Postoperative radiotherapy: 2 Gy/day, 10 Gy/week, for a total dose of 50–66 Gy.
   c. Curative doses per se: 2 Gy/day, 10 Gy/week and total dose of 66–70 Gy.

   Higher total doses may be used in hyperfractionated schedules.

2. *Fractional dose*. This may vary between 1 and 2 Gy in each fraction. Hyperfractionated schedules with two or more fractions each day are generally composed of doses lower than 2 Gy. Hypofractionation with doses above 2 Gy is seldom utilised in curative settings, but may be of value in palliation where short courses of therapy generally is preferred.

3. Overall treatment time

Treatment periods than 7 weeks must be avoided. The total treatment time may be reduced by about a third in accelerated schedules.

9.6.7.5 Side Effects of Radiotherapy and Subsequent Treatment

1. Acute side effects

Acute side effects are associated with the denudation of the epithelia. The mucosal membrane of the upper aerodigestive tract and the skin are rapidly proliferating tissues.

The side effects are dependent on the killing of stem cells in basal layers. Thus the normal loss of the superficial layers is not substituted. The denudation triggers a regenerative response in the stem cells surviving the radiation injury.

Typical acute side effects are redness, soreness, and oedema of the involved mucosa in the throat and pharynx, often accompanied by secondary fungal infections. It is important that patients prior to and during radiotherapy have the support of dentists, dental hygienists and nutritionists in order to preserve quality of life and avoid unwanted breaks of fractionation.

2. Late side effects

Late side effects may occur in almost all tissues in the head and neck region including vascular and connective tissue, bone, endocrine glands and the central nervous system. Because these tissues are actively proliferative, the duration of a course of treatment does not affect their tolerance to radiation therapy. The sensitivity of these tissues is dependent on the size of the dose per fraction. The tolerance is much better for a smaller dose per fraction.

Typical late effects appear more than 3–6 months after radiotherapy, and some of these may be fibrosis of muscles, atrophy of the skin, cataracts, pituitary insufficiency, hypothyroidism and very infrequently, necrosis.

3. Handling of tissue side effects

It is important that patients before start and during radiotherapy have the support of dentists, dental hygienists and nutritionists in order to save the quality of life and avoid unwanted breaks of fractionation.

   a. Acute side effects

   Almost all patients develop mucosal side effects after irradiation; the signs and symptoms general appear a after about a little more than 2 weeks of treatment. Before the start of radiotherapy every patient should see a *dentist* with special interest in the field of radiotherapy. Even patients with upper and lower dental prostheses should be referred to the dentist. The status of the teeth, possible chronic infections of the gums and periodontal diseases should be examined. If necessary, affected teeth with a poor prognosis should be extracted before radiotherapy. All patients should also have scheduled life-long follow-up with their dentists after finishing radiotherapy. Caries may increase because of the xerostomia induced by radiotherapy and thus have to be treated skilfully.

During the radiotherapy the patient needs the support of a *dental hygienist* for dental and mucosal care. Developing mucositis can be quite painful, which makes chewing and swallowing difficult. Local anaesthetics mixed with a fat-based cream before eating may ease the pain. In a majority of cases a secondary fungal infection develops in the affected mucosa. This generally best treated with a course of Nystatin. Most important, however, is the mechanical cleansing of the mucosal surfaces of denuded and infected debris. This cannot effectively be substituted by any medicine.

The aim of the *nutritionists'* work is to prevent catabolism; most easily observed as loss of body weight and reduced serum albumin level. These parameters should be charted every week during radiotherapy. An analysis of the patient's diet should be done before radiotherapy, and supplements be given if necessary during treatment. If pain makes chewing and swallowing impossible, then a nasogastric tube must be put into use. The patient should have full information on the necessity not to lose weight, as it might interfere with the effectiveness of treatment. A patient with advanced catabolism may experience stronger side effects, feel increased fatigue and have longer time for recovery after finishing radiotherapy.

Every patient should be advised to stop smoking as soon as possible. If the patient continues to smoke, then it may harm the efficacy of irradiation; the smoke generally amplifies the mucosal side effects, and the carcinogenic effect of smoking may lead to the development of new tumours in the head and neck, bronchi or lung as a part of a "field cancerisation".

b. Late side effects

A few per cent of patients develop lasting side effects of radiotherapy, as mentioned above. It is the view of this author that the term *radiation damage* should be avoided. The mechanism for the late side effects is not clear in all patients, independent of how cleverly and skilfully the treatment was

planned and performed. In rare cases a necrosis may develop in, e.g. the mandible bone. In some patients repeated exposures to oxygen in a hyperbaric chamber may induce healing. A resection with wide margins around the affected tissue may also be considered. Provided sufficient blood supply can be arranged to a transplanted free flap, a reconstruction of the lost tissue may be possible.

9.6.8 Localisation of Tumours at the Most Common Sites in Head and Neck Region

The incidence, risk factors, histopathology, signs and symptoms, metastasis, examinations, treatment and prognosis for common tumour sites in the head and neck are listed in Table 9.6.1.

9.6.9 Considerations Concerning Neck Lymph Nodes

The lymphatic drainage of different areas of the upper aerodigestive tract occurs along predictable pathways. Tumours from certain areas metastasise to the lymph nodes, following the same pathways, provided the neck has not been treated with surgery or radiotherapy [16].

It is now common to distinguish between certain lymph node levels on the neck. These have defined anatomic borders:

Level I	Divided in a submental and submandibular compartment
Level II	Upper jugular
Level III	Mid-jugular
Level IV	Lower jugular
Level V	Posterior triangle
Level VI	Anterior compartment

The extent of each level may be found in [11].

Oral carcinomas most often metastasise to levels I, II and III; submental, submandibular and upper jugular vein nodes. Carcinomas in the oropharynx, larynx and the hypopharynx metastasise along the jugular vein, levels II, III and IV.

The retropharyngeal nodes may have metastases when the primary tumour is located in the hypopharynx, tonsillar fossa, soft palate, posterior and lateral oropharyngeal walls.

This pattern is of importance both for occult and manifest metastases [17].

The presence of clinically proven lymph node metastasis in general decreases overall survival by at least half. The presence of extracapsular spread worsens the prognosis. In addition, the number of involved lymph nodes affects survival. Multiple involvements are associated with shorter survival. Lymph node involvement usually calls for neck dissection with removal of the metastases. Postoperative radiation of the neck is recommended in a majority of these cases. Radiotherapy may also be applied to the lymph nodes of the neck in patients with advanced primary tumours with high risk of occult metastases [21].

Table 9.6.1 Most common sites for head and neck tumours

Lips	
Incidence	1.8 per 100,000 individuals per year in the United States and 1.3 per 100,000 individuals per year in Sweden
Risk factors	Tobacco and overconsumption of alcohol
Histopathology	Squamous epithelial carcinoma in 95% of the patients. Basal cell carcinoma may occasionally occur in the upper lip. Tumours of the lower lip are five times more common than are tumours of the lower lip
Signs and symptoms	A hard nodule in the lip, induration or a ulcer that does not heal
Metastasis	Lip tumours metastasise relatively late in the course of the disease to submental and submandibular lymph nodes
Examinations	Inspection, palpation and biopsy and CT of the bottom of the mouth and the neck in advanced cases to find possible local node metastasis
Treatment	In patients with small tumours without lymph node metastasis, surgery is the first choice. Advanced cancers, especially those with growth into the oral commissure, are more suited for curative intended irradiation with electrons, or brachytherapy with iridium implants
Prognosis	Patients with tumours of the lower lip have better outcomes than do those with tumours of the upper lip. Tumour size is highly prognostic, with 5-year local control of 90% for T1–T2 tumours and 40% for T4 tumours
Tongue	
Incidence	4.5 per 100,000 individuals per year in the United States, and 2.1 per 100,000 individuals for men and 1.2 per 100,000 individuals per year for woman in Sweden. The world standard rate is 1.3 for men and 0.7 for woman per 100,000 individuals The tongue is the most common site of squamous cell carcinoma of the oral cavity
Risk factors	Tobacco smoking and overconsumption of alcohol. HPV may be involved in carcinogenesis. Plummer-Vinson's syndrome with a combination of sideropenic dysphagia with mucosal atrophy and iron-deficiency anaemia may increase the risk of cancer in the oral cavity
Histopathology	Most cancers are squamous epithelial carcinomas. More infrequent are adenoid-cystic carcinomas, mucoid epidermal carcinomas and sarcomas. Melanomas seldom occur in the tongue mucosa
Signs and symptoms	An ulcer not healing or hard nodule that persists, local pain
Metastasis	Submandibular and cervical nodes on the same side as the tumour. With larger tumours (T3 and T4) metastasis may appear on both of sides of the neck
Examinations	Inspection and endoscopy of the pharynx and larynx. Careful palpation of the tongue, the floor of the mouth and the lymph nodes on the neck. MR or CT. Biopsy of the suspected tumour and involved lymph nodes on the neck
Treatment	Primary surgery followed by postoperative irradiation for small tumours (T1N0–T2N0). In some institutions where brachytherapy is available it is the first choice of treatment. Larger tumour, judged nonresectable, should be treated with radiation at least to a total dose of 70 Gy in 1.8- or 2-Gy fractions. Provided the general condition of the patient allows hyperfractionation and/or concomitant chemotherapy, these alternatives should be considered
Prognosis	Patients with small cancers may display local control close to 90% after 5 years. In advanced cases, however, it may be as low as 25%

Table 9.6.1 *(continued)* Most common sites for head and neck tumours

Floor of the mouth	
Incidence	The standard rate in Sweden is 0.6 per 100,000 individuals for men and 0.3 per 100,000 individuals per year. The world standard rate is 0.4 and 0.2 for men and women, respectively per 100,000 individuals
Risk factors	Tobacco smoking and overconsumption of alcohol. HPV may be involved in carcinogenesis. Plummer–Vinson's syndrome with a combination of sideropenic dysphagia with mucosal atrophy and iron-deficiency anaemia may increase the risk of cancer in the oral cavity
Histopathology	Squamous cell carcinoma is the preponderant type of tumour
Signs and symptoms	An ulcer not healing or hard nodule that persists, local pain
Metastasis	Submandibular and cervical nodes on the same side as the tumour. With larger tumours (T3 and T4) metastasis may appear on both of sides of the neck
Examinations	Inspection and endoscopy of the pharynx and larynx. Careful palpation of the tongue, the floor of the mouth and the lymph nodes on the neck. MR or CT. Biopsy of the suspected tumour and involved lymph nodes on the neck
Treatment	For small lesions surgery is generally preferred. Depending on the routines at the centre, postoperative radiotherapy is given. Patients with larger nonresectable tumours should be recommended radiotherapy and if possible, included in a protocol for hyper- and/or accelerated fractionation with or without concomitant radiotherapy
Prognosis	Five-year survival is dependent on the initial stage of tumour at presentation and varies between 88% for stage I and 0–14% for stage IV. For more advanced stages the effect of postoperative radiotherapy seems to increase compared with earlier stages
Base of tongue	
Incidence	The standard rate is 0.9 per 100,000 individuals for men and 0.3 per 100,000 individuals per year for woman in Sweden. The world standard rate is 0.5 and 0.2 for men and women, respectively, per 100,000 individuals
Risk factors	Tobacco smoking and overconsumption of alcohol. HPV may be involved in the carcinogenesis. Plummer–Vinson's syndrome with a combination of sideropenic dysphagia with mucosal atrophy and iron-deficiency anaemia may increase the risk of cancer in the oral cavity
Histopathology	Squamous cell carcinoma is the preponderant type of tumour. However tumours probably derived from accessory salivary glands may give rise to unusual tumours like adenoidcystic carcinoma
Signs and symptoms	An ulcer not healing or hard nodule that persists, local pain and pain at swallowing
Metastasis	Submandibular and cervical nodes on sides of the neck
Examinations	Inspection and endoscopy of the pharynx and larynx. Careful palpation of the tongue, the floor of the mouth and the lymph nodes on the neck. MR or CT. Biopsy of the suspected tumour and involved lymph nodes on the neck
Treatment	For small lesions surgery is generally preferred. Depending on the routines at the treatment centre, postoperative radiotherapy is generally given. Patients with larger nonresectable tumours should be recommended radiotherapy, and if possible included in a protocol for hyper- and/or accelerated fractionation with or without concomitant radiotherapy. Another alternative is external radiotherapy to a total dose around 50 Gy, dependent on the metastatic involvement of cervical lymph nodes, which is then followed by brachytherapy with iridium implants
Prognosis	Five-year survival is dependent on the initial stage of tumour at presentation
Risk factors	Tobacco smoking and overconsumption of alcohol is strongly associated with the development of tumour
Histopathology	Squamous cell carcinoma is the preponderant type of tumour accounting for more than 90% of the malignant lesions. However tumours probably derived from accessory salivary glands may give rise to unusual tumours like adenoidcystic carcinoma

Table 9.6.1 *(continued)* Most common sites for head and neck tumours

Signs and symptoms	The most common tumour in the oropharynx is tonsillar cancer or cancer derived from the anterior tonsillar pillar. An ulcer not healing or hard nodule that persists, local pain may not be apparent in earlier stages and pain at swallowing. The tonsillar cancer may initially be interpreted as local infection not responding to antibiotic treatment. In some patients a metastatic nodule on the neck may be first sign
Metastasis	Submandibular and cervical nodes on the same side of the neck. Larger tumour that infiltrate the base of tongue may metastasise to the contralateral side of the neck
Examinations	Inspection and endoscopy of the oropharynx and larynx. Careful palpation of the tongue, the floor of the mouth, the tonsillar region and the lymph nodes on the neck. MR or CT. Biopsy of the suspected tumour and involved lymph nodes on the neck
Treatment	Radiotherapy with curative intended doses, e. g. 2-Gy fractions to a total dose of 70 Gy during 7 weeks, or in some centres an accelerated schedule preferred. The primary tumour volumes as well as lymph nodes on the affected side should be included For larger tumours infiltrating the base of tongue, both lymph nodes on both sides of the neck may need irradiation. In some centres surgery followed by postoperative irradiation may be chosen
Prognosis	Local control may vary between 100% for T1 tumours down to 24% for T4 tumours at a 3-year follow-up. Disease-free survival after 5 years may vary in median between 48 and 71%
Nasopharynx	
Incidence	This tumour is uncommon in Europe and the United States. One case per 100,000 individuals per year in these areas, but frequent in southern China, with 50 cases per 100,000 per year. The tumour is infrequent at all ages
Risk factors	EBV seems to be associated with the development of this cancer. In China the consumption of salty fish with a content of nitrosamines has been suggested as a carcinogenic factor
Histopathology	In children, they manifest mostly as sarcomas. In adults, squamous epithelial carcinomas are 90% of the cases including lymphoepithelial carcinomas of the Schmincke type
Signs and symptoms	The primary signs might be swelling of the lymph nodes of the neck. Later on, breathing through the nose in combination with bloody discharge might follow. With involvement of the Eustachian tubes the patient might have involvement of hearing loss and pain from the ears. Involvement of the skull base may lead to involvement of the cranial nerves and headache, especially from the forehead
Metastasis	Lymphogenic to all nodes on the neck along the jugular vein and along the retropharyngeal nodes. Haematogenous spread to the bone, lung and liver
Examinations	The aim is to be able to classify the size and spread of the tumour according to the TNM schedule Palpation of the cervical nodes including the supraclavicularis. Neurological examination, especially the function of the cranial nerves Endoscopic examination of the nasopharynx. Biopsies of the nasopharynx and of affected lymph nodes Radiological examinations preferably with MRI or CT for suspected bone lesions X-ray of the thorax and if clinical signs and symptoms indicate general metastatic spread CT or US of the abdomen may be necessary as well as scintigram of the bones
Treatment	Radiotherapy of the primary tumour and metastatic nodes to 68–70 Gy in 1.8- or 2-Gy fractions. In general the whole neck has to be treated. Radical surgery of the primary tumour is generally not possible because of the anatomical localisation Lymph nodes on the neck that remain after irradiation may be removed by neck dissection
Prognosis	Early development of node metastasis may confer a bad prognosis. The median 5-year survival is about 30–35%

Table 9.6.1 *(continued)* Most common sites for head and neck tumours

Hypopharynx	
Incidence	In Sweden 3.5 new cases per year per 100,000 individuals. Men are more affected than woman are by a ratio of 2:1
Risk factors	Smoking and overconsumption of alcohol
Histopathology	In 90% of patients carcinomas are squamous epithelial. Other tumours like lymphoepithelial tumours, and adenocarcinomas are infrequent
Signs and symptoms	The symptoms may be unspecific, and the first symptom may be come from a metastatic involved lymph node on the neck. Indistinct problems with swallowing, feeling of a foreign body or a tickling feeling in the throat may be experienced
Metastasis	Lymphogenic spread to adjacent lymph nodes on the neck. Haematogenous spread to lungs, liver, bone and the brain (mostly in locally advances cases)
Examinations	Palpation of the cervical lymph nodes. Endoscopic examination of the larynx and hypopharynx with biopsies of the suspected tumour. CT or preferably MRI scans of the neck. X-ray of the thorax and if clinical signs and symptoms indicate general metastatic spread, CT or US of the abdomen may be necessary as well as scintigram of the bones
Treatment	In small tumours (preferably without macroscopic metastasis); primary surgery with reconstruction of the lumen if necessary, followed by radiotherapy to the primary target and the neck to total doses between 60 and 66 Gy in 1.8- or 2-Gy fractions For larger tumours, radiation to doses between 68 and 70 Gy in 1.8- or 2-Gy fractions In advanced cases concomitant radiotherapy with cisplatinum may be of value. Hyperfractionated therapy may also increase the number of patient with local control
Prognosis	Patients with small lesions and no lymph node metastasis have a median 5-year survival of 70%. Patients with advanced diseases have median survival of 20–30%
Larynx	
Incidence	In Sweden 180–200 patients, corresponding to 2.2 per 100,000 individuals per year. The age of peak of incidence is between 50 and 70 years
Risk factors	Most patients are heavy smokers (more than 90%)
Histopathology	Dominance by squamous epithelial carcinomas. Infrequent cases with sarcomas, lymphoepithelial tumours or adenocarcinomas may appear For patients in Western Europe the following distribution of anatomical sites is valid: glottic carcinoma, 60–65%; supraglottic carcinoma, 30–35%; subglottic carcinoma, 5%
Prognosis	The 5-year survival for larynx carcinoma is strongly correlated to the size of the tumour at diagnosis: glottic T1, >90%; glottic T4, <50%; supraglottic T1, ≈80%; supraglottic T4, ≈ 50%
Signs and symptoms	Chronic hoarseness. If the hoarseness has been persistent for more than 3 weeks, then an endoscopic examination should be done. First symptom may also be lymph node swelling from metastasis
Metastasis	Lymphogenic spread to adjacent lymph nodes on the neck. Haematogenous spread to lungs, liver, bone and the brain
Examinations	Palpation of the neck. Endoscopic inspection of the larynx with biopsy. CT or MR of the neck to evaluate possible lymph node metastasis and invasion of the thyroid cartilage. If available, a stroboscopic examination of the vocal cords to decide their mobility should be done
Treatment	For T1 glottic tumours located to the middle, movable part on the vocal cord, microsurgery by an endoscopic approach may be advantageous. Small tumours, T1 or T2 in general, respond nicely to radiotherapy to a total dose 66–70 Gy. For T3 tumours radiotherapy is usually the first choice. Patients with T4 tumours may have laryngectomy as their first treatment or palliative treatment with radiotherapy initially

Table 9.6.1 *(continued)* Most common sites for head and neck tumours

Parotid glands	
Incidence	The incidence is 0.5–1 per 100,000 individuals per year. Men and women experience the disease in the same frequency
Risk factors	Pleomorphic adenomas may transform to malignancy. Ionising radiation has, in some cases 15–20 years after the exposure, been blamed as a causative factor
Histopathology	Mucoepidermoid cancer, adenoid-cystic cancers and other types of adenocarcinomas are the most common
Signs and symptoms	Palpable tumour in the parotid gland. Local pain. Involvement of the facialis nerve, with paralysis of the face on the tumour side. One, two or three of the innervated parts may be affected. Lymph node swelling, preferably on the tumour side
Metastasis	Spread to cervical lymph nodes on the tumour side. Haematogenous spread to the lungs
Examinations	Palpation of the parotid gland and the whole neck. MRI or CT for detailed for information of the tumour growth and metastasis spread
Treatment	Total resection of parotid gland is preferable in most cases. Reconstruction of the facial nerve should be considered in the same surgical session
Prognosis	Dependent on histopathology and initial tumour size and spread. The 5-year survival may vary between 25 and 80%.

Nasal cavity and paranasal sinuses	
Incidence	The standard rate is 1.3 per 100,000 individuals for men and 0.6 per 100,000 individuals per year for woman in Sweden. The world standard rate is 0.6 and 0.4 for men and women, respectively per 100,000 individuals. The age peak is between 60 and 70 years
Risk factors	A classical epidemiological example of hazardous exposure is the increased incidence of adeno-carcinomas in the ethmoid sinuses in workers exposed to wood dust. The incidence is about 1,000 times higher than in the general population. Smoking and overconsumption of alcohol may contribute to the development of cancer
Histopathology	The most predominant diagnoses are squamous epithelial carcinomas. Other not-so-frequent malignant tumours include adenoid-cystic carcinomas, adenocarcinomas, olfactory neuroblastomas, melanomas and sarcomas
Signs and symptoms	Chronic infections of the nose or sinuses, papillary outgrowths in the nasal cavity, repeated epistaxis
Metastasis	May spread to neck nodes, especially in locally advanced cases with invasion of neighbouring structures like the infratemporal fossa or pterytopalatine fossa
Examinations	Endoscopic inspection of the nose. Careful palpation of the lymph nodes on the neck. CT examination of the facial bone, the base of the skull and the neck. Biopsy of the suspected tumour
Treatment	Surgery followed by postoperative radiotherapy. So-called craniofacial resection may be applied
Prognosis	Five-year survival varies between 67% for early stages down to 15% for advanced stages

Modified from [24]

9.6.10 New Development in Cancer Treatment: Molecular Targeted Therapy

A development is taking place in the field of diagnosing and treating patients with head and neck cancer, especially for those in advanced cases: molecular-targeted therapy.

New antitumor agents are greatly needed, particularly for overcoming resistance that may occur with failures of primary therapy. The addition of cetuximab to cisplatinum as a first-line therapy has, in one study, been shown to increase the overall response rate when compared with cisplatinum alone [5].

The search for novel targeted anticancer agents that do not exclusively target the epidermal growth receptor includes the following areas of substances [15]:

- Monoclonal antibodies directed against vascular endothelial growth factor and the HER-2 receptor
- Receptor tyrokinase inhibitors with and without angiogenetic effect
- Intracytoplasmatic proteins inhibitors
- Nuclear protein inhibitors

9.6.10.1 Current Treatment Recommendations

In an excellent overview of the present status in the field of oncological treatments, Corvò [8] draws the following conclusions regarding treatment recommendations:

1. External radiotherapy alone and/or brachytherapy may offer excellent outcomes in early-stage disease.
2. Altered fractionation radiotherapy and concomitant chemoradiation have resulted in improved locoregional control of locally advanced disease.
3. Concomitant chemoradiation appears to confer a reproducible survival benefit in locally advanced disease; the optimal time–dose regimen has not yet been defined for this approach.
4. Altered fractionation radiotherapy and chemoradiation increase the acute toxicity profile.
5. Concomitant chemoradiotherapy should be the gold standard for resected patients at high-risk for failure.
6. 3D CRT is the minimal standard of technique in patients with cancer in the head and neck region.
7. Patient preference, physician expertise and toxicity issues are important factors in determining clinical management for individual treatment.

Acknowledgement

The comments and suggestions of Associate Prof. Anders Montelius are much appreciated.

References

1. Aird EG, Williams JR (1993) Brachytherapy. In: Edsby Williams JR, Thwaites DI (eds) Treatment planning for external beam therapy in radiotherapy physics in practice. Oxford Medical, Oxford, pp 187–226
2. Almond P (1999) Physics of radiotherapy of head and neck tumors. In: Thawley SE, Panje WR, Batsakis JG, Lindberg RD (eds) Comprehensive management of head and neck tumors, vol 1, 2nd edn. Saunders, Philadelphia, pp 124–140
3. Batsakis JG (1999) Pathology of tumors of the oral cavity. In: Thawley SE, Panje WR, Batsakis JG, Lindberg RD (eds) Comprehensive management of head and neck tumors, vol 1, 2nd edn. Saunders, Philadelphia
4. Bonner JA, Harari PM, Giralt J, Azarnia N, Shin DM, Cohen RB, Jones CU, Sur R, Raben D, Jassem J, Ove R, Kies MS, Baselga J, Yuossoufian H, Amellal N, Rowinsky EK, Ang KK (2006) Radiotherapy plus cetuximab for squamous-cell carcinoma of the head and neck. N Engl J Med 354:567–578
5. Burtness B, Goldwasser MA, Flood W, Mattar B, Forastiere AA (2005) Phase III randomized trial of cisplatin plus placebo compared with cisplatin plus cetuximab in metastatic/recurrent head and neck cancer: an Eastern Cooperative Oncology Group study. J Clin Oncol 23:8646–8654
6. Collins SL (1999) Controversies in multimodality therapy for head and neck cancer: clinical and biological perspective. In: Thawley SE, Panje WR, Batsakis JG, Lindberg RD (eds) Comprehensive management of head and neck tumors, vol 1, 2nd edn. Saunders, Philadelphia
7. Collins SL (1999) Smoking cessation and prevention of head and neck cancer. In: Thawley SE, Panje WR, Batsakis JG, Lindberg RD (eds) Comprehensive management of head and neck tumors, vol 1, 2nd edn. Saunders, Philadelphia, pp 346–377
8. Corvò R (2007) Evidence-based radiation oncology in head and neck squamous cell carcinoma. Radiother Oncol 85:156–170
9. DeLacure MD (2004) General principles of reconstructive surgery for head and neck cancer patients. In: Harrison LB, Sessions RB, Hong WK (eds) Head and neck cancer: a multidisciplinary approach, 2nd edn. Lippincott, Williams and Wilkins, Philadelphia, pp 150–164
10. Frank DK and Sessions RB, (2004) Physical examination of the head and neck. In: Harrison LB, Sessions RB, Hong WK (eds) Head and neck cancer: a multidisciplinary approach, 2nd edn. Lippincott, Williams and Wilkins, Philadelphia
11. Grégoire V, Levendag P, Kian K. Ang KK, Bernier J, Braaksmab M, Budach V, Chao C, Coche E, Cooper JS, Cosnard G, Eisbruch A, El-Sayed S, Emami B, Grau C, Hamoir M, Lee N, Maingon P, Muller K, Reychler H (2003) CT-based delineation of lymph node levels and related CTVs in the node-negative neck: DAHANCA, EORTC, GORTEC, NCIC, RTOG consensus guidelines. Radiother Oncol 69:227–336
12. Hao D, Ritter MA, Oliver T, Browman GP (2006) Platinum-based concurrent chemoradiotherapy for tumors of head and neck and the esophagus. Semin Radiat Oncol 1:10–19

13. Harari PM, Shyhmin H (2006) Radiation combined with EGFR signal inhibitors: head and neck cancer focus. Semin in Radiat Oncol 16:38–44

14. International Commission of Radiation Units and Measurements (1999) Prescribing, recording and reporting photon beam therapy. ICRU Report 50. International Commission of Radiation Units and Measurements, Bethesda, Md.

15. Le Tourneau C, Faivre S, Siu LL (2007) Molecular targeted therapy of head and neck cancer: review and clinical development challenges. Eur J Cancer 43:2457–2466

16. Lindberg R (1972) Distribution of cervical lymph node metastases from squamous cell carcinoma of the upper respiratory and digestive tracts. Cancer 29:1446–1449.

17. Medina JE, Houck JR Jr (2004) Surgical management of cervical lymph nodes In: Harrison LB, Sessions RB, Hong WK (eds) Head and neck cancer: a multidisciplinary approach, 2nd edn. Lippincott, Williams and Wilkins, Philadelphia, pp 203–244

18. Milas L, Peters LJ (1999) Biology of radiation therapy. In: Thawley SE, Panje WR, Batsakis JG, Lindberg RD (eds) Comprehensive management of head and neck tumors, vol 1, 2nd edn. Saunders, Philadelphia, pp 99–123

19. Mork J, Lie KL, Glattre E, Hallmans G, Jellum G, Koskela P, Möller B, Pukkala E, Schiller JT, Youngman L, Lehtinen M, Dillner J (2001) Human papilloma infection as a risk factor for squamous-cell carcinoma of the head and neck. N Engl J Med 344:1125–1131

20. Nag S (1994) High-dose-rate brachytherapy: a textbook. Futura, New York

21. O'Brien CJ, Smith JW, Soong SJ et al. (1986) Neck dissection with and without radiotherapy—prognostic patterns of recurrence and survival. Am J Surg 152:456–463

22. Pignon J P, Bourhis J, Designé C, on behalf of the MACH-NC Collaborative Group (2000) Chemotherapy added to locoregional treatment for head and neck squamous cell carcinoma: three meta-analyses of updated individual data. Lancet 355:949–955

23. Redpath AT, Williams JR, Thwaites DI (1993) Treatment planning for external beam therapy. In: Williams JR, Thwaites DI (eds) Radiotherapy physics in practice. Oxford Medical, Oxford, pp 135–185

24. Senn H-J, Drings P, Glaus A, Jungi WF, Pralle HB, Sauer R, Schlag PM (2001) Chapters 21.2–21.8 In: Checkliste Onkologie 5.Thieme, Stuttgart, pp 299–321

25. Shah JP, Zelefsky MJ (2004) Cancer of the oral cavity. In: Harrison LB, Sessions RB, Hong WK (eds) Head and neck cancer: a multidisciplinary approach, 2nd edn. Lippincott, Williams and Wilkins, Philadelphia, pp 266–305

26. Smith BD, Haffty BG (2004) Prognostic factors in patients with head and neck cancer. In: Harrison LB, Sessions RB, Hong WK (eds) Head and neck cancer: a multidisciplinary approach, 2nd edn. Lippincott, Williams and Wilkins, Philadelphia, pp 49–73

27. Stupp R, Vokes EE (1999) Chemotherapy of head and neck cancer. In: Thawley SE, Panje WR, Batsakis JG, Lindberg RD (eds) Comprehensive management of head and neck tumors, vol 1, 2nd edn. Saunders, Philadelphia pp 141–156

28. Wheldon T (1999) Radiobiological principles. In: Dobbs J, Barrett A, Ash D (1999) Practical radiotherapy planning, 3rd edn. Arnold, London, pp 46–59

29. Wilson GD, Bentzen SM, Harari PM (2006) Biological basis for combining drugs with irradiation. Semin in Radiat Oncol 16:2–9

30. Wittekind C, Greene FL, Hutter RVP, Klimpfinger M, Sobin LH (2005) TNM atlas: illustrated guide to the TNM/pTNM classification of malignant tumors, 5th edn. Springer, Berlin Heidelberg New York

9.7 Principles and Techniques of Neck Dissection

REIDAR GRÉNMAN

9.7.1 Basics

Head and neck cancer is primarily a locoregional disease, which usually sends distant metastases late in the course of the disease. Benign lesions of the neck due to unspecific or specific infections, congenital disorders or benign neoplasms are common and often cause diagnostic and differential diagnostic problems. Therefore it is of great importance that every otolaryngologist, and head and neck surgeon be well familiar with the clinical anatomy of the neck in order to be able to make the clinical diagnosis, and plan the necessary additional investigations and the treatment.

9.7.2 Clinical Anatomy of the Neck, with Special Reference to Neck Dissection

9.7.2.1 Fasciae of the Neck

The superficial layer of the cervical fascia is very thin, underlies the skin and is of less importance. In contrast, the deep fascia, which is divided into three layers, forms important compartments of the neck, extending from the base of the skull and oral cavity to the mediastinum. The external layer of the deep fascia underlies the platysma muscle and encircles the superficial neck structures, dividing in the area of the sternocleidomastoid and trapezius muscles, and enveloping them. The middle layer encloses the oesophagus, trachea and thyroid gland. The internal layer of the deep fascia surrounds the deep muscles of the neck, including the splenius, levator scapulae, erector spinae, the scalene, the longus capitus and the longus colli muscles, and the vertebrae. The so-called prevertebral fascia is a part of the internal layer of the deep fascia. The internal layer of the deep fascia envelopes the carotid artery, internal jugular vein, the vagus and some nerves of the cervical plexus (Fig. 9.7.1a).

9.7.2.2 Triangles of the Neck

For practical reasons the neck can be divided into two triangles, the posterior and the anterior. The three layers of the deep fascia forms the boundaries to these triangles.

9.7.2.2.1 The Posterior Triangle

The sternocleidomastoid muscle, the anterior border of the trapezius muscle and the clavicle form the boundaries of the posterior triangle (see Fig. 9.7.4). The external layer of the deep fascia forms its lateral and posterior wall, surrounding the trapezius muscle, and the internal layer forms its medial wall and anterior wall, surrounding the carotid and internal jugular vessels.

The major contents of the posterior triangle are the cutaneous branches of the cervical plexus, the accessory nerve (cranial nerve [CN] XI), two arteries from the subclavian artery with the corresponding veins and the abundant number of lymph nodes associated with them.

The cutaneous branches of the cervical plexus supply the skin of the head from the posterior skull to the supraclavicular region. The nerves contain parts from C2–C4. These cutaneous nerves loop around the posterior part of the sternocleidomastoid muscle at the level where the accessory nerves enter the posterior triangle from among the muscle fibres of the sternocleidomastoid muscle. The greater auricular nerve runs along the sternocleidomastoid muscle in a cranial direction, whereas the lesser occipital nerve runs cranioposteriorly. The supraclavicular nerves run inferiorly, whereas the anterior cutaneous nerve runs anteriorly (Fig. 9.7.2). Before entering the posterior triangle the accessory nerve (CN XI) supplies the sternocleidomastoid muscle with motor fibres. The fibres of the CN XI, which enters the posterior triangle, run through the fat, often close to the superficial fascia, to the trapezius muscle. The accessory nerve is the only motor nerve in the posterior triangle. The other motor nerves, which run medially to the fat of posterior triangle under the internal layer of the deep fascia, include the phrenic nerve and the brachial plexus.

The thyrocervical trunk of the subclavian artery gives rise to the two major arteries of the posterior triangle, the suprascapular and transverse cervical arteries, which are located near the base of the posterior triangle in the supraclavicular fossa, running transversally deep to the sternocleidomastoid muscle. The transverse cervical and suprascapular veins run parallel to the arteries. The external jugular vein runs laterally to the surface of the ster-

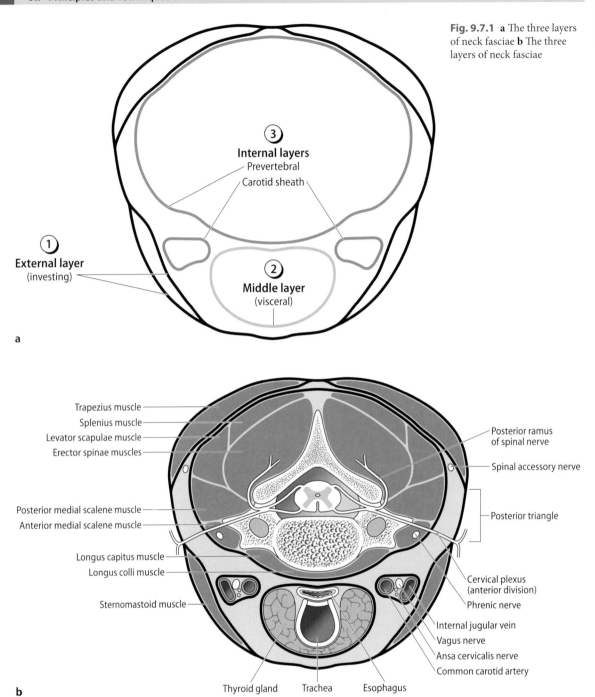

Fig. 9.7.1 a The three layers of neck fasciae **b** The three layers of neck fasciae

③ **Internal layers**
— Prevertebral
— Carotid sheath

① **External layer** (investing)

② **Middle layer** (visceral)

a

Trapezius muscle
Splenius muscle
Levator scapulae muscle
Erector spinae muscles

Posterior ramus of spinal nerve

Spinal accessory nerve

Posterior medial scalene muscle
Anterior medial scalene muscle

Posterior triangle

Longus capitus muscle
Longus colli muscle

Cervical plexus (anterior division)
Phrenic nerve

Sternomastoid muscle

Internal jugular vein
Vagus nerve
Ansa cervicalis nerve
Common carotid artery

Thyroid gland   Trachea   Esophagus

b

nocleidomastoid muscle, parallel to the greater auricular nerve and after entering the posterior fossa, it runs inferiorly to the base of the supraclavicular fossa, where it enters the subclavian vein near to the area where the internal jugular vein joins the vena subclavia (see Fig. 9.7.6a).

The lower border, or the base of the neck, is at the level of the thoracic inlet. It runs from the manubrium along the first rib to the transverse process of the sixth cervical vertebrae. In the midline runs the tracheo-oesophageal tract. It contains among others the subclavian and common carotid arteries, the brachiocephalic vein, the vagus nerve (CN X) and the sympathetic trunk. It is important to note that the described fascial spaces run from the neck into the mediastinum.

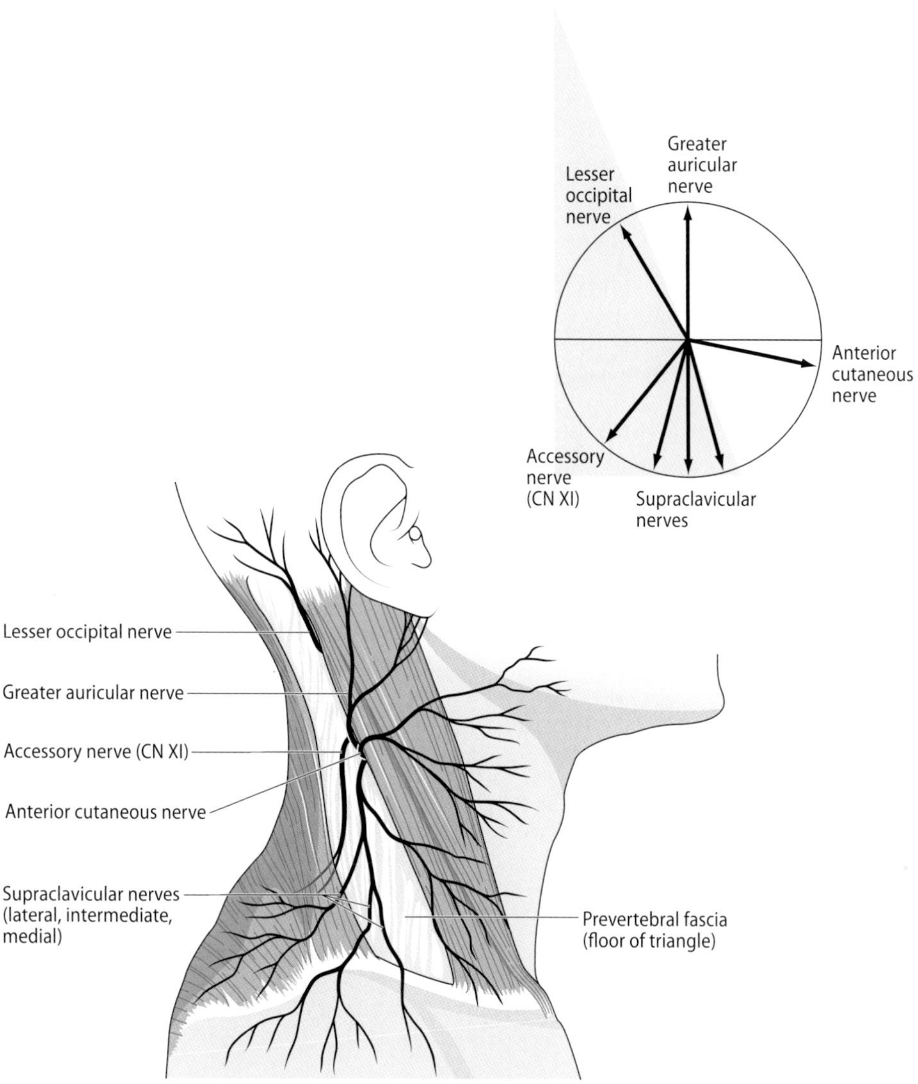

Fig. 9.7.2 The anterior and posterior triangles of the neck

9.7.2.2.2 The Anterior Triangle

The anterior triangle lies forward of the posterior triangle. Superiorly its border is the mandible, laterally the sterno-cleidomastoid muscle and the external layer of the deep cervical fascia, and the midline. The anterior triangle can be further divided into the submandibular triangle, and the supra- and the infrahyoid triangles.

The submandibular triangle is bounded by the two bellies of the digastric muscle and the ramus of the mandible. The mylohyoid and hyoglossus muscles form the medial wall, and the platysma and the skin form the lateral wall. The submandibular gland with its associated lymph nodes, the facial artery and vein, and the motor nerve to the mylohyoideus and digastric muscle lies laterally to the mylohyoideus muscle. The mandibular branch of the facial nerve (CN VII) often runs inferior to the mandible, enters the submandibular triangle and runs

laterally to the submandibular gland before ascending to the face from the anterior part of the triangle. In addition to the submandibular gland duct, the lingual and hypoglossal (CN XII) nerves run in the submandibular space. The lingual nerve runs laterally and superiorly to the submandibular gland duct. The hypoglossal nerve runs in the inferior-most part of the submandibular space (see Fig. 6b).

The triangle bordered by the posterior belly of the digastric muscle, the midportion of the sternocleidomastoid muscle and the posterior belly of the omohyoid muscle is also called the supraomohyoid or the carotid triangle. The lateral wall is formed by the superficial layer of the deep cervical fascia; medially it is bordered by the internal layer of the deep cervical fascia surrounding the vertebral column and the middle layer of the deep cervical fascia surrounding the pharynx and the larynx. The carotid sheath including the carotid artery, internal jugular vein and the vagus nerve (CN X) runs through this triangle. The accessory nerve (CN XI) runs in the upper portion of the carotid sheath, turns backwards and enters the sternocleidomastoid muscle inferior to the area where the posterior belly of the digastric muscle crosses the sternocleidomastoid muscle. The hypoglossal nerve (CN XII) runs anteriorly to the carotid and runs anteroinferiorly until it passes medially to the posterior belly of the digastric muscle to the surface of the hyoglossus muscle in the medial aspect of the submandibular triangle before entering the muscle of the tongue. The vagal nerve (CN X) runs between the internal jugular vein and the carotid artery. The sternohyoid, sternothyroid and omohyoid muscles are innervated by the ansa cervicalis, which is part of the cervical plexus getting fibres from C1–C3. In addition to the motor innervation supplied by the ansa cervicalis, motor filaments from the cervical routes 3 and 4 supply the levator scapulae muscle. They lie deep to the prevertebral fascia. So does the phrenic nerve (C3–C4, sometimes C5), which sends motor and sensory fibres to the diaphragm.

The bifurcation of the common carotid artery lies within this triangle. The internal carotid artery ascends posteriorly to the external carotid artery and runs without branching cranially. The branches of the external carotid artery form important landmarks. Three anterior branches are the superior thyroid, the lingual and the fa-

cial arteries. It is important to note that the superior thyroid artery can also originate from the common carotid artery, inferior to the bifurcation. Therefore it is advisable to ligate the external carotid artery cranial to the lingual artery in the case of severe bleeding from the nose or facial fractures. The medial branch is the ascending pharyngeal artery; the posterior branches in ascending order are the occipital and posterior auricular arteries (Fig. 9.7.3).

The infrahyoid triangle extends from the triangle inferiorly to the level of the clavicle and the thoracic inlet. The omohyoid muscle runs laterally to the carotid sheath, which is the most important structure of this triangle together with the lymphatic vessels and lymph nodes that run along the carotid sheath. Surgically it is important to note that the thoracic duct runs from the mediastinum to the left supraclavicular fossa before entering the venous system in the jugulosubclavian angle (Fig. 9.7.8). Special care must be taken not to damage the thoracic duct when removing metastatic lymph nodes in this region often originating from subclavicular malignancies, the so-called Virchow's nodes.

9.7.2.3 Lymphatic Drainage of the Head and Neck

Lymph drains into either the superficial or the deep system. The skin and mucus membranes of the head and neck contain a network of thin, superficial-running afferent lymphatics, which drain into an outer circle of superficial original lymph nodes and eventually into the deep circle of nodes following the carotid sheaths with the deep cervical lymph nodes. Both the superficial lymph nodes and the lymphatics serving the visceral structures, the pharynx and the larynx drain into these deep cervical lymph nodes.

The anterior part of the scalp drains into the preauricular and sometimes to the infra-auricular or the parotid lymph nodes. The parietal skin drains into the preauricular or infra-auricular lymph nodes. The occipital part of the scalp drains into the superficial occipital nodes or the lateral and cervical nodes.

In the face the lymphatics draining the nose and midface do so for the skin muscles, perichondrium and periosteum, whereas the vessels for the lip, buccal area and orbit also drain the lymphatics from the mucus membranes. Most of the face drains into the submandibular nodes. Some of the lymphatics from the eyelids, the cheek and the nose drain into the parotid lymph nodes. The lymphatics from the skin and the mucus membrane of the middle portion of the lower lip drain into the submental lymph nodes. The lymphatics from the earlobes drain into preauricular, parotid, retro and infra-auricular lymph nodes or directly into the deep jugular nodes. The skin of the neck drains from the posterior part into the

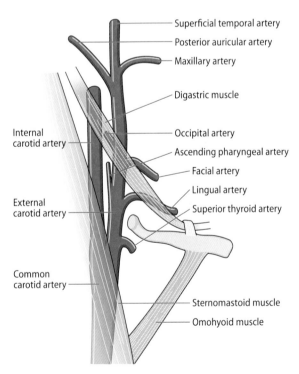

Superficial temporal artery

Posterior auricular artery

Maxillary artery

Digastric muscle

Internal carotid artery

Occipital artery

Ascending pharyngeal artery

Facial artery

Lingual artery

Superior thyroid artery

External carotid artery

Common carotid artery

Sternomastoid muscle

Omohyoid muscle

Fig. 9.7.3 Bifurcation of the common carotid artery in the anterior triangle

occipital and accessory nodes, as do the lateral parts of the skin in addition to the jugular nodes. The skin of the submental and submandibular area drains into the submental, submandibular and even the infra-auricular nodes.

The deep cervical lymph nodes run along the carotid sheath in close association with the internal jugular vein, medially to the sternocleidomastoid muscle. Two groups of nodes are of special interest. The jugulodigastric nodes lie in the area where the posterior belly of the digastric muscle crosses the internal jugular vein, where usually some lymph nodes are palpable. The jugulo-omohyoid nodes are often palpable in the area where the posterior belly of the omohyoid muscle crosses the sternocleidomastoid muscle. Afferent lymphatics from the deep jugular nodes enter the internal jugular trunk and drain into the venous system at the jugular subclavian angle.

9.7.2.3.1 Lymphatic Drainage of the Nasal Cavity, the Oral Cavity, Pharynx and Larynx

The paranasal sinuses have sparse lymphatics compared with the nasal cavity. Most of the lymphatics drain from these regions into the nasopharynx and to the jugulodigastric (subdigastric) nodes. The nasopharynx drains primarily directly into the upper deep cervical lymph nodes along the jugular chain, into the retropharyngeal nodes and into the accessory lymph nodes. The lymphatics commonly cross the midline. The oropharynx and particularly the tonsillar region drain into the parapharyngeal space, and the jugulodigastric nodes into the midportion of the jugular chain. The hypopharynx and the supraglottic larynx drain often into the deep cervical nodes near the bifurcation of the carotid artery. The true vocal folds have sparse lymphatics, and metastases from malignancies of this region usually occur late, when the supra- and/or infraglottic area is affected. The subglottic area drains into the pretracheal region and the low, deep nodes of the jugular chain.

9.7.3 Regions of the Neck

For clinical oncological purposes the neck has been divided into regions. The topographic anatomy of the lymph nodes in the neck has been studied by, among others, Poirer and Sharpy, Trotter and in depth by Rouvier in 1932 [2]. In 1972 Lindberg showed that the head and neck tumours of the various sites had a predilection to metastasise to certain regions (Table 9.7.1) [1]. Based on this information Shy et al. in 1989 classified the neck lymph nodes into seven regions. Based on these the American Academy of Otorhinolaryngology–Head and Neck Surgery published a classification of five levels, which was then revised by the Committee for Neck Dissection Clas-

sification, American Head and Neck Society in 2000, which classification has gained acceptance worldwide (Tables 9.7.2 and 9.7.3).

9.7.3.1 Lymph Node Levels of the Neck

In 1991, the Committee for Head and neck Surgery and Oncology, American Academy of Otorhinolaryngology–Head and Neck Surgery recommended a classification for neck dissection. Recognising the need to standardise the expanding terminology of neck dissection procedures, the Committee worked to define the anatomic boundaries of lymph node dissection and to offer fundamental principles upon which the terminology of neck dissection procedures should be based. The information contained in this report represents an update of the original classification. In essence, few changes have been made since the Committee agreed that the original work had been effective in meeting its goal. The two most important changes relate to the manner in which various selective neck dissection procedures are described, and to the use of anatomical structure–depicted nodes. The information presented is intended to provide an easy reference source for physicians using neck dissection terminology [3, 4].

9.7.3.1.1 Division of Lymph Nodes by Levels

The level system for describing the location of lymph nodes in the neck (Fig. 9.7.4) is as follows:

Level I	Submental and submandibular group
Level II	Upper jugular group
Level III	Middle jugular group
Level IV	Lower jugular group
Level V	Posterior triangle group
Level VI	Anterior compartment

9.7.3.2 Definitions of Lymph Node Groups

9.7.3.2.1 Submental Group

These are the lymph nodes within the triangular boundary of the anterior belly of the digastric muscles and the hyoid bone. These nodes are at greatest risk for harbouring metastases from cancers arising from the floor of mouth, anterior oral tongue, anterior mandibular alveolar ridge and lower lip (Fig. 9.7.4b).

9.7.3.2.2 Submandibular Group

These are the lymph nodes within the boundaries of the anterior and posterior bellies of the digastric muscle, the

Table 9.7.1   Probability of metastasis relative to T stage

Primary site	T stage	N0 (%)	N1 (%)	N2–3 (%)
Tongue	T1	86	10	4
	T2	70	19	11
	T3	52	16	31
	T4	24	10	66
Floor of mouth	T1	89	9	2
	T2	71	18	10
	T3	56	20	24
	T4	46	10	43
Retromolar trigone/anterior tonsillar pillar	T1	88	2	9
	T2	62	18	20
	T3	46	21	33
	T4	32	18	50
Soft palate	T1	92	0	8
	T2	64	12	24
	T3	35	26	39
	T4	33	11	56
Tonsillar fossa	T1	30	41	30
	T2	32	14	54
	T3	30	18	52
	T4	10	13	76
Base of tongue	T1	30	15	55
	T2	29	14	56
	T3	26	23	52
	T4	16	8	76
Oropharyngeal walls	T1	75	0	25
	T2	70	10	20
	T3	33	22	44
	T4	24	24	52
Supraglottic larynx	T1	61	10	29
	T2	58	16	26
	T3	36	25	40
	T4	41	18	41
Hypopharynx	T1	37	21	42
	T2	30	20	49
	T3	21	26	54
	T4	26	15	58
Nasopharynx	T1	8	11	82
	T2	16	12	72
	T3	12	9	80
	T4	17	6	78

Data from Lindberg R (1972) Distribution of cervical lymph node metastases from squamous cell carcinoma of the upper respiratory and digestive tracts. Cancer 29:1446–1449

Table 9.7.2 Division of neck levels by subzones [3, 4]

Level	Subzone	Lymph node location
I	IA	Submental
	IB	Submandibular
II	IIA	Anterior (medial) to the vertical plane, defined by the spinal accessory nerve
	IIB	Posterior (lateral) to the vertical plane, defined by the spinal accessory nerve
V	VA	Above the horizontal plane, defined by the inferior border of the cricoid cartilage. Included are the lymph nodes lying along the spinal accessory nerve
	VB	Below the horizontal plane, defined by the inferior border of the cricoid cartilage. Included are the lymph nodes lying along the transverse cervical artery

Table 9.7.3 Anatomical boundaries of the neck levels [3, 4]

Level	Boundary			
	Superior	Inferior	Anterior (medial)	Posterior (lateral)
IA	Symphysis of mandible	Body of hyoid Anterior belly	Anterior belly of contralateral digastric muscle	Anterior belly of ipsilateral digastric muscle
IB	Body of mandible	Posterior belly of muscle	Anterior belly of digastric muscle	Stylohyoid muscle
IIA	Skull base	Horizontal, defined by the inferior body of the hyoid one	Stylohyoid muscle	Vertical plane, defined by the spinal accessory nerve
IIB	Skull base	Horizontal plane, defined by the inferior hyoid bone	Vertical plane, defined by the spinal accessory	Lateral border of the sternocleidomastoid
III	Horizontal plane, defined by inferior body of hyoid	Horizontal plane, defined by inferior border of cricoid	Lateral border of the sternohyoid muscle	Lateral border of the sternocleidomastoid
V	Horizontal plane, defined by the inferior border of the cricoid cartilage	Clavicle	Lateral border of the sternohyoid muscle	Lateral border of the sternocleidomastoid
VA	Apex of the convergence of the sternocleidomastoid and trapezius muscles	Horizontal plane, defined by the lower border of the cricoid cartilage	Posterior border of the sternocleidomastoid muscle	Anterior border of the trapezius muscle
VB	Horizontal plane, defined by the lower border of cricoid	Clavicle	Posterior border of the sternocleidomastoid muscle	Anterior border of the trapezius muscle
VI	Hyoid bone	Suprasternal	Common carotid artery	Common carotid

stylohyoid muscle and the body of the mandible. It includes the pre- and postglandular nodes, and the pre- and postvascular nodes. The submandibular gland is included in the specimen when the lymph nodes within this triangle are removed. These nodes are at greatest risk for harbouring metastases from cancers arising from the oral cavity, anterior nasal cavity, and soft tissue structures of the mid-face, and submandibular gland (Fig. 9.7.4b).

9.7.3.2.3 Upper Jugular Group

This group includes the lymph nodes located around the upper third of the internal jugular vein and adjacent spinal accessory nerve, extending from the level of the skull base (above) to the level of the inferior border of the hyoid bone (below). The anterior (medial) boundary is the lateral border of the sternohyoid muscle and the stylohyoid muscle, and the posterior (lateral) boundary is the posterior border of the sternocleidomastoid muscle. These nodes are at greatest risk for harbouring metastases from cancers arising from the oral cavity, nasal cavity, nasopharynx, oropharynx, hypopharynx, larynx and parotid gland (Fig 9.7.4b).

9.7.3.2.4 Middle Jugular

The middle jugular lymph nodes are located around the middle third of the internal jugular vein, extending from the inferior border of the hyoid bone (above) to the inferior border of the cricoid bone (below). The anterior (medial) boundary is the lateral border of the sternohyoid muscle, and the posterior (lateral) boundary is the posterior border of the sternocleidomastoid muscle. These nodes are at greatest risk for harbouring metastases from cancers arising from the oral cavity, nasopharynx, oropharynx, hypopharynx and larynx (Fig. 9.7.4b).

9.7.3.2.5 Lower Jugular

These lymph nodes are located around the lower third of the internal jugular vein, extending from the inferior border of the sternohyoid muscle, and the posterior (lateral) boundary is the posterior border of the sternocleidomastoid muscle. These nodes are at greatest risk for harbour-

ing metastases from cancers arising from the hypopharynx, cervical oesophagus and larynx (Fig. 9.7.4b).

9.7.3.2.6 Posterior Triangle Group

This group is composed predominantly of the lymph nodes located along the lower half of the spinal accessory nerve and the transverse cervical artery. The supraclavicular nodes are also included in the posterior triangle group. The superior boundary is the clavicle, the anterior (medial) boundary is the posterior border of the sternocleidomastoid muscle, and the posterior (lateral) boundary is the anterior border of the trapezius muscle. These nodes are at greatest risk for harbouring metastases from cancers arising from the nasopharynx, and oropharynx (Fig. 9.7.4b).

9.7.3.2.7 Anterior Compartment Group

Lymph nodes in this compartment include the pre- and paratracheal nodes, precricoid (Delphian) node, and the perithyroidal nodes including the lymph nodes along the recurrent laryngeal nerves. The superior boundary is the hyoid bone, the inferior boundary is the suprasternal notch, and the lateral boundaries are the common carotid arteries. These nodes are at greatest risk for harbouring

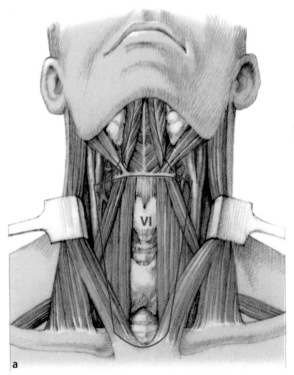

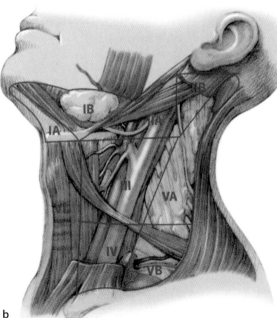

Fig. 9.7.4 a,b Level system for describing the location of lymph nodes in the neck [6]

metastases from cancers arising from the thyroid gland, glottic and subglottic larynx, apex of the piriform sinus, and cervical oesophagus (Fig 9.7.4a).

9.7.4   Neck Dissection

9.7.4.1   Background

George Washington Crile described the radical neck dissection in 1905. However, in 1888 the Polish surgeon Franciszek A. Jawdynski had performed a very similar operation. He reported four cases of a radical en bloc resection [5] in a Polish journal, which gave the work little attention. In the coming decades the technique was further popularised by the well-known American head and neck surgeon Hayes Martin, among others. However, criticism towards the radicality and the morbidity caused by the radical neck dissection was expressed by many surgeons. In 1963 Suarez presented the principles of functional neck dissection, which was based on anatomical work of the lymph node regions in the neck. Suarez pointed out that functional neck dissection is as radical as radical neck dissection is towards the tumour, but is functional with respect of the patient. Ettore Bocca published the operation technique, and his results in the English literature thus popularised the technique.

The indications and type of neck dissection is based on the location, extent of the primary tumour and the metastatic neck nodes or the risk of metastatic disease in the neck. For preoperative decision making, imaging studies like contrast-enhanced CT, MRI, US, US-guided FNA cytology and PET are necessary.

In the sentinel lymph node biopsy, the are surrounding the primary tumour site is injected with a radioactive tracer and/or methylene blue, and thereafter the sentinel lymph node is traced based on the radioactivity and colour, and is excised for histopathological examination. This method has proven valuable in staging and treatment planning of mammary cancer as well as for melanoma in the head and neck region. However, at present there is not sufficient evidence of the usefulness of this method in HNSCC patients to justify its use clinical routine.

Although the clinical and imaging studies are helpful, the ultimate decision as to the type and extent of the neck dissection lies with the surgeon performing the operation. Comorbidity might affect this decision, but chronologic age is not an indication for changing treatment strategies. A bilateral radical neck dissection should be avoided whenever possible. At least one of the internal jugular veins should be saved, and such a procedure should be performed with an interval of 2–4 weeks to minimise morbidity.

When a neck dissection is performed without a larger en bloc procedure extending to the contaminated mucous membranes of the head and neck area, antibiotic prophylaxis is not routinely necessary. It might be considered in special cases, e. g. for immunocompromised patients, diabetics or patients who have received preoperative chemoradiation therapy, in whom there is an increased risk of postoperative infection.

9.7.4.2   Radical Neck Dissection

A radical neck dissection is indicated when a more organ-sparing technique such as a modified radical, functional or selective neck dissection is not sufficient, typically in N3 or some N2 disease or salvage surgery. In particular, metastatic disease at level II very often adheres to the accessory nerve (CN XI), the internal jugular vein, and it might infiltrate the sternocleidomastoid muscle.

Large varieties of incisions have been used for the neck dissection (Fig. 9.7.5). The incision used is primarily by surgeon' choice, which might be influenced by the location of the disease and other procedures performed in conjunction with the neck dissection. The incision should be planned so that good visibility to the entire operative field can be achieved. In addition, the blood supply to the skin flaps and the risk of necrosis as well as a scar formation should be considered. If skin needs to be resected, then the incision should be planned to allow for adequate reconstruction. In the case of a radical neck dissection, one should choose an incision that does not overlie the carotid artery. If a pectoralis major myocutaneous flap is used for reconstruction of the operative field outside the neck region, then two horizontal incisions are useful. If a laryngectomy is performed simultaneously with the neck surgery, then a U-shaped incision is practical. The choice of incision is influenced by other procedures, for example, a tracheostomy performed simultaneously. When choosing the incision the surgeon should also keep in mind the possibility of the necessity of a procedure larger than originally planned. The J-shaped and "hockey-stick" incisions are today fairly common. These can be combined with the forwards-bending S shape, allowing for better visibility of level I. The S curve might also decrease scar formation of the skin and underlying tissue.

9.7.4.2.1   Surgical Technique
A J-shape incision starting from the tip of the mastoid extending closely to the anterior border of the trapezius muscle, bending at the level of the clavicle anteriorly, and extending to the midline gives good visibility (Fig. 9.7.6). The skin flap is elevated with a scissor, scalpel or electric knife (including the platysma) to support the skin blood

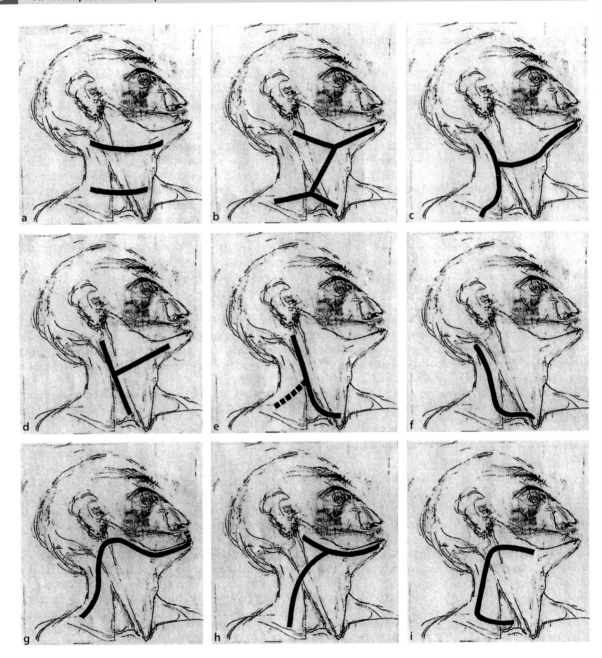

Fig. 9.7.5 a–i Various types of incisions for neck dissection. **a** MacFee incision; **b** Martin incision; **c** three-quarter H incision, according to Hetter; **d** De Quervain incision, modified according to Roux-Berger; **e** Lahey incision; **f** modified hockey-stick incision; **g** inverted hockey-stick incision; **h** Schobinger incision; **i** Dietzel incision

supply. The skin flaps can be fixed with hooks or sutures to the dressing during the operation, allowing good visibility of the operative field. The vena jugularis externa is cut and ligated with a 2-0 or 3-0 resorbable suture. The fat of the anterior triangle is dissected from the caudal end of the parotid gland and from the mandible. Special care has to be taken not to damage the marginal ramus

of the facial nerve. The nerve lies laterally to the external jugular vein, but bends below the mandible in the mid-part of the ramus, and often runs close to the surface of the submandibular gland when the preparation is continued medially and anteriorly to the sternocleidomastoid muscle. The posterior belly of the digastric muscle is identified, and the accessory nerve (CN XI) becomes

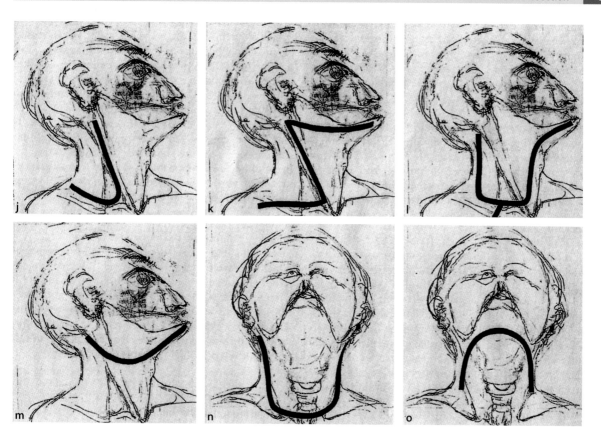

Fig. 9.7.5 *(continued)* **j–o** Various types of incisions for neck dissection. **j** De Quervain incision; **k** Z incision; **l** Latshevsky incision; **m,n** U incision; **o** inverted U incision [6]

visible lateral to the internal jugular vein before it enters the sternocleidomastoid muscle. Further anteriorly runs the hypoglossal nerve (CN XII) along the lower border of the digastric muscle. To dissect level I, the preparation is carried on anteriorly, with careful dissection of the marginal ramus of the facial nerve, which lies laterally to the facial artery and vein. The artery can be saved, but the vein is often cut and ligated. The soft tissue of the anterior triangle is removed anteriorly, the anterior belly of the digastric muscle is left intact and the preparation is continued by mobilising the submandibular gland. The lingual nerve runs laterally to the duct of the submandibular gland, from which it runs cranially. The duct is cut and ligated with a resorbable suture. Several minor vessels in the region of the submandibular gland are cut and either sutured or coagulated with a bipolar coagulation. The fat around the submandibular gland is included in the dissection, but care must be taken not to damage the hypoglossal nerve when it runs medially to the digastric muscle behind the duct on the hyoglossus muscle. The submental fat up to the anterior belly of the contralateral digastric muscle is included in the dissection.

Depending on the location of the bulk of the disease, the dissection can be carried on with a craniocaudal dissection or with a caudocranial dissection. If the dissection is continued in the craniocaudal direction, then the internal jugular vein is resected at this stage. The vein is large in dimension, and the wall of the vein is very thin. Therefore care should be taken in this ligation. The usual method is to place two or three clamps around the vein. It is cut between the two caudal clamps. Commonly a nonresorbable 2-0 or 0 suture is placed cranially to the most cranial clamp. Caudal from the suture another suture is placed and secured with a needle suture through the wall of the vein. This way the location of the first suture is secured, and it cannot slip from the vein. Before clamping and ligation of the internal jugular vein the vagal nerve (CN X) must be identified and left intact. The sternocleidomastoid muscle is cut at its insertion to the mastoid process, and haemostasis is controlled either with a bipolar forceps or the cut is performed with an electrical knife. Now the dissection of level II can continue. The accessory nerve is now readily visible, and the cranial border of the dissection is the posterior belly of the digastric muscle.

Fig. 9.7.6a–d Surgical procedure of radical neck dissection [6]

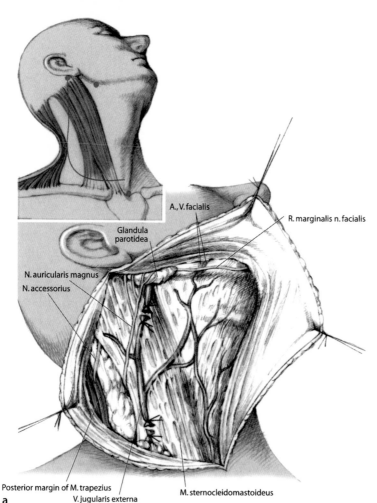

A., V. facialis

R. marginalis n. facialis

Glandula parotidea

N. auricularis magnus

N. accessorius

Posterior margin of M. trapezius

V. jugularis externa

M. sternocleidomastoideus

a

When the preparation is carried out from below (caudocranially) the sternocleidomastoid muscle is cut at its insertion to the clavicle; the common carotid artery, internal jugular vein and the vagus nerve are identified. The internal jugular vein is ligated and cut as described earlier. The omohyoid muscle is included in the dissection. The fat of the anterior triangle including numerous lymph nodes is elevated in the plane of the internal layer of the deep cervical fascia and the middle layer surrounding the larynx. Effort is made to spare the ansa cervicalis.

The dissection of level V is usually done in parallel to the dissection levels II–IV. Special attention has to be paid to the side left of the thoracic duct in the supraclavicular fossa, where it runs to the venous system at the angle of the internal jugular and subclavian veins. The plane of preparation is the internal layer of the deep cervical fascia. This protects the phrenic nerve, which should be left intact. Usually the arteria and vena transversa colli are saved. The lower portion of the external jugular vein is cut and ligated. The resection block is now elevated cranially; the accessory nerve (CN XI) as well as branches of the cervical plexus is resected and often coagulated to avoid neurinomas. If not performed earlier, the sternocleidomastoid muscle and the internal jugular vein are dissected cranially as earlier described.

After the en bloc resection, the operative field is cleaned with saline, and haemostasis is secured. A self-contained suction drain of sufficient size is placed from a separate skin incision and secured with a 2-0 or 3-0 suture. The wound is closed in the subcutaneous layers with resorbable 2-0 or 3-0 sutures. The borders of the wound can be adapted with tape or thin sutures. A dry, sterile pressure dressing is applied.

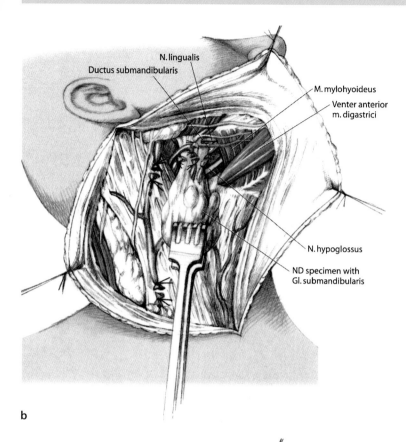

b

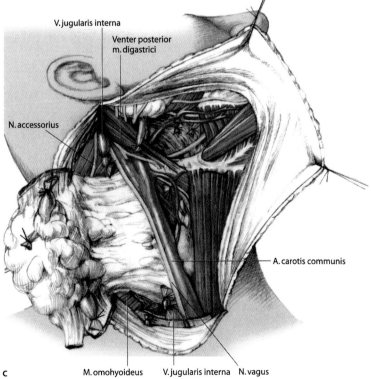

c

Fig. 9.7.6a–d *(continued)* Surgical procedure of radical neck dissection

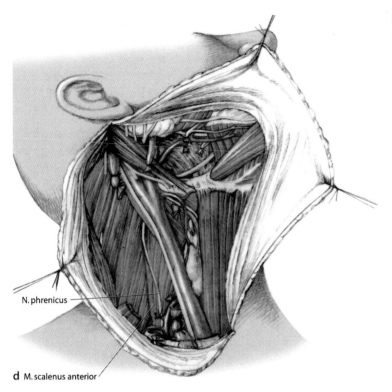

Fig. 9.7.6 a–d *(continued)* Surgical procedure of radical neck dissection

N. phrenicus

d M. scalenus anterior

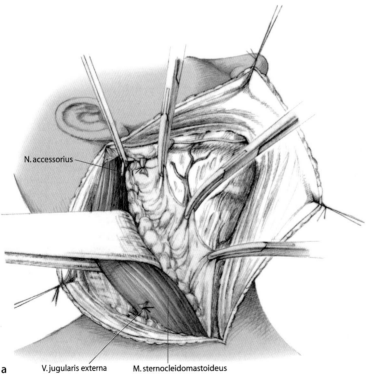

N. accessorius

a   V. jugularis externa   M. sternocleidomastoideus

Fig. 9.7.7a–d Surgical procedure of functional/modified radical neck dissection [6]

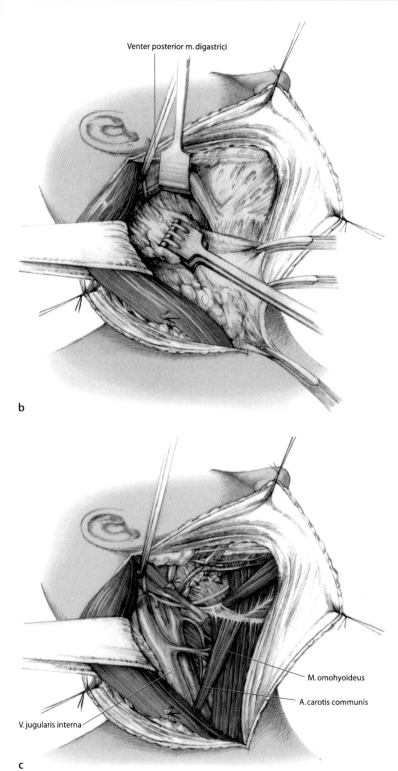

Venter posterior m. digastrici

b

M. omohyoideus

A. carotis communis

V. jugularis interna

c

Fig. 9.7.7a–d *(continued)* Surgical procedure of functional/modified radical neck dissection [6]

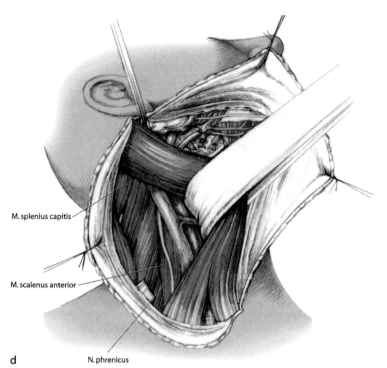

M. splenius capitis

M. scalenus anterior

d   N. phrenicus

Fig. 9.7.7a–d *(continued)* Surgical procedure of functional/modified radical neck dissection [6]

9.7.4.3   Modified Radical Neck Dissection

In the modified radical neck dissection one or two of the three nonlymphatic structures—the accessory nerve (CN XI), the internal jugular vein, the sternocleidomastoid muscle—are saved. If all three structures are saved, but levels I–V are included in the resection, then the neck dissection is called *functional*. The modified radical neck dissection and (especially) the functional neck dissection decrease the morbidity for the patient compared with the radical neck dissection, without decreasing the radicality of the procedure towards the malignant disease; it should therefore be used whenever feasible from the oncologic standpoint. The technique of the functional neck dissection is illustrated in Fig. 9.7.7.

When the sternocleidomastoid muscle is saved, its fascia is included in the resection. The greater auricular nerve can often be saved. By leaving the sternocleidomastoid muscle, a better cosmetic result is achieved, and a good cover is provided for the carotid artery.

The accessory nerve (CN XI) can be identified at the point where it runs into the anterior part of the sternocleidomastoid muscle. The nerve runs from the base of the skull close to the internal jugular vein on its lateral surface, medial to the posterior belly of the digastric muscle, and follows a dorsocaudal direction in the fat. It can be gently dissected from the surrounding fat with scissors. The underlying fat posterior to the jugular vein can be included in the dissection either by raising the nerve and continuing the preparation under the nerve or by completing the dissection posteriorly under the sternocleidomastoid muscle together with the preparation of level VA. When identifying the accessory nerve posterior to the sternocleidomastoid muscle, the greater auricular nerve can be used as a landmark. The branches of the accessory nerve are followed until they enter the trapezius muscle. The dissection of the fat and lymph nodes in levels IIB and VA is continued and extended medially up to the internal layer of the deep cervical fascia. It is once more important to stress that the internal layer of the deep cervical fascia, or the so-called prevertebral fascia should be left intact, and doing so protects the brachial plexus, phrenic nerve, sympathetic trunk and the motor nerves to the deep cervical muscles, which lie under it. To help identify cervical nerves C1–C5, the scalenus anterior and the longus capitis muscles serve as important landmarks where the nerves penetrate the internal layer of the deep cervical fascia.

Often several branches of the cervical plexus have to be sacrificed. It is advisable to coagulate the ends of the nerves to prevent neurinoma formation. Care should be taken to not sever the phrenic nerve, which lies under the internal layer of the deep cervical fascia. The preparation of levels II–IV and V is usually done parallel. When removing the fat in level V with its numerous lymph nodes, special care should be taken to not sever the transverse cervical nor puncture the thoracic duct, which would lead to a severe chylous leak. The vessels and bleedings are controlled by either bipolar coagulation or sutures with resorbable material. Often the thoracic duct can be left intact. The omohyoid muscle is included in the dissection.

After cleaning the operative field with saline and maintaining haemostasis, one or sometimes two self-contained suction drains, one to the anterior the other to the posterior triangle, are placed through a separate skin incision and secured.

The wound is closed in the subcutaneous layer with a 2-0 or 3-0 resorbable suture. The borders of the skin can be adapted with either tape or nonresorbable sutures, which are left in place for 6–8 days. A pressure dressing is applied.

9.7.4.4 Selective Neck Dissection

It is very important from the clinical as well as the research point of view to agree on a universal nomenclature of neck dissection. The classification by the American Academy of Otolaryngology–Head and Neck Surgery (in 2000) gives a good and widely accepted basis for this. The levels (I–VI) outlined in the classification should be used. The radical and modified radical neck dissection has been described earlier. In the modified radical neck dissection, the structures saved should be noted. Functional neck dissection is synonymous with a selective neck dissection including levels I to V. In other selective neck dissections, the regions included in the dissection should also be indicated.

The selective neck dissection I–III, or the so-called supraomohyoid neck dissection, is utilised in patients with cancer of the mobile tongue or floor of the mouth. The J-form incision can be shorter since level IV is not included. The accessory nerve (CN XI) is identified, and the fat around it is dissected as described earlier. The dissection is continued including levels II and III up to the border of level IV at the omohyoid muscle. Level I is resected as earlier described, and the tissue is removed en bloc. The incision is closed as previously described.

Selective neck dissection I–IV, the earlier the so-called anterolateral neck dissection, can often be used in treatment of oral cavity cancer patients, when multiple metastases or metastatic disease extends to the lower part of the jugular chain. Only level V is left intact, and otherwise the dissection is performed as described in the functional neck dissection.

Selective neck dissection II–IV or the lateral neck dissection is often used in treatment of oropharyngeal, hypopharyngeal and laryngeal cancer. The incision follows the posterior border of the sternocleidomastoid muscle from the mastoid to the clavicle, the skin flap is raised and the accessory nerve (CN XI) is identified as earlier described. After elevating the sternocleidomastoid mastoid muscle the fat and lymph nodes are dissected, leaving the

internal jugular vein intact. The omohyoid muscle is usually included, but it can also be saved. The wound closure is as earlier described.

Selective neck dissection II–V, or the earlier so-called posterolateral neck dissection, can often be used in the treatment of patients with cancers involving the posterior scalp, upper neck and pharyngeal cancer. The preparation is carried out as described in the functional neck dissection, and special attention is paid to save the function of the accessory nerve (CN XI).

Selective neck dissection VI or dissection of the anterior compartment is utilised in the treatment of thyroid carcinoma.

One advantage with the selective neck dissections is that they can be performed bilaterally, without significant increase in morbidity. Typically selective neck dissection II–IV is used bilaterally in patients with oral, hypopharyngeal and supraglottic larynx cancer.

The neck dissection can be performed extending to additional lymph node groups when necessary. In patients with cancer of the scalp or postauricular skin, the suboccipital lymph nodes can be removed. Squamous cell cancer of the skin of the face may metastasise to the parotid lymph nodes and make it necessary to include a parotidectomy or/and removal of the buccal lymph nodes together with the selective neck dissection. Paratracheal lymph nodes may be resected in cases of laryngeal carcinoma and retropharyngeal lymph nodes, when indicated, in conjunction with a neck dissection.

- Selective neck dissection I–III: mobile tongue and floor of the mouth
- Selective neck dissection I–IV: mobile tongue, floor of the mouth
- Selective neck dissection II–IV: oropharynx, hypopharynx and laryngeal cancer
- Selective neck dissection II–V: nasopharynx cancer, melanoma of the scalp, sometimes oral and hypopharynx

9.7.4.5 Postoperative Care, Follow-up and Complications of Neck Dissection

The postoperative follow-up of patients who have undergone a neck dissection is similar to that of other patients after major head and neck surgery. Vital signs such as blood pressure, heart rate, postoperative haematoma or bleeding, and excessive pain should be recorded. The function of the drains should be checked because haematoma under the skin flaps increases the risk of flap necrosis. Unilateral swelling, ecchymosis, and facial or neck pain are signs of haematoma. This can be combined with tachycardia and drop in blood pressure as signs of significant postoperative haemorrhage, requiring surgical intervention.

Redness of the skin combined with pain, fever, and increased C-reactive protein and white blood cell counts are signs of infection requiring antibiotic treatment.

The risk of severe postoperative complications after selective neck dissection is low, whereas the risk after radical or modified radical neck dissections is significantly higher. After an uneventful postoperative course the drains can be removed after the secretion is 25 ml or less per day, usually on postoperative days 4–6, whereafter the patient can be discharged from the hospital the following day. The tapes or skin sutures can be removed on days 7–10.

Radical neck dissection has been reported to have perioperative mortality of 1%, and in simultaneous bilateral neck dissection of 10%, whereas as a staged procedure, it has a reduced mortality rate of 3.2%. The complication rate is not only dependent on the procedure, but also very much on the general condition of the patient, other surgical procedures as well as the conservative treatment.

Previous radiotherapy decreases wound healing and increases the risk of postoperative wound problems, which should be considered in postoperative treatment. This is typically true when the radiotherapy has been given several months before surgery. However, immediate preoperative radiotherapy, typically 3–6 weeks before surgery (even to the full dose of 65 Gy), seems to have lesser effect on wound healing and the surgical procedure.

During the surgery the big vessels should be handled with care to avoid intra- and postoperative thrombosis of the internal jugular vein, rupture of the carotid artery as well as air embolus into the venous system during the surgery. Skin necrosis leading to fistula formation over the carotid sheath increases the risk of rupture of the carotid artery. Such a fistula should be surgically treated immediately, using, for example, a pedicled myocutaneous or free microvascular flap.

The damage or sacrifice of the accessory nerve (CN XI) causes a shoulder symptom often leading to moderate or severe pain. The morbidity caused can be decreased with active physical therapy. A careful surgical technique helps avoid damage of the marginal branch of the facial nerve (CN VII), which leads to reduced function of lower lip. Damage to the hypoglossal nerve leads to loss of the motor function of the ipsilateral mobile tongue. A bilateral lesion is particularly devastating and leads to severe nutritional problems. Damage to the brachial plexus, which leads to decreased motor function of the arm, can be avoided by identifying the internal layer of the deep cervical fascia, which covers the brachial plexus. The same is true for the phrenic nerve. Bilateral paresis of the phrenic nerves leads to significant ventilation problems.

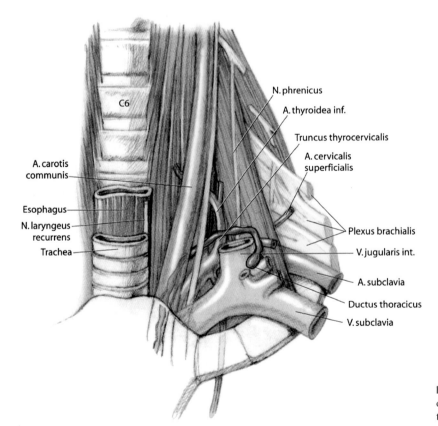

Fig. 9.7.8 Schematic description of the cervical direction of the thoracic duct [6]

When a phrenic nerve lesion is suspected, a chest X-ray should be taken in addition to a careful clinical examination with auscultation of both lungs. The sympathetic trunk runs medially to the carotid artery. Care should be taken during the operation to not damage the sympathetic trunk, which can lead to Horner's syndrome, with the classic symptoms of ptosis, miosis and enophthalmus. Manipulation of the carotid bulb can lead to a vasovagal reflex, causing bradycardia, hypotension and heart arrhythmias. Damage to the vagal nerve (CN X) can lead to an ipsilateral paresis of the recurrent nerve, leading to hoarseness (Fig. 9.7.8).

Damage of the thoracic duct leads to a chylous fistula. To avoid this, careful preparation and good knowledge of the anatomy of the left supraclavicular fossa is important. The thoracic duct runs posteriorly to the common carotid artery and the internal jugular vein. It enters the venous system at the angle of the subclavian and internal jugular veins. Often it also drains directly into the subclavian vein. The thoracic duct runs, as a rule, above the level of the clavicle to the left, whereas the lymphatic vessels run lower to the right in the intrathoracic region and thus inferiorly, and are protected by the subclavian artery. However, damage of the right lymphatic vessels can lead to a chylothorax, requiring surgical draining.

To avoid a chylous fistula a careful preparation of the supraclavicular fossa region should be the rule. The fat contains several blood and lymph vessels, and therefore a liberal ligation before resection is recommended. When the thoracic duct has been identified, it can then be ligated. If a chylous fistula is diagnosed postoperatively, then it can usually be managed conservatively. The drained chylous should be monitored; the serum protein values including the albumin, the electrolytes and liver function should be monitored. A chest X-ray is recommended. A low-fat diet is recommended, and the serum albumin values should be corrected with intravenous administration if necessary. A chylous fistula should close spontaneously within 30 days. If the production of the fistula is over 600 ml day^{-1}, or its spontaneous closure is not observed, then a surgical procedure is recommended. The location of the chylous fistula can be difficult to identify. Care is necessary not to damage important structures while suturing the site of the fistula.

The closure of the internal jugular vein during a radical neck dissection unilaterally or especially bilaterally increases the endocranial pressure, and complications are possible. A blood flow crisis in the vertebral plexus as well as in the emissary and diploid veins, and in the veins of the orbit and the foramina in the base of the skull can result in signs of increased intracranial pressure such as increased blood pressure, bradycardia, headache and nausea.

A ligation of the common or internal carotid artery, for example in conjunction with a neck dissection, leads to a 25–50% risk of hemiparesis and a 40% risk of death.

A neck dissection destroys lymphatic vessels, resects lymph nodes and damages the venous flow, especially if the internal jugular vein is ligated. This can lead to a temporary or permanent lymphoedema of the head, which in the case of bilateral radical neck dissection can be very pronounced and a severe cause of morbidity. A combined treatment of surgery and radiotherapy to the neck increases the risk of lymphoedema. Lymphoedema begins in the first postoperative days and should decrease in approximately 10 days. Care should be taken that severe oedema does not affect the pharynx and the larynx, causing respiratory distress. If necessary a tracheostomy should be performed, which is recommended electively in the case of a simultaneous radical neck dissection.

Scars in the skin can vary from mild to severe. Subcutaneous scaring can lead to painful contractions in addition to aesthetic problems.

9.7.4.6 Preoperative Patient Information

The patient should be informed preoperatively of the morbidity and possible complications resulting from a neck dissection. This should be done in a systematic way and documented in the patient's chart. National legislation and rules should be followed when deciding the extent of the information given the patient. After the provided information, a written or oral consent by the patient should be obtained, again depending on national requirements.

References

1. Lindberg R (1972) Distribution of cervical lymph node metastases from squamous cell carcinoma of the upper respiratory and digestive tracts. Cancer 29:1446–1449
2. Rouvier H (1932) Anatomie des lymphatiques de l'homme. Masson, Paris
3. Robbins KT, Medina JE, Wolfe GT, Levine PA, Sessions RB, Pruet CW (1991) Standardizing neck dissection terminology. Official report of the Academy's Committee for Head and Neck Surgery and Oncology. Arch Otolaryngol Head Neck Surg 117:601–605
4. Robbins KT, Denys D, Committee for Neck dissection classification, American Head and Neck Society (2000) The American Head and Neck Society's revised classification for neck dissection. In: Johnson JT, Shaha AR (eds) Proceedings of the 5th International Conference in Head and Neck Cancer. Omnipress, Madison, Wis., pp 365–370
5. Towpik E (1990) Centennial of the first description of the en bloc neck dissection. Plast Reconstr Surg 85:468–470
6. Werner JA. Lymphknotenerkrankungen im Kopf-Hals-Bereich. Springer-Verlag Berlin Heidelberg 2002

9.8 Carcinoma of Unknown Primary Syndrome

ANDREAS ARNOLD

Carcinoma of unknown primary (CUP) syndrome is also referred to as occult primary tumours of the head and neck.

- Definition
  - Cytologically or histologically proven metastases of a malignant tumour in one or several lymph nodes of one or both sides of the neck
  - The primary tumour is identified sometimes after therapy of metastases, postmortem or not at all.
- Incidence
  - Ten per cent of all cervical lymph node metastases are occult primary tumours.
  - There is increasing incidence.
  - Males are more often affected than females are.
  - The average age of onset is 55–65, but there is an growing tendency in younger patients.
- Histology
  - In most cases, squamous cell carcinoma, undifferentiated carcinoma or lymphoepithelial carcinoma (Schmincke's tumour)
  - Less often, adenocarcinoma, malignant lymphoma, others
- Probable location of the occult primary tumour
  - Seventy per cent of the occult primaries are located in the head and neck region (nasopharynx, oral cavity, tonsillar region, oropharynx, hypopharynx, larynx, thyroid gland) (Fig. 9.8.1). If the metastases are located in the parotid gland, the skin of the head must be inspected carefully. If they are located in the occipital or upper lateral neck region (dorsal to the sternocleidomastoid muscle), the nasopharynx requires cautious examination.
  - Twenty to 30% of occult primaries are situated in the lungs, gastrointestinal tract, breast, urogenital tract (kidney, testes, uterus) or pancreas.
- Symptoms
  - Usually, there are no symptoms or pain, only aesthetic alteration caused by swollen lymph nodes.
- Complications
  - If the occult primary tumour cannot be detected by using the current diagnostic tools as next described, the course is unfavourable.

- Diagnostic procedures (recommended European standard) (Fig. 9.8.2)
  - Search for the occult primary tumour
    - Inspection
      - Skin of the head/scalp
      - Special attention to the back side of the auricles
    - Palpation
      - Lymph nodes of the neck, thyroid gland, salivary glands, tonsils, uvula, base of the tongue
    - Endoscopy
      - Rigid and flexible endoscopy of the nasopharynx, meso- and hypopharynx and larynx, with special attention to the fossa of Rosenmüller, tonsillar region and sinus piriformes
    - Ultrasound
      - Floor of the mouth
      - Neck
      - Thyroid gland
      - Parotid glands
    - Audiogram/tympanogram
      - To exclude malfunction of one or both Eustachian tubes (e.g. caused by an infiltrating nasopharyngeal tumour)
    - MRI, CT
      - Head
      - Neck
      - Thorax
      - Abdomen
      - Whole-body CT
    - Panendoscopy
    - Rigid and flexible panendoscopy of bilateral submucosal biopsy from the fossae of Rosenmüller
    - Bilateral tonsillectomy (right and left tonsil must be separated for histological investigation)
    - Bilateral biopsy from the base of the tongue
  - If no primary tumour can be found
    - Ultrasound-guided fine-needle aspiration cytology (FNAC) is the first step in the invasive diagnostic workup of an unclear neck mass. It is a safe, fast and reliable method to make a diagnosis in an outpatient setting.

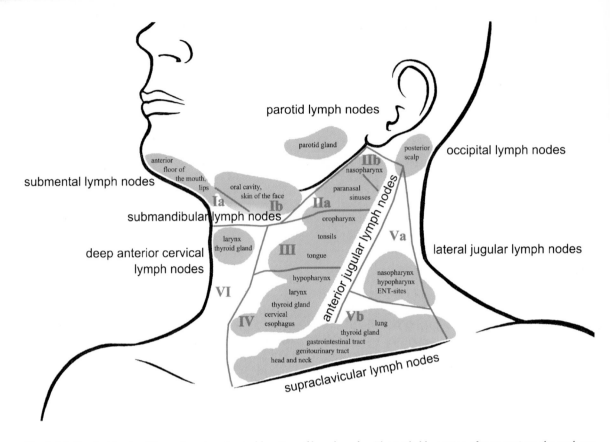

Fig. 9.8.1 Surgical levels of the neck and anatomical location of lymph nodes. The probable origins of metastasis to the neck are indicated for the main groups of lymph nodes

- Punch-needle biopsy has a certain risk of spilling of tumour cells, and it should be avoided.
- If FNAC does not lead to an unequivocal diagnosis, surgical exploration of the suspect neck mass must include total removal of one intact lymph node for histological investigation. However, if frozen sections from the neck mass reveal carcinoma metastasis, and the simultaneously performed panendoscopy (see above) does not show any pathology, lymph node removal should be extended to neck dissection during the same intervention.
  - Note: Excisional biopsy has a high risk of spilling of tumour cells and therefore should only be performed if an infectious cause or a malignant lymphoma is highly suspected.
- Epstein-Barr virus (EBV) serology
  - A search should be done for reliable tumour markers to diagnose an occult undifferentiated (lymphoepithelial) or anaplastic carcinoma of the nasopharynx.
    - EBV antibodies, virus capsid antigens (VCA) immunoglobulin (Ig)G, VCA IgA
    - Early antigens (EA)

  - To exclude a medullary carcinoma of the thyroid gland
    - Immunologic detection of serum calcitonin
  - To exclude a carcinoma of the thyroid gland
    - Investigation of serum thyroglobulin
  - Crucial diagnostic procedures if the investigations to date did not detect the primary tumour
    - FDG-PET-CT(^{18}F-2-deoxyglucose–positron emission tomography–CT)
      - Nowadays, it is the best method to detect the location of primary tumour or of the unknown metastases (sensitivity is ca. 90%). A simultaneous CT reveals the detailed location and extension of the primary tumour, especially when performed with contrast agent. FDG-PET-CT may detect primary tumours undetected by other modalities in approximately 25% of cases.
    - Note: PET has low specificity for tonsillar tumours and low sensitivity for base-of-tongue (area of the lingual tonsil) malignancies (false-positive results).
- Differential diagnosis
  - Branchiogenic carcinoma

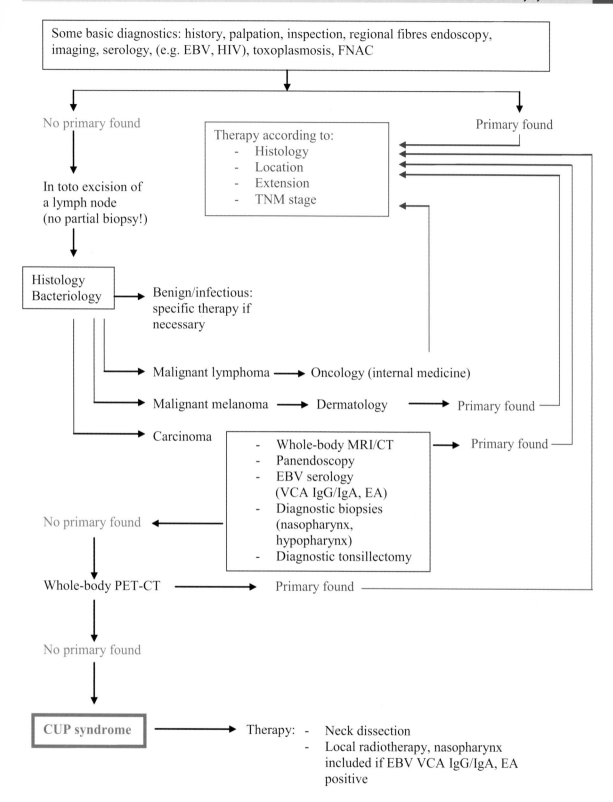

Fig. 9.8.2 Algorithm: persistent indolent swelling of neck lymph node(s)

- A few squamous cell carcinomas may arise from the deep tissues of the neck, presumably from occult branchial, or lateral cervical cysts or clefts. Histologically, remnants of thin-walled cysts lined by squamous or respiratory epithelium indicate branchiogenic carcinoma.
  - Malignant lymphoma
  - Metastasis of a thyroid gland carcinoma
  - Lymph node mass of infectious origin
- Therapeutic strategies (recommended European standard)
  - As long as the occult primary tumour has not been detected by using the diagnostic workup described above, the diagnosis remains "CUP syndrome"
  - In undifferentiated/anaplastic or lymphoepithelial carcinoma with positive EBV serology but without confirmed primary tumour in the nasopharynx
    - Radiotherapy of the nasopharynx and both neck sides
    - Some centres recommend neck dissection, which is then followed by radiotherapy of the nasopharynx and the neck.
  - Other metastases of the neck in cases with negative EBV serology, but occult primary tumour
    - Modified radical neck dissection, which is followed by radiotherapy of the affected neck side
  - Close clinical follow-up of the patient, including endoscopy, every 1–3 months
  - Imaging studies (MRI or PET-CT) every 6–12 months
- Prognosis
  - The overall mean survival of all squamous cell carcinoma metastases of unknown primary tumour is 30 months.
  - The 5-year survival rate is around 30%.

- Overall survival is comparable to that of patients with known primary tumours.
- The prognosis of metastatic cervical CUP adenocarcinoma is poor. Although the optimal treatment strategy is still unclear, surgery that is followed by radiotherapy is the therapy of choice.

Suggested Reading

1. Freudenberg LS, Fischer M, Antoch G, Jentzen W, Gutzelt A, Rosenbaum SJ, Bockisch A, Egelhof T (2005) Dual modality of ^{18}F-fluorodeoxyglucose-positron emission tomography/computed tomography in patients with cervical carcinoma of unknown primary. Med Princ Pract 14:155–160

2. Mistry RC, Qureshi SS, Talole SD, Deshmukh S (2008) Cervical lymph node metastases of squamous cell carcinoma from an unknown primary: outcomes and patterns of failure. Indian J Cancer 45:54–58

3. Pelosi E, Pennone M, Deandreis D, Douroukas A, Mancini M, Bisi GA (2006) Role of whole body positron emission tomography/computed tomography scan with ^{18}F-fluorodeoxyglucose in patients with biopsy proven tumor metastases from unknown primary site. J Nucl Med Mol Imaging 50:15–22

4. Pimiento JM, Teso D, Malkan A, Dudrick SJ, Palesty JA (2007) Cancer of unknown primary origin: a decade of experience in a community-based hospital. Am J Surg 194:833–837

5. Rusthoven KE, Koshy M, Paulino AC (2004) The role of fluorodeoxyglucose positron emission tomography in cervical lymph node metastases from an unknown primary tumor. Cancer 101:2641–2649

6. Weber A, Schmoz S, Bootz F (2001) CUP (carcinoma of unknown primary) syndrome in head and neck: clinic, diagnostic, and therapy. Onkologie 24:38–43

Ear, Nose and Throat Anaestesia

Edited by Matti Anniko

10.1 Ear, Nose and Throat Anaesthesia

LARS WIKLUND

10.1.1 Introduction

In many instances of ENT surgery, the upper airway is "shared" by the surgical and anaesthesia teams. Hence, close cooperation is a necessity. In most cases the airway must be protected by using an endotracheal tube, and the oropharynx must be packed to prevent contamination of the larynx with blood, pus and other debris. Due to both anaesthesiological and surgical interference with the often very reactive airway, great vigilance is required. In these as in other cases, serious complications related to the patient's ventilatory function can arise. This may lead to hypoxaemia, hypercapnia and to unduly light anaesthesia when inhalational agents are used.

This chapter addresses forms of anaesthesia used in ear, nose and throat (ENT) surgery.

10.1.2 General Anaesthesia for Paediatric ENT Surgery

10.1.2.1 Preoperative Considerations for the Paediatric ENT Patient

Approximately 30% of ENT patients are children younger than 6 years of age. A general rule for these paediatric patients is to exercise great care to prevent unnecessary fasting and avoidance of fluids before surgery.

Another very important factor in this kind of surgery is the hyperreactivity of the airway, e.g. an increased sensitivity of the airways after bronchitis with productive cough will last up to 6 weeks. In fact, the incidence of postanaesthesia complications such as laryngospasm, bronchospasm and pneumonia is increased two- to sevenfold during this period. It should be remembered that surgery in the mouth and pharynx in otherwise-healthy patients is complicated by an increased incidence of laryngospasm. With this in mind, elective surgery of this kind is not advisable until freedom from infection has been achieved. On the other hand, it is often not possible to get a child who is scheduled for adenoidectomy free from infection without eliminating this tissue. However, a productive cough is generally seen as a contraindication

to this procedure. In contrast, a child with frequent ear infections can be anaesthetised for microscopy and placement of a tympanic drain even with ongoing rhinitis. For this procedure only mask anaesthesia is required.

Children with congenital malformations such as Pierre Robin, Goldenhar's, Nager, and Treacher Collins syndromes are extremely difficult to intubate, and before administering anaesthesia it is necessary to be well prepared with different laryngoscopes, different guide leaders, endotracheal tubes, a fiberoptic endoscope for intubation and, above all, by maintaining spontaneous ventilation during the intubation procedure. It is also appropriate to seek advice from senior colleagues in such a situation.

10.1.2.2 Considerations for Paediatric ENT Anaesthesia

On placement of an infant or child on the operating table, turning of the head, especially with an extended cervical spine, should be avoided due to the danger of causing subluxation of the cervical spine.

Endotracheal intubation should always be performed with a tube that is the proper size for the patient, especially if the patient is an infant or a child (Table 10.1.1).

In order to prevent blood and secretions from oral and pharyngeal surgery from draining into the lower pharynx, oesophagus and stomach, with the risk of subsequent vomiting, the usual procedure is to place either a moist, heart-shaped foam or gauze pack between the posterior wall of the pharynx and the endotracheal tube. The proximal part of the gauze or an indicator band from the foam pack must be fixed in a prominent position somewhere near the patient's mouth, making it impossible to ignore during the extubation procedure.

Gaseous induction can nowadays preferentially be done with sevoflurane plus nitrous oxide and oxygen. However, intravenous induction with thiopental is currently preferred by most anaesthetists. In the latter case, venipuncture is done in an area where EMLA (eutectic mixture of lidocaine and prilocaine) cream has been applied 1–2 h previously.

For oral or rectal premedication for paediatric patients, a mixture containing 15 mg pethidine, 2.5 mg midazolam and 0.2 atropine per millilitre; paracetamol

Table 10.1.1 Recommended sizes of endotracheal tubes for paediatric patients

Age	Body weight (kg)	Uncuffed tube, inner diameter (mm)	Cuffed tube, inner diameter (mm)
Premature	2.8	2.5	
Newborn	3.0	3.0	
2–3 months	5.4	3.0	3.0
3–6 months	6.6	3.0	3.0
6 months–2 years	10.5	3.5	3.0–3.5
2–4 years	14.5	4.0	3.5–4.0
4–6 years	17	4.5	4.0–4.5
6–8 years	20	5.0	5.0
8–10 years	20	5.5	5.0–5.5
10–14 years	30	6.0	5.5–6.0
14–18 years (females)	48	6.0–7.0	6.0–7.0
14–18 years (males)	48	6.5–7.5	6.0–7.5

syrup containing 24 mg ml^{-1} is used. Infants with less than 5 kg body weight are only given atropine 0.02 mg kg^{-1} (Table 10.1.2).

10.1.2.3 Airway Foreign Bodies

In 75 to 85% of all cases, the patient is a child between the age of 6 months and 4 years. In this age group this foreign-body airway obstructions the sixth most common accidental cause of death. In 10–20% of cases the foreign body is in the larynx or the trachea.

Immediate treatment of a child *younger than 1 year of age* is to keep the child upright and to give the infant four broad slaps between the scapulae with the palm of the hand, followed by four anterior–posterior compressions of the thorax. An effort should be made to visualise the pharynx and larynx, and then the foreign body should be extracted with a common forceps or a Magill forceps. During the entire removal attempt, free-flowing oxygen should be directed at and flood the infant's face. Further surgical treatment is often necessary, and it should be performed in close cooperation with the surgical team (who should be prepared for different types of bronchoscopy). Should this not be successful, then immediate positive-pressure ventilation is necessary. However, this could result in driving the foreign body deeper into the tracheal–bronchial tree.

For *children older than 1 year of age*, 6–10 Heimlich manoeuvres must be performed. An attempt is made visualise the larynx and then extract the foreign body. If not successful, then positive-pressure ventilation with pure oxygen should be given. (This procedure *should not* be performed in a child who is able to breath, cry or talk,

Table 10.1.2 Oral and rectal premedication recommendations for paediatric patients

Body weight (kg)	PMA dose (ml)	+ paracetamol dose (ml)
5	0.5	2.5
6	0.6	3.0
7	0.7	3.5
8	0.8	4.0
9	0.9	4.5
10	1.0	5.0
11	1.1	5.5
12	1.2	6.0
13	1.3	6.5
14	–	7.0
15	1.5	7.5
16	1.6	8.0
17	1.7	8.5
18	1.8	9.0
19	1.9	9.5
20	2.0	10.0
20–24	2.1	11.0
25–28	2.2	12.5
29–32	2.3	15.0
33–36	2.4	17.0
37–40	2.5	20.0

PMA phorbol 12-myristate-13-acetate

but only in situations of respiratory distress.) The more common situation is a child presenting with fever, cough, asthma-like symptoms, and recurring cyanotic attacks. In such cases treatment must comprise joint endoscopic efforts by the surgical and anaesthesia teams, performed under deep general anaesthesia.

There are two main possibilities for ventilating the patient:

1. The oxygen pressure is reduced from an oxygen cylinder or the central gas system to a maximum of 1.5 bar (b) (in children) or 5 b (adults). A Venturi mask is placed on the child and pressurised oxygen enters the bronchoscope in order to expand the thorax at a frequency somewhat similar to that of normal breathing.

2. The second possibility is to use a jet ventilator (e. g. Acutronics Medical System, Barr, Switzerland). The lowest possible driving pressure is used, which is usually 0.5 b for children. The mixer is set at 100% oxygen and a respiratory frequency of 30–60 breaths per minute is utilized, with an inspiratory time of 30%. The hose from the jet ventilator is attached to the side channel of the bronchoscope. In both cases it must be ensured that air trapping does not occur, e. g. in-an-out flow is maintained; otherwise, a barotrauma could occur. The endoscopist should regularly withdraw the endoscope up into the trachea in order to allow ventilation of the greater part of both lungs. If that is not done, then there is a risk of hypoxia and hypercapnia, and subsequent cardiac arrest. On many occasions the foreign body is too big to be extracted in one piece. In fact, in some 5–15% of cases another bronchoscopy must be performed 1 or 2 days later to extract the remainder of the foreign body. In the majority of cases the bronchoscopy is concluded by introducing a 3-mm uncuffed endotracheal tube until the patient has good spontaneous ventilation of his/her own. A pulmonary X-ray is mandatory after such an operation. In addition, antibiotics will often have to be considered post-operatively.

10.1.2.4 Epiglottitis: Treatment with Nasotracheal Intubation

Even before a patient with suspected epiglottitis arrives at the hospital, it is routine to call both the anaesthesia and ENT surgical teams to the operating room (OR). In many cases it is preferable a senior specialist be called to the scene. Both children and adults with a suspected epiglottitis are brought to the operating theatre in the sitting position, leaning slightly forward to facilitate optimal airway expansion. Full preparations for a possible tracheostomy must be undertaken. Remaining calm during this time is highly recommended. After premedication with atropine alone, the patient is put to sleep with sevoflurane in pure

oxygen, but this can also be combined with small dosages of thiopental. Spontaneous ventilation *must* preserved.

During the induction, only when sufficient depth of anaesthesia has been achieved should venipuncture be undertaken. It is *critical* that this not be tried earlier.

Muscle relaxants should never be used.

Intubation *should not* be attempted until there is sufficient depth of anaesthesia. This has been achieved when the frequency of spontaneous ventilation decreases, and the pupils begin to dilate. Great patience is a necessity with this procedure. (Intubation should be done *orally*.)

An endotracheal tube that is 0.5 mm narrower than usual is used. Here is a rough guideline for endotracheal tube sizes for children:

0–2 years	3.0 mm
2–3 years	3.5 mm
3–5 years	4.0 mm
>5 years	4.5 mm

In the case of an emergency with no ventilation, the cricothyroid membrane can be punctured with a 2-mm needle. Correct positioning of the needle is confirmed by aspiration of air from the trachea. Attach a 3-mm adapter taken from a 3-mm (paediatric) endotracheal tube onto this needle. Ventilate with pure oxygen delivered from a Venturi ventilation set or a jet ventilator. The applied pressure must be the lowest possible in order to avoid the risk of barotrauma. Should this technique be considered too hazardous, perform a regular tracheostomy.

Once a good airway has been established, anaesthesia is maintained with the volatile agent of choice, and once the situation is stable, the oral endotracheal tube is exchanged for a nasotracheal tube of the same size. This tube should be well fixed. (Bacterial cultures from the pharynx and blood should be taken before antibiotics are administered.)

The patient is then taken to the intensive care unit, still under anaesthesia and intubated. The patient is kept under continuous light anaesthesia via intravenous infusion of morphine and midazolam. The patient should be cared for under the continuous surveillance of an experienced nurse. *The child should never be left alone.* The inspiratory gas must be well humidified in order to keep the lumen of the nasotracheal tube patent, and before suctioning, 1 ml normal saline should be instilled to rinse the tube. Suction should not be carried out by forcing the narrow end of the suction catheter beyond the end of the endotracheal tube. All equipment necessary for emergency intubation should be stored at the bedside. If the patient shows symptoms of dyspnoea or respiratory distress, then it is usually caused by secretions in the tube. Should respiratory arrest occur when no physician is present and suction of the tube does not help, the nurse should know to remove the tube and place the child in a sitting position, leaning forward, until a physician arrives. Reasons for reintubation should then be re-evaluated. The time needed for having the patient intubated generally varies between 24 and 72 h. Before planned extubation an ENT surgeon should evaluate the patient by fiberoptic endoscopy. A daily pulmonary X-ray is necessary.

10.1.2.5 Adenoidectomy

This procedure is often combined either with microscopic examination of the ears or an occasion tonsillectomy. Premedication is usually advisable, and an oral diazepam dose of 0.2 mg kg^{-1} is common. Anaesthesia is induced either by inhalation or by the intravenous route. Oral tracheal intubation or a laryngeal mask can be used. After the adenoids have been curetted, the postnasal space is packed for a few minutes, after which this pack is removed, and the patient turned to the lateral position and then extubated. Postoperative analgesia can be achieved with rectal paracetamol.

10.1.2.6 Myringectomy: Drainage of the Middle Ear with Transtympanic Tubing

Examination of the ears together with myringectomy and insertion of grommets in children with have secretory otitis is a common day-surgery procedure. Either intravenous induction after application of EMLA cream or inhalational induction is carried out. Anaesthesia is maintained with spontaneous ventilation via a face mask or a laryngeal mask.

10.1.2.7 Tonsillectomy

See Sect. 10.1.3.2 regarding adult tonsillectomy.

10.1.2.8 Postoperative Considerations for Infants and Children

Children born prematurely are prone to apnoea after anaesthesia. Therefore elective surgery is preferably postponed until these infants are 5–6 months of age. In fact, some of them can have periods of asphyxia up to the age of 12 months, so that during this time cautious vigilance and monitoring are recommended in the postoperative period. When caring for these children, as for children with a tracheomalacia, it is sometimes advisable to leave a 3-mm uncuffed endotracheal tube in place until the effects of anaesthesia have worn off.

Symptoms of croup after extubation are common in children, and this is especially so after oro-pharyngo-laryngo-bronchial surgery. This is due in part to the often-sensitive airways, sometimes because of large-bore endotracheal tubes or a traumatic intubation technique, coughing after intubation or surgical manipulations of the tube. Children with a history of pseudocroup seem to be especially sensitive. The oedema that may arise is localised in particular in the narrow subglottic area. The incidence of post-extubation croup in children younger than the age of 6 years seems to be as high as 30%. In order to avoid this, some anaesthetists use 2% lidocaine spray before endotracheal intubation when the body weight of the child is below 10 kg, and 4% when it is more than 10 kg. Alternatively, some recommend lidocaine at 1.25 mg kg^{-1} intravenously before extubation. If lidocaine is used during induction of anaesthesia, then the fact that lidocaine potentiates the action of most anaesthetics should be taken into account.

10.1.3 General Anaesthesia for Adult ENT Surgery: Specific Comments

10.1.3.1 Acute Care for Upper Airway Obstruction (Tumour or Pharyngeal Phlegmon)

An experienced anaesthetist and an experienced ENT surgeon must be present in such situations, assisted by experienced nurses. This collaborative effort requires thorough planning and close attention. The patient sits up and leans slightly forward until a full clinical investigation of the patient has been carried out, intravenous access has been established and alternative ways of guaranteeing a free airway have been considered. A secure, calm atmosphere in the operating room should be the goal. The patient should feel comfortable with and confident in the team. If the team decides to try to intubate, then *no muscular relaxants should be administered*. Intubation is best carried out under deep-inhalational anaesthesia. If this procedure is not fruitful, then fiberoptic intubation is the next alternative. If this procedure is not successful, then the time has come for tracheostomy or transtracheal jet ventilation through a punctured cricothyroid membrane. If the last of these alternatives is selected, then it is important that gas can pass upwards through the airways. Otherwise, there is a risk of air trapping and barotrauma.

10.1.3.2 Tonsillectomy

Tonsillectomies are less common than they used to be, and only about half as many are performed today compared with 20 years ago. Premedication is usually a combination of a sedative (e. g. diazepam 0.2 mg kg^{-1}, up to a total of 10 mg) and atropine (20 µg kg^{-1}, up to a total of 0.5 mg). Intubation is facilitated by muscular relaxation with suxamethonium, deep inhalational anaesthesia or a propofol bolus. After dissection of the tonsils, the patient is usually extubated while still under deep anaesthesia, in a lateral position with the head in a slightly lowered position, after thorough suctioning of the pharynx. In this case the anaesthesiologist must continue to guard and protect the airway until the patient is awake. Postoperative vomiting is common. Oral (administered preoperatively) or rectal analgesics should be given before waking the patient in order to prevent postoperative pain.

Unfortunately, postoperative bleeding is not rare. In severe cases, hypovolaemia can result. Swallowing of blood is common, which is followed by vomiting. Reoperation in these cases must be treated as a surgical emergency and is considered a difficult procedure, and the assistance of an experienced anaesthesiologist must be sought. Intravenous fluid infusion and/or blood transfusion are often necessary. After resuscitation the patient is placed head-down in the lateral position, with a suction apparatus within reach. Atropine is given intravenously to prevent bradycardia. After pre-oxygenation and a small dose of thiopentone, which is followed by cricoid pressure and suxamethonium (1 mg kg^{-1}), the patient is intubated. Alternatively, gaseous induction may be used, after which intubation may be done under deep-inhalational anaesthesia without suxamethonium. After bleeding has been controlled surgically, the stomach is emptied with a nasogastric tube. At the end of the procedure, extubation is performed with the patient in the lateral position. Nowadays tonsillectomy with a CO_2 laser is often performed on children suffering from upper airway obstruction. The anaesthetic induction and the intubation and extubation techniques are the same as in a routine tonsillectomy. Either a specially designed tube for laser surgery should be used, or the ordinary endotracheal tube must be covered with a special copper tape. However, the tape should not be applied on the distal part of the tube and should never be applied on the part of the tube that is adjacent to the vocal cords, as this would constitute a risk for mechanical injury to the vocal cords.

10.1.3.3 Anaesthesia for ENT Endoscopies, Microlaryngoscopy

Diagnostic fiberoptic bronchoscopy can be performed by introducing the bronchoscope through the nose, and injecting local anaesthetic solution through the injection port (under direct vision) as the instrument is advanced. In an anaesthetised patient the bronchoscope may be introduced through an endotracheal tube or a tracheostomy tube through a diaphragm, resulting in minimal leakage of gas into the operating theatre. In the latter case mechanical ventilation must be maintained throughout the bronchoscopy. Ventilation is impaired unless the internal diameter of the tube is at least 2 mm or larger than is the diameter of the bronchoscope. Ventilation techniques using jet devices may be dangerous if expiration through the endotracheal tube is impeded by the presence of the bronchoscope, resulting in high pressures in the lower trachea and bronchi, with an ensuing risk of alveolar rupture, tension pneumothorax, and massive intrathoracic and subcutaneous emphysema.

The rigid bronchoscope remains the preferred instrument for location of bronchial tumours and for removal of foreign bodies or dilatation of strictures. Nowadays this type of bronchoscopy is usually carried out under general anaesthesia with a short-acting muscular relaxant and with positive-pressure ventilation from a jet ventilator or a Venturi set. High-frequency, positive-pressure ventilation may also be employed.

Fiberoptic oesophagoscopy is normally undertaken in a sedated patient. In contrast, the rigid oesophagoscope is inserted under general anaesthesia, including short-acting muscular relaxants. Factors of importance to the anaesthesiologist are the potential for regurgitation on induction of anaesthesia and the risk of damage to the teeth or the cervical spine. A rapid-sequence induction technique is recommended for induction, after which intubation and controlled ventilation are carried out. The cuff of the endotracheal tube might have to be deflated to enable the oesophagoscope to pass down and through the cricopharyngeal area. The most serious complication is perforation of the oesophagus. Therefore a chest X-ray is required after the procedure, before any oral fluids are allowed.

Microlaryngoscopy via the Kleinsasser laryngoscope is, in many cases, the method of choice for investigation of the laryngeal tract. In order to utilise this equipment safely, the most popular technique is to use a long (approximately 30 cm), plastic cuffed endotracheal tube, 5 mm in diameter (e. g. Coplan's microlaryngoscopy tube), which is used for intubation after an induction dose of thiopentone and a non-depolarising muscle relaxant, and spraying the vocal cords with 3 ml 4% lidocaine. The tube is passed either orally or nasally, after which the lungs are ventilated with oxygen/nitrous oxide supplemented with a volatile agent or analgesic drug and ketamine or propofol. This small-diameter tube does not impede the surgeon's view and allows good access to the larynx, and the cuff prevents contamination of the trachea. During the procedure the lungs are mechanically ventilated. At the end of the procedure the pharynx is cleared by suctioning under direct vision, the muscle relaxants are antagonised, and tracheal extubation performed with the patient in the lateral position. Oxygen is administered in order to minimise the risk of hypoxaemia if laryngeal stridor should occur. A CO_2 laser is sometimes used during these procedures.

10.1.4 Head and Neck Surgery

10.1.4.1 Laryngectomy

Cancer of the larynx is treated by surgery and/or laser surgery. Airway obstruction is the major problem during anaesthesia, and alcohol and smoking are aetiological factors that may affect anaesthesia. Respiratory function should therefore be assessed preoperatively. In addition, chest physiotherapy should always be prescribed both pre- and postoperatively to aid in clearance of secretions. Very rarely, intubation might have to be considered while the patient is awake if there are pronounced obstructive problems. In this case topical anaesthesia with 2 or 4% lidocaine is of great help. Anticholinergic agents such as atropine are often also used to decrease the secretions. There is a risk of mechanical obstruction on induction of anaesthesia, and a minimal dose of an intravenous induction agent should therefore be given until consciousness is lost. If the patient's lungs can subsequently be inflated by a face mask, then suxamethonium should be given to facilitate intubation; if not, anaesthesia should be deepened slowly with gas/oxygen and a volatile agent until laryngoscopy is possible. If there is any doubt regarding the patient's ability to maintain a patent airway after loss of consciousness, then the anaesthetist should not use an intravenous induction agent, and an inhalational technique should be used instead. Tracheal intubation might be more difficult if radiotherapy has been given preoperatively. Online monitoring of the electrocardiogram (ECG) and arterial blood pressure should be done, and anaesthesia should be induced and maintained with standard induction and volatile and/or opioid analgesic agents. When the larynx has been opened and the trachea exposed, it is important to check that a sterile tracheal tube and compatible connections are available before the trachea is divided. The patient's lungs are then ventilated with pure oxygen and an inhalational agent for several minutes, after which the endotracheal tube is withdrawn into the larynx, the trachea is divided, and then a second tracheal tube is placed in the trachea and secured firmly. The tube should be positioned carefully within the now-shortened trachea in order to prevent one-lung ventilation. At the end of surgery, remaining neuromuscular blockage is antagonised and the tracheal tube exchanged for a laryngectomy or tracheostomy tube, after which the patient is allowed to recover from anaesthesia. Adequate humidification of inspiratory gases is essential postoperatively.

10.1.4.2 Tracheal and Bronchial YAG Laser Operations Under General Anaesthesia

This type of surgery entails considerable risk, such as rupture of the trachea and bronchi, intense bleeding, pneumomediastinum and subsequent compression of central veins and the right heart, with shutdown of venous return and circulatory failure. Air may also enter pleural and peritoneal cavities as well as the retroperitoneal space. In addition to this, bronchospasm, bronchial oedema and cerebral air emboli may occur. Another risk in this sort of surgery in the airways is damage to the endotracheal tube, either in the form of a hole burnt by the laser beam or a fire igniting in the plastic material in the tube. It is therefore essential that this kind of anaesthesia be handled by experienced anaesthesiologists. Great vigilance as well as very careful preoperative preparations is recommended.

The area of the endotracheal tube that is next to the operating field should be made of metal to avoid the risk of creating holes in the tube with the laser beam. Nitrous oxide should not be used, as this gas mixed with oxygen is flammable, and this accident occurs when the extremely hot laser beam penetrates the anaesthetic gas. The patient should be monitored with indwelling arterial and central venous catheters in addition to ECG, pulse oximetry and capnometry. This author has found that during these procedures it is best to use intravenous anaesthesia with a propofol and a remifentanil infusion. Muscular relaxation with rocuronium is usually advisable. A special double-lumen tube that can both ventilate and measure the airway pressure during the procedure is introduced distally to the operating site. The best ventilation through the special tube is achieved by a jet ventilator that should have a maximum driving pressure of 3b. The respiratory frequency is set at 15–30 cycles per min. During the YAG (yttrium aluminium garnet) laser treatment of the tumour, no more than 30% oxygen can be used, to avoid the risk of a fire in the airway. This laser burning must be interrupted whenever the patient's respiration is endangered. It is common for the anaesthesia team to be forced to accept a PaO_2 of 5 kPa and a SpO_2 of 75% for some time during the procedure. The $PaCO_2$ should not be allowed to be higher than 15 kPa. In cases when intrabronchial bleeding could occur, the patient should be in the lateral position to avoid filling both main bronchi with blood. Direct application of epinephrine to areas with uncontrollable oozing of blood might be necessary.

Closely related, but fortunately less risky, is the placement of a bronchial stent in the trachea or one of the main bronchi for purposes of dilatation when a bronchial tumour threatens to constrict the airway. Intrabronchial bleeding, however, can occur.

10.1.4.3 Reconstruction of the Middle Ear and Translabyrinthine Neurosurgery

This kind of surgery could be considered a sort of neurosurgery for which neuroanaesthesia methods are applicable. As gaseous anaesthesia can result in an expanding gas pocket in the middle ear or intracranially after anaesthesia and surgery, this kind of anaesthesia must be avoided. Instead, infusions of propofol and remifentanil together with a noncompetitive muscular relaxant for endotracheal intubation are now the preferred method. This type of long-lasting anaesthesia also offers an advantage: the anaesthetic can be finished soon after the end of surgery, with minimal "hangover" after initial recovery from the anaesthetic. This also functions well, as pain is not a major complaint in the postoperative period. An intravenous injection of lidocaine (1 mg kg^{-1}) can be recommended before intubation as well as before extubation to minimise the risk of coughing, which might be deleterious to the surgical result.

10.1.4.4 Reconstructive Surgery Secondary to Head and Neck Tumours

Due to the localisation of the tumour and possible fibrosis after previous surgery and radiotherapy, the anatomy of the airway may be changed, making endotracheal intubation difficult. Therefore, the following can be done in order to secure the airway initially: fiberoptic intubation while the patient is conscious or the same kind of intubation carried out after slow intravenous induction with propofol and remifentanil, without muscular relaxation, with the patient still breathing spontaneously. In some cases a tracheostomy must follow. Monitoring consists of online arterial and central venous pressures, ECG, capnometry, measurement of body temperature and urine secretion (an indwelling bladder catheter is necessary). The surgical procedure can be very time-consuming and involve ENT surgeons, oral surgeons and plastic surgeons if free cutaneous flaps and sometimes bone must be used to stabilise and cover the surgical wound. Dissection of the neck, when the surgeons are working close to nerves and the carotid sinus, frequently results in sudden blood pressure instability and bradycardia. This can to some degree be avoided if this region of the surgical site is infiltrated beforehand with 0.5% lidocaine. It is frequently the case that the patients are elderly, with comorbid diseases such as diabetes mellitus, angina pectoris, peripheral vascular disease and left ventricular insufficiency. As the surgery

is time-consuming, special care must be taken to avoid hypothermia (heated humidification of inhalational gas), decubital injury (special mattress) and thromboembolic complications (low-molecular-weight heparin). Sometimes the lungs are ventilated with double the tidal volume (half the respiratory frequency) for 10 min every hour to prevent the development of atelectasis. Most surgeons also use antibiotics for infection prophylaxis.

10.1.5 Local/Regional Anaesthesia for ENT Surgery: Specific Comments

Local administration of local anaesthetics and infiltration of the mucosa in the airways has long been a frequently used method. Cocaine was the classic preferred drug, but it is now used only in the nose. The short-acting amide local anaesthetics (lidocaine, mepivacaine, prilocaine) are currently preferred. They are usually administrated by spray. As indicated above, lidocaine is often favoured, as this drug has the ability to reduce coughing when often-sensitive mucous membranes are subjected to surgical and anaesthesiological manipulations. This anti-cough effect can also be achieved by intravenous injection of lidocaine. Local infiltration by injection of these drugs is also used for surgery more superficial. The use of these methods is restricted by the fact that most ENT surgery is performed in tissues with very rich vascularisation, thereby increasing the risk of injecting the drug into venous and arterial blood, causing very high blood concentrations. This is also why the more long-acting and toxic local anaesthetic drugs (bupivaacaine, levobupivacaine and ropivaciane) are not recommended for this kind of anaesthesia and surgery. The first side effects to appear are usually CNS effects (from mild mental intoxication to generalised seizures), and somewhat later, when the drug concentration is greater, circulatory effects (arrhythmias and cardiac arrest). Seizures are treated by intravenous injection of diazepam or thiopental, arrhythmias preferentially by active monitoring and possibly by bretylium, and cardiac arrest by cardiopulmonary resuscitation (CPR). It must be remembered that cardiac arrest caused by local anaesthetics is sometimes unusually difficult to convert to spontaneous circulation. It may very well take some time, and furthermore, much larger dosages of epinephrine are usually required for anaesthetically induced cardiac arrest CPR than for standard CPR, e.g. those dosages recommended by the American Heart Association and the European Resuscitation Council.

Subject Index